STANDARD
EDITION

2018
ICD-10-PCS

INCLUDES
NETTER'S
ANATOMY
ART

Carol J. Buck
MS, CPC, CCS-P

Former Program Director
Medical Secretary Programs
Northwest Technical College
East Grand Forks, Minnesota

ELSEVIER

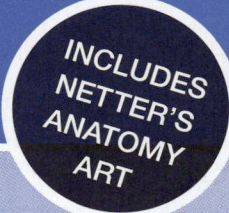

ELSEVIER

3251 Riverport Lane
St. Louis, Missouri 63043

2018 ICD-10-PCS STANDARD EDITION

ISBN:978-0-323-43068-5

Notice

Knowledge and best practice in this field are constantly changing. As new research and experience broaden our understanding, changes in research methods, professional practices, or medical treatment may become necessary.

Practitioners and researchers must always rely on their own experience and knowledge in evaluating and using any information, methods, compounds, or experiments described herein. In using such information or methods they should be mindful of their own safety and the safety of others, including parties for whom they have a professional responsibility.

With respect to any drug or pharmaceutical products identified, readers are advised to check the most current information provided (i) on procedures featured or (ii) by the manufacturer of each product to be administered, to verify the recommended dose or formula, the method and duration of administration, and contraindications. It is the responsibility of practitioners, relying on their own experience and knowledge of their patients, to make diagnoses, to determine dosages and the best treatment for each individual patient, and to take all appropriate safety precautions.

To the fullest extent of the law, neither the Publisher nor the authors, contributors, or editors, assume any liability for any injury and/or damage to persons or property as a matter of products liability, negligence or otherwise, or from any use or operation of any methods, products, instructions, or ideas contained in the material herein.

International Standard Book Number: 978-0-323-43068-5

Content Strategist: Brandi Graham
Content Development Manager: Luke Held
Associate Content Development Specialist: Anna Miller
Publishing Services Manager: Jeffrey Patterson
Project Manager: Lisa A. P. Bushey
Designer: Maggie Reid

Printed in United States of America

Last digit is the print number: 9 8 7 6 5 4 3 2 1

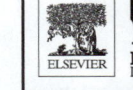

Working together
to grow libraries in
developing countries

www.elsevier.com • www.bookaid.org

DEDICATION

To all the brave medical coders who transitioned the nation into a new coding system.
Decades of waiting finally concluded with the implementation of I-10,
and you have been the pioneers leading the way.

With greatest appreciations for your efforts!

Carol J. Buck, MS, CPC, CCS-P

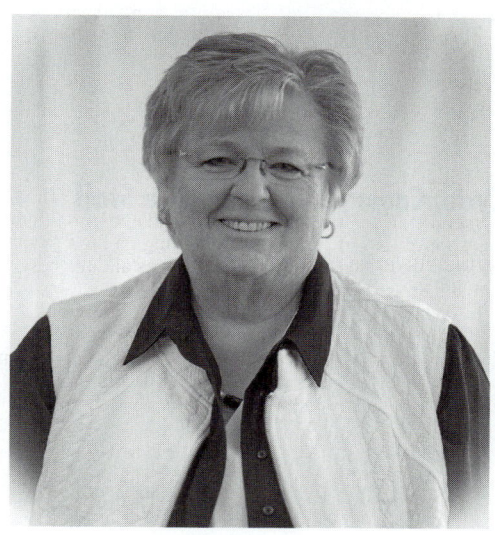

DEVELOPMENT OF THIS EDITION

Editorial Consultant

Jenna Price, CPC
President
Price Editorial Services, LLC
St. Louis, Missouri

Query Team

Patricia Cordy Henricksen, MS, CHCA, CPC-I, CPC, CCP-P, ASC-PM
Auditing and Coding Educator
Soterion Medical Services
Lexington, Kentucky

Jackie Grass Koesterman, CPC
Coding and Reimbursement Specialist
Grand Forks, North Dakota

Kathleen Buchda, CPC, CPMA
Revenue Recognition
New Richmond, Wisconsin

Elsevier/MC Strategies Revenue Cycle, Coding and Compliance Staff

"Experts in providing e-learning on revenue cycle, coding and compliance."

Deborah Neville, RHIA, CCS-P
Director

Lynn-Marie D. Wozniak, MS, RHIT
Content Manager

Sandra L. Macica, MS, RHIA, CCS, ROCC
Content Manager

CONTENTS

ICD-10-PCS SYMBOLS AND CONVENTIONS...vi

GUIDE TO THE 2018 UPDATES...vii

Netter's Anatomy Illustrations NAP-1

INTRODUCTION...1

ICD-10-PCS Official Guidelines for Coding and Reporting..1

TABLES...7

Ø   Medical and Surgical...7

    ØØ   Central Nervous System and Cranial Nerves 8

    Ø1   Peripheral Nervous System..25

    Ø2   Heart and Great Vessels 36

    Ø3   Upper Arteries..55

    Ø4   Lower Arteries..74

    Ø5   Upper Veins..94

    Ø6   Lower Veins..111

    Ø7   Lymphatic and Hemic Systems 128

    Ø8   Eye..139

    Ø9   Ear, Nose, Sinus...156

    ØB   Respiratory System..174

    ØC   Mouth and Throat..191

    ØD   Gastrointestinal System...206

    ØF   Hepatobiliary System and Pancreas..232

    ØG   Endocrine System..247

    ØH   Skin and Breast..255

    ØJ   Subcutaneous Tissue and Fascia 273

    ØK   Muscles...292

    ØL   Tendons..3Ø8

    ØM   Bursae and Ligaments 323

    ØN   Head and Facial Bones 338

    ØP   Upper Bones...354

    ØQ   Lower Bones...371

    ØR   Upper Joints...387

    ØS   Lower Joints...4Ø4

    ØT   Urinary System..421

    ØU   Female Reproductive System..437

    ØV   Male Reproductive System..454

    ØW   Anatomical Regions, General 469

    ØX   Anatomical Regions, Upper Extremities..481

    ØY   Anatomical Regions, Lower Extremities..49Ø

1   Obstetrics..499

2 Placement 504
3 Administration.. 513
4 Measurement and Monitoring 531
5 Extracorporeal or Systemic Assistance and Performance.......................... 537
6 Extracorporeal or Systemic Therapies... 540
7 Osteopathic 544
8 Other Procedures 546
9 Chiropractic.. 549
B Imaging 551
C Nuclear Medicine... 609
D Radiation Therapy.. 630
F Physical Rehabilitation and Diagnostic Audiology 654
G Mental Health... 672
H Substance Abuse Treatment... 676
X New Technology.. 680

INDEX 687
APPENDIX A – Definitions... 801
APPENDIX B – Body Part Key 846
APPENDIX C – Device Key... 875
APPENDIX D – Substance Key... 887
APPENDIX E – Device Aggregation Table.. 888

SYMBOLS AND CONVENTIONS

Annotated

Throughout the manual, revisions, additions, and deleted codes or words are indicated by the following symbols:

New and revised content from the previous edition are indicated by blue font.

~~deleted~~ Deletions from the previous edition are struck through.

ICD-10-PCS Table Symbols

Throughout the manual information is indicated by the following symbols:

OGCR The *Official Guidelines for Coding and Reporting* symbol includes the placement of a portion of a guideline as that guideline pertains to the code by which it is located. The complete OGCR are located in the Introduction.

[ ] Brackets below the tables enclose the alphanumeric options for Non-covered, Limited Coverage, DRG Non-OR, Non-OR, and HAC.

GUIDE TO THE 2018 UPDATES

The ICD-10-PCS codes that have changed are shown in the lists below.
If you would like to see this information in table format, please visit codingupdates.com for a complete listing.

2018 ICD-10-PCS New, Revised, and Deleted Codes.

NEW CODES

00160ZB	00H03YZ	00R607Z	00RL4KZ	00RT4JZ	00UL0JZ	00US4KZ	01R50JZ	01RG07Z	01U54KZ
00163ZB	00H04YZ	00R60JZ	00RM07Z	00RT4KZ	00UL0KZ	00W00YZ	01R50KZ	01RG0JZ	01U60JZ
0016470	00H60YZ	00R60KZ	00RM0JZ	00U607Z	00UL3JZ	00W03YZ	01R547Z	01RG0KZ	01U60KZ
0016471	00H63YZ	00R647Z	00RM0KZ	00U60JZ	00UL3KZ	00W04YZ	01R54JZ	01RG47Z	01U63JZ
0016472	00H64YZ	00R64JZ	00RM47Z	00U60KZ	00UL4JZ	00W60YZ	01R54KZ	01RG4JZ	01U63KZ
0016473	00HE0YZ	00R64KZ	00RM4JZ	00U637Z	00UL4KZ	00W63YZ	01R607Z	01RG4KZ	01U64JZ
0016474	00HE3YZ	00RF07Z	00RM4KZ	00U63JZ	00UM0JZ	00W64YZ	01R60JZ	01RH07Z	01U64KZ
0016475	00HE4YZ	00RF0JZ	00RN07Z	00U63KZ	00UM0KZ	00WE0YZ	01R60KZ	01RH0JZ	01U80JZ
0016476	00HU0YZ	00RF0KZ	00RN0JZ	00U647Z	00UM3JZ	00WE3YZ	01R647Z	01RH0KZ	01U80KZ
0016477	00HU3YZ	00RF47Z	00RN0KZ	00U64JZ	00UM3KZ	00WE4YZ	01R64JZ	01RH47Z	01U83JZ
0016478	00HU4YZ	00RF4JZ	00RN47Z	00U64KZ	00UM4JZ	00WU0YZ	01R64KZ	01RH4JZ	01U83KZ
001647B	00HV0YZ	00RF4KZ	00RN4JZ	00UF0JZ	00UM4KZ	00WU3YZ	01R807Z	01RH4KZ	01U84JZ
00164J0	00HV3YZ	00RG07Z	00RN4KZ	00UF0KZ	00UN0JZ	00WU4YZ	01R80JZ	01RR07Z	01U84KZ
00164J1	00HV4YZ	00RG0JZ	00RP07Z	00UF3JZ	00UN0KZ	00WV0YZ	01R80KZ	01RR0JZ	01UB0JZ
00164J2	00P00YZ	00RG0KZ	00RP0JZ	00UF3KZ	00UN3JZ	00WV3YZ	01R847Z	01RR0KZ	01UB0KZ
00164J3	00P03YZ	00RG47Z	00RP0KZ	00UF4JZ	00UN3KZ	00WV4YZ	01R84JZ	01RR47Z	01UB3JZ
00164J4	00P04YZ	00RG4JZ	00RP47Z	00UF4KZ	00UN4JZ	01HY0YZ	01R84KZ	01RR4JZ	01UB3KZ
00164J5	00P60YZ	00RG4KZ	00RP4JZ	00UG0JZ	00UN4KZ	01HY3YZ	01RB07Z	01RR4KZ	01UB4JZ
00164J6	00P63YZ	00RH07Z	00RP4KZ	00UG0KZ	00UP0JZ	01HY4YZ	01RB0JZ	01U10JZ	01UB4KZ
00164J7	00P64YZ	00RH0JZ	00RQ07Z	00UG3JZ	00UP0KZ	01PY0YZ	01RB0KZ	01U10KZ	01UC0JZ
00164J8	00PE0YZ	00RH0KZ	00RQ0JZ	00UG3KZ	00UP3JZ	01PY3YZ	01RB47Z	01U13JZ	01UC0KZ
00164JB	00PE3YZ	00RH47Z	00RQ0KZ	00UG4JZ	00UP3KZ	01PY4YZ	01RB4JZ	01U13KZ	01UC3JZ
00164K0	00PE4YZ	00RH4JZ	00RQ47Z	00UG4KZ	00UP4JZ	01R107Z	01RB4KZ	01U14JZ	01UC3KZ
00164K1	00PU0YZ	00RH4KZ	00RQ4JZ	00UH0JZ	00UP4KZ	01R10JZ	01RC07Z	01U14KZ	01UC4JZ
00164K2	00PU3YZ	00RJ07Z	00RQ4KZ	00UH0KZ	00UQ0JZ	01R10KZ	01RC0JZ	01U20JZ	01UC4KZ
00164K3	00PU4YZ	00RJ0JZ	00RR07Z	00UH3JZ	00UQ0KZ	01R147Z	01RC0KZ	01U20KZ	01UD0JZ
00164K4	00PV0YZ	00RJ0KZ	00RR0JZ	00UH3KZ	00UQ3JZ	01R14JZ	01RC47Z	01U23JZ	01UD0KZ
00164K5	00PV3YZ	00RJ47Z	00RR0KZ	00UH4JZ	00UQ3KZ	01R14KZ	01RC4JZ	01U23KZ	01UD3JZ
00164K6	00PV4YZ	00RJ4JZ	00RR47Z	00UH4KZ	00UQ4JZ	01R207Z	01RC4KZ	01U24JZ	01UD3KZ
00164K7	00R107Z	00RJ4KZ	00RR4JZ	00UJ0JZ	00UQ4KZ	01R20JZ	01RD07Z	01U24KZ	01UD4JZ
00164K8	00R10JZ	00RK07Z	00RR4KZ	00UJ0KZ	00UR0JZ	01R20KZ	01RD0JZ	01U40JZ	01UD4KZ
00164KB	00R10KZ	00RK0JZ	00RS07Z	00UJ3JZ	00UR0KZ	01R247Z	01RD0KZ	01U40KZ	01UF0JZ
00164ZB	00R147Z	00RK0KZ	00RS0JZ	00UJ3KZ	00UR3JZ	01R24JZ	01RD47Z	01U43JZ	01UF0KZ
00760ZZ	00R14JZ	00RK47Z	00RS0KZ	00UJ4JZ	00UR3KZ	01R24KZ	01RD4JZ	01U43KZ	01UF3JZ
00763ZZ	00R14KZ	00RK4JZ	00RS47Z	00UJ4KZ	00UR4JZ	01R407Z	01RD4KZ	01U44JZ	01UF3KZ
00764ZZ	00R207Z	00RK4KZ	00RS4JZ	00UK0JZ	00UR4KZ	01R40JZ	01RF07Z	01U44KZ	01UF4JZ
00CU0ZZ	00R20JZ	00RL07Z	00RS4KZ	00UK0KZ	00US0JZ	01R40KZ	01RF0JZ	01U50JZ	01UF4KZ
00CU3ZZ	00R20KZ	00RL0JZ	00RT07Z	00UK3JZ	00US0KZ	01R447Z	01RF0KZ	01U50KZ	01UG0JZ
00CU4ZZ	00R247Z	00RL0KZ	00RT0JZ	00UK3KZ	00US3JZ	01R44JZ	01RF47Z	01U53JZ	01UG0KZ
00H004Z	00R24JZ	00RL47Z	00RT0KZ	00UK4JZ	00US3KZ	01R44KZ	01RF4JZ	01U53KZ	01UG3JZ
00H00YZ	00R24KZ	00RL4JZ	00RT47Z	00UK4KZ	00US4JZ	01R507Z	01RF4KZ	01U54JZ	01UG3KZ

01UG4JZ	02HT0YZ	02VG3ZZ	031L0ZJ	041T49S	041V4KP	04733D1	047A4Z1	047P341	047W4D1
01UG4KZ	02HT3YZ	02VG4ZZ	031M09K	041T4AP	041V4KQ	04733Z1	047B041	047P3D1	047W4Z1
01UH0JZ	02HT4YZ	02WA0RS	031M0AK	041T4AQ	041V4KS	0473441	047B0D1	047P3Z1	047Y041
01UH0KZ	02HV0YZ	02WA0YZ	031M0JK	041T4AS	041V4ZP	04734D1	047B0Z1	047P441	047Y0D1
01UH3JZ	02HV3YZ	02WA3RS	031M0KK	041T4JP	041V4ZQ	04734Z1	047B341	047P4D1	047Y0Z1
01UH3KZ	02HV4YZ	02WA3YZ	031M0ZK	041T4JQ	041V4ZS	0474041	047B3D1	047P4Z1	047Y341
01UH4JZ	02HW0YZ	02WA4RS	031N09J	041T4JS	041W09P	04740D1	047B3Z1	047Q041	047Y3D1
01UH4KZ	02HW3YZ	02WA4YZ	031N0AJ	041T4KP	041W09Q	04740Z1	047B441	047Q0D1	047Y3Z1
01UR0JZ	02HW4YZ	02WAXRS	031N0JJ	041T4KQ	041W09S	0474341	047B4D1	047Q0Z1	047Y441
01UR0KZ	02LP0CZ	02WF37Z	031N0KJ	041T4KS	041W0AP	04743D1	047B4Z1	047Q341	047Y4D1
01UR3JZ	02LP0DZ	02WF38Z	031N0ZJ	041T4ZP	041W0AQ	04743Z1	047C041	047Q3D1	047Y4Z1
01UR3KZ	02LP0ZZ	02WF3JZ	03HY0YZ	041T4ZQ	041W0AS	0474441	047C0D1	047Q3Z1	04HY0YZ
01UR4JZ	02LP3CZ	02WF3KZ	03HY3YZ	041T4ZS	041W0JP	04744D1	047C0Z1	047Q441	04HY3YZ
01UR4KZ	02LP3DZ	02WG37Z	03HY4YZ	041U09P	041W0JQ	04744Z1	047C341	047Q4D1	04HY4YZ
01WY0YZ	02LP3ZZ	02WG38Z	03PY0YZ	041U09Q	041W0JS	0475041	047C3D1	047Q4Z1	04L03DJ
01WY3YZ	02LP4CZ	02WG3JZ	03PY3YZ	041U09S	041W0KP	04750D1	047C3Z1	047R041	04PY0YZ
01WY4YZ	02LP4DZ	02WG3KZ	03PY4YZ	041U0AP	041W0KQ	04750Z1	047C441	047R0D1	04PY3YZ
02163Z7	02LP4ZZ	02WH37Z	03WY0YZ	041U0AQ	041W0KS	0475341	047C4D1	047R0Z1	04PY4YZ
021W0JG	02LQ0CZ	02WH38Z	03WY3YZ	041U0AS	041W0ZP	04753D1	047C4Z1	047R341	04WY0YZ
021W0JH	02LQ0DZ	02WH3JZ	03WY4YZ	041U0JP	041W0ZQ	04753Z1	047D041	047R3D1	04WY3YZ
021W0KG	02LQ0ZZ	02WH3KZ	0413093	041U0JQ	041W0ZS	0475441	047D0D1	047R3Z1	04WY4YZ
021W0KH	02LQ3CZ	02WJ37Z	0413094	041U0JS	041W49P	04754D1	047D0Z1	047R441	05HY0YZ
027L04Z	02LQ3DZ	02WJ38Z	0413095	041U0KP	041W49Q	04754Z1	047D341	047R4D1	05HY3YZ
027L0DZ	02LQ3ZZ	02WJ3JZ	04130A3	041U0KQ	041W49S	0476041	047D3D1	047R4Z1	05HY4YZ
027L0ZZ	02LQ4CZ	02WJ3KZ	04130A4	041U0KS	041W4AP	04760D1	047D3Z1	047S041	05PY0YZ
027L34Z	02LQ4DZ	02WY0YZ	04130A5	041U0ZP	041W4AQ	04760Z1	047D441	047S0D1	05PY3YZ
027L3DZ	02LQ4ZZ	02WY3YZ	04130J3	041U0ZQ	041W4AS	0476341	047D4D1	047S0Z1	05PY4YZ
027L3ZZ	02LR0CZ	02WY4YZ	04130J4	041U0ZS	041W4JP	04763D1	047D4Z1	047S341	05WY0YZ
027L44Z	02LR0DZ	031509V	04130J5	041U49P	041W4JQ	04763Z1	047E041	047S3D1	05WY3YZ
027L4DZ	02LR0ZZ	03150AV	04130K3	041U49Q	041W4JS	0476441	047E0D1	047S3Z1	05WY4YZ
027L4ZZ	02LR3CZ	03150JV	04130K4	041U49S	041W4KP	04764D1	047E0Z1	047S441	061007P
02H40YZ	02LR3DZ	03150KV	04130K5	041U4AP	041W4KQ	04764Z1	047E341	047S4D1	061007Q
02H43YZ	02LR3ZZ	03150ZV	04130Z3	041U4AQ	041W4KS	0477041	047E3D1	047S4Z1	061007R
02H44YZ	02LR4CZ	031609V	04130Z4	041U4AS	041W4ZP	04770D1	047E3Z1	047T041	061009P
02H60YZ	02LR4DZ	03160AV	04130Z5	041U4JP	041W4ZQ	04770Z1	047E441	047T0D1	061009Q
02H63YZ	02LR4ZZ	03160JV	0413493	041U4JQ	041W4ZS	0477341	047E4D1	047T0Z1	061009R
02H64YZ	02LW3DJ	03160KV	0413494	041U4JS	0470041	04773D1	047E4Z1	047T341	06100AP
02H70YZ	02N00ZZ	03160ZV	0413495	041U4KP	04700D1	04773Z1	047F041	047T3D1	06100AQ
02H73YZ	02N03ZZ	031709V	04134A3	041U4KQ	04700Z1	0477441	047F0D1	047T3Z1	06100AR
02H74YZ	02N04ZZ	03170AV	04134A4	041U4KS	0470341	04774D1	047F0Z1	047T441	06100JP
02HA0RJ	02N10ZZ	03170JV	04134A5	041U4ZP	04703D1	04774Z1	047F341	047T4D1	06100JQ
02HA0YZ	02N13ZZ	03170KV	04134J3	041U4ZQ	04703Z1	0478041	047F3D1	047T4Z1	06100JR
02HA3RJ	02N14ZZ	03170ZV	04134J4	041U4ZS	0470441	04780D1	047F3Z1	047U041	06100KP
02HA3YZ	02N20ZZ	031809V	04134J5	041V09P	04704D1	04780Z1	047F441	047U0D1	06100KQ
02HA4RJ	02N23ZZ	03180AV	04134K3	041V09Q	04704Z1	0478341	047F4D1	047U0Z1	06100KR
02HA4YZ	02N24ZZ	03180JV	04134K4	041V09S	0471041	04783D1	047F4Z1	047U341	06100ZP
02HK0YZ	02N30ZZ	03180KV	04134K5	041V0AP	04710D1	04783Z1	047H041	047U3D1	06100ZQ
02HK3YZ	02N33ZZ	03180ZV	04134Z3	041V0AQ	04710Z1	0478441	047H0D1	047U3Z1	06100ZR
02HK4YZ	02N34ZZ	031H09K	04134Z4	041V0AS	0471341	04784D1	047H0Z1	047U441	061047P
02HL0YZ	02PA0RS	031H0AK	04134Z5	041V0JP	04713D1	04784Z1	047H341	047U4D1	061047Q
02HL3YZ	02PA0YZ	031H0JK	041T09P	041V0JQ	04713Z1	0479041	047H3D1	047U4Z1	061047R
02HL4YZ	02PA3RS	031H0KK	041T09Q	041V0JS	0471441	04790D1	047H3Z1	047V041	061049P
02HN0YZ	02PA3YZ	031H0ZK	041T09S	041V0KP	04714D1	04790Z1	047H441	047V0D1	061049Q
02HN3YZ	02PA4RS	031J09J	041T0AP	041V0KQ	04714Z1	0479341	047H4D1	047V0Z1	061049R
02HN4YZ	02PA4YZ	031J0AJ	041T0AQ	041V0KS	0472041	04793D1	047H4Z1	047V341	06104AP
02HP0YZ	02PY0YZ	031J0JJ	041T0AS	041V0ZP	04720D1	04793Z1	047J041	047V3D1	06104AQ
02HP3YZ	02PY3YZ	031J0KJ	041T0JP	041V0ZQ	04720Z1	0479441	047J0D1	047V3Z1	06104AR
02HP4YZ	02PY4YZ	031J0ZJ	041T0JQ	041V0ZS	0472341	04794D1	047J0Z1	047V441	06104JP
02HQ0YZ	02RJ37H	031K09K	041T0JS	041V49P	04723D1	04794Z1	047J341	047V4D1	06104JQ
02HQ3YZ	02RJ37Z	031K0AK	041T0KP	041V49Q	04723Z1	047A041	047J3D1	047V4Z1	06104JR
02HQ4YZ	02RJ38H	031K0JK	041T0KQ	041V49S	0472441	047A0D1	047J3Z1	047W041	06104KP
02HR0YZ	02RJ38Z	031K0KK	041T0KS	041V4AP	04724D1	047A0Z1	047J441	047W0D1	06104KQ
02HR3YZ	02RJ3JH	031K0ZK	041T0ZP	041V4AQ	04724Z1	047A341	047J4D1	047W0Z1	06104KR
02HR4YZ	02RJ3JZ	031L09J	041T0ZQ	041V4AS	0473041	047A3D1	047J4Z1	047W341	06104ZP
02HS0YZ	02RJ3KH	031L0AJ	041T0ZS	041V4JP	04730D1	047A3Z1	047P041	047W3D1	06104ZQ
02HS3YZ	02RJ3KZ	031L0JJ	041T49P	041V4JQ	04730Z1	047A441	047P0D1	047W3Z1	06104ZR
02HS4YZ	02VG0ZZ	031L0KJ	041T49Q	041V4JS	0473341	047A4D1	047P0Z1	047W441	06183J4

06183JY	079J8ZZ	07DP4ZX	08H03YZ	09997ZX	099S7ZZ	09BV8ZZ	09PH0YZ	09UA87Z	0BD18ZX
06184J4	079K80Z	07HK0YZ	08H07YZ	09997ZZ	099S80Z	09BW8ZX	09PH3YZ	09UA8JZ	0BD24ZX
06HY0YZ	079K8ZX	07HK3YZ	08H08YZ	099980Z	099S8ZX	09BW8ZZ	09PH4YZ	09UA8KZ	0BD28ZX
06HY3YZ	079K8ZZ	07HK4YZ	08H10YZ	09998ZX	099S8ZZ	09BX8ZX	09PH7YZ	09UD87Z	0BD34ZX
06HY4YZ	079L80Z	07HL0YZ	08H13YZ	09998ZZ	099T70Z	09BX8ZZ	09PH8YZ	09UD8JZ	0BD38ZX
06L37CZ	079L8ZX	07HL3YZ	08H17YZ	099A70Z	099T7ZX	09C58ZZ	09PJ0YZ	09UD8KZ	0BD44ZX
06L37DZ	079L8ZZ	07HL4YZ	08H18YZ	099A7ZX	099T7ZZ	09C68ZZ	09PJ3YZ	09UE87Z	0BD48ZX
06L37ZZ	07D03ZX	07HM0YZ	08P00YZ	099A7ZZ	099T80Z	09C98ZZ	09PJ4YZ	09UE8JZ	0BD54ZX
06L38CZ	07D04ZX	07HM3YZ	08P03YZ	099A80Z	099T8ZX	09CA8ZZ	09PJ7YZ	09UE8KZ	0BD58ZX
06L38DZ	07D08ZX	07HM4YZ	08P07YZ	099A8ZX	099T8ZZ	09CB8ZZ	09PJ8YZ	09UK87Z	0BD64ZX
06L38ZZ	07D13ZX	07HN0YZ	08P08YZ	099A8ZZ	099U70Z	09CC8ZZ	09PK0YZ	09UK8JZ	0BD68ZX
06PY0YZ	07D14ZX	07HN3YZ	08P10YZ	099B70Z	099U7ZX	09CD8ZZ	09PK3YZ	09UK8KZ	0BD74ZX
06PY3YZ	07D18ZX	07HN4YZ	08P13YZ	099B7ZX	099U7ZZ	09CE8ZZ	09PK4YZ	09UM87Z	0BD78ZX
06PY4YZ	07D23ZX	07HP0YZ	08P17YZ	099B7ZZ	099U80Z	09CK8ZZ	09PK7YZ	09UM8JZ	0BD84ZX
06WY0YZ	07D24ZX	07HP3YZ	08P18YZ	099B80Z	099U8ZX	09CM8ZZ	09PK8YZ	09UM8KZ	0BD88ZX
06WY3YZ	07D28ZX	07HP4YZ	08PJ3YZ	099B8ZX	099U8ZZ	09CP8ZZ	09PY0YZ	09WH0YZ	0BD94ZX
06WY4YZ	07D33ZX	07JN8ZZ	08PK3YZ	099B8ZZ	099V70Z	09CQ8ZZ	09PY3YZ	09WH3YZ	0BD98ZX
079080Z	07D34ZX	07PK0YZ	08PL0YZ	099C70Z	099V7ZX	09CR8ZZ	09PY4YZ	09WH4YZ	0BDB4ZX
07908ZX	07D38ZX	07PK3YZ	08PL3YZ	099C7ZX	099V7ZZ	09CS8ZZ	09PY7YZ	09WH7YZ	0BDB8ZX
07908ZZ	07D43ZX	07PK4YZ	08PM0YZ	099C7ZZ	099V80Z	09CT8ZZ	09PY8YZ	09WH8YZ	0BDC4ZX
079180Z	07D44ZX	07PL0YZ	08PM3YZ	099C80Z	099V8ZX	09CU8ZZ	09Q58ZZ	09WJ0YZ	0BDC8ZX
07918ZX	07D48ZX	07PL3YZ	08W00YZ	099C8ZX	099V8ZZ	09CV8ZZ	09Q68ZZ	09WJ3YZ	0BDD4ZX
07918ZZ	07D53ZX	07PL4YZ	08W03YZ	099C8ZZ	099W70Z	09CW8ZZ	09Q98ZZ	09WJ4YZ	0BDD8ZX
079280Z	07D54ZX	07PM0YZ	08W07YZ	099D70Z	099W7ZX	09CX8ZZ	09QA8ZZ	09WJ7YZ	0BDF4ZX
07928ZX	07D58ZX	07PM3YZ	08W08YZ	099D7ZX	099W7ZZ	09HH0YZ	09QB8ZZ	09WJ8YZ	0BDF8ZX
07928ZZ	07D63ZX	07PM4YZ	08W10YZ	099D7ZZ	099W80Z	09HH3YZ	09QC8ZZ	09WK0YZ	0BDG4ZX
079380Z	07D64ZX	07PN0YZ	08W13YZ	099D80Z	099W8ZX	09HH4YZ	09QD8ZZ	09WK3YZ	0BDG8ZX
07938ZX	07D68ZX	07PN3YZ	08W17YZ	099D8ZX	099W8ZZ	09HH7YZ	09QE8ZZ	09WK4YZ	0BDH4ZX
07938ZZ	07D73ZX	07PN4YZ	08W18YZ	099D8ZZ	099X70Z	09HH8YZ	09QK8ZZ	09WK7YZ	0BDH8ZX
079480Z	07D74ZX	07PP0YZ	08WJ3YZ	099E70Z	099X7ZX	09HJ0YZ	09QM8ZZ	09WK8YZ	0BDJ4ZX
07948ZX	07D78ZX	07PP3YZ	08WK3YZ	099E7ZX	099X7ZZ	09HJ3YZ	09QP8ZZ	09WY0YZ	0BDJ8ZX
07948ZZ	07D83ZX	07PP4YZ	08WL0YZ	099E7ZZ	099X80Z	09HJ4YZ	09QQ8ZZ	09WY3YZ	0BDK4ZX
079580Z	07D84ZX	07Q08ZZ	08WL3YZ	099E80Z	099X8ZX	09HJ7YZ	09QR8ZZ	09WY4YZ	0BDK8ZX
07958ZX	07D88ZX	07Q18ZZ	08WM0YZ	099E8ZX	099X8ZZ	09HJ8YZ	09QS8ZZ	09WY7YZ	0BDL4ZX
07958ZZ	07D93ZX	07Q28ZZ	08WM3YZ	099E8ZZ	09B58ZX	09HK0YZ	09QT8ZZ	09WY8YZ	0BDL8ZX
079680Z	07D94ZX	07Q38ZZ	09558ZZ	099K70Z	09B58ZZ	09HK3YZ	09QU8ZZ	0B5T0ZZ	0BDM4ZX
07968ZX	07D98ZX	07Q48ZZ	09568ZZ	099K7ZX	09B68ZX	09HK4YZ	09QV8ZZ	0B5T3ZZ	0BDM8ZX
07968ZZ	07DB3ZX	07Q58ZZ	09598ZZ	099K7ZZ	09B68ZZ	09HK7YZ	09QW8ZZ	0B5T4ZZ	0BH00YZ
079780Z	07DB4ZX	07Q68ZZ	095A8ZZ	099K80Z	09B98ZX	09HK8YZ	09QX8ZZ	0B9N80Z	0BH03YZ
07978ZX	07DB8ZX	07Q78ZZ	095B8ZZ	099K8ZX	09B98ZZ	09HY0YZ	09T58ZZ	0B9N8ZX	0BH04YZ
07978ZZ	07DC3ZX	07Q88ZZ	095C8ZZ	099K8ZZ	09BA8ZX	09HY3YZ	09T68ZZ	0B9N8ZZ	0BH07YZ
079880Z	07DC4ZX	07Q98ZZ	095D8ZZ	099M70Z	09BA8ZZ	09HY4YZ	09T98ZZ	0B9P80Z	0BH08YZ
07988ZX	07DC8ZX	07QB8ZZ	095E8ZZ	099M7ZX	09BB8ZX	09HY7YZ	09TA8ZZ	0B9P8ZX	0BH10YZ
07988ZZ	07DD3ZX	07QC8ZZ	095K8ZZ	099M7ZZ	09BB8ZZ	09HY8YZ	09TB8ZZ	0B9P8ZZ	0BH13YZ
079980Z	07DD4ZX	07QD8ZZ	095M8ZZ	099M80Z	09BC8ZX	09JD8ZZ	09TC8ZZ	0B9T00Z	0BH14YZ
07998ZX	07DD8ZX	07QF8ZZ	095P8ZZ	099M8ZX	09BC8ZZ	09JE8ZZ	09TD8ZZ	0B9T0ZX	0BH17YZ
07998ZZ	07DF3ZX	07QG8ZZ	095Q8ZZ	099M8ZZ	09BD8ZX	09JK8ZZ	09TE8ZZ	0B9T0ZZ	0BH18YZ
079B80Z	07DF4ZX	07QH8ZZ	095R8ZZ	099P70Z	09BD8ZZ	09JY8ZZ	09TK8ZZ	0B9T30Z	0BHK0YZ
079B8ZX	07DF8ZX	07QJ8ZZ	095S8ZZ	099P7ZX	09BE8ZX	09N58ZZ	09TM8ZZ	0B9T3ZX	0BHK3YZ
079B8ZZ	07DG3ZX	07QK8ZZ	095T8ZZ	099P7ZZ	09BE8ZZ	09N68ZZ	09TP8ZZ	0B9T3ZZ	0BHK4YZ
079C80Z	07DG4ZX	07QL8ZZ	095U8ZZ	099P80Z	09BK8ZX	09N98ZZ	09TQ8ZZ	0B9T40Z	0BHK7YZ
079C8ZX	07DG8ZX	07WK0YZ	095V8ZZ	099P8ZX	09BK8ZZ	09NA8ZZ	09TR8ZZ	0B9T4ZX	0BHK8YZ
079C8ZZ	07DH3ZX	07WK3YZ	095W8ZZ	099P8ZZ	09BM8ZX	09NB8ZZ	09TS8ZZ	0B9T4ZZ	0BHL0YZ
079D80Z	07DH4ZX	07WK4YZ	095X8ZZ	099Q70Z	09BM8ZZ	09NC8ZZ	09TT8ZZ	0BBN8ZX	0BHL3YZ
079D8ZX	07DH8ZX	07WL0YZ	099570Z	099Q7ZX	09BP8ZX	09ND8ZZ	09TU8ZZ	0BBN8ZZ	0BHL4YZ
079D8ZZ	07DJ3ZX	07WL3YZ	09957ZX	099Q7ZZ	09BP8ZZ	09NE8ZZ	09TV8ZZ	0BBP8ZX	0BHL7YZ
079F80Z	07DJ4ZX	07WL4YZ	09957ZZ	099Q80Z	09BQ8ZX	09NK8ZZ	09TW8ZZ	0BBP8ZZ	0BHL8YZ
079F8ZX	07DJ8ZX	07WM0YZ	099580Z	099Q8ZX	09BQ8ZZ	09NM8ZZ	09TX8ZZ	0BBT0ZX	0BHQ0YZ
079F8ZZ	07DK3ZX	07WM3YZ	09958ZX	099Q8ZZ	09BR8ZX	09NP8ZZ	09U587Z	0BBT0ZZ	0BHQ3YZ
079G80Z	07DK4ZX	07WM4YZ	09958ZZ	099R70Z	09BR8ZZ	09NQ8ZZ	09U58JZ	0BBT3ZX	0BHQ4YZ
079G8ZX	07DK8ZX	07WN0YZ	099670Z	099R7ZX	09BS8ZZ	09NR8ZZ	09U58KZ	0BBT3ZZ	0BHQ7YZ
079G8ZZ	07DL3ZX	07WN3YZ	09967ZX	099R7ZZ	09BT8ZX	09NS8ZZ	09U687Z	0BBT4ZX	0BHQ8YZ
079H80Z	07DL4ZX	07WN4YZ	09967ZZ	099R80Z	09BT8ZZ	09NT8ZZ	09U68JZ	0BBT4ZZ	0BHT02Z
079H8ZX	07DL8ZX	07WP0YZ	099680Z	099R8ZX	09BU8ZX	09NU8ZZ	09U68KZ	0BCT0ZZ	0BHT0MZ
079H8ZZ	07DM3ZX	07WP3YZ	09968ZX	099R8ZZ	09BU8ZZ	09NV8ZZ	09U987Z	0BCT3ZZ	0BHT0YZ
079J80Z	07DM4ZX	07WP4YZ	09968ZZ	099S70Z	09BV8ZX	09NW8ZZ	09U98JZ	0BCT4ZZ	0BHT32Z
079J8ZX	07DP3ZX	08H00YZ	099970Z	099S7ZX	09BV8ZZ	09NX8ZZ	09U98KZ	0BD14ZX	0BHT3MZ

ØBHT3YZ	ØBR54KZ	ØBUB87Z	ØCWY3YZ	ØDDF3ZX	ØDP67YZ	ØF17ØZ6	ØFB77ZX	ØFP44YZ	ØFU73JZ
ØBHT42Z	ØBR6Ø7Z	ØBUB8JZ	ØCWY7YZ	ØDDF4ZX	ØDP68YZ	ØF17ØZ7	ØFB77ZZ	ØFPBØYZ	ØFU73KZ
ØBHT4MZ	ØBR6ØJZ	ØBUB8KZ	ØCWY8YZ	ØDDF8ZX	ØDPDØYZ	ØF17ØZ8	ØFB78ZX	ØFPB3YZ	ØFU747Z
ØBHT4YZ	ØBR6ØKZ	ØBUTØ7Z	ØD5UØZZ	ØDDG3ZX	ØDPD3YZ	ØF17ØZ9	ØFB78ZZ	ØFPB4YZ	ØFU74JZ
ØBHT7YZ	ØBR647Z	ØBUTØJZ	ØD5U3ZZ	ØDDG4ZX	ØDPD4YZ	ØF17ØZB	ØFBG8ZX	ØFPB7YZ	ØFU74KZ
ØBHT8YZ	ØBR64JZ	ØBUTØKZ	ØD5U4ZZ	ØDDG8ZX	ØDPD7YZ	ØF174D3	ØFBG8ZZ	ØFPB8YZ	ØFU787Z
ØBMTØZZ	ØBR64KZ	ØBUT47Z	ØD9UØØZ	ØDDH3ZX	ØDPD8YZ	ØF174D4	ØFC48ZZ	ØFPDØYZ	ØFU78JZ
ØBNTØZZ	ØBR7Ø7Z	ØBUT4JZ	ØD9UØZX	ØDDH4ZX	ØDQUØZZ	ØF174D5	ØFC7ØZZ	ØFPD3YZ	ØFU78KZ
ØBNT3ZZ	ØBR7ØJZ	ØBUT4KZ	ØD9UØZZ	ØDDH8ZX	ØDQU3ZZ	ØF174D6	ØFC73ZZ	ØFPD4YZ	ØFU887Z
ØBNT4ZZ	ØBR7ØKZ	ØBWØØYZ	ØD9U3ØZ	ØDDJ3ZX	ØDQU4ZZ	ØF174D7	ØFC74ZZ	ØFPD7YZ	ØFU88JZ
ØBPØØYZ	ØBR747Z	ØBWØ3YZ	ØD9U3ZX	ØDDJ4ZX	ØDRUØ7Z	ØF174D8	ØFC77ZZ	ØFPD8YZ	ØFU88KZ
ØBPØ3YZ	ØBR74JZ	ØBWØ4YZ	ØD9U3ZZ	ØDDJ8ZX	ØDRUØJZ	ØF174D9	ØFC78ZZ	ØFPGØYZ	ØFU987Z
ØBPØ4YZ	ØBR74KZ	ØBWØ7YZ	ØD9U4ØZ	ØDDK3ZX	ØDRUØKZ	ØF174DB	ØFCG8ZZ	ØFPG3YZ	ØFU98KZ
ØBPØ7YZ	ØBR8Ø7Z	ØBWØ8YZ	ØD9U4ZX	ØDDK4ZX	ØDRU47Z	ØF174Z3	ØFF7ØZZ	ØFPG4YZ	ØFUC87Z
ØBPØ8YZ	ØBR8ØJZ	ØBWKØYZ	ØD9U4ZZ	ØDDK8ZX	ØDRU4JZ	ØF174Z4	ØFF73ZZ	ØFQ48ZZ	ØFUC8JZ
ØBPKØYZ	ØBR8ØKZ	ØBWK3YZ	ØDBGFZZ	ØDDL3ZX	ØDRU4KZ	ØF174Z5	ØFF74ZZ	ØFQ7ØZZ	ØFUC8KZ
ØBPK3YZ	ØBR847Z	ØBWK4YZ	ØDBLFZZ	ØDDL4ZX	ØDS8ØZZ	ØF174Z6	ØFF77ZZ	ØFQ73ZZ	ØFUD87Z
ØBPK4YZ	ØBR84JZ	ØBWK7YZ	ØDBMFZZ	ØDDL8ZX	ØDS84ZZ	ØF174Z7	ØFF78ZZ	ØFQ74ZZ	ØFUD8JZ
ØBPK7YZ	ØBR84KZ	ØBWK8YZ	ØDBNFZZ	ØDDM3ZX	ØDS87ZZ	ØF174Z8	ØFF7XZZ	ØFQ77ZZ	ØFUD8KZ
ØBPK8YZ	ØBR9Ø7Z	ØBWLØYZ	ØDBUØZX	ØDDM4ZX	ØDS88ZZ	ØF174Z9	ØFHØØYZ	ØFQ78ZZ	ØFUF87Z
ØBPLØYZ	ØBR9ØJZ	ØBWL3YZ	ØDBUØZZ	ØDDM8ZX	ØDSEØZZ	ØF174ZB	ØFHØ3YZ	ØFQG8ZZ	ØFUF8JZ
ØBPL3YZ	ØBR9ØKZ	ØBWL4YZ	ØDBU3ZX	ØDDN3ZX	ØDSE4ZZ	ØF548ZZ	ØFHØ4YZ	ØFR587Z	ØFUF8KZ
ØBPL4YZ	ØBR947Z	ØBWL7YZ	ØDBU3ZZ	ØDDN4ZX	ØDSE7ZZ	ØF57ØZZ	ØFH4ØYZ	ØFR58JZ	ØFV7ØCZ
ØBPL7YZ	ØBR94JZ	ØBWL8YZ	ØDBU4ZX	ØDDN8ZX	ØDSE8ZZ	ØF573ZZ	ØFH43YZ	ØFR58KZ	ØFV7ØDZ
ØBPL8YZ	ØBR94KZ	ØBWQØYZ	ØDBU4ZZ	ØDDP3ZX	ØDTGFZZ	ØF574ZZ	ØFH44YZ	ØFR687Z	ØFV7ØZZ
ØBPQØYZ	ØBRBØ7Z	ØBWQ3YZ	ØDCUØZZ	ØDDP4ZX	ØDTLFZZ	ØF577ZZ	ØFHBØYZ	ØFR68JZ	ØFV73CZ
ØBPQ3YZ	ØBRBØJZ	ØBWQ4YZ	ØDCU3ZZ	ØDDP8ZX	ØDTMFZZ	ØF578ZZ	ØFHB3YZ	ØFR68KZ	ØFV73DZ
ØBPQ4YZ	ØBRBØKZ	ØBWQ7YZ	ØDCU4ZZ	ØDDQ3ZX	ØDTNFZZ	ØF5G8ZZ	ØFHB4YZ	ØFR7Ø7Z	ØFV73ZZ
ØBPQ7YZ	ØBRB47Z	ØBWQ8YZ	ØDD13ZX	ØDDQ4ZX	ØDTUØZZ	ØF77ØDZ	ØFHB7YZ	ØFR7ØJZ	ØFV74CZ
ØBPQ8YZ	ØBRB4JZ	ØBWTØYZ	ØDD14ZX	ØDDQ8ZX	ØDTU4ZZ	ØF77ØZZ	ØFHB8YZ	ØFR7ØKZ	ØFV74DZ
ØBPTØYZ	ØBRB4KZ	ØBWT3YZ	ØDD18ZX	ØDDQXZX	ØDUUØ7Z	ØF773DZ	ØFHDØYZ	ØFR747Z	ØFV74ZZ
ØBPT3YZ	ØBRTØ7Z	ØBWT4YZ	ØDD23ZX	ØDHØØYZ	ØDUUØJZ	ØF773ZZ	ØFHD3YZ	ØFR74JZ	ØFV77DZ
ØBPT4YZ	ØBRTØJZ	ØBWT7YZ	ØDD24ZX	ØDHØ3YZ	ØDUUØKZ	ØF774DZ	ØFHD4YZ	ØFR74KZ	ØFV77ZZ
ØBPT7YZ	ØBRTØKZ	ØBWT8YZ	ØDD28ZX	ØDHØ4YZ	ØDUU47Z	ØF774ZZ	ØFHD7YZ	ØFR787Z	ØFV78DZ
ØBPT8YZ	ØBRT47Z	ØCHAØYZ	ØDD33ZX	ØDHØ7YZ	ØDUU4JZ	ØF777DZ	ØFHD8YZ	ØFR78JZ	ØFV78ZZ
ØBQTØZZ	ØBRT4JZ	ØCHA3YZ	ØDD34ZX	ØDHØ8YZ	ØDUU4KZ	ØF777ZZ	ØFHGØYZ	ØFR78KZ	ØFWØØYZ
ØBQT3ZZ	ØBRT4KZ	ØCHA7YZ	ØDD38ZX	ØDH5ØYZ	ØDWØØYZ	ØF778DZ	ØFHG3YZ	ØFR887Z	ØFWØ3YZ
ØBQT4ZZ	ØBSTØZZ	ØCHA8YZ	ØDD43ZX	ØDH53YZ	ØDWØ3YZ	ØF778ZZ	ØFHG4YZ	ØFR88JZ	ØFWØ4YZ
ØBR1Ø7Z	ØBTTØZZ	ØCHSØYZ	ØDD44ZX	ØDH54YZ	ØDWØ4YZ	ØF948ØZ	ØFJ48ZZ	ØFR88KZ	ØFW4ØYZ
ØBR1ØJZ	ØBTT4ZZ	ØCHS3YZ	ØDD48ZX	ØDH57YZ	ØDWØ7YZ	ØF948ZX	ØFJG8ZZ	ØFR987Z	ØFW43YZ
ØBR1ØKZ	ØBU187Z	ØCHS7YZ	ØDD53ZX	ØDH58YZ	ØDWØ8YZ	ØF948ZZ	ØFL7ØCZ	ØFR98JZ	ØFW44YZ
ØBR147Z	ØBU18JZ	ØCHS8YZ	ØDD54ZX	ØDH6ØYZ	ØDW5ØYZ	ØF97ØØZ	ØFL7ØDZ	ØFR98KZ	ØFWBØYZ
ØBR14JZ	ØBU18KZ	ØCHYØYZ	ØDD58ZX	ØDH63YZ	ØDW53YZ	ØF97ØZX	ØFL7ØZZ	ØFRC87Z	ØFWB3YZ
ØBR14KZ	ØBU287Z	ØCHY3YZ	ØDD63ZX	ØDH64YZ	ØDW54YZ	ØF97ØZZ	ØFL73CZ	ØFRC8JZ	ØFWB4YZ
ØBR2Ø7Z	ØBU28JZ	ØCHY7YZ	ØDD64ZX	ØDH67YZ	ØDW57YZ	ØF973ØZ	ØFL73DZ	ØFRC8KZ	ØFWB7YZ
ØBR2ØJZ	ØBU28KZ	ØCHY8YZ	ØDD68ZX	ØDH68YZ	ØDW58YZ	ØF973ZX	ØFL73ZZ	ØFRD87Z	ØFWB8YZ
ØBR2ØKZ	ØBU387Z	ØCPAØYZ	ØDD73ZX	ØDHDØYZ	ØDW6ØYZ	ØF973ZZ	ØFL74CZ	ØFRD8JZ	ØFWDØYZ
ØBR387Z	ØBU38JZ	ØCPA3YZ	ØDD74ZX	ØDHD3YZ	ØDW63YZ	ØF974ØZ	ØFL74DZ	ØFRD8KZ	ØFWD3YZ
ØBR247Z	ØBU38KZ	ØCPA7YZ	ØDD78ZX	ØDHD4YZ	ØDW64YZ	ØF974ZX	ØFL74ZZ	ØFRF87Z	ØFWD4YZ
ØBR24JZ	ØBU487Z	ØCPA8YZ	ØDD83ZX	ØDHD7YZ	ØDW67YZ	ØF974ZZ	ØFL77DZ	ØFRF8JZ	ØFWD7YZ
ØBR24KZ	ØBU48JZ	ØCPSØYZ	ØDD84ZX	ØDHD8YZ	ØDW68YZ	ØF977ØZ	ØFL77ZZ	ØFRF8KZ	ØFWD8YZ
ØBR3Ø7Z	ØBU48KZ	ØCPS3YZ	ØDD88ZX	ØDNUØZZ	ØDWDØYZ	ØF977ZX	ØFL78DZ	ØFS7ØZZ	ØFWGØYZ
ØBR3ØJZ	ØBU587Z	ØCPS7YZ	ØDD93ZX	ØDNU3ZZ	ØDWD3YZ	ØF977ZZ	ØFL78ZZ	ØFS74ZZ	ØFWG3YZ
ØBR3ØKZ	ØBU58JZ	ØCPS8YZ	ØDD94ZX	ØDNU4ZZ	ØDWD4YZ	ØF978ØZ	ØFM7ØZZ	ØFT7ØZZ	ØFWG4YZ
ØBR347Z	ØBU58KZ	ØCPYØYZ	ØDD98ZX	ØDPØØYZ	ØDWD7YZ	ØF978ZX	ØFM74ZZ	ØFT74ZZ	ØGBJØZX
ØBR34JZ	ØBU687Z	ØCPY3YZ	ØDDA3ZX	ØDPØ3YZ	ØDWD8YZ	ØF978ZZ	ØFN48ZZ	ØFT77ZZ	ØGBJØZZ
ØBR34KZ	ØBU68JZ	ØCPY7YZ	ØDDA4ZX	ØDPØ4YZ	ØF17ØD3	ØF9G8ØZ	ØFN7ØZZ	ØFT78ZZ	ØGBJ3ZX
ØBR4Ø7Z	ØBU68KZ	ØCPY8YZ	ØDDA8ZX	ØDPØ7YZ	ØF17ØD4	ØF9G8ZX	ØFN73ZZ	ØFU587Z	ØGBJ4ZX
ØBR4ØJZ	ØBU787Z	ØCWAØYZ	ØDDB3ZX	ØDPØ8YZ	ØF17ØD5	ØF9G8ZZ	ØFN74ZZ	ØFU58KZ	ØGBJ4ZZ
ØBR4ØKZ	ØBU78JZ	ØCWA3YZ	ØDDB8ZX	ØDP5ØYZ	ØF17ØD6	ØFB48ZX	ØFN77ZZ	ØFU687Z	ØGHSØYZ
ØBR447Z	ØBU78KZ	ØCWA7YZ	ØDDC3ZX	ØDP53YZ	ØF17ØD7	ØFB48ZZ	ØFN78ZZ	ØFU68KZ	ØGHS3YZ
ØBR44JZ	ØBU887Z	ØCWA8YZ	ØDDC4ZX	ØDP54YZ	ØF17ØD8	ØFB7ØZX	ØFNG8ZZ	ØFU7Ø7Z	ØGHS4YZ
ØBR44KZ	ØBU88JZ	ØCWSØYZ	ØDDC8ZX	ØDP57YZ	ØF17ØD9	ØFB7ØZZ	ØFPØØYZ	ØFU7ØJZ	ØGPSØYZ
ØBR5Ø7Z	ØBU88KZ	ØCWS3YZ	ØDDE3ZX	ØDP58YZ	ØF17ØDB	ØFB73ZX	ØFPØ3YZ	ØFU7ØKZ	ØGPS3YZ
ØBR5ØJZ	ØBU987Z	ØCWS7YZ	ØDDE4ZX	ØDP6ØYZ	ØF17ØZ3	ØFB73ZZ	ØFPØ4YZ	ØFU737Z	ØGPS4YZ
ØBR5ØKZ	ØBU98JZ	ØCWS8YZ	ØDDE8ZX	ØDP63YZ	ØF17ØZ4	ØFB74ZX	ØFP4ØYZ		
ØBR547Z	ØBU98KZ	ØCWYØYZ		ØDP64YZ	ØF17ØZ5	ØFB74ZZ	ØFP43YZ		
ØBR54JZ									

ØGTJØZZ	ØKDCØZZ	ØKR6ØKZ	ØKRK47Z	ØKWY3YZ	ØMHYØYZ	ØMR94JZ	ØMRN4KZ	ØNDQØZZ	ØQSPØ42
ØGTJ4ZZ	ØKDDØZZ	ØKR647Z	ØKRK4JZ	ØKWY4YZ	ØMHY3YZ	ØMR94KZ	ØMRPØ7Z	ØNDRØZZ	ØQSPØ52
ØGWSØYZ	ØKDFØZZ	ØKR64JZ	ØKRK4KZ	ØKXFØZ5	ØMHY4YZ	ØMRBØ7Z	ØMRPØJZ	ØNDTØZZ	ØQSPØZ2
ØGWS3YZ	ØKDGØZZ	ØKR64KZ	ØKRLØ7Z	ØKXFØZ7	ØMPXØYZ	ØMRBØJZ	ØMRPØKZ	ØNDVØZZ	ØQSP342
ØGWS4YZ	ØKDHØZZ	ØKR7Ø7Z	ØKRLØJZ	ØKXFØZ8	ØMPX3YZ	ØMRBØKZ	ØMRP47Z	ØNDXØZZ	ØQSP352
ØHHPXYZ	ØKDJØZZ	ØKR7ØJZ	ØKRLØKZ	ØKXFØZ9	ØMPX4YZ	ØMRB47Z	ØMRP4JZ	ØPDØØZZ	ØQSP3Z2
ØHHTØYZ	ØKDKØZZ	ØKR7ØKZ	ØKRL47Z	ØKXF4Z5	ØMPYØYZ	ØMRB4JZ	ØMRP4KZ	ØPD1ØZZ	ØQSP442
ØHHT3YZ	ØKDLØZZ	ØKR747Z	ØKRL4JZ	ØKXF4Z7	ØMPY3YZ	ØMRB4KZ	ØMRQØ7Z	ØPD2ØZZ	ØQSP452
ØHHT7YZ	ØKDMØZZ	ØKR74JZ	ØKRL4KZ	ØKXF4Z8	ØMPY4YZ	ØMRCØ7Z	ØMRQØJZ	ØPD3ØZZ	ØQSP4Z2
ØHHT8YZ	ØKDNØZZ	ØKR74KZ	ØKRMØ7Z	ØKXF4Z9	ØMRØØ7Z	ØMRCØJZ	ØMRQØKZ	ØPD4ØZZ	ØQSPXZ2
ØHHUØYZ	ØKDPØZZ	ØKR8Ø7Z	ØKRMØJZ	ØKXGØZ5	ØMRØØJZ	ØMRCØKZ	ØMRQ47Z	ØPD5ØZZ	ØSR9Ø69
ØHHU3YZ	ØKDQØZZ	ØKR8ØJZ	ØKRMØKZ	ØKXGØZ7	ØMRØØKZ	ØMRC47Z	ØMRQ4JZ	ØPD6ØZZ	ØSR9Ø6A
ØHHU7YZ	ØKDRØZZ	ØKR8ØKZ	ØKRM47Z	ØKXGØZ8	ØMRØ47Z	ØMRC4JZ	ØMRQ4KZ	ØPD7ØZZ	ØSR9Ø6Z
ØHHU8YZ	ØKDSØZZ	ØKR847Z	ØKRM4JZ	ØKXGØZ9	ØMRØ4JZ	ØMRC4KZ	ØMRRØ7Z	ØPD8ØZZ	ØSRBØ69
ØHPPXYZ	ØKDTØZZ	ØKR84JZ	ØKRM4KZ	ØKXG4Z5	ØMRØ4KZ	ØMRDØ7Z	ØMRRØJZ	ØPD9ØZZ	ØSRBØ6A
ØHPTØYZ	ØKDVØZZ	ØKR84KZ	ØKRNØ7Z	ØKXG4Z7	ØMR1Ø7Z	ØMRDØJZ	ØMRRØKZ	ØPDBØZZ	ØSRBØ6Z
ØHPT3YZ	ØKDWØZZ	ØKR9Ø7Z	ØKRNØJZ	ØKXG4Z8	ØMR1ØJZ	ØMRDØKZ	ØMRR47Z	ØPDCØZZ	ØSRCØ69
ØHPT7YZ	ØKHXØYZ	ØKR9ØJZ	ØKRNØKZ	ØKXG4Z9	ØMR1ØKZ	ØMRD47Z	ØMRR4JZ	ØPDDØZZ	ØSRCØ6A
ØHPT8YZ	ØKHX3YZ	ØKR9ØKZ	ØKRN47Z	ØLDØØZZ	ØMR147Z	ØMRD4JZ	ØMRR4KZ	ØPDFØZZ	ØSRCØ6Z
ØHPUØYZ	ØKHX4YZ	ØKR947Z	ØKRN4JZ	ØLD1ØZZ	ØMR14JZ	ØMRD4KZ	ØMRSØ7Z	ØPDGØZZ	ØSRDØ69
ØHPU3YZ	ØKHYØYZ	ØKR94JZ	ØKRN4KZ	ØLD2ØZZ	ØMR14KZ	ØMRFØ7Z	ØMRSØJZ	ØPDHØZZ	ØSRDØ6A
ØHPU7YZ	ØKHY3YZ	ØKR94KZ	ØKRPØ7Z	ØLD3ØZZ	ØMR2Ø7Z	ØMRFØJZ	ØMRSØKZ	ØPDJØZZ	ØSRDØ6Z
ØHPU8YZ	ØKHY4YZ	ØKRBØ7Z	ØKRPØJZ	ØLD4ØZZ	ØMR2ØJZ	ØMRFØKZ	ØMRS47Z	ØPDKØZZ	ØTH5ØYZ
ØHWPXYZ	ØKPXØYZ	ØKRBØJZ	ØKRPØKZ	ØLD5ØZZ	ØMR2ØKZ	ØMRF47Z	ØMRS4JZ	ØPDLØZZ	ØTH53YZ
ØHWTØYZ	ØKPX3YZ	ØKRBØKZ	ØKRP47Z	ØLD6ØZZ	ØMR247Z	ØMRF4JZ	ØMRS4KZ	ØPDMØZZ	ØTH54YZ
ØHWT3YZ	ØKPX4YZ	ØKRB47Z	ØKRP4JZ	ØLD7ØZZ	ØMR24JZ	ØMRF4KZ	ØMRTØ7Z	ØPDNØZZ	ØTH57YZ
ØHWT7YZ	ØKPYØYZ	ØKRB4JZ	ØKRP4KZ	ØLD8ØZZ	ØMR24KZ	ØMRGØ7Z	ØMRTØJZ	ØPDPØZZ	ØTH58YZ
ØHWT8YZ	ØKPY3YZ	ØKRB4KZ	ØKRQØ7Z	ØLD9ØZZ	ØMR3Ø7Z	ØMRGØJZ	ØMRTØKZ	ØPDQØZZ	ØTH9ØYZ
ØHWUØYZ	ØKPY4YZ	ØKRCØ7Z	ØKRQØJZ	ØLDBØZZ	ØMR3ØJZ	ØMRGØKZ	ØMRT47Z	ØPDRØZZ	ØTH93YZ
ØHWU3YZ	ØKRØØ7Z	ØKRCØJZ	ØKRQØKZ	ØLDCØZZ	ØMR3ØKZ	ØMRG47Z	ØMRT4JZ	ØPDSØZZ	ØTH94YZ
ØHWU7YZ	ØKRØØJZ	ØKRCØKZ	ØKRQ47Z	ØLDDØZZ	ØMR347Z	ØMRG4JZ	ØMRT4KZ	ØPDTØZZ	ØTH97YZ
ØHWU8YZ	ØKRØØKZ	ØKRC47Z	ØKRQ4JZ	ØLDFØZZ	ØMR34JZ	ØMRG4KZ	ØMRVØ7Z	ØPDVØZZ	ØTH98YZ
ØJHSØYZ	ØKRØ47Z	ØKRC4JZ	ØKRQ4KZ	ØLDGØZZ	ØMR34KZ	ØMRHØ7Z	ØMRVØJZ	ØQDØØZZ	ØTHBØYZ
ØJHS3YZ	ØKRØ4JZ	ØKRC4KZ	ØKRRØ7Z	ØLDHØZZ	ØMR4Ø7Z	ØMRHØJZ	ØMRVØKZ	ØQD1ØZZ	ØTHB3YZ
ØJHTØYZ	ØKRØ4KZ	ØKRDØ7Z	ØKRRØJZ	ØLDJØZZ	ØMR4ØJZ	ØMRHØKZ	ØMRV47Z	ØQD2ØZZ	ØTHB4YZ
ØJHT3YZ	ØKR1Ø7Z	ØKRDØJZ	ØKRRØKZ	ØLDKØZZ	ØMR4ØKZ	ØMRH47Z	ØMRV4JZ	ØQD3ØZZ	ØTHB7YZ
ØJHVØYZ	ØKR1ØJZ	ØKRDØKZ	ØKRR47Z	ØLDLØZZ	ØMR447Z	ØMRH4JZ	ØMRV4KZ	ØQD4ØZZ	ØTHB8YZ
ØJHV3YZ	ØKR1ØKZ	ØKRD47Z	ØKRR4JZ	ØLDMØZZ	ØMR44JZ	ØMRH4KZ	ØMRWØ7Z	ØQD5ØZZ	ØTHDØYZ
ØJHWØYZ	ØKR147Z	ØKRD4JZ	ØKRR4KZ	ØLDNØZZ	ØMR44KZ	ØMRJØ7Z	ØMRWØJZ	ØQD6ØZZ	ØTHD3YZ
ØJHW3YZ	ØKR14JZ	ØKRD4KZ	ØKRSØ7Z	ØLDPØZZ	ØMR5Ø7Z	ØMRJØJZ	ØMRWØKZ	ØQD7ØZZ	ØTHD4YZ
ØJPSØYZ	ØKR14KZ	ØKRFØ7Z	ØKRSØJZ	ØLDQØZZ	ØMR5ØJZ	ØMRJØKZ	ØMRW47Z	ØQD8ØZZ	ØTHD7YZ
ØJPS3YZ	ØKR2Ø7Z	ØKRFØJZ	ØKRSØKZ	ØLDRØZZ	ØMR5ØKZ	ØMRJ47Z	ØMRW4JZ	ØQD9ØZZ	ØTHD8YZ
ØJPTØYZ	ØKR2ØJZ	ØKRFØKZ	ØKRS47Z	ØLDSØZZ	ØMR547Z	ØMRJ4JZ	ØMRW4KZ	ØQDBØZZ	ØTP5ØYZ
ØJPT3YZ	ØKR2ØKZ	ØKRF47Z	ØKRS4JZ	ØLDTØZZ	ØMR54JZ	ØMRJ4KZ	ØMWXØYZ	ØQDCØZZ	ØTP53YZ
ØJPVØYZ	ØKR247Z	ØKRF4JZ	ØKRS4KZ	ØLDVØZZ	ØMR54KZ	ØMRKØ7Z	ØMWX3YZ	ØQDDØZZ	ØTP54YZ
ØJPV3YZ	ØKR24JZ	ØKRF4KZ	ØKRTØ7Z	ØLDWØZZ	ØMR6Ø7Z	ØMRKØJZ	ØMWX4YZ	ØQDFØZZ	ØTP57YZ
ØJPWØYZ	ØKR24KZ	ØKRGØ7Z	ØKRTØJZ	ØLHXØYZ	ØMR6ØJZ	ØMRKØKZ	ØMWYØYZ	ØQDGØZZ	ØTP58YZ
ØJPW3YZ	ØKR3Ø7Z	ØKRGØJZ	ØKRTØKZ	ØLHX3YZ	ØMR6ØKZ	ØMRK47Z	ØMWY3YZ	ØQDHØZZ	ØTP9ØYZ
ØJWSØYZ	ØKR3ØJZ	ØKRGØKZ	ØKRT47Z	ØLHX4YZ	ØMR647Z	ØMRK4JZ	ØMWY4YZ	ØQDJØZZ	ØTP93YZ
ØJWS3YZ	ØKR3ØKZ	ØKRG47Z	ØKRT4JZ	ØLHYØYZ	ØMR64JZ	ØMRK4KZ	ØNDØØZZ	ØQDKØZZ	ØTP94YZ
ØJWTØYZ	ØKR347Z	ØKRG4JZ	ØKRT4KZ	ØLHY3YZ	ØMR64KZ	ØMRLØ7Z	ØND1ØZZ	ØQDLØZZ	ØTP97YZ
ØJWT3YZ	ØKR34JZ	ØKRG4KZ	ØKRVØ7Z	ØLHY4YZ	ØMR7Ø7Z	ØMRLØJZ	ØND3ØZZ	ØQDMØZZ	ØTP98YZ
ØJWVØYZ	ØKR34KZ	ØKRHØ7Z	ØKRVØJZ	ØLPXØYZ	ØMR7ØJZ	ØMRLØKZ	ØND4ØZZ	ØQDNØZZ	ØTPBØYZ
ØJWV3YZ	ØKR4Ø7Z	ØKRHØJZ	ØKRVØKZ	ØLPX3YZ	ØMR7ØKZ	ØMRL47Z	ØND5ØZZ	ØQDPØZZ	ØTPB3YZ
ØJWWØYZ	ØKR4ØJZ	ØKRHØKZ	ØKRV47Z	ØLPX4YZ	ØMR747Z	ØMRL4JZ	ØND6ØZZ	ØQDQØZZ	ØTPB4YZ
ØJWW3YZ	ØKR4ØKZ	ØKRH47Z	ØKRV4JZ	ØLPYØYZ	ØMR74JZ	ØMRL4KZ	ØND7ØZZ	ØQDRØZZ	ØTPB7YZ
ØKDØØZZ	ØKR447Z	ØKRH4JZ	ØKRV4KZ	ØLPY3YZ	ØMR74KZ	ØMRMØ7Z	ØNDBØZZ	ØQDSØZZ	ØTPB8YZ
ØKD1ØZZ	ØKR44JZ	ØKRH4KZ	ØKRWØ7Z	ØLPY4YZ	ØMR8Ø7Z	ØMRMØJZ	ØNDCØZZ	ØQSNØ42	ØTPDØYZ
ØKD2ØZZ	ØKR44KZ	ØKRJØ7Z	ØKRWØJZ	ØLWXØYZ	ØMR8ØJZ	ØMRMØKZ	ØNDFØZZ	ØQSNØ52	ØTPD3YZ
ØKD3ØZZ	ØKR5Ø7Z	ØKRJØJZ	ØKRWØKZ	ØLWX3YZ	ØMR8ØKZ	ØMRM47Z	ØNDGØZZ	ØQSNØZ2	ØTPD4YZ
ØKD4ØZZ	ØKR5ØJZ	ØKRJØKZ	ØKRW47Z	ØLWX4YZ	ØMR847Z	ØMRM4JZ	ØNDHØZZ	ØQSN342	ØTPD7YZ
ØKD5ØZZ	ØKR5ØKZ	ØKRJ47Z	ØKRW4JZ	ØLWYØYZ	ØMR84JZ	ØMRM4KZ	ØNDJØZZ	ØQSN352	ØTPD8YZ
ØKD6ØZZ	ØKR547Z	ØKRJ4JZ	ØKRW4KZ	ØLWY3YZ	ØMR84KZ	ØMRNØ7Z	ØNDKØZZ	ØQSN3Z2	ØTW5ØYZ
ØKD7ØZZ	ØKR54JZ	ØKRJ4KZ	ØKWXØYZ	ØLWY4YZ	ØMR9Ø7Z	ØMRNØJZ	ØNDLØZZ	ØQSN442	ØTW53YZ
ØKD8ØZZ	ØKR54KZ	ØKRKØ7Z	ØKWX3YZ	ØMHXØYZ	ØMR9ØJZ	ØMRNØKZ	ØNDMØZZ	ØQSN452	ØTW54YZ
ØKD9ØZZ	ØKR6Ø7Z	ØKRKØJZ	ØKWX4YZ	ØMHX3YZ	ØMR9ØKZ	ØMRN47Z	ØNDNØZZ	ØQSN4Z2	ØTW57YZ
ØKDBØZZ	ØKR6ØJZ	ØKRKØKZ	ØKWYØYZ	ØMHX4YZ	ØMR947Z	ØMRN4JZ	ØNDPØZZ	ØQSNXZ2	ØTW58YZ

ØTW9ØYZ	ØUHD4YZ	ØUSG7ZZ	ØVBL8ZZ	ØVLN8DZ	ØVQF8ZZ	ØVUL8KZ	ØWB3XZZ	4AØ27CZ	4A128CZ
ØTW93YZ	ØUHD7YZ	ØUSG8ZZ	ØVBN8ZX	ØVLN8ZZ	ØVQG8ZZ	ØVUN87Z	ØWCHØZZ	4AØ27FZ	4A128FZ
ØTW94YZ	ØUHD8YZ	ØUT9ØZL	ØVBN8ZZ	ØVLP8CZ	ØVQH8ZZ	ØVUN8JZ	ØWCH3ZZ	4AØ27HZ	4A128HZ
ØTW97YZ	ØUHHØYZ	ØUT94ZL	ØVBP8ZX	ØVLP8DZ	ØVQJ8ZZ	ØVUN8KZ	ØWCH4ZZ	4AØ27N6	4A1675Z
ØTW98YZ	ØUHH3YZ	ØUT97ZL	ØVBP8ZZ	ØVLP8ZZ	ØVQK8ZZ	ØVUP87Z	ØWCHXZZ	4AØ27N7	4A167BZ
ØTWBØYZ	ØUHH4YZ	ØUT98ZL	ØVBQ8ZX	ØVLQ8CZ	ØVQL8ZZ	ØVUP8JZ	ØWQ3ØZZ	4AØ27N8	4A1685Z
ØTWB3YZ	ØUHH7YZ	ØUT9FZL	ØVBQ8ZZ	ØVLQ8DZ	ØVQN8ZZ	ØVUP8KZ	ØWQ33ZZ	4AØ27PZ	4A168BZ
ØTWB4YZ	ØUHH8YZ	ØUW3ØYZ	ØVH4ØYZ	ØVLQ8ZZ	ØVQP8ZZ	ØVUQ87Z	ØWQ34ZZ	4AØ284Z	4A1D83Z
ØTWB7YZ	ØUJ38ZZ	ØUW33YZ	ØVH43YZ	ØVNF8ZZ	ØVQQ8ZZ	ØVUQ8JZ	ØWQ3XZZ	4AØ289Z	4A1D85Z
ØTWB8YZ	ØUNØ8ZZ	ØUW34YZ	ØVH44YZ	ØVNG8ZZ	ØVS98ZZ	ØVUQ8KZ	1ØD17Z9	4AØ28CZ	4A1D8BZ
ØTWDØYZ	ØUN18ZZ	ØUW37YZ	ØVH47YZ	ØVNH8ZZ	ØVSB8ZZ	ØVW4ØYZ	1ØD18Z9	4AØ28FZ	4A1D8DZ
ØTWD3YZ	ØUN28ZZ	ØUW38YZ	ØVH48YZ	ØVNJ8ZZ	ØVSC8ZZ	ØVW43YZ	3EØ134Ø	4AØ28HZ	4A1D8LZ
ØTWD4YZ	ØUN48ZZ	ØUW8ØYZ	ØVH8ØYZ	ØVNK8ZZ	ØVSF8ZZ	ØVW44YZ	3EØ74GC	4AØ28N6	5AØ92ØZ
ØTWD7YZ	ØUP3ØYZ	ØUW83YZ	ØVH83YZ	ØVNL8ZZ	ØVSG8ZZ	ØVW47YZ	3EØ84GC	4AØ28N7	5A1D7ØZ
ØTWD8YZ	ØUP33YZ	ØUW84YZ	ØVH84YZ	ØVNN8ZZ	ØVSH8ZZ	ØVW48YZ	3EØE4GC	4AØ28N8	5A1D8ØZ
ØU5Ø8ZZ	ØUP34YZ	ØUW87YZ	ØVH87YZ	ØVNP8ZZ	ØVU187Z	ØVW8ØYZ	3EØF4GC	4AØ28PZ	5A1D9ØZ
ØU518ZZ	ØUP37YZ	ØUW88YZ	ØVH88YZ	ØVNQ8ZZ	ØVU18JZ	ØVW83YZ	3EØG4GC	4AØ675Z	B31UØ1Ø
ØU528ZZ	ØUP38YZ	ØUWDØYZ	ØVHDØYZ	ØVP4ØYZ	ØVU18KZ	ØVW84YZ	3EØH4GC	4AØ67BZ	B31UØZZ
ØU548ZZ	ØUP8ØYZ	ØUWD3YZ	ØVHD3YZ	ØVP43YZ	ØVU287Z	ØVW87YZ	3EØJ4GC	4AØ685Z	B31U11Ø
ØU9Ø8ØZ	ØUP83YZ	ØUWD4YZ	ØVHD4YZ	ØVP44YZ	ØVU28JZ	ØVW88YZ	3EØK4GC	4AØ68BZ	B31UY1Ø
ØU9Ø8ZX	ØUP84YZ	ØUWD7YZ	ØVHD7YZ	ØVP47YZ	ØVU28KZ	ØVWDØYZ	3EØL35Z	4AØD83Z	B31UYZZ
ØU9Ø8ZZ	ØUP87YZ	ØUWD8YZ	ØVHD8YZ	ØVP48YZ	ØVU387Z	ØVWD3YZ	3EØL45Z	4AØD85Z	B31UZZZ
ØU918ØZ	ØUP88YZ	ØUWHØYZ	ØVHMØYZ	ØVP8ØYZ	ØVU38JZ	ØVWD4YZ	3EØL4GC	4AØD8BZ	XKØ23Ø3
ØU918ZX	ØUPDØYZ	ØUWH3YZ	ØVHM3YZ	ØVP83YZ	ØVU38KZ	ØVWD7YZ	3EØM35Z	4AØD8DZ	XNSØ332
ØU918ZZ	ØUPD3YZ	ØUWH4YZ	ØVHM4YZ	ØVP84YZ	ØVU687Z	ØVWD8YZ	3EØM45Z	4AØD8LZ	XNS3332
ØU928ØZ	ØUPD4YZ	ØUWH7YZ	ØVHM7YZ	ØVP87YZ	ØVU68JZ	ØVWMØYZ	3EØM4GC	4A1Ø74G	XNS4332
ØU928ZX	ØUPD7YZ	ØUWH8YZ	ØVHM8YZ	ØVP88YZ	ØVU68KZ	ØVWM3YZ	3EØN4GC	4A1Ø74Z	XRGØØF3
ØU928ZZ	ØUPD8YZ	ØV5F8ZZ	ØVHRØYZ	ØVPDØYZ	ØVU787Z	ØVWM4YZ	3EØP35Z	4A1Ø84G	XRG1ØF3
ØU948ØZ	ØUPHØYZ	ØV5G8ZZ	ØVHR3YZ	ØVPD3YZ	ØVU78JZ	ØVWM7YZ	3EØP3VZ	4A1Ø84Z	XRG2ØF3
ØU948ZX	ØUPH3YZ	ØV5H8ZZ	ØVHR4YZ	ØVPD4YZ	ØVU78KZ	ØVWM8YZ	3EØP45Z	4A1Ø8BD	XRG4ØF3
ØU948ZZ	ØUPH4YZ	ØV5J8ZZ	ØVHR7YZ	ØVPD7YZ	ØVUF87Z	ØVWRØYZ	3EØP4GC	4A1Ø8KD	XRG6ØF3
ØUCØ8ZZ	ØUPH7YZ	ØV5K8ZZ	ØVHR8YZ	ØVPD8YZ	ØVUF8JZ	ØVWR3YZ	3EØP7VZ	4A1Ø8RD	XRG7ØF3
ØUC18ZZ	ØUPH8YZ	ØV5L8ZZ	ØVHSØYZ	ØVPMØYZ	ØVUF8KZ	ØVWR4YZ	3EØU4GC	4A11729	XRG8ØF3
ØUC28ZZ	ØUQØ8ZZ	ØV5N8ZZ	ØVHS3YZ	ØVPM3YZ	ØVUG87Z	ØVWR7YZ	3EØY4GC	4A1172B	XRGAØF3
ØUC48ZZ	ØUQ18ZZ	ØV5P8ZZ	ØVHS4YZ	ØVPM4YZ	ØVUG8JZ	ØVWR8YZ	4AØØ74Z	4A1174G	XRGBØF3
ØUH3ØYZ	ØUQ28ZZ	ØV5Q8ZZ	ØVHS7YZ	ØVPM7YZ	ØVUG8KZ	ØVWSØYZ	4AØØ84Z	4A1174Z	XRGCØF3
ØUH33YZ	ØUQ48ZZ	ØVBF8ZX	ØVHS8YZ	ØVPM8YZ	ØVUH87Z	ØVWS3YZ	4AØØ8BD	4A11829	XRGDØF3
ØUH34YZ	ØUSØ8ZZ	ØVBF8ZZ	ØVLF8CZ	ØVPRØYZ	ØVUH8JZ	ØVWS4YZ	4AØØ8KD	4A1182B	XWØ33A3
ØUH37YZ	ØUS18ZZ	ØVBG8ZX	ØVLF8DZ	ØVPR3YZ	ØVUH8KZ	ØVWS7YZ	4AØØ8RD	4A1184G	XWØ33B3
ØUH38YZ	ØUS28ZZ	ØVBG8ZZ	ØVLF8ZZ	ØVPR4YZ	ØVUJ87Z	ØVWS8YZ	4AØ1729	4A1184Z	XWØ33C3
ØUH8ØYZ	ØUS48ZZ	ØVBH8ZX	ØVLG8CZ	ØVPR7YZ	ØVUJ8JZ	ØWB3ØZX	4AØ172B	4A1274Z	XWØ33F3
ØUH83YZ	ØUS58ZZ	ØVBH8ZZ	ØVLG8DZ	ØVPR8YZ	ØVUJ8KZ	ØWB3ØZZ	4AØ174Z	4A1279Z	XWØ43A3
ØUH84YZ	ØUS68ZZ	ØVBJ8ZX	ØVLG8ZZ	ØVPSØYZ	ØVUK87Z	ØWB33ZX	4AØ1829	4A127CZ	XWØ43B3
ØUH87YZ	ØUS78ZZ	ØVBJ8ZZ	ØVLH8CZ	ØVPS3YZ	ØVUK8JZ	ØWB33ZZ	4AØ182B	4A127FZ	XWØ43C3
ØUH88YZ	ØUS97ZZ	ØVBK8ZX	ØVLH8DZ	ØVPS4YZ	ØVUK8KZ	ØWB34ZX	4AØ184Z	4A127HZ	XWØ43F3
ØUH9ØHZ	ØUS98ZZ	ØVBK8ZZ	ØVLH8ZZ	ØVPS7YZ	ØVUL87Z	ØWB34ZZ	4AØ274Z	4A1284Z	XYØVX83
ØUHDØYZ	ØUSC8ZZ	ØVBL8ZX	ØVLN8CZ	ØVPS8YZ	ØVUL8JZ	ØWB3XZZ	4AØ279Z	4A1289Z	
ØUHD3YZ	ØUSF8ZZ								

REVISED CODES

009300Z	02WA4RZ	069Q40Z	06NP4ZZ	06VQ3DZ	09NKXZZ	09WK37Z	0J940ZZ	0JHM0XZ	0JU53KZ
00930ZX	02WAXRZ	069Q4ZX	06NQ0ZZ	06VQ3ZZ	09PK00Z	09WK3DZ	0J9430Z	0JHM3WZ	0JWT0WZ
00930ZZ	061P07Y	069Q4ZZ	06NQ3ZZ	06VQ4CZ	09PK07Z	09WK3JZ	0J943ZX	0JHM3XZ	0JWT0XZ
009330Z	061P09Y	06BP0ZX	06NQ4ZZ	06VQ4DZ	09PK0DZ	09WK3KZ	0J943ZZ	0JHN0WZ	0JWT3WZ
00933ZX	061P0AY	06BP0ZZ	06QP0ZZ	06VQ4ZZ	09PK0JZ	09WK40Z	0J9500Z	0JHN0XZ	0JWT3XZ
00933ZZ	061P0JY	06BP3ZX	06QP3ZZ	090K07Z	09PK0KZ	09WK47Z	0J950ZX	0JHN3WZ	0JWTXWZ
009340Z	061P0KY	06BP3ZZ	06QP4ZZ	090K0JZ	09PK30Z	09WK4DZ	0J950ZZ	0JHN3XZ	0JWTXXZ
00934ZX	061P0ZY	06BP4ZX	06QQ0ZZ	090K0KZ	09PK37Z	09WK4JZ	0J9530Z	0JHP0WZ	0JWV0WZ
00934ZZ	061P47Y	06BP4ZZ	06QQ3ZZ	090K0ZZ	09PK3DZ	09WK4KZ	0J953ZX	0JHP0XZ	0JWV0XZ
009400Z	061P49Y	06BQ0ZX	06QQ4ZZ	090K37Z	09PK3JZ	09WK70Z	0J953ZZ	0JHP3WZ	0JWV3WZ
00940ZX	061P4AY	06BQ0ZZ	06RP07Z	090K3JZ	09PK3KZ	09WK77Z	0JB40ZX	0JHP3XZ	0JWV3XZ
00940ZZ	061P4JY	06BQ3ZX	06RP0JZ	090K3KZ	09PK40Z	09WK7DZ	0JB40ZZ	0JN40ZZ	0JWVXWZ
009430Z	061P4KY	06BQ3ZZ	06RP0KZ	090K3ZZ	09PK47Z	09WK7JZ	0JB43ZX	0JN43ZZ	0JWVXXZ
00943ZX	061P4ZY	06BQ4ZX	06RP47Z	090K47Z	09PK4DZ	09WK7KZ	0JB43ZZ	0JN4XZZ	0JWW0WZ
00943ZZ	061Q07Y	06BQ4ZZ	06RP4JZ	090K4JZ	09PK4JZ	09WK80Z	0JB50ZX	0JN50ZZ	0JWW0XZ
009440Z	061Q09Y	06CP0ZZ	06RP4KZ	090K4KZ	09PK4KZ	09WK87Z	0JB50ZZ	0JN53ZZ	0JWW3WZ
00944ZX	061Q0AY	06CP3ZZ	06RQ07Z	090K4ZZ	09PK70Z	09WK8DZ	0JB53ZX	0JN5XZZ	0JWW3XZ
00944ZZ	061Q0JY	06CP4ZZ	06RQ0JZ	090KX7Z	09PK77Z	09WK8JZ	0JB53ZZ	0JPT0WZ	0JWWXWZ
009500Z	061Q0KY	06CQ0ZZ	06RQ0KZ	090KXJZ	09PK7DZ	09WK8KZ	0JC40ZZ	0JPT0XZ	0JWWXXZ
00950ZX	061Q0ZY	06CQ3ZZ	06RQ47Z	090KXKZ	09PK7JZ	09WKX0Z	0JC43ZZ	0JPT3WZ	0JX40ZB
00950ZZ	061Q47Y	06CQ4ZZ	06RQ4JZ	090KXZZ	09PK7KZ	09WKX7Z	0JC50ZZ	0JPT3XZ	0JX40ZC
009530Z	061Q49Y	06DP0ZZ	06RQ4KZ	092KX0Z	09PK80Z	09WKXDZ	0JC53ZZ	0JPTXXZ	0JX40ZZ
00953ZX	061Q4AY	06DP3ZZ	06SP0ZZ	092KXYZ	09PK87Z	09WKXJZ	0JD40ZZ	0JPV0WZ	0JX43ZB
00953ZZ	061Q4JY	06DP4ZZ	06SP3ZZ	095K0ZZ	09PK8DZ	09WKXKZ	0JD43ZZ	0JPV0XZ	0JX43ZC
009540Z	061Q4KY	06DQ0ZZ	06SP4ZZ	095K3ZZ	09PK8JZ	0H5AXZD	0JD50ZZ	0JPV3WZ	0JX43ZZ
00954ZX	061Q4ZY	06DQ3ZZ	06SQ0ZZ	095K4ZZ	09PK8KZ	0H5AXZZ	0JD53ZZ	0JPV3XZ	0JX50ZB
00954ZZ	065P0ZZ	06DQ4ZZ	06SQ3ZZ	095KXZZ	09PKX0Z	0H8AXZZ	0JH40NZ	0JPVXXZ	0JX50ZC
00C30ZZ	065P3ZZ	06HP03Z	06SQ4ZZ	099K00Z	09PKX7Z	0H9AX0Z	0JH43NZ	0JPW0WZ	0JX50ZZ
00C33ZZ	065P4ZZ	06HP0DZ	06UP07Z	099K0ZX	09PKXDZ	0H9AXZX	0JH50NZ	0JPW0XZ	0JX53ZB
00C34ZZ	065Q0ZZ	06HP33Z	06UP0JZ	099K0ZZ	09PKXJZ	0H9AXZZ	0JH53NZ	0JPW3WZ	0JX53ZC
00C40ZZ	065Q3ZZ	06HP3DZ	06UP0KZ	099K30Z	09PKXKZ	0HBAXZX	0JH60WZ	0JPW3XZ	0JX53ZZ
00C43ZZ	065Q4ZZ	06HP43Z	06UP37Z	099K3ZX	09QK0ZZ	0HBAXZZ	0JH60XZ	0JPWXXZ	0M5C0ZZ
00C44ZZ	067P0DZ	06HP4DZ	06UP3JZ	099K3ZZ	09QK3ZZ	0HCAXZZ	0JH63WZ	0JQ40ZZ	0M5C3ZZ
00C50ZZ	067P0ZZ	06HQ03Z	06UP3KZ	099K40Z	09QK4ZZ	0HDAXZZ	0JH63XZ	0JQ43ZZ	0M5C4ZZ
00C53ZZ	067P3DZ	06HQ0DZ	06UP47Z	099K4ZX	09QKXZZ	0HMAXZZ	0JH80WZ	0JQ50ZZ	0M5D0ZZ
00C54ZZ	067P3ZZ	06HQ33Z	06UP4JZ	099K4ZZ	09RK07Z	0HNAXZZ	0JH80XZ	0JQ53ZZ	0M5D3ZZ
00F30ZZ	067P4DZ	06HQ3DZ	06UP4KZ	099KX0Z	09RK0JZ	0HQAXZZ	0JH83WZ	0JR407Z	0M5D4ZZ
00F33ZZ	067P4ZZ	06HQ43Z	06UQ07Z	099KXZX	09RK0KZ	0HRAX73	0JH83XZ	0JR40JZ	0M5F0ZZ
00F34ZZ	067Q0DZ	06HQ4DZ	06UQ0JZ	099KXZZ	09RKX7Z	0HRAX74	0JHD0WZ	0JR40KZ	0M5F3ZZ
00F3XZZ	067Q0ZZ	06LP0CZ	06UQ0KZ	09BK0ZX	09RKXJZ	0HRAXJ3	0JHD0XZ	0JR437Z	0M5F4ZZ
00F40ZZ	067Q3DZ	06LP0DZ	06UQ37Z	09BK0ZZ	09RKXKZ	0HRAXJ4	0JHD3WZ	0JR43JZ	0M5G0ZZ
00F43ZZ	067Q3ZZ	06LP0ZZ	06UQ3JZ	09BK3ZX	09SK0ZZ	0HRAXJZ	0JHD3XZ	0JR43KZ	0M5G3ZZ
00F44ZZ	067Q4DZ	06LP3CZ	06UQ3KZ	09BK3ZZ	09SK4ZZ	0HRAXK3	0JHF0WZ	0JR507Z	0M5G4ZZ
00F4XZZ	067Q4ZZ	06LP3DZ	06UQ47Z	09BK4ZX	09SKXZZ	0HRAXK4	0JHF0XZ	0JR50JZ	0M8C0ZZ
00F50ZZ	069P00Z	06LP3ZZ	06UQ4JZ	09BK4ZZ	09TK0ZZ	0HXAXZZ	0JHF3WZ	0JR50KZ	0M8C3ZZ
00F53ZZ	069P0ZX	06LP4CZ	06UQ4KZ	09BKXZX	09TK4ZZ	0J040ZZ	0JHF3XZ	0JR537Z	0M8C4ZZ
00F54ZZ	069P0ZZ	06LP4DZ	06VP0CZ	09BKXZZ	09TKXZZ	0J043ZZ	0JHG0WZ	0JR53JZ	0M8D0ZZ
00F5XZZ	069P30Z	06LP4ZZ	06VP0DZ	09CK0ZZ	09UK07Z	0J050ZZ	0JHG0XZ	0JR53KZ	0M8D3ZZ
02HA0RS	069P3ZX	06LQ0CZ	06VP0ZZ	09CK3ZZ	09UK0JZ	0J053ZZ	0JHG3WZ	0JU407Z	0M8D4ZZ
02HA0RZ	069P3ZZ	06LQ0DZ	06VP3CZ	09CK4ZZ	09UK0KZ	0J540ZZ	0JHG3XZ	0JU40JZ	0M8F0ZZ
02HA3RS	069P40Z	06LQ0ZZ	06VP3DZ	09CKXZZ	09UKX7Z	0J543ZZ	0JHH0WZ	0JU40KZ	0M8F3ZZ
02HA3RZ	069P4ZX	06LQ3CZ	06VP3ZZ	09JK0ZZ	09UKXJZ	0J550ZZ	0JHH0XZ	0JU437Z	0M8F4ZZ
02HA4RS	069P4ZZ	06LQ3DZ	06VP4CZ	09JK3ZZ	09UKXKZ	0J553ZZ	0JHH3WZ	0JU43JZ	0M8G0ZZ
02HA4RZ	069Q00Z	06LQ3ZZ	06VP4DZ	09JK4ZZ	09WK00Z	0J840ZZ	0JHH3XZ	0JU43KZ	0M8G3ZZ
02PA0RZ	069Q0ZX	06LQ4CZ	06VP4ZZ	09JKXZZ	09WK07Z	0J843ZZ	0JHL0WZ	0JU507Z	0M8G4ZZ
02PA3RZ	069Q0ZZ	06LQ4DZ	06VQ0CZ	09MKXZZ	09WK0DZ	0J850ZZ	0JHL0XZ	0JU50JZ	0M9C00Z
02PA4RZ	069Q30Z	06LQ4ZZ	06VQ0DZ	09NK0ZZ	09WK0JZ	0J853ZZ	0JHL3WZ	0JU50KZ	0M9C0ZX
02WA0RZ	069Q3ZX	06NP0ZZ	06VQ0ZZ	09NK3ZZ	09WK0KZ	0J9400Z	0JHL3XZ	0JU537Z	0M9C0ZZ
02WA3RZ	069Q3ZZ	06NP3ZZ	06VQ3CZ	09NK4ZZ	09WK30Z	0J940ZX	0JHM0WZ	0JU53JZ	0M9C30Z

ØM9C3ZX	ØMCD4ZZ	ØMSG0ZZ	ØN8C3ZZ	ØNBR3ZX	ØNR10KZ	ØNSR44Z	ØP913ZZ	ØPP237Z	ØPU20KZ
ØM9C3ZZ	ØMCF0ZZ	ØMSG4ZZ	ØN8C4ZZ	ØNBR3ZZ	ØNR137Z	ØNSR45Z	ØP9140Z	ØPP23JZ	ØPU237Z
ØM9C40Z	ØMCF3ZZ	ØMTC0ZZ	ØN8R0ZZ	ØNBR4ZX	ØNR13JZ	ØNSR4ZZ	ØP914ZX	ØPP23KZ	ØPU23JZ
ØM9C4ZX	ØMCF4ZZ	ØMTC4ZZ	ØN8R3ZZ	ØNBR4ZZ	ØNR13KZ	ØNSRXZZ	ØP914ZZ	ØPP244Z	ØPU23KZ
ØM9C4ZZ	ØMCG0ZZ	ØMTD0ZZ	ØN8R4ZZ	ØNC10ZZ	ØNR147Z	ØNT10ZZ	ØP9200Z	ØPP247Z	ØPU247Z
ØM9D00Z	ØMCG3ZZ	ØMTD4ZZ	ØN9100Z	ØNC13ZZ	ØNR14JZ	ØNT70ZZ	ØP920ZX	ØPP24JZ	ØPU24JZ
ØM9D0ZX	ØMCG4ZZ	ØMTF0ZZ	ØN910ZX	ØNC14ZZ	ØNR14KZ	ØNTC0ZZ	ØP920ZZ	ØPP24KZ	ØPU24KZ
ØM9D0ZZ	ØMDC0ZZ	ØMTF4ZZ	ØN910ZZ	ØNC70ZZ	ØNR707Z	ØNTR0ZZ	ØP9230Z	ØPP2X4Z	ØPW104Z
ØM9D30Z	ØMDC3ZZ	ØMTG0ZZ	ØN9130Z	ØNC73ZZ	ØNR70JZ	ØNU107Z	ØP923ZX	ØPQ10ZZ	ØPW107Z
ØM9D3ZX	ØMDC4ZZ	ØMTG4ZZ	ØN913ZX	ØNC74ZZ	ØNR70KZ	ØNU10JZ	ØP923ZZ	ØPQ13ZZ	ØPW10JZ
ØM9D3ZZ	ØMDD0ZZ	ØMUC07Z	ØN913ZZ	ØNCC0ZZ	ØNR737Z	ØNU10KZ	ØP9240Z	ØPQ14ZZ	ØPW10KZ
ØM9D40Z	ØMDD3ZZ	ØMUC0JZ	ØN9140Z	ØNCC3ZZ	ØNR73JZ	ØNU137Z	ØP924ZX	ØPQ1XZZ	ØPW134Z
ØM9D4ZX	ØMDD4ZZ	ØMUC0KZ	ØN914ZX	ØNCC4ZZ	ØNR73KZ	ØNU13JZ	ØP924ZZ	ØPQ20ZZ	ØPW137Z
ØM9D4ZZ	ØMDF0ZZ	ØMUC47Z	ØN914ZZ	ØNCR0ZZ	ØNR747Z	ØNU13KZ	ØPB10ZX	ØPQ23ZZ	ØPW13JZ
ØM9F00Z	ØMDF3ZZ	ØMUC4JZ	ØN9700Z	ØNCR3ZZ	ØNR74JZ	ØNU147Z	ØPB10ZZ	ØPQ24ZZ	ØPW13KZ
ØM9F0ZX	ØMDF4ZZ	ØMUC4KZ	ØN970ZX	ØNCR4ZZ	ØNR74KZ	ØNU14JZ	ØPB13ZX	ØPQ2XZZ	ØPW144Z
ØM9F0ZZ	ØMDG0ZZ	ØMUD07Z	ØN970ZZ	ØNH104Z	ØNRC07Z	ØNU14KZ	ØPB13ZZ	ØPR107Z	ØPW147Z
ØM9F30Z	ØMDG3ZZ	ØMUD0JZ	ØN9730Z	ØNH134Z	ØNRC0JZ	ØNU707Z	ØPB14ZX	ØPR10JZ	ØPW14JZ
ØM9F3ZX	ØMDG4ZZ	ØMUD0KZ	ØN973ZX	ØNH144Z	ØNRC0KZ	ØNU70JZ	ØPB14ZZ	ØPR10KZ	ØPW14KZ
ØM9F3ZZ	ØMMC0ZZ	ØMUD47Z	ØN973ZZ	ØNH704Z	ØNRC37Z	ØNU70KZ	ØPB20ZX	ØPR137Z	ØPW1X4Z
ØM9F40Z	ØMMC4ZZ	ØMUD4JZ	ØN9740Z	ØNH734Z	ØNRC3JZ	ØNU737Z	ØPB20ZZ	ØPR13JZ	ØPW1X7Z
ØM9F4ZX	ØMMD0ZZ	ØMUD4KZ	ØN974ZX	ØNH744Z	ØNRC3KZ	ØNU73JZ	ØPB23ZX	ØPR13KZ	ØPW1XJZ
ØM9F4ZZ	ØMMD4ZZ	ØMUF07Z	ØN974ZZ	ØNHC04Z	ØNRC47Z	ØNU73KZ	ØPB23ZZ	ØPR147Z	ØPW1XKZ
ØM9G00Z	ØMMF0ZZ	ØMUF0JZ	ØN9C00Z	ØNHC34Z	ØNRC4JZ	ØNU747Z	ØPB24ZX	ØPR14JZ	ØPW204Z
ØM9G0ZX	ØMMF4ZZ	ØMUF0KZ	ØN9C0ZX	ØNHC44Z	ØNRC4KZ	ØNU74JZ	ØPB24ZZ	ØPR14KZ	ØPW207Z
ØM9G0ZZ	ØMMG0ZZ	ØMUF47Z	ØN9C0ZZ	ØNHR04Z	ØNRR07Z	ØNU74KZ	ØPC10ZZ	ØPR207Z	ØPW20JZ
ØM9G30Z	ØMMG4ZZ	ØMUF4JZ	ØN9C30Z	ØNHR05Z	ØNRR0JZ	ØNUC07Z	ØPC13ZZ	ØPR20JZ	ØPW20KZ
ØM9G3ZX	ØMNC0ZZ	ØMUF4KZ	ØN9C3ZX	ØNHR34Z	ØNRR0KZ	ØNUC0JZ	ØPC14ZZ	ØPR20KZ	ØPW234Z
ØM9G3ZZ	ØMNC3ZZ	ØMUG07Z	ØN9C3ZZ	ØNHR35Z	ØNRR37Z	ØNUC0KZ	ØPC20ZZ	ØPR237Z	ØPW237Z
ØM9G40Z	ØMNC4ZZ	ØMUG0JZ	ØN9C40Z	ØNHR44Z	ØNRR3JZ	ØNUC37Z	ØPC23ZZ	ØPR23JZ	ØPW23JZ
ØM9G4ZX	ØMNCXZZ	ØMUG0KZ	ØN9C4ZX	ØNHR45Z	ØNRR3KZ	ØNUC3JZ	ØPC24ZZ	ØPR23KZ	ØPW23KZ
ØM9G4ZZ	ØMND0ZZ	ØMUG47Z	ØN9C4ZZ	ØNN10ZZ	ØNRR47Z	ØNUC3KZ	ØPH104Z	ØPR247Z	ØPW244Z
ØMBC0ZX	ØMND3ZZ	ØMUG4JZ	ØN9R00Z	ØNN13ZZ	ØNRR4JZ	ØNUC47Z	ØPH134Z	ØPR24JZ	ØPW247Z
ØMBC0ZZ	ØMND4ZZ	ØMUG4KZ	ØN9R0ZX	ØNN14ZZ	ØNRR4KZ	ØNUC4JZ	ØPH144Z	ØPR24KZ	ØPW24JZ
ØMBC3ZX	ØMNDXZZ	ØMXC0ZZ	ØN9R0ZZ	ØNN70ZZ	ØNS104Z	ØNUC4KZ	ØPH204Z	ØPS104Z	ØPW24KZ
ØMBC3ZZ	ØMNF0ZZ	ØMXC4ZZ	ØN9R30Z	ØNN73ZZ	ØNS10ZZ	ØNUR07Z	ØPH234Z	ØPS10ZZ	ØPW2X4Z
ØMBC4ZX	ØMNF3ZZ	ØMXD0ZZ	ØN9R3ZX	ØNN74ZZ	ØNS134Z	ØNUR0JZ	ØPH244Z	ØPS134Z	ØPW2X7Z
ØMBC4ZZ	ØMNF4ZZ	ØMXD4ZZ	ØN9R3ZZ	ØNNC0ZZ	ØNS13ZZ	ØNUR0KZ	ØPN10ZZ	ØPS13ZZ	ØPW2XJZ
ØMBD0ZX	ØMNFXZZ	ØMXF0ZZ	ØN9R40Z	ØNNC3ZZ	ØNS144Z	ØNUR37Z	ØPN13ZZ	ØPS144Z	ØPW2XKZ
ØMBD0ZZ	ØMNG0ZZ	ØMXF4ZZ	ØN9R4ZX	ØNNC4ZZ	ØNS14ZZ	ØNUR3JZ	ØPN14ZZ	ØPS14ZZ	ØR5S0ZZ
ØMBD3ZX	ØMNG3ZZ	ØMXG0ZZ	ØN9R4ZZ	ØNNR0ZZ	ØNS1XZZ	ØNUR3KZ	ØPN20ZZ	ØPS1XZZ	ØR5S3ZZ
ØMBD3ZZ	ØMNG4ZZ	ØMXG4ZZ	ØNB10ZX	ØNNR3ZZ	ØNS704Z	ØNUR47Z	ØPN23ZZ	ØPS204Z	ØR5S4ZZ
ØMBD4ZX	ØMNGXZZ	ØN510ZZ	ØNB10ZZ	ØNNR4ZZ	ØNS70ZZ	ØNUR4JZ	ØPN24ZZ	ØPS20ZZ	ØR5T0ZZ
ØMBD4ZZ	ØMQC0ZZ	ØN513ZZ	ØNB13ZX	ØNQ10ZZ	ØNS734Z	ØNUR4KZ	ØPP104Z	ØPS234Z	ØR5T3ZZ
ØMBF0ZX	ØMQC3ZZ	ØN514ZZ	ØNB13ZZ	ØNQ13ZZ	ØNS73ZZ	ØP510ZZ	ØPP107Z	ØPS23ZZ	ØR5T4ZZ
ØMBF0ZZ	ØMQC4ZZ	ØN570ZZ	ØNB14ZX	ØNQ14ZZ	ØNS744Z	ØP513ZZ	ØPP10JZ	ØPS244Z	ØR9S00Z
ØMBF3ZX	ØMQD0ZZ	ØN573ZZ	ØNB14ZZ	ØNQ1XZZ	ØNS74ZZ	ØP514ZZ	ØPP10KZ	ØPS24ZZ	ØR9S0ZX
ØMBF3ZZ	ØMQD3ZZ	ØN574ZZ	ØNB70ZX	ØNQ70ZZ	ØNS7XZZ	ØP520ZZ	ØPP134Z	ØPS2XZZ	ØR9S0ZZ
ØMBF4ZX	ØMQD4ZZ	ØN5C0ZZ	ØNB70ZZ	ØNQ73ZZ	ØNSC04Z	ØP523ZZ	ØPP137Z	ØPT10ZZ	ØR9S30Z
ØMBF4ZZ	ØMQF0ZZ	ØN5C3ZZ	ØNB73ZX	ØNQ74ZZ	ØNSC0ZZ	ØP524ZZ	ØPP13JZ	ØPT20ZZ	ØR9S3ZX
ØMBG0ZX	ØMQF3ZZ	ØN5C4ZZ	ØNB73ZZ	ØNQ7XZZ	ØNSC34Z	ØP810ZZ	ØPP13KZ	ØPU107Z	ØR9S3ZZ
ØMBG0ZZ	ØMQF4ZZ	ØN5R0ZZ	ØNB74ZX	ØNQC0ZZ	ØNSC3ZZ	ØP813ZZ	ØPP144Z	ØPU10JZ	ØR9S40Z
ØMBG3ZX	ØMQG0ZZ	ØN5R3ZZ	ØNB74ZZ	ØNQC3ZZ	ØNSC44Z	ØP814ZZ	ØPP147Z	ØPU10KZ	ØR9S4ZX
ØMBG3ZZ	ØMQG3ZZ	ØN5R4ZZ	ØNBC0ZX	ØNQC4ZZ	ØNSC4ZZ	ØP820ZZ	ØPP14JZ	ØPU137Z	ØR9S4ZZ
ØMBG4ZX	ØMQG4ZZ	ØN810ZZ	ØNBC0ZZ	ØNQCXZZ	ØNSCXZZ	ØP823ZZ	ØPP14KZ	ØPU13JZ	ØR9T00Z
ØMBG4ZZ	ØMSC0ZZ	ØN813ZZ	ØNBC3ZX	ØNQR0ZZ	ØNSR04Z	ØP824ZZ	ØPP1X4Z	ØPU13KZ	ØR9T0ZX
ØMCC0ZZ	ØMSC4ZZ	ØN814ZZ	ØNBC3ZZ	ØNQR3ZZ	ØNSR05Z	ØP9100Z	ØPP204Z	ØPU147Z	ØR9T0ZZ
ØMCC3ZZ	ØMSD0ZZ	ØN870ZZ	ØNBC4ZX	ØNQR4ZZ	ØNSR0ZZ	ØP910ZX	ØPP207Z	ØPU14JZ	ØR9T30Z
ØMCC4ZZ	ØMSD4ZZ	ØN873ZZ	ØNBC4ZZ	ØNQRXZZ	ØNSR34Z	ØP910ZZ	ØPP20JZ	ØPU14KZ	ØR9T3ZX
ØMCD0ZZ	ØMSF0ZZ	ØN874ZZ	ØNBR0ZX	ØNR107Z	ØNSR35Z	ØP9130Z	ØPP20KZ	ØPU207Z	ØR9T3ZZ
ØMCD3ZZ	ØMSF4ZZ	ØN8C0ZZ	ØNBR0ZZ	ØNR10JZ	ØNSR3ZZ	ØP913ZX	ØPP234Z	ØPU20JZ	ØR9T40Z

0R9T4ZX	0RHS38Z	0RPT03Z	0RSTX4Z	0RWT0KZ	0SCK3ZZ	0SHL44Z	0SPL3KZ	0SUL07Z	0SWL48Z
0R9T4ZZ	0RHS43Z	0RPT04Z	0RSTX5Z	0RWT30Z	0SCK4ZZ	0SHL45Z	0SPL40Z	0SUL0JZ	0SWL4JZ
0RBS0ZX	0RHS44Z	0RPT05Z	0RSTXZZ	0RWT33Z	0SCL0ZZ	0SHL48Z	0SPL43Z	0SUL0KZ	0SWL4KZ
0RBS0ZZ	0RHS45Z	0RPT07Z	0RTS0ZZ	0RWT34Z	0SCL3ZZ	0SJK0ZZ	0SPL44Z	0SUL37Z	0SWLX0Z
0RBS3ZX	0RHS48Z	0RPT08Z	0RTT0ZZ	0RWT35Z	0SCL4ZZ	0SJK3ZZ	0SPL45Z	0SUL3JZ	0SWLX3Z
0RBS3ZZ	0RHT03Z	0RPT0JZ	0RUS07Z	0RWT37Z	0SGK04Z	0SJK4ZZ	0SPL47Z	0SUL3KZ	0SWLX4Z
0RBS4ZX	0RHT04Z	0RPT0KZ	0RUS0JZ	0RWT38Z	0SGK05Z	0SJKXZZ	0SPL48Z	0SUL47Z	0SWLX5Z
0RBS4ZZ	0RHT05Z	0RPT30Z	0RUS0KZ	0RWT3JZ	0SGK07Z	0SJL0ZZ	0SPL4JZ	0SUL4JZ	0SWLX7Z
0RBT0ZX	0RHT08Z	0RPT33Z	0RUS37Z	0RWT3KZ	0SGK0JZ	0SJL3ZZ	0SPL4KZ	0SUL4KZ	0SWLX8Z
0RBT0ZZ	0RHT33Z	0RPT34Z	0RUS3JZ	0RWT40Z	0SGK0KZ	0SJL4ZZ	0SPLX0Z	0SWK00Z	0SWLXJZ
0RBT3ZX	0RHT34Z	0RPT35Z	0RUS3KZ	0RWT43Z	0SGK0ZZ	0SJLXZZ	0SPLX3Z	0SWK03Z	0SWLXKZ
0RBT3ZZ	0RHT35Z	0RPT37Z	0RUS47Z	0RWT44Z	0SGK34Z	0SNK0ZZ	0SPLX4Z	0SWK04Z	3E00XBZ
0RBT4ZX	0RHT38Z	0RPT38Z	0RUS4JZ	0RWT45Z	0SGK35Z	0SNK3ZZ	0SPLX5Z	0SWK05Z	3E013BZ
0RBT4ZZ	0RHT43Z	0RPT3JZ	0RUS4KZ	0RWT47Z	0SGK37Z	0SNK4ZZ	0SQK0ZZ	0SWK07Z	3E023BZ
0RCS0ZZ	0RHT44Z	0RPT3KZ	0RUT07Z	0RWT48Z	0SGK3JZ	0SNKXZZ	0SQK3ZZ	0SWK08Z	3E093BZ
0RCS3ZZ	0RHT45Z	0RPT40Z	0RUT0JZ	0RWT4JZ	0SGK3KZ	0SNL0ZZ	0SQK4ZZ	0SWK0JZ	3E097BZ
0RCS4ZZ	0RHT48Z	0RPT43Z	0RUT0KZ	0RWT4KZ	0SGK3ZZ	0SNL3ZZ	0SQKXZZ	0SWK0KZ	3E09XBZ
0RCT0ZZ	0RJS0ZZ	0RPT44Z	0RUT37Z	0RWTX0Z	0SGK44Z	0SNL4ZZ	0SQL0ZZ	0SWK30Z	3E0B3BZ
0RCT3ZZ	0RJS3ZZ	0RPT45Z	0RUT3JZ	0RWTX3Z	0SGK45Z	0SNLXZZ	0SQL3ZZ	0SWK33Z	3E0B7BZ
0RCT4ZZ	0RJS4ZZ	0RPT47Z	0RUT3KZ	0RWTX4Z	0SGK47Z	0SPK00Z	0SQL4ZZ	0SWK34Z	3E0BXBZ
0RGS04Z	0RJSXZZ	0RPT48Z	0RUT47Z	0RWTX5Z	0SGK4JZ	0SPK03Z	0SQLXZZ	0SWK35Z	3E0C3BZ
0RGS05Z	0RJT0ZZ	0RPT4JZ	0RUT4JZ	0RWTX7Z	0SGK4KZ	0SPK04Z	0SRK07Z	0SWK37Z	3E0C7BZ
0RGS07Z	0RJT3ZZ	0RPT4KZ	0RUT4KZ	0RWTX8Z	0SGK4ZZ	0SPK05Z	0SRK0JZ	0SWK38Z	3E0CXBZ
0RGS0JZ	0RJT4ZZ	0RPTX0Z	0RWS00Z	0RWTXJZ	0SGL04Z	0SPK07Z	0SRK0KZ	0SWK3JZ	3E0D3BZ
0RGS0KZ	0RJTXZZ	0RPTX3Z	0RWS03Z	0RWTXKZ	0SGL05Z	0SPK08Z	0SRL07Z	0SWK3KZ	3E0D7BZ
0RGS0ZZ	0RNS0ZZ	0RPTX4Z	0RWS04Z	0S5K0ZZ	0SGL07Z	0SPK0JZ	0SRL0JZ	0SWK40Z	3E0DXBZ
0RGS34Z	0RNS3ZZ	0RPTX5Z	0RWS05Z	0S5K3ZZ	0SGL0JZ	0SPK0KZ	0SRL0KZ	0SWK43Z	3E0E3BZ
0RGS35Z	0RNS4ZZ	0RQS0ZZ	0RWS07Z	0S5K4ZZ	0SGL0KZ	0SPK30Z	0SSK04Z	0SWK44Z	3E0E7BZ
0RGS37Z	0RNSXZZ	0RQS3ZZ	0RWS08Z	0S5L0ZZ	0SGL0ZZ	0SPK33Z	0SSK05Z	0SWK45Z	3E0E8BZ
0RGS3JZ	0RNT0ZZ	0RQS4ZZ	0RWS0JZ	0S5L3ZZ	0SGL34Z	0SPK34Z	0SSK0ZZ	0SWK47Z	3E0F3BZ
0RGS3KZ	0RNT3ZZ	0RQSXZZ	0RWS0KZ	0S5L4ZZ	0SGL35Z	0SPK35Z	0SSK34Z	0SWK48Z	3E0F7BZ
0RGS3ZZ	0RNT4ZZ	0RQT0ZZ	0RWS30Z	0S9K00Z	0SGL37Z	0SPK37Z	0SSK35Z	0SWK4JZ	3E0F8BZ
0RGS44Z	0RNTXZZ	0RQT3ZZ	0RWS33Z	0S9K0ZX	0SGL3JZ	0SPK38Z	0SSK3ZZ	0SWK4KZ	3E0G3BZ
0RGS45Z	0RPS00Z	0RQT4ZZ	0RWS34Z	0S9K0ZZ	0SGL3KZ	0SPK3JZ	0SSK44Z	0SWKX0Z	3E0G7BZ
0RGS47Z	0RPS03Z	0RQTXZZ	0RWS35Z	0S9K30Z	0SGL3ZZ	0SPK3KZ	0SSK45Z	0SWKX3Z	3E0G8BZ
0RGS4JZ	0RPS04Z	0RRS07Z	0RWS37Z	0S9K3ZX	0SGL44Z	0SPK40Z	0SSK4ZZ	0SWKX4Z	3E0H3BZ
0RGS4KZ	0RPS05Z	0RRS0JZ	0RWS38Z	0S9K3ZZ	0SGL45Z	0SPK43Z	0SSKX4Z	0SWKX5Z	3E0H7BZ
0RGS4ZZ	0RPS07Z	0RRS0KZ	0RWS3JZ	0S9K40Z	0SGL47Z	0SPK44Z	0SSKX5Z	0SWKX7Z	3E0H8BZ
0RGT04Z	0RPS08Z	0RRT07Z	0RWS3KZ	0S9K4ZX	0SGL4JZ	0SPK45Z	0SSKXZZ	0SWKX8Z	3E0J3BZ
0RGT05Z	0RPS0JZ	0RRT0JZ	0RWS40Z	0S9K4ZZ	0SGL4KZ	0SPK47Z	0SSL04Z	0SWKXJZ	3E0J7BZ
0RGT07Z	0RPS0KZ	0RRT0KZ	0RWS43Z	0S9L00Z	0SGL4ZZ	0SPK48Z	0SSL05Z	0SWKXKZ	3E0J8BZ
0RGT0JZ	0RPS30Z	0RSS04Z	0RWS44Z	0S9L0ZX	0SHK03Z	0SPK4JZ	0SSL0ZZ	0SWL00Z	3E0K3BZ
0RGT0KZ	0RPS33Z	0RSS05Z	0RWS45Z	0S9L0ZZ	0SHK04Z	0SPK4KZ	0SSL34Z	0SWL03Z	3E0K7BZ
0RGT0ZZ	0RPS34Z	0RSS0ZZ	0RWS47Z	0S9L30Z	0SHK05Z	0SPKX0Z	0SSL35Z	0SWL04Z	3E0K8BZ
0RGT34Z	0RPS35Z	0RSS34Z	0RWS48Z	0S9L3ZX	0SHK08Z	0SPKX3Z	0SSL3ZZ	0SWL05Z	3E0L3BZ
0RGT35Z	0RPS37Z	0RSS35Z	0RWS4JZ	0S9L3ZZ	0SHK33Z	0SPKX4Z	0SSL44Z	0SWL07Z	3E0M3BZ
0RGT37Z	0RPS38Z	0RSS3ZZ	0RWS4KZ	0S9L40Z	0SHK34Z	0SPKX5Z	0SSL45Z	0SWL08Z	3E0N3BZ
0RGT3JZ	0RPS3JZ	0RSS44Z	0RWSX0Z	0S9L4ZX	0SHK35Z	0SPL00Z	0SSL4ZZ	0SWL0JZ	3E0N7BZ
0RGT3KZ	0RPS3KZ	0RSS45Z	0RWSX3Z	0S9L4ZZ	0SHK38Z	0SPL03Z	0SSLX4Z	0SWL0KZ	3E0N8BZ
0RGT3ZZ	0RPS40Z	0RSS4ZZ	0RWSX4Z	0SBK0ZX	0SHK43Z	0SPL04Z	0SSLX5Z	0SWL30Z	3E0P3BZ
0RGT44Z	0RPS43Z	0RSSX4Z	0RWSX5Z	0SBK0ZZ	0SHK44Z	0SPL05Z	0SSLXZZ	0SWL33Z	3E0P7BZ
0RGT45Z	0RPS44Z	0RSSX5Z	0RWSX7Z	0SBK3ZX	0SHK45Z	0SPL07Z	0STK0ZZ	0SWL34Z	3E0P8BZ
0RGT47Z	0RPS45Z	0RSSXZZ	0RWSX8Z	0SBK3ZZ	0SHK48Z	0SPL08Z	0STL0ZZ	0SWL35Z	3E0Q0BZ
0RGT4JZ	0RPS47Z	0RST04Z	0RWSXJZ	0SBK4ZX	0SHL03Z	0SPL0JZ	0SUK07Z	0SWL37Z	3E0Q3BZ
0RGT4KZ	0RPS48Z	0RST05Z	0RWSXKZ	0SBK4ZZ	0SHL04Z	0SPL0KZ	0SUK0JZ	0SWL38Z	3E0R3BZ
0RGT4ZZ	0RPS4JZ	0RST0ZZ	0RWT00Z	0SBL0ZX	0SHL05Z	0SPL30Z	0SUK0KZ	0SWL3JZ	3E0S3BZ
0RHS03Z	0RPS4KZ	0RST34Z	0RWT03Z	0SBL0ZZ	0SHL08Z	0SPL33Z	0SUK37Z	0SWL3KZ	3E0T3BZ
0RHS04Z	0RPSX0Z	0RST35Z	0RWT04Z	0SBL3ZX	0SHL33Z	0SPL34Z	0SUK3JZ	0SWL40Z	3E0U3BZ
0RHS05Z	0RPSX3Z	0RST3ZZ	0RWT05Z	0SBL3ZZ	0SHL34Z	0SPL35Z	0SUK3KZ	0SWL43Z	3E0V3BZ
0RHS08Z	0RPSX4Z	0RST44Z	0RWT07Z	0SBL4ZX	0SHL35Z	0SPL37Z	0SUK47Z	0SWL44Z	3E0W3BZ
0RHS33Z	0RPSX5Z	0RST45Z	0RWT08Z	0SBL4ZZ	0SHL38Z	0SPL38Z	0SUK4JZ	0SWL45Z	3E0X3BZ
0RHS34Z	0RPT00Z	0RST4ZZ	0RWT0JZ	0SCK0ZZ	0SHL43Z	0SPL3JZ	0SUK4KZ	0SWL47Z	3E0Y3BZ
0RHS35Z									

DELETED CODES

04VC0DZ	069P4ZX	06LQ0DZ	06VP0DZ	0BUT0KZ	0N5R4ZZ	0NB70ZZ	0NQ10ZZ	0NS144Z	0NUC4JZ
04VC3DZ	069P4ZZ	06LQ0ZZ	06VP0ZZ	0BUT47Z	0N810ZZ	0NB73ZX	0NQ13ZZ	0NS14ZZ	0NUC4KZ
04VC4DZ	069Q00Z	06LQ3CZ	06VP3CZ	0BUT4JZ	0N813ZZ	0NB73ZZ	0NQ14ZZ	0NS1XZZ	0NUR07Z
04VD0DZ	069Q0ZX	06LQ3DZ	06VP3DZ	0BUT4KZ	0N814ZZ	0NB74ZX	0NQ70ZZ	0NS704Z	0NUR0JZ
04VD3DZ	069Q0ZZ	06LQ3ZZ	06VP3ZZ	0D5U0ZZ	0N870ZZ	0NB74ZZ	0NQ73ZZ	0NS70ZZ	0NUR0KZ
04VD4DZ	069Q30Z	06LQ4CZ	06VP4CZ	0D5U3ZZ	0N873ZZ	0NBC0ZX	0NQ74ZZ	0NS734Z	0NUR37Z
06183JY	069Q3ZX	06LQ4DZ	06VP4DZ	0D5U4ZZ	0N874ZZ	0NBC0ZZ	0NQ7XZZ	0NS73ZZ	0NUR3JZ
06184JY	069Q3ZZ	06LQ4ZZ	06VP4ZZ	0D9U00Z	0N8C0ZZ	0NBC3ZX	0NQC0ZZ	0NS744Z	0NUR3KZ
061P07Y	069Q40Z	06NP0ZZ	06VQ0CZ	0D9U0ZX	0N8C3ZZ	0NBC3ZZ	0NQC3ZZ	0NS74ZZ	0NUR47Z
061P09Y	069Q4ZX	06NP3ZZ	06VQ0DZ	0D9U0ZZ	0N8C4ZZ	0NBC4ZX	0NQC4ZZ	0NS7XZZ	0NUR4JZ
061P0AY	069Q4ZZ	06NP4ZZ	06VQ0ZZ	0D9U30Z	0N8R0ZZ	0NBC4ZZ	0NQCXZZ	0NSC04Z	0NUR4KZ
061P0JY	06BP0ZX	06NQ0ZZ	06VQ3CZ	0D9U3ZX	0N8R3ZZ	0NBR0ZX	0NQR0ZZ	0NSC0ZZ	0RG00AJ
061P0KY	06BP0ZZ	06NQ3ZZ	06VQ3DZ	0D9U3ZZ	0N8R4ZZ	0NBR0ZZ	0NQR3ZZ	0NSC34Z	0RG03AJ
061P0ZY	06BP3ZX	06NQ4ZZ	06VQ3ZZ	0D9U40Z	0N9100Z	0NBR3ZX	0NQR4ZZ	0NSC3ZZ	0RG04AJ
061P47Y	06BP3ZZ	06QP0ZZ	06VQ4CZ	0D9U4ZX	0N910ZX	0NBR3ZZ	0NQRXZZ	0NSC44Z	0RG10AJ
061P49Y	06BP4ZX	06QP3ZZ	06VQ4DZ	0D9U4ZZ	0N910ZZ	0NBR4ZX	0NR107Z	0NSC4ZZ	0RG13AJ
061P4AY	06BP4ZZ	06QP4ZZ	06VQ4ZZ	0DBU0ZX	0N9130Z	0NBR4ZZ	0NR10JZ	0NSCXZZ	0RG14AJ
061P4JY	06BQ0ZX	06QQ0ZZ	0B5T0ZZ	0DBU0ZZ	0N913ZX	0NC10ZZ	0NR10KZ	0NSR04Z	0RG20AJ
061P4KY	06BQ0ZZ	06QQ3ZZ	0B5T3ZZ	0DBU3ZX	0N913ZZ	0NC13ZZ	0NR137Z	0NSR05Z	0RG23AJ
061P4ZY	06BQ3ZX	06QQ4ZZ	0B5T4ZZ	0DBU3ZZ	0N9140Z	0NC14ZZ	0NR13JZ	0NSR0ZZ	0RG24AJ
061Q07Y	06BQ3ZZ	06RP07Z	0B9T00Z	0DBU4ZX	0N914ZX	0NC70ZZ	0NR13KZ	0NSR34Z	0RG40AJ
061Q09Y	06BQ4ZX	06RP0JZ	0B9T0ZZ	0DBU4ZZ	0N914ZZ	0NC73ZZ	0NR147Z	0NSR35Z	0RG43AJ
061Q0AY	06BQ4ZZ	06RP0KZ	0B9T0ZZ	0DCU0ZZ	0N9700Z	0NC74ZZ	0NR14JZ	0NSR3ZZ	0RG44AJ
061Q0JY	06CP0ZZ	06RP47Z	0B9T30Z	0DCU3ZZ	0N970ZX	0NCC0ZZ	0NR14KZ	0NSR44Z	0RG60AJ
061Q0KY	06CP3ZZ	06RP4JZ	0B9T3ZX	0DCU4ZZ	0N970ZZ	0NCC3ZZ	0NR707Z	0NSR45Z	0RG63AJ
061Q0ZY	06CP4ZZ	06RP4KZ	0B9T3ZZ	0DNU0ZZ	0N9730Z	0NCC4ZZ	0NR70JZ	0NSR4ZZ	0RG64AJ
061Q47Y	06CQ0ZZ	06RQ07Z	0B9T40Z	0DNU3ZZ	0N973ZX	0NCR0ZZ	0NR70KZ	0NSRXZZ	0RG70AJ
061Q49Y	06CQ3ZZ	06RQ0JZ	0B9T4ZX	0DNU4ZZ	0N973ZZ	0NCR3ZZ	0NT10ZZ	0NT10ZZ	0RG73AJ
061Q4AY	06CQ4ZZ	06RQ0KZ	0B9T4ZZ	0DQU0ZZ	0N9740Z	0NCR4ZZ	0NR737Z	0NT70ZZ	0RG74AJ
061Q4JY	06DP0ZZ	06RQ47Z	0BBT0ZX	0DQU3ZZ	0N974ZX	0NH104Z	0NR73JZ	0NTC0ZZ	0RG80AJ
061Q4KY	06DP3ZZ	06RQ4JZ	0BBT0ZZ	0DQU4ZZ	0N974ZZ	0NH134Z	0NR73KZ	0NTR0ZZ	0RG83AJ
061Q4ZY	06DP4ZZ	06RQ4KZ	0BBT3ZX	0DRU07Z	0N9C00Z	0NH144Z	0NR747Z	0NU107Z	0RG84AJ
065P0ZZ	06DQ0ZZ	06SP0ZZ	0BBT3ZZ	0DRU0JZ	0N9C0ZX	0NH704Z	0NR74JZ	0NU10JZ	0RGA0AJ
065P3ZZ	06DQ3ZZ	06SP3ZZ	0BBT4ZX	0DRU0KZ	0N9C0ZZ	0NH734Z	0NR74KZ	0NU10KZ	0RGA3AJ
065P4ZZ	06DQ4ZZ	06SP4ZZ	0BBT4ZZ	0DRU47Z	0N9C30Z	0NH744Z	0NRC07Z	0NU137Z	0RGA4AJ
065Q0ZZ	06HP03Z	06SQ0ZZ	0BCT0ZZ	0DRU4JZ	0N9C3ZX	0NHC04Z	0NRC0JZ	0NU13JZ	0SG00AJ
065Q3ZZ	06HP0DZ	06SQ3ZZ	0BCT3ZZ	0DRU4KZ	0N9C3ZZ	0NHC34Z	0NRC0KZ	0NU13KZ	0SG03AJ
065Q4ZZ	06HP33Z	06SQ4ZZ	0BCT4ZZ	0DTU0ZZ	0N9C40Z	0NHC44Z	0NRC37Z	0NU147Z	0SG04AJ
067P0DZ	06HP3DZ	06UP07Z	0BHT02Z	0DTU4ZZ	0N9C4ZX	0NHR04Z	0NRC3JZ	0NU14JZ	0SG10AJ
067P0ZZ	06HP43Z	06UP0JZ	0BHT0MZ	0DUU07Z	0N9C4ZZ	0NHR05Z	0NRC3KZ	0NU14KZ	0SG13AJ
067P3DZ	06HP4DZ	06UP0KZ	0BHT32Z	0DUU0JZ	0N9R00Z	0NHR34Z	0NRC47Z	0NU707Z	0SG14AJ
067P3ZZ	06HQ03Z	06UP37Z	0BHT3MZ	0DUU0KZ	0N9R0ZX	0NHR35Z	0NRC4JZ	0NU70JZ	0SG30AJ
067P4DZ	06HQ0DZ	06UP3JZ	0BHT42Z	0DUU47Z	0N9R0ZZ	0NHR44Z	0NRC4KZ	0NU70KZ	0SG33AJ
067P4ZZ	06HQ33Z	06UP3KZ	0BHT4MZ	0DUU4JZ	0N9R30Z	0NHR45Z	0NRR07Z	0NU737Z	0SG34AJ
067Q0DZ	06HQ3DZ	06UP47Z	0BMT0ZZ	0DUU4KZ	0N9R3ZX	0NN10ZZ	0NRR0JZ	0NU73JZ	3E0F7BZ
067Q0ZZ	06HQ43Z	06UP4JZ	0BNT0ZZ	0N510ZZ	0N9R3ZZ	0NN13ZZ	0NRR0KZ	0NU73KZ	3E0F8BZ
067Q3DZ	06HQ4DZ	06UP4KZ	0BNT3ZZ	0N513ZZ	0N9R40Z	0NN14ZZ	0NRR37Z	0NU747Z	3E0R3BZ
067Q3ZZ	06LP0CZ	06UQ07Z	0BNT4ZZ	0N514ZZ	0N9R4ZX	0NN70ZZ	0NRR3JZ	0NU74JZ	3E0S3BZ
067Q4DZ	06LP0DZ	06UQ0JZ	0BQT0ZZ	0N570ZZ	0N9R4ZZ	0NN73ZZ	0NRR3KZ	0NU74KZ	3E0T3BZ
067Q4ZZ	06LP0ZZ	06UQ0KZ	0BQT3ZZ	0N573ZZ	0NB10ZX	0NN74ZZ	0NRR47Z	0NUC07Z	3E0X3BZ
069P00Z	06LP3CZ	06UQ37Z	0BQT4ZZ	0N574ZZ	0NB10ZZ	0NNC0ZZ	0NRR4JZ	0NUC0JZ	5A1D70Z
069P0ZX	06LP3DZ	06UQ3JZ	0BST0ZZ	0N5C0ZZ	0NB13ZX	0NNC3ZZ	0NRR4KZ	0NUC0KZ	5A1D80Z
069P0ZZ	06LP3ZZ	06UQ3KZ	0BTT0ZZ	0N5C3ZZ	0NB13ZZ	0NNC4ZZ	0NS104Z	0NUC37Z	5A1D90Z
069P30Z	06LP4CZ	06UQ47Z	0BTT4ZZ	0N5C4ZZ	0NB14ZX	0NNR0ZZ	0NS10ZZ	0NUC3JZ	XNS0332
069P3ZX	06LP4DZ	06UQ4JZ	0BUT07Z	0N5R0ZZ	0NB14ZZ	0NNR3ZZ	0NS134Z	0NUC3KZ	XNS3332
069P3ZZ	06LP4ZZ	06UQ4KZ	0BUT0JZ	0N5R3ZZ	0NB70ZX	0NNR4ZZ	0NS13ZZ	0NUC47Z	XNS4332
069P40Z	06LQ0CZ	06VP0CZ							

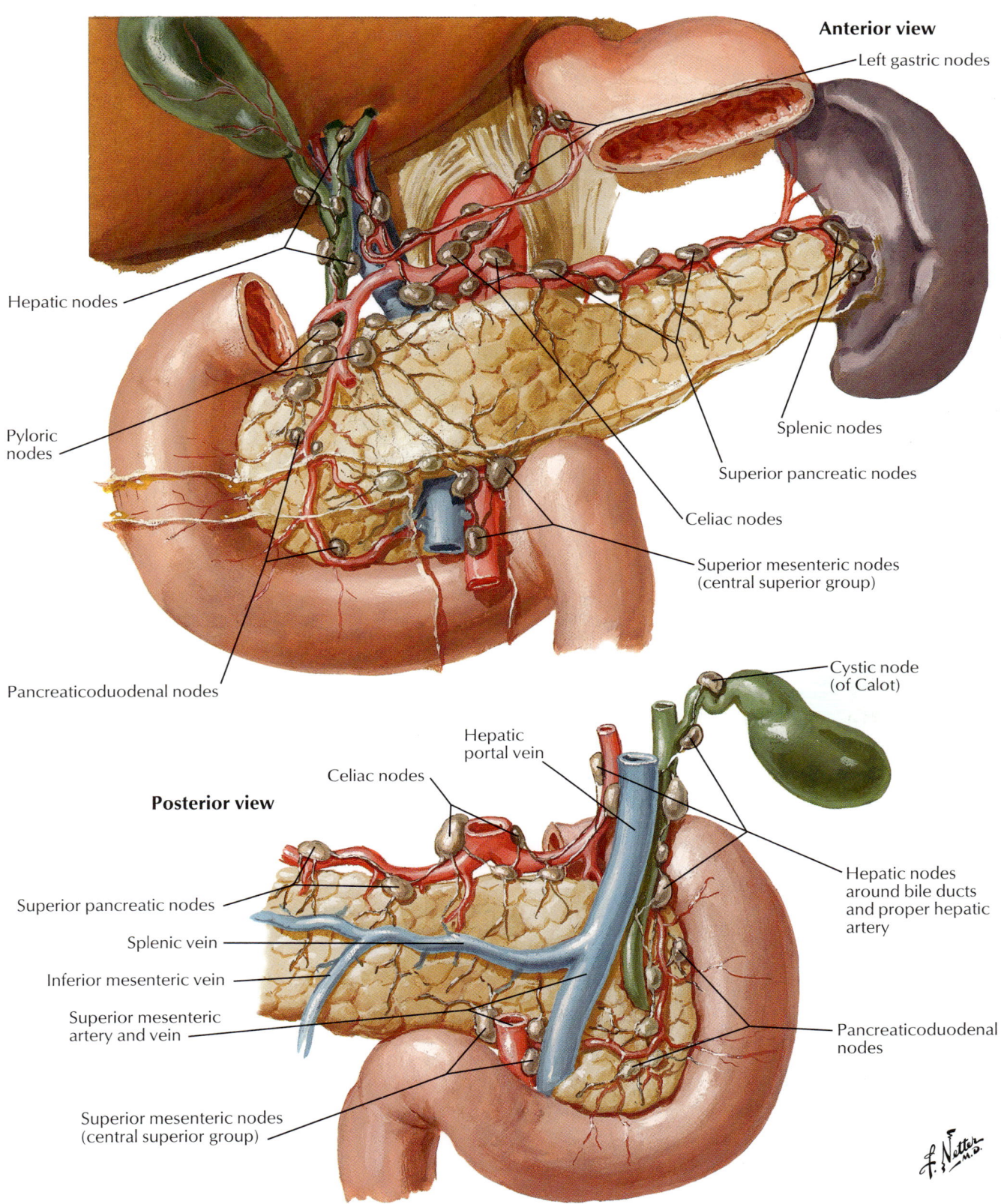

Anterior view

Left gastric nodes

Hepatic nodes

Pyloric nodes

Pancreaticoduodenal nodes

Splenic nodes

Superior pancreatic nodes

Celiac nodes

Superior mesenteric nodes (central superior group)

Cystic node (of Calot)

Hepatic portal vein

Celiac nodes

Posterior view

Hepatic nodes around bile ducts and proper hepatic artery

Superior pancreatic nodes

Splenic vein

Inferior mesenteric vein

Superior mesenteric artery and vein

Pancreaticoduodenal nodes

Superior mesenteric nodes (central superior group)

Plate 315   Lymph Vessels and Nodes of Pancreas. (Netter: Atlas of Human Anatomy, 4 ed, 2006, Saunders.)

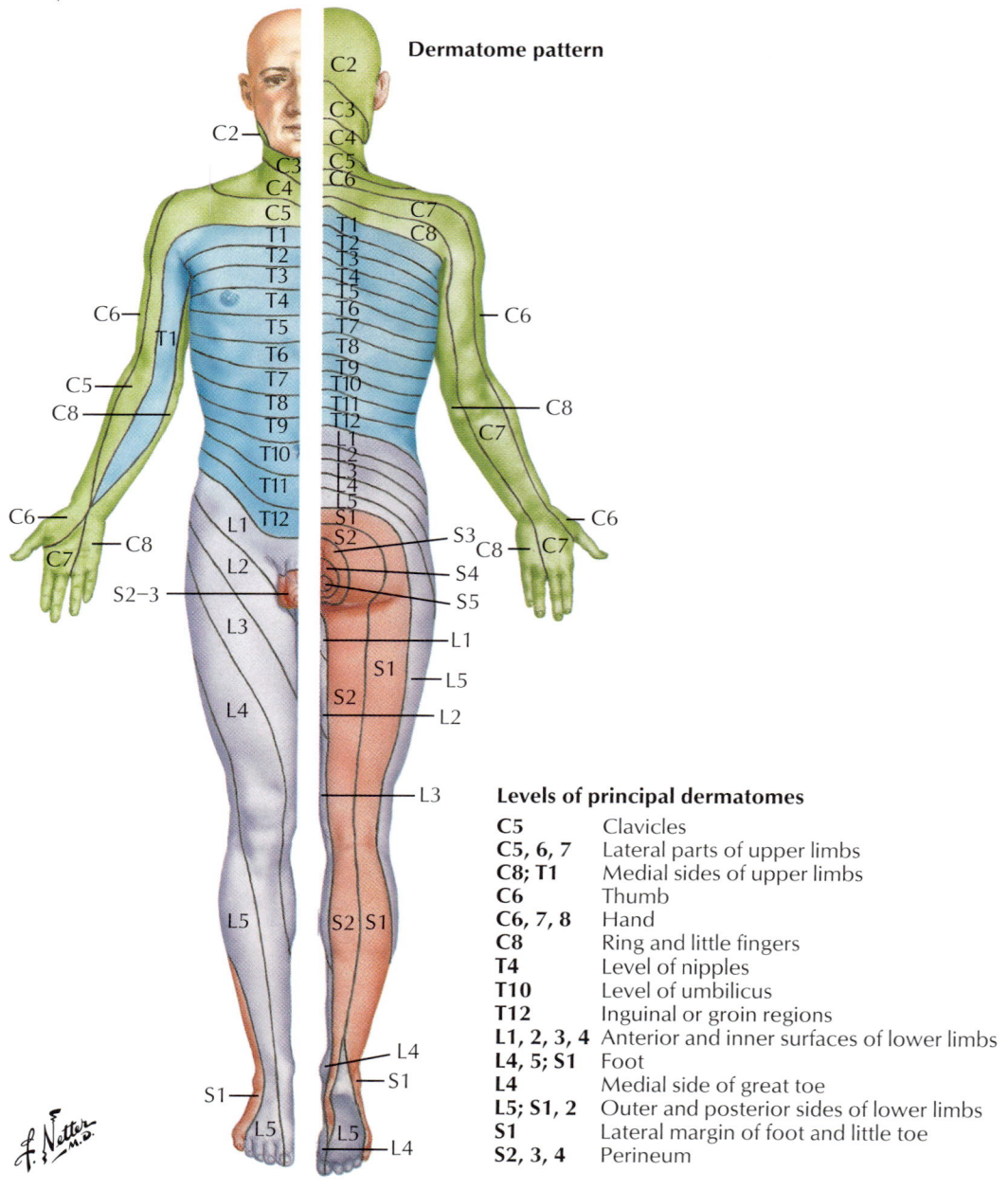

Dermatome pattern

Levels of principal dermatomes

C5	Clavicles
C5, 6, 7	Lateral parts of upper limbs
C8; T1	Medial sides of upper limbs
C6	Thumb
C6, 7, 8	Hand
C8	Ring and little fingers
T4	Level of nipples
T10	Level of umbilicus
T12	Inguinal or groin regions
L1, 2, 3, 4	Anterior and inner surfaces of lower limbs
L4, 5; S1	Foot
L4	Medial side of great toe
L5; S1, 2	Outer and posterior sides of lower limbs
S1	Lateral margin of foot and little toe
S2, 3, 4	Perineum

Plate 164 Dermatomes. (Netter: Atlas of Human Anatomy, 4 ed, 2006, Saunders.)

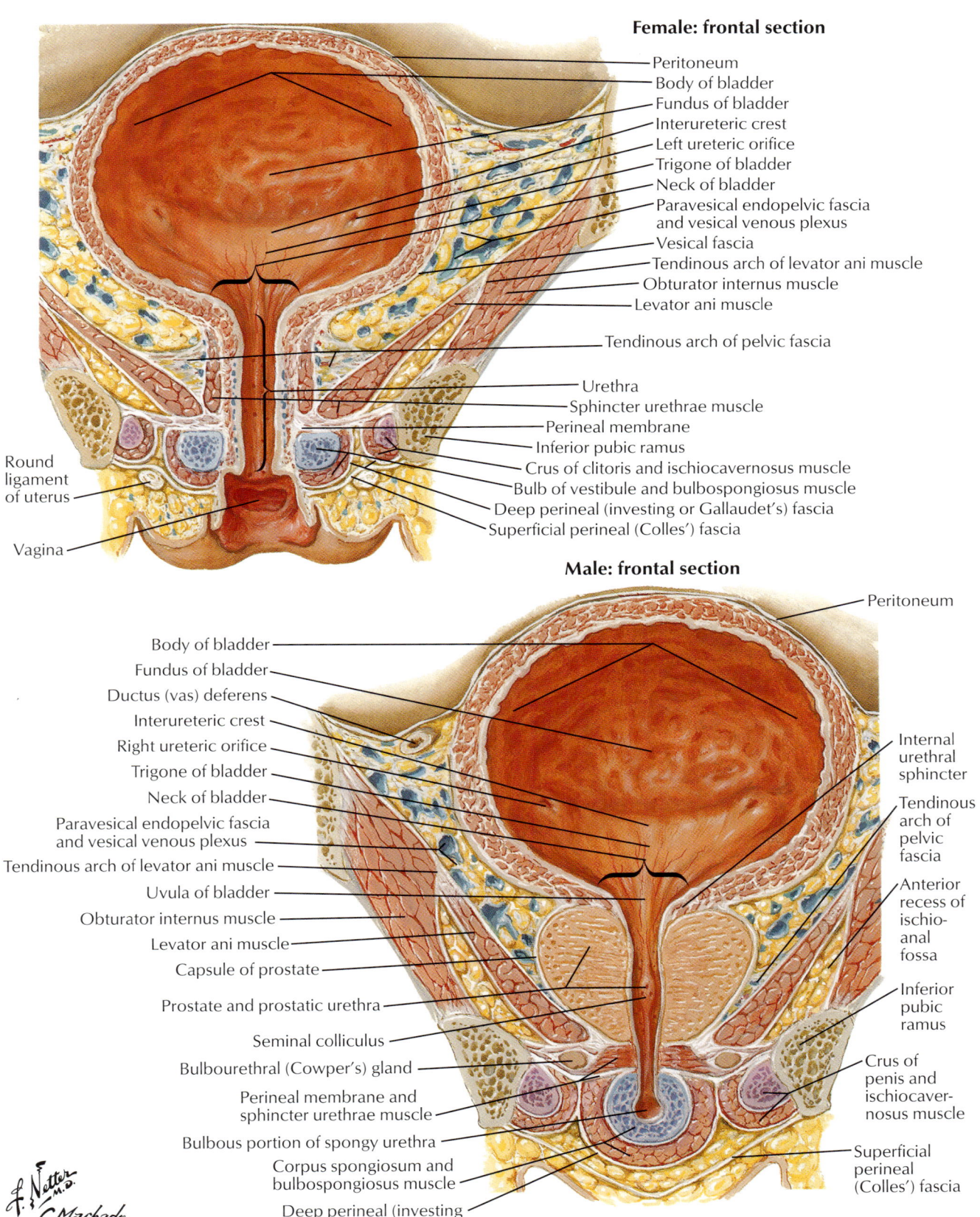

Female: frontal section

- Peritoneum
- Body of bladder
- Fundus of bladder
- Interureteric crest
- Left ureteric orifice
- Trigone of bladder
- Neck of bladder
- Paravesical endopelvic fascia and vesical venous plexus
- Vesical fascia
- Tendinous arch of levator ani muscle
- Obturator internus muscle
- Levator ani muscle
- Tendinous arch of pelvic fascia
- Urethra
- Sphincter urethrae muscle
- Perineal membrane
- Inferior pubic ramus
- Crus of clitoris and ischiocavernosus muscle
- Bulb of vestibule and bulbospongiosus muscle
- Deep perineal (investing or Gallaudet's) fascia
- Superficial perineal (Colles') fascia

Round ligament of uterus

Vagina

Male: frontal section

- Peritoneum
- Body of bladder
- Fundus of bladder
- Ductus (vas) deferens
- Interureteric crest
- Right ureteric orifice
- Trigone of bladder
- Neck of bladder
- Paravesical endopelvic fascia and vesical venous plexus
- Tendinous arch of levator ani muscle
- Uvula of bladder
- Obturator internus muscle
- Levator ani muscle
- Capsule of prostate
- Prostate and prostatic urethra
- Seminal colliculus
- Bulbourethral (Cowper's) gland
- Perineal membrane and sphincter urethrae muscle
- Bulbous portion of spongy urethra
- Corpus spongiosum and bulbospongiosus muscle
- Deep perineal (investing or Gallaudet's) fascia

- Internal urethral sphincter
- Tendinous arch of pelvic fascia
- Anterior recess of ischioanal fossa
- Inferior pubic ramus
- Crus of penis and ischiocavernosus muscle
- Superficial perineal (Colles') fascia

Plate 366 Urinary Bladder: Female and Male. (Netter: Atlas of Human Anatomy, 4 ed, 2006, Saunders.)

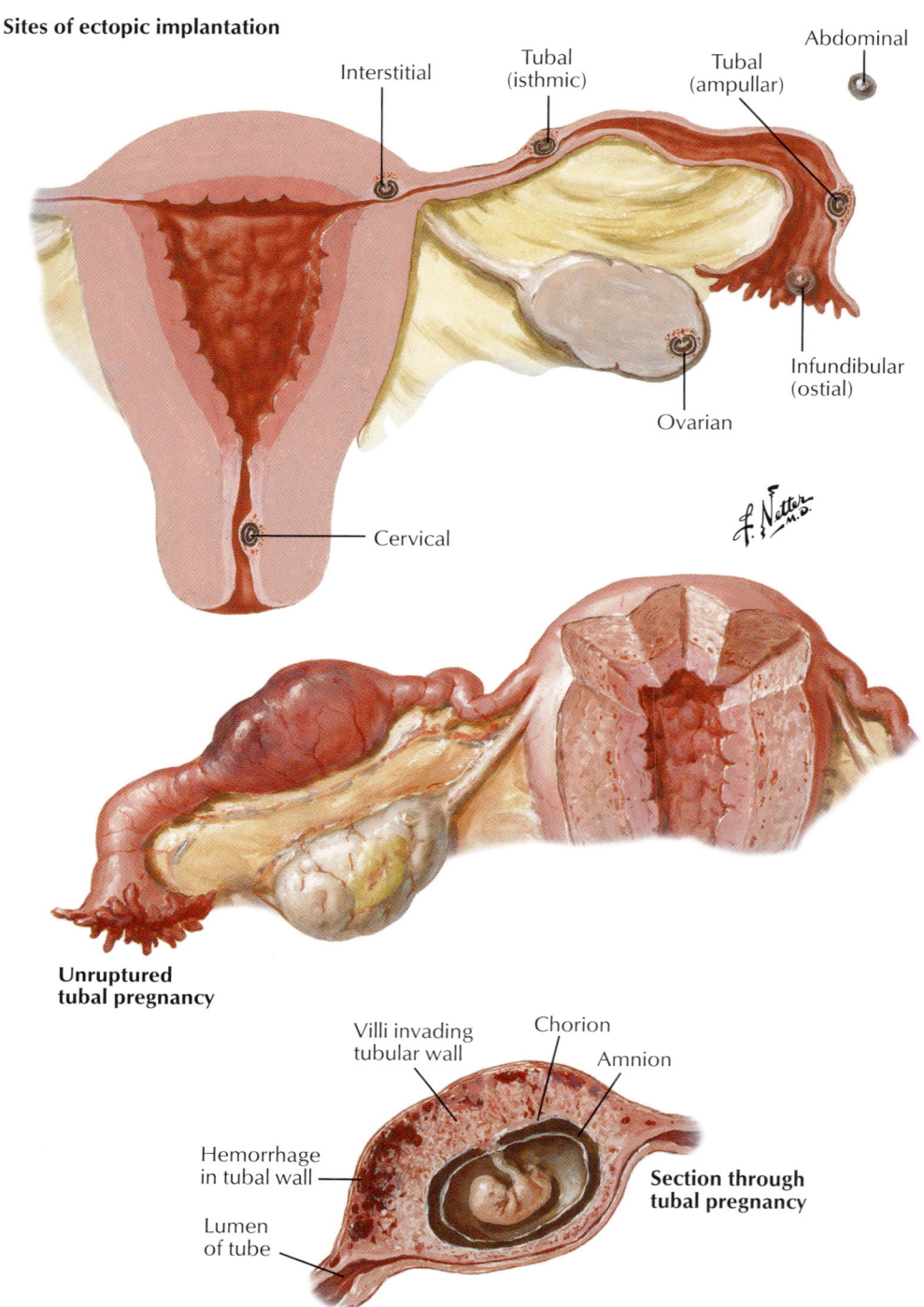

Sites of ectopic implantation

Interstitial

Tubal (isthmic)

Tubal (ampullar)

Abdominal

Infundibular (ostial)

Ovarian

Cervical

f. Netter M.D.

Unruptured tubal pregnancy

Villi invading tubular wall

Chorion

Amnion

Hemorrhage in tubal wall

Section through tubal pregnancy

Lumen of tube

Plate 375 Ectopic Pregnancy. (Netter: Atlas of Human Anatomy, 4 ed, 2006, Saunders.)

NAP-4

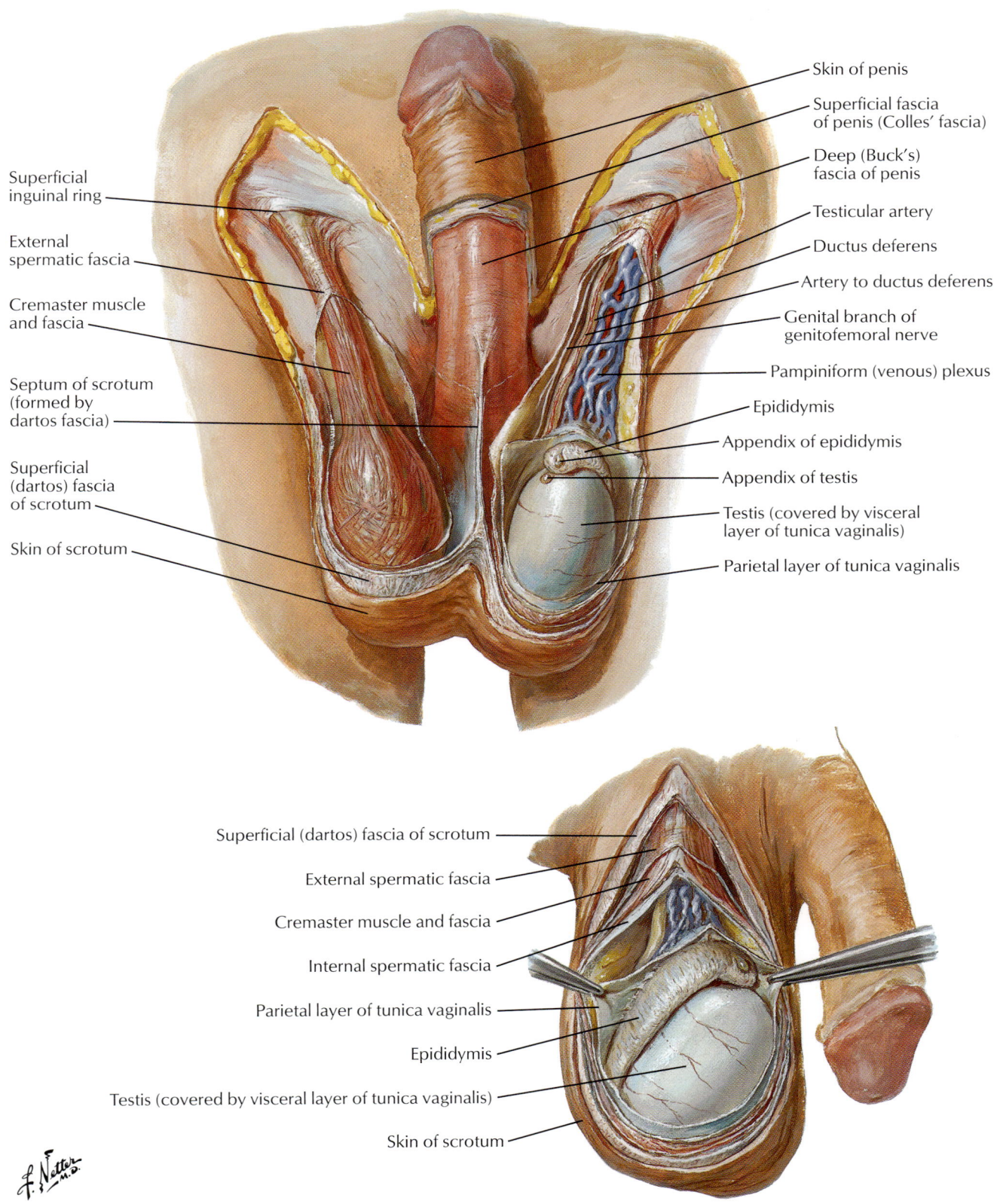

Skin of penis

Superficial fascia
of penis (Colles' fascia)

Deep (Buck's)
fascia of penis

Testicular artery

Ductus deferens

Artery to ductus deferens

Genital branch of
genitofemoral nerve

Pampiniform (venous) plexus

Epididymis

Appendix of epididymis

Appendix of testis

Testis (covered by visceral
layer of tunica vaginalis)

Parietal layer of tunica vaginalis

Superficial
inguinal ring

External
spermatic fascia

Cremaster muscle
and fascia

Septum of scrotum
(formed by
dartos fascia)

Superficial
(dartos) fascia
of scrotum

Skin of scrotum

Superficial (dartos) fascia of scrotum

External spermatic fascia

Cremaster muscle and fascia

Internal spermatic fascia

Parietal layer of tunica vaginalis

Epididymis

Testis (covered by visceral layer of tunica vaginalis)

Skin of scrotum

Plate 387   Scrotum and Contents. (Netter: Atlas of Human Anatomy, 4 ed, 2006, Saunders.)

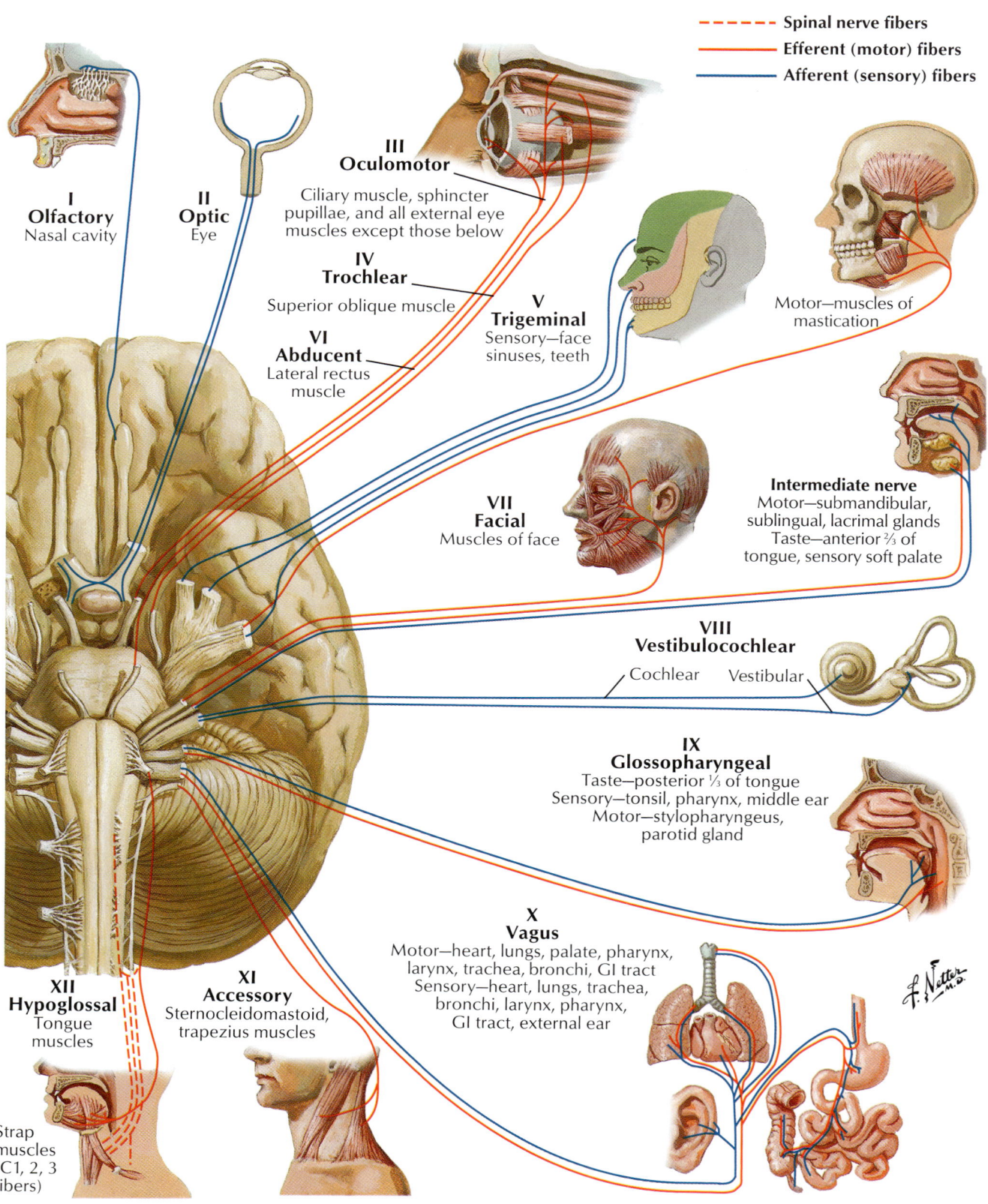

Spinal nerve fibers
Efferent (motor) fibers
Afferent (sensory) fibers

I
Olfactory
Nasal cavity

II
Optic
Eye

III
Oculomotor
Ciliary muscle, sphincter
pupillae, and all external eye
muscles except those below

IV
Trochlear
Superior oblique muscle

VI
Abducent
Lateral rectus
muscle

V
Trigeminal
Sensory—face
sinuses, teeth

Motor—muscles of
mastication

VII
Facial
Muscles of face

Intermediate nerve
Motor—submandibular,
sublingual, lacrimal glands
Taste—anterior ⅔ of
tongue, sensory soft palate

VIII
Vestibulocochlear
Cochlear   Vestibular

IX
Glossopharyngeal
Taste—posterior ⅓ of tongue
Sensory—tonsil, pharynx, middle ear
Motor—stylopharyngeus,
parotid gland

X
Vagus
Motor—heart, lungs, palate, pharynx,
larynx, trachea, bronchi, GI tract
Sensory—heart, lungs, trachea,
bronchi, larynx, pharynx,
GI tract, external ear

XII
Hypoglossal
Tongue
muscles

XI
Accessory
Sternocleidomastoid,
trapezius muscles

Strap
muscles
(C1, 2, 3
fibers)

Plate 118   Cranial Nerves (Motor and Sensory Distribution): Schema. (Netter: Atlas of Human Anatomy, 4 ed, 2006, Saunders.)

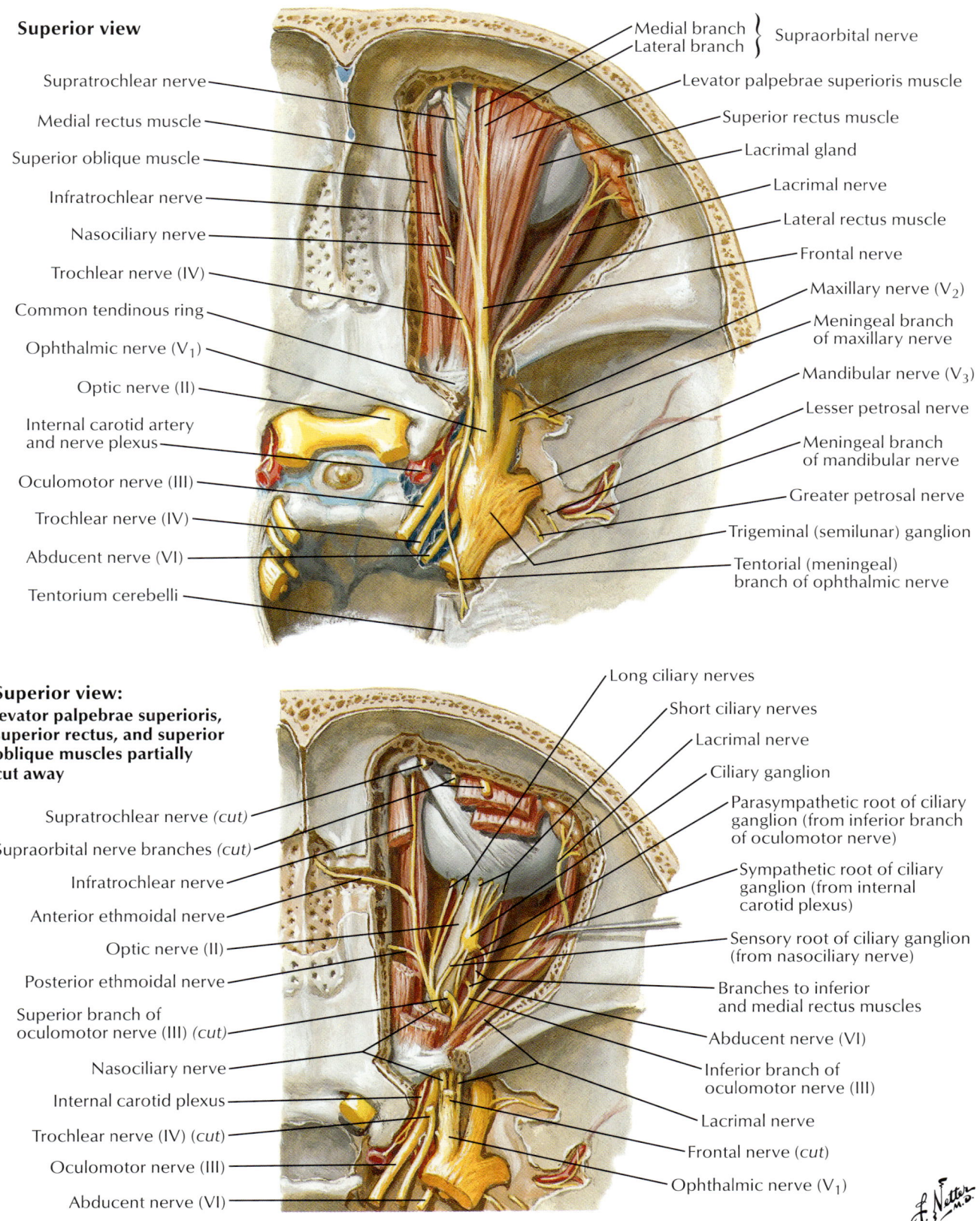

Superior view

- Supratrochlear nerve
- Medial rectus muscle
- Superior oblique muscle
- Infratrochlear nerve
- Nasociliary nerve
- Trochlear nerve (IV)
- Common tendinous ring
- Ophthalmic nerve (V₁)
- Optic nerve (II)
- Internal carotid artery and nerve plexus
- Oculomotor nerve (III)
- Trochlear nerve (IV)
- Abducent nerve (VI)
- Tentorium cerebelli

- Medial branch ⎱ Supraorbital nerve
- Lateral branch ⎰
- Levator palpebrae superioris muscle
- Superior rectus muscle
- Lacrimal gland
- Lacrimal nerve
- Lateral rectus muscle
- Frontal nerve
- Maxillary nerve (V₂)
- Meningeal branch of maxillary nerve
- Mandibular nerve (V₃)
- Lesser petrosal nerve
- Meningeal branch of mandibular nerve
- Greater petrosal nerve
- Trigeminal (semilunar) ganglion
- Tentorial (meningeal) branch of ophthalmic nerve

**Superior view:
levator palpebrae superioris, superior rectus, and superior oblique muscles partially cut away**

- Supratrochlear nerve *(cut)*
- Supraorbital nerve branches *(cut)*
- Infratrochlear nerve
- Anterior ethmoidal nerve
- Optic nerve (II)
- Posterior ethmoidal nerve
- Superior branch of oculomotor nerve (III) *(cut)*
- Nasociliary nerve
- Internal carotid plexus
- Trochlear nerve (IV) *(cut)*
- Oculomotor nerve (III)
- Abducent nerve (VI)

- Long ciliary nerves
- Short ciliary nerves
- Lacrimal nerve
- Ciliary ganglion
- Parasympathetic root of ciliary ganglion (from inferior branch of oculomotor nerve)
- Sympathetic root of ciliary ganglion (from internal carotid plexus)
- Sensory root of ciliary ganglion (from nasociliary nerve)
- Branches to inferior and medial rectus muscles
- Abducent nerve (VI)
- Inferior branch of oculomotor nerve (III)
- Lacrimal nerve
- Frontal nerve *(cut)*
- Ophthalmic nerve (V₁)

Plate 86   Nerves of Orbit. (Netter: Atlas of Human Anatomy, 4 ed, 2006, Saunders.)

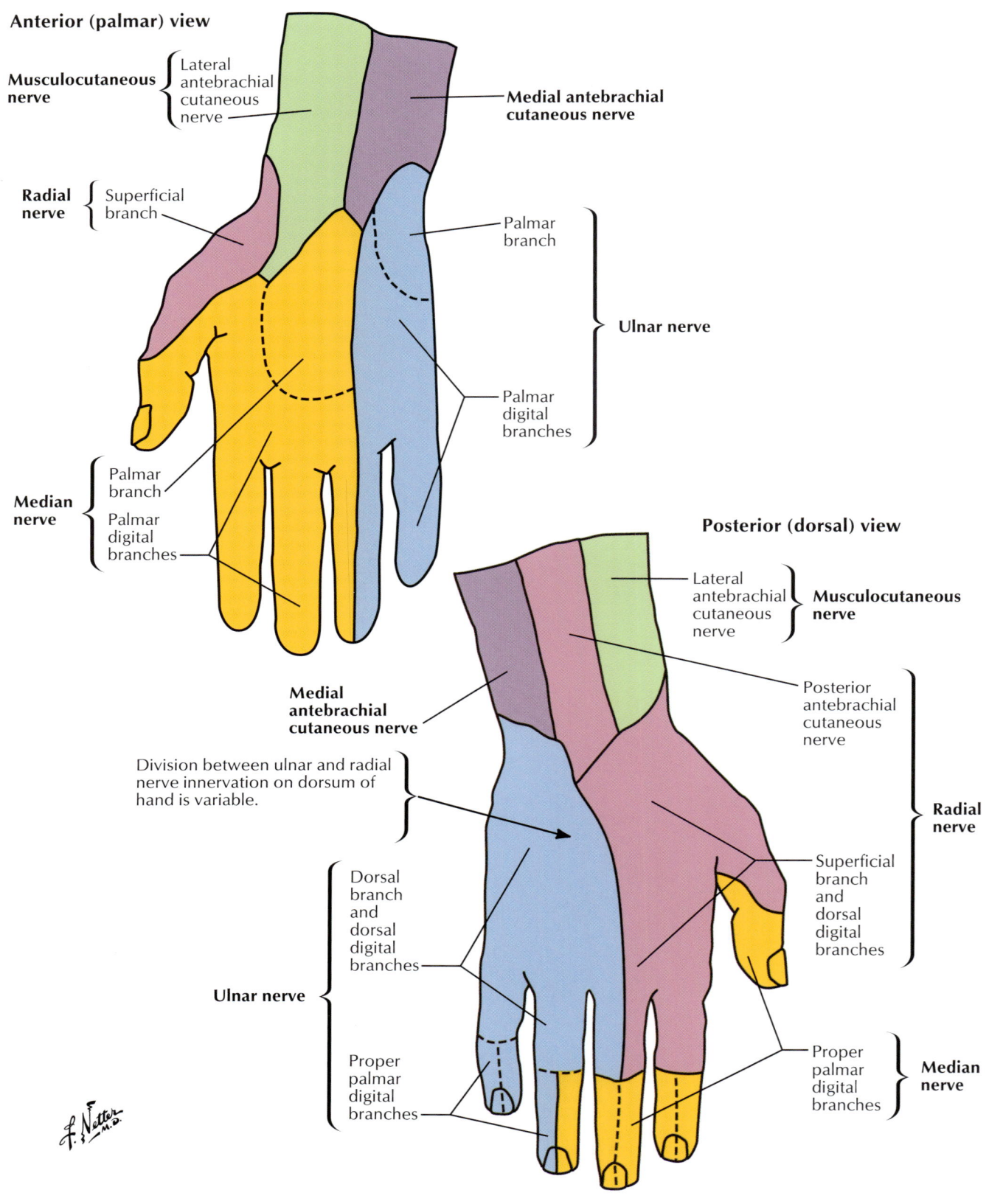

Anterior (palmar) view

Musculocutaneous nerve { Lateral antebrachial cutaneous nerve

Medial antebrachial cutaneous nerve

Radial nerve { Superficial branch

Palmar branch

Ulnar nerve

Palmar digital branches

Median nerve { Palmar branch
Palmar digital branches

Posterior (dorsal) view

Lateral antebrachial cutaneous nerve — **Musculocutaneous nerve**

Medial antebrachial cutaneous nerve

Posterior antebrachial cutaneous nerve

Division between ulnar and radial nerve innervation on dorsum of hand is variable.

Radial nerve

Superficial branch and dorsal digital branches

Ulnar nerve { Dorsal branch and dorsal digital branches

Proper palmar digital branches

Proper palmar digital branches — **Median nerve**

Plate 472   Cutaneous Innervation of Wrist and Hand. (Netter: Atlas of Human Anatomy, 4 ed, 2006, Saunders.)

Anterior view

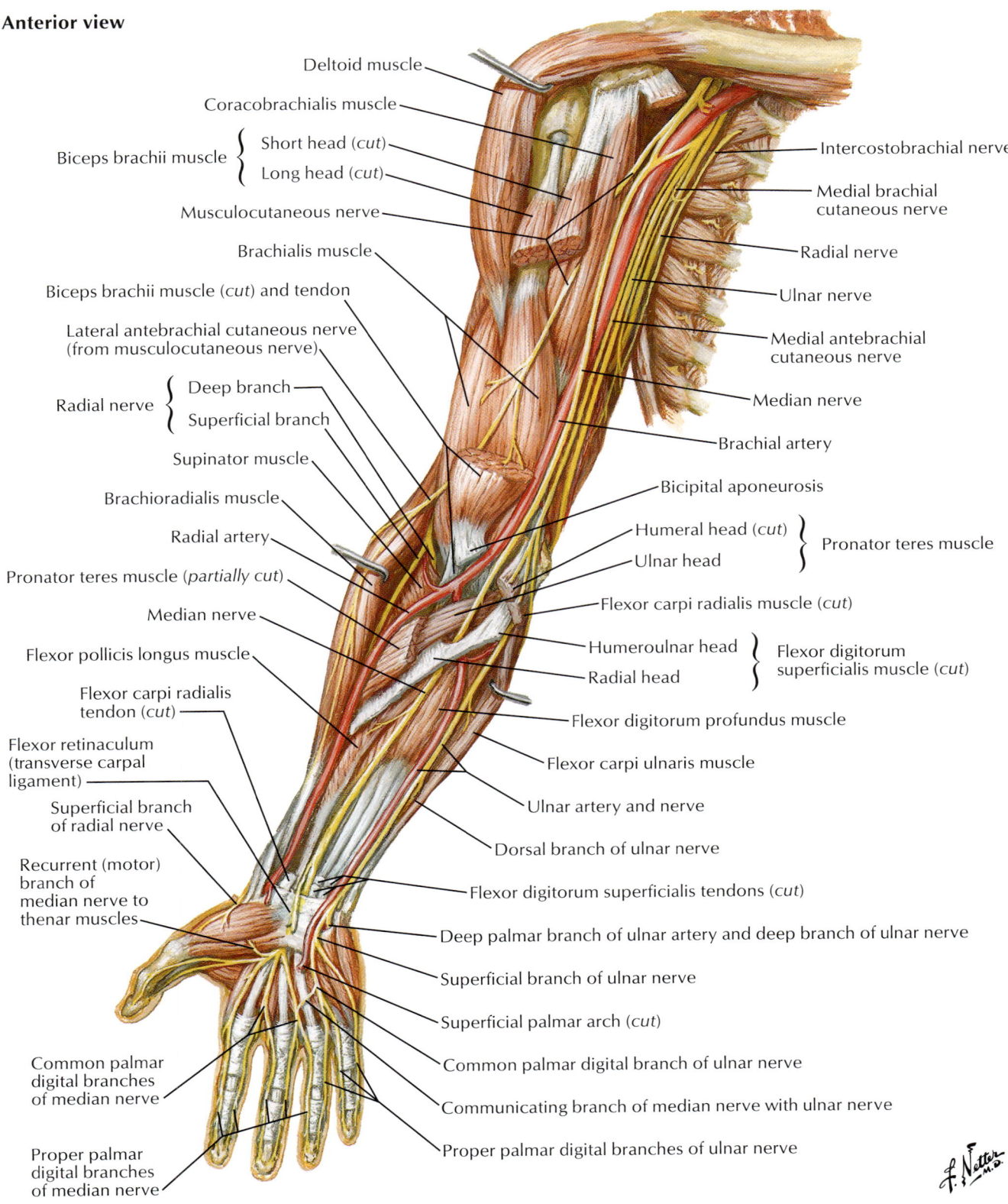

Deltoid muscle

Coracobrachialis muscle

Biceps brachii muscle { Short head (*cut*)
Long head (*cut*)

Musculocutaneous nerve

Brachialis muscle

Biceps brachii muscle (*cut*) and tendon

Lateral antebrachial cutaneous nerve
(from musculocutaneous nerve)

Radial nerve { Deep branch
Superficial branch

Supinator muscle

Brachioradialis muscle

Radial artery

Pronator teres muscle (*partially cut*)

Median nerve

Flexor pollicis longus muscle

Flexor carpi radialis
tendon (*cut*)

Flexor retinaculum
(transverse carpal
ligament)

Superficial branch
of radial nerve

Recurrent (motor)
branch of
median nerve to
thenar muscles

Common palmar
digital branches
of median nerve

Proper palmar
digital branches
of median nerve

Intercostobrachial nerve

Medial brachial
cutaneous nerve

Radial nerve

Ulnar nerve

Medial antebrachial
cutaneous nerve

Median nerve

Brachial artery

Bicipital aponeurosis

Humeral head (*cut*) } Pronator teres muscle
Ulnar head

Flexor carpi radialis muscle (*cut*)

Humeroulnar head } Flexor digitorum
superficialis muscle (*cut*)
Radial head

Flexor digitorum profundus muscle

Flexor carpi ulnaris muscle

Ulnar artery and nerve

Dorsal branch of ulnar nerve

Flexor digitorum superficialis tendons (*cut*)

Deep palmar branch of ulnar artery and deep branch of ulnar nerve

Superficial branch of ulnar nerve

Superficial palmar arch (*cut*)

Common palmar digital branch of ulnar nerve

Communicating branch of median nerve with ulnar nerve

Proper palmar digital branches of ulnar nerve

NETTER'S ANATOMY ILLUSTRATIONS

Plate 473 Arteries and Nerves of Upper Limb. (Netter: Atlas of Human Anatomy, 4 ed, 2006, Saunders.)

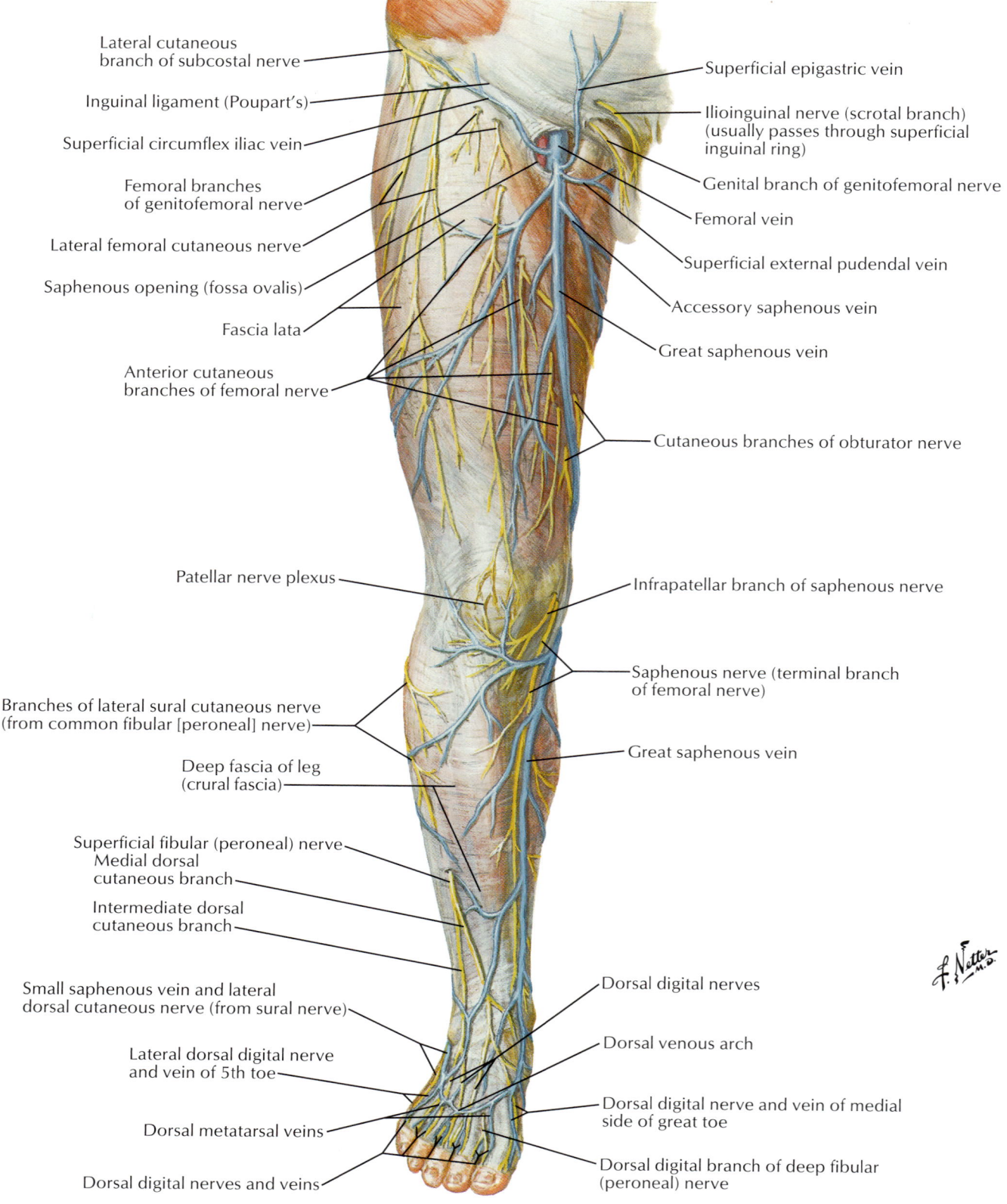

Lateral cutaneous branch of subcostal nerve

Inguinal ligament (Poupart's)

Superficial circumflex iliac vein

Femoral branches of genitofemoral nerve

Lateral femoral cutaneous nerve

Saphenous opening (fossa ovalis)

Fascia lata

Anterior cutaneous branches of femoral nerve

Patellar nerve plexus

Branches of lateral sural cutaneous nerve (from common fibular [peroneal] nerve)

Deep fascia of leg (crural fascia)

Superficial fibular (peroneal) nerve Medial dorsal cutaneous branch

Intermediate dorsal cutaneous branch

Small saphenous vein and lateral dorsal cutaneous nerve (from sural nerve)

Lateral dorsal digital nerve and vein of 5th toe

Dorsal metatarsal veins

Dorsal digital nerves and veins

Superficial epigastric vein

Ilioinguinal nerve (scrotal branch) (usually passes through superficial inguinal ring)

Genital branch of genitofemoral nerve

Femoral vein

Superficial external pudendal vein

Accessory saphenous vein

Great saphenous vein

Cutaneous branches of obturator nerve

Infrapatellar branch of saphenous nerve

Saphenous nerve (terminal branch of femoral nerve)

Great saphenous vein

Dorsal digital nerves

Dorsal venous arch

Dorsal digital nerve and vein of medial side of great toe

Dorsal digital branch of deep fibular (peroneal) nerve

Plate 544   Superficial Nerves and Veins of Lower Limb: Anterior View. (Netter: Atlas of Human Anatomy, 4 ed, 2006, Saunders.)

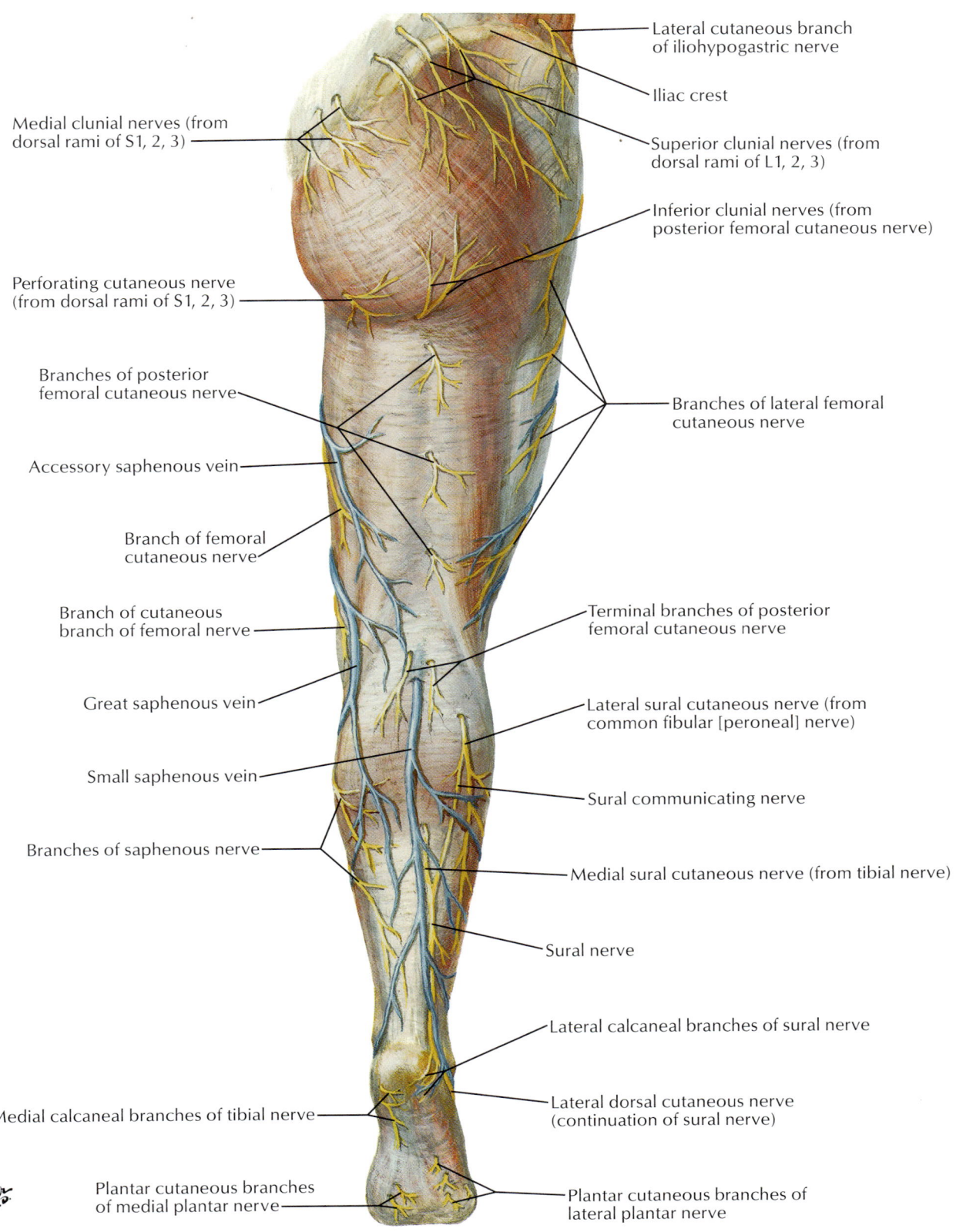

Lateral cutaneous branch of iliohypogastric nerve

Iliac crest

Medial clunial nerves (from dorsal rami of S1, 2, 3)

Superior clunial nerves (from dorsal rami of L1, 2, 3)

Inferior clunial nerves (from posterior femoral cutaneous nerve)

Perforating cutaneous nerve (from dorsal rami of S1, 2, 3)

Branches of posterior femoral cutaneous nerve

Branches of lateral femoral cutaneous nerve

Accessory saphenous vein

Branch of femoral cutaneous nerve

Branch of cutaneous branch of femoral nerve

Terminal branches of posterior femoral cutaneous nerve

Great saphenous vein

Lateral sural cutaneous nerve (from common fibular [peroneal] nerve)

Small saphenous vein

Sural communicating nerve

Branches of saphenous nerve

Medial sural cutaneous nerve (from tibial nerve)

Sural nerve

Lateral calcaneal branches of sural nerve

Medial calcaneal branches of tibial nerve

Lateral dorsal cutaneous nerve (continuation of sural nerve)

Plantar cutaneous branches of medial plantar nerve

Plantar cutaneous branches of lateral plantar nerve

Plate 545 Superficial Nerves and Veins of Lower Limb: Posterior View. (Netter: Atlas of Human Anatomy, 4 ed, 2006, Saunders.)

NAP-11

Superficial dissections

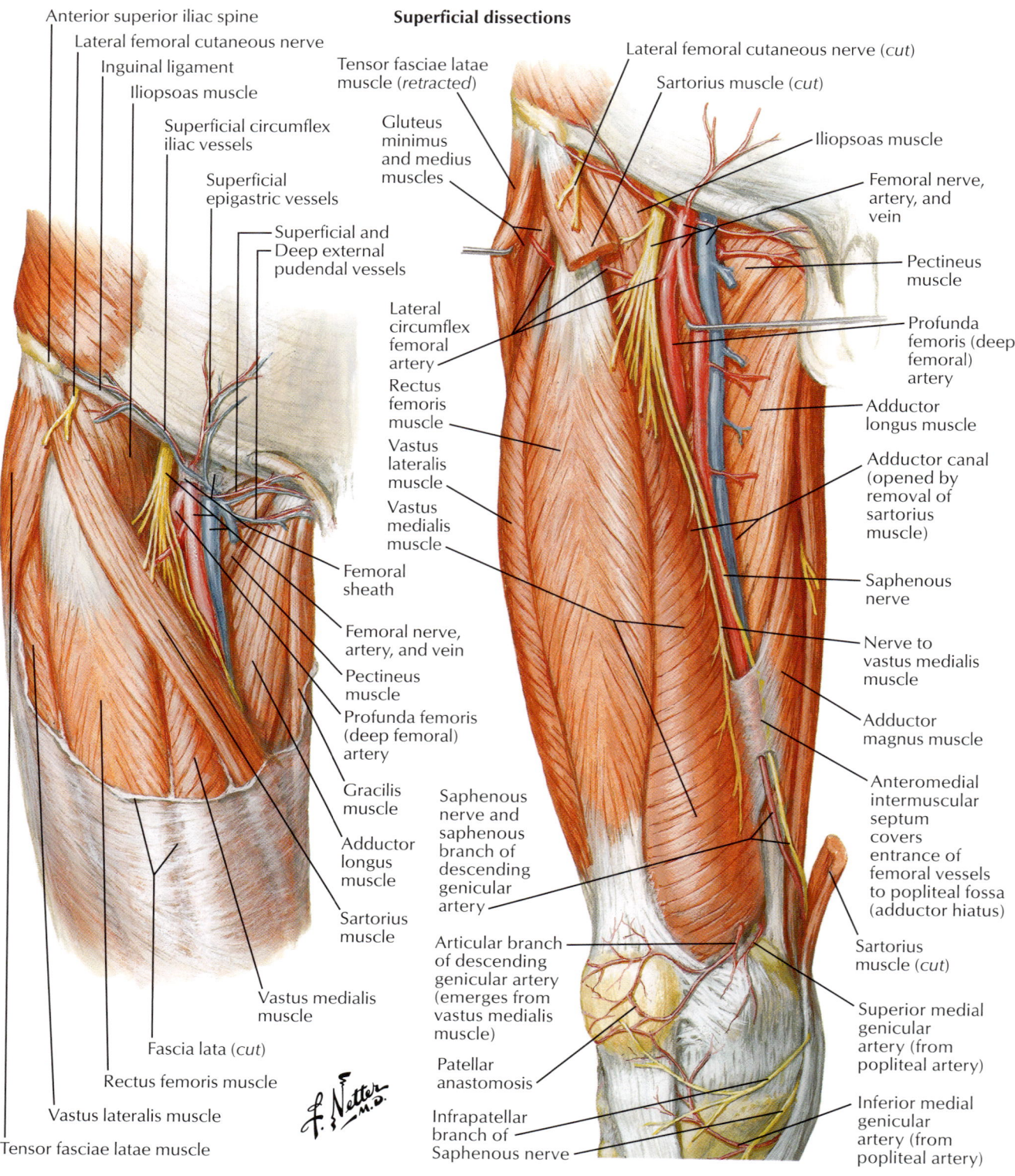

Anterior superior iliac spine

Lateral femoral cutaneous nerve

Inguinal ligament

Iliopsoas muscle

Superficial circumflex iliac vessels

Superficial epigastric vessels

Superficial and Deep external pudendal vessels

Tensor fasciae latae muscle (retracted)

Gluteus minimus and medius muscles

Lateral circumflex femoral artery

Rectus femoris muscle

Vastus lateralis muscle

Vastus medialis muscle

Femoral sheath

Femoral nerve, artery, and vein

Pectineus muscle

Profunda femoris (deep femoral) artery

Gracilis muscle

Adductor longus muscle

Sartorius muscle

Vastus medialis muscle

Fascia lata (cut)

Rectus femoris muscle

Vastus lateralis muscle

Tensor fasciae latae muscle

Lateral femoral cutaneous nerve (cut)

Sartorius muscle (cut)

Iliopsoas muscle

Femoral nerve, artery, and vein

Pectineus muscle

Profunda femoris (deep femoral) artery

Adductor longus muscle

Adductor canal (opened by removal of sartorius muscle)

Saphenous nerve

Nerve to vastus medialis muscle

Adductor magnus muscle

Anteromedial intermuscular septum covers entrance of femoral vessels to popliteal fossa (adductor hiatus)

Sartorius muscle (cut)

Superior medial genicular artery (from popliteal artery)

Inferior medial genicular artery (from popliteal artery)

Saphenous nerve and saphenous branch of descending genicular artery

Articular branch of descending genicular artery (emerges from vastus medialis muscle)

Patellar anastomosis

Infrapatellar branch of Saphenous nerve

Plate 500 Arteries and Nerves of Thigh: Anterior Views. (Netter: Atlas of Human Anatomy, 4 ed, 2006, Saunders.)

Deep dissection

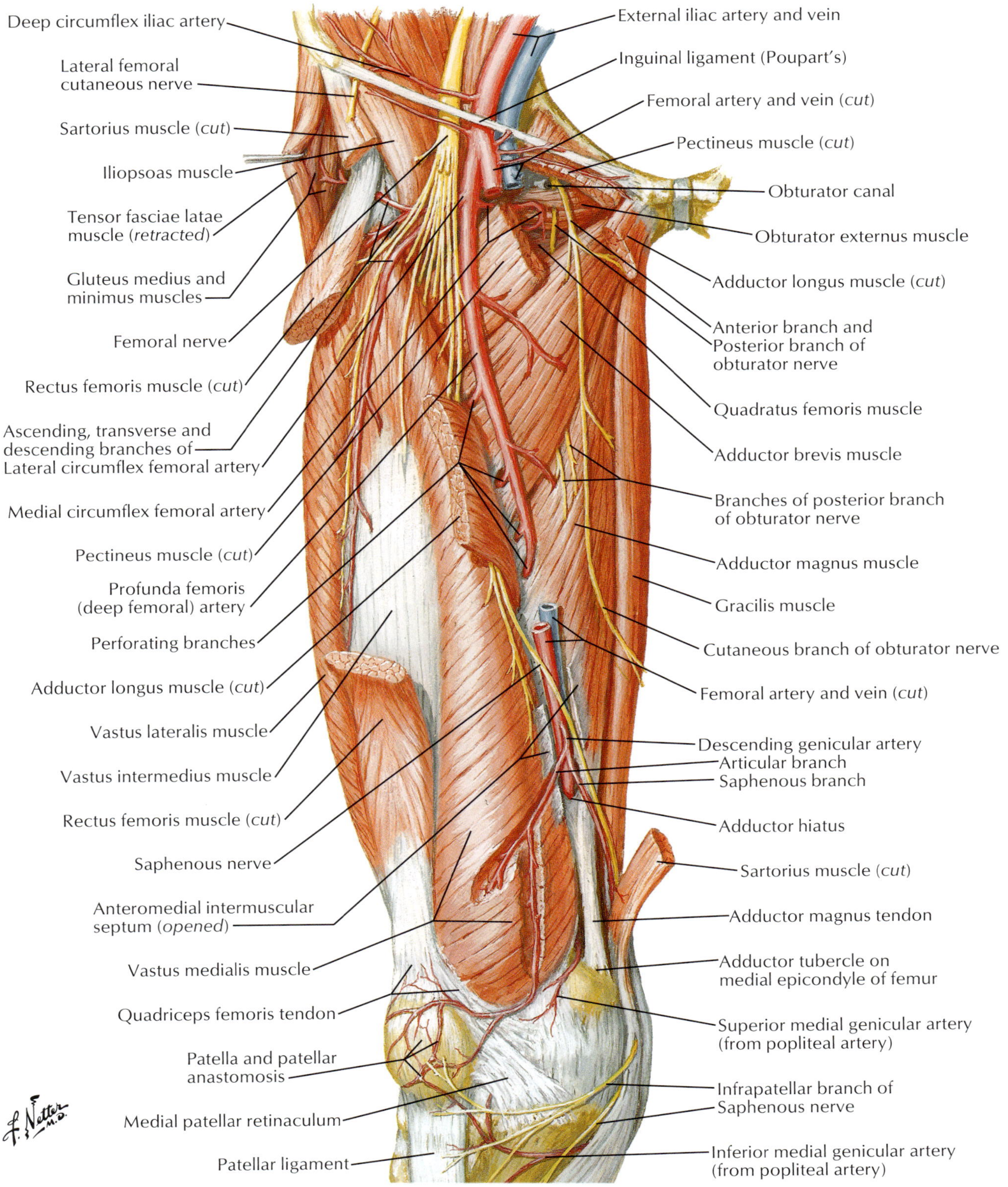

Deep circumflex iliac artery

Lateral femoral cutaneous nerve

Sartorius muscle (*cut*)

Iliopsoas muscle

Tensor fasciae latae muscle (*retracted*)

Gluteus medius and minimus muscles

Femoral nerve

Rectus femoris muscle (*cut*)

Ascending, transverse and descending branches of Lateral circumflex femoral artery

Medial circumflex femoral artery

Pectineus muscle (*cut*)

Profunda femoris (deep femoral) artery

Perforating branches

Adductor longus muscle (*cut*)

Vastus lateralis muscle

Vastus intermedius muscle

Rectus femoris muscle (*cut*)

Saphenous nerve

Anteromedial intermuscular septum (*opened*)

Vastus medialis muscle

Quadriceps femoris tendon

Patella and patellar anastomosis

Medial patellar retinaculum

Patellar ligament

External iliac artery and vein

Inguinal ligament (Poupart's)

Femoral artery and vein (*cut*)

Pectineus muscle (*cut*)

Obturator canal

Obturator externus muscle

Adductor longus muscle (*cut*)

Anterior branch and Posterior branch of obturator nerve

Quadratus femoris muscle

Adductor brevis muscle

Branches of posterior branch of obturator nerve

Adductor magnus muscle

Gracilis muscle

Cutaneous branch of obturator nerve

Femoral artery and vein (*cut*)

Descending genicular artery

Articular branch

Saphenous branch

Adductor hiatus

Sartorius muscle (*cut*)

Adductor magnus tendon

Adductor tubercle on medial epicondyle of femur

Superior medial genicular artery (from popliteal artery)

Infrapatellar branch of Saphenous nerve

Inferior medial genicular artery (from popliteal artery)

Plate 501 Arteries and Nerves of Thigh: Posterior View. (Netter: Atlas of Human Anatomy, 4 ed, 2006, Saunders.)

NAP-13

Deep dissection

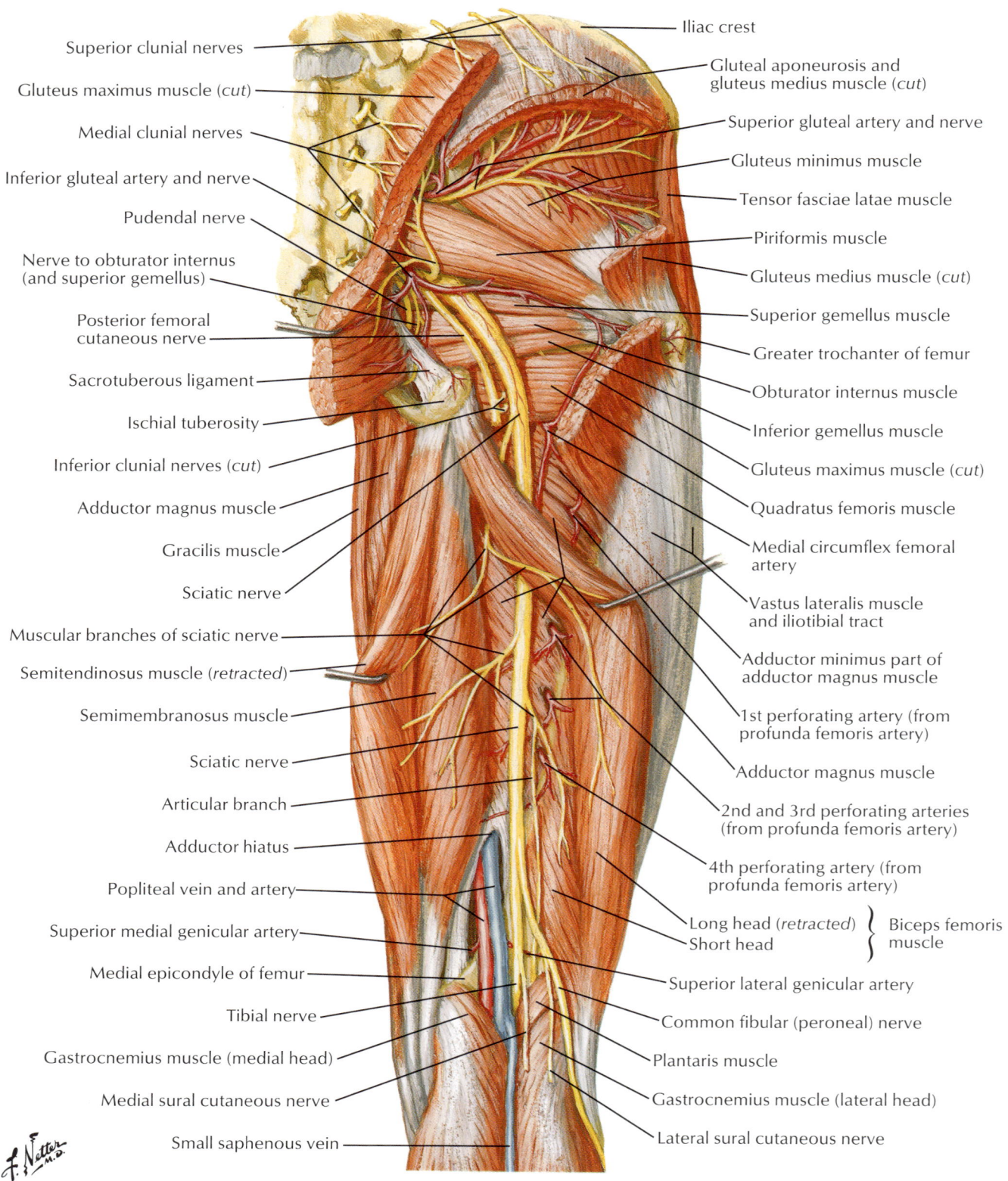

Superior clunial nerves

Gluteus maximus muscle (*cut*)

Medial clunial nerves

Inferior gluteal artery and nerve

Pudendal nerve

Nerve to obturator internus (and superior gemellus)

Posterior femoral cutaneous nerve

Sacrotuberous ligament

Ischial tuberosity

Inferior clunial nerves (*cut*)

Adductor magnus muscle

Gracilis muscle

Sciatic nerve

Muscular branches of sciatic nerve

Semitendinosus muscle (*retracted*)

Semimembranosus muscle

Sciatic nerve

Articular branch

Adductor hiatus

Popliteal vein and artery

Superior medial genicular artery

Medial epicondyle of femur

Tibial nerve

Gastrocnemius muscle (medial head)

Medial sural cutaneous nerve

Small saphenous vein

Iliac crest

Gluteal aponeurosis and gluteus medius muscle (*cut*)

Superior gluteal artery and nerve

Gluteus minimus muscle

Tensor fasciae latae muscle

Piriformis muscle

Gluteus medius muscle (*cut*)

Superior gemellus muscle

Greater trochanter of femur

Obturator internus muscle

Inferior gemellus muscle

Gluteus maximus muscle (*cut*)

Quadratus femoris muscle

Medial circumflex femoral artery

Vastus lateralis muscle and iliotibial tract

Adductor minimus part of adductor magnus muscle

1st perforating artery (from profunda femoris artery)

Adductor magnus muscle

2nd and 3rd perforating arteries (from profunda femoris artery)

4th perforating artery (from profunda femoris artery)

Long head (*retracted*) ⎫ Biceps femoris
Short head ⎭ muscle

Superior lateral genicular artery

Common fibular (peroneal) nerve

Plantaris muscle

Gastrocnemius muscle (lateral head)

Lateral sural cutaneous nerve

Plate 502 Arteries and Nerves of Thigh: Posterior View. (Netter: Atlas of Human Anatomy, 4 ed, 2006, Saunders.)

Horizontal section

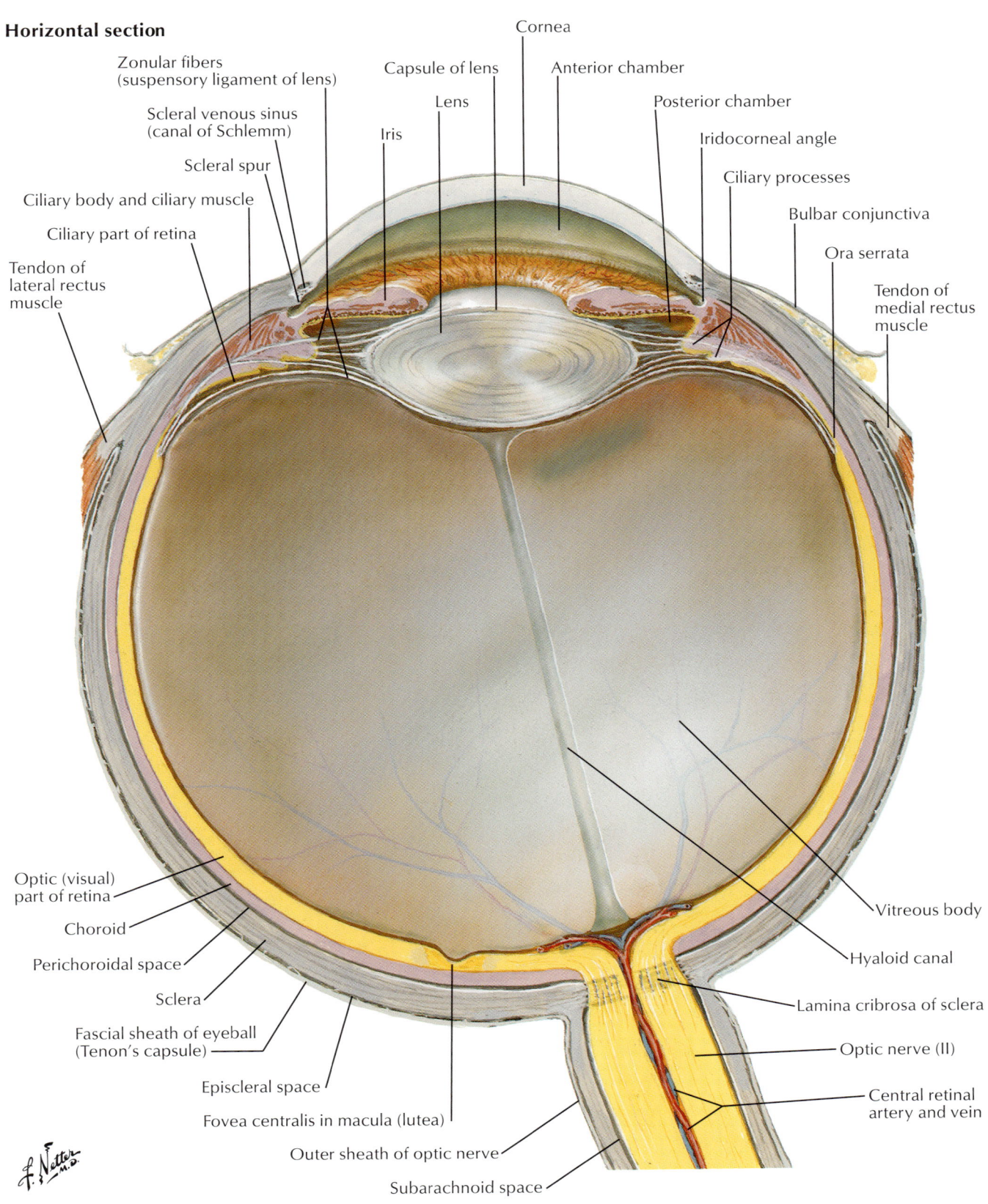

Zonular fibers (suspensory ligament of lens)

Scleral venous sinus (canal of Schlemm)

Scleral spur

Ciliary body and ciliary muscle

Ciliary part of retina

Tendon of lateral rectus muscle

Iris

Capsule of lens

Lens

Cornea

Anterior chamber

Posterior chamber

Iridocorneal angle

Ciliary processes

Bulbar conjunctiva

Ora serrata

Tendon of medial rectus muscle

Optic (visual) part of retina

Choroid

Perichoroidal space

Sclera

Fascial sheath of eyeball (Tenon's capsule)

Episcleral space

Fovea centralis in macula (lutea)

Outer sheath of optic nerve

Subarachnoid space

Vitreous body

Hyaloid canal

Lamina cribrosa of sclera

Optic nerve (II)

Central retinal artery and vein

Plate 87   Eyeball. (Netter: Atlas of Human Anatomy, 4 ed, 2006, Saunders.)

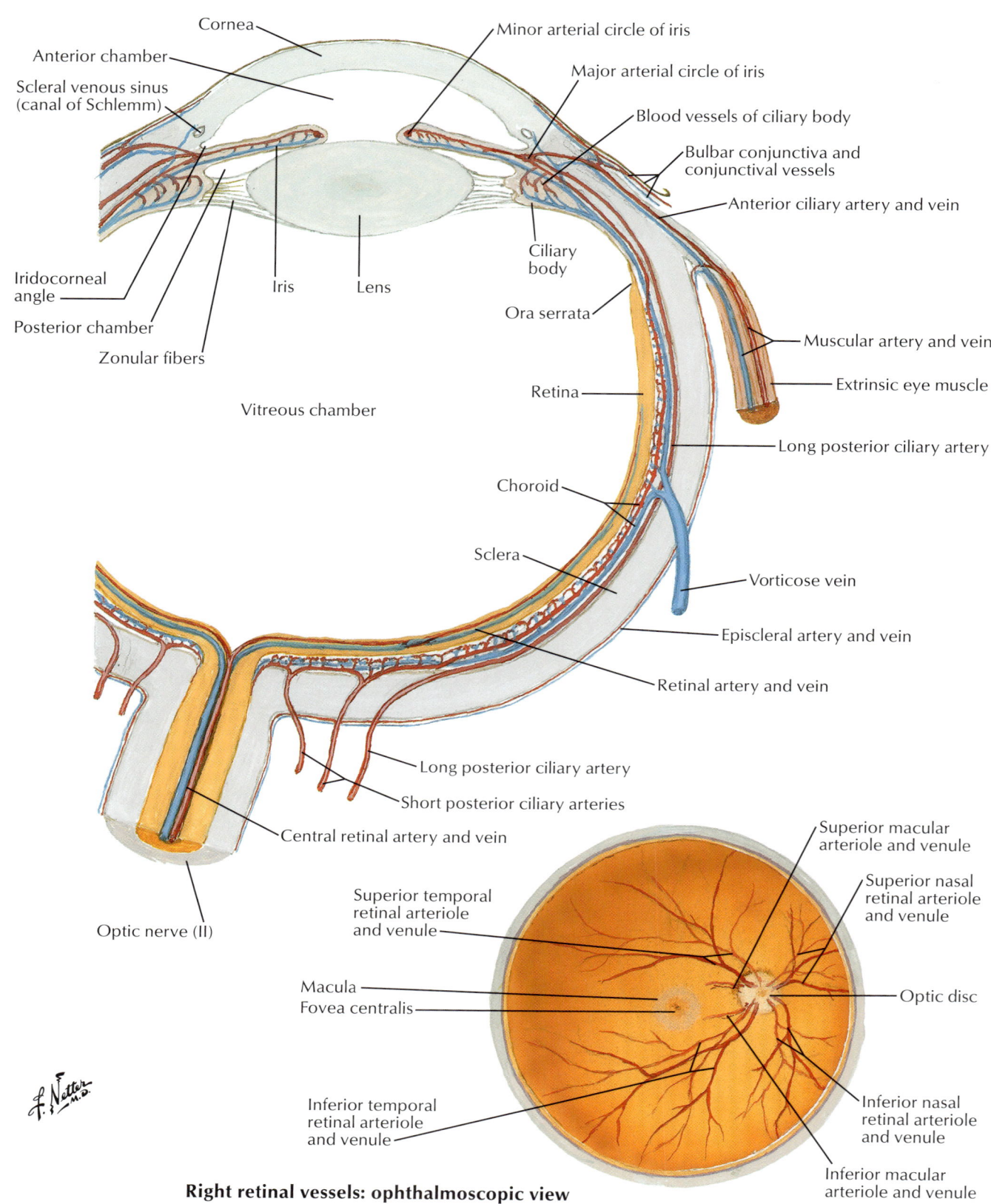

Cornea

Anterior chamber

Scleral venous sinus (canal of Schlemm)

Minor arterial circle of iris

Major arterial circle of iris

Blood vessels of ciliary body

Bulbar conjunctiva and conjunctival vessels

Anterior ciliary artery and vein

Iridocorneal angle

Iris

Lens

Ciliary body

Posterior chamber

Ora serrata

Muscular artery and vein

Zonular fibers

Extrinsic eye muscle

Retina

Long posterior ciliary artery

Vitreous chamber

Choroid

Sclera

Vorticose vein

Episcleral artery and vein

Retinal artery and vein

Long posterior ciliary artery

Short posterior ciliary arteries

Central retinal artery and vein

Optic nerve (II)

Superior macular arteriole and venule

Superior temporal retinal arteriole and venule

Superior nasal retinal arteriole and venule

Macula

Fovea centralis

Optic disc

Inferior temporal retinal arteriole and venule

Inferior nasal retinal arteriole and venule

Inferior macular arteriole and venule

Right retinal vessels: ophthalmoscopic view

Plate 90 Intrinsic Arteries and Veins of Eye. (Netter: Atlas of Human Anatomy, 4 ed, 2006, Saunders.)

NAP-16

NETTER'S ANATOMY ILLUSTRATIONS

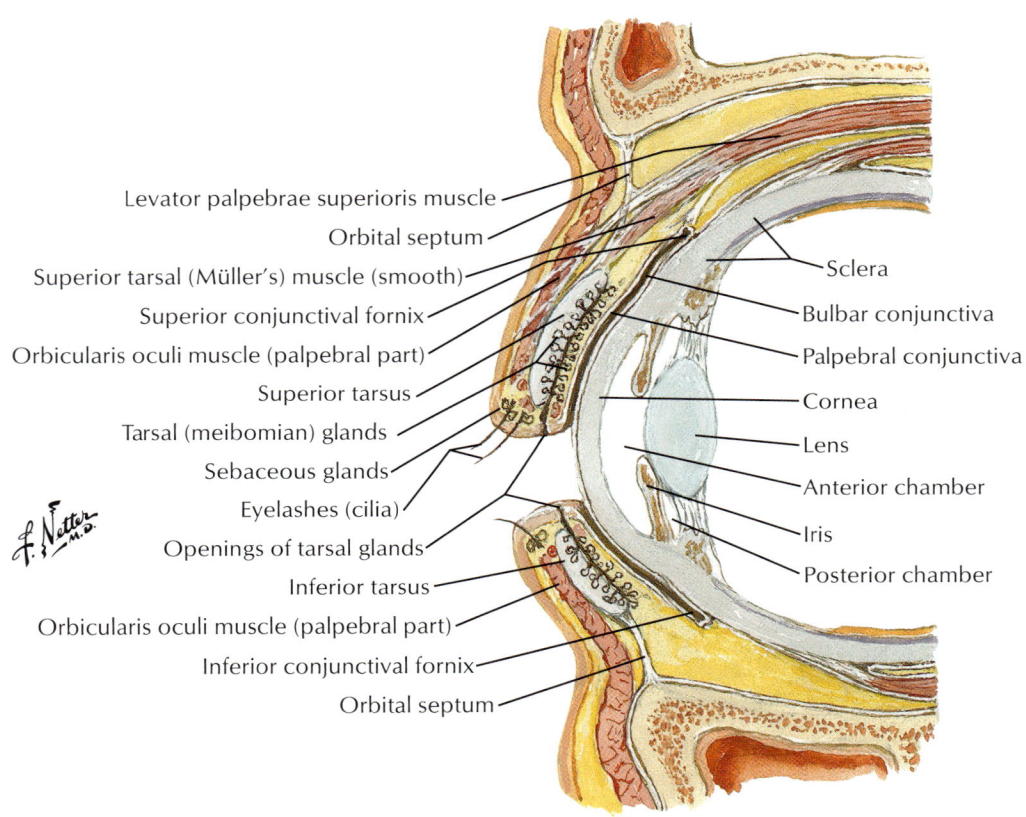

Levator palpebrae superioris muscle

Orbital septum

Superior tarsal (Müller's) muscle (smooth)

Superior conjunctival fornix

Orbicularis oculi muscle (palpebral part)

Superior tarsus

Tarsal (meibomian) glands

Sebaceous glands

Eyelashes (cilia)

Openings of tarsal glands

Inferior tarsus

Orbicularis oculi muscle (palpebral part)

Inferior conjunctival fornix

Orbital septum

Sclera

Bulbar conjunctiva

Palpebral conjunctiva

Cornea

Lens

Anterior chamber

Iris

Posterior chamber

Plate 81, Middle   Eyelids. (Netter: Atlas of Human Anatomy, 4 ed, 2006, Saunders.)

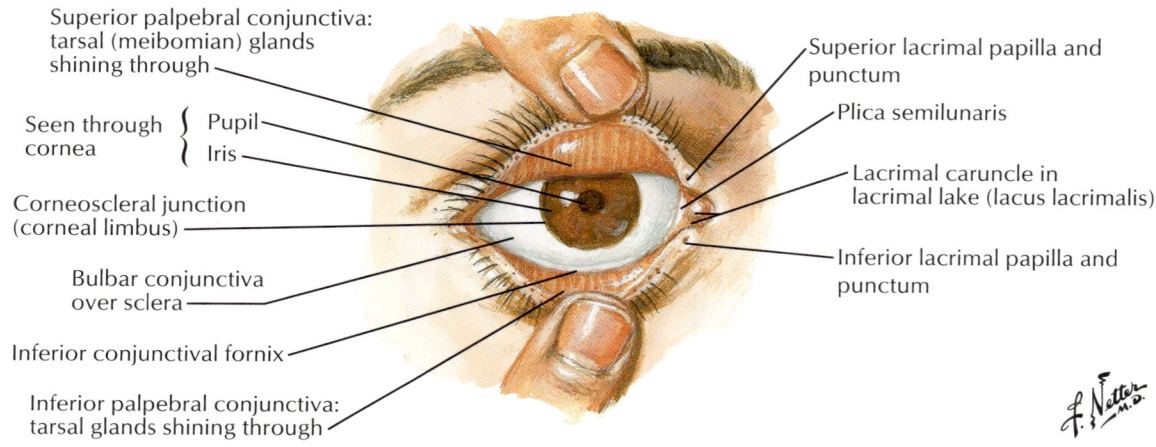

Superior palpebral conjunctiva:
tarsal (meibomian) glands
shining through

Seen through { Pupil
cornea   { Iris

Corneoscleral junction
(corneal limbus)

Bulbar conjunctiva
over sclera

Inferior conjunctival fornix

Inferior palpebral conjunctiva:
tarsal glands shining through

Superior lacrimal papilla and
punctum

Plica semilunaris

Lacrimal caruncle in
lacrimal lake (lacus lacrimalis)

Inferior lacrimal papilla and
punctum

Plate 81, Upper Eyelid. (Netter: Atlas of Human Anatomy, 4 ed, 2006, Saunders.)

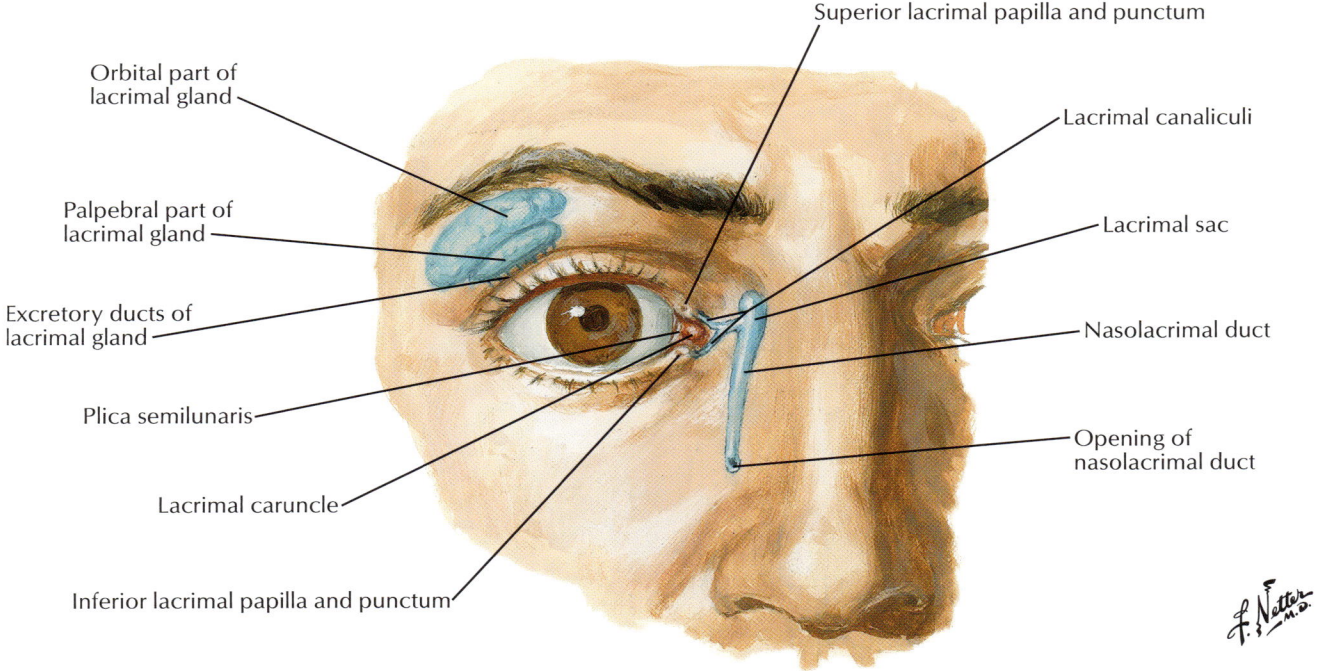

Orbital part of
lacrimal gland

Palpebral part of
lacrimal gland

Excretory ducts of
lacrimal gland

Plica semilunaris

Lacrimal caruncle

Inferior lacrimal papilla and punctum

Superior lacrimal papilla and punctum

Lacrimal canaliculi

Lacrimal sac

Nasolacrimal duct

Opening of
nasolacrimal duct

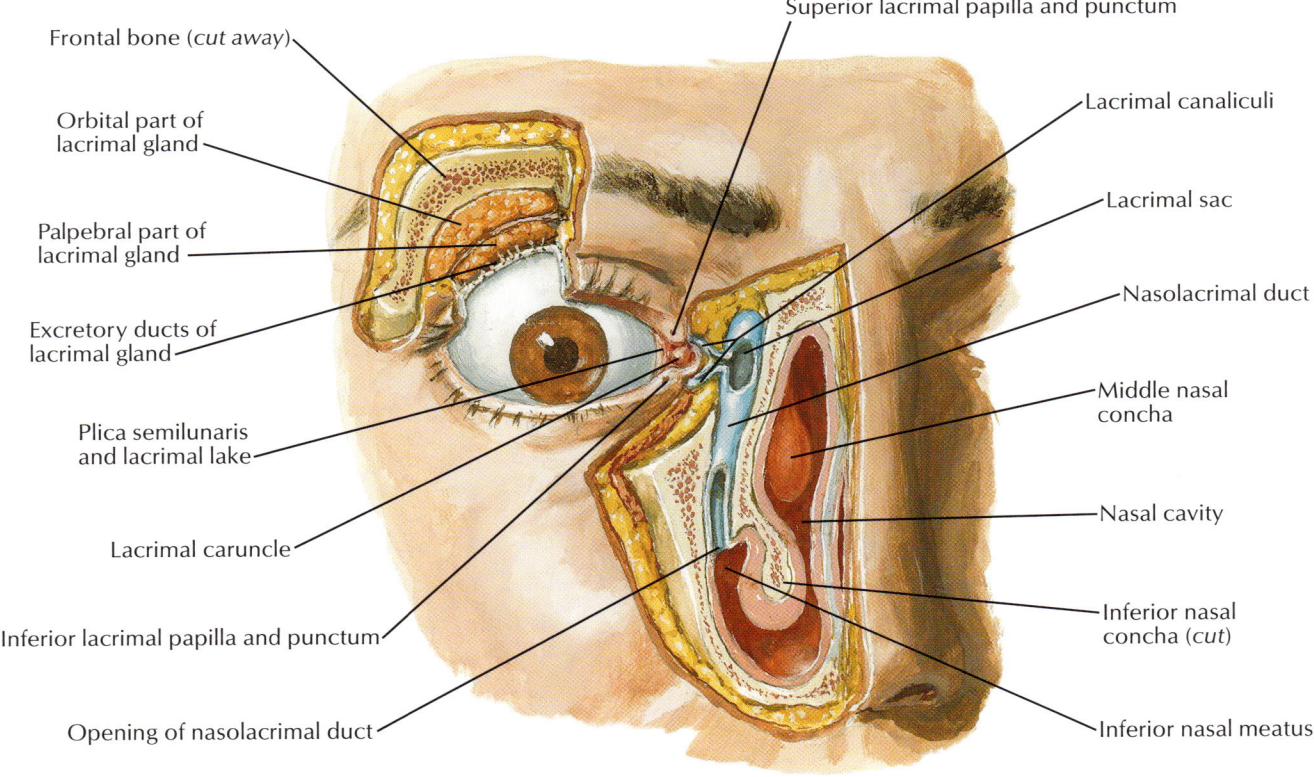

Frontal bone (*cut away*)

Orbital part of
lacrimal gland

Palpebral part of
lacrimal gland

Excretory ducts of
lacrimal gland

Plica semilunaris
and lacrimal lake

Lacrimal caruncle

Inferior lacrimal papilla and punctum

Opening of nasolacrimal duct

Superior lacrimal papilla and punctum

Lacrimal canaliculi

Lacrimal sac

Nasolacrimal duct

Middle nasal
concha

Nasal cavity

Inferior nasal
concha (*cut*)

Inferior nasal meatus

Plate 82   Lacrimal Apparatus. (Netter: Atlas of Human Anatomy, 4 ed, 2006, Saunders.)

Frontal section

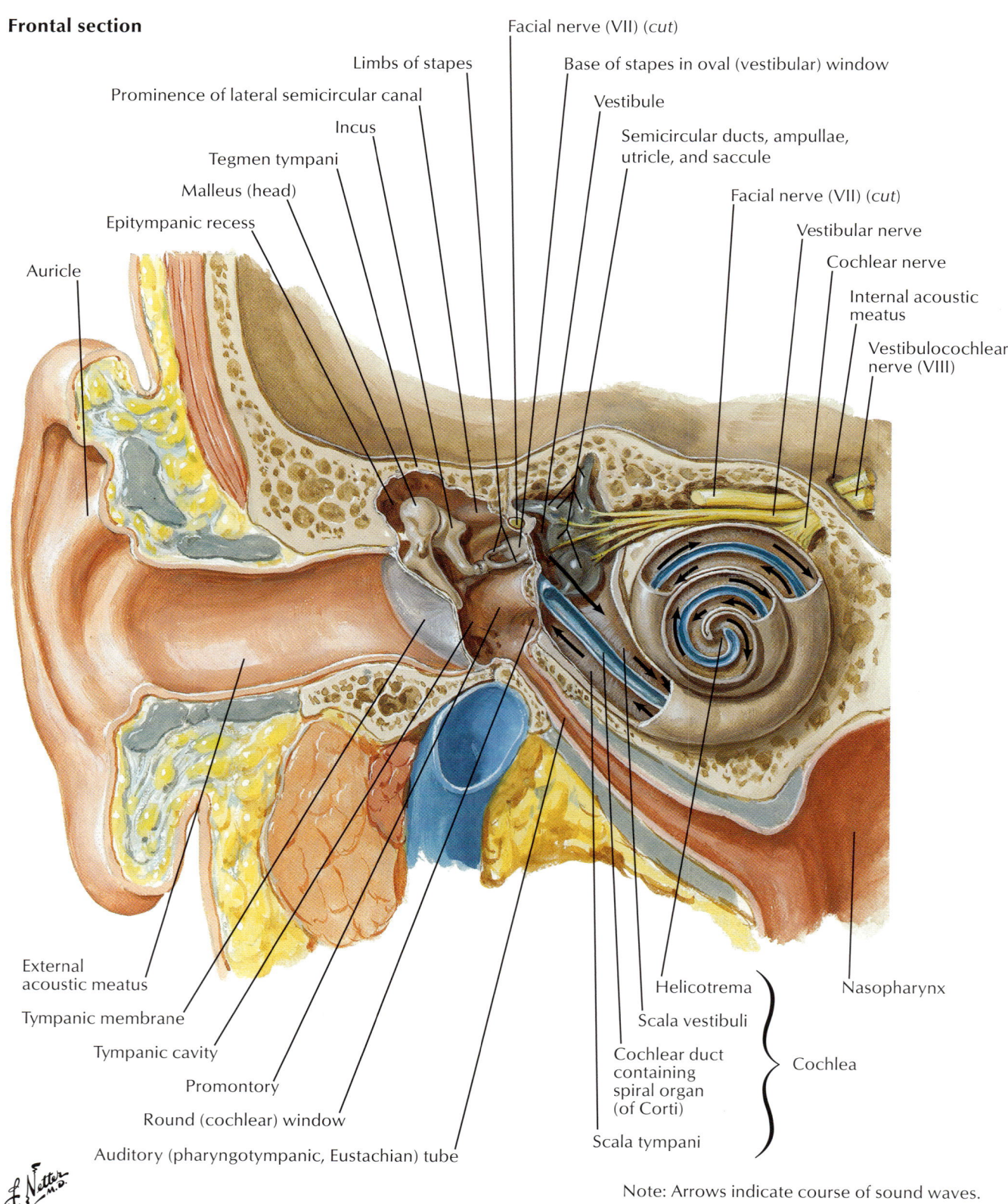

Facial nerve (VII) (*cut*)

Limbs of stapes

Base of stapes in oval (vestibular) window

Prominence of lateral semicircular canal

Vestibule

Incus

Semicircular ducts, ampullae, utricle, and saccule

Tegmen tympani

Malleus (head)

Facial nerve (VII) (*cut*)

Epitympanic recess

Vestibular nerve

Auricle

Cochlear nerve

Internal acoustic meatus

Vestibulocochlear nerve (VIII)

External acoustic meatus

Tympanic membrane

Tympanic cavity

Promontory

Round (cochlear) window

Auditory (pharyngotympanic, Eustachian) tube

Helicotrema

Scala vestibuli

Cochlear duct containing spiral organ (of Corti)

Scala tympani

Nasopharynx

Cochlea

Note: Arrows indicate course of sound waves.

Plate 92 Pathway of Sound Reception. (Netter: Atlas of Human Anatomy, 4 ed, 2006, Saunders.)

Medial wall of tympanic cavity: lateral view

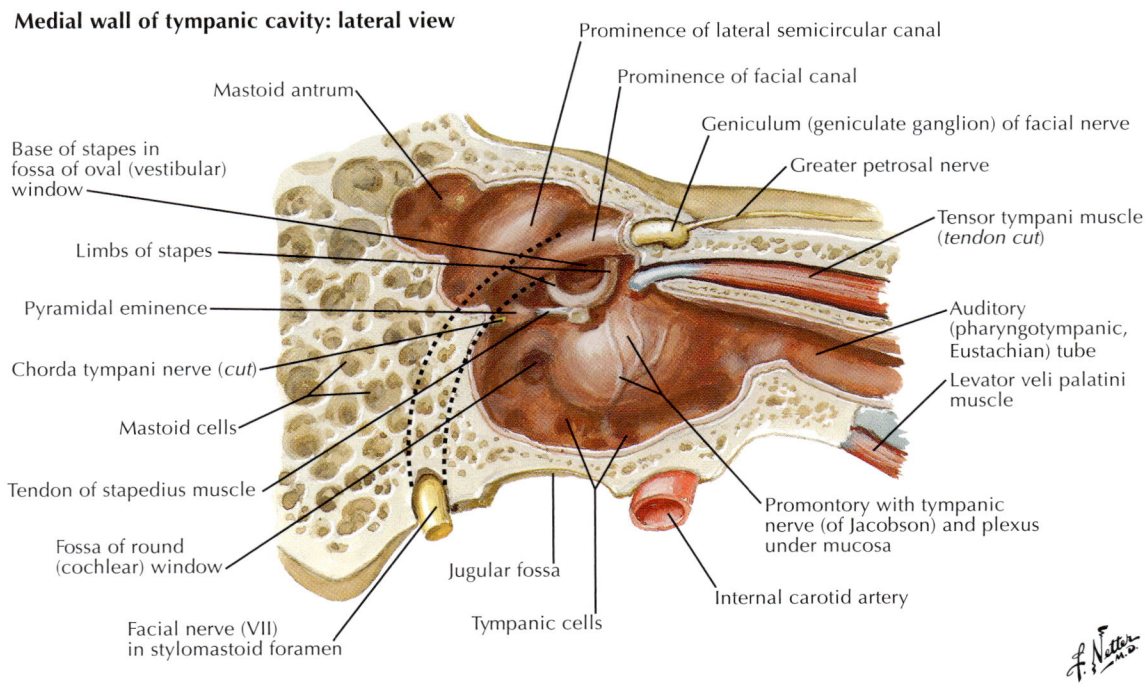

Mastoid antrum

Prominence of lateral semicircular canal

Prominence of facial canal

Geniculum (geniculate ganglion) of facial nerve

Greater petrosal nerve

Base of stapes in fossa of oval (vestibular) window

Tensor tympani muscle (*tendon cut*)

Limbs of stapes

Pyramidal eminence

Auditory (pharyngotympanic, Eustachian) tube

Chorda tympani nerve (*cut*)

Levator veli palatini muscle

Mastoid cells

Tendon of stapedius muscle

Fossa of round (cochlear) window

Promontory with tympanic nerve (of Jacobson) and plexus under mucosa

Jugular fossa

Facial nerve (VII) in stylomastoid foramen

Tympanic cells

Internal carotid artery

Plate 94 Tympanic Cavity. (Netter: Atlas of Human Anatomy, 4 ed, 2006, Saunders.)

Otoscopic view of right tympanic membrane

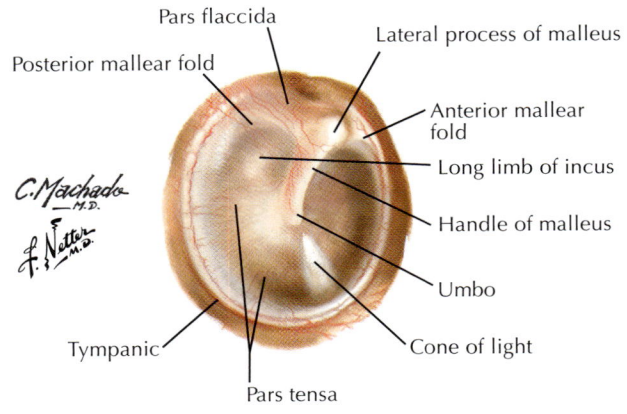

Pars flaccida

Posterior mallear fold

Lateral process of malleus

Anterior mallear fold

Long limb of incus

Handle of malleus

Umbo

Cone of light

Tympanic

Pars tensa

Plate 93 Tympanic Cavity. (Netter: Atlas of Human Anatomy, 4 ed, 2006, Saunders.)

Dissected right bony labyrinth (otic capsule): membranous labyrinth removed

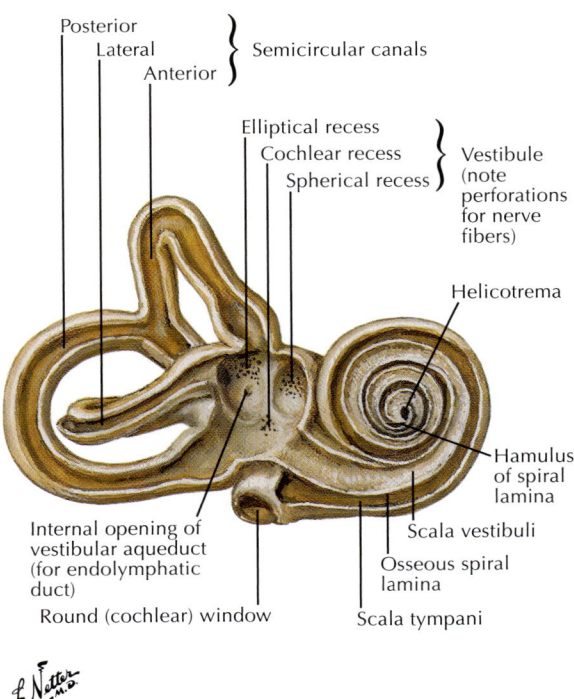

Posterior

Lateral

Anterior

Semicircular canals

Elliptical recess

Cochlear recess

Spherical recess

Vestibule (note perforations for nerve fibers)

Helicotrema

Hamulus of spiral lamina

Scala vestibuli

Osseous spiral lamina

Scala tympani

Internal opening of vestibular aqueduct (for endolymphatic duct)

Round (cochlear) window

Plate 95 Bony Membranous Labyrinth. (Netter: Atlas of Human Anatomy, 4 ed, 2006, Saunders.)

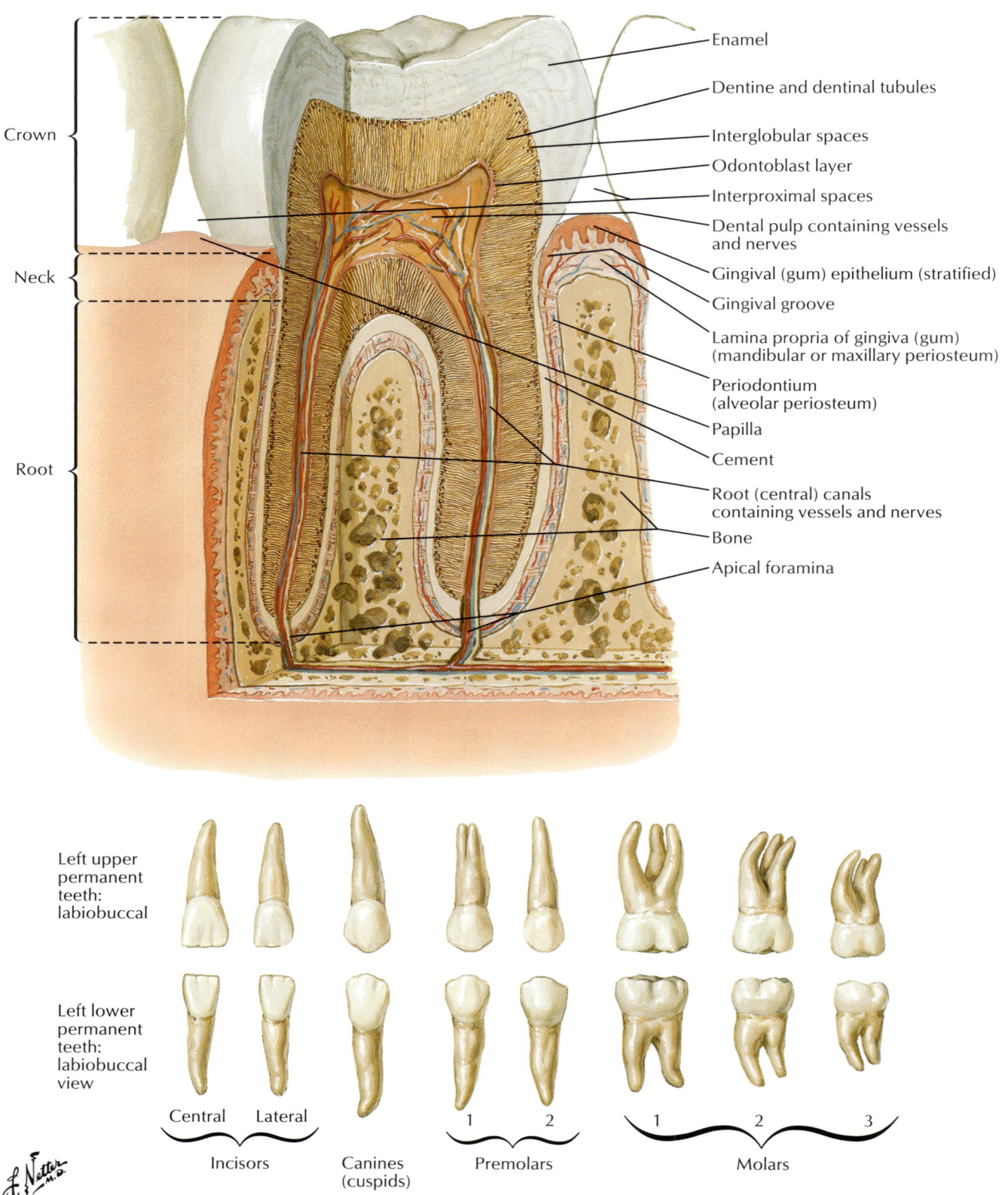

Crown

Enamel

Dentine and dentinal tubules

Interglobular spaces

Odontoblast layer

Interproximal spaces

Dental pulp containing vessels and nerves

Neck

Gingival (gum) epithelium (stratified)

Gingival groove

Lamina propria of gingiva (gum) (mandibular or maxillary periosteum)

Periodontium (alveolar periosteum)

Papilla

Cement

Root

Root (central) canals containing vessels and nerves

Bone

Apical foramina

Left upper permanent teeth: labiobuccal

Left lower permanent teeth: labiobuccal view

Central   Lateral

Incisors

Canines (cuspids)

1   2

Premolars

1   2   3

Molars

Plate 57   Teeth. (Netter: Atlas of Human Anatomy, 4 ed, 2006, Saunders.)

Tongue

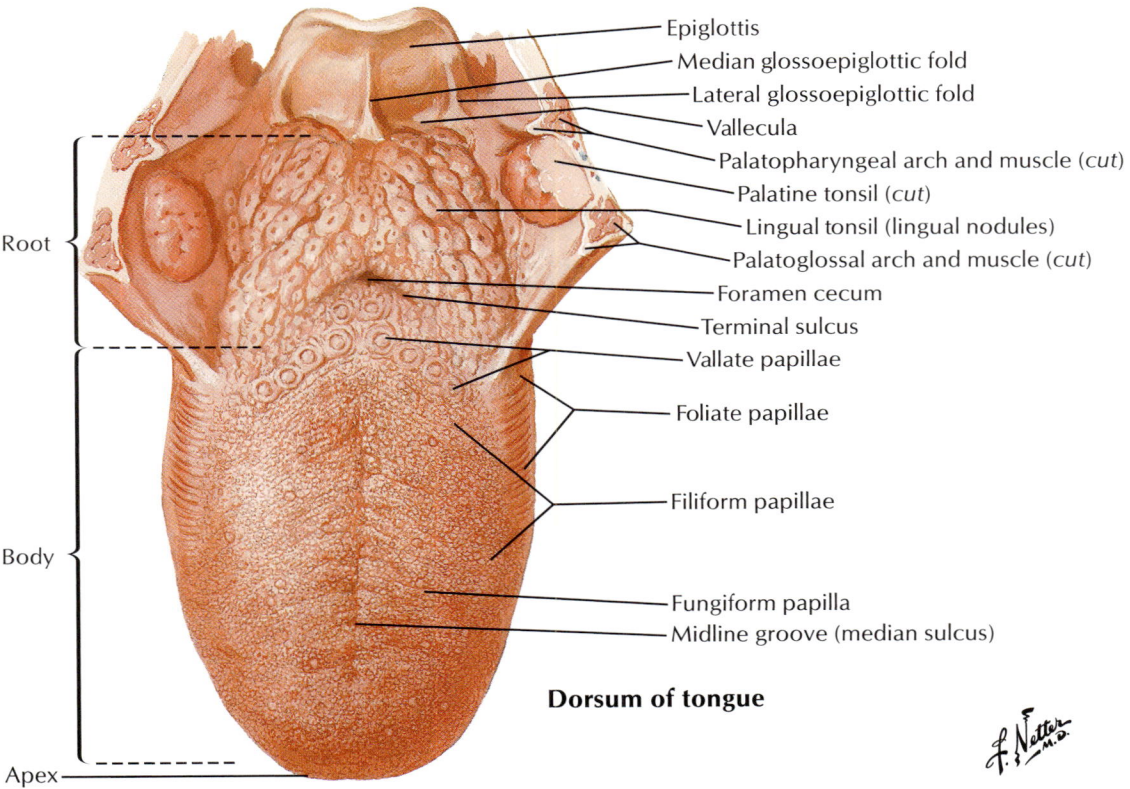

Epiglottis

Median glossoepiglottic fold

Lateral glossoepiglottic fold

Vallecula

Palatopharyngeal arch and muscle (*cut*)

Palatine tonsil (*cut*)

Lingual tonsil (lingual nodules)

Palatoglossal arch and muscle (*cut*)

Foramen cecum

Terminal sulcus

Vallate papillae

Foliate papillae

Filiform papillae

Fungiform papilla

Midline groove (median sulcus)

Root

Body

Apex

Dorsum of tongue

Plate 58   Tongue. (Netter: Atlas of Human Anatomy, 4 ed, 2006, Saunders.)

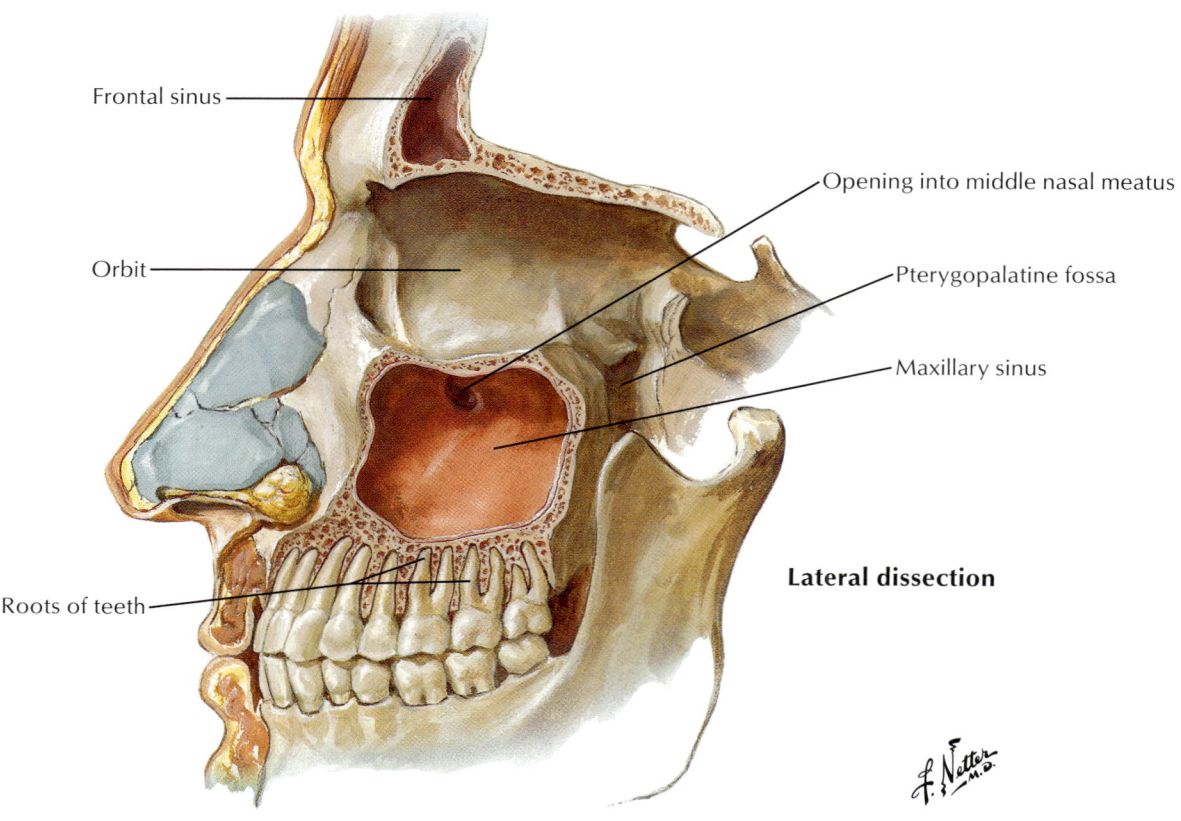

Frontal sinus

Orbit

Roots of teeth

Opening into middle nasal meatus

Pterygopalatine fossa

Maxillary sinus

Lateral dissection

Plate 49 Paranasal Sinuses. (Netter: Atlas of Human Anatomy, 4 ed, 2006, Saunders.)

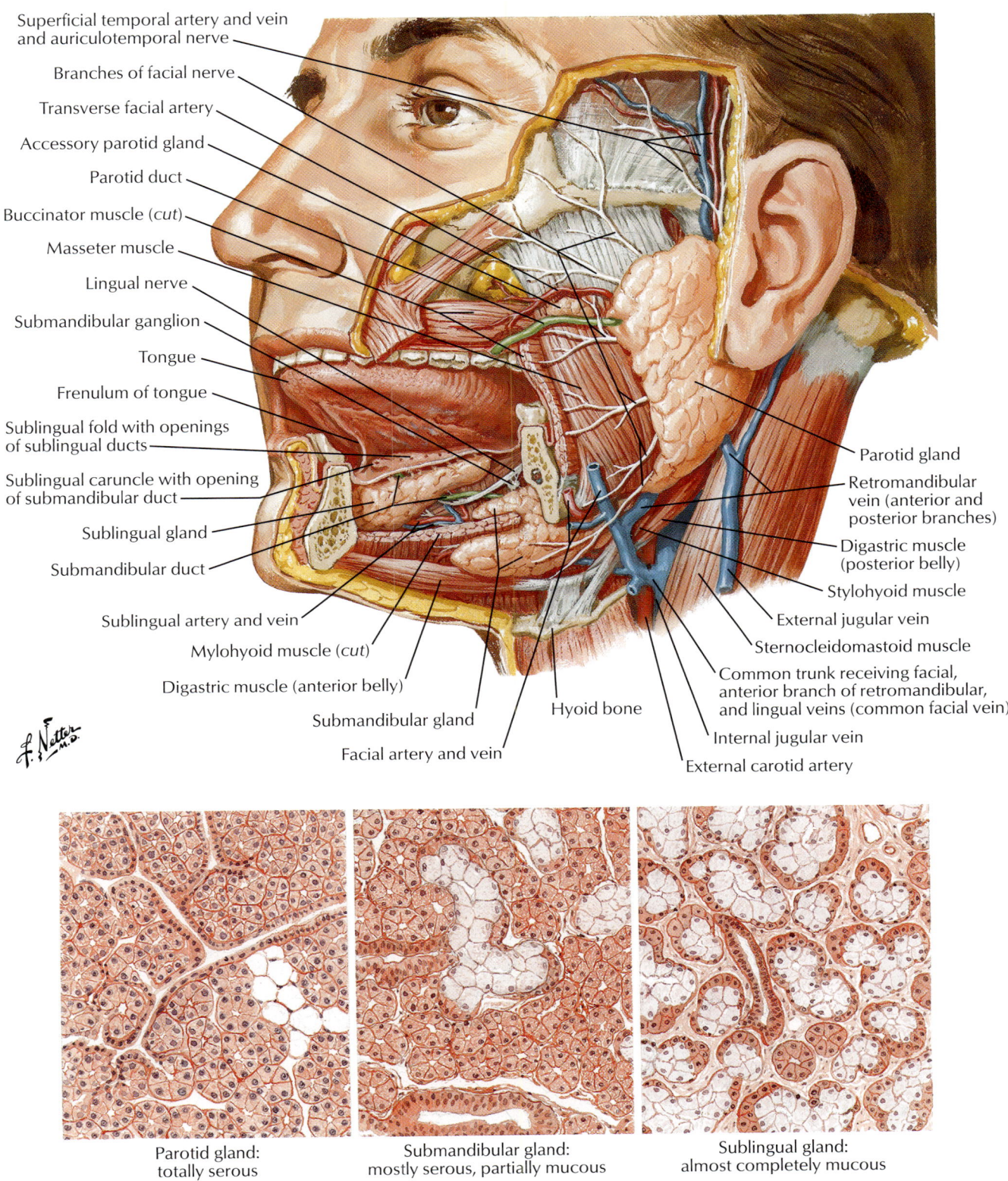

Superficial temporal artery and vein and auriculotemporal nerve

Branches of facial nerve

Transverse facial artery

Accessory parotid gland

Parotid duct

Buccinator muscle (*cut*)

Masseter muscle

Lingual nerve

Submandibular ganglion

Tongue

Frenulum of tongue

Sublingual fold with openings of sublingual ducts

Sublingual caruncle with opening of submandibular duct

Sublingual gland

Submandibular duct

Sublingual artery and vein

Mylohyoid muscle (*cut*)

Digastric muscle (anterior belly)

Submandibular gland

Facial artery and vein

Hyoid bone

Parotid gland

Retromandibular vein (anterior and posterior branches)

Digastric muscle (posterior belly)

Stylohyoid muscle

External jugular vein

Sternocleidomastoid muscle

Common trunk receiving facial, anterior branch of retromandibular, and lingual veins (common facial vein)

Internal jugular vein

External carotid artery

Parotid gland: totally serous

Submandibular gland: mostly serous, partially mucous

Sublingual gland: almost completely mucous

Plate 61   Salivary Glands. (Netter: Atlas of Human Anatomy, 4 ed, 2006, Saunders.)

Coronary Arteries: Arteriographic Views

Right coronary artery: left anterior oblique view

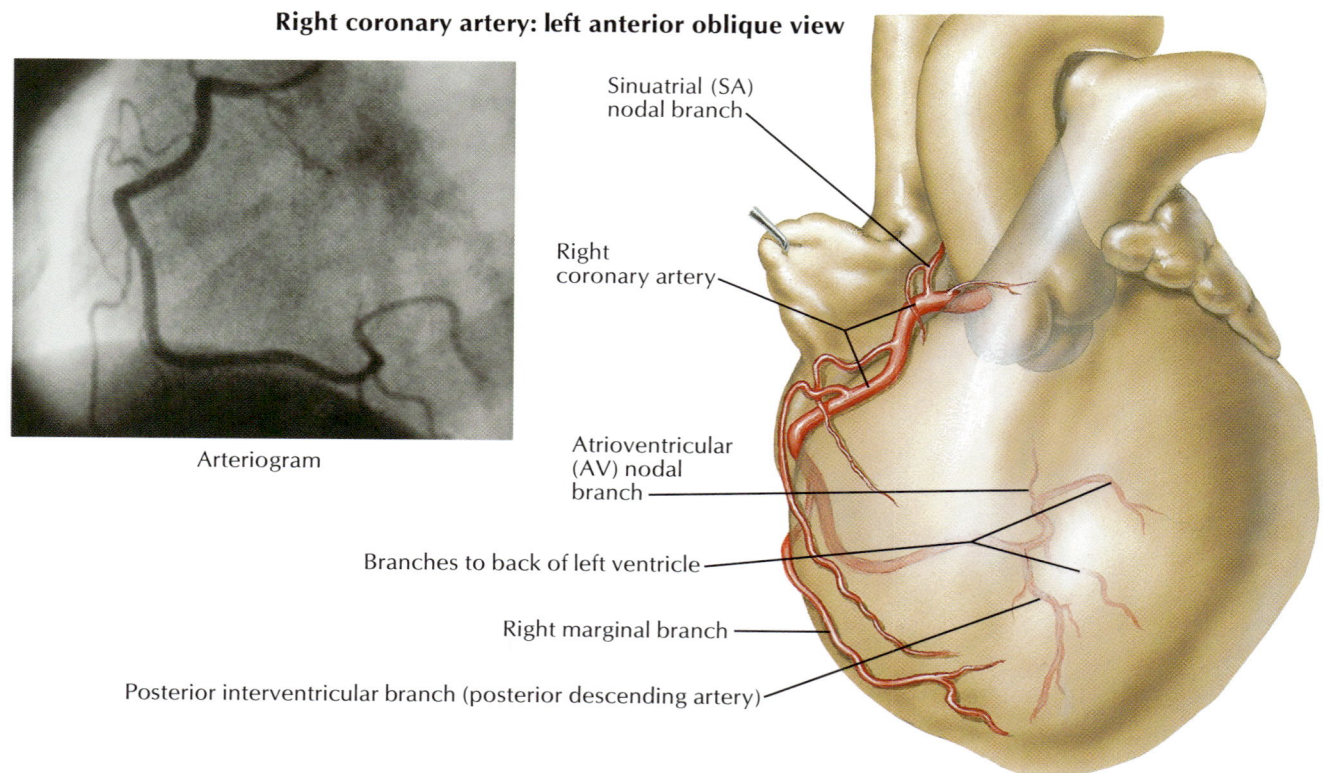

Arteriogram

Sinuatrial (SA) nodal branch

Right coronary artery

Atrioventricular (AV) nodal branch

Branches to back of left ventricle

Right marginal branch

Posterior interventricular branch (posterior descending artery)

Right coronary artery: right anterior oblique view

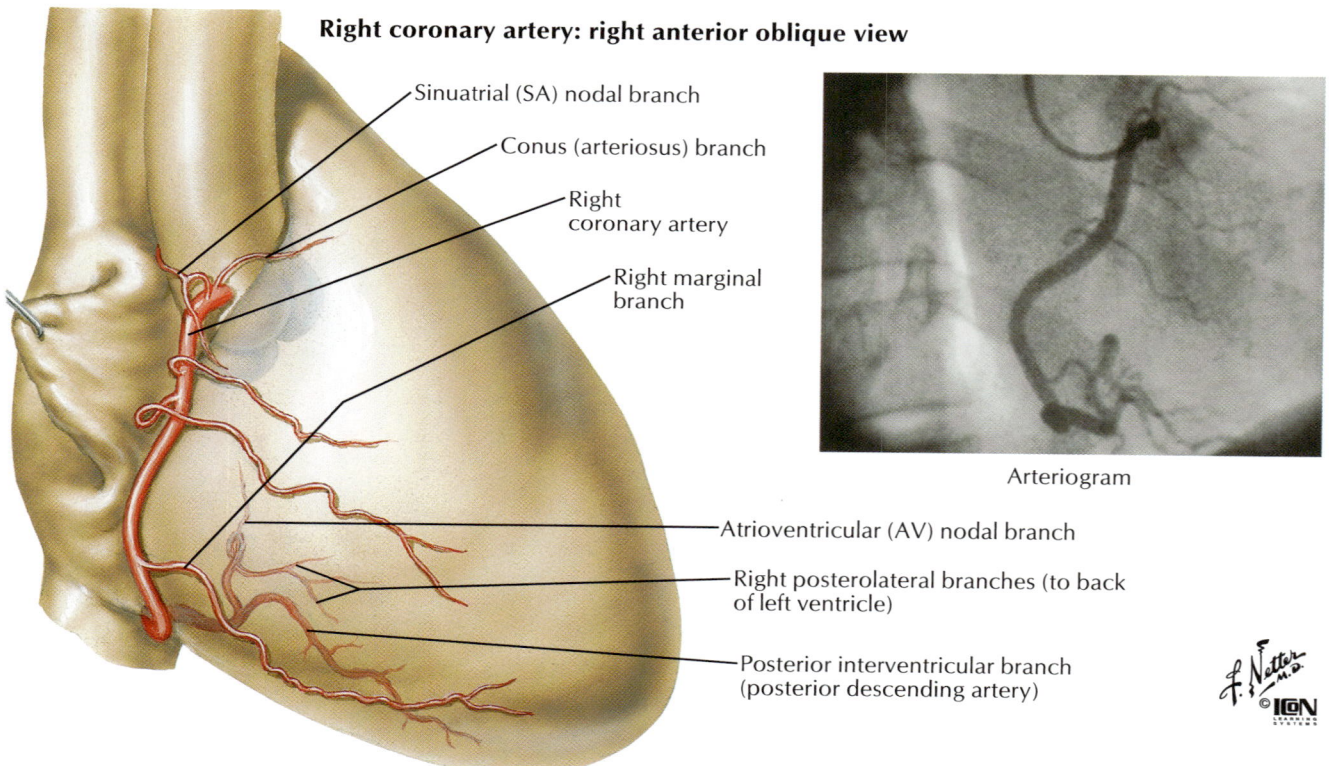

Sinuatrial (SA) nodal branch

Conus (arteriosus) branch

Right coronary artery

Right marginal branch

Arteriogram

Atrioventricular (AV) nodal branch

Right posterolateral branches (to back of left ventricle)

Posterior interventricular branch (posterior descending artery)

Plate 218 Coronary Arteries: Arteriographic Views. (Netter: Atlas of Human Anatomy, 4 ed, 2006, Saunders.)

Left coronary artery: left anterior oblique view

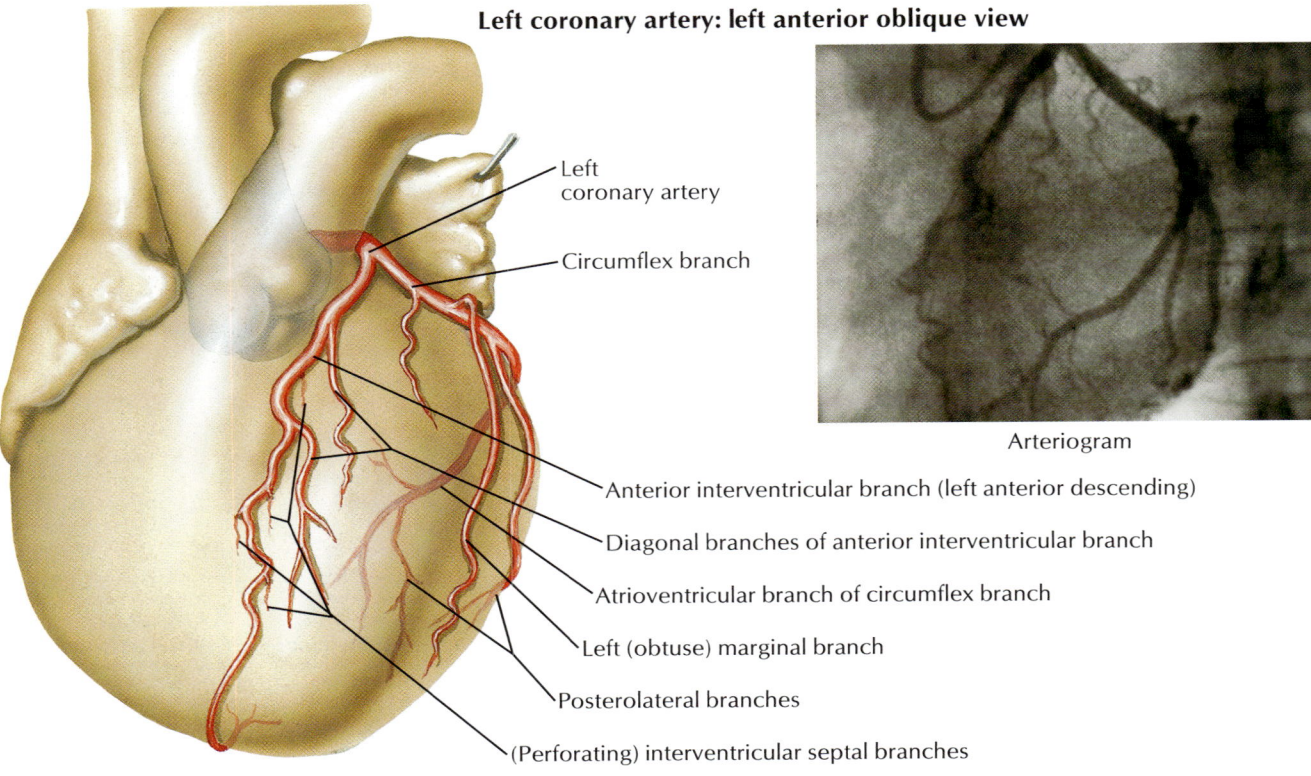

Left coronary artery

Circumflex branch

Arteriogram

Anterior interventricular branch (left anterior descending)

Diagonal branches of anterior interventricular branch

Atrioventricular branch of circumflex branch

Left (obtuse) marginal branch

Posterolateral branches

(Perforating) interventricular septal branches

Left coronary artery: right anterior oblique view

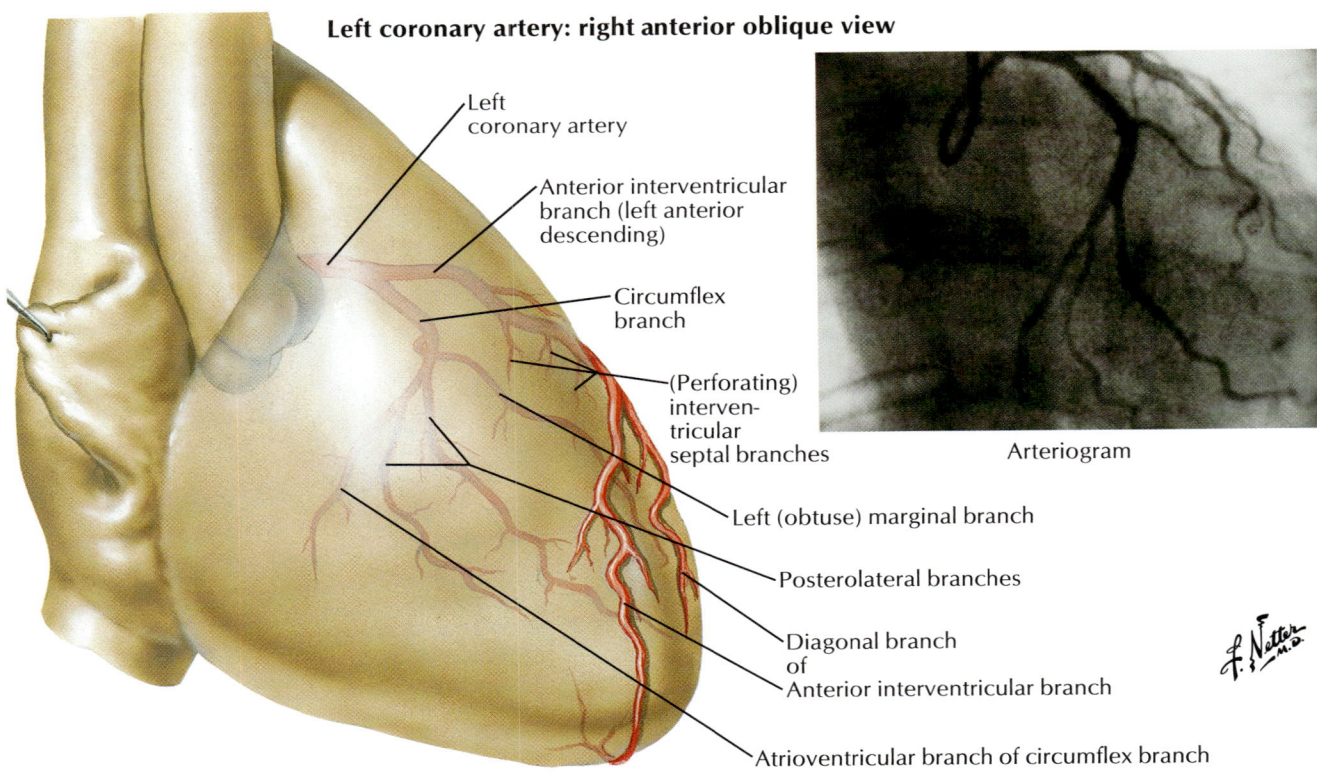

Left coronary artery

Anterior interventricular branch (left anterior descending)

Circumflex branch

(Perforating) interventricular septal branches

Arteriogram

Left (obtuse) marginal branch

Posterolateral branches

Diagonal branch of Anterior interventricular branch

Atrioventricular branch of circumflex branch

Plate 219 Coronary Arteries: Arteriographic Views. (Netter: Atlas of Human Anatomy, 4 ed, 2006, Saunders.)

NAP-27

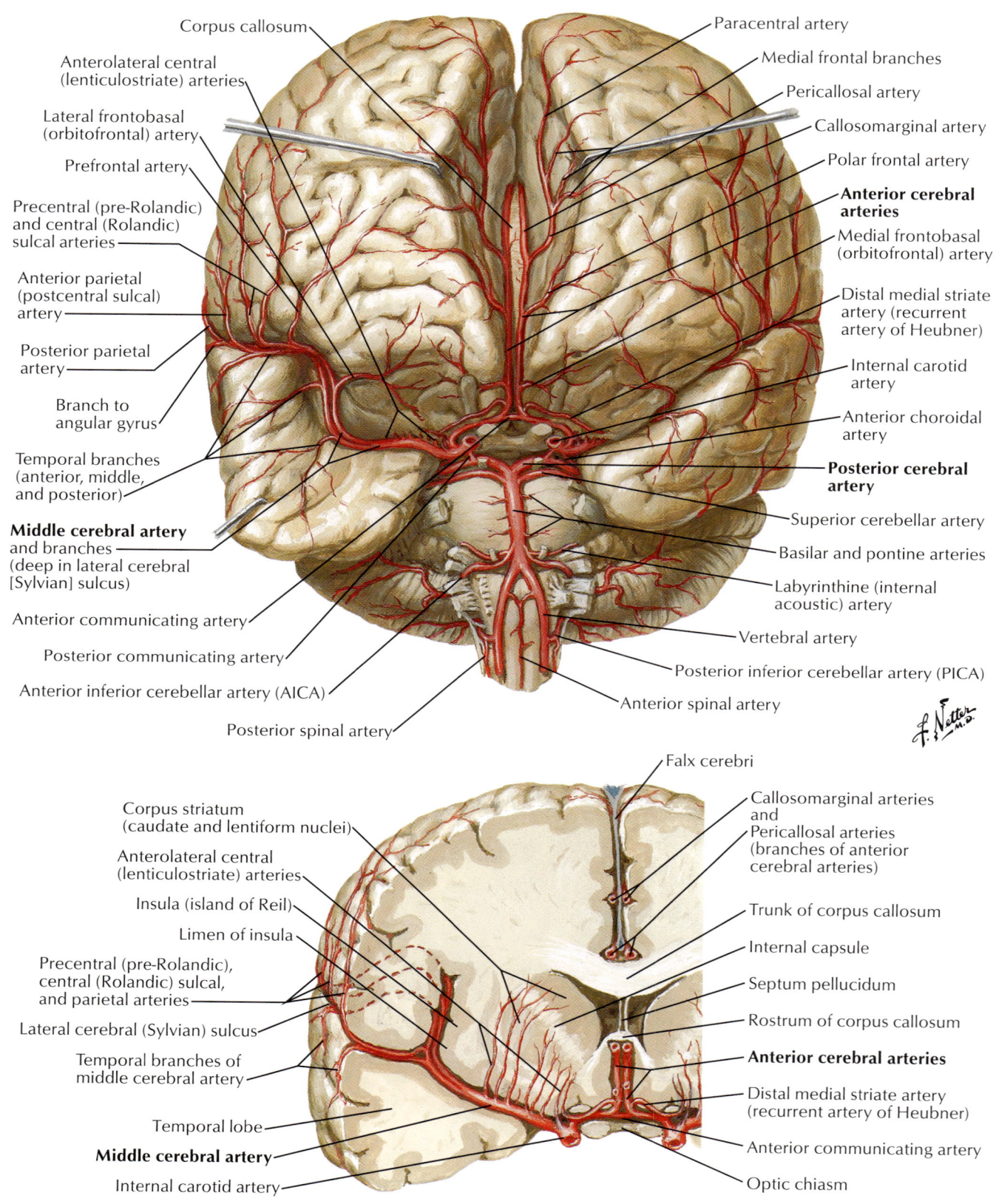

Corpus callosum

Anterolateral central (lenticulostriate) arteries

Lateral frontobasal (orbitofrontal) artery

Prefrontal artery

Precentral (pre-Rolandic) and central (Rolandic) sulcal arteries

Anterior parietal (postcentral sulcal) artery

Posterior parietal artery

Branch to angular gyrus

Temporal branches (anterior, middle, and posterior)

Middle cerebral artery and branches (deep in lateral cerebral [Sylvian] sulcus)

Anterior communicating artery

Posterior communicating artery

Anterior inferior cerebellar artery (AICA)

Posterior spinal artery

Paracentral artery

Medial frontal branches

Pericallosal artery

Callosomarginal artery

Polar frontal artery

Anterior cerebral arteries

Medial frontobasal (orbitofrontal) artery

Distal medial striate artery (recurrent artery of Heubner)

Internal carotid artery

Anterior choroidal artery

Posterior cerebral artery

Superior cerebellar artery

Basilar and pontine arteries

Labyrinthine (internal acoustic) artery

Vertebral artery

Posterior inferior cerebellar artery (PICA)

Anterior spinal artery

Corpus striatum (caudate and lentiform nuclei)

Anterolateral central (lenticulostriate) arteries

Insula (island of Reil)

Limen of insula

Precentral (pre-Rolandic), central (Rolandic) sulcal, and parietal arteries

Lateral cerebral (Sylvian) sulcus

Temporal branches of middle cerebral artery

Temporal lobe

Middle cerebral artery

Internal carotid artery

Falx cerebri

Callosomarginal arteries and Pericallosal arteries (branches of anterior cerebral arteries)

Trunk of corpus callosum

Internal capsule

Septum pellucidum

Rostrum of corpus callosum

Anterior cerebral arteries

Distal medial striate artery (recurrent artery of Heubner)

Anterior communicating artery

Optic chiasm

Plate 141 Arteries of Brain: Frontal View and Section. (Netter: Atlas of Human Anatomy, 4 ed, 2006, Saunders.)

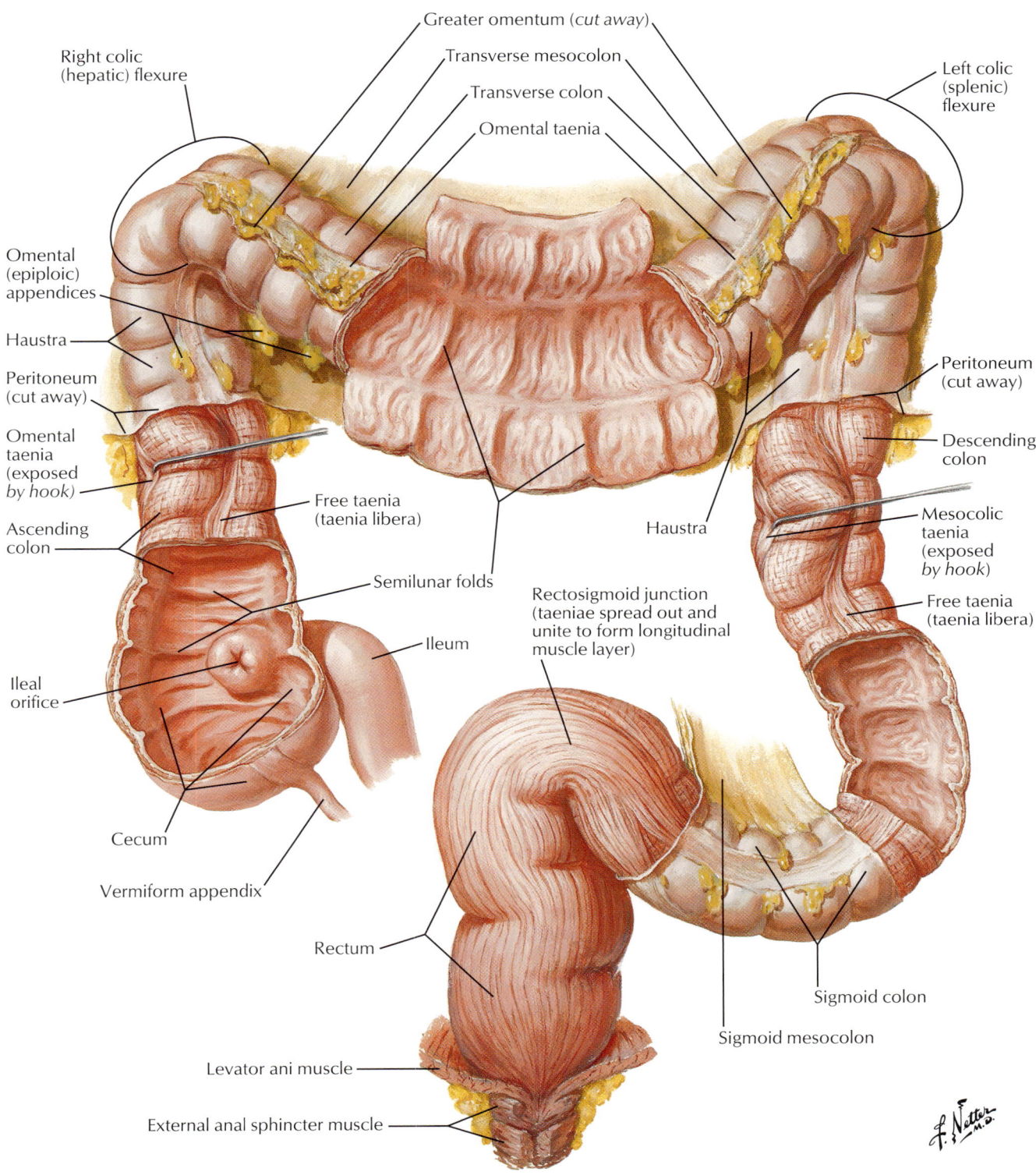

Right colic
(hepatic) flexure

Greater omentum (*cut away*)

Transverse mesocolon

Transverse colon

Omental taenia

Left colic
(splenic)
flexure

Omental
(epiploic)
appendices

Haustra

Peritoneum
(cut away)

Omental
taenia
(exposed
by hook)

Ascending
colon

Ileal
orifice

Cecum

Vermiform appendix

Rectum

Levator ani muscle

External anal sphincter muscle

Free taenia
(taenia libera)

Semilunar folds

Ileum

Haustra

Peritoneum
(cut away)

Descending
colon

Mesocolic
taenia
(exposed
by hook)

Free taenia
(taenia libera)

Rectosigmoid junction
(taeniae spread out and
unite to form longitudinal
muscle layer)

Sigmoid colon

Sigmoid mesocolon

Plate 284 Mucosa and Musculature of Large Intestine. (Netter: Atlas of Human Anatomy, 4 ed, 2006, Saunders.)

Transverse Section: T3–4 Intervertebral Disc, Manubrium

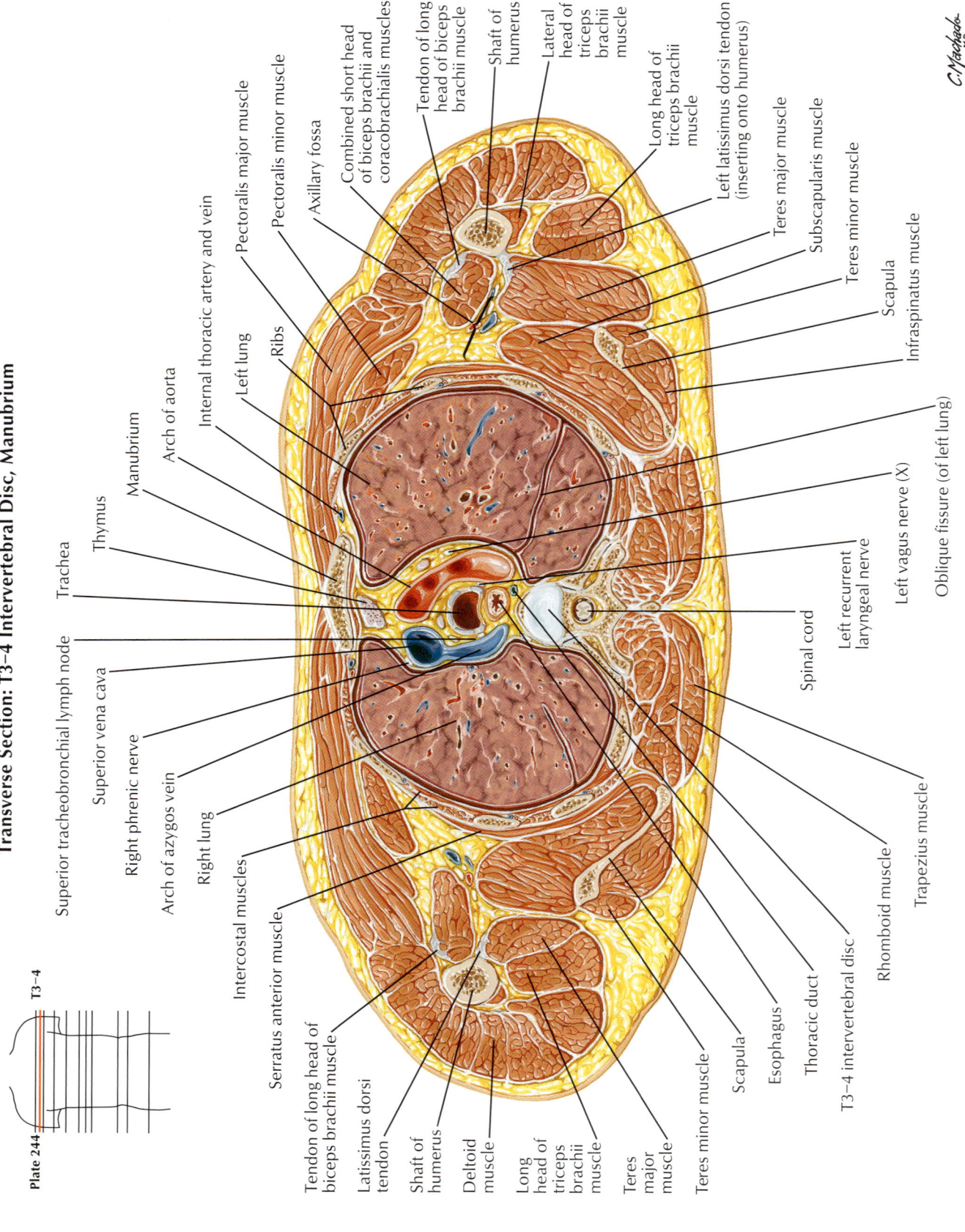

Superior tracheobronchial lymph node

Superior vena cava

Right phrenic nerve

Arch of azygos vein

Right lung

Intercostal muscles

Serratus anterior muscle

Tendon of long head of biceps brachii muscle

Latissimus dorsi tendon

Shaft of humerus

Deltoid muscle

Long head of triceps brachii muscle

Teres major muscle

Teres minor muscle

Trachea

Thymus

Manubrium

Arch of aorta

Internal thoracic artery and vein

Left lung

Ribs

Axillary fossa

Combined short head of biceps brachii and coracobrachialis muscles

Pectoralis minor muscle

Pectoralis major muscle

Tendon of long head of biceps brachii muscle

Shaft of humerus

Lateral head of triceps brachii muscle

Long head of triceps brachii muscle

Left latissimus dorsi tendon (inserting onto humerus)

Teres major muscle

Subscapularis muscle

Teres minor muscle

Scapula

Infraspinatus muscle

Spinal cord

Left recurrent laryngeal nerve

Left vagus nerve (X)

Oblique fissure (of left lung)

Scapula

Esophagus

Thoracic duct

T3–4 intervertebral disc

Rhomboid muscle

Trapezius muscle

Plate 244   Cross Section of Thorax at T3-4 Disc Level. (Netter: Atlas of Human Anatomy, 4 ed, 2006, Saunders.)

Plate 244

T3–4

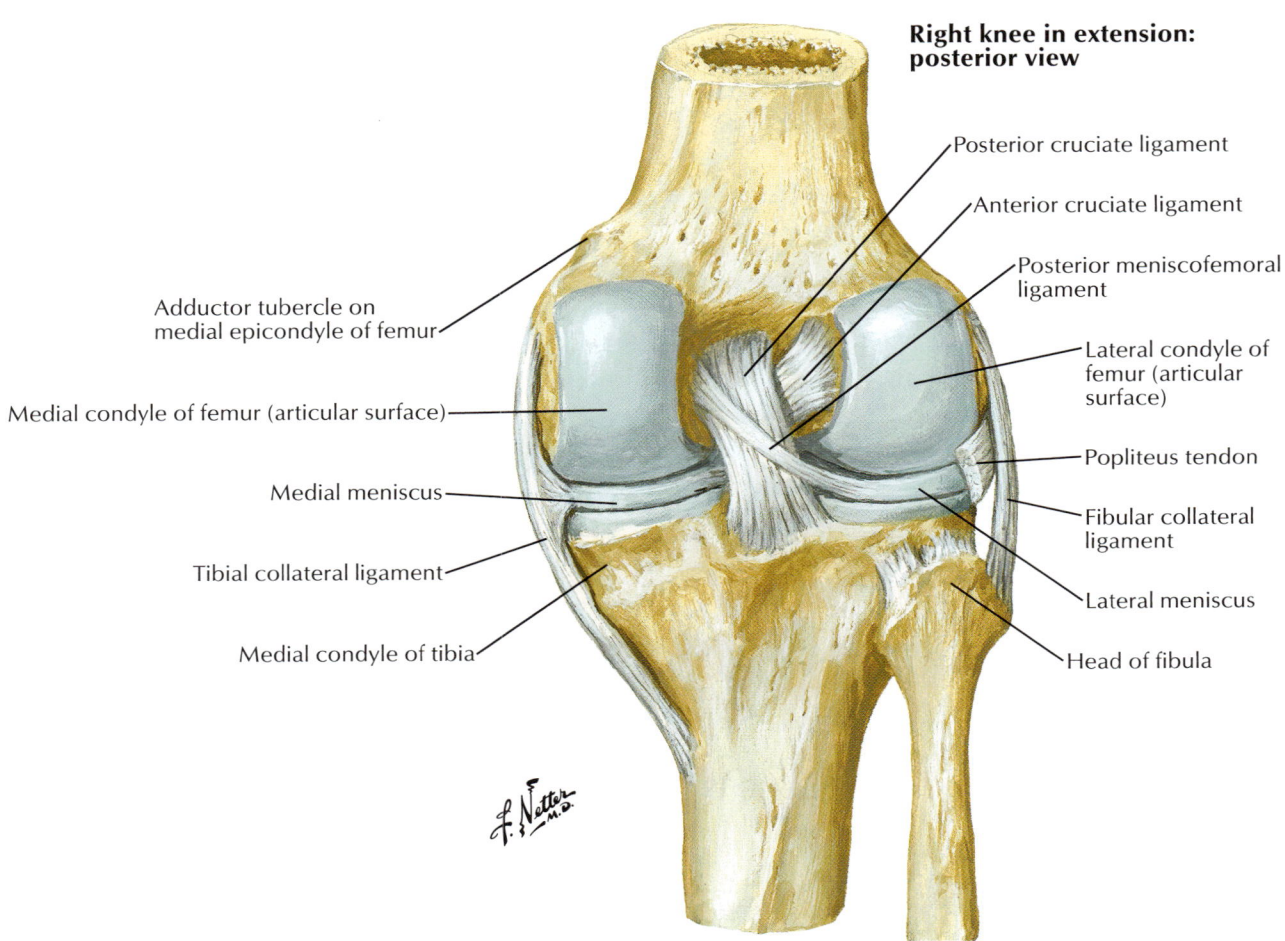

Right knee in extension: posterior view

Adductor tubercle on medial epicondyle of femur

Medial condyle of femur (articular surface)

Medial meniscus

Tibial collateral ligament

Medial condyle of tibia

Posterior cruciate ligament

Anterior cruciate ligament

Posterior meniscofemoral ligament

Lateral condyle of femur (articular surface)

Popliteus tendon

Fibular collateral ligament

Lateral meniscus

Head of fibula

Plate 509 Knee: Cruciate and Collateral Ligaments. (Netter: Atlas of Human Anatomy, 4 ed, 2006, Saunders.)

Paramedian (sagittal) dissection

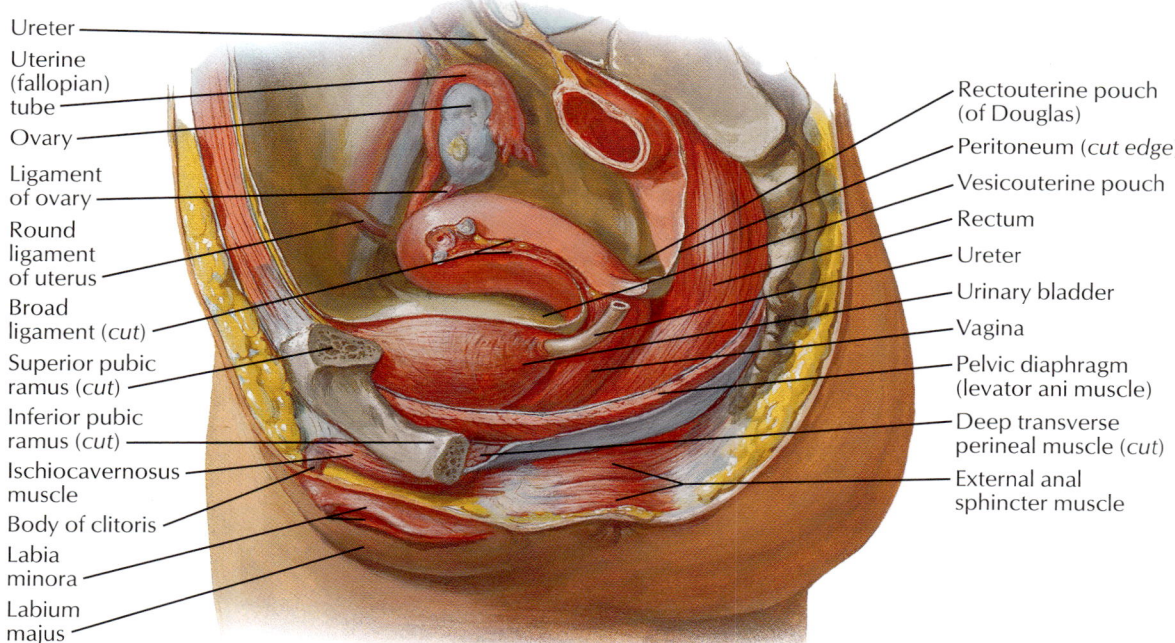

Ureter
Uterine (fallopian) tube
Ovary
Ligament of ovary
Round ligament of uterus
Broad ligament (*cut*)
Superior pubic ramus (*cut*)
Inferior pubic ramus (*cut*)
Ischiocavernosus muscle
Body of clitoris
Labia minora
Labium majus

Rectouterine pouch (of Douglas)
Peritoneum (*cut edge*)
Vesicouterine pouch
Rectum
Ureter
Urinary bladder
Vagina
Pelvic diaphragm (levator ani muscle)
Deep transverse perineal muscle (*cut*)
External anal sphincter muscle

Median (sagittal) section

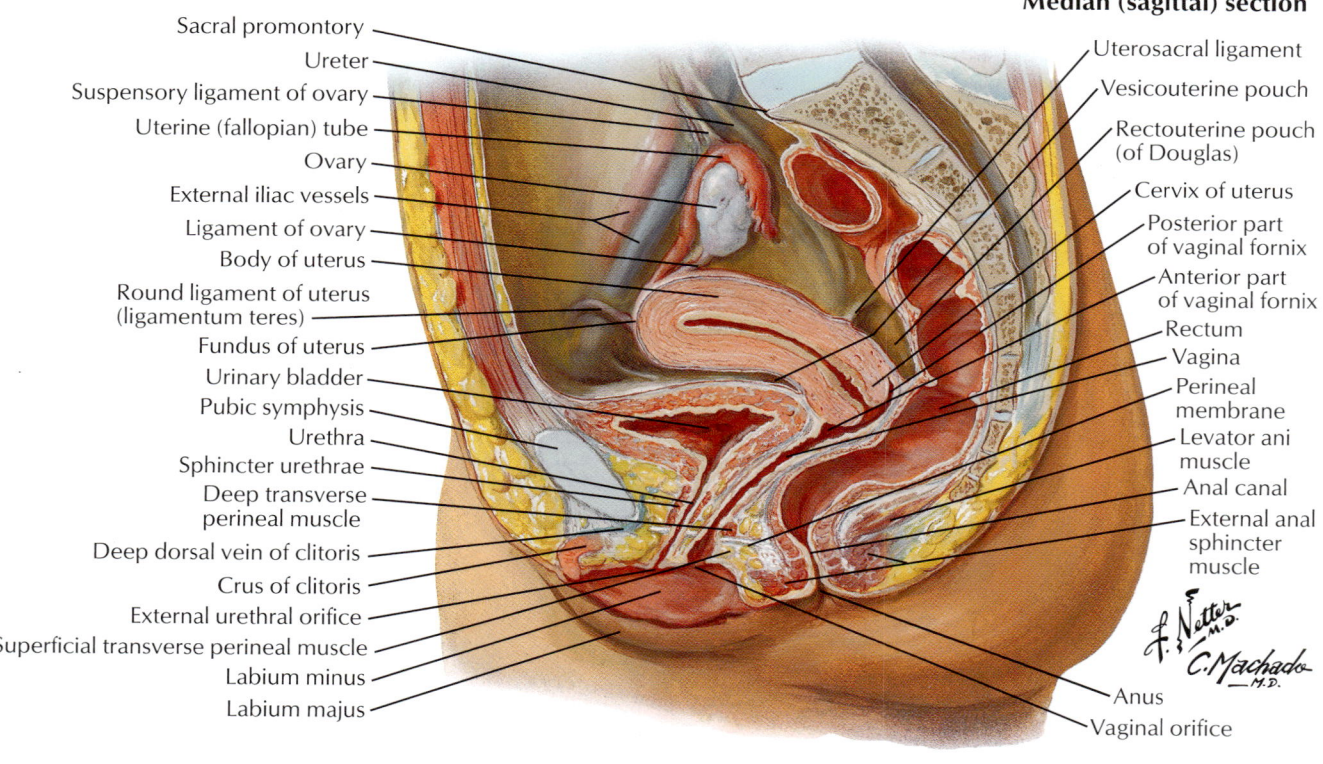

Sacral promontory
Ureter
Suspensory ligament of ovary
Uterine (fallopian) tube
Ovary
External iliac vessels
Ligament of ovary
Body of uterus
Round ligament of uterus (ligamentum teres)
Fundus of uterus
Urinary bladder
Pubic symphysis
Urethra
Sphincter urethrae
Deep transverse perineal muscle
Deep dorsal vein of clitoris
Crus of clitoris
External urethral orifice
Superficial transverse perineal muscle
Labium minus
Labium majus

Uterosacral ligament
Vesicouterine pouch
Rectouterine pouch (of Douglas)
Cervix of uterus
Posterior part of vaginal fornix
Anterior part of vaginal fornix
Rectum
Vagina
Perineal membrane
Levator ani muscle
Anal canal
External anal sphincter muscle
Anus
Vaginal orifice

Plate 360 Pelvic Viscera and Perineum: Female. (Netter: Atlas of Human Anatomy, 4 ed, 2006, Saunders.)

Introduction

ICD-10-PCS Official Guidelines for Coding and Reporting

2018

The Centers for Medicare and Medicaid Services (CMS) and the National Center for Health Statistics (NCHS), two departments within the U.S. Federal Government's Department of Health and Human Services (DHHS) provide the following guidelines for coding and reporting using the International Classification of Diseases, 10th Revision, Procedure Coding System (ICD-10-PCS). These guidelines should be used as a companion document to the official version of the ICD-10-PCS as published on the CMS website. The ICD-10-PCS is a procedure classification published by the United States for classifying procedures performed in hospital inpatient health care settings.

These guidelines have been approved by the four organizations that make up the Cooperating Parties for the ICD-10-PCS: the American Hospital Association (AHA), the American Health Information Management Association (AHIMA), CMS, and NCHS.

These guidelines are a set of rules that have been developed to accompany and complement the official conventions and instructions provided within the ICD-10-PCS itself. The instructions and conventions of the classification take precedence over guidelines. These guidelines are based on the coding and sequencing instructions in the Tables, Index and Definitions of ICD-10-PCS, but provide additional instruction. Adherence to these guidelines when assigning ICD-10-PCS procedure codes is required under the Health Insurance Portability and Accountability Act (HIPAA). The procedure codes have been adopted under HIPAA for hospital inpatient healthcare settings. A joint effort between the healthcare provider and the coder is essential to achieve complete and accurate documentation, code assignment, and reporting of diagnoses and procedures. These guidelines have been developed to assist both the healthcare provider and the coder in identifying those procedures that are to be reported. The importance of consistent, complete documentation in the medical record cannot be overemphasized. Without such documentation accurate coding cannot be achieved.

Table of Contents

A. Conventions
B. Medical and Surgical Section Guidelines
    2. Body System
    3. Root Operation
    4. Body Part
    5. Approach
    6. Device
C. Obstetrics Section Guidelines
D. Selection of Principal Procedure

Conventions

A1

ICD-10-PCS codes are composed of seven characters. Each character is an axis of classification that specifies information about the procedure performed. Within a defined code range, a character specifies the same type of information in that axis of classification.

Example: The fifth axis of classification specifies the approach in sections Ø through 4 and 7 through 9 of the system.

A2

One of 34 possible values can be assigned to each axis of classification in the seven-character code: they are the numbers Ø through 9 and the alphabet (except I and O because they are easily confused with the numbers 1 and Ø). The number of unique values used in an axis of classification differs as needed.

Example: Where the fifth axis of classification specifies the approach, seven different approach values are currently used to specify the approach.

A3

The valid values for an axis of classification can be added to as needed.

Example: If a significantly distinct type of device is used in a new procedure, a new device value can be added to the system.

A4

As with words in their context, the meaning of any single value is a combination of its axis of classification and any preceding values on which it may be dependent.

Example: The meaning of a body part value in the Medical and Surgical section is always dependent on the body system value. The body part value Ø in the Central Nervous body system specifies Brain and the body part value Ø in the Peripheral Nervous body system specifies Cervical Plexus.

A5

As the system is expanded to become increasingly detailed, over time more values will depend on preceding values for their meaning.

Example: In the Lower Joints body system, the device value 3 in the root operation Insertion specifies Infusion Device and the device value 3 in the root operation Replacement specifies Ceramic Synthetic Substitute.

A6

The purpose of the alphabetic index is to locate the appropriate table that contains all information necessary to construct a procedure code. The PCS Tables should always be consulted to find the most appropriate valid code.

A7

It is not required to consult the index first before proceeding to the tables to complete the code. A valid code may be chosen directly from the tables.

A8

All seven characters must be specified to be a valid code. If the documentation is incomplete for coding purposes, the physician should be queried for the necessary information.

A9

Within a PCS table, valid codes include all combinations of choices in characters 4 through 7 contained in the same row of the table. In the example below, ØJHT3VZ is a valid code, and ØJHW3VZ is *not* a valid code.

A1Ø

"And," when used in a code description, means "and/or."

Example: Lower Arm and Wrist Muscle means lower arm and/or wrist muscle.

A11

Many of the terms used to construct PCS codes are defined within the system. It is the coder's responsibility to determine what the documentation in the medical record equates to in the PCS definitions. The physician is not expected to use the terms used in PCS code descriptions, nor is the coder required to query the physician when the correlation between the documentation and the defined PCS terms is clear.

Example: When the physician documents "partial resection" the coder can independently correlate "partial resection" to

the root operation Excision without querying the physician for clarification.

Medical and Surgical Section Guidelines (section Ø)

B2. Body System

General guidelines

B2.1a

The procedure codes in the general anatomical regions body systems can be used when the procedure is performed on an anatomical region rather than a specific body part (e.g., root operations Control and Detachment, Drainage of a body cavity) or on the rare occasion when no information is available to support assignment of a code to a specific body part.

Examples: Control of postoperative hemorrhage is coded to the root operation Control found in the general anatomical regions body systems.

Chest tube drainage of the pleural cavity is coded to the root operation Drainage found in the general anatomical regions body systems. Suture repair of the abdominal wall is coded to the root operation Repair in the general anatomical regions body system.

B2.1b

Where the general body part values "upper" and "lower" are provided as an option in the Upper Arteries, Lower Arteries, Upper Veins, Lower Veins, Muscles and Tendons body systems, "upper" or "lower" specifies body parts located above or below the diaphragm respectively.

Example: Vein body parts above the diaphragm are found in the Upper Veins body system; vein body parts below the diaphragm are found in the Lower Veins body system.

B3. Root Operation

General guidelines

B3.1a

In order to determine the appropriate root operation, the full definition of the root operation as contained in the PCS Tables must be applied.

B3.1b

Components of a procedure specified in the root operation definition and explanation are not coded separately. Procedural steps necessary to reach the operative site and close the operative site, including anastomosis of a tubular body part, are also not coded separately.

Examples: Resection of a joint as part of a joint replacement procedure is included in the root operation definition of Replacement and is not coded separately. Laparotomy performed to reach the site of an open liver biopsy is not coded separately. In a resection of sigmoid colon with anastomosis of descending colon to rectum, the anastomosis is not coded separately.

SECTION: Ø MEDICAL AND SURGICAL

BODY SYSTEM: J SUBCUTANEOUS TISSUE AND FASCIA

OPERATION: H INSERTION: Putting in a nonbiological appliance that monitors, assists, performs, or prevents a physiological function but does not physically take the place of a body part

Body Part	Approach	Device	Qualifier
S Subcutaneous Tissue and Fascia, Head and Neck V Subcutaneous Tissue and Fascia, Upper Extremity W Subcutaneous Tissue and Fascia, Lower Extremity	Ø Open 3 Percutaneous	1 Radioactive Element 3 Infusion Device	Z No Qualifier
T Subcutaneous Tissue and Fascia, Trunk	Ø Open 3 Percutaneous	1 Radioactive Element 3 Infusion Device V Infusion Pump	Z No Qualifier

Multiple procedures
B3.2
During the same operative episode, multiple procedures are coded if:
   a. The same root operation is performed on different body parts as defined by distinct values of the body part character.
      Examples: Diagnostic excision of liver and pancreas are coded separately.
   b. The same root operation is repeated in multiple body parts, and those body parts are separate and distinct body parts classified to a single ICD-10-PCS body part value.
      Examples: Excision of the sartorius muscle and excision of the gracilis muscle are both included in the upper leg muscle body part value, and multiple procedures are coded.
      Extraction of multiple toenails are coded separately.
   c. Multiple root operations with distinct objectives are performed on the same body part.
      Example: Destruction of sigmoid lesion and bypass of sigmoid colon are coded separately.
   d. The intended root operation is attempted using one approach, but is converted to a different approach.
      Example: Laparoscopic cholecystectomy converted to an open cholecystectomy is coded as percutaneous endoscopic Inspection and open Resection.

Discontinued or incomplete procedures
B3.3
If the intended procedure is discontinued or otherwise not completed, code the procedure to the root operation performed. If a procedure is discontinued before any other root operation is performed, code the root operation Inspection of the body part or anatomical region inspected.
Example: A planned aortic valve replacement procedure is discontinued after the initial thoracotomy and before any incision is made in the heart muscle, when the patient becomes hemodynamically unstable. This procedure is coded as an open Inspection of the mediastinum.

Biopsy procedures
B3.4a
Biopsy procedures are coded using the root operations Excision, Extraction, or Drainage and the qualifier Diagnostic.
Examples: Fine needle aspiration biopsy of fluid in the lung is coded to the root operation Drainage with the qualifier Diagnostic. Biopsy of bone marrow is coded to the root operation Extraction with the qualifier Diagnostic. Lymph node sampling for biopsy is coded to the root operation Excision with the qualifier Diagnostic.

Biopsy followed by more definitive treatment
B3.4b
If a diagnostic Excision, Extraction, or Drainage procedure (biopsy) is followed by a more definitive procedure, such as Destruction, Excision or Resection at the same procedure site, both the biopsy and the more definitive treatment are coded.
Example: Biopsy of breast followed by partial mastectomy at the same procedure site, both the biopsy and the partial mastectomy procedure are coded.

Overlapping body layers
B3.5
If the root operations Excision, Repair or Inspection are performed on overlapping layers of the musculoskeletal system, the body part specifying the deepest layer is coded.
Example: Excisional debridement that includes skin and subcutaneous tissue and muscle is coded to the muscle body part.

Bypass procedures
B3.6a
Bypass procedures are coded by identifying the body part bypassed "from" and the body part bypassed "to." The fourth character body part specifies the body part bypassed from, and the qualifier specifies the body part bypassed to.
Example: Bypass from stomach to jejunum, stomach is the body part and jejunum is the qualifier.
B3.6b
Coronary artery bypass procedures are coded differently than other bypass procedures as described in the previous guideline. Rather than identifying the body part bypassed from, the body part identifies the number of coronary arteries bypassed to, and the qualifier specifies the vessel bypassed from.
Example: Aortocoronary artery bypass of the left anterior descending coronary artery and the obtuse marginal coronary artery is classified in the body part axis of classification as two coronary arteries, and the qualifier specifies the aorta as the body part bypassed from.
B3.6c
If multiple coronary arteries are bypassed, a separate procedure is coded for each coronary artery that uses a different device and/or qualifier.
Example: Aortocoronary artery bypass and internal mammary coronary artery bypass are coded separately.

Control vs. more definitive root operations
B3.7
The root operation Control is defined as, "Stopping, or attempting to stop, postprocedural or other acute bleeding." If an attempt to stop postprocedural or other acute bleeding is initially unsuccessful, and to stop the bleeding requires performing a more definitive root operation, such as Bypass, Detachment, Excision, Extraction, Reposition, Replacement, or Resection, then the more definitive root operation is coded instead of Control.
Example: Resection of spleen to stop bleeding is coded to Resection instead of Control.

Excision vs. Resection
B3.8
PCS contains specific body parts for anatomical subdivisions of a body part, such as lobes of the lungs or liver and regions of the intestine. Resection of the specific body part is coded whenever all of the body part is cut out or off, rather than coding Excision of a less specific body part.
Example: Left upper lung lobectomy is coded to Resection of Upper Lung Lobe, Left rather than Excision of Lung, Left.

Excision for graft
B3.9
If an autograft is obtained from a different procedure site in order to complete the objective of the procedure, a separate procedure is coded.
Example: Coronary bypass with excision of saphenous vein graft, excision of saphenous vein is coded separately.

Fusion procedures of the spine
B3.10a
The body part coded for a spinal vertebral joint(s) rendered immobile by a spinal fusion procedure is classified by the level of the spine (e.g. thoracic). There are distinct body part values for a single vertebral joint and for multiple vertebral joints at each spinal level.
Example: Body part values specify Lumbar Vertebral Joint, Lumbar Vertebral Joints, 2 or More and Lumbosacral Vertebral Joint.

B3.10b

If multiple vertebral joints are fused, a separate procedure is coded for each vertebral joint that uses a different device and/or qualifier.

Example: Fusion of lumbar vertebral joint, posterior approach, anterior column and fusion of lumbar vertebral joint, posterior approach, posterior column are coded separately.

B3.10c

Combinations of devices and materials are often used on a vertebral joint to render the joint immobile. When combinations of devices are used on the same vertebral joint, the device value coded for the procedure is as follows:

- If an interbody fusion device is used to render the joint immobile (alone or containing other material like bone graft), the procedure is coded with the device value Interbody Fusion Device
- If bone graft is the *only* device used to render the joint immobile, the procedure is coded with the device value Nonautologous Tissue Substitute or Autologous Tissue Substitute
- If a mixture of autologous and nonautologous bone graft (with or without biological or synthetic extenders or binders) is used to render the joint immobile, code the procedure with the device value Autologous Tissue Substitute

Examples: Fusion of a vertebral joint using a cage style interbody fusion device containing morsellized bone graft is coded to the device Interbody Fusion Device. Fusion of a vertebral joint using a bone dowel interbody fusion device made of cadaver bone and packed with a mixture of local morsellized bone and demineralized bone matrix is coded to the device Interbody Fusion Device.

Fusion of a vertebral joint using both autologous bone graft and bone bank bone graft is coded to the device Autologous Tissue Substitute.

Inspection procedures

B3.11a

Inspection of a body part(s) performed in order to achieve the objective of a procedure is not coded separately.

Example: Fiberoptic bronchoscopy performed for irrigation of bronchus, only the irrigation procedure is coded.

B3.11b

If multiple tubular body parts are inspected, the most distal body part (the body part furthest from the starting point of the inspection) is coded. If multiple non-tubular body parts in a region are inspected, the body part that specifies the entire area inspected is coded.

Examples: Cystoureteroscopy with inspection of bladder and ureters is coded to the ureter body part value. Exploratory laparotomy with general inspection of abdominal contents is coded to the peritoneal cavity body part value.

B3.11c

When both an Inspection procedure and another procedure are performed on the same body part during the same episode, if the Inspection procedure is performed using a different approach than the other procedure, the Inspection procedure is coded separately.

Example: Endoscopic Inspection of the duodenum is coded separately when open

Excision of the duodenum is performed during the same procedural episode.

Occlusion vs. Restriction for vessel embolization procedures

B3.12

If the objective of an embolization procedure is to completely close a vessel, the root operation Occlusion is coded. If the objective of an embolization procedure is to narrow the lumen of a vessel, the root operation Restriction is coded.

Examples: Tumor embolization is coded to the root operation Occlusion, because the objective of the procedure is to cut off the blood supply to the vessel.

Embolization of a cerebral aneurysm is coded to the root operation Restriction, because the objective of the procedure is not to close off the vessel entirely, but to narrow the lumen of the vessel at the site of the aneurysm where it is abnormally wide.

Release procedures

B3.13

In the root operation Release, the body part value coded is the body part being freed and not the tissue being manipulated or cut to free the body part.

Example: Lysis of intestinal adhesions is coded to the specific intestine body part value.

Release vs. Division

B3.14

If the sole objective of the procedure is freeing a body part without cutting the body part, the root operation is Release. If the sole objective of the procedure is separating or transecting a body part, the root operation is Division.

Examples: Freeing a nerve root from surrounding scar tissue to relieve pain is coded to the root operation Release. Severing a nerve root to relieve pain is coded to the root operation Division.

Reposition for fracture treatment

B3.15

Reduction of a displaced fracture is coded to the root operation Reposition and the application of a cast or splint in conjunction with the Reposition procedure is not coded separately. Treatment of a nondisplaced fracture is coded to the procedure performed.

Examples: Casting of a nondisplaced fracture is coded to the root operation Immobilization in the Placement section. Putting a pin in a nondisplaced fracture is coded to the root operation Insertion.

Transplantation vs. Administration

B3.16

Putting in a mature and functioning living body part taken from another individual or animal is coded to the root operation Transplantation. Putting in autologous or nonautologous cells is coded to the Administration section.

Example: Putting in autologous or nonautologous bone marrow, pancreatic islet cells or stem cells is coded to the Administration section.

B4. Body Part

General guidelines

B4.1a

If a procedure is performed on a portion of a body part that does not have a separate body part value, code the body part value corresponding to the whole body part.

Example: A procedure performed on the alveolar process of the mandible is coded to the mandible body part.

B4.1b

If the prefix "peri" is combined with a body part to identify the site of the procedure, and the site of the procedure is not further specified, then the procedure is coded to the body part named. This guideline applies only when a more specific body part value is not available.

Examples: A procedure site identified as perirenal is coded to the kidney body part when the site of the procedure is not further specified. A procedure site described in the documentation as peri-urethral, and the documentation also indicates that it is the vulvar tissue and not the urethral tissue that is the site of the procedure, then the procedure is coded to the vulva body part.

B4.1c
If a procedure is performed on a continuous section of a tubular body part, code the body part value corresponding to the furthest anatomical site from the point of entry.
Example: A procedure performed on a continuous section of artery from the femoral artery to the external iliac artery with the point of entry at the femoral artery is coded to the external iliac body part.

Branches of body parts
B4.2
Where a specific branch of a body part does not have its own body part value in PCS, the body part is typically coded to the closest proximal branch that has a specific body part value. In the cardiovascular body systems, if a general body part is available in the correct root operation table, and coding to a proximal branch would require assigning a code in a different body system, the procedure is coded using the general body part value.
Example: A procedure performed on the mandibular branch of the trigeminal nerve is coded to the trigeminal nerve body part value.

Bilateral body part values
B4.3
Bilateral body part values are available for a limited number of body parts. If the identical procedure is performed on contralateral body parts, and a bilateral body part value exists for that body part, a single procedure is coded using the bilateral body part value. If no bilateral body part value exists, each procedure is coded separately using the appropriate body part value.
Examples: The identical procedure performed on both fallopian tubes is coded once using the body part value Fallopian Tube, Bilateral. The identical procedure performed on both knee joints is coded twice using the body part values Knee Joint, Right and Knee Joint, Left.

Coronary arteries
B4.4
The coronary arteries are classified as a single body part that is further specified by number of arteries treated. One procedure code specifying multiple arteries is used when the same procedure is performed, including the same device and qualifier values.
Examples: Angioplasty of two distinct coronary arteries with placement of two stents is coded as Dilation of Coronary Artery, Two Arteries with Two Intraluminal Devices. Angioplasty of two distinct coronary arteries, one with stent placed and one without, is coded separately as Dilation of Coronary Artery, One Artery with Intraluminal Device, and Dilation of Coronary Artery, One Artery with no device.

Tendons, ligaments, bursae and fascia near a joint
B4.5
Procedures performed on tendons, ligaments, bursae and fascia supporting a joint are coded to the body part in the respective body system that is the focus of the procedure. Procedures performed on joint structures themselves are coded to the body part in the joint body systems.
Examples: Repair of the anterior cruciate ligament of the knee is coded to the knee bursae and ligament body part in the bursae and ligaments body system. Knee arthroscopy with shaving of articular cartilage is coded to the knee joint body part in the Lower Joints body system.

Skin, subcutaneous tissue and fascia overlying a joint
B4.6
If a procedure is performed on the skin, subcutaneous tissue or fascia overlying a joint, the procedure is coded to the following body part:
- Shoulder is coded to Upper Arm
- Elbow is coded to Lower Arm
- Wrist is coded to Lower Arm
- Hip is coded to Upper Leg
- Knee is coded to Lower Leg
- Ankle is coded to Foot

Fingers and toes
B4.7
If a body system does not contain a separate body part value for fingers, procedures performed on the fingers are coded to the body part value for the hand. If a body system does not contain a separate body part value for toes, procedures performed on the toes are coded to the body part value for the foot.
Example: Excision of finger muscle is coded to one of the hand muscle body part values in the Muscles body system.

Upper and lower intestinal tract
B4.8
In the Gastrointestinal body system, the general body part values Upper Intestinal Tract and Lower Intestinal Tract are provided as an option for the root operations Change, Inspection, Removal and Revision. Upper Intestinal Tract includes the portion of the gastrointestinal tract from the esophagus down to and including the duodenum, and Lower Intestinal Tract includes the portion of the gastrointestinal tract from the jejunum down to and including the rectum and anus.
Example: In the root operation Change table, change of a device in the jejunum is coded using the body part Lower Intestinal Tract.

B5. Approach
Open approach with percutaneous endoscopic assistance
B5.2
Procedures performed using the open approach with percutaneous endoscopic assistance are coded to the approach Open.
Example: Laparoscopic-assisted sigmoidectomy is coded to the approach Open.

External approach
B5.3a
Procedures performed within an orifice on structures that are visible without the aid of any instrumentation are coded to the approach External.
Example: Resection of tonsils is coded to the approach External.
B5.3b
Procedures performed indirectly by the application of external force through the intervening body layers are coded to the approach External.
Example: Closed reduction of fracture is coded to the approach External.

Percutaneous procedure via device
B5.4
Procedures performed percutaneously via a device placed for the procedure are coded to the approach Percutaneous.
Example: Fragmentation of kidney stone performed via percutaneous nephrostomy is coded to the approach Percutaneous.

B6. Device
General guidelines
B6.1a
A device is coded only if a device remains after the procedure is completed. If no device remains, the device value No Device is coded. In limited root operations, the classification provides the qualifier values Temporary and Intraoperative, for specific procedures involving clinically significant devices, where the purpose of the device is to be utilized for a brief duration during the procedure or current inpatient stay.
B6.1b
Materials such as sutures, ligatures, radiological markers and temporary post-operative wound drains are considered integral to the performance of a procedure and are not coded as devices.
B6.1c
Procedures performed on a device only and not on a body part are specified in the root operations Change, Irrigation, Removal and Revision, and are coded to the procedure performed.
Example: Irrigation of percutaneous nephrostomy tube is coded to the root operation Irrigation of indwelling device in the Administration section.

Drainage device
B6.2
A separate procedure to put in a drainage device is coded to the root operation Drainage with the device value Drainage Device.

Obstetric Section Guidelines (section 1)

C. Obstetrics Section
Products of conception
C1
Procedures performed on the products of conception are coded to the Obstetrics section. Procedures performed on the pregnant female other than the products of conception are coded to the appropriate root operation in the Medical and Surgical section.
Example: Amniocentesis is coded to the products of conception body part in the Obstetrics section. Repair of obstetric urethral laceration is coded to the urethra body part in the Medical and Surgical section.

Procedures following delivery or abortion
C2
Procedures performed following a delivery or abortion for curettage of the endometrium or evacuation of retained products of conception are all coded in the Obstetrics section, to the root operation Extraction and the body part Products of Conception, Retained. Diagnostic or therapeutic dilation and curettage performed during times other than the postpartum or post-abortion period are all coded in the Medical and Surgical section, to the root operation Extraction and the body part Endometrium.

New Technology Section Guidelines (section X)

D. New Technology Section
General guidelines
D1
Section X codes are standalone codes. They are not supplemental codes. Section X codes fully represent the specific procedure described in the code title, and do not require any additional codes from other sections of ICD-10-PCS. When section X contains a code title which describes a specific new technology procedure, only that X code is reported for the procedure. There is no need to report a broader, non-specific code in another section of ICD-10-PCS.
Example: XW04321 Introduction of Ceftazidime-Avibactam Anti-infective into Central Vein, Percutaneous Approach, New Technology Group 1, can be coded to indicate that Ceftazidime-Avibactam Anti-infective was administered via a central vein. A separate code from table 3E0 in the Administration section of ICD-10-PCS is not coded in addition to this code.

Selection of Principal Procedure
The following instructions should be applied in the selection of principal procedure and clarification on the importance of the relation to the principal diagnosis when more than one procedure is performed:
1. Procedure performed for definitive treatment of both principal diagnosis and secondary diagnosis
   a. Sequence procedure performed for definitive treatment most related to principal diagnosis as principal procedure.
2. Procedure performed for definitive treatment and diagnostic procedures performed for both principal diagnosis and secondary diagnosis
   a. Sequence procedure performed for definitive treatment most related to principal diagnosis as principal procedure
3. A diagnostic procedure was performed for the principal diagnosis and a procedure is performed for definitive treatment of a secondary diagnosis.
   a. Sequence diagnostic procedure as principal procedure, since the procedure most related to the principal diagnosis takes precedence.
4. No procedures performed that are related to principal diagnosis; procedures performed for definitive treatment and diagnostic procedures were performed for secondary diagnosis
   a. Sequence procedure performed for definitive treatment of secondary diagnosis as principal procedure, since there are no procedures (definitive or nondefinitive treatment) related to principal diagnosis.

Medical and Surgical

00. Central Nervous System and Cranial Nerves..8
    001. Bypass..9
    002. Change..9
    005. Destruction...10
    007. Dilation..10
    008. Division...11
    009. Drainage...12
    00B. Excision..14
    00C. Extirpation...15
    00D. Extraction..16
    00F. Fragmentation..16
    00H. Insertion..17
    00J. Inspection...17
    00K. Map..18
    00N. Release...18
    00P. Removal...19
    00Q. Repair..20
    00R. Replacement..21
    00S. Reposition..21
    00T. Resection..22
    00U. Supplement...22
    00W. Revision...23
    00X. Transfer...24

SECTION: Ø MEDICAL AND SURGICAL

BODY SYSTEM: Ø CENTRAL NERVOUS SYSTEM **AND CRANIAL NERVES**

OPERATION: 1 **BYPASS:** Altering the route of passage of the contents of a tubular body part

Body Part	Approach	Device	Qualifier
6 Cerebral Ventricle	Ø Open 3 Percutaneous 4 Percutaneous Endoscopic	7 Autologous Tissue Substitute J Synthetic Substitute K Nonautologous Tissue Substitute	Ø Nasopharynx 1 Mastoid Sinus 2 Atrium 3 Blood Vessel 4 Pleural Cavity 5 Intestine 6 Peritoneal Cavity 7 Urinary Tract 8 Bone Marrow B Cerebral Cisterns
6 Cerebral Ventricle	Ø Open 3 Percutaneous 4 Percutaneous Endoscopic	Z No Device	B Cerebral Cisterns
U Spinal Canal	Ø Open 3 Percutaneous	7 Autologous Tissue Substitute J Synthetic Substitute K Nonautologous Tissue Substitute	4 Pleural Cavity 6 Peritoneal Cavity 7 Urinary Tract 9 Fallopian Tube

SECTION: Ø MEDICAL AND SURGICAL

BODY SYSTEM: Ø CENTRAL NERVOUS SYSTEM **AND CRANIAL NERVES**

OPERATION: 2 **CHANGE:** Taking out or off a device from a body part and putting back an identical or similar device in or on the same body part without cutting or puncturing the skin or a mucous membrane

Body Part	Approach	Device	Qualifier
Ø Brain E Cranial Nerve U Spinal Canal	X External	Ø Drainage Device Y Other Device	Z No Qualifier

0: CENTRAL NERVOUS SYSTEM AND CRANIAL NERVES | **5: DESTRUCTION** | **7: DILATION** | **0: M/S**

SECTION: Ø MEDICAL AND SURGICAL
BODY SYSTEM: Ø CENTRAL NERVOUS SYSTEM **AND CRANIAL NERVES**
OPERATION: 5 DESTRUCTION: Physical eradication of all or a portion of a body part by the direct use of energy, force, or a destructive agent

Body Part	Approach	Device	Qualifier
Ø Brain 1 Cerebral Meninges 2 Dura Mater 6 Cerebral Ventricle 7 Cerebral Hemisphere 8 Basal Ganglia 9 Thalamus A Hypothalamus B Pons C Cerebellum D Medulla Oblongata F Olfactory Nerve G Optic Nerve H Oculomotor Nerve J Trochlear Nerve K Trigeminal Nerve L Abducens Nerve M Facial Nerve N Acoustic Nerve P Glossopharyngeal Nerve Q Vagus Nerve R Accessory Nerve S Hypoglossal Nerve T Spinal Meninges W Cervical Spinal Cord X Thoracic Spinal Cord Y Lumbar Spinal Cord	Ø Open 3 Percutaneous 4 Percutaneous Endoscopic	Z No Device	Z No Qualifier

SECTION: Ø MEDICAL AND SURGICAL
BODY SYSTEM: Ø CENTRAL NERVOUS SYSTEM **AND CRANIAL NERVES**
OPERATION: 7 **DILATION:** Expanding an orifice or the lumen of a tubular body part

Body Part	Approach	Device	Qualifier
6 Cerebral Ventricle	Ø Open 3 Percutaneous 4 Percutaneous Endoscopic	Z No Device	Z No Qualifier

New/Revised Text in Blue   ~~deleted~~ Deleted

SECTION: Ø MEDICAL AND SURGICAL
BODY SYSTEM: Ø CENTRAL NERVOUS SYSTEM AND CRANIAL NERVES
OPERATION: 8 DIVISION: Cutting into a body part, without draining fluids and/or gases from the body part, in order to separate or transect a body part

Body Part	Approach	Device	Qualifier
Ø Brain 7 Cerebral Hemisphere 8 Basal Ganglia F Olfactory Nerve G Optic Nerve H Oculomotor Nerve J Trochlear Nerve K Trigeminal Nerve L Abducens Nerve M Facial Nerve N Acoustic Nerve P Glossopharyngeal Nerve Q Vagus Nerve R Accessory Nerve S Hypoglossal Nerve W Cervical Spinal Cord X Thoracic Spinal Cord Y Lumbar Spinal Cord	Ø Open 3 Percutaneous 4 Percutaneous Endoscopic	Z No Device	Z No Qualifier

SECTION: Ø MEDICAL AND SURGICAL
BODY SYSTEM: Ø CENTRAL NERVOUS SYSTEM AND CRANIAL NERVES
OPERATION: 9 DRAINAGE: *(on multiple pages)*
Taking or letting out fluids and/or gases from a body part

9: DRAINAGE

Ø: CENTRAL NERVOUS SYSTEM AND CRANIAL NERVES

Ø: M/S

Body Part	Approach	Device	Qualifier
Ø Brain 1 Cerebral Meninges 2 Dura Mater 3 Epidural Space, Intracranial 4 Subdural Space, Intracranial 5 Subarachnoid Space, Intracranial 6 Cerebral Ventricle 7 Cerebral Hemisphere 8 Basal Ganglia 9 Thalamus A Hypothalamus B Pons C Cerebellum D Medulla Oblongata F Olfactory Nerve G Optic Nerve H Oculomotor Nerve J Trochlear Nerve K Trigeminal Nerve L Abducens Nerve M Facial Nerve N Acoustic Nerve P Glossopharyngeal Nerve Q Vagus Nerve R Accessory Nerve S Hypoglossal Nerve T Spinal Meninges U Spinal Canal W Cervical Spinal Cord X Thoracic Spinal Cord Y Lumbar Spinal Cord	Ø Open 3 Percutaneous 4 Percutaneous Endoscopic	Ø Drainage Device	Z No Qualifier

SECTION: Ø MEDICAL AND SURGICAL
BODY SYSTEM: Ø CENTRAL NERVOUS SYSTEM AND CRANIAL NERVES
OPERATION: 9 DRAINAGE: *(continued)*

Taking or letting out fluids and/or gases from a body part

Body Part	Approach	Device	Qualifier
Ø Brain 1 Cerebral Meninges 2 Dura Mater 3 Epidural Space, Intracranial 4 Subdural Space, Intracranial 5 Subarachnoid Space, Intracranial 6 Cerebral Ventricle 7 Cerebral Hemisphere 8 Basal Ganglia 9 Thalamus A Hypothalamus B Pons C Cerebellum D Medulla Oblongata F Olfactory Nerve G Optic Nerve H Oculomotor Nerve J Trochlear Nerve K Trigeminal Nerve L Abducens Nerve M Facial Nerve N Acoustic Nerve P Glossopharyngeal Nerve Q Vagus Nerve R Accessory Nerve S Hypoglossal Nerve T Spinal Meninges U Spinal Canal W Cervical Spinal Cord X Thoracic Spinal Cord Y Lumbar Spinal Cord	Ø Open 3 Percutaneous 4 Percutaneous Endoscopic	Z No Device	X Diagnostic Z No Qualifier

SECTION: Ø MEDICAL AND SURGICAL

BODY SYSTEM: Ø **CENTRAL NERVOUS SYSTEM AND CRANIAL NERVES**

OPERATION: B **EXCISION:** Cutting out or off, without replacement, a portion of a body part

Body Part	Approach	Device	Qualifier
Ø Brain 1 Cerebral Meninges 2 Dura Mater 6 Cerebral Ventricle 7 Cerebral Hemisphere 8 Basal Ganglia 9 Thalamus A Hypothalamus B Pons C Cerebellum D Medulla Oblongata F Olfactory Nerve G Optic Nerve H Oculomotor Nerve J Trochlear Nerve K Trigeminal Nerve L Abducens Nerve M Facial Nerve N Acoustic Nerve P Glossopharyngeal Nerve Q Vagus Nerve R Accessory Nerve S Hypoglossal Nerve T Spinal Meninges W Cervical Spinal Cord X Thoracic Spinal Cord Y Lumbar Spinal Cord	Ø Open 3 Percutaneous 4 Percutaneous Endoscopic	Z No Device	X Diagnostic Z No Qualifier

SECTION: Ø MEDICAL AND SURGICAL
BODY SYSTEM: Ø CENTRAL NERVOUS SYSTEM **AND CRANIAL NERVES**
OPERATION: C **EXTIRPATION:** Taking or cutting out solid matter from a body part

Body Part	Approach	Device	Qualifier
Ø Brain 1 Cerebral Meninges 2 Dura Mater 3 Epidural Space, Intracranial 4 Subdural Space, Intracranial 5 Subarachnoid Space, Intracranial 6 Cerebral Ventricle 7 Cerebral Hemisphere 8 Basal Ganglia 9 Thalamus A Hypothalamus B Pons C Cerebellum D Medulla Oblongata F Olfactory Nerve G Optic Nerve H Oculomotor Nerve J Trochlear Nerve K Trigeminal Nerve L Abducens Nerve M Facial Nerve N Acoustic Nerve P Glossopharyngeal Nerve Q Vagus Nerve R Accessory Nerve S Hypoglossal Nerve T Spinal Meninges U Spinal Canal W Cervical Spinal Cord X Thoracic Spinal Cord Y Lumbar Spinal Cord	Ø Open 3 Percutaneous 4 Percutaneous Endoscopic	Z No Device	Z No Qualifier

SECTION: Ø MEDICAL AND SURGICAL
BODY SYSTEM: Ø CENTRAL NERVOUS SYSTEM **AND CRANIAL NERVES**
OPERATION: D EXTRACTION: Pulling or stripping out or off all or a portion of a body part by the use of force

Body Part	Approach	Device	Qualifier
1 Cerebral Meninges 2 Dura Mater F Olfactory Nerve G Optic Nerve H Oculomotor Nerve J Trochlear Nerve K Trigeminal Nerve L Abducens Nerve M Facial Nerve N Acoustic Nerve P Glossopharyngeal Nerve Q Vagus Nerve R Accessory Nerve S Hypoglossal Nerve T Spinal Meninges	Ø Open 3 Percutaneous 4 Percutaneous Endoscopic	Z No Device	Z No Qualifier

SECTION: Ø MEDICAL AND SURGICAL
BODY SYSTEM: Ø CENTRAL NERVOUS SYSTEM **AND CRANIAL NERVES**
OPERATION: F FRAGMENTATION: Breaking solid matter in a body part into pieces

Body Part	Approach	Device	Qualifier
3 Epidural Space, Intracranial 4 Subdural Space, Intracranial 5 Subarachnoid Space, Intracranial 6 Cerebral Ventricle U Spinal Canal	Ø Open 3 Percutaneous 4 Percutaneous Endoscopic X External	Z No Device	Z No Qualifier

SECTION: Ø MEDICAL AND SURGICAL
BODY SYSTEM: Ø CENTRAL NERVOUS SYSTEM AND CRANIAL NERVES
OPERATION: H INSERTION: Putting in a nonbiological appliance that monitors, assists, performs, or prevents a physiological function but does not physically take the place of a body part

Body Part	Approach	Device	Qualifier
Ø Brain	Ø Open	2 Monitoring Device 3 Infusion Device 4 Radioactive Element, Cesium-131 Collagen Implant M Neurostimulator Lead Y Other Device	Z No Qualifier
Ø Brain	3 Percutaneous 4 Percutaneous Endoscopic	2 Monitoring Device 3 Infusion Device M Neurostimulator Lead Y Other Device	Z No Qualifier
~~Ø Brain~~ 6 Cerebral Ventricle E Cranial Nerve U Spinal Canal V Spinal Cord	Ø Open 3 Percutaneous 4 Percutaneous Endoscopic	2 Monitoring Device 3 Infusion Device M Neurostimulator Lead Y Other Device	Z No Qualifier

SECTION: Ø MEDICAL AND SURGICAL
BODY SYSTEM: Ø CENTRAL NERVOUS SYSTEM AND CRANIAL NERVES
OPERATION: J INSPECTION: Visually and/or manually exploring a body part

Body Part	Approach	Device	Qualifier
Ø Brain E Cranial Nerve U Spinal Canal V Spinal Cord	Ø Open 3 Percutaneous 4 Percutaneous Endoscopic	Z No Device	Z No Qualifier

Ø: M/S

Ø: CENTRAL NERVOUS SYSTEM AND CRANIAL NERVES

H: INSERTION   J: INSPECTION

SECTION: Ø MEDICAL AND SURGICAL

BODY SYSTEM: Ø CENTRAL NERVOUS SYSTEM AND CRANIAL NERVES
OPERATION: K MAP: Locating the route of passage of electrical impulses and/or locating functional areas in a body part

Body Part	Approach	Device	Qualifier
Ø Brain 7 Cerebral Hemisphere 8 Basal Ganglia 9 Thalamus A Hypothalamus B Pons C Cerebellum D Medulla Oblongata	Ø Open 3 Percutaneous 4 Percutaneous Endoscopic	Z No Device	Z No Qualifier

SECTION: Ø MEDICAL AND SURGICAL

BODY SYSTEM: Ø CENTRAL NERVOUS SYSTEM AND CRANIAL NERVES
OPERATION: N RELEASE: Freeing a body part from an abnormal physical constraint by cutting or by the use of force

Body Part	Approach	Device	Qualifier
Ø Brain 1 Cerebral Meninges 2 Dura Mater 6 Cerebral Ventricle 7 Cerebral Hemisphere 8 Basal Ganglia 9 Thalamus A Hypothalamus B Pons C Cerebellum D Medulla Oblongata F Olfactory Nerve G Optic Nerve H Oculomotor Nerve J Trochlear Nerve K Trigeminal Nerve L Abducens Nerve M Facial Nerve N Acoustic Nerve P Glossopharyngeal Nerve Q Vagus Nerve R Accessory Nerve S Hypoglossal Nerve T Spinal Meninges W Cervical Spinal Cord X Thoracic Spinal Cord Y Lumbar Spinal Cord	Ø Open 3 Percutaneous 4 Percutaneous Endoscopic	Z No Device	Z No Qualifier

K: MAP   N: RELEASE

Ø: CENTRAL NERVOUS SYSTEM AND CRANIAL NERVES

Ø: M/S

SECTION: Ø MEDICAL AND SURGICAL
BODY SYSTEM: Ø CENTRAL NERVOUS SYSTEM AND CRANIAL NERVES
OPERATION: P REMOVAL: Taking out or off a device from a body part

Body Part	Approach	Device	Qualifier
Ø Brain V Spinal Cord	Ø Open 3 Percutaneous 4 Percutaneous Endoscopic	Ø Drainage Device 2 Monitoring Device 3 Infusion Device 7 Autologous Tissue Substitute J Synthetic Substitute K Nonautologous Tissue Substitute M Neurostimulator Lead Y Other Device	Z No Qualifier
Ø Brain V Spinal Cord	X External	Ø Drainage Device 2 Monitoring Device 3 Infusion Device M Neurostimulator Lead	Z No Qualifier
6 Cerebral Ventricle U Spinal Canal	Ø Open 3 Percutaneous 4 Percutaneous Endoscopic	Ø Drainage Device 2 Monitoring Device 3 Infusion Device J Synthetic Substitute M Neurostimulator Lead Y Other Device	Z No Qualifier
6 Cerebral Ventricle U Spinal Canal	X External	Ø Drainage Device 2 Monitoring Device 3 Infusion Device M Neurostimulator Lead	Z No Qualifier
E Cranial Nerve	Ø Open 3 Percutaneous 4 Percutaneous Endoscopic	Ø Drainage Device 2 Monitoring Device 3 Infusion Device 7 Autologous Tissue Substitute M Neurostimulator Lead Y Other Device	Z No Qualifier
E Cranial Nerve	X External	Ø Drainage Device 2 Monitoring Device 3 Infusion Device M Neurostimulator Lead	Z No Qualifier

Ø: M/S

Ø: CENTRAL NERVOUS SYSTEM AND CRANIAL NERVES

P: REMOVAL

SECTION: Ø MEDICAL AND SURGICAL
BODY SYSTEM: Ø CENTRAL NERVOUS SYSTEM AND CRANIAL NERVES
OPERATION: Q REPAIR: Restoring, to the extent possible, a body part to its normal
anatomic structure and function

Body Part	Approach	Device	Qualifier
Ø Brain	Ø Open	Z No Device	Z No Qualifier
1 Cerebral Meninges	3 Percutaneous		
2 Dura Mater	4 Percutaneous Endoscopic		
6 Cerebral Ventricle			
7 Cerebral Hemisphere			
8 Basal Ganglia			
9 Thalamus			
A Hypothalamus			
B Pons			
C Cerebellum			
D Medulla Oblongata			
F Olfactory Nerve			
G Optic Nerve			
H Oculomotor Nerve			
J Trochlear Nerve			
K Trigeminal Nerve			
L Abducens Nerve			
M Facial Nerve			
N Acoustic Nerve			
P Glossopharyngeal Nerve			
Q Vagus Nerve			
R Accessory Nerve			
S Hypoglossal Nerve			
T Spinal Meninges			
W Cervical Spinal Cord			
X Thoracic Spinal Cord			
Y Lumbar Spinal Cord			

New/Revised Text in Blue   ~~deleted~~ Deleted

SECTION: Ø MEDICAL AND SURGICAL
BODY SYSTEM: Ø CENTRAL NERVOUS SYSTEM AND CRANIAL NERVES
OPERATION: R REPLACEMENT: Putting in or on biological or synthetic material that physically takes the place and/or function of all or a portion of a body part

Body Part	Approach	Device	Qualifier
1 Cerebral Meninges 2 Dura Mater 6 Cerebral Ventricle F Olfactory Nerve G Optic Nerve H Oculomotor Nerve J Trochlear Nerve K Trigeminal Nerve L Abducens Nerve M Facial Nerve N Acoustic Nerve P Glossopharyngeal Nerve Q Vagus Nerve R Accessory Nerve S Hypoglossal Nerve T Spinal Meninges	Ø Open 4 Percutaneous Endoscopic	7 Autologous Tissue Substitute J Synthetic Substitute K Nonautologous Tissue Substitute	Z No Qualifier

SECTION: Ø MEDICAL AND SURGICAL
BODY SYSTEM: Ø CENTRAL NERVOUS SYSTEM AND CRANIAL NERVES
OPERATION: S REPOSITION: Moving to its normal location, or other suitable location, all or a portion of a body part

Body Part	Approach	Device	Qualifier
F Olfactory Nerve G Optic Nerve H Oculomotor Nerve J Trochlear Nerve K Trigeminal Nerve L Abducens Nerve M Facial Nerve N Acoustic Nerve P Glossopharyngeal Nerve Q Vagus Nerve R Accessory Nerve S Hypoglossal Nerve W Cervical Spinal Cord X Thoracic Spinal Cord Y Lumbar Spinal Cord	Ø Open 3 Percutaneous 4 Percutaneous Endoscopic	Z No Device	Z No Qualifier

SECTION: Ø MEDICAL AND SURGICAL
BODY SYSTEM: Ø CENTRAL NERVOUS SYSTEM **AND CRANIAL NERVES**
OPERATION: T RESECTION: Cutting out or off, without replacement, all of a body part

Body Part	Approach	Device	Qualifier
7 Cerebral Hemisphere	Ø Open 3 Percutaneous 4 Percutaneous Endoscopic	Z No Device	Z No Qualifier

SECTION: Ø MEDICAL AND SURGICAL
BODY SYSTEM: Ø CENTRAL NERVOUS SYSTEM **AND CRANIAL NERVES**
OPERATION: U SUPPLEMENT: Putting in or on biological or synthetic material that physically reinforces and/or augments the function of a portion of a body part

Body Part	Approach	Device	Qualifier
1 Cerebral Meninges 2 Dura Mater T Spinal Meninges	Ø Open 3 Percutaneous 4 Percutaneous Endoscopic	7 Autologous Tissue Substitute J Synthetic Substitute K Nonautologous Tissue Substitute	Z No Qualifier
1 Cerebral Meninges 2 Dura Mater 6 Cerebral Ventricle F Olfactory Nerve G Optic Nerve H Oculomotor Nerve J Trochlear Nerve K Trigeminal Nerve L Abducens Nerve M Facial Nerve N Acoustic Nerve P Glossopharyngeal Nerve Q Vagus Nerve R Accessory Nerve S Hypoglossal Nerve T Spinal Meninges	Ø Open 3 Percutaneous 4 Percutaneous Endoscopic	7 Autologous Tissue Substitute J Synthetic Substitute K Nonautologous Tissue Substitute	Z No Qualifier

New/Revised Text in Blue   ~~deleted~~ Deleted

SECTION: Ø MEDICAL AND SURGICAL
BODY SYSTEM: Ø CENTRAL NERVOUS SYSTEM **AND CRANIAL NERVES**
OPERATION: W REVISION: Correcting, to the extent possible, a portion of a malfunctioning device or the position of a displaced device

Body Part	Approach	Device	Qualifier
Ø Brain V Spinal Cord	Ø Open 3 Percutaneous 4 Percutaneous Endoscopic ~~X External~~	Ø Drainage Device 2 Monitoring Device 3 Infusion Device 7 Autologous Tissue Substitute J Synthetic Substitute K Nonautologous Tissue Substitute M Neurostimulator Lead Y Other Device	Z No Qualifier
Ø Brain V Spinal Cord	X External	Ø Drainage Device 2 Monitoring Device 3 Infusion Device 7 Autologous Tissue Substitute J Synthetic Substitute K Nonautologous Tissue Substitute M Neurostimulator Lead	Z No Qualifier
6 Cerebral Ventricle U Spinal Canal	Ø Open 3 Percutaneous 4 Percutaneous Endoscopic ~~X External~~	Ø Drainage Device 2 Monitoring Device 3 Infusion Device J Synthetic Substitute M Neurostimulator Lead Y Other Device	Z No Qualifier
6 Cerebral Ventricle U Spinal Canal	X External	Ø Drainage Device 2 Monitoring Device 3 Infusion Device J Synthetic Substitute M Neurostimulator Lead	Z No Qualifier
E Cranial Nerve	Ø Open 3 Percutaneous 4 Percutaneous Endoscopic ~~X External~~	Ø Drainage Device 2 Monitoring Device 3 Infusion Device 7 Autologous Tissue Substitute M Neurostimulator Lead Y Other Device	Z No Qualifier
E Cranial Nerve	X External	Ø Drainage Device 2 Monitoring Device 3 Infusion Device 7 Autologous Tissue Substitute M Neurostimulator Lead	Z No Qualifier

SECTION: 0 MEDICAL AND SURGICAL
BODY SYSTEM: 0 CENTRAL NERVOUS SYSTEM AND CRANIAL NERVES
OPERATION: X TRANSFER: Moving, without taking out, all or a portion of a body part to another location to take over the function of all or a portion of a body part

Body Part	Approach	Device	Qualifier
F Olfactory Nerve G Optic Nerve H Oculomotor Nerve J Trochlear Nerve K Trigeminal Nerve L Abducens Nerve M Facial Nerve N Acoustic Nerve P Glossopharyngeal Nerve Q Vagus Nerve R Accessory Nerve S Hypoglossal Nerve	0 Open 4 Percutaneous Endoscopic	Z No Device	F Olfactory Nerve G Optic Nerve H Oculomotor Nerve J Trochlear Nerve K Trigeminal Nerve L Abducens Nerve M Facial Nerve N Acoustic Nerve P Glossopharyngeal Nerve Q Vagus Nerve R Accessory Nerve S Hypoglossal Nerve

New/Revised Text in Blue   ~~deleted~~ Deleted

Ø1. Peripheral Nervous System 25
    Ø12. Change 26
    Ø15. Destruction 26
    Ø18. Division 27
    Ø19. Drainage 28
    Ø1B. Excision 29
    Ø1C. Extirpation 3Ø
    Ø1D. Extraction 31
    Ø1H. Insertion 31
    Ø1J. Inspection 31
    Ø1N. Release 32
    Ø1P. Removal 32
    Ø1Q. Repair 33
    Ø1R. Replacement 33
    Ø1S. Reposition 34
    Ø1U. Supplement 34
    Ø1W. Revision 35
    Ø1X. Transfer 35

2: CHANGE   5: DESTRUCTION

1: PERIPHERAL NERVOUS SYSTEM

0: M/S

SECTION: 0   MEDICAL AND SURGICAL
BODY SYSTEM: 1   PERIPHERAL NERVOUS SYSTEM
OPERATION: 2   **CHANGE:** Taking out or off a device from a body part and putting back an identical or similar device in or on the same body part without cutting or puncturing the skin or a mucous membrane

Body Part	Approach	Device	Qualifier
Y Peripheral Nerve	X External	0 Drainage Device Y Other Device	Z No Qualifier

SECTION: 0   MEDICAL AND SURGICAL
BODY SYSTEM: 1   PERIPHERAL NERVOUS SYSTEM
OPERATION: 5   **DESTRUCTION:** Physical eradication of all or a portion of a body part by the direct use of energy, force, or a destructive agent

Body Part	Approach	Device	Qualifier
0 Cervical Plexus 1 Cervical Nerve 2 Phrenic Nerve 3 Brachial Plexus 4 Ulnar Nerve 5 Median Nerve 6 Radial Nerve 8 Thoracic Nerve 9 Lumbar Plexus A Lumbosacral Plexus B Lumbar Nerve C Pudendal Nerve D Femoral Nerve F Sciatic Nerve G Tibial Nerve H Peroneal Nerve K Head and Neck Sympathetic Nerve L Thoracic Sympathetic Nerve M Abdominal Sympathetic Nerve N Lumbar Sympathetic Nerve P Sacral Sympathetic Nerve Q Sacral Plexus R Sacral Nerve	0 Open 3 Percutaneous 4 Percutaneous Endoscopic	Z No Device	Z No Qualifier

New/Revised Text in Blue   ~~deleted~~ Deleted

SECTION: Ø MEDICAL AND SURGICAL
BODY SYSTEM: 1 **PERIPHERAL NERVOUS SYSTEM**
OPERATION: 8 **DIVISION:** Cutting into a body part, without draining fluids and/or gases from the body part, in order to separate or transect a body part

Body Part	Approach	Device	Qualifier
Ø Cervical Plexus 1 Cervical Nerve 2 Phrenic Nerve 3 Brachial Plexus 4 Ulnar Nerve 5 Median Nerve 6 Radial Nerve 8 Thoracic Nerve 9 Lumbar Plexus A Lumbosacral Plexus B Lumbar Nerve C Pudendal Nerve D Femoral Nerve F Sciatic Nerve G Tibial Nerve H Peroneal Nerve K Head and Neck Sympathetic Nerve L Thoracic Sympathetic Nerve M Abdominal Sympathetic Nerve N Lumbar Sympathetic Nerve P Sacral Sympathetic Nerve Q Sacral Plexus R Sacral Nerve	Ø Open 3 Percutaneous 4 Percutaneous Endoscopic	Z No Device	Z No Qualifier

SECTION: Ø MEDICAL AND SURGICAL
BODY SYSTEM: 1 PERIPHERAL NERVOUS SYSTEM
OPERATION: 9 DRAINAGE: Taking or letting out fluids and/or gases from a body part

9: DRAINAGE

1: PERIPHERAL NERVOUS SYSTEM

Ø: M/S

Body Part	Approach	Device	Qualifier
Ø Cervical Plexus 1 Cervical Nerve 2 Phrenic Nerve 3 Brachial Plexus 4 Ulnar Nerve 5 Median Nerve 6 Radial Nerve 8 Thoracic Nerve 9 Lumbar Plexus A Lumbosacral Plexus B Lumbar Nerve C Pudendal Nerve D Femoral Nerve F Sciatic Nerve G Tibial Nerve H Peroneal Nerve K Head and Neck Sympathetic Nerve L Thoracic Sympathetic Nerve M Abdominal Sympathetic Nerve N Lumbar Sympathetic Nerve P Sacral Sympathetic Nerve Q Sacral Plexus R Sacral Nerve	Ø Open 3 Percutaneous 4 Percutaneous Endoscopic	Ø Drainage Device	Z No Qualifier
Ø Cervical Plexus 1 Cervical Nerve 2 Phrenic Nerve 3 Brachial Plexus 4 Ulnar Nerve 5 Median Nerve 6 Radial Nerve 8 Thoracic Nerve 9 Lumbar Plexus A Lumbosacral Plexus B Lumbar Nerve C Pudendal Nerve D Femoral Nerve F Sciatic Nerve G Tibial Nerve H Peroneal Nerve K Head and Neck Sympathetic Nerve L Thoracic Sympathetic Nerve M Abdominal Sympathetic Nerve N Lumbar Sympathetic Nerve P Sacral Sympathetic Nerve Q Sacral Plexus R Sacral Nerve	Ø Open 3 Percutaneous 4 Percutaneous Endoscopic	Z No Device	X Diagnostic Z No Qualifier

New/Revised Text in Blue   ~~deleted~~ Deleted

SECTION: Ø MEDICAL AND SURGICAL
BODY SYSTEM: 1 PERIPHERAL NERVOUS SYSTEM
OPERATION: B EXCISION: Cutting out or off, without replacement, a portion of a body part

Body Part	Approach	Device	Qualifier
Ø Cervical Plexus	Ø Open	Z No Device	X Diagnostic
1 Cervical Nerve	3 Percutaneous		Z No Qualifier
2 Phrenic Nerve	4 Percutaneous Endoscopic		
3 Brachial Plexus			
4 Ulnar Nerve			
5 Median Nerve			
6 Radial Nerve			
8 Thoracic Nerve			
9 Lumbar Plexus			
A Lumbosacral Plexus			
B Lumbar Nerve			
C Pudendal Nerve			
D Femoral Nerve			
F Sciatic Nerve			
G Tibial Nerve			
H Peroneal Nerve			
K Head and Neck Sympathetic Nerve			
L Thoracic Sympathetic Nerve			
M Abdominal Sympathetic Nerve			
N Lumbar Sympathetic Nerve			
P Sacral Sympathetic Nerve			
Q Sacral Plexus			
R Sacral Nerve			

SECTION: Ø MEDICAL AND SURGICAL
BODY SYSTEM: 1 PERIPHERAL NERVOUS SYSTEM
OPERATION: C EXTIRPATION: Taking or cutting out solid matter from a body part

Body Part	Approach	Device	Qualifier
Ø Cervical Plexus	Ø Open	Z No Device	Z No Qualifier
1 Cervical Nerve	3 Percutaneous		
2 Phrenic Nerve	4 Percutaneous Endoscopic		
3 Brachial Plexus			
4 Ulnar Nerve			
5 Median Nerve			
6 Radial Nerve			
8 Thoracic Nerve			
9 Lumbar Plexus			
A Lumbosacral Plexus			
B Lumbar Nerve			
C Pudendal Nerve			
D Femoral Nerve			
F Sciatic Nerve			
G Tibial Nerve			
H Peroneal Nerve			
K Head and Neck Sympathetic Nerve			
L Thoracic Sympathetic Nerve			
M Abdominal Sympathetic Nerve			
N Lumbar Sympathetic Nerve			
P Sacral Sympathetic Nerve			
Q Sacral Plexus			
R Sacral Nerve			

SECTION: Ø MEDICAL AND SURGICAL
BODY SYSTEM: 1 PERIPHERAL NERVOUS SYSTEM
OPERATION: D EXTRACTION: Pulling or stripping out or off all or a portion of a body part by the use of force

Body Part	Approach	Device	Qualifier
Ø Cervical Plexus 1 Cervical Nerve 2 Phrenic Nerve 3 Brachial Plexus 4 Ulnar Nerve 5 Median Nerve 6 Radial Nerve 8 Thoracic Nerve 9 Lumbar Plexus A Lumbosacral Plexus B Lumbar Nerve C Pudendal Nerve D Femoral Nerve F Sciatic Nerve G Tibial Nerve H Peroneal Nerve K Head and Neck Sympathetic Nerve L Thoracic Sympathetic Nerve M Abdominal Sympathetic Nerve N Lumbar Sympathetic Nerve P Sacral Sympathetic Nerve Q Sacral Plexus R Sacral Nerve	Ø Open 3 Percutaneous 4 Percutaneous Endoscopic	Z No Device	Z No Qualifier

SECTION: Ø MEDICAL AND SURGICAL
BODY SYSTEM: 1 PERIPHERAL NERVOUS SYSTEM
OPERATION: H INSERTION: Putting in a nonbiological appliance that monitors, assists, performs, or prevents a physiological function but does not physically take the place of a body part

Body Part	Approach	Device	Qualifier
Y Peripheral Nerve	Ø Open 3 Percutaneous 4 Percutaneous Endoscopic	2 Monitoring Device M Neurostimulator Lead Y Other Device	Z No Qualifier

SECTION: Ø MEDICAL AND SURGICAL
BODY SYSTEM: 1 PERIPHERAL NERVOUS SYSTEM
OPERATION: J INSPECTION: Visually and/or manually exploring a body part

Body Part	Approach	Device	Qualifier
Y Peripheral Nerve	Ø Open 3 Percutaneous 4 Percutaneous Endoscopic	Z No Device	Z No Qualifier

New/Revised Text in Blue   deleted Deleted

SECTION: 0 MEDICAL AND SURGICAL
BODY SYSTEM: 1 PERIPHERAL NERVOUS SYSTEM
OPERATION: N RELEASE: Freeing a body part from an abnormal physical constraint by cutting or by the use of force

Body Part	Approach	Device	Qualifier
0 Cervical Plexus 1 Cervical Nerve 2 Phrenic Nerve 3 Brachial Plexus 4 Ulnar Nerve 5 Median Nerve 6 Radial Nerve 8 Thoracic Nerve 9 Lumbar Plexus A Lumbosacral Plexus B Lumbar Nerve C Pudendal Nerve D Femoral Nerve F Sciatic Nerve G Tibial Nerve H Peroneal Nerve K Head and Neck Sympathetic Nerve L Thoracic Sympathetic Nerve M Abdominal Sympathetic Nerve N Lumbar Sympathetic Nerve P Sacral Sympathetic Nerve Q Sacral Plexus R Sacral Nerve	0 Open 3 Percutaneous 4 Percutaneous Endoscopic	Z No Device	Z No Qualifier

SECTION: 0 MEDICAL AND SURGICAL
BODY SYSTEM: 1 PERIPHERAL NERVOUS SYSTEM
OPERATION: P REMOVAL: Taking out or off a device from a body part

Body Part	Approach	Device	Qualifier
Y Peripheral Nerve	0 Open 3 Percutaneous 4 Percutaneous Endoscopic	0 Drainage Device 2 Monitoring Device 7 Autologous Tissue Substitute M Neurostimulator Lead Y Other Device	Z No Qualifier
Y Peripheral Nerve	X External	0 Drainage Device 2 Monitoring Device M Neurostimulator Lead	Z No Qualifier

SECTION: Ø MEDICAL AND SURGICAL
BODY SYSTEM: 1 PERIPHERAL NERVOUS SYSTEM
OPERATION: **Q REPAIR:** Restoring, to the extent possible, a body part to its normal anatomic structure and function

Body Part	Approach	Device	Qualifier
Ø Cervical Plexus 1 Cervical Nerve 2 Phrenic Nerve 3 Brachial Plexus 4 Ulnar Nerve 5 Median Nerve 6 Radial Nerve 8 Thoracic Nerve 9 Lumbar Plexus A Lumbosacral Plexus B Lumbar Nerve C Pudendal Nerve D Femoral Nerve F Sciatic Nerve G Tibial Nerve H Peroneal Nerve K Head and Neck Sympathetic Nerve L Thoracic Sympathetic Nerve M Abdominal Sympathetic Nerve N Lumbar Sympathetic Nerve P Sacral Sympathetic Nerve Q Sacral Plexus R Sacral Nerve	Ø Open 3 Percutaneous 4 Percutaneous Endoscopic	Z No Device	Z No Qualifier

SECTION: Ø MEDICAL AND SURGICAL
BODY SYSTEM: 1 PERIPHERAL NERVOUS SYSTEM
OPERATION: **R REPLACEMENT:** Putting in or on biological or synthetic material that physically takes the place and/or function of all or a portion of a body part

Body Part	Approach	Device	Qualifier
1 Cervical Nerve 2 Phrenic Nerve 4 Ulnar Nerve 5 Median Nerve 6 Radial Nerve 8 Thoracic Nerve B Lumbar Nerve C Pudendal Nerve D Femoral Nerve F Sciatic Nerve G Tibial Nerve H Peroneal Nerve R Sacral Nerve	Ø Open 4 Percutaneous Endoscopic	7 Autologous Tissue Substitute J Synthetic Substitute K Nonautologous Tissue Substitute	Z No Qualifier

SECTION: Ø MEDICAL AND SURGICAL
BODY SYSTEM: 1 PERIPHERAL NERVOUS SYSTEM
OPERATION: S REPOSITION: Moving to its normal location, or other suitable location, all or a portion of a body part

Body Part	Approach	Device	Qualifier
Ø Cervical Plexus 1 Cervical Nerve 2 Phrenic Nerve 3 Brachial Plexus 4 Ulnar Nerve 5 Median Nerve 6 Radial Nerve 8 Thoracic Nerve 9 Lumbar Plexus A Lumbosacral Plexus B Lumbar Nerve C Pudendal Nerve D Femoral Nerve F Sciatic Nerve G Tibial Nerve H Peroneal Nerve Q Sacral Plexus R Sacral Nerve	Ø Open 3 Percutaneous 4 Percutaneous Endoscopic	Z No Device	Z No Qualifier

SECTION: Ø MEDICAL AND SURGICAL
BODY SYSTEM: 1 PERIPHERAL NERVOUS SYSTEM
OPERATION: U SUPPLEMENT: Putting in or on biological or synthetic material that physically reinforces and/or augments the function of a portion of a body part

Body Part	Approach	Device	Qualifier
1 Cervical Nerve 2 Phrenic Nerve 4 Ulnar Nerve 5 Median Nerve 6 Radial Nerve 8 Thoracic Nerve B Lumbar Nerve C Pudendal Nerve D Femoral Nerve F Sciatic Nerve G Tibial Nerve H Peroneal Nerve R Sacral Nerve	Ø Open 3 Percutaneous 4 Percutaneous Endoscopic	7 Autologous Tissue Substitute J Synthetic Substitute K Nonautologous Tissue Substitute	Z No Qualifier

New/Revised Text in Blue   ~~deleted~~ Deleted

S: REPOSITION   U: SUPPLEMENT

1: PERIPHERAL NERVOUS SYSTEM

Ø: M/S

SECTION: Ø MEDICAL AND SURGICAL
BODY SYSTEM: 1 PERIPHERAL NERVOUS SYSTEM
OPERATION: W REVISION: Correcting, to the extent possible, a portion of a malfunctioning device or the position of a displaced device

Body Part	Approach	Device	Qualifier
Y Peripheral Nerve	Ø Open 3 Percutaneous 4 Percutaneous Endoscopic X External	Ø Drainage Device 2 Monitoring Device 7 Autologous Tissue Substitute M Neurostimulator Lead Y Other Device	Z No Qualifier
Y Peripheral Nerve	X External	Ø Drainage Device 2 Monitoring Device 7 Autologous Tissue Substitute M Neurostimulator Lead	Z No Qualifier

SECTION: Ø MEDICAL AND SURGICAL
BODY SYSTEM: 1 PERIPHERAL NERVOUS SYSTEM
OPERATION: X TRANSFER: Moving, without taking out, all or a portion of a body part to another location to take over the function of all or a portion of a body part

Body Part	Approach	Device	Qualifier
1 Cervical Nerve 2 Phrenic Nerve	Ø Open 4 Percutaneous Endoscopic	Z No Device	1 Cervical Nerve 2 Phrenic Nerve
4 Ulnar Nerve 5 Median Nerve 6 Radial Nerve	Ø Open 4 Percutaneous Endoscopic	Z No Device	4 Ulnar Nerve 5 Median Nerve 6 Radial Nerve
8 Thoracic Nerve	Ø Open 4 Percutaneous Endoscopic	Z No Device	8 Thoracic Nerve
B Lumbar Nerve C Pudendal Nerve	Ø Open 4 Percutaneous Endoscopic	Z No Device	B Lumbar Nerve C Pudendal Nerve
D Femoral Nerve F Sciatic Nerve G Tibial Nerve H Peroneal Nerve	Ø Open 4 Percutaneous Endoscopic	Z No Device	D Femoral Nerve F Sciatic Nerve G Tibial Nerve H Peroneal Nerve

Ø2. Heart and Great Vessels 36
    Ø21. Bypass 37
    Ø24. Creation 39
    Ø25. Destruction 39
    Ø27. Dilation 40
    Ø28. Division 41
    Ø2B. Excision 41
    Ø2C. Extirpation 42
    Ø2F. Fragmentation 42
    Ø2H. Insertion 43
    Ø2J. Inspection 44
    Ø2K. Map 45
    Ø2L. Occlusion 45
    Ø2N. Release 46
    Ø2P. Removal 47
    Ø2Q. Repair 48
    Ø2R. Replacement 49
    Ø2S. Reposition 50
    Ø2T. Resection 50
    Ø2U. Supplement 51
    Ø2V. Restriction 52
    Ø2W. Revision 53
    Ø2Y. Transplantation 54

New/Revised Text in Blue   ~~deleted~~ Deleted

SECTION: Ø MEDICAL AND SURGICAL
BODY SYSTEM: 2 HEART AND GREAT VESSELS
OPERATION: 1 BYPASS: *(on multiple pages)*
Altering the route of passage of the contents of a tubular body part

Body Part	Approach	Device	Qualifier
Ø Coronary Artery, One Artery 1 Coronary Artery, Two Arteries 2 Coronary Artery, Three Arteries 3 Coronary Artery, Four or More Arteries	Ø Open	8 Zooplastic Tissue 9 Autologous Venous Tissue A Autologous Arterial Tissue J Synthetic Substitute K Nonautologous Tissue Substitute	3 Coronary Artery 8 Internal Mammary, Right 9 Internal Mammary, Left C Thoracic Artery F Abdominal Artery W Aorta
Ø Coronary Artery, One Artery 1 Coronary Artery, Two Arteries 2 Coronary Artery, Three Arteries 3 Coronary Artery, Four or More Arteries	Ø Open	Z No Device	3 Coronary Artery 8 Internal Mammary, Right 9 Internal Mammary, Left C Thoracic Artery F Abdominal Artery
Ø Coronary Artery, One Artery 1 Coronary Artery, Two Arteries 2 Coronary Artery, Three Arteries 3 Coronary Artery, Four or More Arteries	3 Percutaneous	4 Drug-eluting Intraluminal Device D Intraluminal Device	4 Coronary Vein
Ø Coronary Artery, One Artery 1 Coronary Artery, Two Arteries 2 Coronary Artery, Three Arteries 3 Coronary Artery, Four or More Arteries	4 Percutaneous Endoscopic	4 Drug-eluting Intraluminal Device D Intraluminal Device	4 Coronary Vein
Ø Coronary Artery, One Artery 1 Coronary Artery, Two Arteries 2 Coronary Artery, Three Arteries 3 Coronary Artery, Four or More Arteries	4 Percutaneous Endoscopic	8 Zooplastic Tissue 9 Autologous Venous Tissue A Autologous Arterial Tissue J Synthetic Substitute K Nonautologous Tissue Substitute	3 Coronary Artery 8 Internal Mammary, Right 9 Internal Mammary, Left C Thoracic Artery F Abdominal Artery W Aorta
Ø Coronary Artery, One Artery 1 Coronary Artery, Two Arteries 2 Coronary Artery, Three Arteries 3 Coronary Artery, Four or More Arteries	4 Percutaneous Endoscopic	Z No Device	3 Coronary Artery 8 Internal Mammary, Right 9 Internal Mammary, Left C Thoracic Artery F Abdominal Artery
6 Atrium, Right	Ø Open 4 Percutaneous Endoscopic	8 Zooplastic Tissue 9 Autologous Venous Tissue A Autologous Arterial Tissue J Synthetic Substitute K Nonautologous Tissue Substitute	P Pulmonary Trunk Q Pulmonary Artery, Right R Pulmonary Artery, Left
6 Atrium, Right	Ø Open 4 Percutaneous Endoscopic	Z No Device	7 Atrium, Left P Pulmonary Trunk Q Pulmonary Artery, Right R Pulmonary Artery, Left
6 Atrium, Right	3 Percutaneous	Z No Device	7 Atrium, Left

SECTION: Ø MEDICAL AND SURGICAL
BODY SYSTEM: 2 HEART AND GREAT VESSELS
OPERATION: 1 BYPASS: *(continued)*
Altering the route of passage of the contents of a tubular body part

Body Part	Approach	Device	Qualifier
7 Atrium, Left V Superior Vena Cava	Ø Open 4 Percutaneous Endoscopic	8 Zooplastic Tissue 9 Autologous Venous Tissue A Autologous Arterial Tissue J Synthetic Substitute K Nonautologous Tissue Substitute Z No Device	P Pulmonary Trunk Q Pulmonary Artery, Right R Pulmonary Artery, Left S Pulmonary Vein, Right T Pulmonary Vein, Left U Pulmonary Vein, Confluence
K Ventricle, Right L Ventricle, Left	Ø Open 4 Percutaneous Endoscopic	8 Zooplastic Tissue 9 Autologous Venous Tissue A Autologous Arterial Tissue J Synthetic Substitute K Nonautologous Tissue Substitute	P Pulmonary Trunk Q Pulmonary Artery, Right R Pulmonary Artery, Left
K Ventricle, Right L Ventricle, Left	Ø Open 4 Percutaneous Endoscopic	Z No Device	5 Coronary Circulation 8 Internal Mammary, Right 9 Internal Mammary, Left C Thoracic Artery F Abdominal Artery P Pulmonary Trunk Q Pulmonary Artery, Right R Pulmonary Artery, Left W Aorta
P Pulmonary Trunk Q Pulmonary Artery, Right R Pulmonary Artery, Left	Ø Open 4 Percutaneous Endoscopic	8 Zooplastic Tissue 9 Autologous Venous Tissue A Autologous Arterial Tissue J Synthetic Substitute K Nonautologous Tissue Substitute Z No Device	A Innominate Artery B Subclavian D Carotid
W Thoracic Aorta, Descending	Ø Open	8 Zooplastic Tissue 9 Autologous Venous Tissue A Autologous Arterial Tissue Z No Device	B Subclavian D Carotid P Pulmonary Trunk Q Pulmonary Artery, Right R Pulmonary Artery, Left
W Thoracic Aorta, Descending	Ø Open	J Synthetic Substitute K Nonautologous Tissue Substitute	B Subclavian D Carotid G Axillary Artery H Brachial Artery P Pulmonary Trunk Q Pulmonary Artery, Right R Pulmonary Artery, Left
W Thoracic Aorta, Descending	4 Percutaneous Endoscopic	8 Zooplastic Tissue 9 Autologous Venous Tissue A Autologous Arterial Tissue J Synthetic Substitute K Nonautologous Tissue Substitute Z No Device	B Subclavian D Carotid P Pulmonary Trunk Q Pulmonary Artery, Right R Pulmonary Artery, Left
~~W Thoracic Aorta, Descending~~ X Thoracic Aorta, Ascending/Arch	Ø Open 4 Percutaneous Endoscopic	8 Zooplastic Tissue 9 Autologous Venous Tissue A Autologous Arterial Tissue J Synthetic Substitute K Nonautologous Tissue Substitute Z No Device	B Subclavian D Carotid P Pulmonary Trunk Q Pulmonary Artery, Right R Pulmonary Artery, Left

1: BYPASS

2: HEART AND GREAT VESSELS

Ø: M/S

        New/Revised Text in Blue   ~~deleted~~ Deleted

SECTION: Ø **MEDICAL AND SURGICAL**
BODY SYSTEM: 2 **HEART AND GREAT VESSELS**
OPERATION: 4 **CREATION:** Putting in or on biological or synthetic material to form a new body part that to the extent possible replicates the anatomic structure or function of an absent body part

Body Part	Approach	Device	Qualifier
F Aortic Valve	Ø Open	7 Autologous Tissue Substitute 8 Zooplastic Tissue J Synthetic Substitute K Nonautologous Tissue Substitute	J Truncal Valve
G Mitral Valve J Tricuspid Valve	Ø Open	7 Autologous Tissue Substitute 8 Zooplastic Tissue J Synthetic Substitute K Nonautologous Tissue Substitute	2 Common Atrioventricular Valve

SECTION: Ø **MEDICAL AND SURGICAL**
BODY SYSTEM: 2 **HEART AND GREAT VESSELS**
OPERATION: 5 **DESTRUCTION:** Physical eradication of all or a portion of a body part by the direct use of energy, force, or a destructive agent

Body Part	Approach	Device	Qualifier
4 Coronary Vein 5 Atrial Septum 6 Atrium, Right 7 Atrium, Left 8 Conduction Mechanism 9 Chordae Tendineae D Papillary Muscle F Aortic Valve G Mitral Valve H Pulmonary Valve J Tricuspid Valve K Ventricle, Right L Ventricle, Left M Ventricular Septum N Pericardium P Pulmonary Trunk Q Pulmonary Artery, Right R Pulmonary Artery, Left S Pulmonary Vein, Right T Pulmonary Vein, Left V Superior Vena Cava W Thoracic Aorta, Descending X Thoracic Aorta, Ascending/Arch	Ø Open 3 Percutaneous 4 Percutaneous Endoscopic	Z No Device	Z No Qualifier
7 Atrium, Left	Ø Open 3 Percutaneous 4 Percutaneous Endoscopic	Z No Device	K Left Atrial Appendage Z No Qualifier

Ø: M/S   2: HEART AND GREAT VESSELS   4: CREATION   5: DESTRUCTION

SECTION: Ø MEDICAL AND SURGICAL
BODY SYSTEM: 2 HEART AND GREAT VESSELS
OPERATION: 7 DILATION: Expanding an orifice or the lumen of a tubular body part

Body Part	Approach	Device	Qualifier
Ø Coronary Artery, One Artery 1 Coronary Artery, Two Arteries 2 Coronary Artery, Three Arteries 3 Coronary Artery, Four or More Arteries	Ø Open 3 Percutaneous 4 Percutaneous Endoscopic	4 Drug-eluting Intraluminal Device 5 Intraluminal Device, Drug-eluting, Two 6 Intraluminal Device, Drug-eluting, Three 7 Intraluminal Device, Drug-eluting, Four or More D Intraluminal Device E Intraluminal Device, Two F Intraluminal Device, Three G Intraluminal Device, Four or More T Radioactive Intraluminal Device Z No Device	6 Bifurcation Z No Qualifier
F Aortic Valve G Mitral Valve H Pulmonary Valve J Tricuspid Valve K Ventricle, Right L Ventricle, Left P Pulmonary Trunk Q Pulmonary Artery, Right S Pulmonary Vein, Right T Pulmonary Vein, Left V Superior Vena Cava W Thoracic Aorta, Descending X Thoracic Aorta, Ascending/Arch	Ø Open 3 Percutaneous 4 Percutaneous Endoscopic	4 Drug-eluting Intraluminal Device D Intraluminal Device Z No Device	Z No Qualifier
R Pulmonary Artery, Left	Ø Open 3 Percutaneous 4 Percutaneous Endoscopic	4 Drug-eluting Intraluminal Device D Intraluminal Device Z No Device	T Ductus Arteriosus Z No Qualifier

7: DILATION

2: HEART AND GREAT VESSELS

Ø: M/S

SECTION: Ø MEDICAL AND SURGICAL
BODY SYSTEM: 2 HEART AND GREAT VESSELS
OPERATION: 8 DIVISION: Cutting into a body part, without draining fluids and/or gases from the body part, in order to separate or transect a body part

Body Part	Approach	Device	Qualifier
8 Conduction Mechanism 9 Chordae Tendineae D Papillary Muscle	Ø Open 3 Percutaneous 4 Percutaneous Endoscopic	Z No Device	Z No Qualifier

SECTION: Ø MEDICAL AND SURGICAL
BODY SYSTEM: 2 HEART AND GREAT VESSELS
OPERATION: B EXCISION: Cutting out or off, without replacement, a portion of a body part

Body Part	Approach	Device	Qualifier
4 Coronary Vein 5 Atrial Septum 6 Atrium, Right 8 Conduction Mechanism 9 Chordae Tendineae D Papillary Muscle F Aortic Valve G Mitral Valve H Pulmonary Valve J Tricuspid Valve K Ventricle, Right L Ventricle, Left M Ventricular Septum N Pericardium P Pulmonary Trunk Q Pulmonary Artery, Right R Pulmonary Artery, Left S Pulmonary Vein, Right T Pulmonary Vein, Left V Superior Vena Cava W Thoracic Aorta, Descending X Thoracic Aorta, Ascending/Arch	Ø Open 3 Percutaneous 4 Percutaneous Endoscopic	Z No Device	X Diagnostic Z No Qualifier
7 Atrium, Left	Ø Open 3 Percutaneous 4 Percutaneous Endoscopic	Z No Device	K Left Atrial Appendage X Diagnostic Z No Qualifier

SECTION: 0 MEDICAL AND SURGICAL
BODY SYSTEM: 2 HEART AND GREAT VESSELS
OPERATION: C EXTIRPATION: Taking or cutting out solid matter from a body part

Body Part	Approach	Device	Qualifier
0 Coronary Artery, One Artery 1 Coronary Artery, Two Arteries 2 Coronary Artery, Three Arteries 3 Coronary Artery, Four or More Arteries	0 Open 3 Percutaneous 4 Percutaneous Endoscopic	Z No Device	6 Bifurcation Z No Qualifier
4 Coronary Vein 5 Atrial Septum 6 Atrium, Right 7 Atrium, Left 8 Conduction Mechanism 9 Chordae Tendineae D Papillary Muscle F Aortic Valve G Mitral Valve H Pulmonary Valve J Tricuspid Valve K Ventricle, Right L Ventricle, Left M Ventricular Septum N Pericardium P Pulmonary Trunk Q Pulmonary Artery, Right R Pulmonary Artery, Left S Pulmonary Vein, Right T Pulmonary Vein, Left V Superior Vena Cava W Thoracic Aorta, Descending X Thoracic Aorta, Ascending/Arch	0 Open 3 Percutaneous 4 Percutaneous Endoscopic	Z No Device	Z No Qualifier

SECTION: 0 MEDICAL AND SURGICAL
BODY SYSTEM: 2 HEART AND GREAT VESSELS
OPERATION: F FRAGMENTATION: Breaking solid matter in a body part into pieces

Body Part	Approach	Device	Qualifier
N Pericardium	0 Open 3 Percutaneous 4 Percutaneous Endoscopic X External	Z No Device	Z No Qualifier

SECTION: Ø MEDICAL AND SURGICAL
BODY SYSTEM: 2 HEART AND GREAT VESSELS
OPERATION: H INSERTION: *(on multiple pages)*

Putting in a nonbiological appliance that monitors, assists, performs, or prevents a physiological function but does not physically take the place of a body part

Body Part	Approach	Device	Qualifier
4 Coronary Vein 6 Atrium, Right 7 Atrium, Left K Ventricle, Right L Ventricle, Left	Ø Open 3 Percutaneous 4 Percutaneous Endoscopic	Ø Monitoring Device, Pressure Sensor 2 Monitoring Device 3 Infusion Device D Intraluminal Device J Cardiac Lead, Pacemaker K Cardiac Lead, Defibrillator M Cardiac Lead N Intracardiac Pacemaker Y Other Device	Z No Qualifier
A Heart	Ø Open 3 Percutaneous 4 Percutaneous Endoscopic	Q Implantable Heart Assist System Y Other Device	Z No Qualifier
A Heart	Ø Open 3 Percutaneous 4 Percutaneous Endoscopic	R Short-term External Heart Assist System	J Intraoperative S Biventricular Z No Qualifier
N Pericardium	Ø Open 3 Percutaneous 4 Percutaneous Endoscopic	Ø Monitoring Device, Pressure Sensor 2 Monitoring Device J Cardiac Lead, Pacemaker K Cardiac Lead, Defibrillator M Cardiac Lead Y Other Device	Z No Qualifier

SECTION: Ø MEDICAL AND SURGICAL
BODY SYSTEM: 2 HEART AND GREAT VESSELS
OPERATION: H INSERTION: *(continued)*
Putting in a nonbiological appliance that monitors, assists, performs, or prevents a physiological function but does not physically take the place of a body part

Body Part	Approach	Device	Qualifier
P Pulmonary Trunk Q Pulmonary Artery, Right R Pulmonary Artery, Left S Pulmonary Vein, Right T Pulmonary Vein, Left V Superior Vena Cava W Thoracic Aorta, Descending X~~ Thoracic Aorta, Ascending/Arch~~	Ø Open 3 Percutaneous 4 Percutaneous Endoscopic	Ø Monitoring Device, Pressure Sensor 2 Monitoring Device 3 Infusion Device D Intraluminal Device Y Other Device	Z No Qualifier
X Thoracic Aorta, Ascending/Arch	Ø Open 3 Percutaneous 4 Percutaneous Endoscopic	Ø Monitoring Device, Pressure Sensor 2 Monitoring Device 3 Infusion Device D Intraluminal Device	Z No Qualifier

SECTION: Ø MEDICAL AND SURGICAL
BODY SYSTEM: 2 HEART AND GREAT VESSELS
OPERATION: J INSPECTION: Visually and/or manually exploring a body part

Body Part	Approach	Device	Qualifier
A Heart Y Great Vessel	Ø Open 3 Percutaneous 4 Percutaneous Endoscopic	Z No Device	Z No Qualifier

SECTION: Ø MEDICAL AND SURGICAL
BODY SYSTEM: 2 HEART AND GREAT VESSELS
OPERATION: **K MAP:** Locating the route of passage of electrical impulses and/or locating functional areas in a body part

Body Part	Approach	Device	Qualifier
8 Conduction Mechanism	Ø Open 3 Percutaneous 4 Percutaneous Endoscopic	Z No Device	Z No Qualifier

SECTION: Ø MEDICAL AND SURGICAL
BODY SYSTEM: 2 HEART AND GREAT VESSELS
OPERATION: **L OCCLUSION:** Completely closing an orifice or the lumen of a tubular body part

Body Part	Approach	Device	Qualifier
7 Atrium, Left	Ø Open 3 Percutaneous 4 Percutaneous Endoscopic	C Extraluminal Device D Intraluminal Device Z No Device	K Left Atrial Appendage
H Pulmonary Valve P Pulmonary Trunk Q Pulmonary Artery, Right S Pulmonary Vein, Right T Pulmonary Vein, Left V Superior Vena Cava	Ø Open 3 Percutaneous 4 Percutaneous Endoscopic	C Extraluminal Device D Intraluminal Device Z No Device	Z No Qualifier
R Pulmonary Artery, Left	Ø Open 3 Percutaneous 4 Percutaneous Endoscopic	C Extraluminal Device D Intraluminal Device Z No Device	T Ductus Arteriosus Z No Qualifier
W Thoracic Aorta, Descending	3 Percutaneous	D Intraluminal Device	J Temporary

SECTION: Ø MEDICAL AND SURGICAL
BODY SYSTEM: 2 HEART AND GREAT VESSELS
OPERATION: N RELEASE: Freeing a body part from an abnormal physical constraint by cutting or by the use of force

Body Part	Approach	Device	Qualifier
Ø Coronary Artery, One Artery	Ø Open	Z No Device	Z No Qualifier
1 Coronary Artery, Two Arteries	3 Percutaneous		
2 Coronary Artery, Three Arteries	4 Percutaneous Endoscopic		
3 Coronary Artery, Four or More Arteries			
4 Coronary Vein			
5 Atrial Septum			
6 Atrium, Right			
7 Atrium, Left			
8 Conduction Mechanism			
9 Chordae Tendineae			
D Papillary Muscle			
F Aortic Valve			
G Mitral Valve			
H Pulmonary Valve			
J Tricuspid Valve			
K Ventricle, Right			
L Ventricle, Left			
M Ventricular Septum			
N Pericardium			
P Pulmonary Trunk			
Q Pulmonary Artery, Right			
R Pulmonary Artery, Left			
S Pulmonary Vein, Right			
T Pulmonary Vein, Left			
V Superior Vena Cava			
W Thoracic Aorta, Descending			
X Thoracic Aorta, Ascending/Arch			

N: RELEASE

2: HEART AND GREAT VESSELS

Ø: M/S

SECTION: Ø MEDICAL AND SURGICAL
BODY SYSTEM: 2 HEART AND GREAT VESSELS
OPERATION: P REMOVAL: Taking out or off a device from a body part

Body Part	Approach	Device	Qualifier
A Heart	Ø Open 3 Percutaneous 4 Percutaneous Endoscopic	2 Monitoring Device 3 Infusion Device 7 Autologous Tissue Substitute 8 Zooplastic Tissue C Extraluminal Device D Intraluminal Device J Synthetic Substitute K Nonautologous Tissue Substitute M Cardiac Lead N Intracardiac Pacemaker Q Implantable Heart Assist System R External Heart Assist System Y Other Device	Z No Qualifier
A Heart	Ø Open 3 Percutaneous 4 Percutaneous Endoscopic	R Short-term External Heart Assist System	S Biventricular Z No Qualifier
A Heart	X External	2 Monitoring Device 3 Infusion Device D Intraluminal Device M Cardiac Lead	Z No Qualifier
Y Great Vessel	Ø Open 3 Percutaneous 4 Percutaneous Endoscopic	2 Monitoring Device 3 Infusion Device 7 Autologous Tissue Substitute 8 Zooplastic Tissue C Extraluminal Device D Intraluminal Device J Synthetic Substitute K Nonautologous Tissue Substitute Y Other Device	Z No Qualifier
Y Great Vessel	X External	2 Monitoring Device 3 Infusion Device D Intraluminal Device	Z No Qualifier

Ø: M/S

2: HEART AND GREAT VESSELS

P: REMOVAL

SECTION: 0 MEDICAL AND SURGICAL
BODY SYSTEM: 2 HEART AND GREAT VESSELS
OPERATION: Q REPAIR: Restoring, to the extent possible, a body part to its normal anatomic structure and function

Body Part	Approach	Device	Qualifier
0 Coronary Artery, One Artery 1 Coronary Artery, Two Arteries 2 Coronary Artery, Three Arteries 3 Coronary Artery, Four or More Arteries 4 Coronary Vein 5 Atrial Septum 6 Atrium, Right 7 Atrium, Left 8 Conduction Mechanism 9 Chordae Tendineae A Heart B Heart, Right C Heart, Left D Papillary Muscle H Pulmonary Valve K Ventricle, Right L Ventricle, Left M Ventricular Septum N Pericardium P Pulmonary Trunk Q Pulmonary Artery, Right R Pulmonary Artery, Left S Pulmonary Vein, Right T Pulmonary Vein, Left V Superior Vena Cava W Thoracic Aorta, Descending X Thoracic Aorta, Ascending/Arch	0 Open 3 Percutaneous 4 Percutaneous Endoscopic	Z No Device	Z No Qualifier
F Aortic Valve	0 Open 3 Percutaneous 4 Percutaneous Endoscopic	Z No Device	J Truncal Valve Z No Qualifier
G Mitral Valve	0 Open 3 Percutaneous 4 Percutaneous Endoscopic	Z No Device	E Atrioventricular Valve, Left Z No Qualifier
J Tricuspid Valve	0 Open 3 Percutaneous 4 Percutaneous Endoscopic	Z No Device	G Atrioventricular Valve, Right Z No Qualifier

New/Revised Text in Blue   ~~deleted~~ Deleted

SECTION: 0 MEDICAL AND SURGICAL
BODY SYSTEM: 2 HEART AND GREAT VESSELS
OPERATION: **R REPLACEMENT:** Putting in or on biological or synthetic material that physically takes the place and/or function of all or a portion of a body part

Body Part	Approach	Device	Qualifier
5 Atrial Septum 6 Atrium, Right 7 Atrium, Left 9 Chordae Tendineae D Papillary Muscle J Tricuspid Valve K Ventricle, Right L Ventricle, Left M Ventricular Septum N Pericardium P Pulmonary Trunk Q Pulmonary Artery, Right R Pulmonary Artery, Left S Pulmonary Vein, Right T Pulmonary Vein, Left V Superior Vena Cava W Thoracic Aorta, Descending X Thoracic Aorta, Ascending/Arch	0 Open 4 Percutaneous Endoscopic	7 Autologous Tissue Substitute 8 Zooplastic Tissue J Synthetic Substitute K Nonautologous Tissue Substitute	Z No Qualifier
F Aortic Valve G Mitral Valve H Pulmonary Valve J Tricuspid Valve	0 Open 4 Percutaneous Endoscopic	7 Autologous Tissue Substitute 8 Zooplastic Tissue J Synthetic Substitute K Nonautologous Tissue Substitute	Z No Qualifier
F Aortic Valve G Mitral Valve H Pulmonary Valve J Tricuspid Valve	3 Percutaneous	7 Autologous Tissue Substitute 8 Zooplastic Tissue J Synthetic Substitute K Nonautologous Tissue Substitute	H Transapical Z No Qualifier

SECTION: Ø MEDICAL AND SURGICAL
BODY SYSTEM: 2 **HEART AND GREAT VESSELS**
OPERATION: S **REPOSITION:** Moving to its normal location, or other suitable location, all or a portion of a body part

Body Part	Approach	Device	Qualifier
Ø Coronary Artery, One Artery 1 Coronary Artery, Two Arteries P Pulmonary Trunk Q Pulmonary Artery, Right R Pulmonary Artery, Left S Pulmonary Vein, Right T Pulmonary Vein, Left V Superior Vena Cava W Thoracic Aorta, Descending X Thoracic Aorta, Ascending/Arch	Ø Open	Z No Device	Z No Qualifier

SECTION: Ø MEDICAL AND SURGICAL
BODY SYSTEM: 2 **HEART AND GREAT VESSELS**
OPERATION: T **RESECTION:** Cutting out or off, without replacement, all of a body part

Body Part	Approach	Device	Qualifier
5 Atrial Septum 8 Conduction Mechanism 9 Chordae Tendineae D Papillary Muscle H Pulmonary Valve M Ventricular Septum N Pericardium	Ø Open 3 Percutaneous 4 Percutaneous Endoscopic	Z No Device	Z No Qualifier

SECTION: Ø MEDICAL AND SURGICAL
BODY SYSTEM: 2 HEART AND GREAT VESSELS
OPERATION: U SUPPLEMENT: Putting in or on biological or synthetic material that physically reinforces and/or augments the function of a portion of a body part

Body Part	Approach	Device	Qualifier
5 Atrial Septum 6 Atrium, Right 7 Atrium, Left 9 Chordae Tendineae A Heart D Papillary Muscle H Pulmonary Valve K Ventricle, Right L Ventricle, Left M Ventricular Septum N Pericardium P Pulmonary Trunk Q Pulmonary Artery, Right R Pulmonary Artery, Left S Pulmonary Vein, Right T Pulmonary Vein, Left V Superior Vena Cava W Thoracic Aorta, Descending X Thoracic Aorta, Ascending/Arch	Ø Open 3 Percutaneous 4 Percutaneous Endoscopic	7 Autologous Tissue Substitute 8 Zooplastic Tissue J Synthetic Substitute K Nonautologous Tissue Substitute	Z No Qualifier
F Aortic Valve	Ø Open 3 Percutaneous 4 Percutaneous Endoscopic	7 Autologous Tissue Substitute 8 Zooplastic Tissue J Synthetic Substitute K Nonautologous Tissue Substitute	J Truncal Valve Z No Qualifier
G Mitral Valve	Ø Open 3 Percutaneous 4 Percutaneous Endoscopic	7 Autologous Tissue Substitute 8 Zooplastic Tissue J Synthetic Substitute K Nonautologous Tissue Substitute	E Atrioventricular Valve, Left Z No Qualifier
J Tricuspid Valve	Ø Open 3 Percutaneous 4 Percutaneous Endoscopic	7 Autologous Tissue Substitute 8 Zooplastic Tissue J Synthetic Substitute K Nonautologous Tissue Substitute	G Atrioventricular Valve, Right Z No Qualifier

SECTION: Ø MEDICAL AND SURGICAL
BODY SYSTEM: 2 HEART AND GREAT VESSELS
OPERATION: V **RESTRICTION:** Partially closing an orifice or the lumen of a tubular body part

Body Part	Approach	Device	Qualifier
A Heart	Ø Open 3 Percutaneous 4 Percutaneous Endoscopic	C Extraluminal Device Z No Device	Z No Qualifier
G Mitral Valve	Ø Open 3 Percutaneous 4 Percutaneous Endoscopic	Z No Device	Z No Qualifier
P Pulmonary Trunk Q Pulmonary Artery, Right S Pulmonary Vein, Right T Pulmonary Vein, Left V Superior Vena Cava	Ø Open 3 Percutaneous 4 Percutaneous Endoscopic	C Extraluminal Device D Intraluminal Device Z No Device	Z No Qualifier
R Pulmonary Artery, Left	Ø Open 3 Percutaneous 4 Percutaneous Endoscopic	C Extraluminal Device D Intraluminal Device Z No Device	T Ductus Arteriosus Z No Qualifier
W Thoracic Aorta, Descending X Thoracic Aorta, Ascending/Arch	Ø Open 3 Percutaneous 4 Percutaneous Endoscopic	C Extraluminal Device D Intraluminal Device E Intraluminal Device, Branched or Fenestrated, One or Two Arteries F Intraluminal Device, Branched or Fenestrated, Three or More Arteries Z No Device	Z No Qualifier

New/Revised Text in Blue   deleted Deleted

V: RESTRICTION

2: HEART AND GREAT VESSELS

Ø: M/S

SECTION: 0 MEDICAL AND SURGICAL
BODY SYSTEM: 2 HEART AND GREAT VESSELS
OPERATION: W REVISION: *(on multiple pages)*

Correcting, to the extent possible, a portion of a malfunctioning device or the position of a displaced device

Body Part	Approach	Device	Qualifier
5 Atrial Septum M Ventricular Septum	0 Open 4 Percutaneous Endoscopic	J Synthetic Substitute	Z No Qualifier
A Heart	0 Open 3 Percutaneous 4 Percutaneous Endoscopic ~~X External~~	2 Monitoring Device 3 Infusion Device 7 Autologous Tissue Substitute 8 Zooplastic Tissue C Extraluminal Device D Intraluminal Device J Synthetic Substitute K Nonautologous Tissue Substitute M Cardiac Lead N Intracardiac Pacemaker Q Implantable Heart Assist System ~~R External Heart Assist System~~ Y Other Device	Z No Qualifier
A Heart	0 Open 3 Percutaneous 4 Percutaneous Endoscopic	R Short-term External Heart Assist System	S Biventricular Z No Qualifier
A Heart	X External	2 Monitoring Device 3 Infusion Device 7 Autologous Tissue Substitute 8 Zooplastic Tissue C Extraluminal Device D Intraluminal Device J Synthetic Substitute K Nonautologous Tissue Substitute M Cardiac Lead N Intracardiac Pacemaker Q Implantable Heart Assist System	Z No Qualifier
A Heart	X External	R Short-term External Heart Assist System	S Biventricular Z No Qualifier
F Aortic Valve G Mitral Valve H Pulmonary Valve J Tricuspid Valve	0 Open 3 Percutaneous 4 Percutaneous Endoscopic	7 Autologous Tissue Substitute 8 Zooplastic Tissue J Synthetic Substitute K Nonautologous Tissue Substitute	Z No Qualifier

0: M/S

2: HEART AND GREAT VESSELS

W: REVISION

SECTION: Ø MEDICAL AND SURGICAL
BODY SYSTEM: 2 HEART AND GREAT VESSELS
OPERATION: W REVISION: *(continued)*
Correcting, to the extent possible, a portion of a malfunctioning device or the position of a displaced device

Body Part	Approach	Device	Qualifier
Y Great Vessel	Ø Open 3 Percutaneous 4 Percutaneous Endoscopic X ~~External~~	2 Monitoring Device 3 Infusion Device 7 Autologous Tissue Substitute 8 Zooplastic Tissue C Extraluminal Device D Intraluminal Device J Synthetic Substitute K Nonautologous Tissue Substitute Y Other Device	Z No Qualifier
Y Great Vessel	X External	2 Monitoring Device 3 Infusion Device 7 Autologous Tissue Substitute 8 Zooplastic Tissue C Extraluminal Device D Intraluminal Device J Synthetic Substitute K Nonautologous Tissue Substitute	Z No Qualifier

SECTION: Ø MEDICAL AND SURGICAL
BODY SYSTEM: 2 HEART AND GREAT VESSELS
OPERATION: Y TRANSPLANTATION: Putting in or on all or a portion of a living body part taken from another individual or animal to physically take the place and/or function of all or a portion of a similar body part

Body Part	Approach	Device	Qualifier
A Heart	Ø Open	Z No Device	Ø Allogeneic 1 Syngeneic 2 Zooplastic

Ø3. Upper Arteries 55
    Ø31. Bypass...56
    Ø35. Destruction..58
    Ø37. Dilation..59
    Ø39. Drainage 6Ø
    Ø3B. Excision 62
    Ø3C. Extirpation..63
    Ø3H. Insertion..64
    Ø3J. Inspection 65
    Ø3L. Occlusion...65
    Ø3N. Release 66
    Ø3P. Removal 67
    Ø3Q. Repair 68
    Ø3R. Replacement 69
    Ø3S. Reposition..7Ø
    Ø3U. Supplement...71
    Ø3V. Restriction...72
    Ø3W. Revision..73

SECTION: Ø MEDICAL AND SURGICAL
BODY SYSTEM: 3 UPPER ARTERIES
OPERATION: 1 BYPASS: *(on multiple pages)*
Altering the route of passage of the contents of a tubular body part

1: BYPASS

3: UPPER ARTERIES

Ø: M/S

Body Part	Approach	Device	Qualifier
2 Innominate Artery ~~5 Axillary Artery, Right~~ ~~6 Axillary Artery, Left~~	Ø Open	9 Autologous Venous Tissue A Autologous Arterial Tissue J Synthetic Substitute K Nonautologous Tissue Substitute Z No Device	Ø Upper Arm Artery, Right 1 Upper Arm Artery, Left 2 Upper Arm Artery, Bilateral 3 Lower Arm Artery, Right 4 Lower Arm Artery, Left 5 Lower Arm Artery, Bilateral 6 Upper Leg Artery, Right 7 Upper Leg Artery, Left 8 Upper Leg Artery, Bilateral 9 Lower Leg Artery, Right B Lower Leg Artery, Left C Lower Leg Artery, Bilateral D Upper Arm Vein F Lower Arm Vein J Extracranial Artery, Right K Extracranial Artery, Left
3 Subclavian Artery, Right 4 Subclavian Artery, Left	Ø Open	9 Autologous Venous Tissue A Autologous Arterial Tissue J Synthetic Substitute K Nonautologous Tissue Substitute Z No Device	Ø Upper Arm Artery, Right 1 Upper Arm Artery, Left 2 Upper Arm Artery, Bilateral 3 Lower Arm Artery, Right 4 Lower Arm Artery, Left 5 Lower Arm Artery, Bilateral 6 Upper Leg Artery, Right 7 Upper Leg Artery, Left 8 Upper Leg Artery, Bilateral 9 Lower Leg Artery, Right B Lower Leg Artery, Left C Lower Leg Artery, Bilateral D Upper Arm Vein F Lower Arm Vein J Extracranial Artery, Right K Extracranial Artery, Left M Pulmonary Artery, Right N Pulmonary Artery, Left
5 Axillary Artery, Right 6 Axillary Artery, Left	Ø Open	9 Autologous Venous Tissue A Autologous Arterial Tissue J Synthetic Substitute K Nonautologous Tissue Substitute Z No Device	Ø Upper Arm Artery, Right 1 Upper Arm Artery, Left 2 Upper Arm Artery, Bilateral 3 Lower Arm Artery, Right 4 Lower Arm Artery, Left 5 Lower Arm Artery, Bilateral 6 Upper Leg Artery, Right 7 Upper Leg Artery, Left 8 Upper Leg Artery, Bilateral 9 Lower Leg Artery, Right B Lower Leg Artery, Left C Lower Leg Artery, Bilateral D Upper Arm Vein F Lower Arm Vein J Extracranial Artery, Right K Extracranial Artery, Left V Superior Vena Cava

New/Revised Text in Blue   ~~deleted~~ Deleted

SECTION: Ø MEDICAL AND SURGICAL
BODY SYSTEM: 3 UPPER ARTERIES
OPERATION: 1 BYPASS: *(continued)*
Altering the route of passage of the contents of a tubular body part

Body Part	Approach	Device	Qualifier
7 Brachial Artery, Right	Ø Open	9 Autologous Venous Tissue A Autologous Arterial Tissue J Synthetic Substitute K Nonautologous Tissue Substitute Z No Device	Ø Upper Arm Artery, Right 3 Lower Arm Artery, Right D Upper Arm Vein F Lower Arm Vein V Superior Vena Cava
8 Brachial Artery, Left	Ø Open	9 Autologous Venous Tissue A Autologous Arterial Tissue J Synthetic Substitute K Nonautologous Tissue Substitute Z No Device	1 Upper Arm Artery, Left 4 Lower Arm Artery, Left D Upper Arm Vein F Lower Arm Vein V Superior Vena Cava
9 Ulnar Artery, Right B Radial Artery, Right	Ø Open	9 Autologous Venous Tissue A Autologous Arterial Tissue J Synthetic Substitute K Nonautologous Tissue Substitute Z No Device	3 Lower Arm Artery, Right F Lower Arm Vein
A Ulnar Artery, Left C Radial Artery, Left	Ø Open	9 Autologous Venous Tissue A Autologous Arterial Tissue J Synthetic Substitute K Nonautologous Tissue Substitute Z No Device	4 Lower Arm Artery, Left F Lower Arm Vein
G Intracranial Artery S Temporal Artery, Right T Temporal Artery, Left	Ø Open	9 Autologous Venous Tissue A Autologous Arterial Tissue J Synthetic Substitute K Nonautologous Tissue Substitute Z No Device	G Intracranial Artery
H Common Carotid Artery, Right J Common Carotid Artery, Left	Ø Open	9 Autologous Venous Tissue A Autologous Arterial Tissue J Synthetic Substitute K Nonautologous Tissue Substitute Z No Device	G Intracranial Artery J Extracranial Artery, Right K Extracranial Artery, Left
~~J Common Carotid Artery, Left~~	~~Ø Open~~	~~9 Autologous Venous Tissue~~ ~~A Autologous Arterial Tissue~~ ~~J Synthetic Substitute~~ ~~K Nonautologous Tissue~~ ~~Substitute~~ ~~Z No Device~~	~~G Intracranial Artery~~ ~~K Extracranial Artery, Left~~

SECTION: Ø MEDICAL AND SURGICAL
BODY SYSTEM: 3 UPPER ARTERIES
OPERATION: 1 BYPASS: *(continued)*
Altering the route of passage of the contents of a tubular body part

Body Part	Approach	Device	Qualifier
K Internal Carotid Artery, Right L Internal Carotid Artery, Left M External Carotid Artery, Right N External Carotid Artery, Left	Ø Open	9 Autologous Venous Tissue A Autologous Arterial Tissue J Synthetic Substitute K Nonautologous Tissue Substitute Z No Device	J Extracranial Artery, Right K Extracranial Artery, Left
~~L Internal Carotid Artery, Left~~ ~~N External Carotid Artery, Left~~	~~Ø Open~~	~~9 Autologous Venous Tissue~~ ~~A Autologous Arterial Tissue~~ ~~J Synthetic Substitute~~ ~~K Nonautologous Tissue Substitute~~ ~~Z No Device~~	~~K Extracranial Artery, Left~~

SECTION: Ø MEDICAL AND SURGICAL
BODY SYSTEM: 3 UPPER ARTERIES
OPERATION: 5 DESTRUCTION: Physical eradication of all or a portion of a body part by the direct use of energy, force, or a destructive agent

Body Part	Approach	Device	Qualifier
Ø Internal Mammary Artery, Right 1 Internal Mammary Artery, Left 2 Innominate Artery 3 Subclavian Artery, Right 4 Subclavian Artery, Left 5 Axillary Artery, Right 6 Axillary Artery, Left 7 Brachial Artery, Right 8 Brachial Artery, Left 9 Ulnar Artery, Right A Ulnar Artery, Left B Radial Artery, Right C Radial Artery, Left D Hand Artery, Right F Hand Artery, Left G Intracranial Artery H Common Carotid Artery, Right J Common Carotid Artery, Left K Internal Carotid Artery, Right L Internal Carotid Artery, Left M External Carotid Artery, Right N External Carotid Artery, Left P Vertebral Artery, Right Q Vertebral Artery, Left R Face Artery S Temporal Artery, Right T Temporal Artery, Left U Thyroid Artery, Right V Thyroid Artery, Left Y Upper Artery	Ø Open 3 Percutaneous 4 Percutaneous Endoscopic	Z No Device	Z No Qualifier

Sidebar: 1: BYPASS 5: DESTRUCTION 3: UPPER ARTERIES Ø: M/S

SECTION: Ø MEDICAL AND SURGICAL

BODY SYSTEM: 3 UPPER ARTERIES

OPERATION: 7 DILATION: Expanding an orifice or the lumen of a tubular body part

Body Part	Approach	Device	Qualifier
Ø Internal Mammary Artery, Right	Ø Open	4 Intraluminal Device, Drug-eluting	6 Bifurcation
1 Internal Mammary Artery, Left	3 Percutaneous	5 Intraluminal Device, Drug-eluting, Two	Z No Qualifier
2 Innominate Artery	4 Percutaneous Endoscopic	6 Intraluminal Device, Drug-eluting, Three	
3 Subclavian Artery, Right		7 Intraluminal Device, Drug-eluting, Four or More	
4 Subclavian Artery, Left		D Intraluminal Device	
5 Axillary Artery, Right		E Intraluminal Device, Two	
6 Axillary Artery, Left		F Intraluminal Device, Three	
7 Brachial Artery, Right		G Intraluminal Device, Four or More	
8 Brachial Artery, Left		Z No Device	
9 Ulnar Artery, Right			
A Ulnar Artery, Left			
B Radial Artery, Right			
C Radial Artery, Left			
D Hand Artery, Right			
F Hand Artery, Left			
G Intracranial Artery			
H Common Carotid Artery, Right			
J Common Carotid Artery, Left			
K Internal Carotid Artery, Right			
L Internal Carotid Artery, Left			
M External Carotid Artery, Right			
N External Carotid Artery, Left			
P Vertebral Artery, Right			
Q Vertebral Artery, Left			
R Face Artery			
S Temporal Artery, Right			
T Temporal Artery, Left			
U Thyroid Artery, Right			
V Thyroid Artery, Left			
Y Upper Artery			

SECTION: Ø MEDICAL AND SURGICAL
BODY SYSTEM: 3 UPPER ARTERIES
OPERATION: 9 DRAINAGE: *(on multiple pages)*

Taking or letting out fluids and/or gases from a body part

Body Part	Approach	Device	Qualifier
Ø Internal Mammary Artery, Right	Ø Open	Ø Drainage Device	Z No Qualifier
1 Internal Mammary Artery, Left	3 Percutaneous		
2 Innominate Artery	4 Percutaneous Endoscopic		
3 Subclavian Artery, Right			
4 Subclavian Artery, Left			
5 Axillary Artery, Right			
6 Axillary Artery, Left			
7 Brachial Artery, Right			
8 Brachial Artery, Left			
9 Ulnar Artery, Right			
A Ulnar Artery, Left			
B Radial Artery, Right			
C Radial Artery, Left			
D Hand Artery, Right			
F Hand Artery, Left			
G Intracranial Artery			
H Common Carotid Artery, Right			
J Common Carotid Artery, Left			
K Internal Carotid Artery, Right			
L Internal Carotid Artery, Left			
M External Carotid Artery, Right			
N External Carotid Artery, Left			
P Vertebral Artery, Right			
Q Vertebral Artery, Left			
R Face Artery			
S Temporal Artery, Right			
T Temporal Artery, Left			
U Thyroid Artery, Right			
V Thyroid Artery, Left			
Y Upper Artery			

9: DRAINAGE

3: UPPER ARTERIES

Ø: M/S

SECTION: Ø MEDICAL AND SURGICAL
BODY SYSTEM: 3 UPPER ARTERIES
OPERATION: 9 DRAINAGE: *(continued)*
Taking or letting out fluids and/or gases from a body part

Body Part	Approach	Device	Qualifier
Ø Internal Mammary Artery, Right 1 Internal Mammary Artery, Left 2 Innominate Artery 3 Subclavian Artery, Right 4 Subclavian Artery, Left 5 Axillary Artery, Right 6 Axillary Artery, Left 7 Brachial Artery, Right 8 Brachial Artery, Left 9 Ulnar Artery, Right A Ulnar Artery, Left B Radial Artery, Right C Radial Artery, Left D Hand Artery, Right F Hand Artery, Left G Intracranial Artery H Common Carotid Artery, Right J Common Carotid Artery, Left K Internal Carotid Artery, Right L Internal Carotid Artery, Left M External Carotid Artery, Right N External Carotid Artery, Left P Vertebral Artery, Right Q Vertebral Artery, Left R Face Artery S Temporal Artery, Right T Temporal Artery, Left U Thyroid Artery, Right V Thyroid Artery, Left Y Upper Artery	Ø Open 3 Percutaneous 4 Percutaneous Endoscopic	Z No Device	X Diagnostic Z No Qualifier

SECTION: Ø MEDICAL AND SURGICAL
BODY SYSTEM: 3 UPPER ARTERIES
OPERATION: B EXCISION: Cutting out or off, without replacement, a portion of a body part

Body Part	Approach	Device	Qualifier
Ø Internal Mammary Artery, Right 1 Internal Mammary Artery, Left 2 Innominate Artery 3 Subclavian Artery, Right 4 Subclavian Artery, Left 5 Axillary Artery, Right 6 Axillary Artery, Left 7 Brachial Artery, Right 8 Brachial Artery, Left 9 Ulnar Artery, Right A Ulnar Artery, Left B Radial Artery, Right C Radial Artery, Left D Hand Artery, Right F Hand Artery, Left G Intracranial Artery H Common Carotid Artery, Right J Common Carotid Artery, Left K Internal Carotid Artery, Right L Internal Carotid Artery, Left M External Carotid Artery, Right N External Carotid Artery, Left P Vertebral Artery, Right Q Vertebral Artery, Left R Face Artery S Temporal Artery, Right T Temporal Artery, Left U Thyroid Artery, Right V Thyroid Artery, Left Y Upper Artery	Ø Open 3 Percutaneous 4 Percutaneous Endoscopic	Z No Device	X Diagnostic Z No Qualifier

SECTION: 0 MEDICAL AND SURGICAL
BODY SYSTEM: 3 UPPER ARTERIES
OPERATION: C EXTIRPATION: Taking or cutting out solid matter from a body part

Body Part	Approach	Device	Qualifier
0 Internal Mammary Artery, Right	0 Open	Z No Device	6 Bifurcation
1 Internal Mammary Artery, Left	3 Percutaneous		Z No Qualifier
2 Innominate Artery	4 Percutaneous Endoscopic		
3 Subclavian Artery, Right			
4 Subclavian Artery, Left			
5 Axillary Artery, Right			
6 Axillary Artery, Left			
7 Brachial Artery, Right			
8 Brachial Artery, Left			
9 Ulnar Artery, Right			
A Ulnar Artery, Left			
B Radial Artery, Right			
C Radial Artery, Left			
D Hand Artery, Right			
F Hand Artery, Left			
G Intracranial Artery			
H Common Carotid Artery, Right			
J Common Carotid Artery, Left			
K Internal Carotid Artery, Right			
L Internal Carotid Artery, Left			
M External Carotid Artery, Right			
N External Carotid Artery, Left			
P Vertebral Artery, Right			
Q Vertebral Artery, Left			
R Face Artery			
S Temporal Artery, Right			
T Temporal Artery, Left			
U Thyroid Artery, Right			
V Thyroid Artery, Left			
Y Upper Artery			

SECTION: Ø MEDICAL AND SURGICAL
BODY SYSTEM: 3 UPPER ARTERIES
OPERATION: **H INSERTION:** Putting in a nonbiological appliance that monitors, assists, performs, or prevents a physiological function but does not physically take the place of a body part

Body Part	Approach	Device	Qualifier
Ø Internal Mammary Artery, Right 1 Internal Mammary Artery, Left 2 Innominate Artery 3 Subclavian Artery, Right 4 Subclavian Artery, Left 5 Axillary Artery, Right 6 Axillary Artery, Left 7 Brachial Artery, Right 8 Brachial Artery, Left 9 Ulnar Artery, Right A Ulnar Artery, Left B Radial Artery, Right C Radial Artery, Left D Hand Artery, Right F Hand Artery, Left G Intracranial Artery H Common Carotid Artery, Right J Common Carotid Artery, Left M External Carotid Artery, Right N External Carotid Artery, Left P Vertebral Artery, Right Q Vertebral Artery, Left R Face Artery S Temporal Artery, Right T Temporal Artery, Left U Thyroid Artery, Right V Thyroid Artery, Left	Ø Open 3 Percutaneous 4 Percutaneous Endoscopic	3 Infusion Device D Intraluminal Device	Z No Qualifier
K Internal Carotid Artery, Right L Internal Carotid Artery, Left	Ø Open 3 Percutaneous 4 Percutaneous Endoscopic	3 Infusion Device D Intraluminal Device M Stimulator Lead	Z No Qualifier
Y Upper Artery	Ø Open 3 Percutaneous 4 Percutaneous Endoscopic	2 Monitoring Device 3 Infusion Device D Intraluminal Device Y Other Device	Z No Qualifier

SECTION: Ø MEDICAL AND SURGICAL
BODY SYSTEM: 3 UPPER ARTERIES
OPERATION: J INSPECTION: Visually and/or manually exploring a body part

Body Part	Approach	Device	Qualifier
Y Upper Artery	Ø Open 3 Percutaneous 4 Percutaneous Endoscopic X External	Z No Device	Z No Qualifier

SECTION: Ø MEDICAL AND SURGICAL
BODY SYSTEM: 3 UPPER ARTERIES
OPERATION: L OCCLUSION: Completely closing an orifice or the lumen of a tubular body part

Body Part	Approach	Device	Qualifier
Ø Internal Mammary Artery, Right 1 Internal Mammary Artery, Left 2 Innominate Artery 3 Subclavian Artery, Right 4 Subclavian Artery, Left 5 Axillary Artery, Right 6 Axillary Artery, Left 7 Brachial Artery, Right 8 Brachial Artery, Left 9 Ulnar Artery, Right A Ulnar Artery, Left B Radial Artery, Right C Radial Artery, Left D Hand Artery, Right F Hand Artery, Left R Face Artery S Temporal Artery, Right T Temporal Artery, Left U Thyroid Artery, Right V Thyroid Artery, Left Y Upper Artery	Ø Open 3 Percutaneous 4 Percutaneous Endoscopic	C Extraluminal Device D Intraluminal Device Z No Device	Z No Qualifier
G Intracranial Artery H Common Carotid Artery, Right J Common Carotid Artery, Left K Internal Carotid Artery, Right L Internal Carotid Artery, Left M External Carotid Artery, Right N External Carotid Artery, Left P Vertebral Artery, Right Q Vertebral Artery, Left	Ø Open 3 Percutaneous 4 Percutaneous Endoscopic	B Intraluminal Device, Bioactive C Extraluminal Device D Intraluminal Device Z No Device	Z No Qualifier

SECTION: Ø MEDICAL AND SURGICAL
BODY SYSTEM: 3 UPPER ARTERIES
OPERATION: N RELEASE: Freeing a body part from an abnormal physical constraint by cutting or by the use of force

Body Part	Approach	Device	Qualifier
Ø Internal Mammary Artery, Right	Ø Open	Z No Device	Z No Qualifier
1 Internal Mammary Artery, Left	3 Percutaneous		
2 Innominate Artery	4 Percutaneous Endoscopic		
3 Subclavian Artery, Right			
4 Subclavian Artery, Left			
5 Axillary Artery, Right			
6 Axillary Artery, Left			
7 Brachial Artery, Right			
8 Brachial Artery, Left			
9 Ulnar Artery, Right			
A Ulnar Artery, Left			
B Radial Artery, Right			
C Radial Artery, Left			
D Hand Artery, Right			
F Hand Artery, Left			
G Intracranial Artery			
H Common Carotid Artery, Right			
J Common Carotid Artery, Left			
K Internal Carotid Artery, Right			
L Internal Carotid Artery, Left			
M External Carotid Artery, Right			
N External Carotid Artery, Left			
P Vertebral Artery, Right			
Q Vertebral Artery, Left			
R Face Artery			
S Temporal Artery, Right			
T Temporal Artery, Left			
U Thyroid Artery, Right			
V Thyroid Artery, Left			
Y Upper Artery			

SECTION: 0 MEDICAL AND SURGICAL
BODY SYSTEM: 3 UPPER ARTERIES
OPERATION: P REMOVAL: Taking out or off a device from a body part

Body Part	Approach	Device	Qualifier
Y Upper Artery	0 Open 3 Percutaneous 4 Percutaneous Endoscopic	0 Drainage Device 2 Monitoring Device 3 Infusion Device 7 Autologous Tissue Substitute C Extraluminal Device D Intraluminal Device J Synthetic Substitute K Nonautologous Tissue Substitute M Stimulator Lead Y Other Device	Z No Qualifier
Y Upper Artery	X External	0 Drainage Device 2 Monitoring Device 3 Infusion Device D Intraluminal Device M Stimulator Lead	Z No Qualifier

SECTION: Ø MEDICAL AND SURGICAL
BODY SYSTEM: 3 UPPER ARTERIES
OPERATION: Q REPAIR: Restoring, to the extent possible, a body part to its normal anatomic structure and function

Body Part	Approach	Device	Qualifier
Ø Internal Mammary Artery, Right 1 Internal Mammary Artery, Left 2 Innominate Artery 3 Subclavian Artery, Right 4 Subclavian Artery, Left 5 Axillary Artery, Right 6 Axillary Artery, Left 7 Brachial Artery, Right 8 Brachial Artery, Left 9 Ulnar Artery, Right A Ulnar Artery, Left B Radial Artery, Right C Radial Artery, Left D Hand Artery, Right F Hand Artery, Left G Intracranial Artery H Common Carotid Artery, Right J Common Carotid Artery, Left K Internal Carotid Artery, Right L Internal Carotid Artery, Left M External Carotid Artery, Right N External Carotid Artery, Left P Vertebral Artery, Right Q Vertebral Artery, Left R Face Artery S Temporal Artery, Right T Temporal Artery, Left U Thyroid Artery, Right V Thyroid Artery, Left Y Upper Artery	Ø Open 3 Percutaneous 4 Percutaneous Endoscopic	Z No Device	Z No Qualifier

SECTION: Ø MEDICAL AND SURGICAL
BODY SYSTEM: 3 UPPER ARTERIES
OPERATION: R REPLACEMENT: Putting in or on biological or synthetic material that physically takes the place and/or function of all or a portion of a body part

Body Part	Approach	Device	Qualifier
Ø Internal Mammary Artery, Right	Ø Open	7 Autologous Tissue Substitute	Z No Qualifier
1 Internal Mammary Artery, Left	4 Percutaneous Endoscopic	J Synthetic Substitute	
2 Innominate Artery		K Nonautologous Tissue Substitute	
3 Subclavian Artery, Right			
4 Subclavian Artery, Left			
5 Axillary Artery, Right			
6 Axillary Artery, Left			
7 Brachial Artery, Right			
8 Brachial Artery, Left			
9 Ulnar Artery, Right			
A Ulnar Artery, Left			
B Radial Artery, Right			
C Radial Artery, Left			
D Hand Artery, Right			
F Hand Artery, Left			
G Intracranial Artery			
H Common Carotid Artery, Right			
J Common Carotid Artery, Left			
K Internal Carotid Artery, Right			
L Internal Carotid Artery, Left			
M External Carotid Artery, Right			
N External Carotid Artery, Left			
P Vertebral Artery, Right			
Q Vertebral Artery, Left			
R Face Artery			
S Temporal Artery, Right			
T Temporal Artery, Left			
U Thyroid Artery, Right			
V Thyroid Artery, Left			
Y Upper Artery			

SECTION: 0 MEDICAL AND SURGICAL
BODY SYSTEM: 3 UPPER ARTERIES
OPERATION: S REPOSITION: Moving to its normal location, or other suitable location, all or a portion of a body part

Body Part	Approach	Device	Qualifier
0 Internal Mammary Artery, Right 1 Internal Mammary Artery, Left 2 Innominate Artery 3 Subclavian Artery, Right 4 Subclavian Artery, Left 5 Axillary Artery, Right 6 Axillary Artery, Left 7 Brachial Artery, Right 8 Brachial Artery, Left 9 Ulnar Artery, Right A Ulnar Artery, Left B Radial Artery, Right C Radial Artery, Left D Hand Artery, Right F Hand Artery, Left G Intracranial Artery H Common Carotid Artery, Right J Common Carotid Artery, Left K Internal Carotid Artery, Right L Internal Carotid Artery, Left M External Carotid Artery, Right N External Carotid Artery, Left P Vertebral Artery, Right Q Vertebral Artery, Left R Face Artery S Temporal Artery, Right T Temporal Artery, Left U Thyroid Artery, Right V Thyroid Artery, Left Y Upper Artery	0 Open 3 Percutaneous 4 Percutaneous Endoscopic	Z No Device	Z No Qualifier

S: REPOSITION

3: UPPER ARTERIES

0: M/S

SECTION: Ø MEDICAL AND SURGICAL
BODY SYSTEM: 3 UPPER ARTERIES

OPERATION: U SUPPLEMENT: Putting in or on biological or synthetic material that physically reinforces and/or augments the function of a portion of a body part

Body Part	Approach	Device	Qualifier
Ø Internal Mammary Artery, Right 1 Internal Mammary Artery, Left 2 Innominate Artery 3 Subclavian Artery, Right 4 Subclavian Artery, Left 5 Axillary Artery, Right 6 Axillary Artery, Left 7 Brachial Artery, Right 8 Brachial Artery, Left 9 Ulnar Artery, Right A Ulnar Artery, Left B Radial Artery, Right C Radial Artery, Left D Hand Artery, Right F Hand Artery, Left G Intracranial Artery H Common Carotid Artery, Right J Common Carotid Artery, Left K Internal Carotid Artery, Right L Internal Carotid Artery, Left M External Carotid Artery, Right N External Carotid Artery, Left P Vertebral Artery, Right Q Vertebral Artery, Left R Face Artery S Temporal Artery, Right T Temporal Artery, Left U Thyroid Artery, Right V Thyroid Artery, Left Y Upper Artery	Ø Open 3 Percutaneous 4 Percutaneous Endoscopic	7 Autologous Tissue Substitute J Synthetic Substitute K Nonautologous Tissue Substitute	Z No Qualifier

SECTION: Ø MEDICAL AND SURGICAL
BODY SYSTEM: 3 UPPER ARTERIES
OPERATION: **V RESTRICTION:** Partially closing an orifice or the lumen of a tubular body part

Body Part	Approach	Device	Qualifier
Ø Internal Mammary Artery, Right 1 Internal Mammary Artery, Left 2 Innominate Artery 3 Subclavian Artery, Right 4 Subclavian Artery, Left 5 Axillary Artery, Right 6 Axillary Artery, Left 7 Brachial Artery, Right 8 Brachial Artery, Left 9 Ulnar Artery, Right A Ulnar Artery, Left B Radial Artery, Right C Radial Artery, Left D Hand Artery, Right F Hand Artery, Left R Face Artery S Temporal Artery, Right T Temporal Artery, Left U Thyroid Artery, Right V Thyroid Artery, Left Y Upper Artery	Ø Open 3 Percutaneous 4 Percutaneous Endoscopic	C Extraluminal Device D Intraluminal Device Z No Device	Z No Qualifier
G Intracranial Artery H Common Carotid Artery, Right J Common Carotid Artery, Left K Internal Carotid Artery, Right L Internal Carotid Artery, Left M External Carotid Artery, Right N External Carotid Artery, Left P Vertebral Artery, Right Q Vertebral Artery, Left	Ø Open 3 Percutaneous 4 Percutaneous Endoscopic	B Intraluminal Device, Bioactive C Extraluminal Device D Intraluminal Device Z No Device	Z No Qualifier

SECTION: Ø MEDICAL AND SURGICAL
BODY SYSTEM: 3 UPPER ARTERIES
OPERATION: W REVISION: Correcting, to the extent possible, a portion of a malfunctioning device or the position of a displaced device

Body Part	Approach	Device	Qualifier
Y Upper Artery	Ø Open 3 Percutaneous 4 Percutaneous Endoscopic ~~X External~~	Ø Drainage Device 2 Monitoring Device 3 Infusion Device 7 Autologous Tissue Substitute C Extraluminal Device D Intraluminal Device J Synthetic Substitute K Nonautologous Tissue Substitute M Stimulator Lead Y Other Device	Z No Qualifier
Y Upper Artery	X External	Ø Drainage Device 2 Monitoring Device 3 Infusion Device 7 Autologous Tissue Substitute C Extraluminal Device D Intraluminal Device J Synthetic Substitute K Nonautologous Tissue Substitute M Stimulator Lead	Z No Qualifier

Ø4. Lower Arteries 74
    Ø41. Bypass...75
    Ø45. Destruction..76
    Ø47. Dilation...77
    Ø49. Drainage 79
    Ø4B. Excision 81
    Ø4C. Extirpation 82
    Ø4H. Insertion 83
    Ø4J. Inspection 84
    Ø4L. Occlusion 85
    Ø4N. Release 86
    Ø4P. Removal 87
    Ø4Q. Repair 88
    Ø4R. Replacement 89
    Ø4S. Reposition...9Ø
    Ø4U. Supplement...91
    Ø4V. Restriction...92
    Ø4W. Revision..93

SECTION: Ø MEDICAL AND SURGICAL
BODY SYSTEM: 4 LOWER ARTERIES
OPERATION: 1 BYPASS: *(on multiple pages)*
Altering the route of passage of the contents of a tubular body part

Body Part	Approach	Device	Qualifier
Ø Abdominal Aorta C Common Iliac Artery, Right D Common Iliac Artery, Left	Ø Open 4 Percutaneous Endoscopic	9 Autologous Venous Tissue A Autologous Arterial Tissue J Synthetic Substitute K Nonautologous Tissue Substitute Z No Device	Ø Abdominal Aorta 1 Celiac Artery 2 Mesenteric Artery 3 Renal Artery, Right 4 Renal Artery, Left 5 Renal Artery, Bilateral 6 Common Iliac Artery, Right 7 Common Iliac Artery, Left 8 Common Iliac Arteries, Bilateral 9 Internal Iliac Artery, Right B Internal Iliac Artery, Left C Internal Iliac Arteries, Bilateral D External Iliac Artery, Right F External Iliac Artery, Left G External Iliac Arteries, Bilateral H Femoral Artery, Right J Femoral Artery, Left K Femoral Arteries, Bilateral Q Lower Extremity Artery R Lower Artery
3 Hepatic Artery 4 Splenic Artery	Ø Open 4 Percutaneous Endoscopic	9 Autologous Venous Tissue A Autologous Arterial Tissue J Synthetic Substitute K Nonautologous Tissue Substitute Z No Device	3 Renal Artery, Right 4 Renal Artery, Left 5 Renal Artery, Bilateral
E Internal Iliac Artery, Right F Internal Iliac Artery, Left H External Iliac Artery, Right J External Iliac Artery, Left	Ø Open 4 Percutaneous Endoscopic	9 Autologous Venous Tissue A Autologous Arterial Tissue J Synthetic Substitute K Nonautologous Tissue Substitute Z No Device	9 Internal Iliac Artery, Right B Internal Iliac Artery, Left C Internal Iliac Arteries, Bilateral D External Iliac Artery, Right F External Iliac Artery, Left G External Iliac Arteries, Bilateral H Femoral Artery, Right J Femoral Artery, Left K Femoral Arteries, Bilateral P Foot Artery Q Lower Extremity Artery
K Femoral Artery, Right L Femoral Artery, Left	Ø Open 4 Percutaneous Endoscopic	9 Autologous Venous Tissue A Autologous Arterial Tissue J Synthetic Substitute K Nonautologous Tissue Substitute Z No Device	H Femoral Artery, Right J Femoral Artery, Left K Femoral Arteries, Bilateral L Popliteal Artery M Peroneal Artery N Posterior Tibial Artery P Foot Artery Q Lower Extremity Artery S Lower Extremity Vein

SECTION: Ø MEDICAL AND SURGICAL

BODY SYSTEM: 4 **LOWER ARTERIES**
OPERATION: 1 **BYPASS:** *(continued)*
Altering the route of passage of the contents of a tubular body part

Body Part	Approach	Device	Qualifier
M Popliteal Artery, Right N Popliteal Artery, Left	Ø Open 4 Percutaneous Endoscopic	9 Autologous Venous Tissue A Autologous Arterial Tissue J Synthetic Substitute K Nonautologous Tissue Substitute Z No Device	L Popliteal Artery M Peroneal Artery P Foot Artery Q Lower Extremity Artery S Lower Extremity Vein
T Peroneal Artery, Right U Peroneal Artery, Left V Foot Artery, Right W Foot Artery, Left	Ø Open 4 Percutaneous Endoscopic	9 Autologous Venous Tissue A Autologous Arterial Tissue J Synthetic Substitute K Nonautologous Tissue Substitute Z No Device	P Foot Artery Q Lower Extremity Artery S Lower Extremity Vein

SECTION: Ø MEDICAL AND SURGICAL

BODY SYSTEM: 4 **LOWER ARTERIES**
OPERATION: 5 **DESTRUCTION:** Physical eradication of all or a portion of a body part by the direct use of energy, force, or a destructive agent

Body Part	Approach	Device	Qualifier
Ø Abdominal Aorta 1 Celiac Artery 2 Gastric Artery 3 Hepatic Artery 4 Splenic Artery 5 Superior Mesenteric Artery 6 Colic Artery, Right 7 Colic Artery, Left 8 Colic Artery, Middle 9 Renal Artery, Right A Renal Artery, Left B Inferior Mesenteric Artery C Common Iliac Artery, Right D Common Iliac Artery, Left E Internal Iliac Artery, Right F Internal Iliac Artery, Left H External Iliac Artery, Right J External Iliac Artery, Left K Femoral Artery, Right L Femoral Artery, Left M Popliteal Artery, Right N Popliteal Artery, Left P Anterior Tibial Artery, Right Q Anterior Tibial Artery, Left R Posterior Tibial Artery, Right S Posterior Tibial Artery, Left T Peroneal Artery, Right U Peroneal Artery, Left V Foot Artery, Right W Foot Artery, Left Y Lower Artery	Ø Open 3 Percutaneous 4 Percutaneous Endoscopic	Z No Device	Z No Qualifier

1: BYPASS   5: DESTRUCTION

4: LOWER ARTERIES   Ø: M/S

SECTION: Ø MEDICAL AND SURGICAL
BODY SYSTEM: 4 LOWER ARTERIES
OPERATION: 7 DILATION: *(on multiple pages)*
Expanding an orifice or the lumen of a tubular body part

Body Part	Approach	Device	Qualifier
Ø Abdominal Aorta 1 Celiac Artery 2 Gastric Artery 3 Hepatic Artery 4 Splenic Artery 5 Superior Mesenteric Artery 6 Colic Artery, Right 7 Colic Artery, Left 8 Colic Artery, Middle 9 Renal Artery, Right A Renal Artery, Left B Inferior Mesenteric Artery C Common Iliac Artery, Right D Common Iliac Artery, Left E Internal Iliac Artery, Right F Internal Iliac Artery, Left H External Iliac Artery, Right J External Iliac Artery, Left K Femoral Carotid Artery, Right L Femoral Carotid Artery, Left M Popliteal Carotid Artery, Right N Popliteal Carotid Artery, Left P Anterior Tibial Artery, Right Q Anterior Tibial Artery, Left R Posterior Tibial Artery, Right S Posterior Tibial Artery, Left T Peroneal Artery, Right U Peroneal Artery, Left V Foot Artery, Right W Foot Artery, Left Y Lower Artery	Ø Open 3 Percutaneous 4 Percutaneous Endoscopic	4 Intraluminal Device, Drug-eluting ~~5 Intraluminal Device, Drug-eluting, Two~~ ~~6 Intraluminal Device, Drug-eluting, Three~~ ~~7 Intraluminal Device, Drug-eluting, Four or More~~ D Intraluminal Device ~~E Intraluminal Device, Two~~ ~~F Intraluminal Device, Three~~ ~~G Intraluminal Device, Four or More~~ Z No Device	1 Drug-Coated Balloon 6 Bifurcation Z No Qualifier
~~K Femoral Artery, Right~~ ~~L Femoral Artery, Left~~ ~~M Popliteal Artery, Right~~ ~~N Popliteal Artery, Left~~	~~Ø Open~~ ~~3 Percutaneous~~ ~~4 Percutaneous Endoscopic~~	~~4 Intraluminal Device, Drug-eluting~~ ~~D Intraluminal Device~~ ~~Z No Device~~	~~1 Drug-Coated Balloon~~ ~~6 Bifurcation~~ ~~Z No Qualifier~~

SECTION: Ø MEDICAL AND SURGICAL
BODY SYSTEM: 4 LOWER ARTERIES
OPERATION: 7 DILATION: *(continued)*
Expanding an orifice or the lumen of a tubular body part

Body Part	Approach	Device	Qualifier
Ø Abdominal Aorta	Ø Open	5 Intraluminal Device, Drug-eluting, Two	6 Bifurcation
1 Celiac Artery	3 Percutaneous	6 Intraluminal Device, Drug-eluting, Three	Z No Qualifier
2 Gastric Artery	4 Percutaneous Endoscopic	7 Intraluminal Device, Drug-eluting, Four or More	
3 Hepatic Artery		E Intraluminal Device, Two	
4 Splenic Artery		F Intraluminal Device, Three	
5 Superior Mesenteric Artery		G Intraluminal Device, Four or More	
6 Colic Artery, Right			
7 Colic Artery, Left			
8 Colic Artery, Middle			
9 Renal Artery, Right			
A Renal Artery, Left			
B Inferior Mesenteric Artery			
C Common Iliac Artery, Right			
D Common Iliac Artery, Left			
E Internal Iliac Artery, Right			
F Internal Iliac Artery, Left			
H External Iliac Artery, Right			
J External Iliac Artery, Left			
K Femoral Carotid Artery, Right			
L Femoral Carotid Artery, Left			
M Popliteal Carotid Artery, Right			
N Popliteal Carotid Artery, Left			
P Anterior Tibial Artery, Right			
Q Anterior Tibial Artery, Left			
R Posterior Tibial Artery, Right			
S Posterior Tibial Artery, Left			
T Peroneal Artery, Right			
U Peroneal Artery, Left			
V Foot Artery, Right			
W Foot Artery, Left			
Y Lower Artery			

7: DILATION

4: LOWER ARTERIES

Ø: M/S

SECTION: Ø MEDICAL AND SURGICAL
BODY SYSTEM: 4 LOWER ARTERIES
OPERATION: 9 DRAINAGE: *(on multiple pages)*
Taking or letting out fluids and/or gases from a body part

Body Part	Approach	Device	Qualifier
Ø Abdominal Aorta	Ø Open	Ø Drainage Device	Z No Qualifier
1 Celiac Artery	3 Percutaneous		
2 Gastric Artery	4 Percutaneous Endoscopic		
3 Hepatic Artery			
4 Splenic Artery			
5 Superior Mesenteric Artery			
6 Colic Artery, Right			
7 Colic Artery, Left			
8 Colic Artery, Middle			
9 Renal Artery, Right			
A Renal Artery, Left			
B Inferior Mesenteric Artery			
C Common Iliac Artery, Right			
D Common Iliac Artery, Left			
E Internal Iliac Artery, Right			
F Internal Iliac Artery, Left			
H External Iliac Artery, Right			
J External Iliac Artery, Left			
K Femoral Artery, Right			
L Femoral Artery, Left			
M Popliteal Artery, Right			
N Popliteal Artery, Left			
P Anterior Tibial Artery, Right			
Q Anterior Tibial Artery, Left			
R Posterior Tibial Artery, Right			
S Posterior Tibial Artery, Left			
T Peroneal Artery, Right			
U Peroneal Artery, Left			
V Foot Artery, Right			
W Foot Artery, Left			
Y Lower Artery			

SECTION: Ø MEDICAL AND SURGICAL
BODY SYSTEM: 4 LOWER ARTERIES
OPERATION: 9 DRAINAGE: *(continued)*
Taking or letting out fluids and/or gases from a body part

Body Part	Approach	Device	Qualifier
Ø Abdominal Aorta	Ø Open	Z No Device	X Diagnostic
1 Celiac Artery	3 Percutaneous		Z No Qualifier
2 Gastric Artery	4 Percutaneous Endoscopic		
3 Hepatic Artery			
4 Splenic Artery			
5 Superior Mesenteric Artery			
6 Colic Artery, Right			
7 Colic Artery, Left			
8 Colic Artery, Middle			
9 Renal Artery, Right			
A Renal Artery, Left			
B Inferior Mesenteric Artery			
C Common Iliac Artery, Right			
D Common Iliac Artery, Left			
E Internal Iliac Artery, Right			
F Internal Iliac Artery, Left			
H External Iliac Artery, Right			
J External Iliac Artery, Left			
K Femoral Artery, Right			
L Femoral Artery, Left			
M Popliteal Artery, Right			
N Popliteal Artery, Left			
P Anterior Tibial Artery, Right			
Q Anterior Tibial Artery, Left			
R Posterior Tibial Artery, Right			
S Posterior Tibial Artery, Left			
T Peroneal Artery, Right			
U Peroneal Artery, Left			
V Foot Artery, Right			
W Foot Artery, Left			
Y Lower Artery			

9: DRAINAGE

4: LOWER ARTERIES

Ø: M/S

SECTION: Ø MEDICAL AND SURGICAL
BODY SYSTEM: 4 LOWER ARTERIES
OPERATION: B EXCISION: Cutting out or off, without replacement, a portion of a body part

Body Part	Approach	Device	Qualifier
Ø Abdominal Aorta	Ø Open	Z No Device	X Diagnostic
1 Celiac Artery	3 Percutaneous		Z No Qualifier
2 Gastric Artery	4 Percutaneous Endoscopic		
3 Hepatic Artery			
4 Splenic Artery			
5 Superior Mesenteric Artery			
6 Colic Artery, Right			
7 Colic Artery, Left			
8 Colic Artery, Middle			
9 Renal Artery, Right			
A Renal Artery, Left			
B Inferior Mesenteric Artery			
C Common Iliac Artery, Right			
D Common Iliac Artery, Left			
E Internal Iliac Artery, Right			
F Internal Iliac Artery, Left			
H External Iliac Artery, Right			
J External Iliac Artery, Left			
K Femoral Artery, Right			
L Femoral Artery, Left			
M Popliteal Artery, Right			
N Popliteal Artery, Left			
P Anterior Tibial Artery, Right			
Q Anterior Tibial Artery, Left			
R Posterior Tibial Artery, Right			
S Posterior Tibial Artery, Left			
T Peroneal Artery, Right			
U Peroneal Artery, Left			
V Foot Artery, Right			
W Foot Artery, Left			
Y Lower Artery			

Ø: M/S   4: LOWER ARTERIES   B: EXCISION

SECTION: Ø MEDICAL AND SURGICAL
BODY SYSTEM: 4 LOWER ARTERIES
OPERATION: C EXTIRPATION: Taking or cutting out solid matter from a body part

Body Part	Approach	Device	Qualifier
Ø Abdominal Aorta	Ø Open	Z No Device	6 Bifurcation
1 Celiac Artery	3 Percutaneous		Z No Qualifier
2 Gastric Artery	4 Percutaneous Endoscopic		
3 Hepatic Artery			
4 Splenic Artery			
5 Superior Mesenteric Artery			
6 Colic Artery, Right			
7 Colic Artery, Left			
8 Colic Artery, Middle			
9 Renal Artery, Right			
A Renal Artery, Left			
B Inferior Mesenteric Artery			
C Common Iliac Artery, Right			
D Common Iliac Artery, Left			
E Internal Iliac Artery, Right			
F Internal Iliac Artery, Left			
H External Iliac Artery, Right			
J External Iliac Artery, Left			
K Femoral Artery, Right			
L Femoral Artery, Left			
M Popliteal Artery, Right			
N Popliteal Artery, Left			
P Anterior Tibial Artery, Right			
Q Anterior Tibial Artery, Left			
R Posterior Tibial Artery, Right			
S Posterior Tibial Artery, Left			
T Peroneal Artery, Right			
U Peroneal Artery, Left			
V Foot Artery, Right			
W Foot Artery, Left			
Y Lower Artery			

SECTION: Ø MEDICAL AND SURGICAL
BODY SYSTEM: 4 **LOWER ARTERIES**

OPERATION: H **INSERTION:** Putting in a nonbiological appliance that monitors, assists, performs, or prevents a physiological function but does not physically take the place of a body part

Body Part	Approach	Device	Qualifier
Ø Abdominal Aorta ~~Y Lower Artery~~	Ø Open 3 Percutaneous 4 Percutaneous Endoscopic	2 Monitoring Device 3 Infusion Device D Intraluminal Device	Z No Qualifier
1 Celiac Artery 2 Gastric Artery 3 Hepatic Artery 4 Splenic Artery 5 Superior Mesenteric Artery 6 Colic Artery, Right 7 Colic Artery, Left 8 Colic Artery, Middle 9 Renal Artery, Right A Renal Artery, Left B Inferior Mesenteric Artery C Common Iliac Artery, Right D Common Iliac Artery, Left E Internal Iliac Artery, Right F Internal Iliac Artery, Left H External Iliac Artery, Right J External Iliac Artery, Left K Femoral Artery, Right L Femoral Artery, Left M Popliteal Artery, Right N Popliteal Artery, Left P Anterior Tibial Artery, Right Q Anterior Tibial Artery, Left R Posterior Tibial Artery, Right S Posterior Tibial Artery, Left T Peroneal Artery, Right U Peroneal Artery, Left V Foot Artery, Right W Foot Artery, Left	Ø Open 3 Percutaneous 4 Percutaneous Endoscopic	3 Infusion Device D Intraluminal Device	Z No Qualifier
Y Lower Artery	Ø Open 3 Percutaneous 4 Percutaneous Endoscopic	2 Monitoring Device 3 Infusion Device D Intraluminal Device Y Other Device	Z No Qualifier

SECTION: Ø MEDICAL AND SURGICAL
BODY SYSTEM: 4 LOWER ARTERIES
OPERATION: J INSPECTION: Visually and/or manually exploring a body part

Body Part	Approach	Device	Qualifier
Y Lower Artery	Ø Open 3 Percutaneous 4 Percutaneous Endoscopic X External	Z No Device	Z No Qualifier

SECTION: Ø MEDICAL AND SURGICAL
BODY SYSTEM: 4 LOWER ARTERIES
OPERATION: L OCCLUSION: Completely closing an orifice or the lumen of a tubular body part

Body Part	Approach	Device	Qualifier
Ø Abdominal Aorta	Ø Open 4 Percutaneous Endoscopic	C Extraluminal Device D Intraluminal Device Z No Device	Z No Qualifier
Ø Abdominal Aorta	3 Percutaneous	C Extraluminal Device Z No Device	Z No Qualifier
Ø Abdominal Aorta	3 Percutaneous	D Intraluminal Device	J Temporary Z No Qualifier
Ø Abdominal Aorta 1 Celiac Artery 2 Gastric Artery 3 Hepatic Artery 4 Splenic Artery 5 Superior Mesenteric Artery 6 Colic Artery, Right 7 Colic Artery, Left 8 Colic Artery, Middle 9 Renal Artery, Right A Renal Artery, Left B Inferior Mesenteric Artery C Common Iliac Artery, Right D Common Iliac Artery, Left H External Iliac Artery, Right J External Iliac Artery, Left K Femoral Artery, Right L Femoral Artery, Left M Popliteal Artery, Right N Popliteal Artery, Left P Anterior Tibial Artery, Right Q Anterior Tibial Artery, Left R Posterior Tibial Artery, Right S Posterior Tibial Artery, Left T Peroneal Artery, Right U Peroneal Artery, Left V Foot Artery, Right W Foot Artery, Left Y Lower Artery	Ø Open 3 Percutaneous 4 Percutaneous Endoscopic	C Extraluminal Device D Intraluminal Device Z No Device	Z No Qualifier
E Internal Iliac Artery, Right	Ø Open 3 Percutaneous 4 Percutaneous Endoscopic	C Extraluminal Device D Intraluminal Device Z No Device	T Uterine Artery, Right Z No Qualifier
F Internal Iliac Artery, Left	Ø Open 3 Percutaneous 4 Percutaneous Endoscopic	C Extraluminal Device D Intraluminal Device Z No Device	U Uterine Artery, Left Z No Qualifier

Ø: M/S

4: LOWER ARTERIES

L: OCCLUSION

SECTION: 0 MEDICAL AND SURGICAL
BODY SYSTEM: 4 LOWER ARTERIES
OPERATION: N RELEASE: Freeing a body part from an abnormal physical constraint by cutting or by the use of force

Body Part	Approach	Device	Qualifier
0 Abdominal Aorta	0 Open	Z No Device	Z No Qualifier
1 Celiac Artery	3 Percutaneous		
2 Gastric Artery	4 Percutaneous Endoscopic		
3 Hepatic Artery			
4 Splenic Artery			
5 Superior Mesenteric Artery			
6 Colic Artery, Right			
7 Colic Artery, Left			
8 Colic Artery, Middle			
9 Renal Artery, Right			
A Renal Artery, Left			
B Inferior Mesenteric Artery			
C Common Iliac Artery, Right			
D Common Iliac Artery, Left			
E Internal Iliac Artery, Right			
F Internal Iliac Artery, Left			
H External Iliac Artery, Right			
J External Iliac Artery, Left			
K Femoral Artery, Right			
L Femoral Artery, Left			
M Popliteal Artery, Right			
N Popliteal Artery, Left			
P Anterior Tibial Artery, Right			
Q Anterior Tibial Artery, Left			
R Posterior Tibial Artery, Right			
S Posterior Tibial Artery, Left			
T Peroneal Artery, Right			
U Peroneal Artery, Left			
V Foot Artery, Right			
W Foot Artery, Left			
Y Lower Artery			

New/Revised Text in Blue   ~~deleted~~ Deleted

SECTION: 0 MEDICAL AND SURGICAL
BODY SYSTEM: 4 LOWER ARTERIES
OPERATION: P REMOVAL: Taking out or off a device from a body part

Body Part	Approach	Device	Qualifier
Y Lower Artery	0 Open 3 Percutaneous 4 Percutaneous Endoscopic	0 Drainage Device 2 Monitoring Device 3 Infusion Device 7 Autologous Tissue Substitute C Extraluminal Device D Intraluminal Device J Synthetic Substitute K Nonautologous Tissue Substitute Y Other Device	Z No Qualifier
Y Lower Artery	X External	0 Drainage Device 1 Radioactive Element 2 Monitoring Device 3 Infusion Device D Intraluminal Device	Z No Qualifier

SECTION: Ø MEDICAL AND SURGICAL

BODY SYSTEM: 4 LOWER ARTERIES

OPERATION: Q REPAIR: Restoring, to the extent possible, a body part to its normal anatomic structure and function

Body Part	Approach	Device	Qualifier
Ø Abdominal Aorta	Ø Open	Z No Device	Z No Qualifier
1 Celiac Artery	3 Percutaneous		
2 Gastric Artery	4 Percutaneous Endoscopic		
3 Hepatic Artery			
4 Splenic Artery			
5 Superior Mesenteric Artery			
6 Colic Artery, Right			
7 Colic Artery, Left			
8 Colic Artery, Middle			
9 Renal Artery, Right			
A Renal Artery, Left			
B Inferior Mesenteric Artery			
C Common Iliac Artery, Right			
D Common Iliac Artery, Left			
E Internal Iliac Artery, Right			
F Internal Iliac Artery, Left			
H External Iliac Artery, Right			
J External Iliac Artery, Left			
K Femoral Artery, Right			
L Femoral Artery, Left			
M Popliteal Artery, Right			
N Popliteal Artery, Left			
P Anterior Tibial Artery, Right			
Q Anterior Tibial Artery, Left			
R Posterior Tibial Artery, Right			
S Posterior Tibial Artery, Left			
T Peroneal Artery, Right			
U Peroneal Artery, Left			
V Foot Artery, Right			
W Foot Artery, Left			
Y Lower Artery			

Q: REPAIR

4: LOWER ARTERIES

Ø: M/S

               New/Revised Text in Blue   ~~deleted~~ Deleted

SECTION: 0 MEDICAL AND SURGICAL

BODY SYSTEM: 4 LOWER ARTERIES

OPERATION: **R REPLACEMENT:** Putting in or on biological or synthetic material that physically takes the place and/or function of all or a portion of a body part

Body Part	Approach	Device	Qualifier
0 Abdominal Aorta	0 Open	7 Autologous Tissue Substitute	Z No Qualifier
1 Celiac Artery	4 Percutaneous Endoscopic	J Synthetic Substitute	
2 Gastric Artery		K Nonautologous Tissue Substitute	
3 Hepatic Artery			
4 Splenic Artery			
5 Superior Mesenteric Artery			
6 Colic Artery, Right			
7 Colic Artery, Left			
8 Colic Artery, Middle			
9 Renal Artery, Right			
A Renal Artery, Left			
B Inferior Mesenteric Artery			
C Common Iliac Artery, Right			
D Common Iliac Artery, Left			
E Internal Iliac Artery, Right			
F Internal Iliac Artery, Left			
H External Iliac Artery, Right			
J External Iliac Artery, Left			
K Femoral Artery, Right			
L Femoral Artery, Left			
M Popliteal Artery, Right			
N Popliteal Artery, Left			
P Anterior Tibial Artery, Right			
Q Anterior Tibial Artery, Left			
R Posterior Tibial Artery, Right			
S Posterior Tibial Artery, Left			
T Peroneal Artery, Right			
U Peroneal Artery, Left			
V Foot Artery, Right			
W Foot Artery, Left			
Y Lower Artery			

SECTION: Ø MEDICAL AND SURGICAL
BODY SYSTEM: 4 LOWER ARTERIES
OPERATION: S REPOSITION: Moving to its normal location, or other suitable location, all or a portion of a body part

Body Part	Approach	Device	Qualifier
Ø Abdominal Aorta	Ø Open	Z No Device	Z No Qualifier
1 Celiac Artery	3 Percutaneous		
2 Gastric Artery	4 Percutaneous Endoscopic		
3 Hepatic Artery			
4 Splenic Artery			
5 Superior Mesenteric Artery			
6 Colic Artery, Right			
7 Colic Artery, Left			
8 Colic Artery, Middle			
9 Renal Artery, Right			
A Renal Artery, Left			
B Inferior Mesenteric Artery			
C Common Iliac Artery, Right			
D Common Iliac Artery, Left			
E Internal Iliac Artery, Right			
F Internal Iliac Artery, Left			
H External Iliac Artery, Right			
J External Iliac Artery, Left			
K Femoral Artery, Right			
L Femoral Artery, Left			
M Popliteal Artery, Right			
N Popliteal Artery, Left			
P Anterior Tibial Artery, Right			
Q Anterior Tibial Artery, Left			
R Posterior Tibial Artery, Right			
S Posterior Tibial Artery, Left			
T Peroneal Artery, Right			
U Peroneal Artery, Left			
V Foot Artery, Right			
W Foot Artery, Left			
Y Lower Artery			

SECTION: Ø **MEDICAL AND SURGICAL**
BODY SYSTEM: 4 **LOWER ARTERIES**
OPERATION: **U SUPPLEMENT:** Putting in or on biological or synthetic material that physically reinforces and/or augments the function of a portion of a body part

Body Part	Approach	Device	Qualifier
Ø Abdominal Aorta 1 Celiac Artery 2 Gastric Artery 3 Hepatic Artery 4 Splenic Artery 5 Superior Mesenteric Artery 6 Colic Artery, Right 7 Colic Artery, Left 8 Colic Artery, Middle 9 Renal Artery, Right A Renal Artery, Left B Inferior Mesenteric Artery C Common Iliac Artery, Right D Common Iliac Artery, Left E Internal Iliac Artery, Right F Internal Iliac Artery, Left H External Iliac Artery, Right J External Iliac Artery, Left K Femoral Artery, Right L Femoral Artery, Left M Popliteal Artery, Right N Popliteal Artery, Left P Anterior Tibial Artery, Right Q Anterior Tibial Artery, Left R Posterior Tibial Artery, Right S Posterior Tibial Artery, Left T Peroneal Artery, Right U Peroneal Artery, Left V Foot Artery, Right W Foot Artery, Left Y Lower Artery	Ø Open 3 Percutaneous 4 Percutaneous Endoscopic	7 Autologous Tissue Substitute J Synthetic Substitute K Nonautologous Tissue Substitute	Z No Qualifier

SECTION:　Ø　MEDICAL AND SURGICAL
BODY SYSTEM: 4　**LOWER ARTERIES**
OPERATION:　V　**RESTRICTION:** Partially closing an orifice or the lumen of a tubular body part

Body Part	Approach	Device	Qualifier
Ø Abdominal Aorta	Ø Open 3 Percutaneous 4 Percutaneous Endoscopic	C Extraluminal Device E Intraluminal Device, Branched or Fenestrated, One or Two Arteries F Intraluminal Device, Branched or Fenestrated, Three or More Arteries Z No Device	6 Bifurcation Z No Qualifier
Ø Abdominal Aorta	Ø Open 3 Percutaneous 4 Percutaneous Endoscopic	D Intraluminal Device	6 Bifurcation J Temporary Z No Qualifier
1 Celiac Artery 2 Gastric Artery 3 Hepatic Artery 4 Splenic Artery 5 Superior Mesenteric Artery 6 Colic Artery, Right 7 Colic Artery, Left 8 Colic Artery, Middle 9 Renal Artery, Right A Renal Artery, Left B Inferior Mesenteric Artery E Internal Iliac Artery, Right F Internal Iliac Artery, Left H External Iliac Artery, Right J External Iliac Artery, Left K Femoral Artery, Right L Femoral Artery, Left M Popliteal Artery, Right N Popliteal Artery, Left P Anterior Tibial Artery, Right Q Anterior Tibial Artery, Left R Posterior Tibial Artery, Right S Posterior Tibial Artery, Left T Peroneal Artery, Right U Peroneal Artery, Left V Foot Artery, Right W Foot Artery, Left Y Lower Artery	Ø Open 3 Percutaneous 4 Percutaneous Endoscopic	C Extraluminal Device D Intraluminal Device Z No Device	Z No Qualifier
C Common Iliac Artery, Right D Common Iliac Artery, Left	Ø Open 3 Percutaneous 4 Percutaneous Endoscopic	C Extraluminal Device D Intraluminal Device E Intraluminal Device, Branched or Fenestrated, One or Two Arteries ~~F Intraluminal Device, Branched or Fenestrated, Three or More Arteries~~ Z No Device	Z No Qualifier

　　　New/Revised Text in Blue　　~~deleted~~ Deleted

V: RESTRICTION　　4: LOWER ARTERIES　　Ø: M/S

SECTION: Ø MEDICAL AND SURGICAL
BODY SYSTEM: 4 LOWER ARTERIES
OPERATION: W REVISION: Correcting, to the extent possible, a portion of a malfunctioning device or the position of a displaced device

Body Part	Approach	Device	Qualifier
Y Lower Artery	Ø Open 3 Percutaneous 4 Percutaneous Endoscopic ~~X External~~	Ø Drainage Device 2 Monitoring Device 3 Infusion Device 7 Autologous Tissue Substitute C Extraluminal Device D Intraluminal Device J Synthetic Substitute K Nonautologous Tissue Substitute Y Other Device	Z No Qualifier
Y Lower Artery	X External	Ø Drainage Device 2 Monitoring Device 3 Infusion Device 7 Autologous Tissue Substitute C Extraluminal Device D Intraluminal Device J Synthetic Substitute K Nonautologous Tissue Substitute	Z No Qualifier

Ø: M/S

4: LOWER ARTERIES

W: REVISION

Ø5. Upper Veins 94
  Ø51. Bypass..95
  Ø55. Destruction 96
  Ø57. Dilation...97
  Ø59. Drainage 98
  Ø5B. Excision 99
  Ø5C. Extirpation 1ØØ
  Ø5D. Extraction 1ØØ
  Ø5H. Insertion 1Ø1
  Ø5J. Inspection 1Ø1
  Ø5L. Occlusion 1Ø2
  Ø5N. Release 1Ø3
  Ø5P. Removal 1Ø4
  Ø5Q. Repair 1Ø5
  Ø5R. Replacement 1Ø6
  Ø5S. Reposition..1Ø7
  Ø5U. Supplement 1Ø8
  Ø5V. Restriction...1Ø9
  Ø5W. Revision..11Ø

SECTION: Ø MEDICAL AND SURGICAL
BODY SYSTEM: 5 UPPER VEINS

OPERATION: **1 BYPASS:** Altering the route of passage of the contents of a tubular body part

Body Part	Approach	Device	Qualifier
Ø Azygos Vein	Ø Open	7 Autologous Tissue Substitute	Y Upper Vein
1 Hemiazygos Vein	4 Percutaneous Endoscopic	9 Autologous Venous Tissue	
3 Innominate Vein, Right		A Autologous Arterial Tissue	
4 Innominate Vein, Left		J Synthetic Substitute	
5 Subclavian Vein, Right		K Nonautologous Tissue	
6 Subclavian Vein, Left		Substitute	
7 Axillary Vein, Right		Z No Device	
8 Axillary Vein, Left			
9 Brachial Vein, Right			
A Brachial Vein, Left			
B Basilic Vein, Right			
C Basilic Vein, Left			
D Cephalic Vein, Right			
F Cephalic Vein, Left			
G Hand Vein, Right			
H Hand Vein, Left			
L Intracranial Vein			
M Internal Jugular Vein, Right			
N Internal Jugular Vein, Left			
P External Jugular Vein, Right			
Q External Jugular Vein, Left			
R Vertebral Vein, Right			
S Vertebral Vein, Left			
T Face Vein, Right			
V Face Vein, Left			

Ø: M/S

5: UPPER VEINS

1: BYPASS

SECTION: Ø MEDICAL AND SURGICAL
BODY SYSTEM: 5 UPPER VEINS
OPERATION: 5 **DESTRUCTION:** Physical eradication of all or a portion of a body part by the direct use of energy, force, or a destructive agent

Body Part	Approach	Device	Qualifier
Ø Azygos Vein	Ø Open	Z No Device	Z No Qualifier
1 Hemiazygos Vein	3 Percutaneous		
3 Innominate Vein, Right	4 Percutaneous Endoscopic		
4 Innominate Vein, Left			
5 Subclavian Vein, Right			
6 Subclavian Vein, Left			
7 Axillary Vein, Right			
8 Axillary Vein, Left			
9 Brachial Vein, Right			
A Brachial Vein, Left			
B Basilic Vein, Right			
C Basilic Vein, Left			
D Cephalic Vein, Right			
F Cephalic Vein, Left			
G Hand Vein, Right			
H Hand Vein, Left			
L Intracranial Vein			
M Internal Jugular Vein, Right			
N Internal Jugular Vein, Left			
P External Jugular Vein, Right			
Q External Jugular Vein, Left			
R Vertebral Vein, Right			
S Vertebral Vein, Left			
T Face Vein, Right			
V Face Vein, Left			
Y Upper Vein			

5: DESTRUCTION

5: UPPER VEINS

Ø: M/S

New/Revised Text in Blue   ~~deleted~~ Deleted

SECTION: Ø MEDICAL AND SURGICAL
BODY SYSTEM: 5 **UPPER VEINS**
OPERATION: 7 **DILATION:** Expanding an orifice or the lumen of a tubular body part

Body Part	Approach	Device	Qualifier
Ø Azygos Vein	Ø Open	D Intraluminal Device	Z No Qualifier
1 Hemiazygos Vein	3 Percutaneous	Z No Device	
3 Innominate Vein, Right	4 Percutaneous Endoscopic		
4 Innominate Vein, Left			
5 Subclavian Vein, Right			
6 Subclavian Vein, Left			
7 Axillary Vein, Right			
8 Axillary Vein, Left			
9 Brachial Vein, Right			
A Brachial Vein, Left			
B Basilic Vein, Right			
C Basilic Vein, Left			
D Cephalic Vein, Right			
F Cephalic Vein, Left			
G Hand Vein, Right			
H Hand Vein, Left			
L Intracranial Vein			
M Internal Jugular Vein, Right			
N Internal Jugular Vein, Left			
P External Jugular Vein, Right			
Q External Jugular Vein, Left			
R Vertebral Vein, Right			
S Vertebral Vein, Left			
T Face Vein, Right			
V Face Vein, Left			
Y Upper Vein			

Ø:M/S

5: UPPER VEINS

7: DILATION

SECTION: Ø MEDICAL AND SURGICAL
BODY SYSTEM: 5 UPPER VEINS
OPERATION: 9 DRAINAGE: Taking or letting out fluids and/or gases from a body part

Body Part	Approach	Device	Qualifier
Ø Azygos Vein 1 Hemiazygos Vein 3 Innominate Vein, Right 4 Innominate Vein, Left 5 Subclavian Vein, Right 6 Subclavian Vein, Left 7 Axillary Vein, Right 8 Axillary Vein, Left 9 Brachial Vein, Right A Brachial Vein, Left B Basilic Vein, Right C Basilic Vein, Left D Cephalic Vein, Right F Cephalic Vein, Left G Hand Vein, Right H Hand Vein, Left L Intracranial Vein M Internal Jugular Vein, Right N Internal Jugular Vein, Left P External Jugular Vein, Right Q External Jugular Vein, Left R Vertebral Vein, Right S Vertebral Vein, Left T Face Vein, Right V Face Vein, Left Y Upper Vein	Ø Open 3 Percutaneous 4 Percutaneous Endoscopic	Ø Drainage Device	Z No Qualifier
Ø Azygos Vein 1 Hemiazygos Vein 3 Innominate Vein, Right 4 Innominate Vein, Left 5 Subclavian Vein, Right 6 Subclavian Vein, Left 7 Axillary Vein, Right 8 Axillary Vein, Left 9 Brachial Vein, Right A Brachial Vein, Left B Basilic Vein, Right C Basilic Vein, Left D Cephalic Vein, Right F Cephalic Vein, Left G Hand Vein, Right H Hand Vein, Left L Intracranial Vein M Internal Jugular Vein, Right N Internal Jugular Vein, Left P External Jugular Vein, Right Q External Jugular Vein, Left R Vertebral Vein, Right S Vertebral Vein, Left T Face Vein, Right V Face Vein, Left Y Upper Vein	Ø Open 3 Percutaneous 4 Percutaneous Endoscopic	Z No Device	X Diagnostic Z No Qualifier

9: DRAINAGE

5: UPPER VEINS

Ø: M/S

SECTION: Ø MEDICAL AND SURGICAL
BODY SYSTEM: 5 UPPER VEINS
OPERATION: B EXCISION: Cutting out or off, without replacement, a portion of a body part

Body Part	Approach	Device	Qualifier
Ø Azygos Vein 1 Hemiazygos Vein 3 Innominate Vein, Right 4 Innominate Vein, Left 5 Subclavian Vein, Right 6 Subclavian Vein, Left 7 Axillary Vein, Right 8 Axillary Vein, Left 9 Brachial Vein, Right A Brachial Vein, Left B Basilic Vein, Right C Basilic Vein, Left D Cephalic Vein, Right F Cephalic Vein, Left G Hand Vein, Right H Hand Vein, Left L Intracranial Vein M Internal Jugular Vein, Right N Internal Jugular Vein, Left P External Jugular Vein, Right Q External Jugular Vein, Left R Vertebral Vein, Right S Vertebral Vein, Left T Face Vein, Right V Face Vein, Left Y Upper Vein	Ø Open 3 Percutaneous 4 Percutaneous Endoscopic	Z No Device	X Diagnostic Z No Qualifier

SECTION: Ø MEDICAL AND SURGICAL
BODY SYSTEM: 5 **UPPER VEINS**
OPERATION: C **EXTIRPATION:** Taking or cutting out solid matter from a body part

Body Part	Approach	Device	Qualifier
Ø Azygos Vein 1 Hemiazygos Vein 3 Innominate Vein, Right 4 Innominate Vein, Left 5 Subclavian Vein, Right 6 Subclavian Vein, Left 7 Axillary Vein, Right 8 Axillary Vein, Left 9 Brachial Vein, Right A Brachial Vein, Left B Basilic Vein, Right C Basilic Vein, Left D Cephalic Vein, Right F Cephalic Vein, Left G Hand Vein, Right H Hand Vein, Left L Intracranial Vein M Internal Jugular Vein, Right N Internal Jugular Vein, Left P External Jugular Vein, Right Q External Jugular Vein, Left R Vertebral Vein, Right S Vertebral Vein, Left T Face Vein, Right V Face Vein, Left Y Upper Vein	Ø Open 3 Percutaneous 4 Percutaneous Endoscopic	Z No Device	Z No Qualifier

SECTION: Ø MEDICAL AND SURGICAL
BODY SYSTEM: 5 **UPPER VEINS**
OPERATION: D **EXTRACTION:** Pulling or stripping out or off all or a portion of a body part by the use of force

Body Part	Approach	Device	Qualifier
9 Brachial Vein, Right A Brachial Vein, Left B Basilic Vein, Right C Basilic Vein, Left D Cephalic Vein, Right F Cephalic Vein, Left G Hand Vein, Right H Hand Vein, Left Y Upper Vein	Ø Open 3 Percutaneous	Z No Device	Z No Qualifier

New/Revised Text in Blue   ~~deleted~~ Deleted

SECTION: Ø MEDICAL AND SURGICAL

BODY SYSTEM: 5 UPPER VEINS

OPERATION:　H INSERTION: Putting in a nonbiological appliance that monitors, assists, performs, or prevents a physiological function but does not physically take the place of a body part

Body Part	Approach	Device	Qualifier
Ø Azygos Vein	Ø Open 3 Percutaneous 4 Percutaneous Endoscopic	2 Monitoring Device 3 Infusion Device D Intraluminal Device M Neurostimulator Lead	Z No Qualifier
1 Hemiazygos Vein 5 Subclavian Vein, Right 6 Subclavian Vein, Left 7 Axillary Vein, Right 8 Axillary Vein, Left 9 Brachial Vein, Right A Brachial Vein, Left B Basilic Vein, Right C Basilic Vein, Left D Cephalic Vein, Right F Cephalic Vein, Left G Hand Vein, Right H Hand Vein, Left L Intracranial Vein M Internal Jugular Vein, Right N Internal Jugular Vein, Left P External Jugular Vein, Right Q External Jugular Vein, Left R Vertebral Vein, Right S Vertebral Vein, Left T Face Vein, Right V Face Vein, Left	Ø Open 3 Percutaneous 4 Percutaneous Endoscopic	3 Infusion Device D Intraluminal Device	Z No Qualifier
3 Innominate Vein, Right 4 Innominate Vein, Left	Ø Open 3 Percutaneous 4 Percutaneous Endoscopic	3 Infusion Device D Intraluminal Device M Neurostimulator Lead	Z No Qualifier
Y Upper Vein	Ø Open 3 Percutaneous 4 Percutaneous Endoscopic	2 Monitoring Device 3 Infusion Device D Intraluminal Device Y Other Device	Z No Qualifier

SECTION: Ø MEDICAL AND SURGICAL

BODY SYSTEM: 5 UPPER VEINS

OPERATION:　J INSPECTION: Visually and/or manually exploring a body part

Body Part	Approach	Device	Qualifier
Y Upper Vein	Ø Open 3 Percutaneous 4 Percutaneous Endoscopic X External	Z No Device	Z No Qualifier

SECTION: Ø MEDICAL AND SURGICAL
BODY SYSTEM: 5 UPPER VEINS
OPERATION: L OCCLUSION: Completely closing an orifice or the lumen of a tubular body part

Body Part	Approach	Device	Qualifier
Ø Azygos Vein	Ø Open	C Extraluminal Device	Z No Qualifier
1 Hemiazygos Vein	3 Percutaneous	D Intraluminal Device	
3 Innominate Vein, Right	4 Percutaneous Endoscopic	Z No Device	
4 Innominate Vein, Left			
5 Subclavian Vein, Right			
6 Subclavian Vein, Left			
7 Axillary Vein, Right			
8 Axillary Vein, Left			
9 Brachial Vein, Right			
A Brachial Vein, Left			
B Basilic Vein, Right			
C Basilic Vein, Left			
D Cephalic Vein, Right			
F Cephalic Vein, Left			
G Hand Vein, Right			
H Hand Vein, Left			
L Intracranial Vein			
M Internal Jugular Vein, Right			
N Internal Jugular Vein, Left			
P External Jugular Vein, Right			
Q External Jugular Vein, Left			
R Vertebral Vein, Right			
S Vertebral Vein, Left			
T Face Vein, Right			
V Face Vein, Left			
Y Upper Vein			

SECTION: Ø MEDICAL AND SURGICAL
BODY SYSTEM: 5 UPPER VEINS
OPERATION: N RELEASE: Freeing a body part from an abnormal physical constraint

Body Part	Approach	Device	Qualifier
Ø Azygos Vein	Ø Open	Z No Device	Z No Qualifier
1 Hemiazygos Vein	3 Percutaneous		
3 Innominate Vein, Right	4 Percutaneous Endoscopic		
4 Innominate Vein, Left			
5 Subclavian Vein, Right			
6 Subclavian Vein, Left			
7 Axillary Vein, Right			
8 Axillary Vein, Left			
9 Brachial Vein, Right			
A Brachial Vein, Left			
B Basilic Vein, Right			
C Basilic Vein, Left			
D Cephalic Vein, Right			
F Cephalic Vein, Left			
G Hand Vein, Right			
H Hand Vein, Left			
L Intracranial Vein			
M Internal Jugular Vein, Right			
N Internal Jugular Vein, Left			
P External Jugular Vein, Right			
Q External Jugular Vein, Left			
R Vertebral Vein, Right			
S Vertebral Vein, Left			
T Face Vein, Right			
V Face Vein, Left			
Y Upper Vein			

SECTION: Ø MEDICAL AND SURGICAL
BODY SYSTEM: 5 UPPER VEINS
OPERATION: P REMOVAL: Taking out or off a device from a body part

Body Part	Approach	Device	Qualifier
Ø Azygos Vein	Ø Open 3 Percutaneous 4 Percutaneous Endoscopic X External	2 Monitoring Device M Neurostimulator Lead	Z No Qualifier
3 Innominate Vein, Right 4 Innominate Vein, Left	Ø Open 3 Percutaneous 4 Percutaneous Endoscopic X External	M Neurostimulator Lead	Z No Qualifier
Y Upper Vein	Ø Open 3 Percutaneous 4 Percutaneous Endoscopic	Ø Drainage Device 2 Monitoring Device 3 Infusion Device 7 Autologous Tissue Substitute C Extraluminal Device D Intraluminal Device J Synthetic Substitute K Nonautologous Tissue Substitute Y Other Device	Z No Qualifier
Y Upper Vein	X External	Ø Drainage Device 2 Monitoring Device 3 Infusion Device D Intraluminal Device	Z No Qualifier

SECTION: Ø MEDICAL AND SURGICAL
BODY SYSTEM: 5 UPPER VEINS
OPERATION: Q REPAIR: Restoring, to the extent possible, a body part to its normal anatomic structure and function

Body Part	Approach	Device	Qualifier
Ø Azygos Vein 1 Hemiazygos Vein 3 Innominate Vein, Right 4 Innominate Vein, Left 5 Subclavian Vein, Right 6 Subclavian Vein, Left 7 Axillary Vein, Right 8 Axillary Vein, Left 9 Brachial Vein, Right A Brachial Vein, Left B Basilic Vein, Right C Basilic Vein, Left D Cephalic Vein, Right F Cephalic Vein, Left G Hand Vein, Right H Hand Vein, Left L Intracranial Vein M Internal Jugular Vein, Right N Internal Jugular Vein, Left P External Jugular Vein, Right Q External Jugular Vein, Left R Vertebral Vein, Right S Vertebral Vein, Left T Face Vein, Right V Face Vein, Left Y Upper Vein	Ø Open 3 Percutaneous 4 Percutaneous Endoscopic	Z No Device	Z No Qualifier

SECTION: Ø MEDICAL AND SURGICAL
BODY SYSTEM: 5 UPPER VEINS
OPERATION: R REPLACEMENT: Putting in or on biological or synthetic material that physically takes the place and/or function of all or a portion of a body part

Body Part	Approach	Device	Qualifier
Ø Azygos Vein 1 Hemiazygos Vein 3 Innominate Vein, Right 4 Innominate Vein, Left 5 Subclavian Vein, Right 6 Subclavian Vein, Left 7 Axillary Vein, Right 8 Axillary Vein, Left 9 Brachial Vein, Right A Brachial Vein, Left B Basilic Vein, Right C Basilic Vein, Left D Cephalic Vein, Right F Cephalic Vein, Left G Hand Vein, Right H Hand Vein, Left L Intracranial Vein M Internal Jugular Vein, Right N Internal Jugular Vein, Left P External Jugular Vein, Right Q External Jugular Vein, Left R Vertebral Vein, Right S Vertebral Vein, Left T Face Vein, Right V Face Vein, Left Y Upper Vein	Ø Open 4 Percutaneous Endoscopic	7 Autologous Tissue Substitute J Synthetic Substitute K Nonautologous Tissue Substitute	Z No Qualifier

SECTION: Ø MEDICAL AND SURGICAL
BODY SYSTEM: 5 UPPER VEINS
OPERATION: S REPOSITION: Moving to its normal location, or other suitable location, all or a portion of a body part

Body Part	Approach	Device	Qualifier
Ø Azygos Vein	Ø Open	Z No Device	Z No Qualifier
1 Hemiazygos Vein	3 Percutaneous		
3 Innominate Vein, Right	4 Percutaneous Endoscopic		
4 Innominate Vein, Left			
5 Subclavian Vein, Right			
6 Subclavian Vein, Left			
7 Axillary Vein, Right			
8 Axillary Vein, Left			
9 Brachial Vein, Right			
A Brachial Vein, Left			
B Basilic Vein, Right			
C Basilic Vein, Left			
D Cephalic Vein, Right			
F Cephalic Vein, Left			
G Hand Vein, Right			
H Hand Vein, Left			
L Intracranial Vein			
M Internal Jugular Vein, Right			
N Internal Jugular Vein, Left			
P External Jugular Vein, Right			
Q External Jugular Vein, Left			
R Vertebral Vein, Right			
S Vertebral Vein, Left			
T Face Vein, Right			
V Face Vein, Left			
Y Upper Vein			

SECTION: Ø MEDICAL AND SURGICAL
BODY SYSTEM: 5 UPPER VEINS
OPERATION: U SUPPLEMENT: Putting in or on biological or synthetic material that physically reinforces and/or augments the function of a portion of a body part

Body Part	Approach	Device	Qualifier
Ø Azygos Vein 1 Hemiazygos Vein 3 Innominate Vein, Right 4 Innominate Vein, Left 5 Subclavian Vein, Right 6 Subclavian Vein, Left 7 Axillary Vein, Right 8 Axillary Vein, Left 9 Brachial Vein, Right A Brachial Vein, Left B Basilic Vein, Right C Basilic Vein, Left D Cephalic Vein, Right F Cephalic Vein, Left G Hand Vein, Right H Hand Vein, Left L Intracranial Vein M Internal Jugular Vein, Right N Internal Jugular Vein, Left P External Jugular Vein, Right Q External Jugular Vein, Left R Vertebral Vein, Right S Vertebral Vein, Left T Face Vein, Right V Face Vein, Left Y Upper Vein	Ø Open 3 Percutaneous 4 Percutaneous Endoscopic	7 Autologous Tissue Substitute J Synthetic Substitute K Nonautologous Tissue Substitute	Z No Qualifier

SECTION: Ø MEDICAL AND SURGICAL
BODY SYSTEM: 5 **UPPER VEINS**
OPERATION: V **RESTRICTION:** Partially closing an orifice or the lumen of a tubular body part

Body Part	Approach	Device	Qualifier
Ø Azygos Vein	Ø Open	C Extraluminal Device	Z No Qualifier
1 Hemiazygos Vein	3 Percutaneous	D Intraluminal Device	
3 Innominate Vein, Right	4 Percutaneous Endoscopic	Z No Device	
4 Innominate Vein, Left			
5 Subclavian Vein, Right			
6 Subclavian Vein, Left			
7 Axillary Vein, Right			
8 Axillary Vein, Left			
9 Brachial Vein, Right			
A Brachial Vein, Left			
B Basilic Vein, Right			
C Basilic Vein, Left			
D Cephalic Vein, Right			
F Cephalic Vein, Left			
G Hand Vein, Right			
H Hand Vein, Left			
L Intracranial Vein			
M Internal Jugular Vein, Right			
N Internal Jugular Vein, Left			
P External Jugular Vein, Right			
Q External Jugular Vein, Left			
R Vertebral Vein, Right			
S Vertebral Vein, Left			
T Face Vein, Right			
V Face Vein, Left			
Y Upper Vein			

SECTION: Ø MEDICAL AND SURGICAL
BODY SYSTEM: 5 UPPER VEINS
OPERATION: **W REVISION:** Correcting, to the extent possible, a portion of a malfunctioning device or the position of a displaced device

Body Part	Approach	Device	Qualifier
Ø Azygos Vein	Ø Open 3 Percutaneous 4 Percutaneous Endoscopic X External	2 Monitoring Device M Neurostimulator Lead	Z No Qualifier
3 Innominate Vein, Right 4 Innominate Vein, Left	Ø Open 3 Percutaneous 4 Percutaneous Endoscopic X External	M Neurostimulator Lead	Z No Qualifier
Y Upper Vein	Ø Open 3 Percutaneous 4 Percutaneous Endoscopic X̶ ̶E̶x̶t̶e̶r̶n̶a̶l̶	Ø Drainage Device 2 Monitoring Device 3 Infusion Device 7 Autologous Tissue Substitute C Extraluminal Device D Intraluminal Device J Synthetic Substitute K Nonautologous Tissue Substitute Y Other Device	Z No Qualifier
Y Upper Vein	X External	Ø Drainage Device 2 Monitoring Device 3 Infusion Device 7 Autologous Tissue Substitute C Extraluminal Device D Intraluminal Device J Synthetic Substitute K Nonautologous Tissue Substitute	Z No Qualifier

Ø6. Lower Veins..111
 Ø61. Bypass...112
 Ø65. Destruction..113
 Ø67. Dilation...114
 Ø69. Drainage 115
 Ø6B. Excision..117
 Ø6C. Extirpation..118
 Ø6D. Extraction...118
 Ø6H. Insertion...119
 Ø6J. Inspection..120
 Ø6L. Occlusion..120
 Ø6N. Release 121
 Ø6P. Removal 121
 Ø6Q. Repair 122
 Ø6R. Replacement...123
 Ø6S. Reposition...124
 Ø6U. Supplement..125
 Ø6V. Restriction..126
 Ø6W. Revision...127

SECTION: Ø MEDICAL AND SURGICAL

BODY SYSTEM: 6 LOWER VEINS
OPERATION: 1 **BYPASS:** Altering the route of passage of the contents of a tubular body part

Body Part	Approach	Device	Qualifier
Ø Inferior Vena Cava	Ø Open 4 Percutaneous Endoscopic	7 Autologous Tissue Substitute 9 Autologous Venous Tissue A Autologous Arterial Tissue J Synthetic Substitute K Nonautologous Tissue Substitute Z No Device	5 Superior Mesenteric Vein 6 Inferior Mesenteric Vein P Pulmonary Trunk Q Pulmonary Artery, Right R Pulmonary Artery, Left Y Lower Vein
1 Splenic Vein	Ø Open 4 Percutaneous Endoscopic	7 Autologous Tissue Substitute 9 Autologous Venous Tissue A Autologous Arterial Tissue J Synthetic Substitute K Nonautologous Tissue Substitute Z No Device	9 Renal Vein, Right B Renal Vein, Left Y Lower Vein
2 Gastric Vein 3 Esophageal Vein 4 Hepatic Vein 5 Superior Mesenteric Vein 6 Inferior Mesenteric Vein 7 Colic Vein 9 Renal Vein, Right B Renal Vein, Left C Common Iliac Vein, Right D Common Iliac Vein, Left F External Iliac Vein, Right G External Iliac Vein, Left H Hypogastric Vein, Right J Hypogastric Vein, Left M Femoral Vein, Right N Femoral Vein, Left P Saphenous Vein, Right Q Saphenous Vein, Left R Lesser Saphenous Vein, Right S Lesser Saphenous Vein, Left T Foot Vein, Right V Foot Vein, Left	Ø Open 4 Percutaneous Endoscopic	7 Autologous Tissue Substitute 9 Autologous Venous Tissue A Autologous Arterial Tissue J Synthetic Substitute K Nonautologous Tissue Substitute Z No Device	Y Lower Vein
8 Portal Vein	Ø Open	7 Autologous Tissue Substitute 9 Autologous Venous Tissue A Autologous Arterial Tissue J Synthetic Substitute K Nonautologous Tissue Substitute Z No Device	9 Renal Vein, Right B Renal Vein, Left Y Lower Vein
8 Portal Vein	3 Percutaneous	D Intraluminal Device J Synthetic Substitute	4 Hepatic Vein Y Lower Vein
8 Portal Vein	4 Percutaneous Endoscopic	7 Autologous Tissue Substitute 9 Autologous Venous Tissue A Autologous Arterial Tissue J Synthetic Substitute K Nonautologous Tissue Substitute Z No Device	9 Renal Vein, Right B Renal Vein, Left Y Lower Vein
8 Portal Vein	4 Percutaneous Endoscopic	D Intraluminal Device J Synthetic Substitute	4 Hepatic Vein 9 Renal Vein, Right B Renal Vein, Left Y Lower Vein

New/Revised Text in Blue   ~~deleted~~ Deleted

SECTION: Ø MEDICAL AND SURGICAL
BODY SYSTEM: 6 LOWER VEINS
OPERATION: 5 **DESTRUCTION:** Physical eradication of all or a portion of a body part by the direct use of energy, force, or a destructive agent

Body Part	Approach	Device	Qualifier
Ø Inferior Vena Cava 1 Splenic Vein 2 Gastric Vein 3 Esophageal Vein 4 Hepatic Vein 5 Superior Mesenteric Vein 6 Inferior Mesenteric Vein 7 Colic Vein 8 Portal Vein 9 Renal Vein, Right B Renal Vein, Left C Common Iliac Vein, Right D Common Iliac Vein, Left F External Iliac Vein, Right G External Iliac Vein, Left H Hypogastric Vein, Right J Hypogastric Vein, Left M Femoral Vein, Right N Femoral Vein, Left P Saphenous Vein, Right Q Saphenous Vein, Left R Lesser Saphenous Vein, Right S Lesser Saphenous Vein, Left T Foot Vein, Right V Foot Vein, Left	Ø Open 3 Percutaneous 4 Percutaneous Endoscopic	Z No Device	Z No Qualifier
Y Lower Vein	Ø Open 3 Percutaneous 4 Percutaneous Endoscopic	Z No Device	C Hemorrhoidal Plexus Z No Qualifier

SECTION: Ø MEDICAL AND SURGICAL
BODY SYSTEM: 6 LOWER VEINS
OPERATION: 7 **DILATION:** Expanding an orifice or the lumen of a tubular body part

Body Part	Approach	Device	Qualifier
Ø Inferior Vena Cava 1 Splenic Vein 2 Gastric Vein 3 Esophageal Vein 4 Hepatic Vein 5 Superior Mesenteric Vein 6 Inferior Mesenteric Vein 7 Colic Vein 8 Portal Vein 9 Renal Vein, Right B Renal Vein, Left C Common Iliac Vein, Right D Common Iliac Vein, Left F External Iliac Vein, Right G External Iliac Vein, Left H Hypogastric Vein, Right J Hypogastric Vein, Left M Femoral Vein, Right N Femoral Vein, Left P Saphenous Vein, Right Q Saphenous Vein, Left R Lesser Saphenous Vein, Right S Lesser Saphenous Vein, Left T Foot Vein, Right V Foot Vein, Left Y Lower Vein	Ø Open 3 Percutaneous 4 Percutaneous Endoscopic	D Intraluminal Device Z No Device	Z No Qualifier

SECTION: Ø MEDICAL AND SURGICAL
BODY SYSTEM: 6 LOWER VEINS
OPERATION: 9 DRAINAGE: *(on multiple pages)*
Taking or letting out fluids and/or gases from a body part

Body Part	Approach	Device	Qualifier
Ø Inferior Vena Cava 1 Splenic Vein 2 Gastric Vein 3 Esophageal Vein 4 Hepatic Vein 5 Superior Mesenteric Vein 6 Inferior Mesenteric Vein 7 Colic Vein 8 Portal Vein 9 Renal Vein, Right B Renal Vein, Left C Common Iliac Vein, Right D Common Iliac Vein, Left F External Iliac Vein, Right G External Iliac Vein, Left H Hypogastric Vein, Right J Hypogastric Vein, Left M Femoral Vein, Right N Femoral Vein, Left P Saphenous Vein, Right Q Saphenous Vein, Left R Lesser Saphenous Vein, Right S Lesser Saphenous Vein, Left T Foot Vein, Right V Foot Vein, Left Y Lower Vein	Ø Open 3 Percutaneous 4 Percutaneous Endoscopic	Ø Drainage Device	Z No Qualifier

SECTION: Ø MEDICAL AND SURGICAL
BODY SYSTEM: 6 LOWER VEINS
OPERATION: 9 DRAINAGE: *(continued)*

Taking or letting out fluids and/or gases from a body part

Body Part	Approach	Device	Qualifier
Ø Inferior Vena Cava	Ø Open	Z No Device	X Diagnostic
1 Splenic Vein	3 Percutaneous		Z No Qualifier
2 Gastric Vein	4 Percutaneous Endoscopic		
3 Esophageal Vein			
4 Hepatic Vein			
5 Superior Mesenteric Vein			
6 Inferior Mesenteric Vein			
7 Colic Vein			
8 Portal Vein			
9 Renal Vein, Right			
B Renal Vein, Left			
C Common Iliac Vein, Right			
D Common Iliac Vein, Left			
F External Iliac Vein, Right			
G External Iliac Vein, Left			
H Hypogastric Vein, Right			
J Hypogastric Vein, Left			
M Femoral Vein, Right			
N Femoral Vein, Left			
P Saphenous Vein, Right			
Q Saphenous Vein, Left			
R Lesser Saphenous Vein, Right			
S Lesser Saphenous Vein, Left			
T Foot Vein, Right			
V Foot Vein, Left			
Y Lower Vein			

9: DRAINAGE

6: LOWER VEINS

Ø: M/S

SECTION: Ø MEDICAL AND SURGICAL
BODY SYSTEM: 6 LOWER VEINS
OPERATION: B **EXCISION:** Cutting out or off, without replacement, a portion of a body part

Body Part	Approach	Device	Qualifier
Ø Inferior Vena Cava 1 Splenic Vein 2 Gastric Vein 3 Esophageal Vein 4 Hepatic Vein 5 Superior Mesenteric Vein 6 Inferior Mesenteric Vein 7 Colic Vein 8 Portal Vein 9 Renal Vein, Right B Renal Vein, Left C Common Iliac Vein, Right D Common Iliac Vein, Left F External Iliac Vein, Right G External Iliac Vein, Left H Hypogastric Vein, Right J Hypogastric Vein, Left M Femoral Vein, Right N Femoral Vein, Left P Saphenous Vein, Right Q Saphenous Vein, Left R Lesser Saphenous Vein, Right S Lesser Saphenous Vein, Left T Foot Vein, Right V Foot Vein, Left	Ø Open 3 Percutaneous 4 Percutaneous Endoscopic	Z No Device	X Diagnostic Z No Qualifier
Y Lower Vein	Ø Open 3 Percutaneous 4 Percutaneous Endoscopic	Z No Device	C Hemorrhoidal Plexus X Diagnostic Z No Qualifier

SECTION: Ø MEDICAL AND SURGICAL
BODY SYSTEM: 6 LOWER VEINS
OPERATION: C EXTIRPATION: Taking or cutting out solid matter from a body part

Body Part	Approach	Device	Qualifier
Ø Inferior Vena Cava	Ø Open	Z No Device	Z No Qualifier
1 Splenic Vein	3 Percutaneous		
2 Gastric Vein	4 Percutaneous Endoscopic		
3 Esophageal Vein			
4 Hepatic Vein			
5 Superior Mesenteric Vein			
6 Inferior Mesenteric Vein			
7 Colic Vein			
8 Portal Vein			
9 Renal Vein, Right			
B Renal Vein, Left			
C Common Iliac Vein, Right			
D Common Iliac Vein, Left			
F External Iliac Vein, Right			
G External Iliac Vein, Left			
H Hypogastric Vein, Right			
J Hypogastric Vein, Left			
M Femoral Vein, Right			
N Femoral Vein, Left			
P Saphenous Vein, Right			
Q Saphenous Vein, Left			
R Lesser Saphenous Vein, Right			
S Lesser Saphenous Vein, Left			
T Foot Vein, Right			
V Foot Vein, Left			
Y Lower Vein			

SECTION: Ø MEDICAL AND SURGICAL
BODY SYSTEM: 6 LOWER VEINS
OPERATION: D EXTRACTION: Pulling or stripping out or off all or a portion of a body part by the use of force

Body Part	Approach	Device	Qualifier
M Femoral Vein, Right	Ø Open	Z No Device	Z No Qualifier
N Femoral Vein, Left	3 Percutaneous		
P Saphenous Vein, Right	4 Percutaneous Endoscopic		
Q Saphenous Vein, Left			
R Lesser Saphenous Vein, Right			
S Lesser Saphenous Vein, Left			
T Foot Vein, Right			
V Foot Vein, Left			
Y Lower Vein			

C: EXTIRPATION   D: EXTRACTION

6: LOWER VEINS

Ø: M/S

New/Revised Text in Blue   ~~deleted~~ Deleted

SECTION: Ø MEDICAL AND SURGICAL
BODY SYSTEM: 6 LOWER VEINS
OPERATION: H INSERTION: Putting in a nonbiological appliance that monitors, assists, performs, or prevents a physiological function but does not physically take the place of a body part

Body Part	Approach	Device	Qualifier
Ø Inferior Vena Cava	Ø Open 3 Percutaneous	3 Infusion Device	T Via Unbilical Vein Z No Qualifier
Ø Inferior Vena Cava	Ø Open 3 Percutaneous	D Intraluminal Device	Z No Qualifier
Ø Inferior Vena Cava	4 Percutaneous Endoscopic	3 Infusion Device D Intraluminal Device	Z No Qualifier
1 Splenic Vein 2 Gastric Vein 3 Esophageal Vein 4 Hepatic Vein 5 Superior Mesenteric Vein 6 Inferior Mesenteric Vein 7 Colic Vein 8 Portal Vein 9 Renal Vein, Right B Renal Vein, Left C Common Iliac Vein, Right D Common Iliac Vein, Left F External Iliac Vein, Right G External Iliac Vein, Left H Hypogastric Vein, Right J Hypogastric Vein, Left M Femoral Vein, Right N Femoral Vein, Left P Saphenous Vein, Right Q Saphenous Vein, Left R Lesser Saphenous Vein, Right S Lesser Saphenous Vein, Left T Foot Vein, Right V Foot Vein, Left	Ø Open 3 Percutaneous 4 Percutaneous Endoscopic	3 Infusion Device D Intraluminal Device	Z No Qualifier
Y Lower Vein	Ø Open 3 Percutaneous 4 Percutaneous Endoscopic	2 Monitoring Device 3 Infusion Device D Intraluminal Device Y Other Device	Z No Qualifier

SECTION: Ø MEDICAL AND SURGICAL
BODY SYSTEM: 6 LOWER VEINS
OPERATION: J INSPECTION: Visually and/or manually exploring a body part

Body Part	Approach	Device	Qualifier
Y Lower Vein	Ø Open 3 Percutaneous 4 Percutaneous Endoscopic X External	Z No Device	Z No Qualifier

SECTION: Ø MEDICAL AND SURGICAL
BODY SYSTEM: 6 LOWER VEINS
OPERATION: L OCCLUSION: Completely closing an orifice or the lumen of a tubular body part

Body Part	Approach	Device	Qualifier
Ø Inferior Vena Cava 1 Splenic Vein 2 Gastric Vein 3 ~~Esophageal Vein~~ 4 Hepatic Vein 5 Superior Mesenteric Vein 6 Inferior Mesenteric Vein 7 Colic Vein 8 Portal Vein 9 Renal Vein, Right B Renal Vein, Left C Common Iliac Vein, Right D Common Iliac Vein, Left F External Iliac Vein, Right G External Iliac Vein, Left H Hypogastric Vein, Right J Hypogastric Vein, Left M Femoral Vein, Right N Femoral Vein, Left P Saphenous Vein, Right Q Saphenous Vein, Left R ~~Lesser Saphenous Vein, Right~~ S ~~Lesser Saphenous Vein, Left~~ T Foot Vein, Right V Foot Vein, Left	Ø Open 3 Percutaneous 4 Percutaneous Endoscopic	C Extraluminal Device D Intraluminal Device Z No Device	Z No Qualifier
3 Esophageal Vein	Ø Open 3 Percutaneous 4 Percutaneous Endoscopic 7 Via Natural or Artificial Opening 8 Via Natural or Artificial Opening Endoscopic	C Extraluminal Device D Intraluminal Device Z No Device	Z No Qualifier
Y Lower Vein	Ø Open 3 Percutaneous 4 Percutaneous Endoscopic	C Extraluminal Device D Intraluminal Device Z No Device	C Hemorrhoidal Plexus Z No Qualifier

SECTION: Ø MEDICAL AND SURGICAL
BODY SYSTEM: 6 LOWER VEINS
OPERATION: N RELEASE: Freeing a body part from an abnormal physical constraint by cutting or by the use of force

Body Part	Approach	Device	Qualifier
Ø Inferior Vena Cava 1 Splenic Vein 2 Gastric Vein 3 Esophageal Vein 4 Hepatic Vein 5 Superior Mesenteric Vein 6 Inferior Mesenteric Vein 7 Colic Vein 8 Portal Vein 9 Renal Vein, Right B Renal Vein, Left C Common Iliac Vein, Right D Common Iliac Vein, Left F External Iliac Vein, Right G External Iliac Vein, Left H Hypogastric Vein, Right J Hypogastric Vein, Left M Femoral Vein, Right N Femoral Vein, Left P Saphenous Vein, Right Q Saphenous Vein, Left R Lesser Saphenous Vein, Right S Lesser Saphenous Vein, Left T Foot Vein, Right V Foot Vein, Left Y Lower Vein	Ø Open 3 Percutaneous 4 Percutaneous Endoscopic	Z No Device	Z No Qualifier

SECTION: Ø MEDICAL AND SURGICAL
BODY SYSTEM: 6 LOWER VEINS
OPERATION: P REMOVAL: Taking out or off a device from a body part

Body Part	Approach	Device	Qualifier
Y Lower Vein	Ø Open 3 Percutaneous 4 Percutaneous Endoscopic	Ø Drainage Device 2 Monitoring Device 3 Infusion Device 7 Autologous Tissue Substitute C Extraluminal Device D Intraluminal Device J Synthetic Substitute K Nonautologous Tissue Substitute Y Other Device	Z No Qualifier
Y Lower Vein	X External	Ø Drainage Device 2 Monitoring Device 3 Infusion Device D Intraluminal Device	Z No Qualifier

SECTION: Ø MEDICAL AND SURGICAL
BODY SYSTEM: 6 **LOWER VEINS**
OPERATION: **Q REPAIR:** Restoring, to the extent possible, a body part to its normal anatomic structure and function

Body Part	Approach	Device	Qualifier
Ø Inferior Vena Cava 1 Splenic Vein 2 Gastric Vein 3 Esophageal Vein 4 Hepatic Vein 5 Superior Mesenteric Vein 6 Inferior Mesenteric Vein 7 Colic Vein 8 Portal Vein 9 Renal Vein, Right B Renal Vein, Left C Common Iliac Vein, Right D Common Iliac Vein, Left F External Iliac Vein, Right G External Iliac Vein, Left H Hypogastric Vein, Right J Hypogastric Vein, Left M Femoral Vein, Right N Femoral Vein, Left P Saphenous Vein, Right Q Saphenous Vein, Left R ~~Lesser Saphenous Vein, Right~~ S ~~Lesser Saphenous Vein, Left~~ T Foot Vein, Right V Foot Vein, Left Y Lower Vein	Ø Open 3 Percutaneous 4 Percutaneous Endoscopic	Z No Device	Z No Qualifier

SECTION: 0 MEDICAL AND SURGICAL
BODY SYSTEM: 6 LOWER VEINS
OPERATION: R REPLACEMENT: Putting in or on biological or synthetic material that physically takes the place and/or function of all or a portion of a body part

Body Part	Approach	Device	Qualifier
0 Inferior Vena Cava	0 Open	7 Autologous Tissue Substitute	Z No Qualifier
1 Splenic Vein	4 Percutaneous Endoscopic	J Synthetic Substitute	
2 Gastric Vein		K Nonautologous Tissue Substitute	
3 Esophageal Vein			
4 Hepatic Vein			
5 Superior Mesenteric Vein			
6 Inferior Mesenteric Vein			
7 Colic Vein			
8 Portal Vein			
9 Renal Vein, Right			
B Renal Vein, Left			
C Common Iliac Vein, Right			
D Common Iliac Vein, Left			
F External Iliac Vein, Right			
G External Iliac Vein, Left			
H Hypogastric Vein, Right			
J Hypogastric Vein, Left			
M Femoral Vein, Right			
N Femoral Vein, Left			
P Saphenous Vein, Right			
Q Saphenous Vein, Left			
R Lesser Saphenous Vein, Right			
S Lesser Saphenous Vein, Left			
T Foot Vein, Right			
V Foot Vein, Left			
Y Lower Vein			

SECTION: Ø MEDICAL AND SURGICAL
BODY SYSTEM: 6 LOWER VEINS
OPERATION: S REPOSITION: Moving to its normal location, or other suitable location, all or a portion of a body part

Body Part	Approach	Device	Qualifier
Ø Inferior Vena Cava	Ø Open	Z No Device	Z No Qualifier
1 Splenic Vein	3 Percutaneous		
2 Gastric Vein	4 Percutaneous Endoscopic		
3 Esophageal Vein			
4 Hepatic Vein			
5 Superior Mesenteric Vein			
6 Inferior Mesenteric Vein			
7 Colic Vein			
8 Portal Vein			
9 Renal Vein, Right			
B Renal Vein, Left			
C Common Iliac Vein, Right			
D Common Iliac Vein, Left			
F External Iliac Vein, Right			
G External Iliac Vein, Left			
H Hypogastric Vein, Right			
J Hypogastric Vein, Left			
M Femoral Vein, Right			
N Femoral Vein, Left			
P Saphenous Vein, Right			
Q Saphenous Vein, Left			
R Lesser Saphenous Vein, Right			
S Lesser Saphenous Vein, Left			
T Foot Vein, Right			
V Foot Vein, Left			
Y Lower Vein			

S: REPOSITION

6: LOWER VEINS

Ø: M/S

SECTION: 0 MEDICAL AND SURGICAL
BODY SYSTEM: 6 LOWER VEINS
OPERATION: U SUPPLEMENT: Putting in or on biological or synthetic material that physically reinforces and/or augments the function of a portion of a body part

Body Part	Approach	Device	Qualifier
0 Inferior Vena Cava	0 Open	7 Autologous Tissue Substitute	Z No Qualifier
1 Splenic Vein	3 Percutaneous	J Synthetic Substitute	
2 Gastric Vein	4 Percutaneous Endoscopic	K Nonautologous Tissue Substitute	
3 Esophageal Vein			
4 Hepatic Vein			
5 Superior Mesenteric Vein			
6 Inferior Mesenteric Vein			
7 Colic Vein			
8 Portal Vein			
9 Renal Vein, Right			
B Renal Vein, Left			
C Common Iliac Vein, Right			
D Common Iliac Vein, Left			
F External Iliac Vein, Right			
G External Iliac Vein, Left			
H Hypogastric Vein, Right			
J Hypogastric Vein, Left			
M Femoral Vein, Right			
N Femoral Vein, Left			
P Saphenous Vein, Right			
Q Saphenous Vein, Left			
R Lesser Saphenous Vein, Right			
S Lesser Saphenous Vein, Left			
T Foot Vein, Right			
V Foot Vein, Left			
Y Lower Vein			

SECTION: Ø MEDICAL AND SURGICAL
BODY SYSTEM: 6 LOWER VEINS
OPERATION: V RESTRICTION: Partially closing an orifice or the lumen of a tubular body part

Body Part	Approach	Device	Qualifier
Ø Inferior Vena Cava	Ø Open	C Extraluminal Device	Z No Qualifier
1 Splenic Vein	3 Percutaneous	D Intraluminal Device	
2 Gastric Vein	4 Percutaneous Endoscopic	Z No Device	
3 Esophageal Vein			
4 Hepatic Vein			
5 Superior Mesenteric Vein			
6 Inferior Mesenteric Vein			
7 Colic Vein			
8 Portal Vein			
9 Renal Vein, Right			
B Renal Vein, Left			
C Common Iliac Vein, Right			
D Common Iliac Vein, Left			
F External Iliac Vein, Right			
G External Iliac Vein, Left			
H Hypogastric Vein, Right			
J Hypogastric Vein, Left			
M Femoral Vein, Right			
N Femoral Vein, Left			
P Saphenous Vein, Right			
Q Saphenous Vein, Left			
R Lesser Saphenous Vein, Right			
S Lesser Saphenous Vein, Left			
T Foot Vein, Right			
V Foot Vein, Left			
Y Lower Vein			

SECTION: Ø MEDICAL AND SURGICAL
BODY SYSTEM: 6 LOWER VEINS
OPERATION: W REVISION: Correcting, to the extent possible, a portion of a malfunctioning device or the position of a displaced device

Body Part	Approach	Device	Qualifier
Y Lower Vein	Ø Open 3 Percutaneous 4 Percutaneous Endoscopic ~~X External~~	Ø Drainage Device 2 Monitoring Device 3 Infusion Device 7 Autologous Tissue Substitute C Extraluminal Device D Intraluminal Device J Synthetic Substitute K Nonautologous Tissue Substitute Y Other Device	Z No Qualifier
Y Lower Vein	X External	Ø Drainage Device 2 Monitoring Device 3 Infusion Device 7 Autologous Tissue Substitute C Extraluminal Device D Intraluminal Device J Synthetic Substitute K Nonautologous Tissue Substitute	Z No Qualifier

Ø: M/S   6: LOWER VEINS   W: REVISION

Ø7. Lymphatic and Hemic Systems 128
    Ø72. Change 129
    Ø75. Destruction 129
    Ø79. Drainage 13Ø
    Ø7B. Excision 131
    Ø7C. Extirpation 131
    Ø7D. Extraction 132
    Ø7H. Insertion 132
    Ø7J. Inspection 133
    Ø7L. Occlusion 133
    Ø7N. Release 134
    Ø7P. Removal 134
    Ø7Q. Repair 135
    Ø7S. Reposition 135
    Ø7T. Resection 136
    Ø7U. Supplement 137
    Ø7V. Restriction 137
    Ø7W. Revision 138
    Ø7Y. Transplantation 138

SECTION: Ø MEDICAL AND SURGICAL
BODY SYSTEM: 7 LYMPHATIC AND HEMIC SYSTEMS
OPERATION: 2 **CHANGE:** Taking out or off a device from a body part and putting back an identical or similar device in or on the same body part without cutting or puncturing the skin or a mucous membrane

Body Part	Approach	Device	Qualifier
K Thoracic Duct L Cisterna Chyli M Thymus N Lymphatic P Spleen T Bone Marrow	X External	Ø Drainage Device Y Other Device	Z No Qualifier

SECTION: Ø MEDICAL AND SURGICAL
BODY SYSTEM: 7 LYMPHATIC AND HEMIC SYSTEMS
OPERATION: 5 **DESTRUCTION:** Physical eradication of all or a portion of a body part by the direct use of energy, force, or a destructive agent

Body Part	Approach	Device	Qualifier
Ø Lymphatic, Head 1 Lymphatic, Right Neck 2 Lymphatic, Left Neck 3 Lymphatic, Right Upper Extremity 4 Lymphatic, Left Upper Extremity 5 Lymphatic, Right Axillary 6 Lymphatic, Left Axillary 7 Lymphatic, Thorax 8 Lymphatic, Internal Mammary, Right 9 Lymphatic, Internal Mammary, Left B Lymphatic, Mesenteric C Lymphatic, Pelvis D Lymphatic, Aortic F Lymphatic, Right Lower Extremity G Lymphatic, Left Lower Extremity H Lymphatic, Right Inguinal J Lymphatic, Left Inguinal K Thoracic Duct L Cisterna Chyli M Thymus P Spleen	Ø Open 3 Percutaneous 4 Percutaneous Endoscopic	Z No Device	Z No Qualifier

SECTION: Ø MEDICAL AND SURGICAL
BODY SYSTEM: 7 LYMPHATIC AND HEMIC SYSTEMS
OPERATION: 9 DRAINAGE: Taking or letting out fluids and/or gases from a body part

9: DRAINAGE

7: LYMPHATIC AND HEMIC SYSTEMS

Ø: M/S

Body Part	Approach	Device	Qualifier
Ø Lymphatic, Head 1 Lymphatic, Right Neck 2 Lymphatic, Left Neck 3 Lymphatic, Right Upper Extremity 4 Lymphatic, Left Upper Extremity 5 Lymphatic, Right Axillary 6 Lymphatic, Left Axillary 7 Lymphatic, Thorax 8 Lymphatic, Internal Mammary, Right 9 Lymphatic, Internal Mammary, Left B Lymphatic, Mesenteric C Lymphatic, Pelvis D Lymphatic, Aortic F Lymphatic, Right Lower Extremity G Lymphatic, Left Lower Extremity H Lymphatic, Right Inguinal J Lymphatic, Left Inguinal K Thoracic Duct L Cisterna Chyli ~~M Thymus~~ ~~P Spleen~~ ~~T Bone Marrow~~	Ø Open 3 Percutaneous 4 Percutaneous Endoscopic 8 Via Natural or Artificial Opening Endoscopic	Ø Drainage Device	Z No Qualifier
Ø Lymphatic, Head 1 Lymphatic, Right Neck 2 Lymphatic, Left Neck 3 Lymphatic, Right Upper Extremity 4 Lymphatic, Left Upper Extremity 5 Lymphatic, Right Axillary 6 Lymphatic, Left Axillary 7 Lymphatic, Thorax 8 Lymphatic, Internal Mammary, Right 9 Lymphatic, Internal Mammary, Left B Lymphatic, Mesenteric C Lymphatic, Pelvis D Lymphatic, Aortic F Lymphatic, Right Lower Extremity G Lymphatic, Left Lower Extremity H Lymphatic, Right Inguinal J Lymphatic, Left Inguinal K Thoracic Duct L Cisterna Chyli ~~M Thymus~~ ~~P Spleen~~ ~~T Bone Marrow~~	Ø Open 3 Percutaneous 4 Percutaneous Endoscopic 8 Via Natural or Artificial Opening Endoscopic	Z No Device	X Diagnostic Z No Qualifier
M Thymus P Spleen T Bone Marrow	Ø Open 3 Percutaneous 4 Percutaneous Endoscopic	Ø Drainage Device	Z No Qualifier
M Thymus P Spleen T Bone Marrow	Ø Open 3 Percutaneous 4 Percutaneous Endoscopic	Z No Device	X Diagnostic Z No Qualifier

SECTION: Ø MEDICAL AND SURGICAL
BODY SYSTEM: 7 LYMPHATIC AND HEMIC SYSTEMS
OPERATION: B EXCISION: Cutting out or off, without replacement, a portion of a body part

Body Part	Approach	Device	Qualifier
Ø Lymphatic, Head 1 Lymphatic, Right Neck 2 Lymphatic, Left Neck 3 Lymphatic, Right Upper Extremity 4 Lymphatic, Left Upper Extremity 5 Lymphatic, Right Axillary 6 Lymphatic, Left Axillary 7 Lymphatic, Thorax 8 Lymphatic, Internal Mammary, Right 9 Lymphatic, Internal Mammary, Left B Lymphatic, Mesenteric C Lymphatic, Pelvis D Lymphatic, Aortic F Lymphatic, Right Lower Extremity G Lymphatic, Left Lower Extremity H Lymphatic, Right Inguinal J Lymphatic, Left Inguinal K Thoracic Duct L Cisterna Chyli M Thymus P Spleen	Ø Open 3 Percutaneous 4 Percutaneous Endoscopic	Z No Device	X Diagnostic Z No Qualifier

SECTION: Ø MEDICAL AND SURGICAL
BODY SYSTEM: 7 LYMPHATIC AND HEMIC SYSTEMS
OPERATION: C EXTIRPATION: Taking or cutting out solid matter from a body part

Body Part	Approach	Device	Qualifier
Ø Lymphatic, Head 1 Lymphatic, Right Neck 2 Lymphatic, Left Neck 3 Lymphatic, Right Upper Extremity 4 Lymphatic, Left Upper Extremity 5 Lymphatic, Right Axillary 6 Lymphatic, Left Axillary 7 Lymphatic, Thorax 8 Lymphatic, Internal Mammary, Right 9 Lymphatic, Internal Mammary, Left B Lymphatic, Mesenteric C Lymphatic, Pelvis D Lymphatic, Aortic F Lymphatic, Right Lower Extremity G Lymphatic, Left Lower Extremity H Lymphatic, Right Inguinal J Lymphatic, Left Inguinal K Thoracic Duct L Cisterna Chyli M Thymus P Spleen	Ø Open 3 Percutaneous 4 Percutaneous Endoscopic	Z No Device	Z No Qualifier

Ø: M/S   7: LYMPHATIC AND HEMIC SYSTEMS   B: EXCISION   C: EXTIRPATION

SECTION: Ø MEDICAL AND SURGICAL
BODY SYSTEM: 7 LYMPHATIC AND HEMIC SYSTEMS
OPERATION: D **EXTRACTION:** Pulling or stripping out or off all or a portion of a body part by the use of force

Body Part	Approach	Device	Qualifier
Ø Lymphatic, Head 1 Lymphatic, Right Neck 2 Lymphatic, Left Neck 3 Lymphatic, Right Upper Extremity 4 Lymphatic, Left Upper Extremity 5 Lymphatic, Right Axillary 6 Lymphatic, Left Axillary 7 Lymphatic, Thorax 8 Lymphatic, Internal Mammary, Right 9 Lymphatic, Internal Mammary, Left B Lymphatic, Mesenteric C Lymphatic, Pelvis D Lymphatic, Aortic F Lymphatic, Right Lower Extremity G Lymphatic, Left Lower Extremity H Lymphatic, Right Inguinal J Lymphatic, Left Inguinal K Thoracic Duct L Cisterna Chyli	3 Percutaneous 4 Percutaneous Endoscopic 8 Via Natural or Artificial Opening Endoscopic	Z No Device	X Diagnostic
M Thymus P Spleen	3 Percutaneous 4 Percutaneous Endoscopic	Z No Device	X Diagnostic
Q Bone Marrow, Sternum R Bone Marrow, Iliac S Bone Marrow, Vertebral	Ø Open 3 Percutaneous	Z No Device	X Diagnostic Z No Qualifier

SECTION: Ø MEDICAL AND SURGICAL
BODY SYSTEM: 7 LYMPHATIC AND HEMIC SYSTEMS
OPERATION: H **INSERTION:** Putting in a nonbiological appliance that monitors, assists, performs, or prevents a physiological function but does not physically take the place of a body part

Body Part	Approach	Device	Qualifier
K Thoracic Duct L Cisterna Chyli M Thymus N Lymphatic P Spleen	Ø Open 3 Percutaneous 4 Percutaneous Endoscopic	3 Infusion Device Y Other Device	Z No Qualifier

SECTION: Ø MEDICAL AND SURGICAL
BODY SYSTEM: 7 LYMPHATIC AND HEMIC SYSTEMS
OPERATION: J INSPECTION: Visually and/or manually exploring a body part

Body Part	Approach	Device	Qualifier
K Thoracic Duct L Cisterna Chyli M Thymus T Bone Marrow	Ø Open 3 Percutaneous 4 Percutaneous Endoscopic	Z No Device	Z No Qualifier
N Lymphatic P Spleen	Ø Open 3 Percutaneous 4 Percutaneous Endoscopic 8 Via Natural or Artificial Opening Endoscopic X External	Z No Device	Z No Qualifier
P Spleen	Ø Open 3 Percutaneous 4 Percutaneous Endoscopic X External	Z No Device	Z No Qualifier

SECTION: Ø MEDICAL AND SURGICAL
BODY SYSTEM: 7 LYMPHATIC AND HEMIC SYSTEMS
OPERATION: L OCCLUSION: Completely closing an orifice or the lumen of a tubular body part

Body Part	Approach	Device	Qualifier
Ø Lymphatic, Head 1 Lymphatic, Right Neck 2 Lymphatic, Left Neck 3 Lymphatic, Right Upper Extremity 4 Lymphatic, Left Upper Extremity 5 Lymphatic, Right Axillary 6 Lymphatic, Left Axillary 7 Lymphatic, Thorax 8 Lymphatic, Internal Mammary, Right 9 Lymphatic, Internal Mammary, Left B Lymphatic, Mesenteric C Lymphatic, Pelvis D Lymphatic, Aortic F Lymphatic, Right Lower Extremity G Lymphatic, Left Lower Extremity H Lymphatic, Right Inguinal J Lymphatic, Left Inguinal K Thoracic Duct L Cisterna Chyli	Ø Open 3 Percutaneous 4 Percutaneous Endoscopic	C Extraluminal Device D Intraluminal Device Z No Device	Z No Qualifier

SECTION: Ø MEDICAL AND SURGICAL
BODY SYSTEM: 7 LYMPHATIC AND HEMIC SYSTEMS
OPERATION: N RELEASE: Freeing a body part from an abnormal physical constraint by cutting or by the use of force

N: RELEASE   P: REMOVAL

7: LYMPHATIC AND HEMIC SYSTEMS

Body Part	Approach	Device	Qualifier
Ø Lymphatic, Head 1 Lymphatic, Right Neck 2 Lymphatic, Left Neck 3 Lymphatic, Right Upper Extremity 4 Lymphatic, Left Upper Extremity 5 Lymphatic, Right Axillary 6 Lymphatic, Left Axillary 7 Lymphatic, Thorax 8 Lymphatic, Internal Mammary, Right 9 Lymphatic, Internal Mammary, Left B Lymphatic, Mesenteric C Lymphatic, Pelvis D Lymphatic, Aortic F Lymphatic, Right Lower Extremity G Lymphatic, Left Lower Extremity H Lymphatic, Right Inguinal J Lymphatic, Left Inguinal K Thoracic Duct L Cisterna Chyli M Thymus P Spleen	Ø Open 3 Percutaneous 4 Percutaneous Endoscopic	Z No Device	Z No Qualifier

SECTION: Ø MEDICAL AND SURGICAL
BODY SYSTEM: 7 LYMPHATIC AND HEMIC SYSTEMS
OPERATION: P REMOVAL: Taking out or off a device from a body part

Ø: M/S

Body Part	Approach	Device	Qualifier
K Thoracic Duct L Cisterna Chyli N Lymphatic	Ø Open 3 Percutaneous 4 Percutaneous Endoscopic	Ø Drainage Device 3 Infusion Device 7 Autologous Tissue Substitute C Extraluminal Device D Intraluminal Device J Synthetic Substitute K Nonautologous Tissue Substitute Y Other Device	Z No Qualifier
K Thoracic Duct L Cisterna Chyli N Lymphatic	X External	Ø Drainage Device 3 Infusion Device D Intraluminal Device	Z No Qualifier
M Thymus P Spleen	Ø Open 3 Percutaneous 4 Percutaneous Endoscopic ~~X External~~	Ø Drainage Device 3 Infusion Device Y Other Device	Z No Qualifier
M Thymus P Spleen	X External	Ø Drainage Device 3 Infusion Device	Z No Qualifier
T Bone Marrow	Ø Open 3 Percutaneous 4 Percutaneous Endoscopic X External	Ø Drainage Device	Z No Qualifier

SECTION: Ø MEDICAL AND SURGICAL
BODY SYSTEM: 7 **LYMPHATIC AND HEMIC SYSTEMS**
OPERATION: Q **REPAIR:** Restoring, to the extent possible, a body part to its normal anatomic structure and function

Body Part	Approach	Device	Qualifier
Ø Lymphatic, Head 1 Lymphatic, Right Neck 2 Lymphatic, Left Neck 3 Lymphatic, Right Upper Extremity 4 Lymphatic, Left Upper Extremity 5 Lymphatic, Right Axillary 6 Lymphatic, Left Axillary 7 Lymphatic, Thorax 8 Lymphatic, Internal Mammary, Right 9 Lymphatic, Internal Mammary, Left B Lymphatic, Mesenteric C Lymphatic, Pelvis D Lymphatic, Aortic F Lymphatic, Right Lower Extremity G Lymphatic, Left Lower Extremity H Lymphatic, Right Inguinal J Lymphatic, Left Inguinal K Thoracic Duct L Cisterna Chyli M Thymus P Spleen	Ø Open 3 Percutaneous 4 Percutaneous Endoscopic 8 Via Natural or Artificial Opening Endoscopic	Z No Device	Z No Qualifier
M Thymus P Spleen	Ø Open 3 Percutaneous 4 Percutaneous Endoscopic	Z No Device	Z No Qualifier

SECTION: Ø MEDICAL AND SURGICAL
BODY SYSTEM: 7 **LYMPHATIC AND HEMIC SYSTEMS**
OPERATION: S **REPOSITION:** Moving to its normal location, or other suitable location, all or a portion of a body part

Body Part	Approach	Device	Qualifier
M Thymus P Spleen	Ø Open	Z No Device	Z No Qualifier

SECTION: Ø MEDICAL AND SURGICAL
BODY SYSTEM: 7 LYMPHATIC AND HEMIC SYSTEMS
OPERATION: T RESECTION: Cutting out or off, without replacement, all of a body part

Body Part	Approach	Device	Qualifier
Ø Lymphatic, Head 1 Lymphatic, Right Neck 2 Lymphatic, Left Neck 3 Lymphatic, Right Upper Extremity 4 Lymphatic, Left Upper Extremity 5 Lymphatic, Right Axillary 6 Lymphatic, Left Axillary 7 Lymphatic, Thorax 8 Lymphatic, Internal Mammary, Right 9 Lymphatic, Internal Mammary, Left B Lymphatic, Mesenteric C Lymphatic, Pelvis D Lymphatic, Aortic F Lymphatic, Right Lower Extremity G Lymphatic, Left Lower Extremity H Lymphatic, Right Inguinal J Lymphatic, Left Inguinal K Thoracic Duct L Cisterna Chyli M Thymus P Spleen	Ø Open 4 Percutaneous Endoscopic	Z No Device	Z No Qualifier

T: RESECTION

7: LYMPHATIC AND HEMIC SYSTEMS

Ø: M/S

SECTION: Ø MEDICAL AND SURGICAL
BODY SYSTEM: 7 LYMPHATIC AND HEMIC SYSTEMS
OPERATION: U SUPPLEMENT: Putting in or on biological or synthetic material that physically reinforces and/or augments the function of a portion of a body part

Body Part	Approach	Device	Qualifier
Ø Lymphatic, Head 1 Lymphatic, Right Neck 2 Lymphatic, Left Neck 3 Lymphatic, Right Upper Extremity 4 Lymphatic, Left Upper Extremity 5 Lymphatic, Right Axillary 6 Lymphatic, Left Axillary 7 Lymphatic, Thorax 8 Lymphatic, Internal Mammary, Right 9 Lymphatic, Internal Mammary, Left B Lymphatic, Mesenteric C Lymphatic, Pelvis D Lymphatic, Aortic F Lymphatic, Right Lower Extremity G Lymphatic, Left Lower Extremity H Lymphatic, Right Inguinal J Lymphatic, Left Inguinal K Thoracic Duct L Cisterna Chyli	Ø Open 4 Percutaneous Endoscopic	7 Autologous Tissue Substitute J Synthetic Substitute K Nonautologous Tissue Substitute	Z No Qualifier

SECTION: Ø MEDICAL AND SURGICAL
BODY SYSTEM: 7 LYMPHATIC AND HEMIC SYSTEMS
OPERATION: V RESTRICTION: Partially closing an orifice or the lumen of a tubular body part

Body Part	Approach	Device	Qualifier
Ø Lymphatic, Head 1 Lymphatic, Right Neck 2 Lymphatic, Left Neck 3 Lymphatic, Right Upper Extremity 4 Lymphatic, Left Upper Extremity 5 Lymphatic, Right Axillary 6 Lymphatic, Left Axillary 7 Lymphatic, Thorax 8 Lymphatic, Internal Mammary, Right 9 Lymphatic, Internal Mammary, Left B Lymphatic, Mesenteric C Lymphatic, Pelvis D Lymphatic, Aortic F Lymphatic, Right Lower Extremity G Lymphatic, Left Lower Extremity H Lymphatic, Right Inguinal J Lymphatic, Left Inguinal K Thoracic Duct L Cisterna Chyli	Ø Open 3 Percutaneous 4 Percutaneous Endoscopic	C Extraluminal Device D Intraluminal Device Z No Device	Z No Qualifier

SECTION: Ø MEDICAL AND SURGICAL
BODY SYSTEM: 7 LYMPHATIC AND HEMIC SYSTEMS
OPERATION: W REVISION: Correcting, to the extent possible, a portion of a malfunctioning device or the position of a displaced device

Body Part	Approach	Device	Qualifier
K Thoracic Duct L Cisterna Chyli N Lymphatic	Ø Open 3 Percutaneous 4 Percutaneous Endoscopic ~~X External~~	Ø Drainage Device 3 Infusion Device 7 Autologous Tissue Substitute C Extraluminal Device D Intraluminal Device J Synthetic Substitute K Nonautologous Tissue Substitute Y Other Device	Z No Qualifier
K Thoracic Duct L Cisterna Chyli N Lymphatic	X External	Ø Drainage Device 3 Infusion Device 7 Autologous Tissue Substitute C Extraluminal Device D Intraluminal Device J Synthetic Substitute K Nonautologous Tissue Substitute	Z No Qualifier
M Thymus P Spleen	Ø Open 3 Percutaneous 4 Percutaneous Endoscopic ~~X External~~	Ø Drainage Device 3 Infusion Device Y Other Device	Z No Qualifier
M Thymus P Spleen	X External	Ø Drainage Device 3 Infusion Device	Z No Qualifier
T Bone Marrow	Ø Open 3 Percutaneous 4 Percutaneous Endoscopic X External	Ø Drainage Device	Z No Qualifier

SECTION: Ø MEDICAL AND SURGICAL
BODY SYSTEM: 7 LYMPHATIC AND HEMIC SYSTEMS
OPERATION: Y TRANSPLANTATION: Putting in or on all or a portion of a living body part taken from another individual or animal to physically take the place and/or function of all or a portion of a similar body part

Body Part	Approach	Device	Qualifier
M Thymus P Spleen	Ø Open	Z No Device	Ø Allogeneic 1 Syngeneic 2 Zooplastic

Ø8. Eye 139
    Ø8Ø. Alteration 140
   Ø81. Bypass 140
   Ø82. Change 140
   Ø85. Destruction 141
   Ø87. Dilation 141
   Ø89. Drainage 142
   Ø8B. Excision 144
   Ø8C. Extirpation 145
   Ø8D. Extraction 145
   Ø8F. Fragmentation 146
   Ø8H. Insertion 146
   Ø8J. Inspection 146
   Ø8L. Occlusion 147
   Ø8M. Reattachment 147
   Ø8N. Release 148
   Ø8P. Removal 149
   Ø8Q. Repair 150
   Ø8R. Replacement 151
   Ø8S. Reposition 152
   Ø8T. Resection 153
   Ø8U. Supplement 154
   Ø8V. Restriction 154
   Ø8W. Revision 155
   Ø8X. Transfer 155

SECTION: Ø MEDICAL AND SURGICAL
BODY SYSTEM: 8 EYE
OPERATION: Ø **ALTERATION:** Modifying the anatomic structure of a body part without affecting the function of the body part

Body Part	Approach	Device	Qualifier
N Upper Eyelid, Right P Upper Eyelid, Left Q Lower Eyelid, Right R Lower Eyelid, Left	Ø Open 3 Percutaneous X External	7 Autologous Tissue Substitute J Synthetic Substitute K Nonautologous Tissue Substitute Z No Device	Z No Qualifier

SECTION: Ø MEDICAL AND SURGICAL
BODY SYSTEM: 8 EYE
OPERATION: 1 **BYPASS:** Altering the route of passage of the contents of a tubular body part

Body Part	Approach	Device	Qualifier
2 Anterior Chamber, Right 3 Anterior Chamber, Left	3 Percutaneous	J Synthetic Substitute K Nonautologous Tissue Substitute Z No Device	4 Sclera
X Lacrimal Duct, Right Y Lacrimal Duct, Left	Ø Open 3 Percutaneous	J Synthetic Substitute K Nonautologous Tissue Substitute Z No Device	3 Nasal Cavity

SECTION: Ø MEDICAL AND SURGICAL
BODY SYSTEM: 8 EYE
OPERATION: 2 **CHANGE:** Taking out or off a device from a body part and putting back an identical or similar device in or on the same body part without cutting or puncturing the skin or a mucous membrane

Body Part	Approach	Device	Qualifier
Ø Eye, Right 1 Eye, Left	X External	Ø Drainage Device Y Other Device	Z No Qualifier

SECTION: Ø MEDICAL AND SURGICAL

BODY SYSTEM: 8 EYE

OPERATION: 5 DESTRUCTION: Physical eradication of all or a portion of a body part by the direct use of energy, force, or a destructive agent

Body Part	Approach	Device	Qualifier
Ø Eye, Right 1 Eye, Left 6 Sclera, Right 7 Sclera, Left 8 Cornea, Right 9 Cornea, Left S Conjunctiva, Right T Conjunctiva, Left	X External	Z No Device	Z No Qualifier
2 Anterior Chamber, Right 3 Anterior Chamber, Left 4 Vitreous, Right 5 Vitreous, Left C Iris, Right D Iris, Left E Retina, Right F Retina, Left G Retinal Vessel, Right H Retinal Vessel, Left J Lens, Right K Lens, Left	3 Percutaneous	Z No Device	Z No Qualifier
A Choroid, Right B Choroid, Left L Extraocular Muscle, Right M Extraocular Muscle, Left V Lacrimal Gland, Right W Lacrimal Gland, Left	Ø Open 3 Percutaneous	Z No Device	Z No Qualifier
N Upper Eyelid, Right P Upper Eyelid, Left Q Lower Eyelid, Right R Lower Eyelid, Left	Ø Open 3 Percutaneous X External	Z No Device	Z No Qualifier
X Lacrimal Duct, Right Y Lacrimal Duct, Left	Ø Open 3 Percutaneous 7 Via Natural or Artificial Opening 8 Via Natural or Artificial Opening Endoscopic	Z No Device	Z No Qualifier

SECTION: Ø MEDICAL AND SURGICAL

BODY SYSTEM: 8 EYE

OPERATION: 7 DILATION: Expanding an orifice or the lumen of a tubular body part

Body Part	Approach	Device	Qualifier
X Lacrimal Duct, Right Y Lacrimal Duct, Left	Ø Open 3 Percutaneous 7 Via Natural or Artificial Opening 8 Via Natural or Artificial Opening Endoscopic	D Intraluminal Device Z No Device	Z No Qualifier

Ø: M/S 8: EYE 5: DESTRUCTION 7: DILATION

SECTION: Ø MEDICAL AND SURGICAL
BODY SYSTEM: 8 EYE
OPERATION: 9 DRAINAGE: *(on multiple pages)*
Taking or letting out fluids and/or gases from a body part

Body Part	Approach	Device	Qualifier
Ø Eye, Right 1 Eye, Left 6 Sclera, Right 7 Sclera, Left 8 Cornea, Right 9 Cornea, Left S Conjunctiva, Right T Conjunctiva, Left	X External	Ø Drainage Device	Z No Qualifier
Ø Eye, Right 1 Eye, Left 6 Sclera, Right 7 Sclera, Left 8 Cornea, Right 9 Cornea, Left S Conjunctiva, Right T Conjunctiva, Left	X External	Z No Device	X Diagnostic Z No Qualifier
2 Anterior Chamber, Right 3 Anterior Chamber, Left 4 Vitreous, Right 5 Vitreous, Left C Iris, Right D Iris, Left E Retina, Right F Retina, Left G Retinal Vessel, Right H Retinal Vessel, Left J Lens, Right K Lens, Left	3 Percutaneous	Ø Drainage Device	Z No Qualifier
2 Anterior Chamber, Right 3 Anterior Chamber, Left 4 Vitreous, Right 5 Vitreous, Left C Iris, Right D Iris, Left E Retina, Right F Retina, Left G Retinal Vessel, Right H Retinal Vessel, Left J Lens, Right K Lens, Left	3 Percutaneous	Z No Device	X Diagnostic Z No Qualifier
A Choroid, Right B Choroid, Left L Extraocular Muscle, Right M Extraocular Muscle, Left V Lacrimal Gland, Right W Lacrimal Gland, Left	Ø Open 3 Percutaneous	Ø Drainage Device	Z No Qualifier

SECTION: Ø MEDICAL AND SURGICAL
BODY SYSTEM: 8 EYE
OPERATION: 9 DRAINAGE: *(continued)*
Taking or letting out fluids and/or gases from a body part

Body Part	Approach	Device	Qualifier
A Choroid, Right B Choroid, Left L Extraocular Muscle, Right M Extraocular Muscle, Left V Lacrimal Gland, Right W Lacrimal Gland, Left	Ø Open 3 Percutaneous	Z No Device	X Diagnostic Z No Qualifier
N Upper Eyelid, Right P Upper Eyelid, Left Q Lower Eyelid, Right R Lower Eyelid, Left	Ø Open 3 Percutaneous X External	Ø Drainage Device	Z No Qualifier
N Upper Eyelid, Right P Upper Eyelid, Left Q Lower Eyelid, Right R Lower Eyelid, Left	Ø Open 3 Percutaneous X External	Z No Device	X Diagnostic Z No Qualifier
X Lacrimal Duct, Right Y Lacrimal Duct, Left	Ø Open 3 Percutaneous 7 Via Natural or Artificial Opening 8 Via Natural or Artificial Opening Endoscopic	Ø Drainage Device	Z No Qualifier
X Lacrimal Duct, Right Y Lacrimal Duct, Left	Ø Open 3 Percutaneous 7 Via Natural or Artificial Opening 8 Via Natural or Artificial Opening Endoscopic	Z No Device	X Diagnostic Z No Qualifier

SECTION: Ø MEDICAL AND SURGICAL
BODY SYSTEM: 8 EYE
OPERATION: B EXCISION: Cutting out or off, without replacement, a portion of a body part

Body Part	Approach	Device	Qualifier
Ø Eye, Right 1 Eye, Left N Upper Eyelid, Right P Upper Eyelid, Left Q Lower Eyelid, Right R Lower Eyelid, Left	Ø Open 3 Percutaneous X External	Z No Device	X Diagnostic Z No Qualifier
4 Vitreous, Right 5 Vitreous, Left C Iris, Right D Iris, Left E Retina, Right F Retina, Left J Lens, Right K Lens, Left	3 Percutaneous	Z No Device	X Diagnostic Z No Qualifier
6 Sclera, Right 7 Sclera, Left 8 Cornea, Right 9 Cornea, Left S Conjunctiva, Right T Conjunctiva, Left	X External	Z No Device	X Diagnostic Z No Qualifier
A Choroid, Right B Choroid, Left L Extraocular Muscle, Right M Extraocular Muscle, Left V Lacrimal Gland, Right W Lacrimal Gland, Left	Ø Open 3 Percutaneous	Z No Device	X Diagnostic Z No Qualifier
X Lacrimal Duct, Right Y Lacrimal Duct, Left	Ø Open 3 Percutaneous 7 Via Natural or Artificial Opening 8 Via Natural or Artificial Opening Endoscopic	Z No Device	X Diagnostic Z No Qualifier

B: EXCISION   8: EYE   Ø: M/S

SECTION: Ø MEDICAL AND SURGICAL
BODY SYSTEM: 8 EYE
OPERATION: C EXTIRPATION: Taking or cutting out solid matter from a body part

Body Part	Approach	Device	Qualifier
Ø Eye, Right 1 Eye, Left 6 Sclera, Right 7 Sclera, Left 8 Cornea, Right 9 Cornea, Left S Conjunctiva, Right T Conjunctiva, Left	X External	Z No Device	Z No Qualifier
2 Anterior Chamber, Right 3 Anterior Chamber, Left 4 Vitreous, Right 5 Vitreous, Left C Iris, Right D Iris, Left E Retina, Right F Retina, Left G Retinal Vessel, Right H Retinal Vessel, Left J Lens, Right K Lens, Left	3 Percutaneous X External	Z No Device	Z No Qualifier
A Choroid, Right B Choroid, Left L Extraocular Muscle, Right M Extraocular Muscle, Left N Upper Eyelid, Right P Upper Eyelid, Left Q Lower Eyelid, Right R Lower Eyelid, Left V Lacrimal Gland, Right W Lacrimal Gland, Left	Ø Open 3 Percutaneous X External	Z No Device	Z No Qualifier
X Lacrimal Duct, Right Y Lacrimal Duct, Left	Ø Open 3 Percutaneous 7 Via Natural or Artificial Opening 8 Via Natural or Artificial Opening Endoscopic	Z No Device	Z No Qualifier

SECTION: Ø MEDICAL AND SURGICAL
BODY SYSTEM: 8 EYE
OPERATION: D EXTRACTION: Pulling or stripping out or off all or a portion of a body part by the use of force

Body Part	Approach	Device	Qualifier
8 Cornea, Right 9 Cornea, Left	X External	Z No Device	X Diagnostic Z No Qualifier
J Lens, Right K Lens, Left	3 Percutaneous	Z No Device	Z No Qualifier

SECTION: Ø MEDICAL AND SURGICAL
BODY SYSTEM: 8 EYE
OPERATION: F FRAGMENTATION: Breaking solid matter in a body part into pieces

Body Part	Approach	Device	Qualifier
4 Vitreous, Right 5 Vitreous, Left	3 Percutaneous X External	Z No Device	Z No Qualifier

SECTION: Ø MEDICAL AND SURGICAL
BODY SYSTEM: 8 EYE
OPERATION: H INSERTION: Putting in a nonbiological appliance that monitors, assists, performs, or prevents a physiological function but does not physically take the place of a body part

Body Part	Approach	Device	Qualifier
Ø Eye, Right 1 Eye, Left	Ø Open	5 Epiretinal Visual Prosthesis Y Other Device	Z No Qualifier
Ø Eye, Right 1 Eye, Left	3 Percutaneous X External	1 Radioactive Element 3 Infusion Device Y Other Device	Z No Qualifier
Ø Eye, Right 1 Eye, Left	7 Via Natural or Artificial Opening 8 Via Natural or Artificial Opening Endoscopic	Y Other Device	Z No Qualifier
Ø Eye, Right 1 Eye, Left	X External	1 Radioactive Element 3 Infusion Device	Z No Qualifier

SECTION: Ø MEDICAL AND SURGICAL
BODY SYSTEM: 8 EYE
OPERATION: J INSPECTION: Visually and/or manually exploring a body part

Body Part	Approach	Device	Qualifier
Ø Eye, Right 1 Eye, Left J Lens, Right K Lens, Left	X External	Z No Device	Z No Qualifier
L Extraocular Muscle, Right M Extraocular Muscle, Left	Ø Open X External	Z No Device	Z No Qualifier

F: FRAGMENTATION   H: INSERTION   J: INSPECTION
8: EYE
Ø: M/S

SECTION: Ø MEDICAL AND SURGICAL
BODY SYSTEM: 8 EYE
OPERATION: L OCCLUSION: Completely closing an orifice or the lumen of a tubular body part

Body Part	Approach	Device	Qualifier
X Lacrimal Duct, Right Y Lacrimal Duct, Left	Ø Open 3 Percutaneous	C Extraluminal Device D Intraluminal Device Z No Device	Z No Qualifier
X Lacrimal Duct, Right Y Lacrimal Duct, Left	7 Via Natural or Artificial Opening 8 Via Natural or Artificial Opening Endoscopic	D Intraluminal Device Z No Device	Z No Qualifier

SECTION: Ø MEDICAL AND SURGICAL
BODY SYSTEM: 8 EYE
OPERATION: M REATTACHMENT: Putting back in or on all or a portion of a separated body part to its normal location or other suitable location

Body Part	Approach	Device	Qualifier
N Upper Eyelid, Right P Upper Eyelid, Left Q Lower Eyelid, Right R Lower Eyelid, Left	X External	Z No Device	Z No Qualifier

SECTION: Ø MEDICAL AND SURGICAL
BODY SYSTEM: 8 EYE
OPERATION: N RELEASE: Freeing a body part from an abnormal physical constraint by cutting or by the use of force

Body Part	Approach	Device	Qualifier
Ø Eye, Right 1 Eye, Left 6 Sclera, Right 7 Sclera, Left 8 Cornea, Right 9 Cornea, Left S Conjunctiva, Right T Conjunctiva, Left	X External	Z No Device	Z No Qualifier
2 Anterior Chamber, Right 3 Anterior Chamber, Left 4 Vitreous, Right 5 Vitreous, Left C Iris, Right D Iris, Left E Retina, Right F Retina, Left G Retinal Vessel, Right H Retinal Vessel, Left J Lens, Right K Lens, Left	3 Percutaneous	Z No Device	Z No Qualifier
A Choroid, Right B Choroid, Left L Extraocular Muscle, Right M Extraocular Muscle, Left V Lacrimal Gland, Right W Lacrimal Gland, Left	Ø Open 3 Percutaneous	Z No Device	Z No Qualifier
N Upper Eyelid, Right P Upper Eyelid, Left Q Lower Eyelid, Right R Lower Eyelid, Left	Ø Open 3 Percutaneous X External	Z No Device	Z No Qualifier
X Lacrimal Duct, Right Y Lacrimal Duct, Left	Ø Open 3 Percutaneous 7 Via Natural or Artificial Opening 8 Via Natural or Artificial Opening Endoscopic	Z No Device	Z No Qualifier

N: RELEASE 8: EYE Ø: M/S

SECTION: Ø MEDICAL AND SURGICAL
BODY SYSTEM: 8 EYE
OPERATION: P REMOVAL: Taking out or off a device from a body part

Body Part	Approach	Device	Qualifier
Ø Eye, Right 1 Eye, Left	Ø Open 3 Percutaneous 7 Via Natural or Artificial Opening 8 Via Natural or Artificial Opening Endoscopic ~~X External~~	Ø Drainage Device 1 Radioactive Element 3 Infusion Device 7 Autologous Tissue Substitute C Extraluminal Device D Intraluminal Device J Synthetic Substitute K Nonautologous Tissue Substitute Y Other Device	Z No Qualifier
Ø Eye, Right 1 Eye, Left	X External	Ø Drainage Device 1 Radioactive Element 3 Infusion Device 7 Autologous Tissue Substitute C Extraluminal Device D Intraluminal Device J Synthetic Substitute K Nonautologous Tissue Substitute	Z No Qualifier
J Lens, Right K Lens, Left	3 Percutaneous	J Synthetic Substitute Y Other Device	Z No Qualifier
L Extraocular Muscle, Right M Extraocular Muscle, Left	Ø Open 3 Percutaneous	Ø Drainage Device 7 Autologous Tissue Substitute J Synthetic Substitute K Nonautologous Tissue Substitute Y Other Device	Z No Qualifier

SECTION: Ø MEDICAL AND SURGICAL
BODY SYSTEM: 8 EYE
OPERATION: **Q REPAIR:** Restoring, to the extent possible, a body part to its normal anatomic structure and function

Body Part	Approach	Device	Qualifier
Ø Eye, Right 1 Eye, Left 6 Sclera, Right 7 Sclera, Left 8 Cornea, Right 9 Cornea, Left S Conjunctiva, Right T Conjunctiva, Left	X External	Z No Device	Z No Qualifier
2 Anterior Chamber, Right 3 Anterior Chamber, Left 4 Vitreous, Right 5 Vitreous, Left C Iris, Right D Iris, Left E Retina, Right F Retina, Left G Retinal Vessel, Right H Retinal Vessel, Left J Lens, Right K Lens, Left	3 Percutaneous	Z No Device	Z No Qualifier
A Choroid, Right B Choroid, Left L Extraocular Muscle, Right M Extraocular Muscle, Left V Lacrimal Gland, Right W Lacrimal Gland, Left	Ø Open 3 Percutaneous	Z No Device	Z No Qualifier
N Upper Eyelid, Right P Upper Eyelid, Left Q Lower Eyelid, Right R Lower Eyelid, Left	Ø Open 3 Percutaneous X External	Z No Device	Z No Qualifier
X Lacrimal Duct, Right Y Lacrimal Duct, Left	Ø Open 3 Percutaneous 7 Via Natural or Artificial Opening 8 Via Natural or Artificial Opening Endoscopic	Z No Device	Z No Qualifier

Q: REPAIR   8: EYE   Ø: M/S

SECTION: Ø MEDICAL AND SURGICAL
BODY SYSTEM: 8 EYE
OPERATION: R REPLACEMENT: Putting in or on biological or synthetic material that physically takes the place and/or function of all or a portion of a body part

Body Part	Approach	Device	Qualifier
Ø Eye, Right 1 Eye, Left A Choroid, Right B Choroid, Left	Ø Open 3 Percutaneous	7 Autologous Tissue Substitute J Synthetic Substitute K Nonautologous Tissue Substitute	Z No Qualifier
4 Vitreous, Right 5 Vitreous, Left C Iris, Right D Iris, Left G Retinal Vessel, Right H Retinal Vessel, Left	3 Percutaneous	7 Autologous Tissue Substitute J Synthetic Substitute K Nonautologous Tissue Substitute	Z No Qualifier
6 Sclera, Right 7 Sclera, Left S Conjunctiva, Right T Conjunctiva, Left	X External	7 Autologous Tissue Substitute J Synthetic Substitute K Nonautologous Tissue Substitute	Z No Qualifier
8 Cornea, Right 9 Cornea, Left	3 Percutaneous X External	7 Autologous Tissue Substitute J Synthetic Substitute K Nonautologous Tissue Substitute	Z No Qualifier
J Lens, Right K Lens, Left	3 Percutaneous	Ø Synthetic Substitute, Intraocular Telescope 7 Autologous Tissue Substitute J Synthetic Substitute K Nonautologous Tissue Substitute	Z No Qualifier
N Upper Eyelid, Right P Upper Eyelid, Left Q Lower Eyelid, Right R Lower Eyelid, Left	Ø Open 3 Percutaneous X External	7 Autologous Tissue Substitute J Synthetic Substitute K Nonautologous Tissue Substitute	Z No Qualifier
X Lacrimal Duct, Right Y Lacrimal Duct, Left	Ø Open 3 Percutaneous 7 Via Natural or Artificial Opening 8 Via Natural or Artificial Opening Endoscopic	7 Autologous Tissue Substitute J Synthetic Substitute K Nonautologous Tissue Substitute	Z No Qualifier

SECTION: Ø MEDICAL AND SURGICAL
BODY SYSTEM: 8 EYE
OPERATION: S REPOSITION: Moving to its normal location, or other suitable location, all or a portion of a body part

Body Part	Approach	Device	Qualifier
C Iris, Right D Iris, Left G Retinal Vessel, Right H Retinal Vessel, Left J Lens, Right K Lens, Left	3 Percutaneous	Z No Device	Z No Qualifier
L Extraocular Muscle, Right M Extraocular Muscle, Left V Lacrimal Gland, Right W Lacrimal Gland, Left	Ø Open 3 Percutaneous	Z No Device	Z No Qualifier
N Upper Eyelid, Right P Upper Eyelid, Left Q Lower Eyelid, Right R Lower Eyelid, Left	Ø Open 3 Percutaneous X External	Z No Device	Z No Qualifier
X Lacrimal Duct, Right Y Lacrimal Duct, Left	Ø Open 3 Percutaneous 7 Via Natural or Artificial Opening 8 Via Natural or Artificial Opening Endoscopic	Z No Device	Z No Qualifier

S: REPOSITION

8: EYE

Ø: M/S

New/Revised Text in Blue   ~~deleted~~ Deleted

SECTION: Ø MEDICAL AND SURGICAL
BODY SYSTEM: 8 EYE
OPERATION: T RESECTION: Cutting out or off, without replacement, all of a body part

Body Part	Approach	Device	Qualifier
Ø Eye, Right 1 Eye, Left 8 Cornea, Right 9 Cornea, Left	X External	Z No Device	Z No Qualifier
4 Vitreous, Right 5 Vitreous, Left C Iris, Right D Iris, Left J Lens, Right K Lens, Left	3 Percutaneous	Z No Device	Z No Qualifier
L Extraocular Muscle, Right M Extraocular Muscle, Left V Lacrimal Gland, Right W Lacrimal Gland, Left	Ø Open 3 Percutaneous	Z No Device	Z No Qualifier
N Upper Eyelid, Right P Upper Eyelid, Left Q Lower Eyelid, Right R Lower Eyelid, Left	Ø Open X External	Z No Device	Z No Qualifier
X Lacrimal Duct, Right Y Lacrimal Duct, Left	Ø Open 3 Percutaneous 7 Via Natural or Artificial Opening 8 Via Natural or Artificial Opening Endoscopic	Z No Device	Z No Qualifier

SECTION: Ø MEDICAL AND SURGICAL
BODY SYSTEM: 8 EYE
OPERATION: U SUPPLEMENT: Putting in or on biological or synthetic material that physically reinforces and/or augments the function of a portion of a body part

Body Part	Approach	Device	Qualifier
Ø Eye, Right 1 Eye, Left C Iris, Right D Iris, Left E Retina, Right F Retina, Left G Retinal Vessel, Right H Retinal Vessel, Left L Extraocular Muscle, Right M Extraocular Muscle, Left	Ø Open 3 Percutaneous	7 Autologous Tissue Substitute J Synthetic Substitute K Nonautologous Tissue Substitute	Z No Qualifier
8 Cornea, Right 9 Cornea, Left N Upper Eyelid, Right P Upper Eyelid, Left Q Lower Eyelid, Right R Lower Eyelid, Left	Ø Open 3 Percutaneous X External	7 Autologous Tissue Substitute J Synthetic Substitute K Nonautologous Tissue Substitute	Z No Qualifier
X Lacrimal Duct, Right Y Lacrimal Duct, Left	Ø Open 3 Percutaneous 7 Via Natural or Artificial Opening 8 Via Natural or Artificial Opening Endoscopic	7 Autologous Tissue Substitute J Synthetic Substitute K Nonautologous Tissue Substitute	Z No Qualifier

SECTION: Ø MEDICAL AND SURGICAL
BODY SYSTEM: 8 EYE
OPERATION: V RESTRICTION: Partially closing an orifice or the lumen of a tubular body part

Body Part	Approach	Device	Qualifier
X Lacrimal Duct, Right Y Lacrimal Duct, Left	Ø Open 3 Percutaneous	C Extraluminal Device D Intraluminal Device Z No Device	Z No Qualifier
X Lacrimal Duct, Right Y Lacrimal Duct, Left	7 Via Natural or Artificial Opening 8 Via Natural or Artificial Opening Endoscopic	D Intraluminal Device Z No Device	Z No Qualifier

U: SUPPLEMENT V: RESTRICTION

8: EYE

Ø: M/S

SECTION: Ø MEDICAL AND SURGICAL
BODY SYSTEM: 8 EYE
OPERATION: W REVISION: Correcting, to the extent possible, a portion of a malfunctioning device or the positon of a displaced device

Body Part	Approach	Device	Qualifier
Ø Eye, Right 1 Eye, Left	Ø Open 3 Percutaneous 7 Via Natural or Artificial Opening 8 Via Natural or Artificial Opening Endoscopic X External	Ø Drainage Device 3 Infusion Device 7 Autologous Tissue Substitute C Extraluminal Device D Intraluminal Device J Synthetic Substitute K Nonautologous Tissue Substitute Y Other Device	Z No Qualifier
Ø Eye, Right 1 Eye, Left	X External	Ø Drainage Device 3 Infusion Device 7 Autologous Tissue Substitute C Extraluminal Device D Intraluminal Device J Synthetic Substitute K Nonautologous Tissue Substitute	Z No Qualifier
J Lens, Right K Lens, Left	3 Percutaneous X External	J Synthetic Substitute Y Other Device	Z No Qualifier
J Lens, Right K Lens, Left	X External	J Synthetic Substitute	Z No Qualifier
L Extraocular Muscle, Right M Extraocular Muscle, Left	Ø Open 3 Percutaneous	Ø Drainage Device 7 Autologous Tissue Substitute J Synthetic Substitute K Nonautologous Tissue Substitute Y Other Device	Z No Qualifier

SECTION: Ø MEDICAL AND SURGICAL
BODY SYSTEM: 8 EYE
OPERATION: X TRANSFER: Moving, without taking out, all or a portion of a body part to another location to take over the function of all or a portion of a body part

Body Part	Approach	Device	Qualifier
L Extraocular Muscle, Right M Extraocular Muscle, Left	Ø Open 3 Percutaneous	Z No Device	Z No Qualifier

Ø9. Ear, Nose, Sinus 156
    Ø9Ø. Alteration 157
    Ø91. Bypass 157
    Ø92. Change 157
    Ø95. Destruction 158
    Ø97. Dilation 159
    Ø98. Division 159
    Ø99. Drainage 16Ø
    Ø9B. Excision 162
    Ø9C. Extirpation 163
    Ø9D. Extraction 164
    Ø9H. Insertion 164
    Ø9J. Inspection 165
    Ø9M. Reattachment 165
    Ø9N. Release 166
    Ø9P. Removal 167
    Ø9Q. Repair 168
    Ø9R. Replacement 169
    Ø9S. Reposition 170
    Ø9T. Resection 171
    Ø9U. Supplement 172
    Ø9W. Revision 173

SECTION: Ø MEDICAL AND SURGICAL
BODY SYSTEM: 9 EAR, NOSE, SINUS
OPERATION: Ø ALTERATION: Modifying the anatomic structure of a body part without affecting the function of the body part

Body Part	Approach	Device	Qualifier
Ø External Ear, Right 1 External Ear, Left 2 External Ear, Bilateral K Nasal Mucosa and Soft Tissue	Ø Open 3 Percutaneous 4 Percutaneous Endoscopic X External	7 Autologous Tissue Substitute J Synthetic Substitute K Nonautologous Tissue Substitute Z No Device	Z No Qualifier

SECTION: Ø MEDICAL AND SURGICAL
BODY SYSTEM: 9 EAR, NOSE, SINUS
OPERATION: 1 BYPASS: Altering the route of passage of the contents of a tubular body part

Body Part	Approach	Device	Qualifier
D Inner Ear, Right E Inner Ear, Left	Ø Open	7 Autologous Tissue Substitute J Synthetic Substitute K Nonautologous Tissue Substitute Z No Device	Ø Endolymphatic

SECTION: Ø MEDICAL AND SURGICAL
BODY SYSTEM: 9 EAR, NOSE, SINUS
OPERATION: 2 CHANGE: Taking out or off a device from a body part and putting back an identical or similar device in or on the same body part without cutting or puncturing the skin or a mucous membrane

Body Part	Approach	Device	Qualifier
H Ear, Right J Ear, Left K Nasal Mucosa and Soft Tissue Y Sinus	X External	Ø Drainage Device Y Other Device	Z No Qualifier

SECTION: Ø MEDICAL AND SURGICAL
BODY SYSTEM: 9 EAR, NOSE, SINUS
OPERATION: 5 DESTRUCTION: Physical eradication of all or a portion of a body part by the direct use of energy, force, or a destructive agent

Body Part	Approach	Device	Qualifier
Ø External Ear, Right 1 External Ear, Left K Nose	Ø Open 3 Percutaneous 4 Percutaneous Endoscopic X External	Z No Device	Z No Qualifier
3 External Auditory Canal, Right 4 External Auditory Canal, Left	Ø Open 3 Percutaneous 4 Percutaneous Endoscopic 7 Via Natural or Artificial Opening 8 Via Natural or Artificial Opening Endoscopic X External	Z No Device	Z No Qualifier
5 Middle Ear, Right 6 Middle Ear, Left 9 Auditory Ossicle, Right A Auditory Ossicle, Left D Inner Ear, Right E Inner Ear, Left	Ø Open 8 Via Natural or Artificial Opening Endoscopic	Z No Device	Z No Qualifier
7 Tympanic Membrane, Right 8 Tympanic Membrane, Left F Eustachian Tube, Right G Eustachian Tube, Left L Nasal Turbinate N Nasopharynx	Ø Open 3 Percutaneous 4 Percutaneous Endoscopic 7 Via Natural or Artificial Opening 8 Via Natural or Artificial Opening Endoscopic	Z No Device	Z No Qualifier
B Mastoid Sinus, Right C Mastoid Sinus, Left M Nasal Septum P Accessory Sinus Q Maxillary Sinus, Right R Maxillary Sinus, Left S Frontal Sinus, Right T Frontal Sinus, Left U Ethmoid Sinus, Right V Ethmoid Sinus, Left W Sphenoid Sinus, Right X Sphenoid Sinus, Left	Ø Open 3 Percutaneous 4 Percutaneous Endoscopic 8 Via Natural or Artificial Opening Endoscopic	Z No Device	Z No Qualifier
K Nasal Mucosa and Soft Tissue	Ø Open 3 Percutaneous 4 Percutaneous Endoscopic 8 Via Natural or Artificial Opening Endoscopic X External	Z No Device	Z No Qualifier

5: DESTRUCTION

9: EAR, NOSE, SINUS

Ø: M/S

SECTION: Ø MEDICAL AND SURGICAL

BODY SYSTEM: 9 EAR, NOSE, SINUS
OPERATION: 7 DILATION: Expanding an orifice or the lumen of a tubular body part

Body Part	Approach	Device	Qualifier
F Eustachian Tube, Right G Eustachian Tube, Left	Ø Open 7 Via Natural or Artificial Opening 8 Via Natural or Artificial Opening Endoscopic	D Intraluminal Device Z No Device	Z No Qualifier
F Eustachian Tube, Right G Eustachian Tube, Left	3 Percutaneous 4 Percutaneous Endoscopic	Z No Device	Z No Qualifier

SECTION: Ø MEDICAL AND SURGICAL

BODY SYSTEM: 9 EAR, NOSE, SINUS
OPERATION: 8 DIVISION: Cutting into a body part, without draining fluids and/or gases from the body part, in order to separate or transect a body part

Body Part	Approach	Device	Qualifier
L Nasal Turbinate	Ø Open 3 Percutaneous 4 Percutaneous Endoscopic 7 Via Natural or Artificial Opening 8 Via Natural or Artificial Opening Endoscopic	Z No Device	Z No Qualifier

SECTION: Ø MEDICAL AND SURGICAL
BODY SYSTEM: 9 **EAR, NOSE, SINUS**
OPERATION: 9 **DRAINAGE:** *(on multiple pages)*
Taking or letting out fluids and/or gases from a body part

Body Part	Approach	Device	Qualifier
Ø External Ear, Right 1 External Ear, Left ~~K Nose~~	Ø Open 3 Percutaneous 4 Percutaneous Endoscopic X External	Ø Drainage Device	Z No Qualifier
Ø External Ear, Right 1 External Ear, Left ~~K Nose~~	Ø Open 3 Percutaneous 4 Percutaneous Endoscopic X External	Z No Device	X Diagnostic Z No Qualifier
3 External Auditory Canal, Right 4 External Auditory Canal, Left K Nasal Mucosa and Soft Tissue	Ø Open 3 Percutaneous 4 Percutaneous Endoscopic 7 Via Natural or Artificial Opening 8 Via Natural or Artificial Opening Endoscopic X External	Ø Drainage Device	Z No Qualifier
3 External Auditory Canal, Right 4 External Auditory Canal, Left K Nasal Mucosa and Soft Tissue	Ø Open 3 Percutaneous 4 Percutaneous Endoscopic 7 Via Natural or Artificial Opening 8 Via Natural or Artificial Opening Endoscopic X External	Z No Device	X Diagnostic Z No Qualifier
5 Middle Ear, Right 6 Middle Ear, Left 9 Auditory Ossicle, Right A Auditory Ossicle, Left D Inner Ear, Right E Inner Ear, Left	Ø Open 7 Via Natural or Artificial Opening 8 Via Natural or Artificial Opening Endoscopic	Ø Drainage Device	Z No Qualifier
5 Middle Ear, Right 6 Middle Ear, Left 9 Auditory Ossicle, Right A Auditory Ossicle, Left D Inner Ear, Right E Inner Ear, Left	Ø Open 7 Via Natural or Artificial Opening 8 Via Natural or Artificial Opening Endoscopic	Z No Device	X Diagnostic Z No Qualifier
~~7 Tympanic Membrane, Right~~ ~~8 Tympanic Membrane, Left~~ ~~F Eustachian Tube, Right~~ ~~G Eustachian Tube, Left~~ ~~L Nasal Turbinate~~ ~~N Nasopharynx~~	~~Ø Open~~ ~~3 Percutaneous~~ ~~4 Percutaneous Endoscopic~~ ~~7 Via Natural or Artificial Opening~~ ~~8 Via Natural or Artificial Opening Endoscopic~~	~~Ø Drainage Device~~	~~Z No Qualifier~~

SECTION: Ø MEDICAL AND SURGICAL
BODY SYSTEM: 9 EAR, NOSE, SINUS
OPERATION: 9 DRAINAGE: *(continued)*
Taking or letting out fluids and/or gases from a body part

Body Part	Approach	Device	Qualifier
~~7 Tympanic Membrane, Right~~ ~~8 Tympanic Membrane, Left~~ ~~F Eustachian Tube, Right~~ ~~G Eustachian Tube, Left~~ ~~L Nasal Turbinate~~ ~~N Nasopharynx~~	~~Ø Open~~ ~~3 Percutaneous~~ ~~4 Percutaneous Endoscopic~~ ~~7 Via Natural or Artificial Opening~~ ~~8 Via Natural or Artificial Opening Endoscopic~~	~~Z No Device~~	~~X Diagnostic~~ ~~Z No Qualifier~~
7 Tympanic Membrane, Right 8 Tympanic Membrane, Left B Mastoid Sinus, Right C Mastoid Sinus, Left F Eustachian Tube, Right G Eustachian Tube, Left L Nasal Turbinate M Nasal Septum N Nasopharynx P Accessory Sinus Q Maxillary Sinus, Right R Maxillary Sinus, Left S Frontal Sinus, Right T Frontal Sinus, Left U Ethmoid Sinus, Right V Ethmoid Sinus, Left W Sphenoid Sinus, Right X Sphenoid Sinus, Left	Ø Open 3 Percutaneous 4 Percutaneous Endoscopic 7 Via Natural or Artificial Opening 8 Via Natural or Artificial Opening Endoscopic	Ø Drainage Device	Z No Qualifier
7 Tympanic Membrane, Right 8 Tympanic Membrane, Left B Mastoid Sinus, Right C Mastoid Sinus, Left F Eustachian Tube, Right G Eustachian Tube, Left L Nasal Turbinate M Nasal Septum N Nasopharynx P Accessory Sinus Q Maxillary Sinus, Right R Maxillary Sinus, Left S Frontal Sinus, Right T Frontal Sinus, Left U Ethmoid Sinus, Right V Ethmoid Sinus, Left W Sphenoid Sinus, Right X Sphenoid Sinus, Left	Ø Open 3 Percutaneous 4 Percutaneous Endoscopic 7 Via Natural or Artificial Opening 8 Via Natural or Artificial Opening Endoscopic	Z No Device	X Diagnostic Z No Qualifier

SECTION: Ø MEDICAL AND SURGICAL
BODY SYSTEM: 9 EAR, NOSE, SINUS
OPERATION: B EXCISION: Cutting out or off, without replacement, a portion of a body part

Body Part	Approach	Device	Qualifier
Ø External Ear, Right 1 External Ear, Left K Nose	Ø Open 3 Percutaneous 4 Percutaneous Endoscopic X External	Z No Device	X Diagnostic Z No Qualifier
3 External Auditory Canal, Right 4 External Auditory Canal, Left	Ø Open 3 Percutaneous 4 Percutaneous Endoscopic 7 Via Natural or Artificial Opening 8 Via Natural or Artificial Opening Endoscopic X External	Z No Device	X Diagnostic Z No Qualifier
5 Middle Ear, Right 6 Middle Ear, Left 9 Auditory Ossicle, Right A Auditory Ossicle, Left D Inner Ear, Right E Inner Ear, Left	Ø Open 8 Via Natural or Artificial Opening Endoscopic	Z No Device	X Diagnostic Z No Qualifier
7 Tympanic Membrane, Right 8 Tympanic Membrane, Left F Eustachian Tube, Right G Eustachian Tube, Left L Nasal Turbinate N Nasopharynx	Ø Open 3 Percutaneous 4 Percutaneous Endoscopic 7 Via Natural or Artificial Opening 8 Via Natural or Artificial Opening Endoscopic	Z No Device	X Diagnostic Z No Qualifier
B Mastoid Sinus, Right C Mastoid Sinus, Left M Nasal Septum P Accessory Sinus Q Maxillary Sinus, Right R Maxillary Sinus, Left S Frontal Sinus, Right T Frontal Sinus, Left U Ethmoid Sinus, Right V Ethmoid Sinus, Left W Sphenoid Sinus, Right X Sphenoid Sinus, Left	Ø Open 3 Percutaneous 4 Percutaneous Endoscopic 8 Via Natural or Artificial Opening Endoscopic	Z No Device	X Diagnostic Z No Qualifier
K Nasal Mucosa and Soft Tissue	Ø Open 3 Percutaneous 4 Percutaneous Endoscopic 8 Via Natural or Artificial Opening Endoscopic X External	Z No Device	X Diagnostic Z No Qualifier

B: EXCISION

9: EAR, NOSE, SINUS

Ø: M/S

SECTION: 0 MEDICAL AND SURGICAL
BODY SYSTEM: 9 EAR, NOSE, SINUS
OPERATION: C EXTIRPATION: Taking or cutting out solid matter from a body part

Body Part	Approach	Device	Qualifier
0 External Ear, Right 1 External Ear, Left ~~K Nose~~	0 Open 3 Percutaneous 4 Percutaneous Endoscopic X External	Z No Device	Z No Qualifier
3 External Auditory Canal, Right 4 External Auditory Canal, Left	0 Open 3 Percutaneous 4 Percutaneous Endoscopic 7 Via Natural or Artificial Opening 8 Via Natural or Artificial Opening Endoscopic X External	Z No Device	Z No Qualifier
5 Middle Ear, Right 6 Middle Ear, Left 9 Auditory Ossicle, Right A Auditory Ossicle, Left D Inner Ear, Right E Inner Ear, Left	0 Open 8 Via Natural or Artificial Opening Endoscopic	Z No Device	Z No Qualifier
7 Tympanic Membrane, Right 8 Tympanic Membrane, Left F Eustachian Tube, Right G Eustachian Tube, Left L Nasal Turbinate N Nasopharynx	0 Open 3 Percutaneous 4 Percutaneous Endoscopic 7 Via Natural or Artificial Opening 8 Via Natural or Artificial Opening Endoscopic	Z No Device	Z No Qualifier
B Mastoid Sinus, Right C Mastoid Sinus, Left M Nasal Septum P Accessory Sinus Q Maxillary Sinus, Right R Maxillary Sinus, Left S Frontal Sinus, Right T Frontal Sinus, Left U Ethmoid Sinus, Right V Ethmoid Sinus, Left W Sphenoid Sinus, Right X Sphenoid Sinus, Left	0 Open 3 Percutaneous 4 Percutaneous Endoscopic 8 Via Natural or Artificial Opening Endoscopic	Z No Device	Z No Qualifier
K Nasal Mucosa and Soft Tissue	0 Open 3 Percutaneous 4 Percutaneous Endoscopic 8 Via Natural or Artificial Opening Endoscopic X External	Z No Device	Z No Qualifier

SECTION: Ø MEDICAL AND SURGICAL

BODY SYSTEM: 9 EAR, NOSE, SINUS
OPERATION: D EXTRACTION: Pulling or stripping out or off all or a portion of a body part by the use of force

Body Part	Approach	Device	Qualifier
7 Tympanic Membrane, Right 8 Tympanic Membrane, Left L Nasal Turbinate	Ø Open 3 Percutaneous 4 Percutaneous Endoscopic 7 Via Natural or Artificial Opening 8 Via Natural or Artificial Opening Endoscopic	Z No Device	Z No Qualifier
9 Auditory Ossicle, Right A Auditory Ossicle, Left	Ø Open	Z No Device	Z No Qualifier
B Mastoid Sinus, Right C Mastoid Sinus, Left M Nasal Septum P Accessory Sinus Q Maxillary Sinus, Right R Maxillary Sinus, Left S Frontal Sinus, Right T Frontal Sinus, Left U Ethmoid Sinus, Right V Ethmoid Sinus, Left W Sphenoid Sinus, Right X Sphenoid Sinus, Left	Ø Open 3 Percutaneous 4 Percutaneous Endoscopic	Z No Device	Z No Qualifier

SECTION: Ø MEDICAL AND SURGICAL

BODY SYSTEM: 9 EAR, NOSE, SINUS
OPERATION: H INSERTION: Putting in a nonbiological appliance that monitors, assists, performs, or prevents a physiological function but does not physically take the place of a body part

Body Part	Approach	Device	Qualifier
D Inner Ear, Right E Inner Ear, Left	Ø Open 3 Percutaneous 4 Percutaneous Endoscopic	4 Hearing Device, Bone Conduction 5 Hearing Device, Single Channel Cochlear Prosthesis 6 Hearing Device, Multiple Channel Cochlear Prosthesis S Hearing Device	Z No Qualifier
H Ear, Right J Ear, Left K Nasal Mucosa and Soft Tissue Y Sinus	Ø Open 3 Percutaneous 4 Percutaneous Endoscopic 7 Via Natural or Artificial Opening 8 Via Natural or Artificial Opening Endoscopic	Y Other Device	Z No Qualifier
N Nasopharynx	7 Via Natural or Artificial Opening 8 Via Natural or Artificial Opening Endoscopic	B Intraluminal Device, Airway	Z No Qualifier

SECTION: Ø MEDICAL AND SURGICAL

BODY SYSTEM: 9 EAR, NOSE, SINUS
OPERATION: J INSPECTION: Visually and/or manually exploring a body part

Body Part	Approach	Device	Qualifier
7 Tympanic Membrane, Right 8 Tympanic Membrane, Left H Ear, Right J Ear, Left	Ø Open 3 Percutaneous 4 Percutaneous Endoscopic 7 Via Natural or Artificial Opening 8 Via Natural or Artificial Opening Endoscopic X External	Z No Device	Z No Qualifier
D Inner Ear, Right E Inner Ear, Left K Nasal Mucosa and Soft Tissue Y Sinus	Ø Open 3 Percutaneous 4 Percutaneous Endoscopic 8 Via Natural or Artificial Opening Endoscopic X External	Z No Device	Z No Qualifier

SECTION: Ø MEDICAL AND SURGICAL

BODY SYSTEM: 9 EAR, NOSE, SINUS
OPERATION: M REATTACHMENT: Putting back in or on all or a portion of a separated body part to its normal location or other suitable location

Body Part	Approach	Device	Qualifier
Ø External Ear, Right 1 External Ear, Left K Nasal Mucosa and Soft Tissue	X External	Z No Device	Z No Qualifier

SECTION: Ø MEDICAL AND SURGICAL
BODY SYSTEM: 9 EAR, NOSE, SINUS
OPERATION: N RELEASE: Freeing a body part from an abnormal physical constraint

Body Part	Approach	Device	Qualifier
Ø External Ear, Right 1 External Ear, Left ~~K Nose~~	Ø Open 3 Percutaneous 4 Percutaneous Endoscopic X External	Z No Device	Z No Qualifier
3 External Auditory Canal, Right 4 External Auditory Canal, Left	Ø Open 3 Percutaneous 4 Percutaneous Endoscopic 7 Via Natural or Artificial Opening 8 Via Natural or Artificial Opening Endoscopic X External	Z No Device	Z No Qualifier
5 Middle Ear, Right 6 Middle Ear, Left 9 Auditory Ossicle, Right A Auditory Ossicle, Left D Inner Ear, Right E Inner Ear, Left	Ø Open 8 Via Natural or Artificial Opening Endoscopic	Z No Device	Z No Qualifier
7 Tympanic Membrane, Right 8 Tympanic Membrane, Left F Eustachian Tube, Right G Eustachian Tube, Left L Nasal Turbinate N Nasopharynx	Ø Open 3 Percutaneous 4 Percutaneous Endoscopic 7 Via Natural or Artificial Opening 8 Via Natural or Artificial Opening Endoscopic	Z No Device	Z No Qualifier
B Mastoid Sinus, Right C Mastoid Sinus, Left M Nasal Septum P Accessory Sinus Q Maxillary Sinus, Right R Maxillary Sinus, Left S Frontal Sinus, Right T Frontal Sinus, Left U Ethmoid Sinus, Right V Ethmoid Sinus, Left W Sphenoid Sinus, Right X Sphenoid Sinus, Left	Ø Open 3 Percutaneous 4 Percutaneous Endoscopic 8 Via Natural or Artificial Opening Endoscopic	Z No Device	Z No Qualifier
K Nasal Mucosa and Soft Tissue	Ø Open 3 Percutaneous 4 Percutaneous Endoscopic 8 Via Natural or Artificial Opening Endoscopic X External	Z No Device	Z No Qualifier

SECTION: Ø MEDICAL AND SURGICAL
BODY SYSTEM: 9 EAR, NOSE, SINUS
OPERATION: P REMOVAL: Taking out or off a device from a body part

Body Part	Approach	Device	Qualifier
7 Tympanic Membrane, Right 8 Tympanic Membrane, Left	Ø Open 7 Via Natural or Artificial Opening 8 Via Natural or Artificial Opening Endoscopic X External	Ø Drainage Device	Z No Qualifier
D Inner Ear, Right E Inner Ear, Left	Ø Open 7 Via Natural or Artificial Opening 8 Via Natural or Artificial Opening Endoscopic	S Hearing Device	Z No Qualifier
H Ear, Right J Ear, Left K Nasal Mucosa and Soft Tissue	Ø Open 3 Percutaneous 4 Percutaneous Endoscopic 7 Via Natural or Artificial Opening 8 Via Natural or Artificial Opening Endoscopic X External	Ø Drainage Device 7 Autologous Tissue Substitute D Intraluminal Device J Synthetic Substitute K Nonautologous Tissue Substitute Y Other Device	Z No Qualifier
H Ear, Right J Ear, Left K Nasal Mucosa and Soft Tissue	X External	Ø Drainage Device 7 Autologous Tissue Substitute D Intraluminal Device J Synthetic Substitute K Nonautologous Tissue Substitute	Z No Qualifier
Y Sinus	Ø Open 3 Percutaneous 4 Percutaneous Endoscopic X External	Ø Drainage Device Y Other Device	Z No Qualifier
Y Sinus	7 Via Natural or Artificial Opening 8 Via Natural or Artificial Opening Endoscopic	Y Other Device	Z No Qualifier
Y Sinus	X External	Ø Drainage Device	Z No Qualifier

SECTION: Ø MEDICAL AND SURGICAL
BODY SYSTEM: 9 EAR, NOSE, SINUS
OPERATION: Q REPAIR: Restoring, to the extent possible, a body part to its normal anatomic structure and function

Body Part	Approach	Device	Qualifier
Ø External Ear, Right 1 External Ear, Left 2 External Ear, Bilateral ~~K Nose~~	Ø Open 3 Percutaneous 4 Percutaneous Endoscopic X External	Z No Device	Z No Qualifier
3 External Auditory Canal, Right 4 External Auditory Canal, Left F Eustachian Tube, Right G Eustachian Tube, Left	Ø Open 3 Percutaneous 4 Percutaneous Endoscopic 7 Via Natural or Artificial Opening 8 Via Natural or Artificial Opening Endoscopic X External	Z No Device	Z No Qualifier
5 Middle Ear, Right 6 Middle Ear, Left 9 Auditory Ossicle, Right A Auditory Ossicle, Left D Inner Ear, Right E Inner Ear, Left	Ø Open 8 Via Natural or Artificial Opening Endoscopic	Z No Device	Z No Qualifier
7 Tympanic Membrane, Right 8 Tympanic Membrane, Left L Nasal Turbinate N Nasopharynx	Ø Open 3 Percutaneous 4 Percutaneous Endoscopic 7 Via Natural or Artificial Opening 8 Via Natural or Artificial Opening Endoscopic	Z No Device	Z No Qualifier
B Mastoid Sinus, Right C Mastoid Sinus, Left M Nasal Septum P Accessory Sinus Q Maxillary Sinus, Right R Maxillary Sinus, Left S Frontal Sinus, Right T Frontal Sinus, Left U Ethmoid Sinus, Right V Ethmoid Sinus, Left W Sphenoid Sinus, Right X Sphenoid Sinus, Left	Ø Open 3 Percutaneous 4 Percutaneous Endoscopic 8 Via Natural or Artificial Opening Endoscopic	Z No Device	Z No Qualifier
K Nasal Mucosa and Soft Tissue	Ø Open 3 Percutaneous 4 Percutaneous Endoscopic 8 Via Natural or Artificial Opening Endoscopic X External	Z No Device	Z No Qualifier

SECTION: Ø MEDICAL AND SURGICAL
BODY SYSTEM: 9 EAR, NOSE, SINUS
OPERATION: R REPLACEMENT: Putting in or on biological or synthetic material that physically takes the place and/or function of all or a portion of a body part

Body Part	Approach	Device	Qualifier
Ø External Ear, Right 1 External Ear, Left 2 External Ear, Bilateral K Nasal Mucosa and Soft Tissue	Ø Open X External	7 Autologous Tissue Substitute J Synthetic Substitute K Nonautologous Tissue Substitute	Z No Qualifier
5 Middle Ear, Right 6 Middle Ear, Left 9 Auditory Ossicle, Right A Auditory Ossicle, Left D Inner Ear, Right E Inner Ear, Left	Ø Open	7 Autologous Tissue Substitute J Synthetic Substitute K Nonautologous Tissue Substitute	Z No Qualifier
7 Tympanic Membrane, Right 8 Tympanic Membrane, Left N Nasopharynx	Ø Open 7 Via Natural or Artificial Opening 8 Via Natural or Artificial Opening Endoscopic	7 Autologous Tissue Substitute J Synthetic Substitute K Nonautologous Tissue Substitute	Z No Qualifier
L Nasal Turbinate	Ø Open 3 Percutaneous 4 Percutaneous Endoscopic 7 Via Natural or Artificial Opening 8 Via Natural or Artificial Opening Endoscopic	7 Autologous Tissue Substitute J Synthetic Substitute K Nonautologous Tissue Substitute	Z No Qualifier
M Nasal Septum	Ø Open 3 Percutaneous 4 Percutaneous Endoscopic	7 Autologous Tissue Substitute J Synthetic Substitute K Nonautologous Tissue Substitute	Z No Qualifier

Ø: M/S

9: EAR, NOSE, SINUS

R: REPLACEMENT

SECTION: Ø MEDICAL AND SURGICAL
BODY SYSTEM: 9 EAR, NOSE, SINUS
OPERATION: S REPOSITION: Moving to its normal location, or other suitable location, all or a portion of a body part

Body Part	Approach	Device	Qualifier
Ø External Ear, Right 1 External Ear, Left 2 External Ear, Bilateral K Nasal Mucosa and Soft Tissue	Ø Open 4 Percutaneous Endoscopic X External	Z No Device	Z No Qualifier
7 Tympanic Membrane, Right 8 Tympanic Membrane, Left F Eustachian Tube, Right G Eustachian Tube, Left L Nasal Turbinate	Ø Open 4 Percutaneous Endoscopic 7 Via Natural or Artificial Opening 8 Via Natural or Artificial Opening Endoscopic	Z No Device	Z No Qualifier
9 Auditory Ossicle, Right A Auditory Ossicle, Left M Nasal Septum	Ø Open 4 Percutaneous Endoscopic	Z No Device	Z No Qualifier

S: REPOSITION 9: EAR, NOSE, SINUS Ø: M/S

SECTION: Ø MEDICAL AND SURGICAL
BODY SYSTEM: 9 EAR, NOSE, SINUS
OPERATION: T RESECTION: Cutting out or off, without replacement, all of a body part

Body Part	Approach	Device	Qualifier
Ø External Ear, Right 1 External Ear, Left ~~K Nose~~	Ø Open 4 Percutaneous Endoscopic X External	Z No Device	Z No Qualifier
5 Middle Ear, Right 6 Middle Ear, Left 9 Auditory Ossicle, Right A Auditory Ossicle, Left D Inner Ear, Right E Inner Ear, Left	Ø Open 8 Via Natural or Artificial Opening Endoscopic	Z No Device	Z No Qualifier

7 Tympanic Membrane, Right
8 Tympanic Membrane, Left
F Eustachian Tube, Right
G Eustachian Tube, Left
L Nasal Turbinate
N Nasopharynx
	Ø Open
	4 Percutaneous Endoscopic
	7 Via Natural or Artificial
	  Opening
	8 Via Natural or Artificial
	  Opening Endoscopic
		Z No Device	Z No Qualifier

B Mastoid Sinus, Right C Mastoid Sinus, Left M Nasal Septum P Accessory Sinus Q Maxillary Sinus, Right R Maxillary Sinus, Left S Frontal Sinus, Right T Frontal Sinus, Left U Ethmoid Sinus, Right V Ethmoid Sinus, Left W Sphenoid Sinus, Right X Sphenoid Sinus, Left	Ø Open 4 Percutaneous Endoscopic 8 Via Natural or Artificial Opening Endoscopic	Z No Device	Z No Qualifier
K Nasal Mucosa and Soft Tissue	Ø Open 4 Percutaneous Endoscopic 8 Via Natural or Artificial Opening Endoscopic X External	Z No Device	Z No Qualifier

SECTION: Ø MEDICAL AND SURGICAL
BODY SYSTEM: 9 EAR, NOSE, SINUS
OPERATION: U SUPPLEMENT: Putting in or on biological or synthetic material that physically reinforces and/or augments the function of a portion of a body part

Body Part	Approach	Device	Qualifier
Ø External Ear, Right 1 External Ear, Left 2 External Ear, Bilateral ~~K Nose~~	Ø Open X External	7 Autologous Tissue Substitute J Synthetic Substitute K Nonautologous Tissue Substitute	Z No Qualifier
5 Middle Ear, Right 6 Middle Ear, Left 9 Auditory Ossicle, Right A Auditory Ossicle, Left D Inner Ear, Right E Inner Ear, Left	Ø Open 8 Via Natural or Artificial Opening Endoscopic	7 Autologous Tissue Substitute J Synthetic Substitute K Nonautologous Tissue Substitute	Z No Qualifier
7 Tympanic Membrane, Right 8 Tympanic Membrane, Left N Nasopharynx	Ø Open 7 Via Natural or Artificial Opening 8 Via Natural or Artificial Opening Endoscopic	7 Autologous Tissue Substitute J Synthetic Substitute K Nonautologous Tissue Substitute	Z No Qualifier
K Nasal Mucosa and Soft Tissue	Ø Open 8 Via Natural or Artificial Opening Endoscopic X External	7 Autologous Tissue Substitute J Synthetic Substitute K Nonautologous Tissue Substitute	Z No Qualifier
L Nasal Turbinate	Ø Open 3 Percutaneous 4 Percutaneous Endoscopic 7 Via Natural or Artificial Opening 8 Via Natural or Artificial Opening Endoscopic	7 Autologous Tissue Substitute J Synthetic Substitute K Nonautologous Tissue Substitute	Z No Qualifier
M Nasal Septum	Ø Open 3 Percutaneous 4 Percutaneous Endoscopic 8 Via Natural or Artificial Opening Endoscopic	7 Autologous Tissue Substitute J Synthetic Substitute K Nonautologous Tissue Substitute	Z No Qualifier

SECTION: Ø MEDICAL AND SURGICAL
BODY SYSTEM: 9 EAR, NOSE, SINUS
OPERATION: W REVISION: Correcting, to the extent possible, a portion of a malfunctioning device or the position of a displaced device

Body Part	Approach	Device	Qualifier
7 Tympanic Membrane, Right 8 Tympanic Membrane, Left 9 Auditory Ossicle, Right A Auditory Ossicle, Left	Ø Open 7 Via Natural or Artificial Opening 8 Via Natural or Artificial Opening Endoscopic	7 Autologous Tissue Substitute J Synthetic Substitute K Nonautologous Tissue Substitute	Z No Qualifier
D Inner Ear, Right E Inner Ear, Left	Ø Open 7 Via Natural or Artificial Opening 8 Via Natural or Artificial Opening Endoscopic	S Hearing Device	Z No Qualifier
H Ear, Right J Ear, Left K Nasal Mucosa and Soft Tissue	Ø Open 3 Percutaneous 4 Percutaneous Endoscopic 7 Via Natural or Artificial Opening 8 Via Natural or Artificial Opening Endoscopic X External	Ø Drainage Device 7 Autologous Tissue Substitute D Intraluminal Device J Synthetic Substitute K Nonautologous Tissue Substitute Y Other Device	Z No Qualifier
H Ear, Right J Ear, Left K Nasal Mucosa and Soft Tissue	X External	Ø Drainage Device 7 Autologous Tissue Substitute D Intraluminal Device J Synthetic Substitute K Nonautologous Tissue Substitute	Z No Qualifier
Y Sinus	Ø Open 3 Percutaneous 4 Percutaneous Endoscopic X External	Ø Drainage Device Y Other Device	Z No Qualifier
Y Sinus	7 Via Natural or Artificial Opening 8 Via Natural or Artificial Opening Endoscopic	Y Other Device	Z No Qualifier
Y Sinus	X External	Ø Drainage Device	Z No Qualifier

ØB. Respiratory System...174
   ØB1. Bypass..175
   ØB2. Change 175
   ØB5. Destruction...176
   ØB7. Dilation..176
   ØB9. Drainage 177
   ØBB. Excision 178
   ØBC. Extirpation...179
   ØBD. Extraction...179
   ØBF. Fragmentation...18Ø
   ØBH. Insertion...18Ø
   ØBJ. Inspection..182
   ØBL. Occlusion..182
   ØBM. Reattachment...183
   ØBN. Release 183
   ØBP. Removal..184
   ØBQ. Repair 186
   ØBR. Replacement 186
   ØBS. Reposition...187
   ØBT. Resection..187
   ØBU. Supplement...188
   ØBV. Restriction..188
   ØBW. Revision...189
   ØBY. Transplantation...19Ø

SECTION: Ø MEDICAL AND SURGICAL

BODY SYSTEM: B RESPIRATORY SYSTEM
OPERATION: 1 BYPASS: Altering the route of passage of the contents of a tubular body part

Body Part	Approach	Device	Qualifier
1 Trachea	Ø Open	D Intraluminal Device	6 Esophagus
1 Trachea	Ø Open	F Tracheostomy Device Z No Device	4 Cutaneous
1 Trachea	3 Percutaneous 4 Percutaneous Endoscopic	F Tracheostomy Device Z No Device	4 Cutaneous

SECTION: Ø MEDICAL AND SURGICAL

BODY SYSTEM: B RESPIRATORY SYSTEM
OPERATION: 2 CHANGE: Taking out or off a device from a body part and putting back an identical or similar device in or on the same body part without cutting or puncturing the skin or a mucous membrane

Body Part	Approach	Device	Qualifier
Ø Tracheobronchial Tree K Lung, Right L Lung, Left Q Pleura T Diaphragm	X External	Ø Drainage Device Y Other Device	Z No Qualifier
1 Trachea	X External	Ø Drainage Device E Intraluminal Device, Endotracheal Airway F Tracheostomy Device Y Other Device	Z No Qualifier

SECTION: Ø MEDICAL AND SURGICAL
BODY SYSTEM: B RESPIRATORY SYSTEM
OPERATION: 5 DESTRUCTION: Physical eradication of all or a portion of a body part by the direct use of energy, force, or a destructive agent

Body Part	Approach	Device	Qualifier
1 Trachea 2 Carina 3 Main Bronchus, Right 4 Upper Lobe Bronchus, Right 5 Middle Lobe Bronchus, Right 6 Lower Lobe Bronchus, Right 7 Main Bronchus, Left 8 Upper Lobe Bronchus, Left 9 Lingula Bronchus B Lower Lobe Bronchus, Left C Upper Lung Lobe, Right D Middle Lung Lobe, Right F Lower Lung Lobe, Right G Upper Lung Lobe, Left H Lung Lingula J Lower Lung Lobe, Left K Lung, Right L Lung, Left M Lungs, Bilateral	Ø Open 3 Percutaneous 4 Percutaneous Endoscopic 7 Via Natural or Artificial Opening 8 Via Natural or Artificial Opening Endoscopic	Z No Device	Z No Qualifier
N Pleura, Right P Pleura, Left T Diaphragm S Diaphragm, Left	Ø Open 3 Percutaneous 4 Percutaneous Endoscopic	Z No Device	Z No Qualifier

SECTION: Ø MEDICAL AND SURGICAL
BODY SYSTEM: B RESPIRATORY SYSTEM
OPERATION: 7 DILATION: Expanding an orifice or the lumen of a tubular body part

Body Part	Approach	Device	Qualifier
1 Trachea 2 Carina 3 Main Bronchus, Right 4 Upper Lobe Bronchus, Right 5 Middle Lobe Bronchus, Right 6 Lower Lobe Bronchus, Right 7 Main Bronchus, Left 8 Upper Lobe Bronchus, Left 9 Lingula Bronchus B Lower Lobe Bronchus, Left	Ø Open 3 Percutaneous 4 Percutaneous Endoscopic 7 Via Natural or Artificial Opening 8 Via Natural or Artificial Opening Endoscopic	D Intraluminal Device Z No Device	Z No Qualifier

SECTION: Ø MEDICAL AND SURGICAL
BODY SYSTEM: B RESPIRATORY SYSTEM
OPERATION: 9 DRAINAGE: *(on multiple pages)*

Taking or letting out fluids and/or gases from a body part

Body Part	Approach	Device	Qualifier
1 Trachea 2 Carina 3 Main Bronchus, Right 4 Upper Lobe Bronchus, Right 5 Middle Lobe Bronchus, Right 6 Lower Lobe Bronchus, Right 7 Main Bronchus, Left 8 Upper Lobe Bronchus, Left 9 Lingula Bronchus B Lower Lobe Bronchus, Left C Upper Lung Lobe, Right D Middle Lung Lobe, Right F Lower Lung Lobe, Right G Upper Lung Lobe, Left H Lung Lingula J Lower Lung Lobe, Left K Lung, Right L Lung, Left M Lungs, Bilateral	Ø Open 3 Percutaneous 4 Percutaneous Endoscopic 7 Via Natural or Artificial Opening 8 Via Natural or Artificial Opening Endoscopic	Ø Drainage Device	Z No Qualifier
1 Trachea 2 Carina 3 Main Bronchus, Right 4 Upper Lobe Bronchus, Right 5 Middle Lobe Bronchus, Right 6 Lower Lobe Bronchus, Right 7 Main Bronchus, Left 8 Upper Lobe Bronchus, Left 9 Lingula Bronchus B Lower Lobe Bronchus, Left C Upper Lung Lobe, Right D Middle Lung Lobe, Right F Lower Lung Lobe, Right G Upper Lung Lobe, Left H Lung Lingula J Lower Lung Lobe, Left K Lung, Right L Lung, Left M Lungs, Bilateral	Ø Open 3 Percutaneous 4 Percutaneous Endoscopic 7 Via Natural or Artificial Opening 8 Via Natural or Artificial Opening Endoscopic	Z No Device	X Diagnostic Z No Qualifier
N Pleura, Right P Pleura, Left R Diaphragm, Right S Diaphragm, Left	Ø Open 3 Percutaneous 4 Percutaneous Endoscopic 8 Via Natural or Artificial Opening Endoscopic	Ø Drainage Device	Z No Qualifier

Ø: M/S

B: RESPIRATORY SYSTEM

9: DRAINAGE

SECTION:　Ø　MEDICAL AND SURGICAL
BODY SYSTEM: B　RESPIRATORY SYSTEM
OPERATION:　9　DRAINAGE: *(continued)*
　　　　　　　　　Taking or letting out fluids and/or gases from a body part

Body Part	Approach	Device	Qualifier
N Pleura, Right P Pleura, Left R ~~Diaphragm, Right~~ S ~~Diaphragm, Left~~	Ø Open 3 Percutaneous 4 Percutaneous Endoscopic 8 Via Natural or Artificial Opening Endoscopic	Z No Device	X Diagnostic Z No Qualifier
T Diaphragm	Ø Open 3 Percutaneous 4 Percutaneous Endoscopic	Ø Drainage	Z No Qualifier
T Diaphragm	Ø Open 3 Percutaneous 4 Percutaneous Endoscopic	Z No Device	X Diagnostic Z No Qualifier

SECTION:　Ø　MEDICAL AND SURGICAL
BODY SYSTEM: B　RESPIRATORY SYSTEM
OPERATION:　　B　EXCISION: Cutting out or off, without replacement, a portion of a body part

Body Part	Approach	Device	Qualifier
1 Trachea 2 Carina 3 Main Bronchus, Right 4 Upper Lobe Bronchus, Right 5 Middle Lobe Bronchus, Right 6 Lower Lobe Bronchus, Right 7 Main Bronchus, Left 8 Upper Lobe Bronchus, Left 9 Lingula Bronchus B Lower Lobe Bronchus, Left C Upper Lung Lobe, Right D Middle Lung Lobe, Right F Lower Lung Lobe, Right G Upper Lung Lobe, Left H Lung Lingula J Lower Lung Lobe, Left K Lung, Right L Lung, Left M Lungs, Bilateral	Ø Open 3 Percutaneous 4 Percutaneous Endoscopic 7 Via Natural or Artificial Opening 8 Via Natural or Artificial Opening Endoscopic	Z No Device	X Diagnostic Z No Qualifier
N Pleura, Right P Pleura, Left R ~~Diaphragm, Right~~ S ~~Diaphragm, Left~~	Ø Open 3 Percutaneous 4 Percutaneous Endoscopic 8 Via Natural or Artificial Opening Endoscopic	Z No Device	X Diagnostic Z No Qualifier
T Diaphragm	Ø Open 3 Percutaneous 4 Percutaneous Endoscopic	Z No Device	X Diagnostic Z No Qualifier

New/Revised Text in Blue　　~~deleted~~ Deleted

SECTION: Ø MEDICAL AND SURGICAL
BODY SYSTEM: B RESPIRATORY SYSTEM
OPERATION: C EXTIRPATION: Taking or cutting out solid matter from a body part

Body Part	Approach	Device	Qualifier
1 Trachea 2 Carina 3 Main Bronchus, Right 4 Upper Lobe Bronchus, Right 5 Middle Lobe Bronchus, Right 6 Lower Lobe Bronchus, Right 7 Main Bronchus, Left 8 Upper Lobe Bronchus, Left 9 Lingula Bronchus B Lower Lobe Bronchus, Left C Upper Lung Lobe, Right D Middle Lung Lobe, Right F Lower Lung Lobe, Right G Upper Lung Lobe, Left H Lung Lingula J Lower Lung Lobe, Left K Lung, Right L Lung, Left M Lungs, Bilateral	Ø Open 3 Percutaneous 4 Percutaneous Endoscopic 7 Via Natural or Artificial Opening 8 Via Natural or Artificial Opening Endoscopic	Z No Device	Z No Qualifier
N Pleura, Right P Pleura, Left T Diaphragm ~~S Diaphragm, Left~~	Ø Open 3 Percutaneous 4 Percutaneous Endoscopic	Z No Device	Z No Qualifier

SECTION: Ø MEDICAL AND SURGICAL
BODY SYSTEM: B RESPIRATORY SYSTEM
OPERATION: D EXTRACTION: Pulling or stripping out or off all or a portion of a body part by the use of force

Body Part	Approach	Device	Qualifier
1 Trachea 2 Carina 3 Main Bronchus, Right 4 Upper Lobe Bronchus, Right 5 Middle Lobe Bronchus, Right 6 Lower Lobe Bronchus, Right 7 Main Bronchus, Left 8 Upper Lobe Bronchus, Left 9 Lingula Bronchus B Lower Lobe Bronchus, Left C Upper Lung Lobe, Right D Middle Lung Lobe, Right F Lower Lung Lobe, Right G Upper Lung Lobe, Left H Lung Lingula J Lower Lung Lobe, Left K Lung, Right L Lung, Left M Lungs, Bilateral	4 Percutaneous Endoscopic 8 Via Natural or Artificial Opening Endoscopic	Z No Device	X Diagnostic
N Pleura, Right P Pleura, Left	Ø Open 3 Percutaneous 4 Percutaneous Endoscopic	Z No Device	X Diagnostic Z No Qualifier

SECTION: Ø MEDICAL AND SURGICAL
BODY SYSTEM: B RESPIRATORY SYSTEM
OPERATION: F FRAGMENTATION: Breaking solid matter in a body part into pieces

Body Part	Approach	Device	Qualifier

1 Trachea
2 Carina
3 Main Bronchus, Right
4 Upper Lobe Bronchus, Right
5 Middle Lobe Bronchus, Right
6 Lower Lobe Bronchus, Right
7 Main Bronchus, Left
8 Upper Lobe Bronchus, Left
9 Lingula Bronchus
B Lower Lobe Bronchus, Left
	Ø Open
	3 Percutaneous
	4 Percutaneous Endoscopic
	7 Via Natural or Artificial
	   Opening
	8 Via Natural or Artificial
	   Opening Endoscopic
	X External
		Z No Device	Z No Qualifier

SECTION: Ø MEDICAL AND SURGICAL
BODY SYSTEM: B RESPIRATORY SYSTEM
OPERATION: H INSERTION: *(on multiple pages)*
Putting in a nonbiological appliance that monitors, assists, performs, or prevents a physiological function but does not physically take the place of a body part

Body Part	Approach	Device	Qualifier

Ø Tracheobronchial Tree	Ø Open
	3 Percutaneous
	4 Percutaneous Endoscopic
	7 Via Natural or Artificial
	   Opening
	8 Via Natural or Artificial
	   Opening Endoscopic
		1 Radioactive Element
		2 Monitoring Device
		3 Infusion Device
		D Intraluminal Device
		Y Other Device
			Z No Qualifier

1 Trachea	Ø Open	2 Monitoring Device D Intraluminal Device Y Other Device	Z No Qualifier
1 Trachea	3 Percutaneous	D Intraluminal Device E Intraluminal Device, Endotracheal Airway Y Other Device	Z No Qualifier
1 Trachea	4 Percutaneous Endoscopic	D Intraluminal Device Y Other Device	Z No Qualifier

SECTION: Ø MEDICAL AND SURGICAL
BODY SYSTEM: B RESPIRATORY SYSTEM
OPERATION: H INSERTION: *(continued)*

Putting in a nonbiological appliance that monitors, assists, performs, or prevents a physiological function but does not physically take the place of a body part

Body Part	Approach	Device	Qualifier
1 Trachea	7 Via Natural or Artificial Opening 8 Via Natural or Artificial Opening Endoscopic	2 Monitoring Device D Intraluminal Device E Intraluminal Device, Endotracheal Airway Y Other Device	Z No Qualifier
3 Main Bronchus, Right 4 Upper Lobe Bronchus, Right 5 Middle Lobe Bronchus, Right 6 Lower Lobe Bronchus, Right 7 Main Bronchus, Left 8 Upper Lobe Bronchus, Left 9 Lingula Bronchus B Lower Lobe Bronchus, Left	Ø Open 3 Percutaneous 4 Percutaneous Endoscopic 7 Via Natural or Artificial Opening 8 Via Natural or Artificial Opening Endoscopic	G Endobronchial Device, Endobronchial Valve	Z No Qualifier
K Lung, Right L Lung, Left	Ø Open 3 Percutaneous 4 Percutaneous Endoscopic 7 Via Natural or Artificial Opening 8 Via Natural or Artificial Opening Endoscopic	1 Radioactive Element 2 Monitoring Device 3 Infusion Device Y Other Device	Z No Qualifier
~~R Diaphragm, Right~~ ~~S Diaphragm, Left~~	~~Ø Open~~ ~~3 Percutaneous~~ ~~4 Percutaneous Endoscopic~~	~~2 Monitoring Device~~ ~~M Diaphragmatic Pacemaker Lead~~	~~Z No Qualifier~~
Q Pleura	Ø Open 3 Percutaneous 4 Percutaneous Endoscopic 7 Via Natural or Artificial Opening 8 Via Natural or Artificial Opening Endoscopic	Y Other Device	Z No Qualifier
T Diaphragm	Ø Open 3 Percutaneous 4 Percutaneous Endoscopic	2 Monitoring Device M Diaphragmatic Pacemaker Lead Y Other Device	Z No Qualifier
T Diaphragm	7 Via Natural or Artificial Opening 8 Via Natural or Artificial Opening Endoscopic	Y Other Device	Z No Qualifier

SECTION: Ø MEDICAL AND SURGICAL
BODY SYSTEM: B RESPIRATORY SYSTEM
OPERATION: J INSPECTION: Visually and/or manually exploring a body part

Body Part	Approach	Device	Qualifier
Ø Tracheobronchial Tree 1 Trachea K Lung, Right L Lung, Left Q Pleura T Diaphragm	Ø Open 3 Percutaneous 4 Percutaneous Endoscopic 7 Via Natural or Artificial Opening 8 Via Natural or Artificial Opening Endoscopic X External	Z No Device	Z No Qualifier

SECTION: Ø MEDICAL AND SURGICAL
BODY SYSTEM: B RESPIRATORY SYSTEM
OPERATION: L OCCLUSION: Completely closing an orifice or the lumen of a tubular body part

Body Part	Approach	Device	Qualifier
1 Trachea 2 Carina 3 Main Bronchus, Right 4 Upper Lobe Bronchus, Right 5 Middle Lobe Bronchus, Right 6 Lower Lobe Bronchus, Right 7 Main Bronchus, Left 8 Upper Lobe Bronchus, Left 9 Lingula Bronchus B Lower Lobe Bronchus, Left	Ø Open 3 Percutaneous 4 Percutaneous Endoscopic	C Extraluminal Device D Intraluminal Device Z No Device	Z No Qualifier
1 Trachea 2 Carina 3 Main Bronchus, Right 4 Upper Lobe Bronchus, Right 5 Middle Lobe Bronchus, Right 6 Lower Lobe Bronchus, Right 7 Main Bronchus, Left 8 Upper Lobe Bronchus, Left 9 Lingula Bronchus B Lower Lobe Bronchus, Left	7 Via Natural or Artificial Opening 8 Via Natural or Artificial Opening Endoscopic	D Intraluminal Device Z No Device	Z No Qualifier

SECTION: Ø MEDICAL AND SURGICAL

BODY SYSTEM: B RESPIRATORY SYSTEM

OPERATION: M REATTACHMENT: Putting back in or on all or a portion of a separated body part to its normal location or other suitable location

Body Part	Approach	Device	Qualifier
1 Trachea	Ø Open	Z No Device	Z No Qualifier
2 Carina			
3 Main Bronchus, Right			
4 Upper Lobe Bronchus, Right			
5 Middle Lobe Bronchus, Right			
6 Lower Lobe Bronchus, Right			
7 Main Bronchus, Left			
8 Upper Lobe Bronchus, Left			
9 Lingula Bronchus			
B Lower Lobe Bronchus, Left			
C Upper Lung Lobe, Right			
D Middle Lung Lobe, Right			
F Lower Lung Lobe, Right			
G Upper Lung Lobe, Left			
H Lung Lingula			
J Lower Lung Lobe, Left			
K Lung, Right			
L Lung, Left			
T Diaphragm			
~~S Diaphragm, Left~~			

SECTION: Ø MEDICAL AND SURGICAL

BODY SYSTEM: B RESPIRATORY SYSTEM

OPERATION: N RELEASE: Freeing a body part from an abnormal physical constraint by cutting or by the use of force

Body Part	Approach	Device	Qualifier
1 Trachea	Ø Open	Z No Device	Z No Qualifier
2 Carina	3 Percutaneous		
3 Main Bronchus, Right	4 Percutaneous Endoscopic		
4 Upper Lobe Bronchus, Right	7 Via Natural or Artificial Opening		
5 Middle Lobe Bronchus, Right	8 Via Natural or Artificial Opening Endoscopic		
6 Lower Lobe Bronchus, Right			
7 Main Bronchus, Left			
8 Upper Lobe Bronchus, Left			
9 Lingula Bronchus			
B Lower Lobe Bronchus, Left			
C Upper Lung Lobe, Right			
D Middle Lung Lobe, Right			
F Lower Lung Lobe, Right			
G Upper Lung Lobe, Left			
H Lung Lingula			
J Lower Lung Lobe, Left			
K Lung, Right			
L Lung, Left			
M Lungs, Bilateral			
N Pleura, Right	Ø Open	Z No Device	Z No Qualifier
P Pleura, Left	3 Percutaneous		
T Diaphragm	4 Percutaneous Endoscopic		
~~S Diaphragm, Left~~			

SECTION: Ø MEDICAL AND SURGICAL
BODY SYSTEM: B RESPIRATORY SYSTEM
OPERATION: P REMOVAL: *(on multiple pages)*
Taking out or off a device from a body part

Body Part	Approach	Device	Qualifier
Ø Tracheobronchial Tree	Ø Open 3 Percutaneous 4 Percutaneous Endoscopic 7 Via Natural or Artificial Opening 8 Via Natural or Artificial Opening Endoscopic	Ø Drainage Device 1 Radioactive Element 2 Monitoring Device 3 Infusion Device 7 Autologous Tissue Substitute C Extraluminal Device D Intraluminal Device J Synthetic Substitute K Nonautologous Tissue Substitute Y Other Device	Z No Qualifier
Ø Tracheobronchial Tree	X External	Ø Drainage Device 1 Radioactive Element 2 Monitoring Device 3 Infusion Device D Intraluminal Device	Z No Qualifier
1 Trachea	Ø Open 3 Percutaneous 4 Percutaneous Endoscopic 7 Via Natural or Artificial Opening 8 Via Natural or Artificial Opening Endoscopic	Ø Drainage Device 2 Monitoring Device 7 Autologous Tissue Substitute C Extraluminal Device D Intraluminal Device F Tracheostomy Device J Synthetic Substitute K Nonautologous Tissue Substitute	Z No Qualifier
1 Trachea	X External	Ø Drainage Device 2 Monitoring Device D Intraluminal Device F Tracheostomy Device	Z No Qualifier
K Lung, Right L Lung, Left	Ø Open 3 Percutaneous 4 Percutaneous Endoscopic 7 Via Natural or Artificial Opening 8 Via Natural or Artificial Opening Endoscopic ~~X External~~	Ø Drainage Device 1 Radioactive Element 2 Monitoring Device 3 Infusion Device Y Other Device	Z No Qualifier

New/Revised Text in Blue   ~~deleted~~ Deleted

SECTION: Ø MEDICAL AND SURGICAL
BODY SYSTEM: B RESPIRATORY SYSTEM
OPERATION: P REMOVAL: *(continued)*
Taking out or off a device from a body part

Body Part	Approach	Device	Qualifier
K Lung, Right L Lung, Left	X External	Ø Drainage Device 1 Radioactive Element 2 Monitoring Device 3 Infusion Device	Z No Qualifier
Q Pleura	Ø Open 3 Percutaneous 4 Percutaneous Endoscopic 7 Via Natural or Artificial Opening 8 Via Natural or Artificial Opening Endoscopic ~~X External~~	Ø Drainage Device 1 Radioactive Element 2 Monitoring Device Y Other Device	Z No Qualifier
Q Pleura	X External	Ø Drainage Device 1 Radioactive Element 2 Monitoring Device	Z No Qualifier
T Diaphragm	Ø Open 3 Percutaneous 4 Percutaneous Endoscopic 7 Via Natural or Artificial Opening 8 Via Natural or Artificial Opening Endoscopic	Ø Drainage Device 2 Monitoring Device 7 Autologous Tissue Substitute J Synthetic Substitute K Nonautologous Tissue Substitute M Diaphragmatic Pacemaker Lead Y Other Device	Z No Qualifier
T Diaphragm	X External	Ø Drainage Device 2 Monitoring Device M Diaphragmatic Pacemaker Lead	Z No Qualifier

SECTION: Ø MEDICAL AND SURGICAL
BODY SYSTEM: B RESPIRATORY SYSTEM
OPERATION: Q REPAIR: Restoring, to the extent possible, a body part to its normal anatomic structure and function

Body Part	Approach	Device	Qualifier
1 Trachea 2 Carina 3 Main Bronchus, Right 4 Upper Lobe Bronchus, Right 5 Middle Lobe Bronchus, Right 6 Lower Lobe Bronchus, Right 7 Main Bronchus, Left 8 Upper Lobe Bronchus, Left 9 Lingula Bronchus B Lower Lobe Bronchus, Left C Upper Lung Lobe, Right D Middle Lung Lobe, Right F Lower Lung Lobe, Right G Upper Lung Lobe, Left H Lung Lingula J Lower Lung Lobe, Left K Lung, Right L Lung, Left M Lungs, Bilateral	Ø Open 3 Percutaneous 4 Percutaneous Endoscopic 7 Via Natural or Artificial Opening 8 Via Natural or Artificial Opening Endoscopic	Z No Device	Z No Qualifier
N Pleura, Right P Pleura, Left T Diaphragm S~~ Diaphragm, Left~~	Ø Open 3 Percutaneous 4 Percutaneous Endoscopic	Z No Device	Z No Qualifier

SECTION: Ø MEDICAL AND SURGICAL
BODY SYSTEM: B RESPIRATORY SYSTEM
OPERATION: R REPLACEMENT: Putting in or on biological or synthetic material that physically takes the place and/or function of all or a portion of a body part

Body Part	Approach	Device	Qualifier
1 Trachea 2 Carina 3 Main Bronchus, Right 4 Upper Lobe Bronchus, Right 5 Middle Lobe Bronchus, Right 6 Lower Lobe Bronchus, Right 7 Main Bronchus, Left 8 Upper Lobe Bronchus, Left 9 Lingula Bronchus B Lower Lobe Bronchus, Left T Diaphragm	Ø Open 4 Percutaneous Endoscopic	7 Autologous Tissue Substitute J Synthetic Substitute K Nonautologous Tissue Substitute	Z No Qualifier

SECTION: Ø MEDICAL AND SURGICAL
BODY SYSTEM: B RESPIRATORY SYSTEM
OPERATION: S REPOSITION: Moving to its normal location, or other suitable location, all or a portion of a body part

Body Part	Approach	Device	Qualifier
1 Trachea	Ø Open	Z No Device	Z No Qualifier
2 Carina			
3 Main Bronchus, Right			
4 Upper Lobe Bronchus, Right			
5 Middle Lobe Bronchus, Right			
6 Lower Lobe Bronchus, Right			
7 Main Bronchus, Left			
8 Upper Lobe Bronchus, Left			
9 Lingula Bronchus			
B Lower Lobe Bronchus, Left			
C Upper Lung Lobe, Right			
D Middle Lung Lobe, Right			
F Lower Lung Lobe, Right			
G Upper Lung Lobe, Left			
H Lung Lingula			
J Lower Lung Lobe, Left			
K Lung, Right			
L Lung, Left			
T Diaphragm			
~~S Diaphragm, Left~~			

SECTION: Ø MEDICAL AND SURGICAL
BODY SYSTEM: B RESPIRATORY SYSTEM
OPERATION: T RESECTION: Cutting out or off, without replacement, all of a body part

Body Part	Approach	Device	Qualifier
1 Trachea	Ø Open	Z No Device	Z No Qualifier
2 Carina	4 Percutaneous Endoscopic		
3 Main Bronchus, Right			
4 Upper Lobe Bronchus, Right			
5 Middle Lobe Bronchus, Right			
6 Lower Lobe Bronchus, Right			
7 Main Bronchus, Left			
8 Upper Lobe Bronchus, Left			
9 Lingula Bronchus			
B Lower Lobe Bronchus, Left			
C Upper Lung Lobe, Right			
D Middle Lung Lobe, Right			
F Lower Lung Lobe, Right			
G Upper Lung Lobe, Left			
H Lung Lingula			
J Lower Lung Lobe, Left			
K Lung, Right			
L Lung, Left			
M Lungs, Bilateral			
T Diaphragm			
~~S Diaphragm, Left~~			

SECTION: Ø MEDICAL AND SURGICAL
BODY SYSTEM: B RESPIRATORY SYSTEM
OPERATION: U SUPPLEMENT: Putting in or on biological or synthetic material that physically reinforces and/or augments the function of a portion of a body part

Body Part	Approach	Device	Qualifier
1 Trachea 2 Carina 3 Main Bronchus, Right 4 Upper Lobe Bronchus, Right 5 Middle Lobe Bronchus, Right 6 Lower Lobe Bronchus, Right 7 Main Bronchus, Left 8 Upper Lobe Bronchus, Left 9 Lingula Bronchus B Lower Lobe Bronchus, Left R Diaphragm, Right S Diaphragm, Left	Ø Open 4 Percutaneous Endoscopic 8 Via Natural or Artificial Opening Endoscopic	7 Autologous Tissue Substitute J Synthetic Substitute K Nonautologous Tissue Substitute	Z No Qualifier
T Diaphragm	Ø Open 4 Percutaneous Endoscopic	7 Autologous Tissue Substitute J Synthetic Substitute K Nonautologous Tissue Substitute	Z No Qualifier

SECTION: Ø MEDICAL AND SURGICAL
BODY SYSTEM: B RESPIRATORY SYSTEM
OPERATION: V RESTRICTION: Partially closing an orifice or the lumen of a tubular body part

Body Part	Approach	Device	Qualifier
1 Trachea 2 Carina 3 Main Bronchus, Right 4 Upper Lobe Bronchus, Right 5 Middle Lobe Bronchus, Right 6 Lower Lobe Bronchus, Right 7 Main Bronchus, Left 8 Upper Lobe Bronchus, Left 9 Lingula Bronchus B Lower Lobe Bronchus, Left	Ø Open 3 Percutaneous 4 Percutaneous Endoscopic	C Extraluminal Device D Intraluminal Device Z No Device	Z No Qualifier
1 Trachea 2 Carina 3 Main Bronchus, Right 4 Upper Lobe Bronchus, Right 5 Middle Lobe Bronchus, Right 6 Lower Lobe Bronchus, Right 7 Main Bronchus, Left 8 Upper Lobe Bronchus, Left 9 Lingula Bronchus B Lower Lobe Bronchus, Left	7 Via Natural or Artificial Opening 8 Via Natural or Artificial Opening Endoscopic	D Intraluminal Device Z No Device	Z No Qualifier

U: SUPPLEMENT   V: RESTRICTION

B: RESPIRATORY SYSTEM

Ø: M/S

SECTION: Ø MEDICAL AND SURGICAL
BODY SYSTEM: B RESPIRATORY SYSTEM
OPERATION: W REVISION: *(on multiple pages)*
Correcting, to the extent possible, a portion of a malfunctioning device or the position of a displaced device

Body Part	Approach	Device	Qualifier
Ø Tracheobronchial Tree	Ø Open 3 Percutaneous 4 Percutaneous Endoscopic 7 Via Natural or Artificial Opening 8 Via Natural or Artificial Opening Endoscopic X̶ E̶x̶t̶e̶r̶n̶a̶l̶	Ø Drainage Device 2 Monitoring Device 3 Infusion Device 7 Autologous Tissue Substitute C Extraluminal Device D Intraluminal Device J Synthetic Substitute K Nonautologous Tissue Substitute Y Other Device	Z No Qualifier
Ø Tracheobronchial Tree	X External	Ø Drainage Device 2 Monitoring Device 3 Infusion Device 7 Autologous Tissue Substitute C Extraluminal Device D Intraluminal Device J Synthetic Substitute K Nonautologous Tissue Substitute	Z No Qualifier
1 Trachea	Ø Open 3 Percutaneous 4 Percutaneous Endoscopic 7 Via Natural or Artificial Opening 8 Via Natural or Artificial Opening Endoscopic X External	Ø Drainage Device 2 Monitoring Device 7 Autologous Tissue Substitute C Extraluminal Device D Intraluminal Device F Tracheostomy Device J Synthetic Substitute K Nonautologous Tissue Substitute	Z No Qualifier
K Lung, Right L Lung, Left	Ø Open 3 Percutaneous 4 Percutaneous Endoscopic 7 Via Natural or Artificial Opening 8 Via Natural or Artificial Opening Endoscopic X̶ E̶x̶t̶e̶r̶n̶a̶l̶	Ø Drainage Device 2 Monitoring Device 3 Infusion Device Y Other Device	Z No Qualifier
K Lung, Right L Lung, Left	X External	Ø Drainage Device 2 Monitoring Device 3 Infusion Device	Z No Qualifier
Q Pleura	Ø Open 3 Percutaneous 4 Percutaneous Endoscopic 7 Via Natural or Artificial Opening 8 Via Natural or Artificial Opening Endoscopic X̶ E̶x̶t̶e̶r̶n̶a̶l̶	Ø Drainage Device 2 Monitoring Device Y Other Device	Z No Qualifier
Q Pleura	X External	Ø Drainage Device 2 Monitoring Device	Z No Qualifier

SECTION: Ø MEDICAL AND SURGICAL
BODY SYSTEM: B RESPIRATORY SYSTEM
OPERATION: W REVISION: *(continued)*
Correcting, to the extent possible, a portion of a malfunctioning device or the position of a displaced device

Body Part	Approach	Device	Qualifier
T Diaphragm	Ø Open 3 Percutaneous 4 Percutaneous Endoscopic 7 Via Natural or Artificial Opening 8 Via Natural or Artificial Opening Endoscopic ~~X External~~	Ø Drainage Device 2 Monitoring Device 7 Autologous Tissue Substitute J Synthetic Substitute K Nonautologous Tissue Substitute M Diaphragmatic Pacemaker Lead Y Other Device	Z No Qualifier
T Diaphragm	X External	Ø Drainage Device 2 Monitoring Device 7 Autologous Tissue Substitute J Synthetic Substitute K Nonautologous Tissue Substitute M Diaphragmatic Pacemaker Lead	Z No Qualifier

SECTION: Ø MEDICAL AND SURGICAL
BODY SYSTEM: B RESPIRATORY SYSTEM
OPERATION: Y TRANSPLANTATION: Putting in or on all or a portion of a living body part taken from another individual or animal to physically take the place and/or function of all or a portion of a similar body part

Body Part	Approach	Device	Qualifier
C Upper Lung Lobe, Right D Middle Lung Lobe, Right F Lower Lung Lobe, Right G Upper Lung Lobe, Left H Lung Lingula J Lower Lung Lobe, Left K Lung, Right L Lung, Left M Lungs, Bilateral	Ø Open	Z No Device	Ø Allogeneic 1 Syngeneic 2 Zooplastic

ØC. Mouth and Throat..191
   ØCØ. Alteration...192
   ØC2. Change 192
   ØC5. Destruction..192
   ØC7. Dilation...193
   ØC9. Drainage 194
   ØCB. Excision 195
   ØCC. Extirpation 196
   ØCD. Extraction 196
   ØCF. Fragmentation...197
   ØCH. Insertion 197
   ØCJ. Inspection 197
   ØCL. Occlusion 198
   ØCM. Reattachment 198
   ØCN. Release 199
   ØCP. Removal 200
   ØCQ. Repair 201
   ØCR. Replacement 202
   ØCS. Reposition 202
   ØCT. Resection...203
   ØCU. Supplement..203
   ØCV. Restriction...204
   ØCW. Revision..204
   ØCX. Transfer 205

SECTION: Ø MEDICAL AND SURGICAL
BODY SYSTEM: C MOUTH AND THROAT
OPERATION: Ø ALTERATION: Modifying the anatomic structure of a body part without affecting the function of the body part

Body Part	Approach	Device	Qualifier
Ø Upper Lip 1 Lower Lip	X External	7 Autologous Tissue Substitute J Synthetic Substitute K Nonautologous Tissue Substitute Z No Device	Z No Qualifier

SECTION: Ø MEDICAL AND SURGICAL
BODY SYSTEM: C MOUTH AND THROAT
OPERATION: 2 CHANGE: Taking out or off a device from a body part and putting back an identical or similar device in or on the same body part without cutting or puncturing the skin or a mucous membrane

Body Part	Approach	Device	Qualifier
A Salivary Gland S Larynx Y Mouth and Throat	X External	Ø Drainage Device Y Other Device	Z No Qualifier

SECTION: Ø MEDICAL AND SURGICAL
BODY SYSTEM: C MOUTH AND THROAT
OPERATION: 5 DESTRUCTION: *(on multiple pages)*
Physical eradication of all or a portion of a body part by the use of direct energy, force, or a destructive agent

Body Part	Approach	Device	Qualifier
Ø Upper Lip 1 Lower Lip 2 Hard Palate 3 Soft Palate 4 Buccal Mucosa 5 Upper Gingiva 6 Lower Gingiva 7 Tongue N Uvula P Tonsils Q Adenoids	Ø Open 3 Percutaneous X External	Z No Device	Z No Qualifier

SECTION: Ø MEDICAL AND SURGICAL
BODY SYSTEM: C MOUTH AND THROAT
OPERATION: 5 DESTRUCTION: *(continued)*
Physical eradication of all or a portion of a body part by the use of direct energy, force, or a destructive agent

Body Part	Approach	Device	Qualifier
8 Parotid Gland, Right 9 Parotid Gland, Left B Parotid Duct, Right C Parotid Duct, Left D Sublingual Gland, Right F Sublingual Gland, Left G Submaxillary Gland, Right H Submaxillary Gland, Left J Minor Salivary Gland	Ø Open 3 Percutaneous	Z No Device	Z No Qualifier
M Pharynx R Epiglottis S Larynx T Vocal Cord, Right V Vocal Cord, Left	Ø Open 3 Percutaneous 4 Percutaneous Endoscopic 7 Via Natural or Artificial Opening 8 Via Natural or Artificial Opening Endoscopic	Z No Device	Z No Qualifier
W Upper Tooth X Lower Tooth	Ø Open X External	Z No Device	Ø Single 1 Multiple 2 All

SECTION: Ø MEDICAL AND SURGICAL
BODY SYSTEM: C MOUTH AND THROAT
OPERATION: 7 DILATION: Expanding an orifice or the lumen of a tubular body part

Body Part	Approach	Device	Qualifier
B Parotid Duct, Right C Parotid Duct, Left	Ø Open 3 Percutaneous 7 Via Natural or Artificial Opening	D Intraluminal Device Z No Device	Z No Qualifier
M Pharynx	7 Via Natural or Artificial Opening 8 Via Natural or Artificial Opening Endoscopic	D Intraluminal Device Z No Device	Z No Qualifier
S Larynx	Ø Open 3 Percutaneous 4 Percutaneous Endoscopic 7 Via Natural or Artificial Opening 8 Via Natural or Artificial Opening Endoscopic	D Intraluminal Device Z No Device	Z No Qualifier

Ø: M/S   C: MOUTH AND THROAT   5: DESTRUCTION   7: DILATION

SECTION: 0 MEDICAL AND SURGICAL
BODY SYSTEM: C MOUTH AND THROAT
OPERATION: 9 DRAINAGE: *(on multiple pages)*
Taking or letting out fluids and/or gases from a body part

Body Part	Approach	Device	Qualifier
0 Upper Lip 1 Lower Lip 2 Hard Palate 3 Soft Palate 4 Buccal Mucosa 5 Upper Gingiva 6 Lower Gingiva 7 Tongue N Uvula P Tonsils Q Adenoids	0 Open 3 Percutaneous X External	0 Drainage Device	Z No Qualifier
0 Upper Lip 1 Lower Lip 2 Hard Palate 3 Soft Palate 4 Buccal Mucosa 5 Upper Gingiva 6 Lower Gingiva 7 Tongue N Uvula P Tonsils Q Adenoids	0 Open 3 Percutaneous X External	Z No Device	X Diagnostic Z No Qualifier
8 Parotid Gland, Right 9 Parotid Gland, Left B Parotid Duct, Right C Parotid Duct, Left D Sublingual Gland, Right F Sublingual Gland, Left G Submaxillary Gland, Right H Submaxillary Gland, Left J Minor Salivary Gland	0 Open 3 Percutaneous	0 Drainage Device	Z No Qualifier
8 Parotid Gland, Right 9 Parotid Gland, Left B Parotid Duct, Right C Parotid Duct, Left D Sublingual Gland, Right F Sublingual Gland, Left G Submaxillary Gland, Right H Submaxillary Gland, Left J Minor Salivary Gland	0 Open 3 Percutaneous	Z No Device	X Diagnostic Z No Qualifier
M Pharynx R Epiglottis S Larynx T Vocal Cord, Right V Vocal Cord, Left	0 Open 3 Percutaneous 4 Percutaneous Endoscopic 7 Via Natural or Artificial Opening 8 Via Natural or Artificial Opening Endoscopic	0 Drainage Device	Z No Qualifier

9: DRAINAGE
C: MOUTH AND THROAT
0: M/S

SECTION: Ø MEDICAL AND SURGICAL
BODY SYSTEM: C MOUTH AND THROAT
OPERATION: 9 DRAINAGE: *(continued)*
Taking or letting out fluids and/or gases from a body part

Body Part	Approach	Device	Qualifier
M Pharynx R Epiglottis S Larynx T Vocal Cord, Right V Vocal Cord, Left	Ø Open 3 Percutaneous 4 Percutaneous Endoscopic 7 Via Natural or Artificial Opening 8 Via Natural or Artificial Opening Endoscopic	Z No Device	X Diagnostic Z No Qualifier
W Upper Tooth X Lower Tooth	Ø Open X External	Ø Drainage Device Z No Device	Ø Single 1 Multiple 2 All

SECTION: Ø MEDICAL AND SURGICAL
BODY SYSTEM: C MOUTH AND THROAT
OPERATION: B EXCISION: Cutting out or off, without replacement, a portion of a body part

Body Part	Approach	Device	Qualifier
Ø Upper Lip 1 Lower Lip 2 Hard Palate 3 Soft Palate 4 Buccal Mucosa 5 Upper Gingiva 6 Lower Gingiva 7 Tongue N Uvula P Tonsils Q Adenoids	Ø Open 3 Percutaneous X External	Z No Device	X Diagnostic Z No Qualifier
8 Parotid Gland, Right 9 Parotid Gland, Left B Parotid Duct, Right C Parotid Duct, Left D Sublingual Gland, Right F Sublingual Gland, Left G Submaxillary Gland, Right H Submaxillary Gland, Left J Minor Salivary Gland	Ø Open 3 Percutaneous	Z No Device	X Diagnostic Z No Qualifier
M Pharynx R Epiglottis S Larynx T Vocal Cord, Right V Vocal Cord, Left	Ø Open 3 Percutaneous 4 Percutaneous Endoscopic 7 Via Natural or Artificial Opening 8 Via Natural or Artificial Opening Endoscopic	Z No Device	X Diagnostic Z No Qualifier
W Upper Tooth X Lower Tooth	Ø Open X External	Z No Device	Ø Single 1 Multiple 2 All

SECTION: Ø MEDICAL AND SURGICAL
BODY SYSTEM: C MOUTH AND THROAT
OPERATION: C EXTIRPATION: Taking or cutting out solid matter from a body part

Body Part	Approach	Device	Qualifier
Ø Upper Lip 1 Lower Lip 2 Hard Palate 3 Soft Palate 4 Buccal Mucosa 5 Upper Gingiva 6 Lower Gingiva 7 Tongue N Uvula P Tonsils Q Adenoids	Ø Open 3 Percutaneous X External	Z No Device	Z No Qualifier
8 Parotid Gland, Right 9 Parotid Gland, Left B Parotid Duct, Right C Parotid Duct, Left D Sublingual Gland, Right F Sublingual Gland, Left G Submaxillary Gland, Right H Submaxillary Gland, Left J Minor Salivary Gland	Ø Open 3 Percutaneous	Z No Device	Z No Qualifier
M Pharynx R Epiglottis S Larynx T Vocal Cord, Right V Vocal Cord, Left	Ø Open 3 Percutaneous 4 Percutaneous Endoscopic 7 Via Natural or Artificial Opening 8 Via Natural or Artificial Opening Endoscopic	Z No Device	Z No Qualifier
W Upper Tooth X Lower Tooth	Ø Open X External	Z No Device	Ø Single 1 Multiple 2 All

SECTION: Ø MEDICAL AND SURGICAL
BODY SYSTEM: C MOUTH AND THROAT
OPERATION: D EXTRACTION: Pulling or stripping out or off all or a portion of a body part by the use of force

Body Part	Approach	Device	Qualifier
T Vocal Cord, Right V Vocal Cord, Left	Ø Open 3 Percutaneous 4 Percutaneous Endoscopic 7 Via Natural or Artificial Opening 8 Via Natural or Artificial Opening Endoscopic	Z No Device	Z No Qualifier
W Upper Tooth X Lower Tooth	X External	Z No Device	Ø Single 1 Multiple 2 All

SECTION: Ø MEDICAL AND SURGICAL
BODY SYSTEM: C MOUTH AND THROAT
OPERATION: F FRAGMENTATION: Breaking solid matter in a body part into pieces

Body Part	Approach	Device	Qualifier
B Parotid Duct, Right C Parotid Duct, Left	Ø Open 3 Percutaneous 7 Via Natural or Artificial Opening X External	Z No Device	Z No Qualifier

SECTION: Ø MEDICAL AND SURGICAL
BODY SYSTEM: C MOUTH AND THROAT
OPERATION: H INSERTION: Putting in a nonbiological appliance that monitors, assists, performs, or prevents a physiological function but does not physically take the place of a body part

Body Part	Approach	Device	Qualifier
7 Tongue	Ø Open 3 Percutaneous X External	1 Radioactive Element	Z No Qualifier
A Salivary Gland S Larynx	Ø Open 3 Percutaneous 7 Via Natural or Artificial Opening 8 Via Natural or Artificial Opening Endoscopic	Y Other Device	Z No Qualifier
Y Mouth and Throat	Ø Open 3 Percutaneous	Y Other Device	Z No Qualifier
Y Mouth and Throat	7 Via Natural or Artificial Opening 8 Via Natural or Artificial Opening Endoscopic	B Intraluminal Device, Airway Y Other Device	Z No Qualifier

SECTION: Ø MEDICAL AND SURGICAL
BODY SYSTEM: C MOUTH AND THROAT
OPERATION: J INSPECTION: Visually and/or manually exploring a body part

Body Part	Approach	Device	Qualifier
A Salivary Gland	Ø Open 3 Percutaneous X External	Z No Device	Z No Qualifier
S Larynx Y Mouth and Throat	Ø Open 3 Percutaneous 4 Percutaneous Endoscopic 7 Via Natural or Artificial Opening 8 Via Natural or Artificial Opening Endoscopic X External	Z No Device	Z No Qualifier

L: OCCLUSION   M: REATTACHMENT

C: MOUTH AND THROAT

Ø: M/S

SECTION: Ø MEDICAL AND SURGICAL
BODY SYSTEM: C MOUTH AND THROAT
OPERATION: L OCCLUSION: Completely closing an orifice or the lumen of a tubular body part

Body Part	Approach	Device	Qualifier
B Parotid Duct, Right C Parotid Duct, Left	Ø Open 3 Percutaneous 4 Percutaneous Endoscopic	C Extraluminal Device D Intraluminal Device Z No Device	Z No Qualifier
B Parotid Duct, Right C Parotid Duct, Left	7 Via Natural or Artificial Opening 8 Via Natural or Artificial Opening Endoscopic	D Intraluminal Device Z No Device	Z No Qualifier

SECTION: Ø MEDICAL AND SURGICAL
BODY SYSTEM: C MOUTH AND THROAT
OPERATION: M REATTACHMENT: Putting back in or on all or a portion of a separated body part to its normal location or other suitable location

Body Part	Approach	Device	Qualifier
Ø Upper Lip 1 Lower Lip 3 Soft Palate 7 Tongue N Uvula	Ø Open	Z No Device	Z No Qualifier
W Upper Tooth X Lower Tooth	Ø Open X External	Z No Device	Ø Single 1 Multiple 2 All

SECTION: Ø MEDICAL AND SURGICAL
BODY SYSTEM: C MOUTH AND THROAT
OPERATION: N RELEASE: Freeing a body part from an abnormal physical constraint by cutting or by the use of force

Body Part	Approach	Device	Qualifier
Ø Upper Lip 1 Lower Lip 2 Hard Palate 3 Soft Palate 4 Buccal Mucosa 5 Upper Gingiva 6 Lower Gingiva 7 Tongue N Uvula P Tonsils Q Adenoids	Ø Open 3 Percutaneous X External	Z No Device	Z No Qualifier
8 Parotid Gland, Right 9 Parotid Gland, Left B Parotid Duct, Right C Parotid Duct, Left D Sublingual Gland, Right F Sublingual Gland, Left G Submaxillary Gland, Right H Submaxillary Gland, Left J Minor Salivary Gland	Ø Open 3 Percutaneous	Z No Device	Z No Qualifier
M Pharynx R Epiglottis S Larynx T Vocal Cord, Right V Vocal Cord, Left	Ø Open 3 Percutaneous 4 Percutaneous Endoscopic 7 Via Natural or Artificial Opening 8 Via Natural or Artificial Opening Endoscopic	Z No Device	Z No Qualifier
W Upper Tooth X Lower Tooth	Ø Open X External	Z No Device	Ø Single 1 Multiple 2 All

SECTION: Ø MEDICAL AND SURGICAL
BODY SYSTEM: C MOUTH AND THROAT
OPERATION: **P REMOVAL:** Taking out or off a device from a body part

Body Part	Approach	Device	Qualifier
A Salivary Gland	Ø Open 3 Percutaneous	Ø Drainage Device C Extraluminal Device Y Other Device	Z No Qualifier
A Salivary Gland	7 Via Natural or Artificial Opening 8 Via Natural or Artificial Opening Endoscopic	Y Other Device	Z No Qualifier
S Larynx	Ø Open 3 Percutaneous 7 Via Natural or Artificial Opening 8 Via Natural or Artificial Opening Endoscopic X External	Ø Drainage Device 7 Autologous Tissue Substitute D Intraluminal Device J Synthetic Substitute K Nonautologous Tissue Substitute Y Other Device	Z No Qualifier
S Larynx	X External	Ø Drainage Device 7 Autologous Tissue Substitute D Intraluminal Device J Synthetic Substitute K Nonautologous Tissue Substitute	Z No Qualifier
Y Mouth and Throat	Ø Open 3 Percutaneous 7 Via Natural or Artificial Opening 8 Via Natural or Artificial Opening Endoscopic X External	Ø Drainage Device 1 Radioactive Element 7 Autologous Tissue Substitute D Intraluminal Device J Synthetic Substitute K Nonautologous Tissue Substitute Y Other Device	Z No Qualifier
Y Mouth and Throat	X External	Ø Drainage Device 1 Radioactive Element 7 Autologous Tissue Substitute D Intraluminal Device J Synthetic Substitute K Nonautologous Tissue Substitute	Z No Qualifier

SECTION: 0 MEDICAL AND SURGICAL
BODY SYSTEM: C MOUTH AND THROAT
OPERATION: Q **REPAIR:** Restoring, to the extent possible, a body part to its normal anatomic structure and function

Body Part	Approach	Device	Qualifier
0 Upper Lip 1 Lower Lip 2 Hard Palate 3 Soft Palate 4 Buccal Mucosa 5 Upper Gingiva 6 Lower Gingiva 7 Tongue N Uvula P Tonsils Q Adenoids	0 Open 3 Percutaneous X External	Z No Device	Z No Qualifier
8 Parotid Gland, Right 9 Parotid Gland, Left B Parotid Duct, Right C Parotid Duct, Left D Sublingual Gland, Right F Sublingual Gland, Left G Submaxillary Gland, Right H Submaxillary Gland, Left J Minor Salivary Gland	0 Open 3 Percutaneous	Z No Device	Z No Qualifier
M Pharynx R Epiglottis S Larynx T Vocal Cord, Right V Vocal Cord, Left	0 Open 3 Percutaneous 4 Percutaneous Endoscopic 7 Via Natural or Artificial Opening 8 Via Natural or Artificial Opening Endoscopic	Z No Device	Z No Qualifier
W Upper Tooth X Lower Tooth	0 Open X External	Z No Device	0 Single 1 Multiple 2 All

SECTION: Ø MEDICAL AND SURGICAL
BODY SYSTEM: C MOUTH AND THROAT
OPERATION: R REPLACEMENT: Putting in or on biological or synthetic material that physically takes the place and/or function of all or a portion of a body part

Body Part	Approach	Device	Qualifier
Ø Upper Lip 1 Lower Lip 2 Hard Palate 3 Soft Palate 4 Buccal Mucosa 5 Upper Gingiva 6 Lower Gingiva 7 Tongue N Uvula	Ø Open 3 Percutaneous X External	7 Autologous Tissue Substitute J Synthetic Substitute K Nonautologous Tissue Substitute	Z No Qualifier
B Parotid Duct, Right C Parotid Duct, Left	Ø Open 3 Percutaneous	7 Autologous Tissue Substitute J Synthetic Substitute K Nonautologous Tissue Substitute	Z No Qualifier
M Pharynx R Epiglottis S Larynx T Vocal Cord, Right V Vocal Cord, Left	Ø Open 7 Via Natural or Artificial Opening 8 Via Natural or Artificial Opening Endoscopic	7 Autologous Tissue Substitute J Synthetic Substitute K Nonautologous Tissue Substitute	Z No Qualifier
W Upper Tooth X Lower Tooth	Ø Open X External	7 Autologous Tissue Substitute J Synthetic Substitute K Nonautologous Tissue Substitute	Ø Single 1 Multiple 2 All

SECTION: Ø MEDICAL AND SURGICAL
BODY SYSTEM: C MOUTH AND THROAT
OPERATION: S REPOSITION: Moving to its normal location, or other suitable location, all or a portion of a body part

Body Part	Approach	Device	Qualifier
Ø Upper Lip 1 Lower Lip 2 Hard Palate 3 Soft Palate 7 Tongue N Uvula	Ø Open X External	Z No Device	Z No Qualifier
B Parotid Duct, Right C Parotid Duct, Left	Ø Open 3 Percutaneous	Z No Device	Z No Qualifier
R Epiglottis T Vocal Cord, Right V Vocal Cord, Left	Ø Open 7 Via Natural or Artificial Opening 8 Via Natural or Artificial Opening Endoscopic	Z No Device	Z No Qualifier
W Upper Tooth X Lower Tooth	Ø Open X External	5 External Fixation Device Z No Device	Ø Single 1 Multiple 2 All

SECTION: Ø MEDICAL AND SURGICAL
BODY SYSTEM: C MOUTH AND THROAT
OPERATION: T RESECTION: Cutting out or off, without replacement, all of a body part

Body Part	Approach	Device	Qualifier
Ø Upper Lip 1 Lower Lip 2 Hard Palate 3 Soft Palate 7 Tongue N Uvula P Tonsils Q Adenoids	Ø Open X External	Z No Device	Z No Qualifier
8 Parotid Gland, Right 9 Parotid Gland, Left B Parotid Duct, Right C Parotid Duct, Left D Sublingual Gland, Right F Sublingual Gland, Left G Submaxillary Gland, Right H Submaxillary Gland, Left J Minor Salivary Gland	Ø Open	Z No Device	Z No Qualifier
M Pharynx R Epiglottis S Larynx T Vocal Cord, Right V Vocal Cord, Left	Ø Open 4 Percutaneous Endoscopic 7 Via Natural or Artificial Opening 8 Via Natural or Artificial Opening Endoscopic	Z No Device	Z No Qualifier
W Upper Tooth X Lower Tooth	Ø Open	Z No Device	Ø Single 1 Multiple 2 All

SECTION: Ø MEDICAL AND SURGICAL
BODY SYSTEM: C MOUTH AND THROAT
OPERATION: U SUPPLEMENT: Putting in or on biological or synthetic material that physically reinforces and/or augments the function of a portion of a body part

Body Part	Approach	Device	Qualifier
Ø Upper Lip 1 Lower Lip 2 Hard Palate 3 Soft Palate 4 Buccal Mucosa 5 Upper Gingiva 6 Lower Gingiva 7 Tongue N Uvula	Ø Open 3 Percutaneous X External	7 Autologous Tissue Substitute J Synthetic Substitute K Nonautologous Tissue Substitute	Z No Qualifier
M Pharynx R Epiglottis S Larynx T Vocal Cord, Right V Vocal Cord, Left	Ø Open 7 Via Natural or Artificial Opening 8 Via Natural or Artificial Opening Endoscopic	7 Autologous Tissue Substitute J Synthetic Substitute K Nonautologous Tissue Substitute	Z No Qualifier

SECTION: 0 MEDICAL AND SURGICAL
BODY SYSTEM: C MOUTH AND THROAT
OPERATION: V RESTRICTION: Partially closing an orifice or the lumen of a tubular body part

Body Part	Approach	Device	Qualifier
B Parotid Duct, Right C Parotid Duct, Left	0 Open 3 Percutaneous	C Extraluminal Device D Intraluminal Device Z No Device	Z No Qualifier
B Parotid Duct, Right C Parotid Duct, Left	7 Via Natural or Artificial Opening 8 Via Natural or Artificial Opening Endoscopic	D Intraluminal Device Z No Device	Z No Qualifier

SECTION: 0 MEDICAL AND SURGICAL
BODY SYSTEM: C MOUTH AND THROAT
OPERATION: W REVISION: *(on multiple pages)*
Correcting, to the extent possible, a portion of a malfunctioning device or the position of a displaced device

Body Part	Approach	Device	Qualifier
A Salivary Gland	0 Open 3 Percutaneous X External	0 Drainage Device C Extraluminal Device Y Other Device	Z No Qualifier
A Salivary Gland	7 Via Natural or Artificial Opening 8 Via Natural or Artificial Opening Endoscopic	Y Other Device	Z No Qualifier
A Salivary Gland	X External	0 Drainage Device C Extraluminal Device	Z No Qualifier
S Larynx	0 Open 3 Percutaneous 7 Via Natural or Artificial Opening 8 Via Natural or Artificial Opening Endoscopic X External	0 Drainage Device 7 Autologous Tissue Substitute D Intraluminal Device J Synthetic Substitute K Nonautologous Tissue Substitute Y Other Device	Z No Qualifier
S Larynx	X External	0 Drainage Device 7 Autologous Tissue Substitute D Intraluminal Device J Synthetic Substitute K Nonautologous Tissue Substitute	Z No Qualifier

SECTION: 0 MEDICAL AND SURGICAL
BODY SYSTEM: C MOUTH AND THROAT
OPERATION: W REVISION: *(continued)*
Correcting, to the extent possible, a portion of a malfunctioning device or the position of a displaced device

Body Part	Approach	Device	Qualifier
Y Mouth and Throat	0 Open 3 Percutaneous 7 Via Natural or Artificial Opening 8 Via Natural or Artificial Opening Endoscopic ~~X External~~	0 Drainage Device 1 Radioactive Element 7 Autologous Tissue Substitute D Intraluminal Device J Synthetic Substitute K Nonautologous Tissue Substitute Y Other Device	Z No Qualifier
Y Mouth and Throat	X External	0 Drainage Device 1 Radioactive Element 7 Autologous Tissue Substitute D Intraluminal Device J Synthetic Substitute K Nonautologous Tissue Substitute	Z No Qualifier

SECTION: 0 MEDICAL AND SURGICAL
BODY SYSTEM: C MOUTH AND THROAT
OPERATION: X TRANSFER: Moving, without taking out, all or a portion of a body part to another location to take over the function of all or a portion of a body part

Body Part	Approach	Device	Qualifier
0 Upper Lip 1 Lower Lip 3 Soft Palate 4 Buccal Mucosa 5 Upper Gingiva 6 Lower Gingiva 7 Tongue	0 Open X External	Z No Device	Z No Qualifier

ØD. Gastrointestinal System 206
   ØD1. Bypass 207
   ØD2. Change 208
   ØD5. Destruction 209
   ØD7. Dilation 210
   ØD8. Division 210
   ØD9. Drainage 211
   ØDB. Excision 213
   ØDC. Extirpation 215
   ØDD. Extraction 216
   ØDF. Fragmentation 216
   ØDH. Insertion 217
   ØDJ. Inspection 218
   ØDL. Occlusion 219
   ØDM. Reattachment 220
   ØDN. Release 221
   ØDP. Removal 222
   ØDQ. Repair 224
   ØDR. Replacement 225
   ØDS. Reposition 225
   ØDT. Resection 226
   ØDU. Supplement 227
   ØDV. Restriction 228
   ØDW. Revision 229
   ØDX. Transfer 231
   ØDY. Transplantation 231

SECTION: Ø MEDICAL AND SURGICAL
BODY SYSTEM: D GASTROINTESTINAL SYSTEM
OPERATION: 1 BYPASS: *(on multiple pages)*
Altering the route of passage of the contents of a tubular body part

Body Part	Approach	Device	Qualifier

1 Esophagus, Upper
2 Esophagus, Middle
3 Esophagus, Lower
5 Esophagus
	Ø Open
	4 Percutaneous Endoscopic
	8 Via Natural or Artificial
	  Opening Endoscopic
		7 Autologous Tissue Substitute
		J Synthetic Substitute
		K Nonautologous Tissue
		  Substitute
		Z No Device
			4 Cutaneous
			6 Stomach
			9 Duodenum
			A Jejunum
			B Ileum

1 Esophagus, Upper 2 Esophagus, Middle 3 Esophagus, Lower 5 Esophagus	3 Percutaneous	J Synthetic Substitute	4 Cutaneous

6 Stomach
9 Duodenum
	Ø Open
	4 Percutaneous Endoscopic
	8 Via Natural or Artificial
	  Opening Endoscopic
		7 Autologous Tissue Substitute
		J Synthetic Substitute
		K Nonautologous Tissue
		  Substitute
		Z No Device
			4 Cutaneous
			9 Duodenum
			A Jejunum
			B Ileum
			L Transverse Colon

6 Stomach 9 Duodenum	3 Percutaneous	J Synthetic Substitute	4 Cutaneous

A Jejunum	Ø Open
	4 Percutaneous Endoscopic
	8 Via Natural or Artificial
	  Opening Endoscopic
		7 Autologous Tissue Substitute
		J Synthetic Substitute
		K Nonautologous Tissue
		  Substitute
		Z No Device
			4 Cutaneous
			A Jejunum
			B Ileum
			H Cecum
			K Ascending Colon
			L Transverse Colon
			M Descending Colon
			N Sigmoid Colon
			P Rectum
			Q Anus

A Jejunum	3 Percutaneous	J Synthetic Substitute	4 Cutaneous

B Ileum	Ø Open
	4 Percutaneous Endoscopic
	8 Via Natural or Artificial
	  Opening Endoscopic
		7 Autologous Tissue Substitute
		J Synthetic Substitute
		K Nonautologous Tissue
		  Substitute
		Z No Device
			4 Cutaneous
			B Ileum
			H Cecum
			K Ascending Colon
			L Transverse Colon
			M Descending Colon
			N Sigmoid Colon
			P Rectum
			Q Anus

B Ileum	3 Percutaneous	J Synthetic Substitute	4 Cutaneous

H Cecum	Ø Open
	4 Percutaneous Endoscopic
	8 Via Natural or Artificial
	  Opening Endoscopic
		7 Autologous Tissue Substitute
		J Synthetic Substitute
		K Nonautologous Tissue
		  Substitute
		Z No Device
			4 Cutaneous
			H Cecum
			K Ascending Colon
			L Transverse Colon
			M Descending Colon
			N Sigmoid Colon
			P Rectum

H Cecum	3 Percutaneous	J Synthetic Substitute	4 Cutaneous

SECTION: Ø MEDICAL AND SURGICAL
BODY SYSTEM: D GASTROINTESTINAL SYSTEM
OPERATION: 1 BYPASS: *(continued)*
Altering the route of passage of the contents of a tubular body part

Body Part	Approach	Device	Qualifier
K Ascending Colon	Ø Open 4 Percutaneous Endoscopic 8 Via Natural or Artificial Opening Endoscopic	7 Autologous Tissue Substitute J Synthetic Substitute K Nonautologous Tissue Substitute Z No Device	4 Cutaneous K Ascending Colon L Transverse Colon M Descending Colon N Sigmoid Colon P Rectum
K Ascending Colon	3 Percutaneous	J Synthetic Substitute	4 Cutaneous
L Transverse Colon	Ø Open 4 Percutaneous Endoscopic 8 Via Natural or Artificial Opening Endoscopic	7 Autologous Tissue Substitute J Synthetic Substitute K Nonautologous Tissue Substitute Z No Device	4 Cutaneous L Transverse Colon M Descending Colon N Sigmoid Colon P Rectum
L Transverse Colon	3 Percutaneous	J Synthetic Substitute	4 Cutaneous
M Descending Colon	Ø Open 4 Percutaneous Endoscopic 8 Via Natural or Artificial Opening Endoscopic	7 Autologous Tissue Substitute J Synthetic Substitute K Nonautologous Tissue Substitute Z No Device	4 Cutaneous M Descending Colon N Sigmoid Colon P Rectum
M Descending Colon	3 Percutaneous	J Synthetic Substitute	4 Cutaneous
N Sigmoid Colon	Ø Open 4 Percutaneous Endoscopic 8 Via Natural or Artificial Opening Endoscopic	7 Autologous Tissue Substitute J Synthetic Substitute K Nonautologous Tissue Substitute Z No Device	4 Cutaneous N Sigmoid Colon P Rectum
N Sigmoid Colon	3 Percutaneous	J Synthetic Substitute	4 Cutaneous

SECTION: Ø MEDICAL AND SURGICAL
BODY SYSTEM: D GASTROINTESTINAL SYSTEM
OPERATION: 2 CHANGE: Taking out or off a device from a body part and putting back an identical or similar device in or on the same body part without cutting or puncturing the skin or a mucous membrane

Body Part	Approach	Device	Qualifier
Ø Upper Intestinal Tract D Lower Intestinal Tract	X External	Ø Drainage Device U Feeding Device Y Other Device	Z No Qualifier
U Omentum V Mesentery W Peritoneum	X External	Ø Drainage Device Y Other Device	Z No Qualifier

SECTION: Ø MEDICAL AND SURGICAL
BODY SYSTEM: D GASTROINTESTINAL SYSTEM
OPERATION: 5 DESTRUCTION: Physical eradication of all or a portion of a body part by the direct use of energy, force, or a destructive agent

Body Part	Approach	Device	Qualifier
1 Esophagus, Upper 2 Esophagus, Middle 3 Esophagus, Lower 4 Esophagogastric Junction 5 Esophagus 6 Stomach 7 Stomach, Pylorus 8 Small Intestine 9 Duodenum A Jejunum B Ileum C Ileocecal Valve E Large Intestine F Large Intestine, Right G Large Intestine, Left H Cecum J Appendix K Ascending Colon L Transverse Colon M Descending Colon N Sigmoid Colon P Rectum	Ø Open 3 Percutaneous 4 Percutaneous Endoscopic 7 Via Natural or Artificial Opening 8 Via Natural or Artificial Opening Endoscopic	Z No Device	Z No Qualifier
Q Anus	Ø Open 3 Percutaneous 4 Percutaneous Endoscopic 7 Via Natural or Artificial Opening 8 Via Natural or Artificial Opening Endoscopic X External	Z No Device	Z No Qualifier
R Anal Sphincter U Omentum T Lesser Omentum V Mesentery W Peritoneum	Ø Open 3 Percutaneous 4 Percutaneous Endoscopic	Z No Device	Z No Qualifier

SECTION: Ø MEDICAL AND SURGICAL
BODY SYSTEM: D GASTROINTESTINAL SYSTEM
OPERATION: 7 DILATION: Expanding an orifice or the lumen of a tubular body part

Body Part	Approach	Device	Qualifier
1 Esophagus, Upper 2 Esophagus, Middle 3 Esophagus, Lower 4 Esophagogastric Junction 5 Esophagus 6 Stomach 7 Stomach, Pylorus 8 Small Intestine 9 Duodenum A Jejunum B Ileum C Ileocecal Valve E Large Intestine F Large Intestine, Right G Large Intestine, Left H Cecum K Ascending Colon L Transverse Colon M Descending Colon N Sigmoid Colon P Rectum Q Anus	Ø Open 3 Percutaneous 4 Percutaneous Endoscopic 7 Via Natural or Artificial Opening 8 Via Natural or Artificial Opening Endoscopic	D Intraluminal Device Z No Device	Z No Qualifier

SECTION: Ø MEDICAL AND SURGICAL
BODY SYSTEM: D GASTROINTESTINAL SYSTEM
OPERATION: 8 DIVISION: Cutting into a body part, without draining fluids and/or gases from the body part, in order to separate or transect a body part

Body Part	Approach	Device	Qualifier
4 Esophagogastric Junction 7 Stomach, Pylorus	Ø Open 3 Percutaneous 4 Percutaneous Endoscopic 7 Via Natural or Artificial Opening 8 Via Natural or Artificial Opening Endoscopic	Z No Device	Z No Qualifier
R Anal Sphincter	Ø Open 3 Percutaneous	Z No Device	Z No Qualifier

SECTION: Ø MEDICAL AND SURGICAL
BODY SYSTEM: D GASTROINTESTINAL SYSTEM
OPERATION: 9 DRAINAGE: *(on multiple pages)*

Taking or letting out fluids and/or gases from a body part

Body Part	Approach	Device	Qualifier
1 Esophagus, Upper 2 Esophagus, Middle 3 Esophagus, Lower 4 Esophagogastric Junction 5 Esophagus 6 Stomach 7 Stomach, Pylorus 8 Small Intestine 9 Duodenum A Jejunum B Ileum C Ileocecal Valve E Large Intestine F Large Intestine, Right G Large Intestine, Left H Cecum J Appendix K Ascending Colon L Transverse Colon M Descending Colon N Sigmoid Colon P Rectum	Ø Open 3 Percutaneous 4 Percutaneous Endoscopic 7 Via Natural or Artificial Opening 8 Via Natural or Artificial Opening Endoscopic	Ø Drainage Device	Z No Qualifier
1 Esophagus, Upper 2 Esophagus, Middle 3 Esophagus, Lower 4 Esophagogastric Junction 5 Esophagus 6 Stomach 7 Stomach, Pylorus 8 Small Intestine 9 Duodenum A Jejunum B Ileum C Ileocecal Valve E Large Intestine F Large Intestine, Right G Large Intestine, Left H Cecum J Appendix K Ascending Colon L Transverse Colon M Descending Colon N Sigmoid Colon P Rectum	Ø Open 3 Percutaneous 4 Percutaneous Endoscopic 7 Via Natural or Artificial Opening 8 Via Natural or Artificial Opening Endoscopic	Z No Device	X Diagnostic Z No Qualifier

SECTION: Ø MEDICAL AND SURGICAL
BODY SYSTEM: D GASTROINTESTINAL SYSTEM
OPERATION: 9 DRAINAGE: *(continued)*
Taking or letting out fluids and/or gases from a body part

Body Part	Approach	Device	Qualifier
Q Anus	Ø Open 3 Percutaneous 4 Percutaneous Endoscopic 7 Via Natural or Artificial Opening 8 Via Natural or Artificial Opening Endoscopic X External	Ø Drainage Device	Z No Qualifier
Q Anus	Ø Open 3 Percutaneous 4 Percutaneous Endoscopic 7 Via Natural or Artificial Opening 8 Via Natural or Artificial Opening Endoscopic X External	Z No Device	X Diagnostic Z No Qualifier
R Anal Sphincter U Omentum T Lesser Omentum V Mesentery W Peritoneum	Ø Open 3 Percutaneous 4 Percutaneous Endoscopic	Ø Drainage Device	Z No Qualifier
R Anal Sphincter U Omentum T Lesser Omentum V Mesentery W Peritoneum	Ø Open 3 Percutaneous 4 Percutaneous Endoscopic	Z No Device	X Diagnostic Z No Qualifier

New/Revised Text in Blue   ~~deleted~~ Deleted

SECTION: Ø MEDICAL AND SURGICAL
BODY SYSTEM: D GASTROINTESTINAL SYSTEM
OPERATION: B EXCISION: *(on multiple pages)*
Cutting out or off, without replacement, a portion of a body part

Body Part	Approach	Device	Qualifier
1 Esophagus, Upper 2 Esophagus, Middle 3 Esophagus, Lower 4 Esophagogastric Junction 5 Esophagus 7 Stomach, Pylorus 8 Small Intestine 9 Duodenum A Jejunum B Ileum C Ileocecal Valve E Large Intestine F Large Intestine, Right G Large Intestine, Left H Cecum J Appendix K Ascending Colon L Transverse Colon M Descending Colon N Sigmoid Colon P Rectum	Ø Open 3 Percutaneous 4 Percutaneous Endoscopic 7 Via Natural or Artificial Opening 8 Via Natural or Artificial Opening Endoscopic	Z No Device	X Diagnostic Z No Qualifier
6 Stomach	Ø Open 3 Percutaneous 4 Percutaneous Endoscopic 7 Via Natural or Artificial Opening 8 Via Natural or Artificial Opening Endoscopic	Z No Device	3 Vertical X Diagnostic Z No Qualifier
G Large Intestine, Left L Transverse Colon M Descending Colon N Sigmoid Colon	Ø Open 3 Percutaneous 4 Percutaneous Endoscopic 7 Via Natural or Artificial Opening 8 Via Natural or Artificial Opening Endoscopic	Z No Device	X Diagnostic Z No Qualifier

SECTION: Ø MEDICAL AND SURGICAL
BODY SYSTEM: D GASTROINTESTINAL SYSTEM
OPERATION: B **EXCISION:** *(continued)* Cutting out or off, without replacement, a portion of a body part

Body Part	Approach	Device	Qualifier
G Large Intestine, Left L Transverse Colon M Descending Colon N Sigmoid Colon	F Via Natural or Artificial Opening With Percutaneous Endoscopic Assistance	Z No Device	Z No Qualifier
Q Anus	Ø Open 3 Percutaneous 4 Percutaneous Endoscopic 7 Via Natural or Artificial Opening 8 Via Natural or Artificial Opening Endoscopic X External	Z No Device	X Diagnostic Z No Qualifier
R Anal Sphincter U Omentum T Lesser Omentum V Mesentery W Peritoneum	Ø Open 3 Percutaneous 4 Percutaneous Endoscopic	Z No Device	X Diagnostic Z No Qualifier

New/Revised Text in Blue   ~~deleted~~ Deleted

SECTION: Ø MEDICAL AND SURGICAL
BODY SYSTEM: D GASTROINTESTINAL SYSTEM
OPERATION: C EXTIRPATION: Taking or cutting out solid matter from a body part

Body Part	Approach	Device	Qualifier
1 Esophagus, Upper 2 Esophagus, Middle 3 Esophagus, Lower 4 Esophagogastric Junction 5 Esophagus 6 Stomach 7 Stomach, Pylorus 8 Small Intestine 9 Duodenum A Jejunum B Ileum C Ileocecal Valve E Large Intestine F Large Intestine, Right G Large Intestine, Left H Cecum J Appendix K Ascending Colon L Transverse Colon M Descending Colon N Sigmoid Colon P Rectum	Ø Open 3 Percutaneous 4 Percutaneous Endoscopic 7 Via Natural or Artificial Opening 8 Via Natural or Artificial Opening Endoscopic	Z No Device	Z No Qualifier
Q Anus	Ø Open 3 Percutaneous 4 Percutaneous Endoscopic 7 Via Natural or Artificial Opening 8 Via Natural or Artificial Opening Endoscopic X External	Z No Device	Z No Qualifier
R Anal Sphincter U Omentum T Lesser Omentum V Mesentery W Peritoneum	Ø Open 3 Percutaneous 4 Percutaneous Endoscopic	Z No Device	Z No Qualifier

SECTION: Ø MEDICAL AND SURGICAL
BODY SYSTEM: D GASTROINTESTINAL SYSTEM
OPERATION: D **EXTRACTION:** Pulling or stripping out or off all or a portion of a body part by the use of force

Body Part	Approach	Device	Qualifier
1 Esophagus, Upper 2 Esophagus, Middle 3 Esophagus, Lower 4 Esophagogastric Junction 5 Esophagus 6 Stomach 7 Stomach, Pylorus 8 Small Intestine 9 Duodenum A Jejunum B Ileum C Ileocecal Valve E Large Intestine F Large Intestine, Right G Large Intestine, Left H Cecum J Appendix K Ascending Colon L Transverse Colon M Descending Colon N Sigmoid Colon P Rectum	3 Percutaneous 4 Percutaneous Endoscopic 8 Via Natural or Artificial Opening Endoscopic	Z No Device	X Diagnostic
Q Anus	3 Percutaneous 4 Percutaneous Endoscopic 8 Via Natural or Artificial Opening Endoscopic X External	Z No Device	X Diagnostic

SECTION: Ø MEDICAL AND SURGICAL
BODY SYSTEM: D GASTROINTESTINAL SYSTEM
OPERATION: F **FRAGMENTATION:** Breaking solid matter in a body part into pieces

Body Part	Approach	Device	Qualifier

5 Esophagus
6 Stomach
8 Small Intestine
9 Duodenum
A Jejunum
B Ileum
E Large Intestine
F Large Intestine, Right
G Large Intestine, Left
H Cecum
J Appendix
K Ascending Colon
L Transverse Colon
M Descending Colon
N Sigmoid Colon
P Rectum
Q Anus
	Ø Open
	3 Percutaneous
	4 Percutaneous Endoscopic
	7 Via Natural or Artificial
	   Opening
	8 Via Natural or Artificial
	   Opening Endoscopic
	X External
		Z No Device	Z No Qualifier

Side tab text: D: GASTROINTESTINAL SYSTEM | D: EXTRACTION F: FRAGMENTATION | Ø: M/S

SECTION: Ø MEDICAL AND SURGICAL
BODY SYSTEM: D GASTROINTESTINAL SYSTEM
OPERATION: H INSERTION: *(on multiple pages)*

Putting in a nonbiological appliance that monitors, assists, performs, or prevents a physiological function but does not physically take the place of a body part

Body Part	Approach	Device	Qualifier
Ø Upper Intestinal Tract D Lower Intestinal Tract	Ø Open 3 Percutaneous 4 Percutaneous Endoscopic 7 Via Natural or Artificial Opening 8 Via Natural or Artificial Opening Endoscopic	Y Other Device	Z No Qualifier
5 Esophagus	Ø Open 3 Percutaneous 4 Percutaneous Endoscopic	1 Radioactive Element 2 Monitoring Device 3 Infusion Device D Intraluminal Device U Feeding Device Y Other Device	Z No Qualifier
5 Esophagus	7 Via Natural or Artificial Opening 8 Via Natural or Artificial Opening Endoscopic	1 Radioactive Element 2 Monitoring Device 3 Infusion Device B Airway D Intraluminal Device U Feeding Device Y Other Device	Z No Qualifier
6 Stomach	Ø Open 3 Percutaneous 4 Percutaneous Endoscopic	2 Monitoring Device 3 Infusion Device D Intraluminal Device M Stimulator Lead U Feeding Device Y Other Device	Z No Qualifier
6 Stomach	7 Via Natural or Artificial Opening 8 Via Natural or Artificial Opening Endoscopic	2 Monitoring Device 3 Infusion Device D Intraluminal Device U Feeding Device Y Other Device	Z No Qualifier
8 Small Intestine 9 Duodenum A Jejunum B Ileum	Ø Open 3 Percutaneous 4 Percutaneous Endoscopic 7 Via Natural or Artificial Opening 8 Via Natural or Artificial Opening Endoscopic	2 Monitoring Device 3 Infusion Device D Intraluminal Device U Feeding Device	Z No Qualifier
E Large Intestine	Ø Open 3 Percutaneous 4 Percutaneous Endoscopic 7 Via Natural or Artificial Opening 8 Via Natural or Artificial Opening Endoscopic	D Intraluminal Device	Z No Qualifier

SECTION: Ø MEDICAL AND SURGICAL
BODY SYSTEM: D GASTROINTESTINAL SYSTEM
OPERATION: H INSERTION: *(continued)*
Putting in a nonbiological appliance that monitors, assists, performs, or prevents a physiological function but does not physically take the place of a body part

Body Part	Approach	Device	Qualifier
P Rectum	Ø Open 3 Percutaneous 4 Percutaneous Endoscopic 7 Via Natural or Artificial Opening 8 Via Natural or Artificial Opening Endoscopic	1 Radioactive Element D Intraluminal Device	Z No Qualifier
Q Anus	Ø Open 3 Percutaneous 4 Percutaneous Endoscopic	D Intraluminal Device L Artificial Sphincter	Z No Qualifier
Q Anus	7 Via Natural or Artificial Opening 8 Via Natural or Artificial Opening Endoscopic	D Intraluminal Device	Z No Qualifier
R Anal Sphincter	Ø Open 3 Percutaneous 4 Percutaneous Endoscopic	M Stimulator Lead	Z No Qualifier

SECTION: Ø MEDICAL AND SURGICAL
BODY SYSTEM: D GASTROINTESTINAL SYSTEM
OPERATION: J INSPECTION: Visually and/or manually exploring a body part

Body Part	Approach	Device	Qualifier
Ø Upper Intestinal Tract 6 Stomach D Lower Intestinal Tract	Ø Open 3 Percutaneous 4 Percutaneous Endoscopic 7 Via Natural or Artificial Opening 8 Via Natural or Artificial Opening Endoscopic X External	Z No Device	Z No Qualifier
U Omentum V Mesentery W Peritoneum	Ø Open 3 Percutaneous 4 Percutaneous Endoscopic X External	Z No Device	Z No Qualifier

H: INSERTION J: INSPECTION

D: GASTROINTESTINAL SYSTEM

Ø: M/S

SECTION: Ø MEDICAL AND SURGICAL
BODY SYSTEM: D GASTROINTESTINAL SYSTEM
OPERATION: L OCCLUSION: Completely closing an orifice or the lumen of a tubular body part

Body Part	Approach	Device	Qualifier
1 Esophagus, Upper 2 Esophagus, Middle 3 Esophagus, Lower 4 Esophagogastric Junction 5 Esophagus 6 Stomach 7 Stomach, Pylorus 8 Small Intestine 9 Duodenum A Jejunum B Ileum C Ileocecal Valve E Large Intestine F Large Intestine, Right G Large Intestine, Left H Cecum K Ascending Colon L Transverse Colon M Descending Colon N Sigmoid Colon P Rectum	Ø Open 3 Percutaneous 4 Percutaneous Endoscopic	C Extraluminal Device D Intraluminal Device Z No Device	Z No Qualifier
1 Esophagus, Upper 2 Esophagus, Middle 3 Esophagus, Lower 4 Esophagogastric Junction 5 Esophagus 6 Stomach 7 Stomach, Pylorus 8 Small Intestine 9 Duodenum A Jejunum B Ileum C Ileocecal Valve E Large Intestine F Large Intestine, Right G Large Intestine, Left H Cecum K Ascending Colon L Transverse Colon M Descending Colon N Sigmoid Colon P Rectum	7 Via Natural or Artificial Opening 8 Via Natural or Artificial Opening Endoscopic	D Intraluminal Device Z No Device	Z No Qualifier
Q Anus	Ø Open 3 Percutaneous 4 Percutaneous Endoscopic X External	C Extraluminal Device D Intraluminal Device Z No Device	Z No Qualifier
Q Anus	7 Via Natural or Artificial Opening 8 Via Natural or Artificial Opening Endoscopic	D Intraluminal Device Z No Device	Z No Qualifier

SECTION: Ø MEDICAL AND SURGICAL
BODY SYSTEM: D GASTROINTESTINAL SYSTEM
OPERATION: M REATTACHMENT: Putting back in or on all or a portion of a separated body part to its normal location or other suitable location

Body Part	Approach	Device	Qualifier
5 Esophagus 6 Stomach 8 Small Intestine 9 Duodenum A Jejunum B Ileum E Large Intestine F Large Intestine, Right G Large Intestine, Left H Cecum K Ascending Colon L Transverse Colon M Descending Colon N Sigmoid Colon P Rectum	Ø Open 4 Percutaneous Endoscopic	Z No Device	Z No Qualifier

New/Revised Text in Blue ~~deleted~~ Deleted

SECTION: Ø MEDICAL AND SURGICAL
BODY SYSTEM: D GASTROINTESTINAL SYSTEM
OPERATION: N RELEASE: Freeing a body part from an abnormal physical constraint by cutting or by the use of force

Body Part	Approach	Device	Qualifier
1 Esophagus, Upper 2 Esophagus, Middle 3 Esophagus, Lower 4 Esophagogastric Junction 5 Esophagus 6 Stomach 7 Stomach, Pylorus 8 Small Intestine 9 Duodenum A Jejunum B Ileum C Ileocecal Valve E Large Intestine F Large Intestine, Right G Large Intestine, Left H Cecum J Appendix K Ascending Colon L Transverse Colon M Descending Colon N Sigmoid Colon P Rectum	Ø Open 3 Percutaneous 4 Percutaneous Endoscopic 7 Via Natural or Artificial Opening 8 Via Natural or Artificial Opening Endoscopic	Z No Device	Z No Qualifier
Q Anus	Ø Open 3 Percutaneous 4 Percutaneous Endoscopic 7 Via Natural or Artificial Opening 8 Via Natural or Artificial Opening Endoscopic X External	Z No Device	Z No Qualifier
R Anal Sphincter U Omentum ~~T Lesser Omentum~~ V Mesentery W Peritoneum	Ø Open 3 Percutaneous 4 Percutaneous Endoscopic	Z No Device	Z No Qualifier

SECTION: Ø MEDICAL AND SURGICAL
BODY SYSTEM: D GASTROINTESTINAL SYSTEM
OPERATION: P REMOVAL: *(on multiple pages)*

Taking out or off a device from a body part

Body Part	Approach	Device	Qualifier
Ø Upper Intestinal Tract D Lower Intestinal Tract	Ø Open 3 Percutaneous 4 Percutaneous Endoscopic 7 Via Natural or Artificial Opening 8 Via Natural or Artificial Opening Endoscopic	Ø Drainage Device 2 Monitoring Device 3 Infusion Device 7 Autologous Tissue Substitute C Extraluminal Device D Intraluminal Device J Synthetic Substitute K Nonautologous Tissue Substitute U Feeding Device Y Other Device	Z No Qualifier
Ø Upper Intestinal Tract D Lower Intestinal Tract	X External	Ø Drainage Device 2 Monitoring Device 3 Infusion Device D Intraluminal Device U Feeding Device	Z No Qualifier
5 Esophagus	Ø Open 3 Percutaneous 4 Percutaneous Endoscopic	1 Radioactive Element 2 Monitoring Device 3 Infusion Device U Feeding Device Y Other Device	Z No Qualifier
5 Esophagus	7 Via Natural or Artificial Opening 8 Via Natural or Artificial Opening Endoscopic	1 Radioactive Element D Intraluminal Device Y Other Device	Z No Qualifier
5 Esophagus	X External	1 Radioactive Element 2 Monitoring Device 3 Infusion Device D Intraluminal Device U Feeding Device	Z No Qualifier
6 Stomach	Ø Open 3 Percutaneous 4 Percutaneous Endoscopic	Ø Drainage Device 2 Monitoring Device 3 Infusion Device 7 Autologous Tissue Substitute C Extraluminal Device D Intraluminal Device J Synthetic Substitute K Nonautologous Tissue Substitute M Stimulator Lead U Feeding Device Y Other Device	Z No Qualifier

New/Revised Text in Blue ~~deleted~~ Deleted

SECTION: Ø MEDICAL AND SURGICAL
BODY SYSTEM: D GASTROINTESTINAL SYSTEM
OPERATION: P REMOVAL: *(continued)*
Taking out or off a device from a body part

Body Part	Approach	Device	Qualifier
6 Stomach	7 Via Natural or Artificial Opening 8 Via Natural or Artificial Opening Endoscopic	Ø Drainage Device 2 Monitoring Device 3 Infusion Device 7 Autologous Tissue Substitute C Extraluminal Device D Intraluminal Device J Synthetic Substitute K Nonautologous Tissue Substitute U Feeding Device Y Other Device	Z No Qualifier
6 Stomach	X External	Ø Drainage Device 2 Monitoring Device 3 Infusion Device D Intraluminal Device U Feeding Device	Z No Qualifier
P Rectum	Ø Open 3 Percutaneous 4 Percutaneous Endoscopic 7 Via Natural or Artificial Opening 8 Via Natural or Artificial Opening Endoscopic X External	1 Radioactive Element	Z No Qualifier
Q Anus	Ø Open 3 Percutaneous 4 Percutaneous Endoscopic 7 Via Natural or Artificial Opening 8 Via Natural or Artificial Opening Endoscopic	L Artificial Sphincter	Z No Qualifier
R Anal Sphincter	Ø Open 3 Percutaneous 4 Percutaneous Endoscopic	M Stimulator Lead	Z No Qualifier
U Omentum V Mesentery W Peritoneum	Ø Open 3 Percutaneous 4 Percutaneous Endoscopic	Ø Drainage Device 1 Radioactive Element 7 Autologous Tissue Substitute J Synthetic Substitute K Nonautologous Tissue Substitute	Z No Qualifier

SECTION: Ø MEDICAL AND SURGICAL
BODY SYSTEM: D GASTROINTESTINAL SYSTEM
OPERATION: Q **REPAIR:** Restoring, to the extent possible, a body part to its normal anatomic structure and function

Body Part	Approach	Device	Qualifier
1 Esophagus, Upper 2 Esophagus, Middle 3 Esophagus, Lower 4 Esophagogastric Junction 5 Esophagus 6 Stomach 7 Stomach, Pylorus 8 Small Intestine 9 Duodenum A Jejunum B Ileum C Ileocecal Valve E Large Intestine F Large Intestine, Right G Large Intestine, Left H Cecum J Appendix K Ascending Colon L Transverse Colon M Descending Colon N Sigmoid Colon P Rectum	Ø Open 3 Percutaneous 4 Percutaneous Endoscopic 7 Via Natural or Artificial Opening 8 Via Natural or Artificial Opening Endoscopic	Z No Device	Z No Qualifier
Q Anus	Ø Open 3 Percutaneous 4 Percutaneous Endoscopic 7 Via Natural or Artificial Opening 8 Via Natural or Artificial Opening Endoscopic X External	Z No Device	Z No Qualifier
R Anal Sphincter U Omentum T Lesser Omentum V Mesentery W Peritoneum	Ø Open 3 Percutaneous 4 Percutaneous Endoscopic	Z No Device	Z No Qualifier

New/Revised Text in Blue   ~~deleted~~ Deleted

SECTION: Ø MEDICAL AND SURGICAL
BODY SYSTEM: D GASTROINTESTINAL SYSTEM
OPERATION: R REPLACEMENT: Putting in or on biological or synthetic material that physically takes the place and/or function of all or a portion of a body part

Body Part	Approach	Device	Qualifier
5 Esophagus	Ø Open 4 Percutaneous Endoscopic 7 Via Natural or Artificial Opening 8 Via Natural or Artificial Opening Endoscopic	7 Autologous Tissue Substitute J Synthetic Substitute K Nonautologous Tissue Substitute	Z No Qualifier
R Anal Sphincter U Omentum T Lesser Omentum V Mesentery W Peritoneum	Ø Open 4 Percutaneous Endoscopic	7 Autologous Tissue Substitute J Synthetic Substitute K Nonautologous Tissue Substitute	Z No Qualifier

SECTION: Ø MEDICAL AND SURGICAL
BODY SYSTEM: D GASTROINTESTINAL SYSTEM
OPERATION: S REPOSITION: Moving to its normal location, or other suitable location, all or a portion of a body part

Body Part	Approach	Device	Qualifier
5 Esophagus 6 Stomach 9 Duodenum A Jejunum B Ileum H Cecum K Ascending Colon L Transverse Colon M Descending Colon N Sigmoid Colon P Rectum Q Anus	Ø Open 4 Percutaneous Endoscopic 7 Via Natural or Artificial Opening 8 Via Natural or Artificial Opening Endoscopic X External	Z No Device	Z No Qualifier
8 Small Intestine E Large Intestine	Ø Open 4 Percutaneous Endoscopic 7 Via Natural or Artificial Opening 8 Via Natural or Artificial Opening Endoscopic	Z No Device	Z No Qualifier

SECTION: **Ø MEDICAL AND SURGICAL**
BODY SYSTEM: **D GASTROINTESTINAL SYSTEM**
OPERATION: **T RESECTION:** Cutting out or off, without replacement, all of a body part

Body Part	Approach	Device	Qualifier
1 Esophagus, Upper 2 Esophagus, Middle 3 Esophagus, Lower 4 Esophagogastric Junction 5 Esophagus 6 Stomach 7 Stomach, Pylorus 8 Small Intestine 9 Duodenum A Jejunum B Ileum C Ileocecal Valve E Large Intestine F Large Intestine, Right ~~G Large Intestine, Left~~ H Cecum J Appendix K Ascending Colon ~~L Transverse Colon~~ ~~M Descending Colon~~ ~~N Sigmoid Colon~~ P Rectum Q Anus	Ø Open 4 Percutaneous Endoscopic 7 Via Natural or Artificial 　 Opening 8 Via Natural or Artificial 　 Opening Endoscopic	Z No Device	Z No Qualifier
G Large Intestine, Left L Transverse Colon M Descending Colon N Sigmoid Colon	Ø Open 4 Percutaneous Endoscopic 7 Via Natural or Artificial 　 Opening 8 Via Natural or Artificial 　 Opening Endoscopic F Via Natural or Artificial 　 Opening With Percutaneous 　 Endoscopic Assistance	Z No Device	Z No Qualifier
R Anal Sphincter U Omentum ~~T Lesser Omentum~~	Ø Open 4 Percutaneous Endoscopic	Z No Device	Z No Qualifier

SECTION: Ø MEDICAL AND SURGICAL
BODY SYSTEM: D GASTROINTESTINAL SYSTEM
OPERATION: U SUPPLEMENT: Putting in or on biological or synthetic material that physically reinforces and/or augments the function of a portion of a body part

Body Part	Approach	Device	Qualifier
1 Esophagus, Upper 2 Esophagus, Middle 3 Esophagus, Lower 4 Esophagogastric Junction 5 Esophagus 6 Stomach 7 Stomach, Pylorus 8 Small Intestine 9 Duodenum A Jejunum B Ileum C Ileocecal Valve E Large Intestine F Large Intestine, Right G Large Intestine, Left H Cecum K Ascending Colon L Transverse Colon M Descending Colon N Sigmoid Colon P Rectum	Ø Open 4 Percutaneous Endoscopic 7 Via Natural or Artificial Opening 8 Via Natural or Artificial Opening Endoscopic	7 Autologous Tissue Substitute J Synthetic Substitute K Nonautologous Tissue Substitute	Z No Qualifier
Q Anus	Ø Open 4 Percutaneous Endoscopic 7 Via Natural or Artificial Opening 8 Via Natural or Artificial Opening Endoscopic X External	7 Autologous Tissue Substitute J Synthetic Substitute K Nonautologous Tissue Substitute	Z No Qualifier
R Anal Sphincter U Omentum T Lesser Omentum V Mesentery W Peritoneum	Ø Open 4 Percutaneous Endoscopic	7 Autologous Tissue Substitute J Synthetic Substitute K Nonautologous Tissue Substitute	Z No Qualifier

SECTION: Ø MEDICAL AND SURGICAL
BODY SYSTEM: D GASTROINTESTINAL SYSTEM
OPERATION: V RESTRICTION: Partially closing an orifice or the lumen of a tubular body part

V: RESTRICTION

D: GASTROINTESTINAL SYSTEM

Ø: M/S

Body Part	Approach	Device	Qualifier
1 Esophagus, Upper 2 Esophagus, Middle 3 Esophagus, Lower 4 Esophagogastric Junction 5 Esophagus 6 Stomach 7 Stomach, Pylorus 8 Small Intestine 9 Duodenum A Jejunum B Ileum C Ileocecal Valve E Large Intestine F Large Intestine, Right G Large Intestine, Left H Cecum K Ascending Colon L Transverse Colon M Descending Colon N Sigmoid Colon P Rectum	Ø Open 3 Percutaneous 4 Percutaneous Endoscopic	C Extraluminal Device D Intraluminal Device Z No Device	Z No Qualifier
1 Esophagus, Upper 2 Esophagus, Middle 3 Esophagus, Lower 4 Esophagogastric Junction 5 Esophagus 6 Stomach 7 Stomach, Pylorus 8 Small Intestine 9 Duodenum A Jejunum B Ileum C Ileocecal Valve E Large Intestine F Large Intestine, Right G Large Intestine, Left H Cecum K Ascending Colon L Colon M Descending Colon N Sigmoid Colon P Rectum	7 Via Natural or Artificial Opening 8 Via Natural or Artificial Opening Endoscopic	D Intraluminal Device Z No Device	Z No Qualifier
Q Anus	Ø Open 3 Percutaneous 4 Percutaneous Endoscopic X External	C Extraluminal Device D Intraluminal Device Z No Device	Z No Qualifier
Q Anus	7 Via Natural or Artificial Opening 8 Via Natural or Artificial Opening Endoscopic	D Intraluminal Device Z No Device	Z No Qualifier

SECTION: Ø MEDICAL AND SURGICAL
BODY SYSTEM: D GASTROINTESTINAL SYSTEM
OPERATION: W REVISION: *(on multiple pages)*
Correcting, to the extent possible, a portion of a malfunctioning device or the position of a displaced device

Body Part	Approach	Device	Qualifier
Ø Upper Intestinal Tract D Lower Intestinal Tract	Ø Open 3 Percutaneous 4 Percutaneous Endoscopic 7 Via Natural or Artificial Opening 8 Via Natural or Artificial Opening Endoscopic X External	Ø Drainage Device 2 Monitoring Device 3 Infusion Device 7 Autologous Tissue Substitute C Extraluminal Device D Intraluminal Device J Synthetic Substitute K Nonautologous Tissue Substitute U Feeding Device Y Other Device	Z No Qualifier
Ø Upper Intestinal Tract D Lower Intestinal Tract	X External	Ø Drainage Device 2 Monitoring Device 3 Infusion Device 7 Autologous Tissue Substitute C Extraluminal Device D Intraluminal Device J Synthetic Substitute K Nonautologous Tissue Substitute U Feeding Device	Z No Qualifier
5 Esophagus	Ø Open 3 Percutaneous 4 Percutaneous Endoscopic	Y Other Device	Z No Qualifier
5 Esophagus	7 Via Natural or Artificial Opening 8 Via Natural or Artificial Opening Endoscopic X External	D Intraluminal Device Y Other Device	Z No Qualifier
5 Esophagus	X External	D Intraluminal Device	Z No Qualifier
6 Stomach	Ø Open 3 Percutaneous 4 Percutaneous Endoscopic	Ø Drainage Device 2 Monitoring Device 3 Infusion Device 7 Autologous Tissue Substitute C Extraluminal Device D Intraluminal Device J Synthetic Substitute K Nonautologous Tissue Substitute M Stimulator Lead U Feeding Device Y Other Device	Z No Qualifier
6 Stomach	7 Via Natural or Artificial Opening 8 Via Natural or Artificial Opening Endoscopic X External	Ø Drainage Device 2 Monitoring Device 3 Infusion Device 7 Autologous Tissue Substitute C Extraluminal Device D Intraluminal Device J Synthetic Substitute K Nonautologous Tissue Substitute U Feeding Device Y Other Device	Z No Qualifier

SECTION: Ø MEDICAL AND SURGICAL
BODY SYSTEM: D GASTROINTESTINAL SYSTEM
OPERATION: W REVISION: *(continued)*

Correcting, to the extent possible, a portion of a malfunctioning device or the position of a displaced device

Body Part	Approach	Device	Qualifier
6 Stomach	X External	0 Drainage Device 2 Monitoring Device 3 Infusion Device 7 Autologous Tissue Substitute C Extraluminal Device D Intraluminal Device J Synthetic Substitute K Nonautologous Tissue Substitute U Feeding Device	Z No Qualifier
8 Small Intestine E Large Intestine	0 Open 4 Percutaneous Endoscopic 7 Via Natural or Artificial Opening 8 Via Natural or Artificial Opening Endoscopic	7 Autologous Tissue Substitute J Synthetic Substitute K Nonautologous Tissue Substitute	Z No Qualifier
Q Anus	0 Open 3 Percutaneous 4 Percutaneous Endoscopic 7 Via Natural or Artificial Opening 8 Via Natural or Artificial Opening Endoscopic	L Artificial Sphincter	Z No Qualifier
R Anal Sphincter	0 Open 3 Percutaneous 4 Percutaneous Endoscopic	M Stimulator Lead	Z No Qualifier
U Omentum V Mesentery W Peritoneum	0 Open 3 Percutaneous 4 Percutaneous Endoscopic	0 Drainage Device 7 Autologous Tissue Substitute J Synthetic Substitute K Nonautologous Tissue Substitute	Z No Qualifier

New/Revised Text in Blue   ~~deleted~~ Deleted

SECTION: Ø MEDICAL AND SURGICAL

BODY SYSTEM: D GASTROINTESTINAL SYSTEM

OPERATION: X TRANSFER: Moving, without taking out, all or a portion of a body part to another location to take over the function of all or a portion of a body part

Body Part	Approach	Device	Qualifier
6 Stomach 8 Small Intestine E Large Intestine	Ø Open 4 Percutaneous Endoscopic	Z No Device	5 Esophagus

SECTION: Ø MEDICAL AND SURGICAL

BODY SYSTEM: D GASTROINTESTINAL SYSTEM

OPERATION: Y TRANSPLANTATION: Putting in or on all or a portion of a living body part taken from another individual or animal to physically take the place and/or function of all or a portion of a similar body part

Body Part	Approach	Device	Qualifier
5 Esophagus 6 Stomach 8 Small Intestine E Large Intestine	Ø Open	Z No Device	0 Allogeneic 1 Syngeneic 2 Zooplastic

ØF. Hepatobiliary System and Pancreas 232
   ØF1. Bypass 233
   ØF2. Change 233
   ØF5. Destruction 234
   ØF7. Dilation 235
   ØF8. Division 235
   ØF9. Drainage 236
   ØFB. Excision 237
   ØFC. Extirpation 237
   ØFF. Fragmentation 238
   ØFH. Insertion 238
   ØFJ. Inspection 239
   ØFL. Occlusion 239
   ØFM. Reattachment 240
   ØFN. Release 240
   ØFP. Removal 241
   ØFQ. Repair 242
   ØFR. Replacement 242
   ØFS. Reposition 243
   ØFT. Resection 243
   ØFU. Supplement 244
   ØFV. Restriction 244
   ØFW. Revision 245
   ØFY. Transplantation 246

New/Revised Text in Blue   ~~deleted~~ Deleted

SECTION: Ø MEDICAL AND SURGICAL
BODY SYSTEM: F HEPATOBILIARY SYSTEM AND PANCREAS
OPERATION: 1 BYPASS: Altering the route of passage of the contents of a tubular body part

Body Part	Approach	Device	Qualifier
4 Gallbladder 5 Hepatic Duct, Right 6 Hepatic Duct, Left 7 Hepatic Duct, Common 8 Cystic Duct 9 Common Bile Duct	Ø Open 4 Percutaneous Endoscopic	D Intraluminal Device Z No Device	3 Duodenum 4 Stomach 5 Hepatic Duct, Right 6 Hepatic Duct, Left 7 Hepatic Duct, Caudate 8 Cystic Duct 9 Common Bile Duct B Small Intestine
D Pancreatic Duct F Pancreatic Duct, Accessory G Pancreas	Ø Open 4 Percutaneous Endoscopic	D Intraluminal Device Z No Device	3 Duodenum B Small Intestine C Large Intestine

SECTION: Ø MEDICAL AND SURGICAL
BODY SYSTEM: F HEPATOBILIARY SYSTEM AND PANCREAS
OPERATION: 2 CHANGE: Taking out or off a device from a body part and putting back an identical or similar device in or on the same body part without cutting or puncturing the skin or a mucous membrane

Body Part	Approach	Device	Qualifier
Ø Liver 4 Gallbladder B Hepatobiliary Duct D Pancreatic Duct G Pancreas	X External	Ø Drainage Device Y Other Device	Z No Qualifier

SECTION: Ø MEDICAL AND SURGICAL
BODY SYSTEM: F HEPATOBILIARY SYSTEM AND PANCREAS
OPERATION: 5 **DESTRUCTION:** Physical eradication of all or a portion of a body part by the direct use of energy, force, or a destructive agent

Body Part	Approach	Device	Qualifier
Ø Liver 1 Liver, Right Lobe 2 Liver, Left Lobe 4 ~~Gallbladder~~ G ~~Pancreas~~	Ø Open 3 Percutaneous 4 Percutaneous Endoscopic	Z No Device	Z No Qualifier
4 Gallbladder G Pancreas	Ø Open 3 Percutaneous 4 Percutaneous Endoscopic 8 Via Natural or Artificial Opening Endoscopic	Z No Device	Z No Qualifier
5 Hepatic Duct, Right 6 Hepatic Duct, Left 7 Hepatic Duct, Common 8 Cystic Duct 9 Common Bile Duct C Ampulla of Vater D Pancreatic Duct F Pancreatic Duct, Accessory	Ø Open 3 Percutaneous 4 Percutaneous Endoscopic 7 Via Natural or Artificial Opening 8 Via Natural or Artificial Opening Endoscopic	Z No Device	Z No Qualifier

5: DESTRUCTION

F: HEPATOBILIARY SYSTEM AND PANCREAS

Ø: M/S

SECTION: Ø MEDICAL AND SURGICAL
BODY SYSTEM: F HEPATOBILIARY SYSTEM AND PANCREAS
OPERATION: 7 **DILATION:** Expanding an orifice or the lumen of a tubular body part

Body Part	Approach	Device	Qualifier
5 Hepatic Duct, Right 6 Hepatic Duct, Left 7 Hepatic Duct, Common 8 Cystic Duct 9 Common Bile Duct C Ampulla of Vater D Pancreatic Duct F Pancreatic Duct, Accessory	Ø Open 3 Percutaneous 4 Percutaneous Endoscopic 7 Via Natural or Artificial Opening 8 Via Natural or Artificial Opening Endoscopic	D Intraluminal Device Z No Device	Z No Qualifier

SECTION: Ø MEDICAL AND SURGICAL
BODY SYSTEM: F HEPATOBILIARY SYSTEM AND PANCREAS
OPERATION: 8 **DIVISION:** Cutting into a body part, without draining fluids and/or gases from the body part, in order to separate or transect a body part

Body Part	Approach	Device	Qualifier
G Pancreas	Ø Open 3 Percutaneous 4 Percutaneous Endoscopic	Z No Device	Z No Qualifier

SECTION: Ø MEDICAL AND SURGICAL
BODY SYSTEM: F HEPATOBILIARY SYSTEM AND PANCREAS
OPERATION: 9 DRAINAGE: Taking or letting out fluids and/or gases from a body part

Body Part	Approach	Device	Qualifier
Ø Liver 1 Liver, Right Lobe 2 Liver, Left Lobe ~~4 Gallbladder~~ ~~G Pancreas~~	Ø Open 3 Percutaneous 4 Percutaneous Endoscopic	Ø Drainage Device	Z No Qualifier
Ø Liver 1 Liver, Right Lobe 2 Liver, Left Lobe ~~4 Gallbladder~~ ~~G Pancreas~~	Ø Open 3 Percutaneous 4 Percutaneous Endoscopic	Z No Device	X Diagnostic Z No Qualifier
4 Gallbladder G Pancreas	Ø Open 3 Percutaneous 4 Percutaneous Endoscopic 8 Via Natural or Artificial Opening Endoscopic	Ø Drainage Device	Z No Qualifier
4 Gallbladder G Pancreas	Ø Open 3 Percutaneous 4 Percutaneous Endoscopic 8 Via Natural or Artificial Opening Endoscopic	Z No Device	X Diagnostic Z No Qualifier
5 Hepatic Duct, Right 6 Hepatic Duct, Left 7 Hepatic Duct, Common 8 Cystic Duct 9 Common Bile Duct C Ampulla of Vater D Pancreatic Duct F Pancreatic Duct, Accessory	Ø Open 3 Percutaneous 4 Percutaneous Endoscopic 7 Via Natural or Artificial Opening 8 Via Natural or Artificial Opening Endoscopic	Ø Drainage Device	Z No Qualifier
5 Hepatic Duct, Right 6 Hepatic Duct, Left 7 Hepatic Duct, Common 8 Cystic Duct 9 Common Bile Duct C Ampulla of Vater D Pancreatic Duct F Pancreatic Duct, Accessory	Ø Open 3 Percutaneous 4 Percutaneous Endoscopic 7 Via Natural or Artificial Opening 8 Via Natural or Artificial Opening Endoscopic	Z No Device	X Diagnostic Z No Qualifier

New/Revised Text in Blue ~~deleted~~ Deleted

SECTION: Ø MEDICAL AND SURGICAL
BODY SYSTEM: F HEPATOBILIARY SYSTEM AND PANCREAS
OPERATION: B EXCISION: Cutting out or off, without replacement, a portion of a body part

Body Part	Approach	Device	Qualifier
Ø Liver 1 Liver, Right Lobe 2 Liver, Left Lobe 4 ~~Gallbladder~~ G ~~Pancreas~~	Ø Open 3 Percutaneous 4 Percutaneous Endoscopic	Z No Device	X Diagnostic Z No Qualifier
4 Gallbladder G Pancreas	Ø Open 3 Percutaneous 4 Percutaneous Endoscopic 8 Via Natural or Artificial Opening Endoscopic	Z No Device	X Diagnostic Z No Qualifier
5 Hepatic Duct, Right 6 Hepatic Duct, Left 7 Hepatic Duct, Common 8 Cystic Duct 9 Common Bile Duct C Ampulla of Vater D Pancreatic Duct F Pancreatic Duct, Accessory	Ø Open 3 Percutaneous 4 Percutaneous Endoscopic 7 Via Natural or Artificial Opening 8 Via Natural or Artificial Opening Endoscopic	Z No Device	X Diagnostic Z No Qualifier

SECTION: Ø MEDICAL AND SURGICAL
BODY SYSTEM: F HEPATOBILIARY SYSTEM AND PANCREAS
OPERATION: C EXTIRPATION: Taking or cutting out solid matter from a body part

Body Part	Approach	Device	Qualifier
Ø Liver 1 Liver, Right Lobe 2 Liver, Left Lobe 4 ~~Gallbladder~~ G ~~Pancreas~~	Ø Open 3 Percutaneous 4 Percutaneous Endoscopic	Z No Device	Z No Qualifier
4 Gallbladder G Pancreas	Ø Open 3 Percutaneous 4 Percutaneous Endoscopic 8 Via Natural or Artificial Opening Endoscopic	Z No Device	Z No Qualifier
5 Hepatic Duct, Right 6 Hepatic Duct, Left 7 Hepatic Duct, Common 8 Cystic Duct 9 Common Bile Duct C Ampulla of Vater D Pancreatic Duct F Pancreatic Duct, Accessory	Ø Open 3 Percutaneous 4 Percutaneous Endoscopic 7 Via Natural or Artificial Opening 8 Via Natural or Artificial Opening Endoscopic	Z No Device	Z No Qualifier

Ø: M/S

F: HEPATOBILIARY SYSTEM AND PANCREAS

B: EXCISION   C: EXTIRPATION

SECTION: Ø MEDICAL AND SURGICAL
BODY SYSTEM: F HEPATOBILIARY SYSTEM AND PANCREAS
OPERATION: F FRAGMENTATION: Breaking solid matter in a body part into pieces

Body Part	Approach	Device	Qualifier
4 Gallbladder 5 Hepatic Duct, Right 6 Hepatic Duct, Left 7 Hepatic Duct, Common 8 Cystic Duct 9 Common Bile Duct C Ampulla of Vater D Pancreatic Duct F Pancreatic Duct, Acessory	Ø Open 3 Percutaneous 4 Percutaneous Endoscopic 7 Via Natural or Artificial Opening 8 Via Natural or Artificial Opening Endoscopic X External	Z No Device	Z No Qualifier

SECTION: Ø MEDICAL AND SURGICAL
BODY SYSTEM: F HEPATOBILIARY SYSTEM AND PANCREAS
OPERATION: H INSERTION: Putting in a nonbiological appliance that monitors, assists, performs, or prevents a physiological function but does not physically take the place of a body part

Body Part	Approach	Device	Qualifier
Ø Liver 1 Liver, Right Lobe 2 Liver, Left Lobe 4 Gallbladder G Pancreas	Ø Open 3 Percutaneous 4 Percutaneous Endoscopic	2 Monitoring Device 3 Infusion Device Y Other Device	Z No Qualifier
1 Liver, Right Lobe 2 Liver, Left Lobe	Ø Open 3 Percutaneous 4 Percutaneous Endoscopic	2 Monitoring Device 3 Infusion Device	Z No Qualifier
B Hepatobiliary Duct D Pancreatic Duct	Ø Open 3 Percutaneous 4 Percutaneous Endoscopic 7 Via Natural or Artificial Opening 8 Via Natural or Artificial Opening Endoscopic	1 Radioactive Element 2 Monitoring Device 3 Infusion Device D Intraluminal Device Y Other Device	Z No Qualifier

SECTION: Ø MEDICAL AND SURGICAL
BODY SYSTEM: F HEPATOBILIARY SYSTEM AND PANCREAS
OPERATION: J INSPECTION: Visually and/or manually exploring a body part

Body Part	Approach	Device	Qualifier
Ø Liver	Ø Open 3 Percutaneous 4 Percutaneous Endoscopic X External	Z No Device	Z No Qualifier
~~Ø Liver~~ 4 Gallbladder G Pancreas	Ø Open 3 Percutaneous 4 Percutaneous Endoscopic 8 Via Natural or Artificial Opening Endoscopic X External	Z No Device	Z No Qualifier
B Hepatobiliary Duct D Pancreatic Duct	Ø Open 3 Percutaneous 4 Percutaneous Endoscopic 7 Via Natural or Artificial Opening 8 Via Natural or Artificial Opening Endoscopic	Z No Device	Z No Qualifier

SECTION: Ø MEDICAL AND SURGICAL
BODY SYSTEM: F HEPATOBILIARY SYSTEM AND PANCREAS
OPERATION: L OCCLUSION: Completely closing an orifice or the lumen of a tubular body part

Body Part	Approach	Device	Qualifier
5 Hepatic Duct, Right 6 Hepatic Duct, Left 7 Hepatic Duct, Common 8 Cystic Duct 9 Common Bile Duct C Ampulla of Vater D Pancreatic Duct F Pancreatic Duct, Accessory	Ø Open 3 Percutaneous 4 Percutaneous Endoscopic	C Extraluminal Device D Intraluminal Device Z No Device	Z No Qualifier
5 Hepatic Duct, Right 6 Hepatic Duct, Left 7 Hepatic Duct, Common 8 Cystic Duct 9 Common Bile Duct C Ampulla of Vater D Pancreatic Duct F Pancreatic Duct, Accessory	7 Via Natural or Artificial Opening 8 Via Natural or Artificial Opening Endoscopic	D Intraluminal Device Z No Device	Z No Qualifier

SECTION: Ø MEDICAL AND SURGICAL
BODY SYSTEM: F HEPATOBILIARY SYSTEM AND PANCREAS
OPERATION: M **REATTACHMENT:** Putting back in or on all or a portion of a separated body part to its normal location or other suitable location

Body Part	Approach	Device	Qualifier
Ø Liver 1 Liver, Right Lobe 2 Liver, Left Lobe 4 Gallbladder 5 Hepatic Duct, Right 6 Hepatic Duct, Left 7 Hepatic Duct, Common 8 Cystic Duct 9 Common Bile Duct C Ampulla of Vater D Pancreatic Duct F Pancreatic Duct, Accessory G Pancreas	Ø Open 4 Percutaneous Endoscopic	Z No Device	Z No Qualifier

SECTION: Ø MEDICAL AND SURGICAL
BODY SYSTEM: F HEPATOBILIARY SYSTEM AND PANCREAS
OPERATION: N **RELEASE:** Freeing a body part from an abnormal physical constraint by cutting or by the use of force

Body Part	Approach	Device	Qualifier
Ø Liver 1 Liver, Right Lobe 2 Liver, Left Lobe 4 Gallbladder G Pancreas	Ø Open 3 Percutaneous 4 Percutaneous Endoscopic	Z No Device	Z No Qualifier
4 Gallbladder G Pancreas	Ø Open 3 Percutaneous 4 Percutaneous Endoscopic 8 Via Natural or Artificial Opening Endoscopic	Z No Device	Z No Qualifier
5 Hepatic Duct, Right 6 Hepatic Duct, Left 7 Hepatic Duct, Common 8 Cystic Duct 9 Common Bile Duct C Ampulla of Vater D Pancreatic Duct F Pancreatic Duct, Accessory	Ø Open 3 Percutaneous 4 Percutaneous Endoscopic 7 Via Natural or Artificial Opening 8 Via Natural or Artificial Opening Endoscopic	Z No Device	Z No Qualifier

SECTION: Ø MEDICAL AND SURGICAL
BODY SYSTEM: F HEPATOBILIARY SYSTEM AND PANCREAS
OPERATION: P REMOVAL: Taking out or off a device from a body part

Body Part	Approach	Device	Qualifier
Ø Liver	Ø Open 3 Percutaneous 4 Percutaneous Endoscopic ~~X External~~	Ø Drainage Device 2 Monitoring Device 3 Infusion Device Y Other Device	Z No Qualifier
Ø Liver	X External	Ø Drainage Device 2 Monitoring Device 3 Infusion Device	Z No Qualifier
4 Gallbladder G Pancreas	Ø Open 3 Percutaneous 4 Percutaneous Endoscopic ~~X External~~	Ø Drainage Device 2 Monitoring Device 3 Infusion Device D Intraluminal Device Y Other Device	Z No Qualifier
4 Gallbladder G Pancreas	X External	Ø Drainage Device 2 Monitoring Device 3 Infusion Device D Intraluminal Device	Z No Qualifier
B Hepatobiliary Duct D Pancreatic Duct	Ø Open 3 Percutaneous 4 Percutaneous Endoscopic 7 Via Natural or Artificial Opening 8 Via Natural or Artificial Opening Endoscopic	Ø Drainage Device 1 Radioactive Element 2 Monitoring Device 3 Infusion Device 7 Autologous Tissue Substitute C Extraluminal Device D Intraluminal Device J Synthetic Substitute K Nonautologous Tissue Substitute Y Other Device	Z No Qualifier
B Hepatobiliary Duct D Pancreatic Duct	X External	Ø Drainage Device 1 Radioactive Element 2 Monitoring Device 3 Infusion Device D Intraluminal Device	Z No Qualifier

SECTION: Ø MEDICAL AND SURGICAL
BODY SYSTEM: F HEPATOBILIARY SYSTEM AND PANCREAS
OPERATION: Q REPAIR: Restoring, to the extent possible, a body part to its normal anatomic structure and function

Body Part	Approach	Device	Qualifier
Ø Liver 1 Liver, Right Lobe 2 Liver, Left Lobe 4 ~~Gallbladder~~ G ~~Pancreas~~	Ø Open 3 Percutaneous 4 Percutaneous Endoscopic	Z No Device	Z No Qualifier
4 Gallbladder G Pancreas	Ø Open 3 Percutaneous 4 Percutaneous Endoscopic 8 Via Natural or Artificial Opening Endoscopic	Z No Device	Z No Qualifier
5 Hepatic Duct, Right 6 Hepatic Duct, Left 7 Hepatic Duct, Common 8 Cystic Duct 9 Common Bile Duct C Ampulla of Vater D Pancreatic Duct F Pancreatic Duct, Accessory	Ø Open 3 Percutaneous 4 Percutaneous Endoscopic 7 Via Natural or Artificial Opening 8 Via Natural or Artificial Opening Endoscopic	Z No Device	Z No Qualifier

SECTION: Ø MEDICAL AND SURGICAL
BODY SYSTEM: F HEPATOBILIARY SYSTEM AND PANCREAS
OPERATION: R REPLACEMENT: Putting in or on biological or synthetic material that physically takes the place and/or function of all or a portion of a body part

Body Part	Approach	Device	Qualifier
5 Hepatic Duct, Right 6 Hepatic Duct, Left 7 Hepatic Duct, Common 8 Cystic Duct 9 Common Bile Duct C Ampulla of Vater D Pancreatic Duct F Pancreatic Duct, Accessory	Ø Open 4 Percutaneous Endoscopic 8 Via Natural or Artificial Opening Endoscopic	7 Autologous Tissue Substitute J Synthetic Substitute K Nonautologous Tissue Substitute	Z No Qualifier

New/Revised Text in Blue   ~~deleted~~ Deleted

SECTION: Ø MEDICAL AND SURGICAL
BODY SYSTEM: F HEPATOBILIARY SYSTEM AND PANCREAS
OPERATION: S REPOSITION: Moving to its normal location, or other suitable location, all or a portion of a body part

Body Part	Approach	Device	Qualifier
Ø Liver 4 Gallbladder 5 Hepatic Duct, Right 6 Hepatic Duct, Left 7 Hepatic Duct, Common 8 Cystic Duct 9 Common Bile Duct C Ampulla of Vater D Pancreatic Duct F Pancreatic Duct, Accessory G Pancreas	Ø Open 4 Percutaneous Endoscopic	Z No Device	Z No Qualifier

SECTION: Ø MEDICAL AND SURGICAL
BODY SYSTEM: F HEPATOBILIARY SYSTEM AND PANCREAS
OPERATION: T RESECTION: Cutting out or off, without replacement, all of a body part

Body Part	Approach	Device	Qualifier
Ø Liver 1 Liver, Right Lobe 2 Liver, Left Lobe 4 Gallbladder G Pancreas	Ø Open 4 Percutaneous Endoscopic	Z No Device	Z No Qualifier
5 Hepatic Duct, Right 6 Hepatic Duct, Left 7 Hepatic Duct, Common 8 Cystic Duct 9 Common Bile Duct C Ampulla of Vater D Pancreatic Duct F Pancreatic Duct, Accessory	Ø Open 4 Percutaneous Endoscopic 7 Via Natural or Artificial Opening 8 Via Natural or Artificial Opening Endoscopic	Z No Device	Z No Qualifier

SECTION: Ø MEDICAL AND SURGICAL
BODY SYSTEM: F HEPATOBILIARY SYSTEM AND PANCREAS
OPERATION: U SUPPLEMENT: Putting in or on biological or synthetic material that physically reinforces and/or augments the function of a portion of a body part

Body Part	Approach	Device	Qualifier
5 Hepatic Duct, Right 6 Hepatic Duct, Left 7 Hepatic Duct, Common 8 Cystic Duct 9 Common Bile Duct C Ampulla of Vater D Pancreatic Duct F Pancreatic Duct, Accessory	Ø Open 3 Percutaneous 4 Percutaneous Endoscopic 8 Via Natural or Artificial Opening Endoscopic	7 Autologous Tissue Substitute J Synthetic Substitute K Nonautologous Tissue Substitute	Z No Qualifier

SECTION: Ø MEDICAL AND SURGICAL
BODY SYSTEM: F HEPATOBILIARY SYSTEM AND PANCREAS
OPERATION: V RESTRICTION: Partially closing an orifice or the lumen of a tubular body part

Body Part	Approach	Device	Qualifier
5 Hepatic Duct, Right 6 Hepatic Duct, Left 7 Hepatic Duct, Common 8 Cystic Duct 9 Common Bile Duct C Ampulla of Vater D Pancreatic Duct F Pancreatic Duct, Accessory	Ø Open 3 Percutaneous 4 Percutaneous Endoscopic	C Extraluminal Device D Intraluminal Device Z No Device	Z No Qualifier
5 Hepatic Duct, Right 6 Hepatic Duct, Left 7 Hepatic Duct, Common 8 Cystic Duct 9 Common Bile Duct C Ampulla of Vater D Pancreatic Duct F Pancreatic Duct, Accessory	7 Via Natural or Artificial Opening 8 Via Natural or Artificial Opening Endoscopic	D Intraluminal Device Z No Device	Z No Qualifier

SECTION: Ø MEDICAL AND SURGICAL
BODY SYSTEM: F HEPATOBILIARY SYSTEM AND PANCREAS
OPERATION: W REVISION: Correcting, to the extent possible, a portion of a malfunctioning device or the position of a displaced device

Body Part	Approach	Device	Qualifier
Ø Liver	Ø Open 3 Percutaneous 4 Percutaneous Endoscopic ~~X External~~	Ø Drainage Device 2 Monitoring Device 3 Infusion Device Y Other Device	Z No Qualifier
Ø Liver	X External	Ø Drainage Device 2 Monitoring Device 3 Infusion Device	Z No Qualifier
4 Gallbladder G Pancreas	Ø Open 3 Percutaneous 4 Percutaneous Endoscopic ~~X External~~	Ø Drainage Device 2 Monitoring Device 3 Infusion Device D Intraluminal Device Y Other Device	Z No Qualifier
4 Gallbladder G Pancreas	X External	Ø Drainage Device 2 Monitoring Device 3 Infusion Device D Intraluminal Device	Z No Qualifier
B Hepatobiliary Duct D Pancreatic Duct	Ø Open 3 Percutaneous 4 Percutaneous Endoscopic 7 Via Natural or Artificial Opening 8 Via Natural or Artificial Opening Endoscopic ~~X External~~	Ø Drainage Device 2 Monitoring Device 3 Infusion Device 7 Autologous Tissue Substitute C Extraluminal Device D Intraluminal Device J Synthetic Substitute K Nonautologous Tissue Substitute Y Other Device	Z No Qualifier
B Hepatobiliary Duct D Pancreatic Duct	X External	Ø Drainage Device 2 Monitoring Device 3 Infusion Device 7 Autologous Tissue Substitute C Extraluminal Device D Intraluminal Device J Synthetic Substitute K Nonautologous Tissue Substitute	Z No Qualifier

SECTION: Ø MEDICAL AND SURGICAL
BODY SYSTEM: F HEPATOBILIARY SYSTEM AND PANCREAS
OPERATION: Y TRANSPLANTATION: Putting in or on all or a portion of a living body part taken from another individual or animal to physically take the place and/or function of all or a portion of a similar body part

Body Part	Approach	Device	Qualifier
Ø Liver G Pancreas	Ø Open	Z No Device	Ø Allogeneic 1 Syngeneic 2 Zooplastic

ØG. Endocrine System 247
    ØG2. Change 248
    ØG5. Destruction 248
    ØG8. Division 248
    ØG9. Drainage 249
    ØGB. Excision 250
    ØGC. Extirpation 250
    ØGH. Insertion 251
    ØGJ. Inspection 251
    ØGM. Reattachment 251
    ØGN. Release 252
    ØGP. Removal 252
    ØGQ. Repair 253
    ØGS. Reposition 253
    ØGT. Resection 254
    ØGW. Revision.. 254

SECTION: Ø MEDICAL AND SURGICAL
BODY SYSTEM: G ENDOCRINE SYSTEM
OPERATION: 2 CHANGE: Taking out or off a device from a body part and putting back an identical or similar device in or on the same body part without cutting or puncturing the skin or a mucous membrane

Body Part	Approach	Device	Qualifier
Ø Pituitary Gland 1 Pineal Body 5 Adrenal Gland K Thyroid Gland R Parathyroid Gland S Endocrine Gland	X External	Ø Drainage Device Y Other Device	Z No Qualifier

SECTION: Ø MEDICAL AND SURGICAL
BODY SYSTEM: G ENDOCRINE SYSTEM
OPERATION: 5 DESTRUCTION: Physical eradication of all or a portion of a body part by the direct use of energy, force, or a destructive agent

Body Part	Approach	Device	Qualifier
Ø Pituitary Gland 1 Pineal Body 2 Adrenal Gland, Left 3 Adrenal Gland, Right 4 Adrenal Glands, Bilateral 6 Carotid Body, Left 7 Carotid Body, Right 8 Carotid Bodies, Bilateral 9 Para-aortic Body B Coccygeal Glomus C Glomus Jugulare D Aortic Body F Paraganglion Extremity G Thyroid Gland Lobe, Left H Thyroid Gland Lobe, Right K Thyroid Gland L Superior Parathyroid Gland, Right M Superior Parathyroid Gland, Left N Inferior Parathyroid Gland, Right P Inferior Parathyroid Gland, Left Q Parathyroid Glands, Multiple R Parathyroid Gland	Ø Open 3 Percutaneous 4 Percutaneous Endoscopic	Z No Device	Z No Qualifier

SECTION: Ø MEDICAL AND SURGICAL
BODY SYSTEM: G ENDOCRINE SYSTEM
OPERATION: 8 DIVISION: Cutting into a body part, without draining fluids and/or gases from the body part, in order to separate or transect a body part

Body Part	Approach	Device	Qualifier
Ø Pituitary Gland J Thyroid Gland Isthmus	Ø Open 3 Percutaneous 4 Percutaneous Endoscopic	Z No Device	Z No Qualifier

SECTION: Ø MEDICAL AND SURGICAL
BODY SYSTEM: G ENDOCRINE SYSTEM
OPERATION: 9 DRAINAGE: Taking or letting out fluids and/or gases from a body part

Body Part	Approach	Device	Qualifier
Ø Pituitary Gland 1 Pineal Body 2 Adrenal Gland, Left 3 Adrenal Gland, Right 4 Adrenal Glands, Bilateral 6 Carotid Body, Left 7 Carotid Body, Right 8 Carotid Bodies, Bilateral 9 Para-aortic Body B Coccygeal Glomus C Glomus Jugulare D Aortic Body F Paraganglion Extremity G Thyroid Gland Lobe, Left H Thyroid Gland Lobe, Right K Thyroid Gland L Superior Parathyroid Gland, Right M Superior Parathyroid Gland, Left N Inferior Parathyroid Gland, Right P Inferior Parathyroid Gland, Left Q Parathyroid Glands, Multiple R Parathyroid Gland	Ø Open 3 Percutaneous 4 Percutaneous Endoscopic	Ø Drainage Device	Z No Qualifier
Ø Pituitary Gland 1 Pineal Body 2 Adrenal Gland, Left 3 Adrenal Gland, Right 4 Adrenal Glands, Bilateral 6 Carotid Body, Left 7 Carotid Body, Right 8 Carotid Bodies, Bilateral 9 Para-aortic Body B Coccygeal Glomus C Glomus Jugulare D Aortic Body F Paraganglion Extremity G Thyroid Gland Lobe, Left H Thyroid Gland Lobe, Right K Thyroid Gland L Superior Parathyroid Gland, Right M Superior Parathyroid Gland, Left N Inferior Parathyroid Gland, Right P Inferior Parathyroid Gland, Left Q Parathyroid Glands, Multiple R Parathyroid Gland	Ø Open 3 Percutaneous 4 Percutaneous Endoscopic	Z No Device	X Diagnostic Z No Qualifier

SECTION: Ø MEDICAL AND SURGICAL
BODY SYSTEM: G ENDOCRINE SYSTEM
OPERATION: B EXCISION: Cutting out or off, without replacement, a portion of a body part

Body Part	Approach	Device	Qualifier
Ø Pituitary Gland 1 Pineal Body 2 Adrenal Gland, Left 3 Adrenal Gland, Right 4 Adrenal Glands, Bilateral 6 Carotid Body, Left 7 Carotid Body, Right 8 Carotid Bodies, Bilateral 9 Para-aortic Body B Coccygeal Glomus C Glomus Jugulare D Aortic Body F Paraganglion Extremity G Thyroid Gland Lobe, Left H Thyroid Gland Lobe, Right J Thyroid Gland Isthmus L Superior Parathyroid Gland, Right M Superior Parathyroid Gland, Left N Inferior Parathyroid Gland, Right P Inferior Parathyroid Gland, Left Q Parathyroid Glands, Multiple R Parathyroid Gland	Ø Open 3 Percutaneous 4 Percutaneous Endoscopic	Z No Device	X Diagnostic Z No Qualifier

SECTION: Ø MEDICAL AND SURGICAL
BODY SYSTEM: G ENDOCRINE SYSTEM
OPERATION: C EXTIRPATION: Taking or cutting out solid matter from a body part

Body Part	Approach	Device	Qualifier
Ø Pituitary Gland 1 Pineal Body 2 Adrenal Gland, Left 3 Adrenal Gland, Right 4 Adrenal Glands, Bilateral 6 Carotid Body, Left 7 Carotid Body, Right 8 Carotid Bodies, Bilateral 9 Para-aortic Body B Coccygeal Glomus C Glomus Jugulare D Aortic Body F Paraganglion Extremity G Thyroid Gland Lobe, Left H Thyroid Gland Lobe, Right K Thyroid Gland L Superior Parathyroid Gland, Right M Superior Parathyroid Gland, Left N Inferior Parathyroid Gland, Right P Inferior Parathyroid Gland, Left Q Parathyroid Glands, Multiple R Parathyroid Gland	Ø Open 3 Percutaneous 4 Percutaneous Endoscopic	Z No Device	Z No Qualifier

B: EXCISION   C: EXTIRPATION
G: ENDOCRINE SYSTEM
Ø: M/S

SECTION: Ø MEDICAL AND SURGICAL
BODY SYSTEM: G ENDOCRINE SYSTEM
OPERATION: H INSERTION: Putting in a nonbiological appliance that monitors, assists, performs, or prevents a physiological function but does not physically take the place of a body part

Body Part	Approach	Device	Qualifier
S Endocrine Gland	Ø Open 3 Percutaneous 4 Percutaneous Endoscopic	2 Monitoring Device 3 Infusion Device Y Other Device	Z No Qualifier

SECTION: Ø MEDICAL AND SURGICAL
BODY SYSTEM: G ENDOCRINE SYSTEM
OPERATION: J INSPECTION: Visually and/or manually exploring a body part

Body Part	Approach	Device	Qualifier
Ø Pituitary Gland 1 Pineal Body 5 Adrenal Gland K Thyroid Gland R Parathyroid Gland S Endocrine Gland	Ø Open 3 Percutaneous 4 Percutaneous Endoscopic	Z No Device	Z No Qualifier

SECTION: Ø MEDICAL AND SURGICAL
BODY SYSTEM: G ENDOCRINE SYSTEM
OPERATION: M REATTACHMENT: Putting back in or on all or a portion of a separated body part to its normal location or other suitable location

Body Part	Approach	Device	Qualifier
2 Adrenal Gland, Left 3 Adrenal Gland, Right G Thyroid Gland Lobe, Left H Thyroid Gland Lobe, Right L Superior Parathyroid Gland, Right M Superior Parathyroid Gland, Left N Inferior Parathyroid Gland, Right P Inferior Parathyroid Gland, Left Q Parathyroid Glands, Multiple R Parathyroid Gland	Ø Open 4 Percutaneous Endoscopic	Z No Device	Z No Qualifier

N: RELEASE   P: REMOVAL

G: ENDOCRINE SYSTEM   Ø: M/S

SECTION: Ø MEDICAL AND SURGICAL
BODY SYSTEM: G ENDOCRINE SYSTEM
OPERATION: N RELEASE: Freeing a body part from an abnormal physical constraint by cutting or by the use of force

Body Part	Approach	Device	Qualifier
Ø Pituitary Gland 1 Pineal Body 2 Adrenal Gland, Left 3 Adrenal Gland, Right 4 Adrenal Glands, Bilateral 6 Carotid Body, Left 7 Carotid Body, Right 8 Carotid Bodies, Bilateral 9 Para-aortic Body B Coccygeal Glomus C Glomus Jugulare D Aortic Body F Paraganglion Extremity G Thyroid Gland Lobe, Left H Thyroid Gland Lobe, Right K Thyroid Gland L Superior Parathyroid Gland, Right M Superior Parathyroid Gland, Left N Inferior Parathyroid Gland, Right P Inferior Parathyroid Gland, Left Q Parathyroid Glands, Multiple R Parathyroid Gland	Ø Open 3 Percutaneous 4 Percutaneous Endoscopic	Z No Device	Z No Qualifier

SECTION: Ø MEDICAL AND SURGICAL
BODY SYSTEM: G ENDOCRINE SYSTEM
OPERATION: P REMOVAL: Taking out or off a device from a body part

Body Part	Approach	Device	Qualifier
Ø Pituitary Gland 1 Pineal Body 5 Adrenal Gland K Thyroid Gland R Parathyroid Gland	Ø Open 3 Percutaneous 4 Percutaneous Endoscopic X External	Ø Drainage Device	Z No Qualifier
S Endocrine Gland	Ø Open 3 Percutaneous 4 Percutaneous Endoscopic ~~X External~~	Ø Drainage Device 2 Monitoring Device 3 Infusion Device Y Other Device	Z No Qualifier
S Endocrine Gland	X External	Ø Drainage Device 2 Monitoring Device 3 Infusion Device	Z No Qualifier

SECTION: Ø MEDICAL AND SURGICAL

BODY SYSTEM: G ENDOCRINE SYSTEM

OPERATION: Q REPAIR: Restoring, to the extent possible, a body part to its normal anatomic structure and function

Body Part	Approach	Device	Qualifier
Ø Pituitary Gland 1 Pineal Body 2 Adrenal Gland, Left 3 Adrenal Gland, Right 4 Adrenal Glands, Bilateral 6 Carotid Body, Left 7 Carotid Body, Right 8 Carotid Bodies, Bilateral 9 Para-aortic Body B Coccygeal Glomus C Glomus Jugulare D Aortic Body F Paraganglion Extremity G Thyroid Gland Lobe, Left H Thyroid Gland Lobe, Right J Thyroid Gland Isthmus K Thyroid Gland L Superior Parathyroid Gland, Right M Superior Parathyroid Gland, Left N Inferior Parathyroid Gland, Right P Inferior Parathyroid Gland, Left Q Parathyroid Glands, Multiple R Parathyroid Gland	Ø Open 3 Percutaneous 4 Percutaneous Endoscopic	Z No Device	Z No Qualifier

SECTION: Ø MEDICAL AND SURGICAL

BODY SYSTEM: G ENDOCRINE SYSTEM

OPERATION: S REPOSITION: Moving to its normal location, or other suitable location, all or a portion of a body part

Body Part	Approach	Device	Qualifier
2 Adrenal Gland, Left 3 Adrenal Gland, Right G Thyroid Gland Lobe, Left H Thyroid Gland Lobe, Right L Superior Parathyroid Gland, Right M Superior Parathyroid Gland, Left N Inferior Parathyroid Gland, Right P Inferior Parathyroid Gland, Left Q Parathyroid Glands, Multiple R Parathyroid Gland	Ø Open 4 Percutaneous Endoscopic	Z No Device	Z No Qualifier

SECTION: Ø MEDICAL AND SURGICAL
BODY SYSTEM: G ENDOCRINE SYSTEM
OPERATION: T RESECTION: Cutting out or off, without replacement, all of a body part

Body Part	Approach	Device	Qualifier
Ø Pituitary Gland 1 Pineal Body 2 Adrenal Gland, Left 3 Adrenal Gland, Right 4 Adrenal Glands, Bilateral 6 Carotid Body, Left 7 Carotid Body, Right 8 Carotid Bodies, Bilateral 9 Para-aortic Body B Coccygeal Glomus C Glomus Jugulare D Aortic Body F Paraganglion Extremity G Thyroid Gland Lobe, Left H Thyroid Gland Lobe, Right J Thyroid Gland Isthmus K Thyroid Gland L Superior Parathyroid Gland, Right M Superior Parathyroid Gland, Left N Inferior Parathyroid Gland, Right P Inferior Parathyroid Gland, Left Q Parathyroid Glands, Multiple R Parathyroid Gland	Ø Open 4 Percutaneous Endoscopic	Z No Device	Z No Qualifier

SECTION: Ø MEDICAL AND SURGICAL
BODY SYSTEM: G ENDOCRINE SYSTEM
OPERATION: W REVISION: Correcting, to the extent possible, a portion of a malfunctioning device or the position of a displaced device

Body Part	Approach	Device	Qualifier
Ø Pituitary Gland 1 Pineal Body 5 Adrenal Gland K Thyroid Gland R Parathyroid Gland	Ø Open 3 Percutaneous 4 Percutaneous Endoscopic X External	Ø Drainage Device	Z No Qualifier
S Endocrine Gland	Ø Open 3 Percutaneous 4 Percutaneous Endoscopic X External	Ø Drainage Device 2 Monitoring Device 3 Infusion Device Y Other Device	Z No Qualifier
S Endocrine Gland	X External	Ø Drainage Device 2 Monitoring Device 3 Infusion Device	Z No Qualifier

ØH. Skin and Breast.. 255
    ØHØ. Alteration.. 256
    ØH2. Change... 256
    ØH5. Destruction.. 257
    ØH8. Division... 258
    ØH9. Drainage.. 259
    ØHB. Excision.. 260
    ØHC. Extirpation.. 261
    ØHD. Extraction... 262
    ØHH. Insertion... 263
    ØHJ. Inspection.. 263
    ØHM. Reattachment... 264
    ØHN. Release... 265
    ØHP. Removal.. 266
    ØHQ. Repair.. 267
    ØHR. Replacement... 268
    ØHS. Reposition... 269
    ØHT. Resection.. 270
    ØHU. Supplement.. 270
    ØHW. Revision... 271
    ØHX. Transfer... 272

SECTION: Ø MEDICAL AND SURGICAL
BODY SYSTEM: H SKIN AND BREAST
OPERATION: Ø **ALTERATION:** Modifying the anatomic structure of a body part without affecting the function of the body part

Body Part	Approach	Device	Qualifier
T Breast, Right U Breast, Left V Breast, Bilateral	Ø Open 3 Percutaneous X External	7 Autologous Tissue Substitute J Synthetic Substitute K Nonautologous Tissue Substitute Z No Device	Z No Qualifier

SECTION: Ø MEDICAL AND SURGICAL
BODY SYSTEM: H SKIN AND BREAST
OPERATION: 2 **CHANGE:** Taking out or off a device from a body part and putting back an identical or similar device in or on the same body part without cutting or puncturing the skin or a mucous membrane

Body Part	Approach	Device	Qualifier
P Skin T Breast, Right U Breast, Left	X External	Ø Drainage Device Y Other Device	Z No Qualifier

SECTION: Ø MEDICAL AND SURGICAL
BODY SYSTEM: H SKIN AND BREAST
OPERATION: 5 DESTRUCTION: Physical eradication of all or a portion of a body part by the direct use of energy, force, or a destructive agent

Body Part	Approach	Device	Qualifier
Ø Skin, Scalp 1 Skin, Face 2 Skin, Right Ear 3 Skin, Left Ear 4 Skin, Neck 5 Skin, Chest 6 Skin, Back 7 Skin, Abdomen 8 Skin, Buttock 9 Skin, Perineum A Skin, Inguinal B Skin, Right Upper Arm C Skin, Left Upper Arm D Skin, Right Lower Arm E Skin, Left Lower Arm F Skin, Right Hand G Skin, Left Hand H Skin, Right Upper Leg J Skin, Left Upper Leg K Skin, Right Lower Leg L Skin, Left Lower Leg M Skin, Right Foot N Skin, Left Foot	X External	Z No Device	D Multiple Z No Qualifier
Q Finger Nail R Toe Nail	X External	Z No Device	Z No Qualifier
T Breast, Right U Breast, Left V Breast, Bilateral W Nipple, Right X Nipple, Left	Ø Open 3 Percutaneous 7 Via Natural or Artificial Opening 8 Via Natural or Artificial Opening Endoscopic X External	Z No Device	Z No Qualifier

SECTION: Ø MEDICAL AND SURGICAL
BODY SYSTEM: H SKIN AND BREAST
OPERATION: 8 DIVISION: Cutting into a body part, without draining fluids and/or gases from the body part, in order to separate or transect a body part

Body Part	Approach	Device	Qualifier
Ø Skin, Scalp	X External	Z No Device	Z No Qualifier
1 Skin, Face			
2 Skin, Right Ear			
3 Skin, Left Ear			
4 Skin, Neck			
5 Skin, Chest			
6 Skin, Back			
7 Skin, Abdomen			
8 Skin, Buttock			
9 Skin, Perineum			
A Skin, Inguinal			
B Skin, Right Upper Arm			
C Skin, Left Upper Arm			
D Skin, Right Lower Arm			
E Skin, Left Lower Arm			
F Skin, Right Hand			
G Skin, Left Hand			
H Skin, Right Upper Leg			
J Skin, Left Upper Leg			
K Skin, Right Lower Leg			
L Skin, Left Lower Leg			
M Skin, Right Foot			
N Skin, Left Foot			

8: DIVISION

H: SKIN AND BREAST

Ø: M/S

New/Revised Text in Blue   ~~deleted~~ Deleted

SECTION: Ø MEDICAL AND SURGICAL
BODY SYSTEM: H SKIN AND BREAST
OPERATION: 9 DRAINAGE: *(on multiple pages)*
Taking or letting out fluids and/or gases from a body part

Body Part	Approach	Device	Qualifier
Ø Skin, Scalp	X External	Ø Drainage Device	Z No Qualifier
1 Skin, Face			
2 Skin, Right Ear			
3 Skin, Left Ear			
4 Skin, Neck			
5 Skin, Chest			
6 Skin, Back			
7 Skin, Abdomen			
8 Skin, Buttock			
9 Skin, Perineum			
A Skin, Inguinal			
B Skin, Right Upper Arm			
C Skin, Left Upper Arm			
D Skin, Right Lower Arm			
E Skin, Left Lower Arm			
F Skin, Right Hand			
G Skin, Left Hand			
H Skin, Right Upper Leg			
J Skin, Left Upper Leg			
K Skin, Right Lower Leg			
L Skin, Left Lower Leg			
M Skin, Right Foot			
N Skin, Left Foot			
Q Finger Nail			
R Toe Nail			
Ø Skin, Scalp	X External	Z No Device	X Diagnostic
1 Skin, Face			Z No Qualifier
2 Skin, Right Ear			
3 Skin, Left Ear			
4 Skin, Neck			
5 Skin, Chest			
6 Skin, Back			
7 Skin, Abdomen			
8 Skin, Buttock			
9 Skin, Perineum			
A Skin, Inguinal			
B Skin, Right Upper Arm			
C Skin, Left Upper Arm			
D Skin, Right Lower Arm			
E Skin, Left Lower Arm			
F Skin, Right Hand			
G Skin, Left Hand			
H Skin, Right Upper Leg			
J Skin, Left Upper Leg			
K Skin, Right Lower Leg			
L Skin, Left Lower Leg			
M Skin, Right Foot			
N Skin, Left Foot			
Q Finger Nail			
R Toe Nail			

SECTION: Ø MEDICAL AND SURGICAL
BODY SYSTEM: H SKIN AND BREAST
OPERATION: 9 DRAINAGE: *(continued)*
Taking or letting out fluids and/or gases from a body part

Body Part	Approach	Device	Qualifier
T Breast, Right U Breast, Left V Breast, Bilateral W Nipple, Right X Nipple, Left	Ø Open 3 Percutaneous 7 Via Natural or Artificial Opening 8 Via Natural or Artificial Opening Endoscopic X External	Ø Drainage Device	Z No Qualifier
T Breast, Right U Breast, Left V Breast, Bilateral W Nipple, Right X Nipple, Left	Ø Open 3 Percutaneous 7 Via Natural or Artificial Opening 8 Via Natural or Artificial Opening Endoscopic X External	Z No Device	X Diagnostic Z No Qualifier

SECTION: Ø MEDICAL AND SURGICAL
BODY SYSTEM: H SKIN AND BREAST
OPERATION: B EXCISION: *(on multiple pages)*
Cutting out or off, without replacement, a portion of a body part

Body Part	Approach	Device	Qualifier
Ø Skin, Scalp 1 Skin, Face 2 Skin, Right Ear 3 Skin, Left Ear 4 Skin, Neck 5 Skin, Chest 6 Skin, Back 7 Skin, Abdomen 8 Skin, Buttock 9 Skin, Perineum A Skin, Inguinal B Skin, Right Upper Arm C Skin, Left Upper Arm D Skin, Right Lower Arm E Skin, Left Lower Arm F Skin, Right Hand G Skin, Left Hand H Skin, Right Upper Leg J Skin, Left Upper Leg K Skin, Right Lower Leg L Skin, Left Lower Leg M Skin, Right Foot N Skin, Left Foot Q Finger Nail R Toe Nail	X External	Z No Device	X Diagnostic Z No Qualifier

SECTION: Ø MEDICAL AND SURGICAL

BODY SYSTEM: H SKIN AND BREAST

OPERATION: B EXCISION: *(continued)*

Cutting out or off, without replacement, a portion of a body part

Body Part	Approach	Device	Qualifier
T Breast, Right U Breast, Left V Breast, Bilateral W Nipple, Right X Nipple, Left Y Supernumerary Breast	Ø Open 3 Percutaneous 7 Via Natural or Artificial Opening 8 Via Natural or Artificial Opening Endoscopic X External	Z No Device	X Diagnostic Z No Qualifier

SECTION: Ø MEDICAL AND SURGICAL

BODY SYSTEM: H SKIN AND BREAST

OPERATION: C EXTIRPATION: Taking or cutting out solid matter from a body part

Body Part	Approach	Device	Qualifier
Ø Skin, Scalp 1 Skin, Face 2 Skin, Right Ear 3 Skin, Left Ear 4 Skin, Neck 5 Skin, Chest 6 Skin, Back 7 Skin, Abdomen 8 Skin, Buttock 9 Skin, Perineum A Skin, Inguinal B Skin, Right Upper Arm C Skin, Left Upper Arm D Skin, Right Lower Arm E Skin, Left Lower Arm F Skin, Right Hand G Skin, Left Hand H Skin, Right Upper Leg J Skin, Left Upper Leg K Skin, Right Lower Leg L Skin, Left Lower Leg M Skin, Right Foot N Skin, Left Foot Q Finger Nail R Toe Nail	X External	Z No Device	Z No Qualifier
T Breast, Right U Breast, Left V Breast, Bilateral W Nipple, Right X Nipple, Left	Ø Open 3 Percutaneous 7 Via Natural or Artificial Opening 8 Via Natural or Artificial Opening Endoscopic X External	Z No Device	Z No Qualifier

SECTION: Ø MEDICAL AND SURGICAL
BODY SYSTEM: H SKIN AND BREAST
OPERATION: D EXTRACTION: Pulling or stripping out or off all or a portion of a body part by the use of force

Body Part	Approach	Device	Qualifier
Ø Skin, Scalp	X External	Z No Device	Z No Qualifier
1 Skin, Face			
2 Skin, Right Ear			
3 Skin, Left Ear			
4 Skin, Neck			
5 Skin, Chest			
6 Skin, Back			
7 Skin, Abdomen			
8 Skin, Buttock			
9 Skin, Perineum			
A Skin, Inguinal			
B Skin, Right Upper Arm			
C Skin, Left Upper Arm			
D Skin, Right Lower Arm			
E Skin, Left Lower Arm			
F Skin, Right Hand			
G Skin, Left Hand			
H Skin, Right Upper Leg			
J Skin, Left Upper Leg			
K Skin, Right Lower Leg			
L Skin, Left Lower Leg			
M Skin, Right Foot			
N Skin, Left Foot			
Q Finger Nail			
R Toe Nail			
S Hair			

D: EXTRACTION

H: SKIN AND BREAST

Ø: M/S

     New/Revised Text in Blue ~~deleted~~ Deleted

SECTION: Ø MEDICAL AND SURGICAL
BODY SYSTEM: H SKIN AND BREAST
OPERATION: H INSERTION: Putting in a nonbiological appliance that monitors, assists, performs, or prevents a physiological function but does not physically take the place of a body part

Body Part	Approach	Device	Qualifier
P Skin	X External	Y Other Device	Z No Qualifier
T Breast, Right U Breast, Left ~~V Breast, Bilateral~~ ~~W Nipple, Right~~ ~~X Nipple, Left~~	Ø Open 3 Percutaneous 7 Via Natural or Artificial Opening 8 Via Natural or Artificial Opening Endoscopic	1 Radioactive Element N Tissue Expander Y Other Device	Z No Qualifier
T Breast, Right U Breast, Left	X External	1 Radioactive Element	Z No Qualifier
V Breast, Bilateral W Nipple, Right X Nipple, Left	Ø Open 3 Percutaneous 7 Via Natural or Artificial Opening 8 Via Natural or Artificial Opening Endoscopic	1 Radioactive Element N Tissue Expander	Z No Qualifier
~~T Breast, Right~~ ~~U Breast, Left~~ V Breast, Bilateral W Nipple, Right X Nipple, Left	X External	1 Radioactive Element	Z No Qualifier

SECTION: Ø MEDICAL AND SURGICAL
BODY SYSTEM: H SKIN AND BREAST
OPERATION: J INSPECTION: Visually and/or manually exploring a body part

Body Part	Approach	Device	Qualifier
P Skin Q Finger Nail R Toe Nail	X External	Z No Device	Z No Qualifier
T Breast, Right U Breast, Left	Ø Open 3 Percutaneous 7 Via Natural or Artificial Opening 8 Via Natural or Artificial Opening Endoscopic X External	Z No Device	Z No Qualifier

SECTION: Ø MEDICAL AND SURGICAL
BODY SYSTEM: H SKIN AND BREAST
OPERATION: M REATTACHMENT: Putting back in or on all or a portion of a separated body part to its normal location or other suitable location

Body Part	Approach	Device	Qualifier
Ø Skin, Scalp	X External	Z No Device	Z No Qualifier
1 Skin, Face			
2 Skin, Right Ear			
3 Skin, Left Ear			
4 Skin, Neck			
5 Skin, Chest			
6 Skin, Back			
7 Skin, Abdomen			
8 Skin, Buttock			
9 Skin, Perineum			
A Skin, Inguinal			
B Skin, Right Upper Arm			
C Skin, Left Upper Arm			
D Skin, Right Lower Arm			
E Skin, Left Lower Arm			
F Skin, Right Hand			
G Skin, Left Hand			
H Skin, Right Upper Leg			
J Skin, Left Upper Leg			
K Skin, Right Lower Leg			
L Skin, Left Lower Leg			
M Skin, Right Foot			
N Skin, Left Foot			
T Breast, Right			
U Breast, Left			
V Breast, Bilateral			
W Nipple, Right			
X Nipple, Left			

SECTION: Ø MEDICAL AND SURGICAL
BODY SYSTEM: H SKIN AND BREAST
OPERATION: N RELEASE: Freeing a body part from an abnormal physical constraint by cutting or by the use of force

Body Part	Approach	Device	Qualifier
Ø Skin, Scalp 1 Skin, Face 2 Skin, Right Ear 3 Skin, Left Ear 4 Skin, Neck 5 Skin, Chest 6 Skin, Back 7 Skin, Abdomen 8 Skin, Buttock 9 Skin, Perineum A Skin, Inguinal B Skin, Right Upper Arm C Skin, Left Upper Arm D Skin, Right Lower Arm E Skin, Left Lower Arm F Skin, Right Hand G Skin, Left Hand H Skin, Right Upper Leg J Skin, Left Upper Leg K Skin, Right Lower Leg L Skin, Left Lower Leg M Skin, Right Foot N Skin, Left Foot Q Finger Nail R Toe Nail	X External	Z No Device	Z No Qualifier
T Breast, Right U Breast, Left V Breast, Bilateral W Nipple, Right X Nipple, Left	Ø Open 3 Percutaneous 7 Via Natural or Artificial Opening 8 Via Natural or Artificial Opening Endoscopic X External	Z No Device	Z No Qualifier

SECTION: Ø MEDICAL AND SURGICAL
BODY SYSTEM: H SKIN AND BREAST
OPERATION: P REMOVAL: Taking out or off a device from a body part

Body Part	Approach	Device	Qualifier
P Skin	X External	Ø Drainage Device 7 Autologous Tissue Substitute J Synthetic Substitute K Nonautologous Tissue Substitute Y Other Device	Z No Qualifier
P Skin Q Finger Nail R Toe Nail	X External	Ø Drainage Device 7 Autologous Tissue Substitute J Synthetic Substitute K Nonautologous Tissue Substitute	Z No Qualifier
S Hair	X External	7 Autologous Tissue Substitute J Synthetic Substitute K Nonautologous Tissue Substitute	Z No Qualifier
T Breast, Right U Breast, Left	Ø Open 3 Percutaneous 7 Via Natural or Artificial Opening 8 Via Natural or Artificial Opening Endoscopic	Ø Drainage Device 1 Radioactive Element 7 Autologous Tissue Substitute J Synthetic Substitute K Nonautologous Tissue Substitute N Tissue Expander Y Other Device	Z No Qualifier
T Breast, Right U Breast, Left	X External	Ø Drainage Device 1 Radioactive Element 7 Autologous Tissue Substitute J Synthetic Substitute K Nonautologous Tissue Substitute	Z No Qualifier

P: REMOVAL

H: SKIN AND BREAST

Ø: M/S

New/Revised Text in Blue   ~~deleted~~ Deleted

SECTION: Ø MEDICAL AND SURGICAL
BODY SYSTEM: H SKIN AND BREAST
OPERATION: Q REPAIR: Restoring, to the extent possible, a body part to its normal anatomic structure and function

Body Part	Approach	Device	Qualifier
Ø Skin, Scalp 1 Skin, Face 2 Skin, Right Ear 3 Skin, Left Ear 4 Skin, Neck 5 Skin, Chest 6 Skin, Back 7 Skin, Abdomen 8 Skin, Buttock 9 Skin, Perineum A Skin, Inguinal B Skin, Right Upper Arm C Skin, Left Upper Arm D Skin, Right Lower Arm E Skin, Left Lower Arm F Skin, Right Hand G Skin, Left Hand H Skin, Right Upper Leg J Skin, Left Upper Leg K Skin, Right Lower Leg L Skin, Left Lower Leg M Skin, Right Foot N Skin, Left Foot Q Finger Nail R Toe Nail	X External	Z No Device	Z No Qualifier
T Breast, Right U Breast, Left V Breast, Bilateral W Nipple, Right X Nipple, Left Y Supernumerary Breast	Ø Open 3 Percutaneous 7 Via Natural or Artificial Opening 8 Via Natural or Artificial Opening Endoscopic X External	Z No Device	Z No Qualifier

SECTION: Ø MEDICAL AND SURGICAL
BODY SYSTEM: H SKIN AND BREAST
OPERATION: R REPLACEMENT: *(on multiple pages)*

Putting in or on biological or synthetic material that physically takes the place and/or function of all or a portion of a body part

Body Part	Approach	Device	Qualifier
Ø Skin, Scalp 1 Skin, Face 2 Skin, Right Ear 3 Skin, Left Ear 4 Skin, Neck 5 Skin, Chest 6 Skin, Back 7 Skin, Abdomen 8 Skin, Buttock 9 Skin, Perineum A Skin, Inguinal B Skin, Right Upper Arm C Skin, Left Upper Arm D Skin, Right Lower Arm E Skin, Left Lower Arm F Skin, Right Hand G Skin, Left Hand H Skin, Right Upper Leg J Skin, Left Upper Leg K Skin, Right Lower Leg L Skin, Left Lower Leg M Skin, Right Foot N Skin, Left Foot	X External	7 Autologous Tissue Substitute K Nonautologous Tissue Substitute	3 Full Thickness 4 Partial Thickness
Ø Skin, Scalp 1 Skin, Face 2 Skin, Right Ear 3 Skin, Left Ear 4 Skin, Neck 5 Skin, Chest 6 Skin, Back 7 Skin, Abdomen 8 Skin, Buttock 9 Skin, Perineum A Skin, Inguinal B Skin, Right Upper Arm C Skin, Left Upper Arm D Skin, Right Lower Arm E Skin, Left Lower Arm F Skin, Right Hand G Skin, Left Hand H Skin, Right Upper Leg J Skin, Left Upper Leg K Skin, Right Lower Leg L Skin, Left Lower Leg M Skin, Right Foot N Skin, Left Foot	X External	J Synthetic Substitute	3 Full Thickness 4 Partial Thickness Z No Qualifier
Q Finger Nail R Toe Nail S Hair	X External	7 Autologous Tissue Substitute J Synthetic Substitute K Nonautologous Tissue Substitute	Z No Qualifier

New/Revised Text in Blue   ~~deleted~~ Deleted

SECTION: Ø MEDICAL AND SURGICAL
BODY SYSTEM: H SKIN AND BREAST
OPERATION: R REPLACEMENT: *(continued)*
Putting in or on biological or synthetic material that physically takes the place and/or function of all or a portion of a body part

Body Part	Approach	Device	Qualifier
T Breast, Right U Breast, Left V Breast, Bilateral	Ø Open	7 Autologous Tissue Substitute	5 Latissimus Dorsi Myocutaneous Flap 6 Transverse Rectus Abdominis Myocutaneous Flap 7 Deep Inferior Epigastric Artery Perforator Flap 8 Superficial Inferior Epigastric Artery Flap 9 Gluteal Artery Perforator Flap Z No Qualifier
T Breast, Right U Breast, Left V Breast, Bilateral	Ø Open	J Synthetic Substitute K Nonautologous Tissue Substitute	Z No Qualifier
T Breast, Right U Breast, Left V Breast, Bilateral	3 Percutaneous X External	7 Autologous Tissue Substitute J Synthetic Substitute K Nonautologous Tissue Substitute	Z No Qualifier
W Nipple, Right X Nipple, Left	Ø Open 3 Percutaneous X External	7 Autologous Tissue Substitute J Synthetic Substitute K Nonautologous Tissue Substitute	Z No Qualifier

SECTION: Ø MEDICAL AND SURGICAL
BODY SYSTEM: H SKIN AND BREAST
OPERATION: S REPOSITION: Moving to its normal location, or other suitable location, all or a portion of a body part

Body Part	Approach	Device	Qualifier
S Hair W Nipple, Right X Nipple, Left	X External	Z No Device	Z No Qualifier
T Breast, Right U Breast, Left V Breast, Bilateral	Ø Open	Z No Device	Z No Qualifier

SECTION: Ø MEDICAL AND SURGICAL
BODY SYSTEM: H SKIN AND BREAST
OPERATION: T RESECTION: Cutting out or off, without replacement, all of a body part

Body Part	Approach	Device	Qualifier
Q Finger Nail R Toe Nail W Nipple, Right X Nipple, Left	X External	Z No Device	Z No Qualifier
T Breast, Right U Breast, Left V Breast, Bilateral Y Supernumerary Breast	Ø Open	Z No Device	Z No Qualifier

SECTION: Ø MEDICAL AND SURGICAL
BODY SYSTEM: H SKIN AND BREAST
OPERATION: U SUPPLEMENT: Putting in or on biological or synthetic material that physically reinforces and/or augments the function of a portion of a body part

Body Part	Approach	Device	Qualifier
T Breast, Right U Breast, Left V Breast, Bilateral W Nipple, Right X Nipple, Left	Ø Open 3 Percutaneous 7 Via Natural of Artificial Opening 8 Via Natural or Artificial Opening Endoscopic X External	7 Autologous Tissue Substitute J Synthetic Substitute K Nonautologous Tissue Substitute	Z No Qualifier

SECTION: Ø MEDICAL AND SURGICAL
BODY SYSTEM: H SKIN AND BREAST
OPERATION: **W REVISION:** Correcting, to the extent possible, a portion of a malfunctioning device or the position of a displaced device

Body Part	Approach	Device	Qualifier
P Skin	X External	Ø Drainage Device 7 Autologous Tissue Substitute J Synthetic Substitute K Nonautologous Tissue Substitute Y Other Device	Z No Qualifier
~~P Skin~~ Q Finger Nail R Toe Nail	X External	Ø Drainage Device 7 Autologous Tissue Substitute J Synthetic Substitute K Nonautologous Tissue Substitute	Z No Qualifier
S Hair	X External	7 Autologous Tissue Substitute J Synthetic Substitute K Nonautologous Tissue Substitute	Z No Qualifier
T Breast, Right U Breast, Left	Ø Open 3 Percutaneous 7 Via Natural or Artificial Opening 8 Via Natural or Artificial Opening Endoscopic	Ø Drainage Device 7 Autologous Tissue Substitute J Synthetic Substitute K Nonautologous Tissue Substitute N Tissue Expander Y Other Device	Z No Qualifier
T Breast, Right U Breast, Left	X External	Ø Drainage Device 7 Autologous Tissue Substitute J Synthetic Substitute K Nonautologous Tissue Substitute	Z No Qualifier

SECTION: Ø MEDICAL AND SURGICAL
BODY SYSTEM: H SKIN AND BREAST
OPERATION: X **TRANSFER:** Moving, without taking out, all or a portion of a body part to another location to take over the function of all or a portion of a body part

Body Part	Approach	Device	Qualifier
Ø Skin, Scalp	X External	Z No Device	Z No Qualifier
1 Skin, Face			
2 Skin, Right Ear			
3 Skin, Left Ear			
4 Skin, Neck			
5 Skin, Chest			
6 Skin, Back			
7 Skin, Abdomen			
8 Skin, Buttock			
9 Skin, Perineum			
A Skin, Inguinal			
B Skin, Right Upper Arm			
C Skin, Left Upper Arm			
D Skin, Right Lower Arm			
E Skin, Left Lower Arm			
F Skin, Right Hand			
G Skin, Left Hand			
H Skin, Right Upper Leg			
J Skin, Left Upper Leg			
K Skin, Right Lower Leg			
L Skin, Left Lower Leg			
M Skin, Right Foot			
N Skin, Left Foot			

X: TRANSFER

H: SKIN AND BREAST

Ø: M/S

New/Revised Text in Blue   ~~deleted~~ Deleted

ØJ. Subcutaneous Tissue and Fascia 273
 ØJØ. Alteration 274
 ØJ2. Change 274
 ØJ5. Destruction 275
 ØJ8. Division 276
 ØJ9. Drainage 277
 ØJB. Excision 279
 ØJC. Extirpation 280
 ØJD. Extraction 281
 ØJH. Insertion 282
 ØJJ. Inspection 284
 ØJN. Release 284
 ØJP. Removal 285
 ØJQ. Repair 286
 ØJR. Replacement 287
 ØJU. Supplement 288
 ØJW. Revision 289
 ØJX. Transfer 291

SECTION: Ø MEDICAL AND SURGICAL

BODY SYSTEM: J SUBCUTANEOUS TISSUE AND FASCIA

OPERATION: Ø **ALTERATION:** Modifying the anatomic structure of a body part without affecting the function of the body part

Body Part	Approach	Device	Qualifier
1 Subcutaneous Tissue and Fascia, Face 4 Subcutaneous Tissue and Fascia, Right Neck 5 Subcutaneous Tissue and Fascia, Left Neck 6 Subcutaneous Tissue and Fascia, Chest 7 Subcutaneous Tissue and Fascia, Back 8 Subcutaneous Tissue and Fascia, Abdomen 9 Subcutaneous Tissue and Fascia, Buttock D Subcutaneous Tissue and Fascia, Right Upper Arm F Subcutaneous Tissue and Fascia, Left Upper Arm G Subcutaneous Tissue and Fascia, Right Lower Arm H Subcutaneous Tissue and Fascia, Left Lower Arm L Subcutaneous Tissue and Fascia, Right Upper Leg M Subcutaneous Tissue and Fascia, Left Upper Leg N Subcutaneous Tissue and Fascia, Right Lower Leg P Subcutaneous Tissue and Fascia, Left Lower Leg	Ø Open 3 Percutaneous	Z No Device	Z No Qualifier

SECTION: Ø MEDICAL AND SURGICAL

BODY SYSTEM: J SUBCUTANEOUS TISSUE AND FASCIA

OPERATION: 2 **CHANGE:** Taking out or off a device from a body part and putting back an identical or similar device in or on the same body part without cutting or puncturing the skin or a mucous membrane

Body Part	Approach	Device	Qualifier
S Subcutaneous Tissue and Fascia, Head and Neck T Subcutaneous Tissue and Fascia, Trunk V Subcutaneous Tissue and Fascia, Upper Extremity W Subcutaneous Tissue and Fascia, Lower Extremity	X External	Ø Drainage Device Y Other Device	Z No Qualifier

SECTION: Ø MEDICAL AND SURGICAL
BODY SYSTEM: J SUBCUTANEOUS TISSUE AND FASCIA
OPERATION: 5 DESTRUCTION: Physical eradication of all or a portion of a body part by the direct use of energy, force, or a destructive agent

Body Part	Approach	Device	Qualifier
Ø Subcutaneous Tissue and Fascia, Scalp 1 Subcutaneous Tissue and Fascia, Face 4 Subcutaneous Tissue and Fascia, Right Neck 5 Subcutaneous Tissue and Fascia, Left Neck 6 Subcutaneous Tissue and Fascia, Chest 7 Subcutaneous Tissue and Fascia, Back 8 Subcutaneous Tissue and Fascia, Abdomen 9 Subcutaneous Tissue and Fascia, Buttock B Subcutaneous Tissue and Fascia, Perineum C Subcutaneous Tissue and Fascia, Pelvic Region D Subcutaneous Tissue and Fascia, Right Upper Arm F Subcutaneous Tissue and Fascia, Left Upper Arm G Subcutaneous Tissue and Fascia, Right Lower Arm H Subcutaneous Tissue and Fascia, Left Lower Arm J Subcutaneous Tissue and Fascia, Right Hand K Subcutaneous Tissue and Fascia, Left Hand L Subcutaneous Tissue and Fascia, Right Upper Leg M Subcutaneous Tissue and Fascia, Left Upper Leg N Subcutaneous Tissue and Fascia, Right Lower Leg P Subcutaneous Tissue and Fascia, Left Lower Leg Q Subcutaneous Tissue and Fascia, Right Foot R Subcutaneous Tissue and Fascia, Left Foot	Ø Open 3 Percutaneous	Z No Device	Z No Qualifier

SECTION: Ø MEDICAL AND SURGICAL
BODY SYSTEM: J SUBCUTANEOUS TISSUE AND FASCIA
OPERATION: 8 **DIVISION:** Cutting into a body part, without draining fluids and/or gases from the body part, in order to separate or transect a body part

Body Part	Approach	Device	Qualifier
Ø Subcutaneous Tissue and Fascia, Scalp	Ø Open	Z No Device	Z No Qualifier
1 Subcutaneous Tissue and Fascia, Face	3 Percutaneous		
4 Subcutaneous Tissue and Fascia, Right Neck			
5 Subcutaneous Tissue and Fascia, Left Neck			
6 Subcutaneous Tissue and Fascia, Chest			
7 Subcutaneous Tissue and Fascia, Back			
8 Subcutaneous Tissue and Fascia, Abdomen			
9 Subcutaneous Tissue and Fascia, Buttock			
B Subcutaneous Tissue and Fascia, Perineum			
C Subcutaneous Tissue and Fascia, Pelvic Region			
D Subcutaneous Tissue and Fascia, Right Upper Arm			
F Subcutaneous Tissue and Fascia, Left Upper Arm			
G Subcutaneous Tissue and Fascia, Right Lower Arm			
H Subcutaneous Tissue and Fascia, Left Lower Arm			
J Subcutaneous Tissue and Fascia, Right Hand			
K Subcutaneous Tissue and Fascia, Left Hand			
L Subcutaneous Tissue and Fascia, Right Upper Leg			
M Subcutaneous Tissue and Fascia, Left Upper Leg			
N Subcutaneous Tissue and Fascia, Right Lower Leg			
P Subcutaneous Tissue and Fascia, Left Lower Leg			
Q Subcutaneous Tissue and Fascia, Right Foot			
R Subcutaneous Tissue and Fascia, Left Foot			
S Subcutaneous Tissue and Fascia, Head and Neck			
T Subcutaneous Tissue and Fascia, Trunk			
V Subcutaneous Tissue and Fascia, Upper Extremity			
W Subcutaneous Tissue and Fascia, Lower Extremity			

SECTION: Ø MEDICAL AND SURGICAL

BODY SYSTEM: J SUBCUTANEOUS TISSUE AND FASCIA
OPERATION: 9 DRAINAGE: *(on multiple pages)*
Taking or letting out fluids and/or gases from a body part

Body Part	Approach	Device	Qualifier
Ø Subcutaneous Tissue and Fascia, Scalp	Ø Open	Ø Drainage Device	Z No Qualifier
1 Subcutaneous Tissue and Fascia, Face	3 Percutaneous		
4 Subcutaneous Tissue and Fascia, Right Neck			
5 Subcutaneous Tissue and Fascia, Left Neck			
6 Subcutaneous Tissue and Fascia, Chest			
7 Subcutaneous Tissue and Fascia, Back			
8 Subcutaneous Tissue and Fascia, Abdomen			
9 Subcutaneous Tissue and Fascia, Buttock			
B Subcutaneous Tissue and Fascia, Perineum			
C Subcutaneous Tissue and Fascia, Pelvic Region			
D Subcutaneous Tissue and Fascia, Right Upper Arm			
F Subcutaneous Tissue and Fascia, Left Upper Arm			
G Subcutaneous Tissue and Fascia, Right Lower Arm			
H Subcutaneous Tissue and Fascia, Left Lower Arm			
J Subcutaneous Tissue and Fascia, Right Hand			
K Subcutaneous Tissue and Fascia, Left Hand			
L Subcutaneous Tissue and Fascia, Right Upper Leg			
M Subcutaneous Tissue and Fascia, Left Upper Leg			
N Subcutaneous Tissue and Fascia, Right Lower Leg			
P Subcutaneous Tissue and Fascia, Left Lower Leg			
Q Subcutaneous Tissue and Fascia, Right Foot			
R Subcutaneous Tissue and Fascia, Left Foot			

Ø: M/S

J: SUBCUTANEOUS TISSUE AND FASCIA

9: DRAINAGE

SECTION: Ø MEDICAL AND SURGICAL
BODY SYSTEM: J SUBCUTANEOUS TISSUE AND FASCIA
OPERATION: 9 DRAINAGE: *(continued)*
Taking or letting out fluids and/or gases from a body part

Body Part	Approach	Device	Qualifier
Ø Subcutaneous Tissue and Fascia, Scalp	Ø Open	Z No Device	X Diagnostic
1 Subcutaneous Tissue and Fascia, Face	3 Percutaneous		Z No Qualifier
4 Subcutaneous Tissue and Fascia, Right Neck			
5 Subcutaneous Tissue and Fascia, Left Neck			
6 Subcutaneous Tissue and Fascia, Chest			
7 Subcutaneous Tissue and Fascia, Back			
8 Subcutaneous Tissue and Fascia, Abdomen			
9 Subcutaneous Tissue and Fascia, Buttock			
B Subcutaneous Tissue and Fascia, Perineum			
C Subcutaneous Tissue and Fascia, Pelvic Region			
D Subcutaneous Tissue and Fascia, Right Upper Arm			
F Subcutaneous Tissue and Fascia, Left Upper Arm			
G Subcutaneous Tissue and Fascia, Right Lower Arm			
H Subcutaneous Tissue and Fascia, Left Lower Arm			
J Subcutaneous Tissue and Fascia, Right Hand			
K Subcutaneous Tissue and Fascia, Left Hand			
L Subcutaneous Tissue and Fascia, Right Upper Leg			
M Subcutaneous Tissue and Fascia, Left Upper Leg			
N Subcutaneous Tissue and Fascia, Right Lower Leg			
P Subcutaneous Tissue and Fascia, Left Lower Leg			
Q Subcutaneous Tissue and Fascia, Right Foot			
R Subcutaneous Tissue and Fascia, Left Foot			

SECTION: Ø MEDICAL AND SURGICAL
BODY SYSTEM: J SUBCUTANEOUS TISSUE AND FASCIA
OPERATION: B EXCISION: Cutting out or off, without replacement, a portion of a body part

Body Part	Approach	Device	Qualifier
Ø Subcutaneous Tissue and Fascia, Scalp	Ø Open	Z No Device	X Diagnostic
1 Subcutaneous Tissue and Fascia, Face	3 Percutaneous		Z No Qualifier
4 Subcutaneous Tissue and Fascia, Right Neck			
5 Subcutaneous Tissue and Fascia, Left Neck			
6 Subcutaneous Tissue and Fascia, Chest			
7 Subcutaneous Tissue and Fascia, Back			
8 Subcutaneous Tissue and Fascia, Abdomen			
9 Subcutaneous Tissue and Fascia, Buttock			
B Subcutaneous Tissue and Fascia, Perineum			
C Subcutaneous Tissue and Fascia, Pelvic Region			
D Subcutaneous Tissue and Fascia, Right Upper Arm			
F Subcutaneous Tissue and Fascia, Left Upper Arm			
G Subcutaneous Tissue and Fascia, Right Lower Arm			
H Subcutaneous Tissue and Fascia, Left Lower Arm			
J Subcutaneous Tissue and Fascia, Right Hand			
K Subcutaneous Tissue and Fascia, Left Hand			
L Subcutaneous Tissue and Fascia, Right Upper Leg			
M Subcutaneous Tissue and Fascia, Left Upper Leg			
N Subcutaneous Tissue and Fascia, Right Lower Leg			
P Subcutaneous Tissue and Fascia, Left Lower Leg			
Q Subcutaneous Tissue and Fascia, Right Foot			
R Subcutaneous Tissue and Fascia, Left Foot			

SECTION: Ø MEDICAL AND SURGICAL
BODY SYSTEM: J SUBCUTANEOUS TISSUE AND FASCIA
OPERATION: C EXTIRPATION: Taking or cutting out solid matter from a body part

Body Part	Approach	Device	Qualifier
Ø Subcutaneous Tissue and Fascia, Scalp	Ø Open	Z No Device	Z No Qualifier
1 Subcutaneous Tissue and Fascia, Face	3 Percutaneous		
4 Subcutaneous Tissue and Fascia, Right Neck			
5 Subcutaneous Tissue and Fascia, Left Neck			
6 Subcutaneous Tissue and Fascia, Chest			
7 Subcutaneous Tissue and Fascia, Back			
8 Subcutaneous Tissue and Fascia, Abdomen			
9 Subcutaneous Tissue and Fascia, Buttock			
B Subcutaneous Tissue and Fascia, Perineum			
C Subcutaneous Tissue and Fascia, Pelvic Region			
D Subcutaneous Tissue and Fascia, Right Upper Arm			
F Subcutaneous Tissue and Fascia, Left Upper Arm			
G Subcutaneous Tissue and Fascia, Right Lower Arm			
H Subcutaneous Tissue and Fascia, Left Lower Arm			
J Subcutaneous Tissue and Fascia, Right Hand			
K Subcutaneous Tissue and Fascia, Left Hand			
L Subcutaneous Tissue and Fascia, Right Upper Leg			
M Subcutaneous Tissue and Fascia, Left Upper Leg			
N Subcutaneous Tissue and Fascia, Right Lower Leg			
P Subcutaneous Tissue and Fascia, Left Lower Leg			
Q Subcutaneous Tissue and Fascia, Right Foot			
R Subcutaneous Tissue and Fascia, Left Foot			

SECTION: Ø MEDICAL AND SURGICAL
BODY SYSTEM: J SUBCUTANEOUS TISSUE AND FASCIA
OPERATION: D EXTRACTION: Pulling or stripping out or off all or a portion of a body part by the use of force

Body Part	Approach	Device	Qualifier
Ø Subcutaneous Tissue and Fascia, Scalp	Ø Open	Z No Device	Z No Qualifier
1 Subcutaneous Tissue and Fascia, Face	3 Percutaneous		
4 Subcutaneous Tissue and Fascia, Right Neck			
5 Subcutaneous Tissue and Fascia, Left Neck			
6 Subcutaneous Tissue and Fascia, Chest			
7 Subcutaneous Tissue and Fascia, Back			
8 Subcutaneous Tissue and Fascia, Abdomen			
9 Subcutaneous Tissue and Fascia, Buttock			
B Subcutaneous Tissue and Fascia, Perineum			
C Subcutaneous Tissue and Fascia, Pelvic Region			
D Subcutaneous Tissue and Fascia, Right Upper Arm			
F Subcutaneous Tissue and Fascia, Left Upper Arm			
G Subcutaneous Tissue and Fascia, Right Lower Arm			
H Subcutaneous Tissue and Fascia, Left Lower Arm			
J Subcutaneous Tissue and Fascia, Right Hand			
K Subcutaneous Tissue and Fascia, Left Hand			
L Subcutaneous Tissue and Fascia, Right Upper Leg			
M Subcutaneous Tissue and Fascia, Left Upper Leg			
N Subcutaneous Tissue and Fascia, Right Lower Leg			
P Subcutaneous Tissue and Fascia, Left Lower Leg			
Q Subcutaneous Tissue and Fascia, Right Foot			
R Subcutaneous Tissue and Fascia, Left Foot			

SECTION: Ø MEDICAL AND SURGICAL
BODY SYSTEM: J SUBCUTANEOUS TISSUE AND FASCIA
OPERATION: H INSERTION: *(on multiple pages)*

Putting in a nonbiological appliance that monitors, assists, performs, or prevents a physiological function but does not physically take the place of a body part

Body Part	Approach	Device	Qualifier
Ø Subcutaneous Tissue and Fascia, Scalp 1 Subcutaneous Tissue and Fascia, Face 4 Subcutaneous Tissue and Fascia, Right Neck 5 Subcutaneous Tissue and Fascia, Left Neck 9 Subcutaneous Tissue and Fascia, Buttock B Subcutaneous Tissue and Fascia, Perineum C Subcutaneous Tissue and Fascia, Pelvic Region J Subcutaneous Tissue and Fascia, Right Hand K Subcutaneous Tissue and Fascia, Left Hand Q Subcutaneous Tissue and Fascia, Right Foot R Subcutaneous Tissue and Fascia, Left Foot	Ø Open 3 Percutaneous	N Tissue Expander	Z No Qualifer
6 Subcutaneous Tissue and Fascia, Chest 8 Subcutaneous Tissue and Fascia, Abdomen	Ø Open 3 Percutaneous	Ø Monitoring Device, Hemodynamic 2 Monitoring Device 4 Pacemaker, Single Chamber 5 Pacemaker, Single Chamber Rate Responsive 6 Pacemaker, Dual Chamber 7 Cardiac Resynchronization Pacemaker Pulse Generator 8 Defibrillator Generator 9 Cardiac Resynchronization Defibrillator Pulse Generator A Contractility Modulation Device B Stimulator Generator, Single Array C Stimulator Generator, Single Array Rechargeable D Stimulator Generator, Multiple Array E Stimulator Generator, Multiple Array Rechargeable H Contraceptive Device M Stimulator Generator N Tissue Expander P Cardiac Rhythm Related Device V Infusion Device, Pump W Vascular Access Device, Totally Implantable X Vascular Access Device, Tunneled	Z No Qualifer

SECTION: Ø MEDICAL AND SURGICAL
BODY SYSTEM: J SUBCUTANEOUS TISSUE AND FASCIA
OPERATION: H INSERTION: *(continued)*

Putting in a nonbiological appliance that monitors, assists, performs, or prevents a physiological function but does not physically take the place of a body part

Body Part	Approach	Device	Qualifier
7 Subcutaneous Tissue and Fascia, Back	Ø Open 3 Percutaneous	B Stimulator Generator, Single Array C Stimulator Generator, Single Array Rechargeable D Stimulator Generator, Multiple Array E Stimulator Generator, Multiple Array Rechargeable M Stimulator Generator N Tissue Expander V Infusion Device, Pump	Z No Qualifier
D Subcutaneous Tissue and Fascia, Right Upper Arm F Subcutaneous Tissue and Fascia, Left Upper Arm G Subcutaneous Tissue and Fascia, Right Lower Arm H Subcutaneous Tissue and Fascia, Left Lower Arm L Subcutaneous Tissue and Fascia, Right Upper Leg M Subcutaneous Tissue and Fascia, Left Upper Leg N Subcutaneous Tissue and Fascia, Right Lower Leg P Subcutaneous Tissue and Fascia, Left Lower Leg	Ø Open 3 Percutaneous	H Contraceptive Device N Tissue Expander V Infusion Device, Pump W Vascular Access Device, Totally Implantable X Vascular Access Device, Tunneled	Z No Qualifier
S Subcutaneous Tissue and Fascia, Head and Neck V Subcutaneous Tissue and Fascia, Upper Extremity W Subcutaneous Tissue and Fascia, Lower Extremity	Ø Open 3 Percutaneous	1 Radioactive Element 3 Infusion Device Y Other Device	Z No Qualifier
T Subcutaneous Tissue and Fascia, Trunk	Ø Open 3 Percutaneous	1 Radioactive Element 3 Infusion Device V Infusion Device, Pump Y Other Device	Z No Qualifier

SECTION: Ø MEDICAL AND SURGICAL
BODY SYSTEM: J SUBCUTANEOUS TISSUE AND FASCIA
OPERATION: J INSPECTION: Visually and/or manually exploring a body part

Body Part	Approach	Device	Qualifier
S Subcutaneous Tissue and Fascia, Head and Neck T Subcutaneous Tissue and Fascia, Trunk V Subcutaneous Tissue and Fascia, Upper Extremity W Subcutaneous Tissue and Fascia, Lower Extremity	Ø Open 3 Percutaneous X External	Z No Device	Z No Qualifier

SECTION: Ø MEDICAL AND SURGICAL
BODY SYSTEM: J SUBCUTANEOUS TISSUE AND FASCIA
OPERATION: N RELEASE: Freeing a body part from an abnormal physical constraint by cutting or by the use of force

Body Part	Approach	Device	Qualifier
Ø Subcutaneous Tissue and Fascia, Scalp 1 Subcutaneous Tissue and Fascia, Face 4 Subcutaneous Tissue and Fascia, Right Neck 5 Subcutaneous Tissue and Fascia, Left Neck 6 Subcutaneous Tissue and Fascia, Chest 7 Subcutaneous Tissue and Fascia, Back 8 Subcutaneous Tissue and Fascia, Abdomen 9 Subcutaneous Tissue and Fascia, Buttock B Subcutaneous Tissue and Fascia, Perineum C Subcutaneous Tissue and Fascia, Pelvic Region D Subcutaneous Tissue and Fascia, Right Upper Arm F Subcutaneous Tissue and Fascia, Left Upper Arm G Subcutaneous Tissue and Fascia, Right Lower Arm H Subcutaneous Tissue and Fascia, Left Lower Arm J Subcutaneous Tissue and Fascia, Right Hand K Subcutaneous Tissue and Fascia, Left Hand L Subcutaneous Tissue and Fascia, Right Upper Leg M Subcutaneous Tissue and Fascia, Left Upper Leg N Subcutaneous Tissue and Fascia, Right Lower Leg P Subcutaneous Tissue and Fascia, Left Lower Leg Q Subcutaneous Tissue and Fascia, Right Foot R Subcutaneous Tissue and Fascia, Left Foot	Ø Open 3 Percutaneous X External	Z No Device	Z No Qualifier

New/Revised Text in Blue ~~deleted~~ Deleted

SECTION: Ø MEDICAL AND SURGICAL
BODY SYSTEM: J SUBCUTANEOUS TISSUE AND FASCIA
OPERATION: P REMOVAL: Taking out or off a device from a body part

Body Part	Approach	Device	Qualifier
S Subcutaneous Tissue and Fascia, Head and Neck	Ø Open 3 Percutaneous	Ø Drainage Device 1 Radioactive Element 3 Infusion Device 7 Autologous Tissue Substitute J Synthetic Substitute K Nonautologous Tissue Substitute N Tissue Expander Y Other Device	Z No Qualifier
S Subcutaneous Tissue and Fascia, Head and Neck	X External	Ø Drainage Device 1 Radioactive Element 3 Infusion Device	Z No Qualifier
T Subcutaneous Tissue and Fascia, Trunk	Ø Open 3 Percutaneous	Ø Drainage Device 1 Radioactive Element 2 Monitoring Device 3 Infusion Device 7 Autologous Tissue Substitute H Contraceptive Device J Synthetic Substitute K Nonautologous Tissue Substitute M Stimulator Generator N Tissue Expander P Cardiac Rhythm Related Device V Infusion Device, Pump W Vascular Access Device, Totally Implantable X Vascular Access Device, Tunneled Y Other Device	Z No Qualifier
T Subcutaneous Tissue and Fascia, Trunk	X External	Ø Drainage Device 1 Radioactive Element 2 Monitoring Device 3 Infusion Device H Contraceptive Device V Infusion Device, Pump X Vascular Access Device, Tunneled	Z No Qualifier
V Subcutaneous Tissue and Fascia, Upper Extremity W Subcutaneous Tissue and Fascia, Lower Extremity	Ø Open 3 Percutaneous	Ø Drainage Device 1 Radioactive Element 3 Infusion Device 7 Autologous Tissue Substitute H Contraceptive Device J Synthetic Substitute K Nonautologous Tissue Substitute N Tissue Expander V Infusion Device, Pump W Vascular Access Device, Totally Implantable X Vascular Access Device, Tunneled Y Other Device	Z No Qualifier
V Subcutaneous Tissue and Fascia, Upper Extremity W Subcutaneous Tissue and Fascia, Lower Extremity	X External	Ø Drainage Device 1 Radioactive Element 3 Infusion Device H Contraceptive Device V Infusion Pump X Vascular Access Device, Tunneled	Z No Qualifier

SECTION: Ø MEDICAL AND SURGICAL
BODY SYSTEM: J SUBCUTANEOUS TISSUE AND FASCIA
OPERATION: Q REPAIR: Restoring, to the extent possible, a body part to its normal anatomic structure and function

Body Part	Approach	Device	Qualifier
Ø Subcutaneous Tissue and Fascia, Scalp	Ø Open	Z No Device	Z No Qualifier
1 Subcutaneous Tissue and Fascia, Face	3 Percutaneous		
4 Subcutaneous Tissue and Fascia, Right Neck			
5 Subcutaneous Tissue and Fascia, Left Neck			
6 Subcutaneous Tissue and Fascia, Chest			
7 Subcutaneous Tissue and Fascia, Back			
8 Subcutaneous Tissue and Fascia, Abdomen			
9 Subcutaneous Tissue and Fascia, Buttock			
B Subcutaneous Tissue and Fascia, Perineum			
C Subcutaneous Tissue and Fascia, Pelvic Region			
D Subcutaneous Tissue and Fascia, Right Upper Arm			
F Subcutaneous Tissue and Fascia, Left Upper Arm			
G Subcutaneous Tissue and Fascia, Right Lower Arm			
H Subcutaneous Tissue and Fascia, Left Lower Arm			
J Subcutaneous Tissue and Fascia, Right Hand			
K Subcutaneous Tissue and Fascia, Left Hand			
L Subcutaneous Tissue and Fascia, Right Upper Leg			
M Subcutaneous Tissue and Fascia, Left Upper Leg			
N Subcutaneous Tissue and Fascia, Right Lower Leg			
P Subcutaneous Tissue and Fascia, Left Lower Leg			
Q Subcutaneous Tissue and Fascia, Right Foot			
R Subcutaneous Tissue and Fascia, Left Foot			

SECTION: Ø MEDICAL AND SURGICAL
BODY SYSTEM: J SUBCUTANEOUS TISSUE AND FASCIA
OPERATION: R REPLACEMENT: Putting in or on biological or synthetic material that physically takes the place and/or function of all or a portion of a body part

Body Part	Approach	Device	Qualifier
Ø Subcutaneous Tissue and Fascia, Scalp 1 Subcutaneous Tissue and Fascia, Face 4 Subcutaneous Tissue and Fascia, Right Neck 5 Subcutaneous Tissue and Fascia, Left Neck 6 Subcutaneous Tissue and Fascia, Chest 7 Subcutaneous Tissue and Fascia, Back 8 Subcutaneous Tissue and Fascia, Abdomen 9 Subcutaneous Tissue and Fascia, Buttock B Subcutaneous Tissue and Fascia, Perineum C Subcutaneous Tissue and Fascia, Pelvic Region D Subcutaneous Tissue and Fascia, Right Upper Arm F Subcutaneous Tissue and Fascia, Left Upper Arm G Subcutaneous Tissue and Fascia, Right Lower Arm H Subcutaneous Tissue and Fascia, Left Lower Arm J Subcutaneous Tissue and Fascia, Right Hand K Subcutaneous Tissue and Fascia, Left Hand L Subcutaneous Tissue and Fascia, Right Upper Leg M Subcutaneous Tissue and Fascia, Left Upper Leg N Subcutaneous Tissue and Fascia, Right Lower Leg P Subcutaneous Tissue and Fascia, Left Lower Leg Q Subcutaneous Tissue and Fascia, Right Foot R Subcutaneous Tissue and Fascia, Left Foot	Ø Open 3 Percutaneous	7 Autologous Tissue Substitute J Synthetic Substitute K Nonautologous Tissue Substitute	Z No Qualifier

SECTION: Ø MEDICAL AND SURGICAL
BODY SYSTEM: J SUBCUTANEOUS TISSUE AND FASCIA
OPERATION: U SUPPLEMENT: Putting in or on biological or synthetic material that physically reinforces and/or augments the function of a portion of a body part

Body Part	Approach	Device	Qualifier
Ø Subcutaneous Tissue and Fascia, Scalp	Ø Open	7 Autologous Tissue Substitute	Z No Qualifier
1 Subcutaneous Tissue and Fascia, Face	3 Percutaneous	J Synthetic Substitute	
4 Subcutaneous Tissue and Fascia, Right Neck		K Nonautologous Tissue Substitute	
5 Subcutaneous Tissue and Fascia, Left Neck			
6 Subcutaneous Tissue and Fascia, Chest			
7 Subcutaneous Tissue and Fascia, Back			
8 Subcutaneous Tissue and Fascia, Abdomen			
9 Subcutaneous Tissue and Fascia, Buttock			
B Subcutaneous Tissue and Fascia, Perineum			
C Subcutaneous Tissue and Fascia, Pelvic Region			
D Subcutaneous Tissue and Fascia, Right Upper Arm			
F Subcutaneous Tissue and Fascia, Left Upper Arm			
G Subcutaneous Tissue and Fascia, Right Lower Arm			
H Subcutaneous Tissue and Fascia, Left Lower Arm			
J Subcutaneous Tissue and Fascia, Right Hand			
K Subcutaneous Tissue and Fascia, Left Hand			
L Subcutaneous Tissue and Fascia, Right Upper Leg			
M Subcutaneous Tissue and Fascia, Left Upper Leg			
N Subcutaneous Tissue and Fascia, Right Lower Leg			
P Subcutaneous Tissue and Fascia, Left Lower Leg			
Q Subcutaneous Tissue and Fascia, Right Foot			
R Subcutaneous Tissue and Fascia, Left Foot			

SECTION: Ø MEDICAL AND SURGICAL
BODY SYSTEM: J SUBCUTANEOUS TISSUE AND FASCIA
OPERATION: W REVISION: *(on multiple pages)*
Correcting, to the extent possible, a portion of a malfunctioning device or the position of a displaced device

Body Part	Approach	Device	Qualifier
S Subcutaneous Tissue and Fascia, Head and Neck	Ø Open 3 Percutaneous ~~X External~~	Ø Drainage Device 3 Infusion Device 7 Autologous Tissue Substitute J Synthetic Substitute K Nonautologous Tissue Substitute N Tissue Expander Y Other Device	Z No Qualifier
S Subcutaneous Tissue and Fascia, Head and Neck	X External	Ø Drainage Device 3 Infusion Device 7 Autologous Tissue Substitute J Synthetic Substitute K Nonautologous Tissue Substitute N Tissue Expander	Z No Qualifier
T Subcutaneous Tissue and Fascia, Trunk	Ø Open 3 Percutaneous ~~X External~~	Ø Drainage Device 2 Monitoring Device 3 Infusion Device 7 Autologous Tissue Substitute H Contraceptive Device J Synthetic Substitute K Nonautologous Tissue Substitute M Stimulator Generator N Tissue Expander P Cardiac Rhythm Related Device V Infusion Device, Pump W Vascular Access Device, Totally Implantable X Vascular Access Device, Tunneled Y Other Device	Z No Qualifier
T Subcutaneous Tissue and Fascia, Trunk	X External	Ø Drainage Device 2 Monitoring Device 3 Infusion Device 7 Autologous Tissue Substitute H Contraceptive Device J Synthetic Substitute K Nonautologous Tissue Substitute M Stimulator Generator N Tissue Expander P Cardiac Rhythm Related Device V Infusion Device, Pump W Vascular Access Device, Totally Implantable X Vascular Access Device, Tunneled	Z No Qualifier

SECTION: Ø   MEDICAL AND SURGICAL
BODY SYSTEM: J   SUBCUTANEOUS TISSUE AND FASCIA
OPERATION: W   REVISION: *(continued)*
Correcting, to the extent possible, a portion of a malfunctioning device or the position of a displaced device

Body Part	Approach	Device	Qualifier
V Subcutaneous Tissue and Fascia, Upper Extremity W Subcutaneous Tissue and Fascia, Lower Extremity	Ø Open 3 Percutaneous ~~X External~~	Ø Drainage Device 3 Infusion Device 7 Autologous Tissue Substitute H Contraceptive Device J Synthetic Substitute K Nonautologous Tissue Substitute N Tissue Expander V Infusion Device, Pump W Vascular Access Device, Totally Implantable X Vascular Access Device, Tunneled Y Other Device	Z No Qualifier
V Subcutaneous Tissue and Fascia, Upper Extremity W Subcutaneous Tissue and Fascia, Lower Extremity	X External	Ø Drainage Device 3 Infusion Device 7 Autologous Tissue Substitute H Contraceptive Device J Synthetic Substitute K Nonautologous Tissue Substitute N Tissue Expander V Infusion Device, Pump W Vascular Access Device, Totally Implantable X Vascular Access Device, Tunneled	Z No Qualifier

W: REVISION

J: SUBCUTANEOUS TISSUE AND FASCIA

Ø: M/S

SECTION: Ø MEDICAL AND SURGICAL
BODY SYSTEM: J SUBCUTANEOUS TISSUE AND FASCIA
OPERATION: X TRANSFER: Moving, without taking out, all or a portion of a body part to another location to take over the function of all or a portion of a body part

Body Part	Approach	Device	Qualifier
Ø Subcutaneous Tissue and Fascia, Scalp 1 Subcutaneous Tissue and Fascia, Face 4 Subcutaneous Tissue and Fascia, Right Neck 5 Subcutaneous Tissue and Fascia, Left Neck 6 Subcutaneous Tissue and Fascia, Chest 7 Subcutaneous Tissue and Fascia, Back 8 Subcutaneous Tissue and Fascia, Abdomen 9 Subcutaneous Tissue and Fascia, Buttock B Subcutaneous Tissue and Fascia, Perineum C Subcutaneous Tissue and Fascia, Pelvic Region D Subcutaneous Tissue and Fascia, Right Upper Arm F Subcutaneous Tissue and Fascia, Left Upper Arm G Subcutaneous Tissue and Fascia, Right Lower Arm H Subcutaneous Tissue and Fascia, Left Lower Arm J Subcutaneous Tissue and Fascia, Right Hand K Subcutaneous Tissue and Fascia, Left Hand L Subcutaneous Tissue and Fascia, Right Upper Leg M Subcutaneous Tissue and Fascia, Left Upper Leg N Subcutaneous Tissue and Fascia, Right Lower Leg P Subcutaneous Tissue and Fascia, Left Lower Leg Q Subcutaneous Tissue and Fascia, Right Foot R Subcutaneous Tissue and Fascia, Left Foot	Ø Open 3 Percutaneous	Z No Device	B Skin and Subcutaneous Tissue C Skin, Subcutaneous Tissue and Fascia Z No Qualifier

ØK. Muscles 292
    ØK2. Change 293
    ØK5. Destruction 293
    ØK8. Division 294
    ØK9. Drainage 295
    ØKB. Excision 297
    ØKC. Extirpation 298
    ØKD. Extraction 299
    ØKH. Insertion 299
    ØKJ. Inspection 300
    ØKM. Reattachment 300
    ØKN. Release 301
    ØKP. Removal 301
    ØKQ. Repair 302
    ØKR. Replacement 303
    ØKS. Reposition 304
    ØKT. Resection 305
    ØKU. Supplement 306
    ØKW. Revision 306
    ØKX. Transfer 307

SECTION: Ø MEDICAL AND SURGICAL
BODY SYSTEM: K MUSCLES
OPERATION: 2 CHANGE: Taking out or off a device from a body part and putting back an identical or similar device in or on the same body part without cutting or puncturing the skin or a mucous membrane

Body Part	Approach	Device	Qualifier
X Upper Muscle Y Lower Muscle	X External	Ø Drainage Device Y Other Device	Z No Qualifier

SECTION: Ø MEDICAL AND SURGICAL
BODY SYSTEM: K MUSCLES
OPERATION: 5 DESTRUCTION: Physical eradication of all or a portion of a body part by the direct use of energy, force, or a destructive agent

Body Part	Approach	Device	Qualifier
Ø Head Muscle 1 Facial Muscle 2 Neck Muscle, Right 3 Neck Muscle, Left 4 Tongue, Palate, Pharynx Muscle 5 Shoulder Muscle, Right 6 Shoulder Muscle, Left 7 Upper Arm Muscle, Right 8 Upper Arm Muscle, Left 9 Lower Arm and Wrist Muscle, Right B Lower Arm and Wrist Muscle, Left C Hand Muscle, Right D Hand Muscle, Left F Trunk Muscle, Right G Trunk Muscle, Left H Thorax Muscle, Right J Thorax Muscle, Left K Abdomen Muscle, Right L Abdomen Muscle, Left M Perineum Muscle N Hip Muscle, Right P Hip Muscle, Left Q Upper Leg Muscle, Right R Upper Leg Muscle, Left S Lower Leg Muscle, Right T Lower Leg Muscle, Left V Foot Muscle, Right W Foot Muscle, Left	Ø Open 3 Percutaneous 4 Percutaneous Endoscopic	Z No Device	Z No Qualifier

SECTION: Ø MEDICAL AND SURGICAL
BODY SYSTEM: K MUSCLES
OPERATION: 8 DIVISION: Cutting into a body part, without draining fluids and/or gases from the body part, in order to separate or transect a body part

Body Part	Approach	Device	Qualifier
Ø Head Muscle 1 Facial Muscle 2 Neck Muscle, Right 3 Neck Muscle, Left 4 Tongue, Palate, Pharynx Muscle 5 Shoulder Muscle, Right 6 Shoulder Muscle, Left 7 Upper Arm Muscle, Right 8 Upper Arm Muscle, Left 9 Lower Arm and Wrist Muscle, Right B Lower Arm and Wrist Muscle, Left C Hand Muscle, Right D Hand Muscle, Left F Trunk Muscle, Right G Trunk Muscle, Left H Thorax Muscle, Right J Thorax Muscle, Left K Abdomen Muscle, Right L Abdomen Muscle, Left M Perineum Muscle N Hip Muscle, Right P Hip Muscle, Left Q Upper Leg Muscle, Right R Upper Leg Muscle, Left S Lower Leg Muscle, Right T Lower Leg Muscle, Left V Foot Muscle, Right W Foot Muscle, Left	Ø Open 3 Percutaneous 4 Percutaneous Endoscopic	Z No Device	Z No Qualifier

SECTION: Ø MEDICAL AND SURGICAL
BODY SYSTEM: K MUSCLES
OPERATION: 9 DRAINAGE: *(on multiple pages)*
Taking or letting out fluids and/or gases from a body part

Body Part	Approach	Device	Qualifier
Ø Head Muscle 1 Facial Muscle 2 Neck Muscle, Right 3 Neck Muscle, Left 4 Tongue, Palate, Pharynx Muscle 5 Shoulder Muscle, Right 6 Shoulder Muscle, Left 7 Upper Arm Muscle, Right 8 Upper Arm Muscle, Left 9 Lower Arm and Wrist Muscle, Right B Lower Arm and Wrist Muscle, Left C Hand Muscle, Right D Hand Muscle, Left F Trunk Muscle, Right G Trunk Muscle, Left H Thorax Muscle, Right J Thorax Muscle, Left K Abdomen Muscle, Right L Abdomen Muscle, Left M Perineum Muscle N Hip Muscle, Right P Hip Muscle, Left Q Upper Leg Muscle, Right R Upper Leg Muscle, Left S Lower Leg Muscle, Right T Lower Leg Muscle, Left V Foot Muscle, Right W Foot Muscle, Left	Ø Open 3 Percutaneous 4 Percutaneous Endoscopic	Ø Drainage Device	Z No Qualifier

SECTION: Ø MEDICAL AND SURGICAL
BODY SYSTEM: K MUSCLES
OPERATION: 9 DRAINAGE: *(continued)*

Taking or letting out fluids and/or gases from a body part

Body Part	Approach	Device	Qualifier
Ø Head Muscle 1 Facial Muscle 2 Neck Muscle, Right 3 Neck Muscle, Left 4 Tongue, Palate, Pharynx Muscle 5 Shoulder Muscle, Right 6 Shoulder Muscle, Left 7 Upper Arm Muscle, Right 8 Upper Arm Muscle, Left 9 Lower Arm and Wrist Muscle, Right B Lower Arm and Wrist Muscle, Left C Hand Muscle, Right D Hand Muscle, Left F Trunk Muscle, Right G Trunk Muscle, Left H Thorax Muscle, Right J Thorax Muscle, Left K Abdomen Muscle, Right L Abdomen Muscle, Left M Perineum Muscle N Hip Muscle, Right P Hip Muscle, Left Q Upper Leg Muscle, Right R Upper Leg Muscle, Left S Lower Leg Muscle, Right T Lower Leg Muscle, Left V Foot Muscle, Right W Foot Muscle, Left	Ø Open 3 Percutaneous 4 Percutaneous Endoscopic	Z No Device	X Diagnostic Z No Qualifier

New/Revised Text in Blue   ~~deleted~~ Deleted

SECTION: Ø MEDICAL AND SURGICAL
BODY SYSTEM: K MUSCLES
OPERATION: B EXCISION: Cutting out or off, without replacement, a portion of a body part

Body Part	Approach	Device	Qualifier
Ø Head Muscle 1 Facial Muscle 2 Neck Muscle, Right 3 Neck Muscle, Left 4 Tongue, Palate, Pharynx Muscle 5 Shoulder Muscle, Right 6 Shoulder Muscle, Left 7 Upper Arm Muscle, Right 8 Upper Arm Muscle, Left 9 Lower Arm and Wrist Muscle, Right B Lower Arm and Wrist Muscle, Left C Hand Muscle, Right D Hand Muscle, Left F Trunk Muscle, Right G Trunk Muscle, Left H Thorax Muscle, Right J Thorax Muscle, Left K Abdomen Muscle, Right L Abdomen Muscle, Left M Perineum Muscle N Hip Muscle, Right P Hip Muscle, Left Q Upper Leg Muscle, Right R Upper Leg Muscle, Left S Lower Leg Muscle, Right T Lower Leg Muscle, Left V Foot Muscle, Right W Foot Muscle, Left	Ø Open 3 Percutaneous 4 Percutaneous Endoscopic	Z No Device	X Diagnostic Z No Qualifier

SECTION: Ø MEDICAL AND SURGICAL
BODY SYSTEM: K MUSCLES
OPERATION: C EXTIRPATION: Taking or cutting out solid matter from a body part

Body Part	Approach	Device	Qualifier
Ø Head Muscle 1 Facial Muscle 2 Neck Muscle, Right 3 Neck Muscle, Left 4 Tongue, Palate, Pharynx Muscle 5 Shoulder Muscle, Right 6 Shoulder Muscle, Left 7 Upper Arm Muscle, Right 8 Upper Arm Muscle, Left 9 Lower Arm and Wrist Muscle, Right B Lower Arm and Wrist Muscle, Left C Hand Muscle, Right D Hand Muscle, Left F Trunk Muscle, Right G Trunk Muscle, Left H Thorax Muscle, Right J Thorax Muscle, Left K Abdomen Muscle, Right L Abdomen Muscle, Left M Perineum Muscle N Hip Muscle, Right P Hip Muscle, Left Q Upper Leg Muscle, Right R Upper Leg Muscle, Left S Lower Leg Muscle, Right T Lower Leg Muscle, Left V Foot Muscle, Right W Foot Muscle, Left	Ø Open 3 Percutaneous 4 Percutaneous Endoscopic	Z No Device	Z No Qualifier

SECTION: Ø MEDICAL AND SURGICAL
BODY SYSTEM: K MUSCLES
OPERATION: D EXTRACTION: Pulling or stripping out or off all or a portion of a body part by the use of force

Body Part	Approach	Device	Qualifier
Ø Head Muscle	Ø Open	Z No Device	Z No Qualifier
1 Facial Muscle			
2 Neck Muscle, Right			
3 Neck Muscle, Left			
4 Tongue, Palate, Pharynx Muscle			
5 Shoulder Muscle, Right			
6 Shoulder Muscle, Left			
7 Upper Arm Muscle, Right			
8 Upper Arm Muscle, Left			
9 Lower Arm and Wrist Muscle, Right			
B Lower Arm and Wrist Muscle, Left			
C Hand Muscle, Right			
D Hand Muscle, Left			
F Trunk Muscle, Right			
G Trunk Muscle, Left			
H Thorax Muscle, Right			
J Thorax Muscle, Left			
K Abdomen Muscle, Right			
L Abdomen Muscle, Left			
M Perineum Muscle			
N Hip Muscle, Right			
P Hip Muscle, Left			
Q Upper Leg Muscle, Right			
R Upper Leg Muscle, Left			
S Lower Leg Muscle, Right			
T Lower Leg Muscle, Left			
V Foot Muscle, Right			
W Foot Muscle, Left			

SECTION: Ø MEDICAL AND SURGICAL
BODY SYSTEM: K MUSCLES
OPERATION: H INSERTION: Putting in a nonbiological appliance that monitors, assists, performs, or prevents a physiological function but does not physically take the place of a body part

Body Part	Approach	Device	Qualifier
X Upper Muscle	Ø Open	M Stimulator Lead	Z No Qualifier
Y Lower Muscle	3 Percutaneous	Y Other Device	
	4 Percutaneous Endoscopic		

SECTION: Ø MEDICAL AND SURGICAL
BODY SYSTEM: K MUSCLES
OPERATION: J INSPECTION: Visually and/or manually exploring a body part

Body Part	Approach	Device	Qualifier
X Upper Muscle Y Lower Muscle	Ø Open 3 Percutaneous 4 Percutaneous Endoscopic X External	Z No Device	Z No Qualifier

SECTION: Ø MEDICAL AND SURGICAL
BODY SYSTEM: K MUSCLES
OPERATION: M REATTACHMENT: Putting back in or on all or a portion of a separated body part to its normal location or other suitable location

Body Part	Approach	Device	Qualifier
Ø Head Muscle 1 Facial Muscle 2 Neck Muscle, Right 3 Neck Muscle, Left 4 Tongue, Palate, Pharynx Muscle 5 Shoulder Muscle, Right 6 Shoulder Muscle, Left 7 Upper Arm Muscle, Right 8 Upper Arm Muscle, Left 9 Lower Arm and Wrist Muscle, Right B Lower Arm and Wrist Muscle, Left C Hand Muscle, Right D Hand Muscle, Left F Trunk Muscle, Right G Trunk Muscle, Left H Thorax Muscle, Right J Thorax Muscle, Left K Abdomen Muscle, Right L Abdomen Muscle, Left M Perineum Muscle N Hip Muscle, Right P Hip Muscle, Left Q Upper Leg Muscle, Right R Upper Leg Muscle, Left S Lower Leg Muscle, Right T Lower Leg Muscle, Left V Foot Muscle, Right W Foot Muscle, Left	Ø Open 4 Percutaneous Endoscopic	Z No Device	Z No Qualifier

SECTION: Ø MEDICAL AND SURGICAL
BODY SYSTEM: K MUSCLES
OPERATION: N RELEASE: Freeing a body part from an abnormal physical constraint by cutting or by the use of force

Body Part	Approach	Device	Qualifier
Ø Head Muscle 1 Facial Muscle 2 Neck Muscle, Right 3 Neck Muscle, Left 4 Tongue, Palate, Pharynx Muscle 5 Shoulder Muscle, Right 6 Shoulder Muscle, Left 7 Upper Arm Muscle, Right 8 Upper Arm Muscle, Left 9 Lower Arm and Wrist Muscle, Right B Lower Arm and Wrist Muscle, Left C Hand Muscle, Right D Hand Muscle, Left F Trunk Muscle, Right G Trunk Muscle, Left H Thorax Muscle, Right J Thorax Muscle, Left K Abdomen Muscle, Right L Abdomen Muscle, Left M Perineum Muscle N Hip Muscle, Right P Hip Muscle, Left Q Upper Leg Muscle, Right R Upper Leg Muscle, Lefta S Lower Leg Muscle, Right T Lower Leg Muscle, Left V Foot Muscle, Right W Foot Muscle, Left	Ø Open 3 Percutaneous 4 Percutaneous Endoscopic X External	Z No Device	Z No Qualifier

SECTION: Ø MEDICAL AND SURGICAL
BODY SYSTEM: K MUSCLES
OPERATION: P REMOVAL: Taking out or off a device from a body part

Body Part	Approach	Device	Qualifier
X Upper Muscle Y Lower Muscle	Ø Open 3 Percutaneous 4 Percutaneous Endoscopic	Ø Drainage Device 7 Autologous Tissue Substitute J Synthetic Substitute K Nonautologous Tissue Substitute M Stimulator Lead Y Other Device	Z No Qualifier
X Upper Muscle Y Lower Muscle	X External	Ø Drainage Device M Stimulator Lead	Z No Qualifier

SECTION: Ø MEDICAL AND SURGICAL
BODY SYSTEM: K MUSCLES
OPERATION: Q REPAIR: Restoring, to the extent possible, a body part to its normal anatomic structure and function

Body Part	Approach	Device	Qualifier
Ø Head Muscle 1 Facial Muscle 2 Neck Muscle, Right 3 Neck Muscle, Left 4 Tongue, Palate, Pharynx Muscle 5 Shoulder Muscle, Right 6 Shoulder Muscle, Left 7 Upper Arm Muscle, Right 8 Upper Arm Muscle, Left 9 Lower Arm and Wrist Muscle, Right B Lower Arm and Wrist Muscle, Left C Hand Muscle, Right D Hand Muscle, Left F Trunk Muscle, Right G Trunk Muscle, Left H Thorax Muscle, Right J Thorax Muscle, Left K Abdomen Muscle, Right L Abdomen Muscle, Left M Perineum Muscle N Hip Muscle, Right P Hip Muscle, Left Q Upper Leg Muscle, Right R Upper Leg Muscle, Left S Lower Leg Muscle, Right T Lower Leg Muscle, Left V Foot Muscle, Right W Foot Muscle, Left	Ø Open 3 Percutaneous 4 Percutaneous Endoscopic	Z No Device	Z No Qualifier

Q: REPAIR
K: MUSCLES
Ø: M/S

SECTION: Ø MEDICAL AND SURGICAL
BODY SYSTEM: K MUSCLES
OPERATION: R REPLACEMENT: Putting in or on biological or synthetic material that physically takes the place and/or function of all or a portion of a body part

Body Part	Approach	Device	Qualifier
Ø Head Muscle 1 Facial Muscle 2 Neck Muscle, Right 3 Neck Muscle, Left 4 Tongue, Palate, Pharynx Muscle 5 Shoulder Muscle, Right 6 Shoulder Muscle, Left 7 Upper Arm Muscle, Right 8 Upper Arm Muscle, Left 9 Lower Arm and Wrist Muscle, Right B Lower Arm and Wrist Muscle, Left C Hand Muscle, Right D Hand Muscle, Left F Trunk Muscle, Right G Trunk Muscle, Left H Thorax Muscle, Right J Thorax Muscle, Left K Abdomen Muscle, Right L Abdomen Muscle, Left M Perineum Muscle N Hip Muscle, Right P Hip Muscle, Left Q Upper Leg Muscle, Right R Upper Leg Muscle, Left S Lower Leg Muscle, Right T Lower Leg Muscle, Left V Foot Muscle, Right W Foot Muscle, Left	Ø Open 4 Percutaneous Endoscopic	7 Autologous Tissue Substitute J Synthetic Substitute K Nonautologous Tissue Substitute	Z No Qualifier

SECTION: Ø MEDICAL AND SURGICAL
BODY SYSTEM: K MUSCLES
OPERATION: S REPOSITION: Moving to its normal location, or other suitable location, all or a portion of a body part

Body Part	Approach	Device	Qualifier
Ø Head Muscle 1 Facial Muscle 2 Neck Muscle, Right 3 Neck Muscle, Left 4 Tongue, Palate, Pharynx Muscle 5 Shoulder Muscle, Right 6 Shoulder Muscle, Left 7 Upper Arm Muscle, Right 8 Upper Arm Muscle, Left 9 Lower Arm and Wrist Muscle, Right B Lower Arm and Wrist Muscle, Left C Hand Muscle, Right D Hand Muscle, Left F Trunk Muscle, Right G Trunk Muscle, Left H Thorax Muscle, Right J Thorax Muscle, Left K Abdomen Muscle, Right L Abdomen Muscle, Left M Perineum Muscle N Hip Muscle, Right P Hip Muscle, Left Q Upper Leg Muscle, Right R Upper Leg Muscle, Left S Lower Leg Muscle, Right T Lower Leg Muscle, Left V Foot Muscle, Right W Foot Muscle, Left	Ø Open 4 Percutaneous Endoscopic	Z No Device	Z No Qualifier

SECTION: Ø MEDICAL AND SURGICAL
BODY SYSTEM: K MUSCLES
OPERATION: T RESECTION: Cutting out or off, without replacement, all of a body part

Body Part	Approach	Device	Qualifier
Ø Head Muscle 1 Facial Muscle 2 Neck Muscle, Right 3 Neck Muscle, Left 4 Tongue, Palate, Pharynx Muscle 5 Shoulder Muscle, Right 6 Shoulder Muscle, Left 7 Upper Arm Muscle, Right 8 Upper Arm Muscle, Left 9 Lower Arm and Wrist Muscle, Right B Lower Arm and Wrist Muscle, Left C Hand Muscle, Right D Hand Muscle, Left F Trunk Muscle, Right G Trunk Muscle, Left H Thorax Muscle, Right J Thorax Muscle, Left K Abdomen Muscle, Right L Abdomen Muscle, Left M Perineum Muscle N Hip Muscle, Right P Hip Muscle, Left Q Upper Leg Muscle, Right R Upper Leg Muscle, Left S Lower Leg Muscle, Right T Lower Leg Muscle, Left V Foot Muscle, Right W Foot Muscle, Left	Ø Open 4 Percutaneous Endoscopic	Z No Device	Z No Qualifier

SECTION: Ø MEDICAL AND SURGICAL
BODY SYSTEM: K MUSCLES
OPERATION: U SUPPLEMENT: Putting in or on biological or synthetic material that physically reinforces and/or augments the function of a portion of a body part

Body Part	Approach	Device	Qualifier
Ø Head Muscle 1 Facial Muscle 2 Neck Muscle, Right 3 Neck Muscle, Left 4 Tongue, Palate, Pharynx Muscle 5 Shoulder Muscle, Right 6 Shoulder Muscle, Left 7 Upper Arm Muscle, Right 8 Upper Arm Muscle, Left 9 Lower Arm and Wrist Muscle, Right B Lower Arm and Wrist Muscle, Left C Hand Muscle, Right D Hand Muscle, Left F Trunk Muscle, Right G Trunk Muscle, Left H Thorax Muscle, Right J Thorax Muscle, Left K Abdomen Muscle, Right L Abdomen Muscle, Left M Perineum Muscle N Hip Muscle, Right P Hip Muscle, Left Q Upper Leg Muscle, Right R Upper Leg Muscle, Left S Lower Leg Muscle, Right T Lower Leg Muscle, Left V Foot Muscle, Right W Foot Muscle, Left	Ø Open 4 Percutaneous Endoscopic	7 Autologous Tissue Substitute J Synthetic Substitute K Nonautologous Tissue Substitute	Z No Qualifier

SECTION: Ø MEDICAL AND SURGICAL
BODY SYSTEM: K MUSCLES
OPERATION: W REVISION: Correcting, to the extent possible, a portion of a malfunctioning device or the position of a displaced device

Body Part	Approach	Device	Qualifier
X Upper Muscle Y Lower Muscle	Ø Open 3 Percutaneous 4 Percutaneous Endoscopic X External	Ø Drainage Device 7 Autologous Tissue Substitute J Synthetic Substitute K Nonautologous Tissue Substitute M Stimulator Lead Y Other device	Z No Qualifier
X Upper Muscle Y Lower Muscle	X External	Ø Drainage Device 7 Autologous Tissue Substitute J Synthetic Substitute K Nonautologous Tissue Substitute M Stimulator Lead	Z No Qualifier

SECTION: Ø MEDICAL AND SURGICAL
BODY SYSTEM: K MUSCLES
OPERATION: X TRANSFER: Moving, without taking out, all or a portion of a body part to another location to take over the function of all or a portion of a body part

Body Part	Approach	Device	Qualifier
Ø Head Muscle 1 Facial Muscle 2 Neck Muscle, Right 3 Neck Muscle, Left 4 Tongue, Palate, Pharynx Muscle 5 Shoulder Muscle, Right 6 Shoulder Muscle, Left 7 Upper Arm Muscle, Right 8 Upper Arm Muscle, Left 9 Lower Arm and Wrist Muscle, Right B Lower Arm and Wrist Muscle, Left C Hand Muscle, Right D Hand Muscle, Left ~~F Trunk Muscle, Right~~ ~~G Trunk Muscle, Left~~ H Thorax Muscle, Right J Thorax Muscle, Left M Perineum Muscle N Hip Muscle, Right P Hip Muscle, Left Q Upper Leg Muscle, Right R Upper Leg Muscle, Left S Lower Leg Muscle, Right T Lower Leg Muscle, Left V Foot Muscle, Right W Foot Muscle, Left	Ø Open 4 Percutaneous Endoscopic	Z No Device	Ø Skin 1 Subcutaneous Tissue 2 Skin and Subcutaneous Tissue Z No Qualifier
F Trunk Muscle, Right G Trunk Muscle, Left	Ø Open 4 Percutaneous Endoscopic	Z No Device	Ø Skin 1 Subcutaneous Tissue 2 Skin and Subcutaneous Tissue 5 Latissimus Dorsi Myocutaneous Flap 7 Deep Inferior Epigastric Artery Perforator Flap 8 Superficial Inferior Epigastric Artery Flap 9 Gluteal Artery Perforator Flap Z No Qualifier
K Abdomen Muscle, Right L Abdomen Muscle, Left	Ø Open 4 Percutaneous Endoscopic	Z No Device	Ø Skin 1 Subcutaneous Tissue 2 Skin and Subcutaneous Tissue 6 Transverse Rectus Abdominis Myocutaneous Flap Z No Qualifier

ØL. Tendons 3Ø8
    ØL2. Change 3Ø9
    ØL5. Destruction 3Ø9
    ØL8. Division 31Ø
    ØL9. Drainage 311
    ØLB. Excision 312
    ØLC. Extirpation 313
    ØLD. Extraction 314
    ØLH. Insertion 314
    ØLJ. Inspection 315
    ØLM. Reattachment 315
    ØLN. Release 316
    ØLP. Removal 316
    ØLQ. Repair 317
    ØLR. Replacement 318
    ØLS. Reposition 319
    ØLT. Resection 32Ø
    ØLU. Supplement 321
    ØLW. Revision 321
    ØLX. Transfer 322

SECTION: Ø MEDICAL AND SURGICAL
BODY SYSTEM: L TENDONS
OPERATION: 2 **CHANGE:** Taking out or off a device from a body part and putting back an identical or similar device in or on the same body part without cutting or puncturing the skin or a mucous membrane

Body Part	Approach	Device	Qualifier
X Upper Tendon Y Lower Tendon	X External	Ø Drainage Device Y Other Device	Z No Qualifier

SECTION: Ø MEDICAL AND SURGICAL
BODY SYSTEM: L TENDONS
OPERATION: 5 **DESTRUCTION:** Physical eradication of all or a portion of a body part by the direct use of energy, force, or a destructive agent

Body Part	Approach	Device	Qualifier
Ø Head and Neck Tendon 1 Shoulder Tendon, Right 2 Shoulder Tendon, Left 3 Upper Arm Tendon, Right 4 Upper Arm Tendon, Left 5 Lower Arm and Wrist Tendon, Right 6 Lower Arm and Wrist Tendon, Left 7 Hand Tendon, Right 8 Hand Tendon, Left 9 Trunk Tendon, Right B Trunk Tendon, Left C Thorax Tendon, Right D Thorax Tendon, Left F Abdomen Tendon, Right G Abdomen Tendon, Left H Perineum Tendon J Hip Tendon, Right K Hip Tendon, Left L Upper Leg Tendon, Right M Upper Leg Tendon, Left N Lower Leg Tendon, Right P Lower Leg Tendon, Left Q Knee Tendon, Right R Knee Tendon, Left S Ankle Tendon, Right T Ankle Tendon, Left V Foot Tendon, Right W Foot Tendon, Left	Ø Open 3 Percutaneous 4 Percutaneous Endoscopic	Z No Device	Z No Qualifier

SECTION: Ø MEDICAL AND SURGICAL

BODY SYSTEM: L TENDONS

OPERATION: 8 DIVISION: Cutting into a body part, without draining fluids and/or gases from the body part, in order to separate or transect a body part

Body Part	Approach	Device	Qualifier
Ø Head and Neck Tendon 1 Shoulder Tendon, Right 2 Shoulder Tendon, Left 3 Upper Arm Tendon, Right 4 Upper Arm Tendon, Left 5 Lower Arm and Wrist Tendon, Right 6 Lower Arm and Wrist Tendon, Left 7 Hand Tendon, Right 8 Hand Tendon, Left 9 Trunk Tendon, Right B Trunk Tendon, Left C Thorax Tendon, Right D Thorax Tendon, Left F Abdomen Tendon, Right G Abdomen Tendon, Left H Perineum Tendon J Hip Tendon, Right K Hip Tendon, Left L Upper Leg Tendon, Right M Upper Leg Tendon, Left N Lower Leg Tendon, Right P Lower Leg Tendon, Left Q Knee Tendon, Right R Knee Tendon, Left S Ankle Tendon, Right T Ankle Tendon, Left V Foot Tendon, Right W Foot Tendon, Left	Ø Open 3 Percutaneous 4 Percutaneous Endoscopic	Z No Device	Z No Qualifier

8: DIVISION

L: TENDONS

Ø: M/S

SECTION: Ø MEDICAL AND SURGICAL
BODY SYSTEM: L TENDONS
OPERATION: 9 DRAINAGE: Taking or letting out fluids and/or gases from a body part

Body Part	Approach	Device	Qualifier
Ø Head and Neck Tendon 1 Shoulder Tendon, Right 2 Shoulder Tendon, Left 3 Upper Arm Tendon, Right 4 Upper Arm Tendon, Left 5 Lower Arm and Wrist Tendon, Right 6 Lower Arm and Wrist Tendon, Left 7 Hand Tendon, Right 8 Hand Tendon, Left 9 Trunk Tendon, Right B Trunk Tendon, Left C Thorax Tendon, Right D Thorax Tendon, Left F Abdomen Tendon, Right G Abdomen Tendon, Left H Perineum Tendon J Hip Tendon, Right K Hip Tendon, Left L Upper Leg Tendon, Right M Upper Leg Tendon, Left N Lower Leg Tendon, Right P Lower Leg Tendon, Left Q Knee Tendon, Right R Knee Tendon, Left S Ankle Tendon, Right T Ankle Tendon, Left V Foot Tendon, Right W Foot Tendon, Left	Ø Open 3 Percutaneous 4 Percutaneous Endoscopic	Ø Drainage Device	Z No Qualifier
Ø Head and Neck Tendon 1 Shoulder Tendon, Right 2 Shoulder Tendon, Left 3 Upper Arm Tendon, Right 4 Upper Arm Tendon, Left 5 Lower Arm and Wrist Tendon, Right 6 Lower Arm and Wrist Tendon, Left 7 Hand Tendon, Right 8 Hand Tendon, Left 9 Trunk Tendon, Right B Trunk Tendon, Left C Thorax Tendon, Right D Thorax Tendon, Left F Abdomen Tendon, Right G Abdomen Tendon, Left H Perineum Tendon J Hip Tendon, Right K Hip Tendon, Left L Upper Leg Tendon, Right M Upper Leg Tendon, Left N Lower Leg Tendon, Right P Lower Leg Tendon, Left Q Knee Tendon, Right R Knee Tendon, Left S Ankle Tendon, Right T Ankle Tendon, Left V Foot Tendon, Right W Foot Tendon, Left	Ø Open 3 Percutaneous 4 Percutaneous Endoscopic	Z No Device	X Diagnostic Z No Qualifier

Ø: M/S   L: TENDONS   9: DRAINAGE

SECTION: Ø MEDICAL AND SURGICAL
BODY SYSTEM: L TENDONS
OPERATION: B EXCISION: Cutting out or off, without replacement, a portion of a body part

Body Part	Approach	Device	Qualifier
Ø Head and Neck Tendon	Ø Open	Z No Device	X Diagnostic
1 Shoulder Tendon, Right	3 Percutaneous		Z No Qualifier
2 Shoulder Tendon, Left	4 Percutaneous Endoscopic		
3 Upper Arm Tendon, Right			
4 Upper Arm Tendon, Left			
5 Lower Arm and Wrist Tendon, Right			
6 Lower Arm and Wrist Tendon, Left			
7 Hand Tendon, Right			
8 Hand Tendon, Left			
9 Trunk Tendon, Right			
B Trunk Tendon, Left			
C Thorax Tendon, Right			
D Thorax Tendon, Left			
F Abdomen Tendon, Right			
G Abdomen Tendon, Left			
H Perineum Tendon			
J Hip Tendon, Right			
K Hip Tendon, Left			
L Upper Leg Tendon, Right			
M Upper Leg Tendon, Left			
N Lower Leg Tendon, Right			
P Lower Leg Tendon, Left			
Q Knee Tendon, Right			
R Knee Tendon, Left			
S Ankle Tendon, Right			
T Ankle Tendon, Left			
V Foot Tendon, Right			
W Foot Tendon, Left			

B: EXCISION

L: TENDONS

Ø: M/S

New/Revised Text in Blue   ~~deleted~~ Deleted

SECTION:　Ø MEDICAL AND SURGICAL
BODY SYSTEM: **L　TENDONS**
OPERATION:　**C EXTIRPATION:** Taking or cutting out solid matter from a body part

Body Part	Approach	Device	Qualifier
Ø　Head and Neck Tendon	Ø　Open	Z　No Device	Z　No Qualifier
1　Shoulder Tendon, Right	3　Percutaneous		
2　Shoulder Tendon, Left	4　Percutaneous Endoscopic		
3　Upper Arm Tendon, Right			
4　Upper Arm Tendon, Left			
5　Lower Arm and Wrist Tendon, Right			
6　Lower Arm and Wrist Tendon, Left			
7　Hand Tendon, Right			
8　Hand Tendon, Left			
9　Trunk Tendon, Right			
B　Trunk Tendon, Left			
C　Thorax Tendon, Right			
D　Thorax Tendon, Left			
F　Abdomen Tendon, Right			
G　Abdomen Tendon, Left			
H　Perineum Tendon			
J　Hip Tendon, Right			
K　Hip Tendon, Left			
L　Upper Leg Tendon, Right			
M　Upper Leg Tendon, Left			
N　Lower Leg Tendon, Right			
P　Lower Leg Tendon, Left			
Q　Knee Tendon, Right			
R　Knee Tendon, Left			
S　Ankle Tendon, Right			
T　Ankle Tendon, Left			
V　Foot Tendon, Right			
W　Foot Tendon, Left			

D: EXTRACTION   H: INSERTION

L: TENDONS

Ø: M/S

SECTION: Ø MEDICAL AND SURGICAL
BODY SYSTEM: L TENDONS
OPERATION: D **EXTRACTION:** Pulling or stripping out or off all or a portion of a body part by the use of force

Body Part	Approach	Device	Qualifier
Ø Head and Neck Tendon	Ø Open	Z No Device	Z No Qualifier
1 Shoulder Tendon, Right			
2 Shoulder Tendon, Left			
3 Upper Arm Tendon, Right			
4 Upper Arm Tendon, Left			
5 Lower Arm and Wrist Tendon, Right			
6 Lower Arm and Wrist Tendon, Left			
7 Hand Tendon, Right			
8 Hand Tendon, Left			
9 Trunk Tendon, Right			
B Trunk Tendon, Left			
C Thorax Tendon, Right			
D Thorax Tendon, Left			
F Abdomen Tendon, Right			
G Abdomen Tendon, Left			
H Perineum Tendon			
J Hip Tendon, Right			
K Hip Tendon, Left			
L Upper Leg Tendon, Right			
M Upper Leg Tendon, Left			
N Lower Leg Tendon, Right			
P Lower Leg Tendon, Left			
Q Knee Tendon, Right			
R Knee Tendon, Left			
S Ankle Tendon, Right			
T Ankle Tendon, Left			
V Foot Tendon, Right			
W Foot Tendon, Left			

SECTION: Ø MEDICAL AND SURGICAL
BODY SYSTEM: L TENDONS
OPERATION: H **INSERTION:** Putting in a nonbiological appliance that monitors, assists, performs, or prevents a physiological function but does not physically take the place of a body part

Body Part	Approach	Device	Qualifier
X Upper Tendon	Ø Open	Y Other Device	Z No Qualifier
Y Lower Tendon	3 Percutaneous		
	4 Percutaneous Endoscopic		

SECTION: Ø MEDICAL AND SURGICAL
BODY SYSTEM: L TENDONS
OPERATION: J INSPECTION: Visually and/or manually exploring a body part

Body Part	Approach	Device	Qualifier
X Upper Tendon Y Lower Tendon	Ø Open 3 Percutaneous 4 Percutaneous Endoscopic X External	Z No Device	Z No Qualifier

SECTION: Ø MEDICAL AND SURGICAL
BODY SYSTEM: L TENDONS
OPERATION: M REATTACHMENT: Putting back in or on all or a portion of a separated body part to its normal location or other suitable location

Body Part	Approach	Device	Qualifier
Ø Head and Neck Tendon 1 Shoulder Tendon, Right 2 Shoulder Tendon, Left 3 Upper Arm Tendon, Right 4 Upper Arm Tendon, Left 5 Lower Arm and Wrist Tendon, Right 6 Lower Arm and Wrist Tendon, Left 7 Hand Tendon, Right 8 Hand Tendon, Left 9 Trunk Tendon, Right B Trunk Tendon, Left C Thorax Tendon, Right D Thorax Tendon, Left F Abdomen Tendon, Right G Abdomen Tendon, Left H Perineum Tendon J Hip Tendon, Right K Hip Tendon, Left L Upper Leg Tendon, Right M Upper Leg Tendon, Left N Lower Leg Tendon, Right P Lower Leg Tendon, Left Q Knee Tendon, Right R Knee Tendon, Left S Ankle Tendon, Right T Ankle Tendon, Left V Foot Tendon, Right W Foot Tendon, Left	Ø Open 4 Percutaneous Endoscopic	Z No Device	Z No Qualifier

SECTION: Ø MEDICAL AND SURGICAL
BODY SYSTEM: L TENDONS
OPERATION: N RELEASE: Freeing a body part from an abnormal physical constraint by cutting or by the use of force

Body Part	Approach	Device	Qualifier
Ø Head and Neck Tendon 1 Shoulder Tendon, Right 2 Shoulder Tendon, Left 3 Upper Arm Tendon, Right 4 Upper Arm Tendon, Left 5 Lower Arm and Wrist Tendon, Right 6 Lower Arm and Wrist Tendon, Left 7 Hand Tendon, Right 8 Hand Tendon, Left 9 Trunk Tendon, Right B Trunk Tendon, Left C Thorax Tendon, Right D Thorax Tendon, Left F Abdomen Tendon, Right G Abdomen Tendon, Left H Perineum Tendon J Hip Tendon, Right K Hip Tendon, Left L Upper Leg Tendon, Right M Upper Leg Tendon, Left N Lower Leg Tendon, Right P Lower Leg Tendon, Left Q Knee Tendon, Right R Knee Tendon, Left S Ankle Tendon, Right T Ankle Tendon, Left V Foot Tendon, Right W Foot Tendon, Left	Ø Open 3 Percutaneous 4 Percutaneous Endoscopic X External	Z No Device	Z No Qualifier

SECTION: Ø MEDICAL AND SURGICAL
BODY SYSTEM: L TENDONS
OPERATION: P REMOVAL: Taking out or off a device from a body part

Body Part	Approach	Device	Qualifier
X Upper Tendon Y Lower Tendon	Ø Open 3 Percutaneous 4 Percutaneous Endoscopic	Ø Drainage Device 7 Autologous Tissue Substitute J Synthetic Substitute K Nonautologous Tissue Substitute Y Other Device	Z No Qualifier
X Upper Tendon Y Lower Tendon	X External	Ø Drainage Device	Z No Qualifier

SECTION: Ø MEDICAL AND SURGICAL
BODY SYSTEM: L TENDONS
OPERATION: Q REPAIR: Restoring, to the extent possible, a body part to its normal anatomic structure and function

Body Part	Approach	Device	Qualifier
Ø Head and Neck Tendon 1 Shoulder Tendon, Right 2 Shoulder Tendon, Left 3 Upper Arm Tendon, Right 4 Upper Arm Tendon, Left 5 Lower Arm and Wrist Tendon, Right 6 Lower Arm and Wrist Tendon, Left 7 Hand Tendon, Right 8 Hand Tendon, Left 9 Trunk Tendon, Right B Trunk Tendon, Left C Thorax Tendon, Right D Thorax Tendon, Left F Abdomen Tendon, Right G Abdomen Tendon, Left H Perineum Tendon J Hip Tendon, Right K Hip Tendon, Left L Upper Leg Tendon, Right M Upper Leg Tendon, Left N Lower Leg Tendon, Right P Lower Leg Tendon, Left Q Knee Tendon, Right R Knee Tendon, Left S Ankle Tendon, Right T Ankle Tendon, Left V Foot Tendon, Right W Foot Tendon, Left	Ø Open 3 Percutaneous 4 Percutaneous Endoscopic	Z No Device	Z No Qualifier

SECTION: Ø MEDICAL AND SURGICAL
BODY SYSTEM: L TENDONS
OPERATION: R REPLACEMENT: Putting in or on biological or synthetic material that physically takes the place and/or function of all or a portion of a body part

Body Part	Approach	Device	Qualifier
Ø Head and Neck Tendon	Ø Open	7 Autologous Tissue Substitute	Z No Qualifier
1 Shoulder Tendon, Right	4 Percutaneous Endoscopic	J Synthetic Substitute	
2 Shoulder Tendon, Left		K Nonautologous Tissue Substitute	
3 Upper Arm Tendon, Right			
4 Upper Arm Tendon, Left			
5 Lower Arm and Wrist Tendon, Right			
6 Lower Arm and Wrist Tendon, Left			
7 Hand Tendon, Right			
8 Hand Tendon, Left			
9 Trunk Tendon, Right			
B Trunk Tendon, Left			
C Thorax Tendon, Right			
D Thorax Tendon, Left			
F Abdomen Tendon, Right			
G Abdomen Tendon, Left			
H Perineum Tendon			
J Hip Tendon, Right			
K Hip Tendon, Left			
L Upper Leg Tendon, Right			
M Upper Leg Tendon, Left			
N Lower Leg Tendon, Right			
P Lower Leg Tendon, Left			
Q Knee Tendon, Right			
R Knee Tendon, Left			
S Ankle Tendon, Right			
T Ankle Tendon, Left			
V Foot Tendon, Right			
W Foot Tendon, Left			

R: REPLACEMENT

L: TENDONS

Ø: M/S

SECTION: Ø MEDICAL AND SURGICAL
BODY SYSTEM: L TENDONS
OPERATION: S REPOSITION: Moving to its normal location, or other suitable location, all or a portion of a body part

Body Part	Approach	Device	Qualifier
Ø Head and Neck Tendon	Ø Open	Z No Device	Z No Qualifier
1 Shoulder Tendon, Right	4 Percutaneous Endoscopic		
2 Shoulder Tendon, Left			
3 Upper Arm Tendon, Right			
4 Upper Arm Tendon, Left			
5 Lower Arm and Wrist Tendon, Right			
6 Lower Arm and Wrist Tendon, Left			
7 Hand Tendon, Right			
8 Hand Tendon, Left			
9 Trunk Tendon, Right			
B Trunk Tendon, Left			
C Thorax Tendon, Right			
D Thorax Tendon, Left			
F Abdomen Tendon, Right			
G Abdomen Tendon, Left			
H Perineum Tendon			
J Hip Tendon, Right			
K Hip Tendon, Left			
L Upper Leg Tendon, Right			
M Upper Leg Tendon, Left			
N Lower Leg Tendon, Right			
P Lower Leg Tendon, Left			
Q Knee Tendon, Right			
R Knee Tendon, Left			
S Ankle Tendon, Right			
T Ankle Tendon, Left			
V Foot Tendon, Right			
W Foot Tendon, Left			

SECTION: Ø MEDICAL AND SURGICAL
BODY SYSTEM: L TENDONS
OPERATION: T RESECTION: Cutting out or off, without replacement, all of a body part

Body Part	Approach	Device	Qualifier
Ø Head and Neck Tendon	Ø Open	Z No Device	Z No Qualifier
1 Shoulder Tendon, Right	4 Percutaneous Endoscopic		
2 Shoulder Tendon, Left			
3 Upper Arm Tendon, Right			
4 Upper Arm Tendon, Left			
5 Lower Arm and Wrist Tendon, Right			
6 Lower Arm and Wrist Tendon, Left			
7 Hand Tendon, Right			
8 Hand Tendon, Left			
9 Trunk Tendon, Right			
B Trunk Tendon, Left			
C Thorax Tendon, Right			
D Thorax Tendon, Left			
F Abdomen Tendon, Right			
G Abdomen Tendon, Left			
H Perineum Tendon			
J Hip Tendon, Right			
K Hip Tendon, Left			
L Upper Leg Tendon, Right			
M Upper Leg Tendon, Left			
N Lower Leg Tendon, Right			
P Lower Leg Tendon, Left			
Q Knee Tendon, Right			
R Knee Tendon, Left			
S Ankle Tendon, Right			
T Ankle Tendon, Left			
V Foot Tendon, Right			
W Foot Tendon, Left			

T: RESECTION

L: TENDONS

Ø: M/S

SECTION: Ø MEDICAL AND SURGICAL
BODY SYSTEM: L TENDONS
OPERATION: U SUPPLEMENT: Putting in or on biological or synthetic material that physically reinforces and/or augments the function of a portion of a body part

Body Part	Approach	Device	Qualifier
Ø Head and Neck Tendon 1 Shoulder Tendon, Right 2 Shoulder Tendon, Left 3 Upper Arm Tendon, Right 4 Upper Arm Tendon, Left 5 Lower Arm and Wrist Tendon, Right 6 Lower Arm and Wrist Tendon, Left 7 Hand Tendon, Right 8 Hand Tendon, Left 9 Trunk Tendon, Right B Trunk Tendon, Left C Thorax Tendon, Right D Thorax Tendon, Left F Abdomen Tendon, Right G Abdomen Tendon, Left H Perineum Tendon J Hip Tendon, Right K Hip Tendon, Left L Upper Leg Tendon, Right M Upper Leg Tendon, Left N Lower Leg Tendon, Right P Lower Leg Tendon, Left Q Knee Tendon, Right R Knee Tendon, Left S Ankle Tendon, Right T Ankle Tendon, Left V Foot Tendon, Right W Foot Tendon, Left	Ø Open 4 Percutaneous Endoscopic	7 Autologous Tissue Substitute J Synthetic Substitute K Nonautologous Tissue Substitute	Z No Qualifier

SECTION: Ø MEDICAL AND SURGICAL
BODY SYSTEM: L TENDONS
OPERATION: W REVISION: Correcting, to the extent possible, a portion of a malfunctioning device or the position of a displaced device

Body Part	Approach	Device	Qualifier
X Upper Tendon Y Lower Tendon	Ø Open 3 Percutaneous 4 Percutaneous Endoscopic X External	Ø Drainage Device 7 Autologous Tissue Substitute J Synthetic Substitute K Nonautologous Tissue Substitute Y Other Device	Z No Qualifier
X Upper Tendon Y Lower Tendon	X External	Ø Drainage Device 7 Autologous Tissue Substitute J Synthetic Substitute K Nonautologous Tissue Substitute	Z No Qualifier

SECTION: Ø MEDICAL AND SURGICAL
BODY SYSTEM: L TENDONS
OPERATION: X TRANSFER: Moving, without taking out, all or a portion of a body part to another location to take over the function of all or a portion of a body part

Body Part	Approach	Device	Qualifier
Ø Head and Neck Tendon 1 Shoulder Tendon, Right 2 Shoulder Tendon, Left 3 Upper Arm Tendon, Right 4 Upper Arm Tendon, Left 5 Lower Arm and Wrist Tendon, Right 6 Lower Arm and Wrist Tendon, Left 7 Hand Tendon, Right 8 Hand Tendon, Left 9 Trunk Tendon, Right B Trunk Tendon, Left C Thorax Tendon, Right D Thorax Tendon, Left F Abdomen Tendon, Right G Abdomen Tendon, Left H Perineum Tendon J Hip Tendon, Right K Hip Tendon, Left L Upper Leg Tendon, Right M Upper Leg Tendon, Left N Lower Leg Tendon, Right P Lower Leg Tendon, Left Q Knee Tendon, Right R Knee Tendon, Left S Ankle Tendon, Right T Ankle Tendon, Left V Foot Tendon, Right W Foot Tendon, Left	Ø Open 4 Percutaneous Endoscopic	Z No Device	Z No Qualifier

ØM. Bursae and Ligaments 323
    ØM2. Change 324
    ØM5. Destruction 324
    ØM8. Division 325
    ØM9. Drainage 326
    ØMB. Excision 327
    ØMC. Extirpation 328
    ØMD. Extraction 329
    ØMH. Insertion 329
    ØMJ. Inspection 330
    ØMM. Reattachment 330
    ØMN. Release 331
    ØMP. Removal 331
    ØMQ. Repair 332
    ØMR. Replacement 333
    ØMS. Reposition 334
    ØMT. Resection 335
    ØMU. Supplement 336
    ØMW. Revision 336
    ØMX. Transfer 337

SECTION: Ø MEDICAL AND SURGICAL

BODY SYSTEM: M BURSAE AND LIGAMENTS

OPERATION: 2 CHANGE: Taking out or off a device from a body part and putting back an identical or similar device in or on the same body part without cutting or puncturing the skin or a mucous membrane

Body Part	Approach	Device	Qualifier
X Upper Bursa and Ligament Y Lower Bursa and Ligament	X External	Ø Drainage Device Y Other Device	Z No Qualifier

SECTION: Ø MEDICAL AND SURGICAL

BODY SYSTEM: M BURSAE AND LIGAMENTS

OPERATION: 5 DESTRUCTION: Physical eradication of all or a portion of a body part by the direct use of energy, force, or a destructive agent

Body Part	Approach	Device	Qualifier
Ø Head and Neck Bursa and Ligament 1 Shoulder Bursa and Ligament, Right 2 Shoulder Bursa and Ligament, Left 3 Elbow Bursa and Ligament, Right 4 Elbow Bursa and Ligament, Left 5 Wrist Bursa and Ligament, Right 6 Wrist Bursa and Ligament, Left 7 Hand Bursa and Ligament, Right 8 Hand Bursa and Ligament, Left 9 Upper Extremity Bursa and Ligament, Right B Upper Extremity Bursa and Ligament, Left C Upper Spine Bursa and Ligament D Lower Spine Bursa and Ligament F Sternum Bursa and Ligament G Rib(s) Bursa and Ligament H Abdomen Bursa and Ligament, Right J Abdomen Bursa and Ligament, Left K Perineum Bursa and Ligament L Hip Bursa and Ligament, Right M Hip Bursa and Ligament, Left N Knee Bursa and Ligament, Right P Knee Bursa and Ligament, Left Q Ankle Bursa and Ligament, Right R Ankle Bursa and Ligament, Left S Foot Bursa and Ligament, Right T Foot Bursa and Ligament, Left V Lower Extremity Bursa and Ligament, Right W Lower Extremity Bursa and Ligament, Left	Ø Open 3 Percutaneous 4 Percutaneous Endoscopic	Z No Device	Z No Qualifier

SECTION: Ø MEDICAL AND SURGICAL
BODY SYSTEM: M BURSAE AND LIGAMENTS
OPERATION: 8 DIVISION: Cutting into a body part, without draining fluids and/or gases from the body part, in order to separate or transect a body part

Body Part	Approach	Device	Qualifier
Ø Head and Neck Bursa and Ligament 1 Shoulder Bursa and Ligament, Right 2 Shoulder Bursa and Ligament, Left 3 Elbow Bursa and Ligament, Right 4 Elbow Bursa and Ligament, Left 5 Wrist Bursa and Ligament, Right 6 Wrist Bursa and Ligament, Left 7 Hand Bursa and Ligament, Right 8 Hand Bursa and Ligament, Left 9 Upper Extremity Bursa and Ligament, Right B Upper Extremity Bursa and Ligament, Left C Upper Spine Bursa and Ligament D Lower Spine Bursa and Ligament F Sternum Bursa and Ligament G Rib(s) Bursa and Ligament H Abdomen Bursa and Ligament, Right J Abdomen Bursa and Ligament, Left K Perineum Bursa and Ligament L Hip Bursa and Ligament, Right M Hip Bursa and Ligament, Left N Knee Bursa and Ligament, Right P Knee Bursa and Ligament, Left Q Ankle Bursa and Ligament, Right R Ankle Bursa and Ligament, Left S Foot Bursa and Ligament, Right T Foot Bursa and Ligament, Left V Lower Extremity Bursa and Ligament, Right W Lower Extremity Bursa and Ligament, Left	Ø Open 3 Percutaneous 4 Percutaneous Endoscopic	Z No Device	Z No Qualifier

SECTION: Ø **MEDICAL AND SURGICAL**
BODY SYSTEM: M **BURSAE AND LIGAMENTS**
OPERATION: 9 **DRAINAGE:** Taking or letting out fluids and/or gases from a body part

9: DRAINAGE · **M: BURSAE AND LIGAMENTS** · **Ø: M/S**

Body Part	Approach	Device	Qualifier
Ø Head and Neck Bursa and Ligament 1 Shoulder Bursa and Ligament, Right 2 Shoulder Bursa and Ligament, Left 3 Elbow Bursa and Ligament, Right 4 Elbow Bursa and Ligament, Left 5 Wrist Bursa and Ligament, Right 6 Wrist Bursa and Ligament, Left 7 Hand Bursa and Ligament, Right 8 Hand Bursa and Ligament, Left 9 Upper Extremity Bursa and Ligament, Right B Upper Extremity Bursa and Ligament, Left C Upper Spine Bursa and Ligament D Lower Spine Bursa and Ligament F Sternum Bursa and Ligament G Rib(s) Bursa and Ligament H Abdomen Bursa and Ligament, Right J Abdomen Bursa and Ligament, Left K Perineum Bursa and Ligament L Hip Bursa and Ligament, Right M Hip Bursa and Ligament, Left N Knee Bursa and Ligament, Right P Knee Bursa and Ligament, Left Q Ankle Bursa and Ligament, Right R Ankle Bursa and Ligament, Left S Foot Bursa and Ligament, Right T Foot Bursa and Ligament, Left V Lower Extremity Bursa and Ligament, Right W Lower Extremity Bursa and Ligament, Left	Ø Open 3 Percutaneous 4 Percutaneous Endoscopic	Ø Drainage Device	Z No Qualifier
Ø Head and Neck Bursa and Ligament 1 Shoulder Bursa and Ligament, Right 2 Shoulder Bursa and Ligament, Left 3 Elbow Bursa and Ligament, Right 4 Elbow Bursa and Ligament, Left 5 Wrist Bursa and Ligament, Right 6 Wrist Bursa and Ligament, Left 7 Hand Bursa and Ligament, Right 8 Hand Bursa and Ligament, Left 9 Upper Extremity Bursa and Ligament, Right B Upper Extremity Bursa and Ligament, Left C Upper Spine Bursa and Ligament D Lower Spine Bursa and Ligament F Sternum Bursa and Ligament G Rib(s) Bursa and Ligament H Abdomen Bursa and Ligament, Right J Abdomen Bursa and Ligament, Left K Perineum Bursa and Ligament L Hip Bursa and Ligament, Right M Hip Bursa and Ligament, Left N Knee Bursa and Ligament, Right P Knee Bursa and Ligament, Left Q Ankle Bursa and Ligament, Right R Ankle Bursa and Ligament, Left S Foot Bursa and Ligament, Right T Foot Bursa and Ligament, Left V Lower Extremity Bursa and Ligament, Right W Lower Extremity Bursa and Ligament, Left	Ø Open 3 Percutaneous 4 Percutaneous Endoscopic	Z No Device	X Diagnostic Z No Qualifier

SECTION: Ø MEDICAL AND SURGICAL
BODY SYSTEM: M BURSAE AND LIGAMENTS
OPERATION: B EXCISION: Cutting out or off, without replacement, a portion of a body part

Body Part	Approach	Device	Qualifier
Ø Head and Neck Bursa and Ligament 1 Shoulder Bursa and Ligament, Right 2 Shoulder Bursa and Ligament, Left 3 Elbow Bursa and Ligament, Right 4 Elbow Bursa and Ligament, Left 5 Wrist Bursa and Ligament, Right 6 Wrist Bursa and Ligament, Left 7 Hand Bursa and Ligament, Right 8 Hand Bursa and Ligament, Left 9 Upper Extremity Bursa and Ligament, Right B Upper Extremity Bursa and Ligament, Left C Upper Spine Bursa and Ligament D Lower Spine Bursa and Ligament F Sternum Bursa and Ligament G Rib(s) Bursa and Ligament H Abdomen Bursa and Ligament, Right J Abdomen Bursa and Ligament, Left K Perineum Bursa and Ligament L Hip Bursa and Ligament, Right M Hip Bursa and Ligament, Left N Knee Bursa and Ligament, Right P Knee Bursa and Ligament, Left Q Ankle Bursa and Ligament, Right R Ankle Bursa and Ligament, Left S Foot Bursa and Ligament, Right T Foot Bursa and Ligament, Left V Lower Extremity Bursa and Ligament, Right W Lower Extremity Bursa and Ligament, Left	Ø Open 3 Percutaneous 4 Percutaneous Endoscopic	Z No Device	X Diagnostic Z No Qualifier

SECTION: Ø MEDICAL AND SURGICAL
BODY SYSTEM: M BURSAE AND LIGAMENTS
OPERATION: C EXTIRPATION: Taking or cutting out solid matter from a body part

Body Part	Approach	Device	Qualifier
Ø Head and Neck Bursa and Ligament 1 Shoulder Bursa and Ligament, Right 2 Shoulder Bursa and Ligament, Left 3 Elbow Bursa and Ligament, Right 4 Elbow Bursa and Ligament, Left 5 Wrist Bursa and Ligament, Right 6 Wrist Bursa and Ligament, Left 7 Hand Bursa and Ligament, Right 8 Hand Bursa and Ligament, Left 9 Upper Extremity Bursa and Ligament, Right B Upper Extremity Bursa and Ligament, Left C Upper Spine Bursa and Ligament D Lower Spine Bursa and Ligament F Sternum Bursa and Ligament G Rib(s) Bursa and Ligament H Abdomen Bursa and Ligament, Right J Abdomen Bursa and Ligament, Left K Perineum Bursa and Ligament L Hip Bursa and Ligament, Right M Hip Bursa and Ligament, Left N Knee Bursa and Ligament, Right P Knee Bursa and Ligament, Left Q Ankle Bursa and Ligament, Right R Ankle Bursa and Ligament, Left S Foot Bursa and Ligament, Right T Foot Bursa and Ligament, Left V Lower Extremity Bursa and Ligament, Right W Lower Extremity Bursa and Ligament, Left	Ø Open 3 Percutaneous 4 Percutaneous Endoscopic	Z No Device	Z No Qualifier

SECTION: Ø MEDICAL AND SURGICAL
BODY SYSTEM: M BURSAE AND LIGAMENTS
OPERATION: D EXTRACTION: Pulling or stripping out or off all or a portion of a body part by the use of force

Body Part	Approach	Device	Qualifier
Ø Head and Neck Bursa and Ligament 1 Shoulder Bursa and Ligament, Right 2 Shoulder Bursa and Ligament, Left 3 Elbow Bursa and Ligament, Right 4 Elbow Bursa and Ligament, Left 5 Wrist Bursa and Ligament, Right 6 Wrist Bursa and Ligament, Left 7 Hand Bursa and Ligament, Right 8 Hand Bursa and Ligament, Left 9 Upper Extremity Bursa and Ligament, Right B Upper Extremity Bursa and Ligament, Left C Upper Spine Bursa and Ligament D Lower Spine Bursa and Ligament F Sternum Bursa and Ligament G Rib(s) Bursa and Ligament H Abdomen Bursa and Ligament, Right J Abdomen Bursa and Ligament, Left K Perineum Bursa and Ligament L Hip Bursa and Ligament, Right M Hip Bursa and Ligament, Left N Knee Bursa and Ligament, Right P Knee Bursa and Ligament, Left Q Ankle Bursa and Ligament, Right R Ankle Bursa and Ligament, Left S Foot Bursa and Ligament, Right T Foot Bursa and Ligament, Left V Lower Extremity Bursa and Ligament, Right W Lower Extremity Bursa and Ligament, Left	Ø Open 3 Percutaneous 4 Percutaneous Endoscopic	Z No Device	Z No Qualifier

SECTION: Ø MEDICAL AND SURGICAL
BODY SYSTEM: M BURSAE AND LIGAMENTS
OPERATION: H INSERTION: Putting in a nonbiological appliance that monitors, assists, performs, or prevents a physiological function but does not physically take the place of a body part

Body Part	Approach	Device	Qualifier
X Upper Bursa and Ligament Y Lower Bursa and Ligament	Ø Open 3 Percutaneous 4 Percutaneous Endoscopic	Y Other Device	Z No Qualifier

SECTION: Ø MEDICAL AND SURGICAL
BODY SYSTEM: M BURSAE AND LIGAMENTS
OPERATION: J INSPECTION: Visually and/or manually exploring a body part

Body Part	Approach	Device	Qualifier
X Upper Bursa and Ligament Y Lower Bursa and Ligament	Ø Open 3 Percutaneous 4 Percutaneous Endoscopic X External	Z No Device	Z No Qualifier

SECTION: Ø MEDICAL AND SURGICAL
BODY SYSTEM: M BURSAE AND LIGAMENTS
OPERATION: M REATTACHMENT: Putting back in or on all or a portion of a separated body part to its normal location or other suitable location

Body Part	Approach	Device	Qualifier
Ø Head and Neck Bursa and Ligament 1 Shoulder Bursa and Ligament, Right 2 Shoulder Bursa and Ligament, Left 3 Elbow Bursa and Ligament, Right 4 Elbow Bursa and Ligament, Left 5 Wrist Bursa and Ligament, Right 6 Wrist Bursa and Ligament, Left 7 Hand Bursa and Ligament, Right 8 Hand Bursa and Ligament, Left 9 Upper Extremity Bursa and Ligament, Right B Upper Extremity Bursa and Ligament, Left C Upper Spine Bursa and Ligament D Lower Spine Bursa and Ligament F Sternum Bursa and Ligament G Rib(s) Bursa and Ligament H Abdomen Bursa and Ligament, Right J Abdomen Bursa and Ligament, Left K Perineum Bursa and Ligament L Hip Bursa and Ligament, Right M Hip Bursa and Ligament, Left N Knee Bursa and Ligament, Right P Knee Bursa and Ligament, Left Q Ankle Bursa and Ligament, Right R Ankle Bursa and Ligament, Left S Foot Bursa and Ligament, Right T Foot Bursa and Ligament, Left V Lower Extremity Bursa and Ligament, Right W Lower Extremity Bursa and Ligament, Left	Ø Open 4 Percutaneous Endoscopic	Z No Device	Z No Qualifier

SECTION: Ø MEDICAL AND SURGICAL
BODY SYSTEM: M BURSAE AND LIGAMENTS
OPERATION: N RELEASE: Freeing a body part from an abnormal physical constraint by cutting or by the use of force

Body Part	Approach	Device	Qualifier
Ø Head and Neck Bursa and Ligament 1 Shoulder Bursa and Ligament, Right 2 Shoulder Bursa and Ligament, Left 3 Elbow Bursa and Ligament, Right 4 Elbow Bursa and Ligament, Left 5 Wrist Bursa and Ligament, Right 6 Wrist Bursa and Ligament, Left 7 Hand Bursa and Ligament, Right 8 Hand Bursa and Ligament, Left 9 Upper Extremity Bursa and Ligament, Right B Upper Extremity Bursa and Ligament, Left C Upper Spine Bursa and Ligament D Lower Spine Bursa and Ligament F Sternum Bursa and Ligament G Rib(s) Bursa and Ligament H Abdomen Bursa and Ligament, Right J Abdomen Bursa and Ligament, Left K Perineum Bursa and Ligament L Hip Bursa and Ligament, Right M Hip Bursa and Ligament, Left N Knee Bursa and Ligament, Right P Knee Bursa and Ligament, Left Q Ankle Bursa and Ligament, Right R Ankle Bursa and Ligament, Left S Foot Bursa and Ligament, Right T Foot Bursa and Ligament, Left V Lower Extremity Bursa and Ligament, Right W Lower Extremity Bursa and Ligament, Left	Ø Open 3 Percutaneous 4 Percutaneous Endoscopic X External	Z No Device	Z No Qualifier

SECTION: Ø MEDICAL AND SURGICAL
BODY SYSTEM: M BURSAE AND LIGAMENTS
OPERATION: P REMOVAL: Taking out or off a device from a body part

Body Part	Approach	Device	Qualifier
X Upper Bursa and Ligament Y Lower Bursa and Ligament	Ø Open 3 Percutaneous 4 Percutaneous Endoscopic	Ø Drainage Device 7 Autologous Tissue Substitute J Synthetic Substitute K Nonautologous Tissue Substitute Y Other Device	Z No Qualifier
X Upper Bursa and Ligament Y Lower Bursa and Ligament	X External	Ø Drainage Device	Z No Qualifier

SECTION: Ø MEDICAL AND SURGICAL
BODY SYSTEM: M BURSAE AND LIGAMENTS
OPERATION: Q **REPAIR:** Restoring, to the extent possible, a body part to its normal anatomic structure and function

Body Part	Approach	Device	Qualifier
Ø Head and Neck Bursa and Ligament 1 Shoulder Bursa and Ligament, Right 2 Shoulder Bursa and Ligament, Left 3 Elbow Bursa and Ligament, Right 4 Elbow Bursa and Ligament, Left 5 Wrist Bursa and Ligament, Right 6 Wrist Bursa and Ligament, Left 7 Hand Bursa and Ligament, Right 8 Hand Bursa and Ligament, Left 9 Upper Extremity Bursa and Ligament, Right B Upper Extremity Bursa and Ligament, Left C Upper Spine Bursa and Ligament D Lower Spine Bursa and Ligament F Sternum Bursa and Ligament G Rib(s) Bursa and Ligament H Abdomen Bursa and Ligament, Right J Abdomen Bursa and Ligament, Left K Perineum Bursa and Ligament L Hip Bursa and Ligament, Right M Hip Bursa and Ligament, Left N Knee Bursa and Ligament, Right P Knee Bursa and Ligament, Left Q Ankle Bursa and Ligament, Right R Ankle Bursa and Ligament, Left S Foot Bursa and Ligament, Right T Foot Bursa and Ligament, Left V Lower Extremity Bursa and Ligament, Right W Lower Extremity Bursa and Ligament, Left	Ø Open 3 Percutaneous 4 Percutaneous Endoscopic	Z No Device	Z No Qualifier

SECTION: Ø MEDICAL AND SURGICAL
BODY SYSTEM: M BURSAE AND LIGAMENTS
OPERATION: R REPLACEMENT: Putting in or on biological or synthetic material that physically takes the place and/or function of all or a portion of a body part

Body Part	Approach	Device	Qualifier
Ø Head and Neck Bursa and Ligament	Ø Open	7 Autologous Tissue Substitute	Z No Qualifier
1 Shoulder Bursa and Ligament, Right	4 Percutaneous Endoscopic	J Synthetic Substitute	
2 Shoulder Bursa and Ligament, Left		K Nonautologous Tissue Substitute	
3 Elbow Bursa and Ligament, Right			
4 Elbow Bursa and Ligament, Left			
5 Wrist Bursa and Ligament, Right			
6 Wrist Bursa and Ligament, Left			
7 Hand Bursa and Ligament, Right			
8 Hand Bursa and Ligament, Left			
9 Upper Extremity Bursa and Ligament, Right			
B Upper Extremity Bursa and Ligament, Left			
C Upper Spine Bursa and Ligament			
D Lower Spine Bursa and Ligament			
F Sternum Bursa and Ligament			
G Rib(s) Bursa and Ligament			
H Abdomen Bursa and Ligament, Right			
J Abdomen Bursa and Ligament, Left			
K Perineum Bursa and Ligament			
L Hip Bursa and Ligament, Right			
M Hip Bursa and Ligament, Left			
N Knee Bursa and Ligament, Right			
P Knee Bursa and Ligament, Left			
Q Ankle Bursa and Ligament, Right			
R Ankle Bursa and Ligament, Left			
S Foot Bursa and Ligament, Right			
T Foot Bursa and Ligament, Left			
V Lower Extremity Bursa and Ligament, Right			
W Lower Extremity Bursa and Ligament, Left			

Ø: M/S

M: BURSAE AND LIGAMENTS

R: REPLACEMENT

SECTION: Ø MEDICAL AND SURGICAL
BODY SYSTEM: M BURSAE AND LIGAMENTS
OPERATION: S REPOSITION: Moving to its normal location, or other suitable location, all or a portion of a body part

Body Part	Approach	Device	Qualifier
Ø Head and Neck Bursa and Ligament 1 Shoulder Bursa and Ligament, Right 2 Shoulder Bursa and Ligament, Left 3 Elbow Bursa and Ligament, Right 4 Elbow Bursa and Ligament, Left 5 Wrist Bursa and Ligament, Right 6 Wrist Bursa and Ligament, Left 7 Hand Bursa and Ligament, Right 8 Hand Bursa and Ligament, Left 9 Upper Extremity Bursa and Ligament, Right B Upper Extremity Bursa and Ligament, Left C Upper Spine Bursa and Ligament D Lower Spine Bursa and Ligament F Sternum Bursa and Ligament G Rib(s) Bursa and Ligament H Abdomen Bursa and Ligament, Right J Abdomen Bursa and Ligament, Left K Perineum Bursa and Ligament L Hip Bursa and Ligament, Right M Hip Bursa and Ligament, Left N Knee Bursa and Ligament, Right P Knee Bursa and Ligament, Left Q Ankle Bursa and Ligament, Right R Ankle Bursa and Ligament, Left S Foot Bursa and Ligament, Right T Foot Bursa and Ligament, Left V Lower Extremity Bursa and Ligament, Right W Lower Extremity Bursa and Ligament, Left	Ø Open 4 Percutaneous Endoscopic	Z No Device	Z No Qualifier

SECTION: Ø MEDICAL AND SURGICAL
BODY SYSTEM: M BURSAE AND LIGAMENTS
OPERATION: T RESECTION: Cutting out or off, without replacement, all of a body part

Body Part	Approach	Device	Qualifier
Ø Head and Neck Bursa and Ligament	Ø Open	Z No Device	Z No Qualifier
1 Shoulder Bursa and Ligament, Right	4 Percutaneous Endoscopic		
2 Shoulder Bursa and Ligament, Left			
3 Elbow Bursa and Ligament, Right			
4 Elbow Bursa and Ligament, Left			
5 Wrist Bursa and Ligament, Right			
6 Wrist Bursa and Ligament, Left			
7 Hand Bursa and Ligament, Right			
8 Hand Bursa and Ligament, Left			
9 Upper Extremity Bursa and Ligament, Right			
B Upper Extremity Bursa and Ligament, Left			
C Upper Spine Bursa and Ligament			
D Lower Spine Bursa and Ligament			
F Sternum Bursa and Ligament			
G Rib(s) Bursa and Ligament			
H Abdomen Bursa and Ligament, Right			
J Abdomen Bursa and Ligament, Left			
K Perineum Bursa and Ligament			
L Hip Bursa and Ligament, Right			
M Hip Bursa and Ligament, Left			
N Knee Bursa and Ligament, Right			
P Knee Bursa and Ligament, Left			
Q Ankle Bursa and Ligament, Right			
R Ankle Bursa and Ligament, Left			
S Foot Bursa and Ligament, Right			
T Foot Bursa and Ligament, Left			
V Lower Extremity Bursa and Ligament, Right			
W Lower Extremity Bursa and Ligament, Left			

SECTION: Ø MEDICAL AND SURGICAL
BODY SYSTEM: M BURSAE AND LIGAMENTS
OPERATION: **U SUPPLEMENT:** Putting in or on biological or synthetic material that physically reinforces and/or augments the function of a portion of a body part

Body Part	Approach	Device	Qualifier
Ø Head and Neck Bursa and Ligament 1 Shoulder Bursa and Ligament, Right 2 Shoulder Bursa and Ligament, Left 3 Elbow Bursa and Ligament, Right 4 Elbow Bursa and Ligament, Left 5 Wrist Bursa and Ligament, Right 6 Wrist Bursa and Ligament, Left 7 Hand Bursa and Ligament, Right 8 Hand Bursa and Ligament, Left 9 Upper Extremity Bursa and Ligament, Right B Upper Extremity Bursa and Ligament, Left C Upper Spine Bursa and Ligament D Lower Spine Bursa and Ligament F Sternum Bursa and Ligament G Rib(s) Bursa and Ligament H Abdomen Bursa and Ligament, Right J Abdomen Bursa and Ligament, Left K Perineum Bursa and Ligament L Hip Bursa and Ligament, Right M Hip Bursa and Ligament, Left N Knee Bursa and Ligament, Right P Knee Bursa and Ligament, Left Q Ankle Bursa and Ligament, Right R Ankle Bursa and Ligament, Left S Foot Bursa and Ligament, Right T Foot Bursa and Ligament, Left V Lower Extremity Bursa and Ligament, Right W Lower Extremity Bursa and Ligament, Left	Ø Open 4 Percutaneous Endoscopic	7 Autologous Tissue Substitute J Synthetic Substitute K Nonautologous Tissue Substitute	Z No Qualifier

SECTION: Ø MEDICAL AND SURGICAL
BODY SYSTEM: M BURSAE AND LIGAMENTS
OPERATION: **W REVISION:** Correcting, to the extent possible, a portion of a malfunctioning device or the position of a displaced device

Body Part	Approach	Device	Qualifier
X Upper Bursa and Ligament Y Lower Bursa and Ligament	Ø Open 3 Percutaneous 4 Percutaneous Endoscopic X External	Ø Drainage Device 7 Autologous Tissue Substitute J Synthetic Substitute K Nonautologous Tissue Substitute Y Other Device	Z No Qualifier
X Upper Bursa and Ligament Y Lower Bursa and Ligament	X External	Ø Drainage Device 7 Autologous Tissue Substitute J Synthetic Substitute K Nonautologous Tissue Substitute	Z No Qualifier

New/Revised Text in Blue   ~~deleted~~ Deleted

SECTION: Ø MEDICAL AND SURGICAL
BODY SYSTEM: M BURSAE AND LIGAMENTS
OPERATION: X TRANSFER: Moving, without taking out, all or a portion of a body part to another location to take over the function of all or a portion of a body part

Body Part	Approach	Device	Qualifier
Ø Head and Neck Bursa and Ligament 1 Shoulder Bursa and Ligament, Right 2 Shoulder Bursa and Ligament, Left 3 Elbow Bursa and Ligament, Right 4 Elbow Bursa and Ligament, Left 5 Wrist Bursa and Ligament, Right 6 Wrist Bursa and Ligament, Left 7 Hand Bursa and Ligament, Right 8 Hand Bursa and Ligament, Left 9 Upper Extremity Bursa and Ligament, Right B Upper Extremity Bursa and Ligament, Left C Upper Spine Bursa and Ligament D Lower Spine Bursa and Ligament F Sternum Bursa and Ligament G Rib(s) Bursa and Ligament H Abdomen Bursa and Ligament, Right J Abdomen Bursa and Ligament, Left K Perineum Bursa and Ligament L Hip Bursa and Ligament, Right M Hip Bursa and Ligament, Left N Knee Bursa and Ligament, Right P Knee Bursa and Ligament, Left Q Ankle Bursa and Ligament, Right R Ankle Bursa and Ligament, Left S Foot Bursa and Ligament, Right T Foot Bursa and Ligament, Left V Lower Extremity Bursa and Ligament, Right W Lower Extremity Bursa and Ligament, Left	Ø Open 4 Percutaneous Endoscopic	Z No Device	Z No Qualifier

ØN. Head and Facial Bones 338
    ØN2. Change 339
    ØN5. Destruction 339
    ØN8. Division 34Ø
    ØN9. Drainage 341
    ØNB. Excision 342
    ØNC. Extirpation 343
    ØND. Extraction 344
    ØNH. Insertion 345
    ØNJ. Inspection 346
    ØNN. Release 346
    ØNP. Removal 347
    ØNQ. Repair 348
    ØNR. Replacement 349
    ØNS. Reposition 349
    ØNT. Resection 351
    ØNU. Supplement 352
    ØNW. Revision 353

SECTION: 0 MEDICAL AND SURGICAL
BODY SYSTEM: N HEAD AND FACIAL BONES
OPERATION: 2 CHANGE: Taking out or off a device from a body part and putting back an identical or similar device in or on the same body part without cutting or puncturing the skin or a mucous membrane

Body Part	Approach	Device	Qualifier
0 Skull B Nasal Bone W Facial Bone	X External	0 Drainage Device Y Other Device	Z No Qualifier

SECTION: 0 MEDICAL AND SURGICAL
BODY SYSTEM: N HEAD AND FACIAL BONES
OPERATION: 5 DESTRUCTION: Physical eradication of all or a portion of a body part by the direct use of energy, force, or a destructive agent

Body Part	Approach	Device	Qualifier
0 Skull 1 Frontal Bone 2 Frontal Bone, Left 3 Parietal Bone, Right 4 Parietal Bone, Left 5 Temporal Bone, Right 6 Temporal Bone, Left 7 Occipital Bone 8 Occipital Bone, Left B Nasal Bone C Sphenoid Bone D Sphenoid Bone, Left F Ethmoid Bone, Right G Ethmoid Bone, Left H Lacrimal Bone, Right J Lacrimal Bone, Left K Palatine Bone, Right L Palatine Bone, Left M Zygomatic Bone, Right N Zygomatic Bone, Left P Orbit, Right Q Orbit, Left R Maxilla S Maxilla, Left T Mandible, Right V Mandible, Left X Hyoid Bone	0 Open 3 Percutaneous 4 Percutaneous Endoscopic	Z No Device	Z No Qualifier

SECTION: Ø MEDICAL AND SURGICAL
BODY SYSTEM: N HEAD AND FACIAL BONES
OPERATION: 8 DIVISION: Cutting into a body part, without draining fluids and/or gases from the body part, in order to separate or transect a body part

Body Part	Approach	Device	Qualifier
Ø Skull	Ø Open	Z No Device	Z No Qualifier
1 Frontal Bone	3 Percutaneous		
2 Frontal Bone, Left	4 Percutaneous Endoscopic		
3 Parietal Bone, Right			
4 Parietal Bone, Left			
5 Temporal Bone, Right			
6 Temporal Bone, Left			
7 Occipital Bone			
8 Occipital Bone, Left			
B Nasal Bone			
C Sphenoid Bone			
D Sphenoid Bone, Left			
F Ethmoid Bone, Right			
G Ethmoid Bone, Left			
H Lacrimal Bone, Right			
J Lacrimal Bone, Left			
K Palatine Bone, Right			
L Palatine Bone, Left			
M Zygomatic Bone, Right			
N Zygomatic Bone, Left			
P Orbit, Right			
Q Orbit, Left			
R Maxilla			
S Maxilla, Left			
T Mandible, Right			
V Mandible, Left			
X Hyoid Bone			

New/Revised Text in Blue   ~~deleted~~ Deleted

SECTION: Ø MEDICAL AND SURGICAL
BODY SYSTEM: N HEAD AND FACIAL BONES
OPERATION: 9 DRAINAGE: Taking or letting out fluids and/or gases from a body part

Body Part	Approach	Device	Qualifier
Ø Skull 1 Frontal Bone 2 Frontal Bone, Left 3 Parietal Bone, Right 4 Parietal Bone, Left 5 Temporal Bone, Right 6 Temporal Bone, Left 7 Occipital Bone 8 Occipital Bone, Left B Nasal Bone C Sphenoid Bone D Sphenoid Bone, Left F Ethmoid Bone, Right G Ethmoid Bone, Left H Lacrimal Bone, Right J Lacrimal Bone, Left K Palatine Bone, Right L Palatine Bone, Left M Zygomatic Bone, Right N Zygomatic Bone, Left P Orbit, Right Q Orbit, Left R Maxilla S Maxilla, Left T Mandible, Right V Mandible, Left X Hyoid Bone	Ø Open 3 Percutaneous 4 Percutaneous Endoscopic	Ø Drainage Device	Z No Qualifier
Ø Skull 1 Frontal Bone 2 Frontal Bone, Left 3 Parietal Bone, Right 4 Parietal Bone, Left 5 Temporal Bone, Right 6 Temporal Bone, Left 7 Occipital Bone 8 Occipital Bone, Left B Nasal Bone C Sphenoid Bone D Sphenoid Bone, Left F Ethmoid Bone, Right G Ethmoid Bone, Left H Lacrimal Bone, Right J Lacrimal Bone, Left K Palatine Bone, Right L Palatine Bone, Left M Zygomatic Bone, Right N Zygomatic Bone, Left P Orbit, Right Q Orbit, Left R Maxilla S Maxilla, Left T Mandible, Right V Mandible, Left X Hyoid Bone	Ø Open 3 Percutaneous 4 Percutaneous Endoscopic	Z No Device	X Diagnostic Z No Qualifier

SECTION: Ø MEDICAL AND SURGICAL
BODY SYSTEM: N HEAD AND FACIAL BONES
OPERATION: B EXCISION: Cutting out or off, without replacement, a portion of a body part

Body Part	Approach	Device	Qualifier
Ø Skull	Ø Open	Z No Device	X Diagnostic
1 Frontal Bone	3 Percutaneous		Z No Qualifier
2 Frontal Bone, Left	4 Percutaneous Endoscopic		
3 Parietal Bone, Right			
4 Parietal Bone, Left			
5 Temporal Bone, Right			
6 Temporal Bone, Left			
7 Occipital Bone			
8 Occipital Bone, Left			
B Nasal Bone			
C Sphenoid Bone			
D Sphenoid Bone, Left			
F Ethmoid Bone, Right			
G Ethmoid Bone, Left			
H Lacrimal Bone, Right			
J Lacrimal Bone, Left			
K Palatine Bone, Right			
L Palatine Bone, Left			
M Zygomatic Bone, Right			
N Zygomatic Bone, Left			
P Orbit, Right			
Q Orbit, Left			
R Maxilla			
S Maxilla, Left			
T Mandible, Right			
V Mandible, Left			
X Hyoid Bone			

New/Revised Text in Blue ~~deleted~~ Deleted

SECTION: Ø MEDICAL AND SURGICAL
BODY SYSTEM: N HEAD AND FACIAL BONES
OPERATION: C EXTIRPATION: Taking or cutting out solid matter from a body part

Body Part	Approach	Device	Qualifier
1 Frontal Bone 2 Frontal Bone, Left 3 Parietal Bone, Right 4 Parietal Bone, Left 5 Temporal Bone, Right 6 Temporal Bone, Left 7 Occipital Bone 8 Occipital Bone, Left B Nasal Bone C Sphenoid Bone D Sphenoid Bone, Left F Ethmoid Bone, Right G Ethmoid Bone, Left H Lacrimal Bone, Right J Lacrimal Bone, Left K Palatine Bone, Right L Palatine Bone, Left M Zygomatic Bone, Right N Zygomatic Bone, Left P Orbit, Right Q Orbit, Left R Maxilla S Maxilla, Left T Mandible, Right V Mandible, Left X Hyoid Bone	Ø Open 3 Percutaneous 4 Percutaneous Endoscopic	Z No Device	Z No Qualifier

SECTION: Ø MEDICAL AND SURGICAL
BODY SYSTEM: N HEAD AND FACIAL BONES
OPERATION: D EXTRACTION: Pulling or stripping out or off all or a portion of a body part by the use of force

Body Part	Approach	Device	Qualifier
Ø Skull	Ø Open	Z No Device	Z No Qualifier
1 Frontal Bone			
3 Parietal Bone, Right			
4 Parietal Bone, Left			
5 Temporal Bone, Right			
6 Temporal Bone, Left			
7 Occipital Bone			
B Nasal Bone			
C Sphenoid Bone			
F Ethmoid Bone, Right			
G Ethmoid Bone, Left			
H Lacrimal Bone, Right			
J Lacrimal Bone, Left			
K Palatine Bone, Right			
L Palatine Bone, Left			
M Zygomatic Bone, Right			
N Zygomatic Bone, Left			
P Orbit, Right			
Q Orbit, Left			
R Maxilla			
T Mandible, Right			
V Mandible, Left			
X Hyoid Bone			

D: EXTRACTION

N: HEAD AND FACIAL BONES

Ø: M/S

SECTION: Ø MEDICAL AND SURGICAL
BODY SYSTEM: N HEAD AND FACIAL BONES
OPERATION: H INSERTION: Putting in a nonbiological appliance that monitors, assists, performs, or prevents a physiological function but does not physically take the place of a body part

Body Part	Approach	Device	Qualifier
Ø Skull	Ø Open	4 Internal Fixation Device 5 External Fixation Device M Bone Growth Stimulator N Neurostimulator Generator	Z No Qualifier
Ø Skull	3 Percutaneous 4 Percutaneous Endoscopic	4 Internal Fixation Device 5 External Fixation Device M Bone Growth Stimulator	Z No Qualifier
1 Frontal Bone 2 Frontal Bone, Left 3 Parietal Bone, Right 4 Parietal Bone, Left 7 Occipital Bone 8 Occipital Bone, Left C Sphenoid Bone D Sphenoid Bone, Left F Ethmoid Bone, Right G Ethmoid Bone, Left H Lacrimal Bone, Right J Lacrimal Bone, Left K Palatine Bone, Right L Palatine Bone, Left M Zygomatic Bone, Right N Zygomatic Bone, Left P Orbit, Right Q Orbit, Left X Hyoid Bone	Ø Open 3 Percutaneous 4 Percutaneous Endoscopic	4 Internal Fixation Device	Z No Qualifier
5 Temporal Bone, Right 6 Temporal Bone, Left	Ø Open 3 Percutaneous 4 Percutaneous Endoscopic	4 Internal Fixation Device S Hearing Device	Z No Qualifier
B Nasal Bone	Ø Open 3 Percutaneous 4 Percutaneous Endoscopic	4 Internal Fixation Device M Bone Growth Stimulator	Z No Qualifier
R Maxilla S Maxilla, Left T Mandible, Right V Mandible, Left	Ø Open 3 Percutaneous 4 Percutaneous Endoscopic	4 Internal Fixation Device 5 External Fixation Device	Z No Qualifier
W Facial Bone	Ø Open 3 Percutaneous 4 Percutaneous Endoscopic	M Bone Growth Stimulator	Z No Qualifier

SECTION: Ø MEDICAL AND SURGICAL
BODY SYSTEM: N HEAD AND FACIAL BONES
OPERATION: J INSPECTION: Visually and/or manually exploring a body part

Body Part	Approach	Device	Qualifier
Ø Skull B Nasal Bone W Facial Bone	Ø Open 3 Percutaneous 4 Percutaneous Endoscopic X External	Z No Device	Z No Qualifier

SECTION: Ø MEDICAL AND SURGICAL
BODY SYSTEM: N HEAD AND FACIAL BONES
OPERATION: N RELEASE: Freeing a body part from an abnormal physical constraint by cutting or by the use of force

Body Part	Approach	Device	Qualifier
1 Frontal Bone 2 Frontal Bone, Left 3 Parietal Bone, Right 4 Parietal Bone, Left 5 Temporal Bone, Right 6 Temporal Bone, Left 7 Occipital Bone 8 Occipital Bone, Left B Nasal Bone C Sphenoid Bone D Sphenoid Bone, Left F Ethmoid Bone, Right G Ethmoid Bone, Left H Lacrimal Bone, Right J Lacrimal Bone, Left K Palatine Bone, Right L Palatine Bone, Left M Zygomatic Bone, Right N Zygomatic Bone, Left P Orbit, Right Q Orbit, Left R Maxilla S Maxilla, Left T Mandible, Right V Mandible, Left X Hyoid Bone	Ø Open 3 Percutaneous 4 Percutaneous Endoscopic	Z No Device	Z No Qualifier

Side tabs: J: INSPECTION N: RELEASE N: HEAD AND FACIAL BONES Ø: M/S

SECTION: Ø MEDICAL AND SURGICAL
BODY SYSTEM: N HEAD AND FACIAL BONES
OPERATION: P REMOVAL: Taking out or off a device from a body part

Body Part	Approach	Device	Qualifier
Ø Skull	Ø Open	Ø Drainage Device 4 Internal Fixation Device 5 External Fixation Device 7 Autologous Tissue Substitute J Synthetic Substitute K Nonautologous Tissue Substitute M Bone Growth Stimulator N Neurostimulator Generator S Hearing Device	Z No Qualifier
Ø Skull	3 Percutaneous 4 Percutaneous Endoscopic	Ø Drainage Device 4 Internal Fixation Device 5 External Fixation Device 7 Autologous Tissue Substitute J Synthetic Substitute K Nonautologous Tissue Substitute M Bone Growth Stimulator S Hearing Device	Z No Qualifier
Ø Skull	X External	Ø Drainage Device 4 Internal Fixation Device 5 External Fixation Device M Bone Growth Stimulator S Hearing Device	Z No Qualifier
B Nasal Bone W Facial Bone	Ø Open 3 Percutaneous 4 Percutaneous Endoscopic	Ø Drainage Device 4 Internal Fixation Device 7 Autologous Tissue Substitute J Synthetic Substitute K Nonautologous Tissue Substitute M Bone Growth Stimulator	Z No Qualifier
B Nasal Bone W Facial Bone	X External	Ø Drainage Device 4 Internal Fixation Device M Bone Growth Stimulator	Z No Qualifier

SECTION: Ø MEDICAL AND SURGICAL
BODY SYSTEM: N HEAD AND FACIAL BONES
OPERATION: Q REPAIR: Restoring, to the extent possible, a body part to its normal anatomic structure and function

Body Part	Approach	Device	Qualifier
Ø Skull	Ø Open	Z No Device	Z No Qualifier
1 Frontal Bone	3 Percutaneous		
2 Frontal Bone, Left	4 Percutaneous Endoscopic		
3 Parietal Bone, Right	X External		
4 Parietal Bone, Left			
5 Temporal Bone, Right			
6 Temporal Bone, Left			
7 Occipital Bone			
8 Occipital Bone, Left			
B Nasal Bone			
C Sphenoid Bone			
D Sphenoid Bone, Left			
F Ethmoid Bone, Right			
G Ethmoid Bone, Left			
H Lacrimal Bone, Right			
J Lacrimal Bone, Left			
K Palatine Bone, Right			
L Palatine Bone, Left			
M Zygomatic Bone, Right			
N Zygomatic Bone, Left			
P Orbit, Right			
Q Orbit, Left			
R Maxilla			
S Maxilla, Left			
T Mandible, Right			
V Mandible, Left			
X Hyoid Bone			

SECTION: Ø MEDICAL AND SURGICAL
BODY SYSTEM: N HEAD AND FACIAL BONES
OPERATION: R REPLACEMENT: Putting in or on biological or synthetic material that physically takes the place and/or function of all or a portion of a body part

Body Part	Approach	Device	Qualifier
Ø Skull	Ø Open	7 Autologous Tissue Substitute	Z No Qualifier
1 Frontal Bone	3 Percutaneous	J Synthetic Substitute	
2 Frontal Bone, Left	4 Percutaneous Endoscopic	K Nonautologous Tissue	
3 Parietal Bone, Right		Substitute	
4 Parietal Bone, Left			
5 Temporal Bone, Right			
6 Temporal Bone, Left			
7 Occipital Bone			
8 Occipital Bone, Left			
B Nasal Bone			
C Sphenoid Bone			
D Sphenoid Bone, Left			
F Ethmoid Bone, Right			
G Ethmoid Bone, Left			
H Lacrimal Bone, Right			
J Lacrimal Bone, Left			
K Palatine Bone, Right			
L Palatine Bone, Left			
M Zygomatic Bone, Right			
N Zygomatic Bone, Left			
P Orbit, Right			
Q Orbit, Left			
R Maxilla			
S Maxilla, Left			
T Mandible, Right			
V Mandible, Left			
X Hyoid Bone			

SECTION: Ø MEDICAL AND SURGICAL
BODY SYSTEM: N HEAD AND FACIAL BONES
OPERATION: S REPOSITION: *(on multiple pages)*
Moving to its normal location, or other suitable location, all or a portion of a body part

Body Part	Approach	Device	Qualifier
Ø Skull	Ø Open	4 Internal Fixation Device	Z No Qualifier
R Maxilla	3 Percutaneous	5 External Fixation Device	
S Maxilla, Left	4 Percutaneous Endoscopic	Z No Device	
T Mandible, Right			
V Mandible, Left			
Ø Skull	X External	Z No Device	Z No Qualifier
R Maxilla			
S Maxilla, Left			
T Mandible, Right			
V Mandible, Left			

Ø: M/S   N: HEAD AND FACIAL BONES   R: REPLACEMENT   S: REPOSITION

SECTION: Ø **MEDICAL AND SURGICAL**
BODY SYSTEM: N **HEAD AND FACIAL BONES**
OPERATION: S **REPOSITION:** *(continued)*
Moving to its normal location, or other suitable location, all or a portion of a body part

Body Part	Approach	Device	Qualifier
1 Frontal Bone 2 Frontal Bone, Left 3 Parietal Bone, Right 4 Parietal Bone, Left 5 Temporal Bone, Right 6 Temporal Bone, Left 7 Occipital Bone 8 Occipital Bone, Left B Nasal Bone C Sphenoid Bone D Sphenoid Bone, Left F Ethmoid Bone, Right G Ethmoid Bone, Left H Lacrimal Bone, Right J Lacrimal Bone, Left K Palatine Bone, Right L Palatine Bone, Left M Zygomatic Bone, Right N Zygomatic Bone, Left P Orbit, Right Q Orbit, Left X Hyoid Bone	Ø Open 3 Percutaneous 4 Percutaneous Endoscopic	4 Internal Fixation Device Z No Device	Z No Qualifier
1 Frontal Bone 2 Frontal Bone, Left 3 Parietal Bone, Right 4 Parietal Bone, Left 5 Temporal Bone, Right 6 Temporal Bone, Left 7 Occipital Bone 8 Occipital Bone, Left B Nasal Bone C Sphenoid Bone D Sphenoid Bone, Left F Ethmoid Bone, Right G Ethmoid Bone, Left H Lacrimal Bone, Right J Lacrimal Bone, Left K Palatine Bone, Right L Palatine Bone, Left M Zygomatic Bone, Right N Zygomatic Bone, Left P Orbit, Right Q Orbit, Left X Hyoid Bone	X External	Z No Device	Z No Qualifier

S: REPOSITION

N: HEAD AND FACIAL BONES

Ø: M/S

SECTION: Ø MEDICAL AND SURGICAL
BODY SYSTEM: N HEAD AND FACIAL BONES
OPERATION: T **RESECTION:** Cutting out or off, without replacement, all of a body part

Body Part	Approach	Device	Qualifier
1 Frontal Bone	Ø Open	Z No Device	Z No Qualifier
2 Frontal Bone, Left			
3 Parietal Bone, Right			
4 Parietal Bone, Left			
5 Temporal Bone, Right			
6 Temporal Bone, Left			
7 Occipital Bone			
8 Occipital Bone, Left			
B Nasal Bone			
C Sphenoid Bone			
D Sphenoid Bone, Left			
F Ethmoid Bone, Right			
G Ethmoid Bone, Left			
H Lacrimal Bone, Right			
J Lacrimal Bone, Left			
K Palatine Bone, Right			
L Palatine Bone, Left			
M Zygomatic Bone, Right			
N Zygomatic Bone, Left			
P Orbit, Right			
Q Orbit, Left			
R Maxilla			
S Maxilla, Left			
T Mandible, Right			
V Mandible, Left			
X Hyoid Bone			

SECTION: Ø MEDICAL AND SURGICAL
BODY SYSTEM: N HEAD AND FACIAL BONES
OPERATION: U SUPPLEMENT: Putting in or on biological or synthetic material that physically reinforces and/or augments the function of a portion of a body part

Body Part	Approach	Device	Qualifier
Ø Skull	Ø Open	7 Autologous Tissue Substitute	Z No Qualifier
1 Frontal Bone	3 Percutaneous	J Synthetic Substitute	
2 Frontal Bone, Left	4 Percutaneous Endoscopic	K Nonautologous Tissue Substitute	
3 Parietal Bone, Right			
4 Parietal Bone, Left			
5 Temporal Bone, Right			
6 Temporal Bone, Left			
7 Occipital Bone			
8 Occipital Bone, Left			
B Nasal Bone			
C Sphenoid Bone			
D Sphenoid Bone, Left			
F Ethmoid Bone, Right			
G Ethmoid Bone, Left			
H Lacrimal Bone, Right			
J Lacrimal Bone, Left			
K Palatine Bone, Right			
L Palatine Bone, Left			
M Zygomatic Bone, Right			
N Zygomatic Bone, Left			
P Orbit, Right			
Q Orbit, Left			
R Maxilla			
S Maxilla, Left			
T Mandible, Right			
V Mandible, Left			
X Hyoid Bone			

SECTION: Ø MEDICAL AND SURGICAL
BODY SYSTEM: N HEAD AND FACIAL BONES
OPERATION: W REVISION: Correcting, to the extent possible, a portion of a malfunctioning device or the position of a displaced device

Body Part	Approach	Device	Qualifier
Ø Skull	Ø Open	Ø Drainage Device 4 Internal Fixation Device 5 External Fixation Device 7 Autologous Tissue Substitute J Synthetic Substitute K Nonautologous Tissue Substitute M Bone Growth Stimulator N Neurostimulator Generator S Hearing Device	Z No Qualifier
Ø Skull	3 Percutaneous 4 Percutaneous Endoscopic X External	Ø Drainage Device 4 Internal Fixation Device 5 External Fixation Device 7 Autologous Tissue Substitute J Synthetic Substitute K Nonautologous Tissue Substitute M Bone Growth Stimulator S Hearing Device	Z No Qualifier
B Nasal Bone W Facial Bone	Ø Open 3 Percutaneous 4 Percutaneous Endoscopic X External	Ø Drainage Device 4 Internal Fixation Device 7 Autologous Tissue Substitute J Synthetic Substitute K Nonautologous Tissue Substitute M Bone Growth Stimulator	Z No Qualifier

ØP. Upper Bones 354
    ØP2. Change 355
    ØP5. Destruction 355
    ØP8. Division 356
    ØP9. Drainage 357
    ØPB. Excision 358
    ØPC. Extirpation 359
    ØPD. Extraction 36Ø
    ØPH. Insertion 361
    ØPJ. Inspection 362
    ØPN. Release 362
    ØPP. Removal 363
    ØPQ. Repair 365
    ØPR. Replacement 366
    ØPS. Reposition 366
    ØPT. Resection 368
    ØPU. Supplement 369
    ØPW. Revision 37Ø

SECTION: Ø MEDICAL AND SURGICAL
BODY SYSTEM: P UPPER BONES

OPERATION: 2 **CHANGE:** Taking out or off a device from a body part and putting back an identical or similar device in or on the same body part without cutting or puncturing the skin or a mucous membrane

Body Part	Approach	Device	Qualifier
Y Upper Bone	X External	Ø Drainage Device Y Other Device	Z No Qualifier

SECTION: Ø MEDICAL AND SURGICAL
BODY SYSTEM: P UPPER BONES

OPERATION: 5 **DESTRUCTION:** Physical eradication of all or a portion of a body part by the direct use of energy, force, or a destructive agent

Body Part	Approach	Device	Qualifier
Ø Sternum 1 Rib, 1 to 2 2 Rib, 3 or More 3 Cervical Vertebra 4 Thoracic Vertebra 5 Scapula, Right 6 Scapula, Left 7 Glenoid Cavity, Right 8 Glenoid Cavity, Left 9 Clavicle, Right B Clavicle, Left C Humeral Head, Right D Humeral Head, Left F Humeral Shaft, Right G Humeral Shaft, Left H Radius, Right J Radius, Left K Ulna, Right L Ulna, Left M Carpal, Right N Carpal, Left P Metacarpal, Right Q Metacarpal, Left R Thumb Phalanx, Right S Thumb Phalanx, Left T Finger Phalanx, Right V Finger Phalanx, Left	Ø Open 3 Percutaneous 4 Percutaneous Endoscopic	Z No Device	Z No Qualifier

Ø: M/S   P: UPPER BONES   2: CHANGE   5: DESTRUCTION

SECTION: Ø MEDICAL AND SURGICAL
BODY SYSTEM: P UPPER BONES
OPERATION: 8 DIVISION: Cutting into a body part, without draining fluids and/or gases from the body part, in order to separate or transect a body part

Body Part	Approach	Device	Qualifier
Ø Sternum 1 Rib, 1 to 2 2 Rib, 3 or More 3 Cervical Vertebra 4 Thoracic Vertebra 5 Scapula, Right 6 Scapula, Left 7 Glenoid Cavity, Right 8 Glenoid Cavity, Left 9 Clavicle, Right B Clavicle, Left C Humeral Head, Right D Humeral Head, Left F Humeral Shaft, Right G Humeral Shaft, Left H Radius, Right J Radius, Left K Ulna, Right L Ulna, Left M Carpal, Right N Carpal, Left P Metacarpal, Right Q Metacarpal, Left R Thumb Phalanx, Right S Thumb Phalanx, Left T Finger Phalanx, Right V Finger Phalanx, Left	Ø Open 3 Percutaneous 4 Percutaneous Endoscopic	Z No Device	Z No Qualifier

SECTION: Ø MEDICAL AND SURGICAL
BODY SYSTEM: P UPPER BONES
OPERATION: 9 DRAINAGE: Taking or letting out fluids and/or gases from a body part

Body Part	Approach	Device	Qualifier
Ø Sternum 1 Rib, 1 to 2 2 Rib, 3 or More 3 Cervical Vertebra 4 Thoracic Vertebra 5 Scapula, Right 6 Scapula, Left 7 Glenoid Cavity, Right 8 Glenoid Cavity, Left 9 Clavicle, Right B Clavicle, Left C Humeral Head, Right D Humeral Head, Left F Humeral Shaft, Right G Humeral Shaft, Left H Radius, Right J Radius, Left K Ulna, Right L Ulna, Left M Carpal, Right N Carpal, Left P Metacarpal, Right Q Metacarpal, Left R Thumb Phalanx, Right S Thumb Phalanx, Left T Finger Phalanx, Right V Finger Phalanx, Left	Ø Open 3 Percutaneous 4 Percutaneous Endoscopic	Ø Drainage Device	Z No Qualifier
Ø Sternum 1 Rib, 1 to 2 2 Rib, 3 or More 3 Cervical Vertebra 4 Thoracic Vertebra 5 Scapula, Right 6 Scapula, Left 7 Glenoid Cavity, Right 8 Glenoid Cavity, Left 9 Clavicle, Right B Clavicle, Left C Humeral Head, Right D Humeral Head, Left F Humeral Shaft, Right G Humeral Shaft, Left H Radius, Right J Radius, Left K Ulna, Right L Ulna, Left M Carpal, Right N Carpal, Left P Metacarpal, Right Q Metacarpal, Left R Thumb Phalanx, Right S Thumb Phalanx, Left T Finger Phalanx, Right V Finger Phalanx, Left	Ø Open 3 Percutaneous 4 Percutaneous Endoscopic	Z No Device	X Diagnostic Z No Qualifier

SECTION: Ø MEDICAL AND SURGICAL
BODY SYSTEM: P UPPER BONES
OPERATION: B **EXCISION:** Cutting out or off, without replacement, a portion of a body part

Body Part	Approach	Device	Qualifier
Ø Sternum 1 Rib, 1 to 2 2 Rib, 3 or More 3 Cervical Vertebra 4 Thoracic Vertebra 5 Scapula, Right 6 Scapula, Left 7 Glenoid Cavity, Right 8 Glenoid Cavity, Left 9 Clavicle, Right B Clavicle, Left C Humeral Head, Right D Humeral Head, Left F Humeral Shaft, Right G Humeral Shaft, Left H Radius, Right J Radius, Left K Ulna, Right L Ulna, Left M Carpal, Right N Carpal, Left P Metacarpal, Right Q Metacarpal, Left R Thumb Phalanx, Right S Thumb Phalanx, Left T Finger Phalanx, Right V Finger Phalanx, Left	Ø Open 3 Percutaneous 4 Percutaneous Endoscopic	Z No Device	X Diagnostic Z No Qualifier

B: EXCISION
P: UPPER BONES
Ø: M/S

SECTION: Ø MEDICAL AND SURGICAL
BODY SYSTEM: P UPPER BONES
OPERATION: **C EXTIRPATION:** Taking or cutting out solid matter from a body part

Body Part	Approach	Device	Qualifier
Ø Sternum	Ø Open	Z No Device	Z No Qualifier
1 Rib, 1 to 2	3 Percutaneous		
2 Rib, 3 or More	4 Percutaneous Endoscopic		
3 Cervical Vertebra			
4 Thoracic Vertebra			
5 Scapula, Right			
6 Scapula, Left			
7 Glenoid Cavity, Right			
8 Glenoid Cavity, Left			
9 Clavicle, Right			
B Clavicle, Left			
C Humeral Head, Right			
D Humeral Head, Left			
F Humeral Shaft, Right			
G Humeral Shaft, Left			
H Radius, Right			
J Radius, Left			
K Ulna, Right			
L Ulna, Left			
M Carpal, Right			
N Carpal, Left			
P Metacarpal, Right			
Q Metacarpal, Left			
R Thumb Phalanx, Right			
S Thumb Phalanx, Left			
T Finger Phalanx, Right			
V Finger Phalanx, Left			

SECTION: Ø MEDICAL AND SURGICAL
BODY SYSTEM: P UPPER BONES
OPERATION: D **EXTRACTION:** Pulling or stripping out or off all or a portion of a body part by the use of force

Body Part	Approach	Device	Qualifier
Ø Sternum	Ø Open	Z No Device	Z No Qualifier
1 Rib, 1 to 2			
2 Rib, 3 or More			
3 Cervical Vertebra			
4 Thoracic Vertebra			
5 Scapula, Right			
6 Scapula, Left			
7 Glenoid Cavity, Right			
8 Glenoid Cavity, Left			
9 Clavicle, Right			
B Clavicle, Left			
C Humeral Head, Right			
D Humeral Head, Left			
F Humeral Shaft, Right			
G Humeral Shaft, Left			
H Radius, Right			
J Radius, Left			
K Ulna, Right			
L Ulna, Left			
M Carpal, Right			
N Carpal, Left			
P Metacarpal, Right			
Q Metacarpal, Left			
R Thumb Phalanx, Right			
S Thumb Phalanx, Left			
T Finger Phalanx, Right			
V Finger Phalanx, Left			

New/Revised Text in Blue ~~deleted~~ Deleted

SECTION: Ø MEDICAL AND SURGICAL
BODY SYSTEM: P UPPER BONES

OPERATION: H INSERTION: Putting in a nonbiological appliance that monitors, assists, performs, or prevents a physiological function but does not physically take the place of a body part

Body Part	Approach	Device	Qualifier
Ø Sternum	Ø Open 3 Percutaneous 4 Percutaneous Endoscopic	Ø Internal Fixation Device, Rigid Plate 4 Internal Fixation Device	Z No Qualifier
1 Rib, 1 to 2 2 Rib, 3 or More 3 Cervical Vertebra 4 Thoracic Vertebra 5 Scapula, Right 6 Scapula, Left 7 Glenoid Cavity, Right 8 Glenoid Cavity, Left 9 Clavicle, Right B Clavicle, Left	Ø Open 3 Percutaneous 4 Percutaneous Endoscopic	4 Internal Fixation Device	Z No Qualifier
C Humeral Head, Right D Humeral Head, Left F Humeral Shaft, Right G Humeral Shaft, Left H Radius, Right J Radius, Left K Ulna, Right L Ulna, Left	Ø Open 3 Percutaneous 4 Percutaneous Endoscopic	4 Internal Fixation Device 5 External Fixation Device 6 Internal Fixation Device, Intramedullary 8 External Fixation Device, Limb Lengthening B External Fixation Device, Monoplanar C External Fixation Device, Ring D External Fixation Device, Hybrid	Z No Qualifier
M Carpal, Right N Carpal, Left P Metacarpal, Right Q Metacarpal, Left R Thumb Phalanx, Right S Thumb Phalanx, Left T Finger Phalanx, Right V Finger Phalanx, Left	Ø Open 3 Percutaneous 4 Percutaneous Endoscopic	4 Internal Fixation Device 5 External Fixation Device	Z No Qualifier
Y Upper Bone	Ø Open 3 Percutaneous 4 Percutaneous Endoscopic	M Bone Growth Stimulator	Z No Qualifier
Y Upper Bone	Ø Open 3 Percutaneous 4 Percutaneous Endoscopic X External	Z No Device	Z No Qualifier

SECTION: Ø MEDICAL AND SURGICAL
BODY SYSTEM: **P UPPER BONES**
OPERATION: **J INSPECTION:** Visually and/or manually exploring a body part

Body Part	Approach	Device	Qualifier
Y Upper Bone	Ø Open 3 Percutaneous 4 Percutaneous Endoscopic X External	Z No Device	Z No Qualifier

SECTION: Ø MEDICAL AND SURGICAL
BODY SYSTEM: **P UPPER BONES**
OPERATION: **N RELEASE:** Freeing a body part from an abnormal physical constraint by cutting or by the use of force

Body Part	Approach	Device	Qualifier
Ø Sternum 1 Rib, 1 to 2 2 Rib, 3 or More 3 Cervical Vertebra 4 Thoracic Vertebra 5 Scapula, Right 6 Scapula, Left 7 Glenoid Cavity, Right 8 Glenoid Cavity, Left 9 Clavicle, Right B Clavicle, Left C Humeral Head, Right D Humeral Head, Left F Humeral Shaft, Right G Humeral Shaft, Left H Radius, Right J Radius, Left K Ulna, Right L Ulna, Left M Carpal, Right N Carpal, Left P Metacarpal, Right Q Metacarpal, Left R Thumb Phalanx, Right S Thumb Phalanx, Left T Finger Phalanx, Right V Finger Phalanx, Left	Ø Open 3 Percutaneous 4 Percutaneous Endoscopic	Z No Device	Z No Qualifier

New/Revised Text in Blue   ~~deleted~~ Deleted

SECTION: Ø MEDICAL AND SURGICAL
BODY SYSTEM: P UPPER BONES
OPERATION: P REMOVAL: *(on multiple pages)*
Taking out or off a device from a body part

Body Part	Approach	Device	Qualifier
Ø Sternum 1 Rib, 1 to 2 2 Rib, 3 or More 3 Cervical Vertebra 4 Thoracic Vertebra 5 Scapula, Right 6 Scapula, Left 7 Glenoid Cavity, Right 8 Glenoid Cavity, Left 9 Clavicle, Right B Clavicle, Left	Ø Open 3 Percutaneous 4 Percutaneous Endoscopic	4 Internal Fixation Device 7 Autologous Tissue Substitute J Synthetic Substitute K Nonautologous Tissue Substitute	Z No Qualifier
Ø Sternum 1 Rib, 1 to 2 2 Rib, 3 or More 3 Cervical Vertebra 4 Thoracic Vertebra 5 Scapula, Right 6 Scapula, Left 7 Glenoid Cavity, Right 8 Glenoid Cavity, Left 9 Clavicle, Right B Clavicle, Left	X External	4 Internal Fixation Device	Z No Qualifier
C Humeral Head, Right D Humeral Head, Left F Humeral Shaft, Right G Humeral Shaft, Left H Radius, Right J Radius, Left K Ulna, Right L Ulna, Left M Carpal, Right N Carpal, Left P Metacarpal, Right Q Metacarpal, Left R Thumb Phalanx, Right S Thumb Phalanx, Left T Finger Phalanx, Right V Finger Phalanx, Left	Ø Open 3 Percutaneous 4 Percutaneous Endoscopic	4 Internal Fixation Device 5 External Fixation Device 7 Autologous Tissue Substitute J Synthetic Substitute K Nonautologous Tissue Substitute	Z No Qualifier

SECTION: Ø MEDICAL AND SURGICAL
BODY SYSTEM: P UPPER BONES
OPERATION: P REMOVAL: *(continued)*
Taking out or off a device from a body part

Body Part	Approach	Device	Qualifier
C Humeral Head, Right D Humeral Head, Left F Humeral Shaft, Right G Humeral Shaft, Left H Radius, Right J Radius, Left K Ulna, Right L Ulna, Left M Carpal, Right N Carpal, Left P Metacarpal, Right Q Metacarpal, Left R Thumb Phalanx, Right S Thumb Phalanx, Left T Finger Phalanx, Right V Finger Phalanx, Left	X External	4 Internal Fixation Device 5 External Fixation Device	Z No Qualifier
Y Upper Bone	Ø Open 3 Percutaneous 4 Percutaneous Endoscopic X External	Ø Drainage Device M Bone Growth Stimulator	Z No Qualifier

SECTION: Ø MEDICAL AND SURGICAL
BODY SYSTEM: P UPPER BONES
OPERATION: Q **REPAIR:** Restoring, to the extent possible, a body part to its normal anatomic structure and function

Body Part	Approach	Device	Qualifier
Ø Sternum	Ø Open	Z No Device	Z No Qualifier
1 Rib, 1 to 2	3 Percutaneous		
2 Rib, 3 or More	4 Percutaneous Endoscopic		
3 Cervical Vertebra	X External		
4 Thoracic Vertebra			
5 Scapula, Right			
6 Scapula, Left			
7 Glenoid Cavity, Right			
8 Glenoid Cavity, Left			
9 Clavicle, Right			
B Clavicle, Left			
C Humeral Head, Right			
D Humeral Head, Left			
F Humeral Shaft, Right			
G Humeral Shaft, Left			
H Radius, Right			
J Radius, Left			
K Ulna, Right			
L Ulna, Left			
M Carpal, Right			
N Carpal, Left			
P Metacarpal, Right			
Q Metacarpal, Left			
R Thumb Phalanx, Right			
S Thumb Phalanx, Left			
T Finger Phalanx, Right			
V Finger Phalanx, Left			

R: REPLACEMENT   S: REPOSITION

P: UPPER BONES   Ø: M/S

SECTION: Ø MEDICAL AND SURGICAL
BODY SYSTEM: P UPPER BONES
OPERATION: R REPLACEMENT: Putting in or on biological or synthetic material that physically takes the place and/or function of all or a portion of a body part

Body Part	Approach	Device	Qualifier
Ø Sternum 1 Rib, 1 to 2 2 Rib, 3 or More 3 Cervical Vertebra 4 Thoracic Vertebra 5 Scapula, Right 6 Scapula, Left 7 Glenoid Cavity, Right 8 Glenoid Cavity, Left 9 Clavicle, Right B Clavicle, Left C Humeral Head, Right D Humeral Head, Left F Humeral Shaft, Right G Humeral Shaft, Left H Radius, Right J Radius, Left K Ulna, Right L Ulna, Left M Carpal, Right N Carpal, Left P Metacarpal, Right Q Metacarpal, Left R Thumb Phalanx, Right S Thumb Phalanx, Left T Finger Phalanx, Right V Finger Phalanx, Left	Ø Open 3 Percutaneous 4 Percutaneous Endoscopic	7 Autologous Tissue Substitute J Synthetic Substitute K Nonautologous Tissue Substitute	Z No Qualifier

SECTION: Ø MEDICAL AND SURGICAL
BODY SYSTEM: P UPPER BONES
OPERATION: S REPOSITION: *(on multiple pages)*
Moving to its normal location, or other suitable location, all or a portion of a body part

Body Part	Approach	Device	Qualifier
Ø Sternum	Ø Open 3 Percutaneous 4 Percutaneous Endoscopic	Ø Internal Fixation Device, Rigid Plate 4 Internal Fixation Device Z No Device	Z No Qualifier
Ø Sternum	X External	Z No Device	Z No Qualifier
1 Rib, 1 to 2 2 Rib, 3 or More 3 Cervical Vertebra 4 Thoracic Vertebra 5 Scapula, Right 6 Scapula, Left 7 Glenoid Cavity, Right 8 Glenoid Cavity, Left 9 Clavicle, Right B Clavicle, Left	Ø Open 3 Percutaneous 4 Percutaneous Endoscopic	4 Internal Fixation Device Z No Device	Z No Qualifier

SECTION: Ø MEDICAL AND SURGICAL
BODY SYSTEM: P UPPER BONES
OPERATION: S REPOSITION: *(continued)*

Moving to its normal location, or other suitable location, all or a portion of a body part

Body Part	Approach	Device	Qualifier
1 Rib, 1 to 2 2 Rib, 3 or More 3 Cervical Vertebra 4 Thoracic Vertebra 5 Scapula, Right 6 Scapula, Left 7 Glenoid Cavity, Right 8 Glenoid Cavity, Left 9 Clavicle, Right B Clavicle, Left	X External	Z No Device	Z No Qualifier
C Humeral Head, Right D Humeral Head, Left F Humeral Shaft, Right G Humeral Shaft, Left H Radius, Right J Radius, Left K Ulna, Right L Ulna, Left	Ø Open 3 Percutaneous 4 Percutaneous Endoscopic	4 Internal Fixation Device 5 External Fixation Device 6 Internal Fixation Device, Intramedullary B External Fixation Device, Monoplanar C External Fixation Device, Ring D External Fixation Device, Hybrid Z No Device	Z No Qualifier
C Humeral Head, Right D Humeral Head, Left F Humeral Shaft, Right G Humeral Shaft, Left H Radius, Right J Radius, Left K Ulna, Right L Ulna, Left	X External	Z No Device	Z No Qualifier
M Carpal, Right N Carpal, Left P Metacarpal, Right Q Metacarpal, Left R Thumb Phalanx, Right S Thumb Phalanx, Left T Finger Phalanx, Right V Finger Phalanx, Left	Ø Open 3 Percutaneous 4 Percutaneous Endoscopic	4 Internal Fixation Device 5 External Fixation Device Z No Device	Z No Qualifier
M Carpal, Right N Carpal, Left P Metacarpal, Right Q Metacarpal, Left R Thumb Phalanx, Right S Thumb Phalanx, Left T Finger Phalanx, Right V Finger Phalanx, Left	X External	Z No Device	Z No Qualifier

Ø: M/S
P: UPPER BONES
S: REPOSITION

SECTION: Ø MEDICAL AND SURGICAL
BODY SYSTEM: P UPPER BONES
OPERATION: T RESECTION: Cutting out or off, without replacement, all of a body part

Body Part	Approach	Device	Qualifier
Ø Sternum	Ø Open	Z No Device	Z No Qualifier
1 Rib, 1 to 2			
2 Rib, 3 or More			
5 Scapula, Right			
6 Scapula, Left			
7 Glenoid Cavity, Right			
8 Glenoid Cavity, Left			
9 Clavicle, Right			
B Clavicle, Left			
C Humeral Head, Right			
D Humeral Head, Left			
F Humeral Shaft, Right			
G Humeral Shaft, Left			
H Radius, Right			
J Radius, Left			
K Ulna, Right			
L Ulna, Left			
M Carpal, Right			
N Carpal, Left			
P Metacarpal, Right			
Q Metacarpal, Left			
R Thumb Phalanx, Right			
S Thumb Phalanx, Left			
T Finger Phalanx, Right			
V Finger Phalanx, Left			

New/Revised Text in Blue   deleted Deleted

SECTION: Ø MEDICAL AND SURGICAL
BODY SYSTEM: P UPPER BONES
OPERATION: U SUPPLEMENT: Putting in or on biological or synthetic material that physically reinforces and/or augments the function of a portion of a body part

Body Part	Approach	Device	Qualifier
Ø Sternum	Ø Open	7 Autologous Tissue Substitute	Z No Qualifier
1 Rib, 1 to 2	3 Percutaneous	J Synthetic Substitute	
2 Rib, 3 or More	4 Percutaneous Endoscopic	K Nonautologous Tissue Substitute	
3 Cervical Vertebra			
4 Thoracic Vertebra			
5 Scapula, Right			
6 Scapula, Left			
7 Glenoid Cavity, Right			
8 Glenoid Cavity, Left			
9 Clavicle, Right			
B Clavicle, Left			
C Humeral Head, Right			
D Humeral Head, Left			
F Humeral Shaft, Right			
G Humeral Shaft, Left			
H Radius, Right			
J Radius, Left			
K Ulna, Right			
L Ulna, Left			
M Carpal, Right			
N Carpal, Left			
P Metacarpal, Right			
Q Metacarpal, Left			
R Thumb Phalanx, Right			
S Thumb Phalanx, Left			
T Finger Phalanx, Right			
V Finger Phalanx, Left			

SECTION: Ø MEDICAL AND SURGICAL
BODY SYSTEM: P UPPER BONES
OPERATION: W REVISION: Correcting, to the extent possible, a portion of a malfunctioning device or the position of a displaced device

Body Part	Approach	Device	Qualifier
Ø Sternum 1 Rib, 1 to 2 2 Rib, 3 or More 3 Cervical Vertebra 4 Thoracic Vertebra 5 Scapula, Right 6 Scapula, Left 7 Glenoid Cavity, Right 8 Glenoid Cavity, Left 9 Clavicle, Right B Clavicle, Left	Ø Open 3 Percutaneous 4 Percutaneous Endoscopic X External	4 Internal Fixation Device 7 Autologous Tissue Substitute J Synthetic Substitute K Nonautologous Tissue Substitute	Z No Qualifier
C Humeral Head, Right D Humeral Head, Left F Humeral Shaft, Right G Humeral Shaft, Left H Radius, Right J Radius, Left K Ulna, Right L Ulna, Left M Carpal, Right N Carpal, Left P Metacarpal, Right Q Metacarpal, Left R Thumb Phalanx, Right S Thumb Phalanx, Left T Finger Phalanx, Right V Finger Phalanx, Left	Ø Open 3 Percutaneous 4 Percutaneous Endoscopic X External	4 Internal Fixation Device 5 External Fixation Device 7 Autologous Tissue Substitute J Synthetic Substitute K Nonautologous Tissue Substitute	Z No Qualifier
Y Upper Bone	Ø Open 3 Percutaneous 4 Percutaneous Endoscopic X External	Ø Drainage Device M Bone Growth Stimulator	Z No Qualifier

ØQ. Lower Bones.. 371
    ØQ2. Change 372
    ØQ5. Destruction.. 372
    ØQ8. Division... 373
    ØQ9. Drainage 374
    ØQB. Excision 375
    ØQC. Extirpation.. 376
    ØQD. Extraction.. 377
    ØQH. Insertion 378
    ØQJ. Inspection 379
    ØQN. Release 379
    ØQP. Removal 380
    ØQQ. Repair 381
    ØQR. Replacement 382
    ØQS. Reposition... 383
    ØQT. Resection... 384
    ØQU. Supplement 385
    ØQW. Revision.. 386

SECTION: **0 MEDICAL AND SURGICAL**
BODY SYSTEM: **Q LOWER BONES**
OPERATION: **2 CHANGE:** Taking out or off a device from a body part and putting back an identical or similar device in or on the same body part without cutting or puncturing the skin or a mucous membrane

Body Part	Approach	Device	Qualifier
Y Lower Bone	X External	0 Drainage Device Y Other Device	Z No Qualifier

SECTION: **0 MEDICAL AND SURGICAL**
BODY SYSTEM: **Q LOWER BONES**
OPERATION: **5 DESTRUCTION:** Physical eradication of all or a portion of a body part by the direct use of energy, force, or a destructive agent

Body Part	Approach	Device	Qualifier
0 Lumbar Vertebra 1 Sacrum 2 Pelvic Bone, Right 3 Pelvic Bone, Left 4 Acetabulum, Right 5 Acetabulum, Left 6 Upper Femur, Right 7 Upper Femur, Left 8 Femoral Shaft, Right 9 Femoral Shaft, Left B Lower Femur, Right C Lower Femur, Left D Patella, Right F Patella, Left G Tibia, Right H Tibia, Left J Fibula, Right K Fibula, Left L Tarsal, Right M Tarsal, Left N Metatarsal, Right P Metatarsal, Left Q Toe Phalanx, Right R Toe Phalanx, Left S Coccyx	0 Open 3 Percutaneous 4 Percutaneous Endoscopic	Z No Device	Z No Qualifier

SECTION: Ø MEDICAL AND SURGICAL
BODY SYSTEM: Q LOWER BONES
OPERATION: 8 DIVISION: Cutting into a body part, without draining fluids and/or gases from the body part, in order to separate or transect a body part

Body Part	Approach	Device	Qualifier
Ø Lumbar Vertebra 1 Sacrum 2 Pelvic Bone, Right 3 Pelvic Bone, Left 4 Acetabulum, Right 5 Acetabulum, Left 6 Upper Femur, Right 7 Upper Femur, Left 8 Femoral Shaft, Right 9 Femoral Shaft, Left B Lower Femur, Right C Lower Femur, Left D Patella, Right F Patella, Left G Tibia, Right H Tibia, Left J Fibula, Right K Fibula, Left L Tarsal, Right M Tarsal, Left N Metatarsal, Right P Metatarsal, Left Q Toe Phalanx, Right R Toe Phalanx, Left S Coccyx	Ø Open 3 Percutaneous 4 Percutaneous Endoscopic	Z No Device	Z No Qualifier

SECTION: Ø MEDICAL AND SURGICAL
BODY SYSTEM: Q LOWER BONES
OPERATION: 9 **DRAINAGE:** Taking or letting out fluids and/or gases from a body part

Body Part	Approach	Device	Qualifier
Ø Lumbar Vertebra 1 Sacrum 2 Pelvic Bone, Right 3 Pelvic Bone, Left 4 Acetabulum, Right 5 Acetabulum, Left 6 Upper Femur, Right 7 Upper Femur, Left 8 Femoral Shaft, Right 9 Femoral Shaft, Left B Lower Femur, Right C Lower Femur, Left D Patella, Right F Patella, Left G Tibia, Right H Tibia, Left J Fibula, Right K Fibula, Left L Tarsal, Right M Tarsal, Left N Metatarsal, Right P Metatarsal, Left Q Toe Phalanx, Right R Toe Phalanx, Left S Coccyx	Ø Open 3 Percutaneous 4 Percutaneous Endoscopic	Ø Drainage Device	Z No Qualifier
Ø Lumbar Vertebra 1 Sacrum 2 Pelvic Bone, Right 3 Pelvic Bone, Left 4 Acetabulum, Right 5 Acetabulum, Left 6 Upper Femur, Right 7 Upper Femur, Left 8 Femoral Shaft, Right 9 Femoral Shaft, Left B Lower Femur, Right C Lower Femur, Left D Patella, Right F Patella, Left G Tibia, Right H Tibia, Left J Fibula, Right K Fibula, Left L Tarsal, Right M Tarsal, Left N Metatarsal, Right P Metatarsal, Left Q Toe Phalanx, Right R Toe Phalanx, Left S Coccyx	Ø Open 3 Percutaneous 4 Percutaneous Endoscopic	Z No Device	X Diagnostic Z No Qualifier

9: DRAINAGE   Q: LOWER BONES   Ø: M/S

SECTION: 0 MEDICAL AND SURGICAL
BODY SYSTEM: Q LOWER BONES
OPERATION: B **EXCISION:** Cutting out or off, without replacement, a portion of a body part

Body Part	Approach	Device	Qualifier
0 Lumbar Vertebra	0 Open	Z No Device	X Diagnostic
1 Sacrum	3 Percutaneous		Z No Qualifier
2 Pelvic Bone, Right	4 Percutaneous Endoscopic		
3 Pelvic Bone, Left			
4 Acetabulum, Right			
5 Acetabulum, Left			
6 Upper Femur, Right			
7 Upper Femur, Left			
8 Femoral Shaft, Right			
9 Femoral Shaft, Left			
B Lower Femur, Right			
C Lower Femur, Left			
D Patella, Right			
F Patella, Left			
G Tibia, Right			
H Tibia, Left			
J Fibula, Right			
K Fibula, Left			
L Tarsal, Right			
M Tarsal, Left			
N Metatarsal, Right			
P Metatarsal, Left			
Q Toe Phalanx, Right			
R Toe Phalanx, Left			
S Coccyx			

SECTION: Ø MEDICAL AND SURGICAL
BODY SYSTEM: Q LOWER BONES
OPERATION: C EXTIRPATION: Taking or cutting out solid matter from a body part

Body Part	Approach	Device	Qualifier
Ø Lumbar Vertebra	Ø Open	Z No Device	Z No Qualifier
1 Sacrum	3 Percutaneous		
2 Pelvic Bone, Right	4 Percutaneous Endoscopic		
3 Pelvic Bone, Left			
4 Acetabulum, Right			
5 Acetabulum, Left			
6 Upper Femur, Right			
7 Upper Femur, Left			
8 Femoral Shaft, Right			
9 Femoral Shaft, Left			
B Lower Femur, Right			
C Lower Femur, Left			
D Patella, Right			
F Patella, Left			
G Tibia, Right			
H Tibia, Left			
J Fibula, Right			
K Fibula, Left			
L Tarsal, Right			
M Tarsal, Left			
N Metatarsal, Right			
P Metatarsal, Left			
Q Toe Phalanx, Right			
R Toe Phalanx, Left			
S Coccyx			

SECTION: Ø MEDICAL AND SURGICAL
BODY SYSTEM: Q LOWER BONES
OPERATION: D **EXTRACTION:** Pulling or stripping out or off all or a portion of a body part by the use of force

Body Part	Approach	Device	Qualifier
Ø Lumbar Vertebra	Ø Open	Z No Device	Z No Qualifier
1 Sacrum			
2 Pelvic Bone, Right			
3 Pelvic Bone, Left			
4 Acetabulum, Right			
5 Acetabulum, Left			
6 Upper Femur, Right			
7 Upper Femur, Left			
8 Femoral Shaft, Right			
9 Femoral Shaft, Left			
B Lower Femur, Right			
C Lower Femur, Left			
D Patella, Right			
F Patella, Left			
G Tibia, Right			
H Tibia, Left			
J Fibula, Right			
K Fibula, Left			
L Tarsal, Right			
M Tarsal, Left			
N Metatarsal, Right			
P Metatarsal, Left			
Q Toe Phalanx, Right			
R Toe Phalanx, Left			
S Coccyx			

Ø: M/S

Q: LOWER BONES

D: EXTRACTION

SECTION:　Ø MEDICAL AND SURGICAL
BODY SYSTEM: Q LOWER BONES
OPERATION:　　H INSERTION: Putting in a nonbiological appliance that monitors, assists, performs, or prevents a physiological function but does not physically take the place of a body part

Body Part	Approach	Device	Qualifier
Ø Lumbar Vertebra 1 Sacrum 2 Pelvic Bone, Right 3 Pelvic Bone, Left 4 Acetabulum, Right 5 Acetabulum, Left D Patella, Right F Patella, Left L Tarsal, Right M Tarsal, Left N Metatarsal, Right P Metatarsal, Left Q Toe Phalanx, Right R Toe Phalanx, Left S Coccyx	Ø Open 3 Percutaneous 4 Percutaneous Endoscopic	4 Internal Fixation Device 5 External Fixation Device	Z No Qualifier
6 Upper Femur, Right 7 Upper Femur, Left 8 Femoral Shaft, Right 9 Femoral Shaft, Left B Lower Femur, Right C Lower Femur, Left G Tibia, Right H Tibia, Left J Fibula, Right K Fibula, Left	Ø Open 3 Percutaneous 4 Percutaneous Endoscopic	4 Internal Fixation Device 5 External Fixation Device 6 Internal Fixation Device, Intramedullary 8 External Fixation Device, Limb Lengthening B External Fixation Device, Monoplanar C External Fixation Device, Ring D External Fixation Device, Hybrid	Z No Qualifier
Y Lower Bone	Ø Open 3 Percutaneous 4 Percutaneous Endoscopic	M Bone Growth Stimulator	Z No Qualifier

H: INSERTION

Q: LOWER BONES

Ø: M/S

　　　　　New/Revised Text in Blue　~~deleted~~ Deleted

SECTION: Ø MEDICAL AND SURGICAL
BODY SYSTEM: Q LOWER BONES
OPERATION: J INSPECTION: Visually and/or manually exploring a body part

Body Part	Approach	Device	Qualifier
Y Lower Bone	Ø Open 3 Percutaneous 4 Percutaneous Endoscopic X External	Z No Device	Z No Qualifier

SECTION: Ø MEDICAL AND SURGICAL
BODY SYSTEM: Q LOWER BONES
OPERATION: N RELEASE: Freeing a body part from an abnormal physical constraint by cutting or by the use of force

Body Part	Approach	Device	Qualifier
Ø Lumbar Vertebra 1 Sacrum 2 Pelvic Bone, Right 3 Pelvic Bone, Left 4 Acetabulum, Right 5 Acetabulum, Left 6 Upper Femur, Right 7 Upper Femur, Left 8 Femoral Shaft, Right 9 Femoral Shaft, Left B Lower Femur, Right C Lower Femur, Left D Patella, Right F Patella, Left G Tibia, Right H Tibia, Left J Fibula, Right K Fibula, Left L Tarsal, Right M Tarsal, Left N Metatarsal, Right P Metatarsal, Left Q Toe Phalanx, Right R Toe Phalanx, Left S Coccyx	Ø Open 3 Percutaneous 4 Percutaneous Endoscopic	Z No Device	Z No Qualifier

SECTION: Ø MEDICAL AND SURGICAL
BODY SYSTEM: Q LOWER BONES
OPERATION: P REMOVAL: *(on multiple pages)*
Taking out or off a device from a body part

Body Part	Approach	Device	Qualifier
Ø Lumbar Vertebra 1 Sacrum 4 Acetabulum, Right 5 Acetabulum, Left S Coccyx	Ø Open 3 Percutaneous 4 Percutaneous Endoscopic	4 Internal Fixation Device 7 Autologous Tissue Substitute J Synthetic Substitute K Nonautologous Tissue Substitute	Z No Qualifier
Ø Lumbar Vertebra 1 Sacrum 4 Acetabulum, Right 5 Acetabulum, Left S Coccyx	X External	4 Internal Fixation Device	Z No Qualifier
2 Pelvic Bone, Right 3 Pelvic Bone, Left 6 Upper Femur, Right 7 Upper Femur, Left 8 Femoral Shaft, Right 9 Femoral Shaft, Left B Lower Femur, Right C Lower Femur, Left D Patella, Right F Patella, Left G Tibia, Right H Tibia, Left J Fibula, Right K Fibula, Left L Tarsal, Right M Tarsal, Left N Metatarsal, Right P Metatarsal, Left Q Toe Phalanx, Right R Toe Phalanx, Left	Ø Open 3 Percutaneous 4 Percutaneous Endoscopic	4 Internal Fixation Device 5 External Fixation Device 7 Autologous Tissue Substitute J Synthetic Substitute K Nonautologous Tissue Substitute	Z No Qualifier
2 Pelvic Bone, Right 3 Pelvic Bone, Left 6 Upper Femur, Right 7 Upper Femur, Left 8 Femoral Shaft, Right 9 Femoral Shaft, Left B Lower Femur, Right C Lower Femur, Left D Patella, Right F Patella, Left G Tibia, Right H Tibia, Left J Fibula, Right K Fibula, Left L Tarsal, Right M Tarsal, Left N Metatarsal, Right P Metatarsal, Left Q Toe Phalanx, Right R Toe Phalanx, Left	X External	4 Internal Fixation Device 5 External Fixation Device	Z No Qualifier

P: REMOVAL
Q: LOWER BONES
Ø: M/S

New/Revised Text in Blue ~~deleted~~ Deleted

SECTION: Ø MEDICAL AND SURGICAL
BODY SYSTEM: Q LOWER BONES
OPERATION: P REMOVAL: *(continued)*
Taking out or off a device from a body part

Body Part	Approach	Device	Qualifier
Y Lower Bone	Ø Open 3 Percutaneous 4 Percutaneous Endoscopic X External	Ø Drainage Device M Bone Growth Stimulator	Z No Qualifier

SECTION: Ø MEDICAL AND SURGICAL
BODY SYSTEM: Q LOWER BONES
OPERATION: Q REPAIR: Restoring, to the extent possible, a body part to its normal anatomic structure and function

Body Part	Approach	Device	Qualifier
Ø Lumbar Vertebra 1 Sacrum 2 Pelvic Bone, Right 3 Pelvic Bone, Left 4 Acetabulum, Right 5 Acetabulum, Left 6 Upper Femur, Right 7 Upper Femur, Left 8 Femoral Shaft, Right 9 Femoral Shaft, Left B Lower Femur, Right C Lower Femur, Left D Patella, Right F Patella, Left G Tibia, Right H Tibia, Left J Fibula, Right K Fibula, Left L Tarsal, Right M Tarsal, Left N Metatarsal, Right P Metatarsal, Left Q Toe Phalanx, Right R Toe Phalanx, Left S Coccyx	Ø Open 3 Percutaneous 4 Percutaneous Endoscopic X External	Z No Device	Z No Qualifier

Ø: M/S

Q: LOWER BONES

P: REMOVAL   Q: REPAIR

SECTION: Ø MEDICAL AND SURGICAL
BODY SYSTEM: Q LOWER BONES
OPERATION: R REPLACEMENT: Putting in or on biological or synthetic material that physically takes the place and/or function of all or a portion of a body part

Body Part	Approach	Device	Qualifier
Ø Lumbar Vertebra 1 Sacrum 2 Pelvic Bone, Right 3 Pelvic Bone, Left 4 Acetabulum, Right 5 Acetabulum, Left 6 Upper Femur, Right 7 Upper Femur, Left 8 Femoral Shaft, Right 9 Femoral Shaft, Left B Lower Femur, Right C Lower Femur, Left D Patella, Right F Patella, Left G Tibia, Right H Tibia, Left J Fibula, Right K Fibula, Left L Tarsal, Right M Tarsal, Left N Metatarsal, Right P Metatarsal, Left Q Toe Phalanx, Right R Toe Phalanx, Left S Coccyx	Ø Open 3 Percutaneous 4 Percutaneous Endoscopic	7 Autologous Tissue Substitute J Synthetic Substitute K Nonautologous Tissue Substitute	Z No Qualifier

SECTION: Ø MEDICAL AND SURGICAL
BODY SYSTEM: Q LOWER BONES
OPERATION: S REPOSITION: *(on multiple pages)*

Moving to its normal location, or other suitable location, all or a portion of a body part

Body Part	Approach	Device	Qualifier
Ø Lumbar Vertebra 1 Sacrum 4 Acetabulum, Right 5 Acetabulum, Left S Coccyx	Ø Open 3 Percutaneous 4 Percutaneous Endoscopic	4 Internal Fixation Device Z No Device	Z No Qualifier
Ø Lumbar Vertebra 1 Sacrum 4 Acetabulum, Right 5 Acetabulum, Left S Coccyx	X External	Z No Device	Z No Qualifier
2 Pelvic Bone, Right 3 Pelvic Bone, Left D Patella, Right F Patella, Left L Tarsal, Right M Tarsal, Left N Metatarsal, Right P Metatarsal, Left Q Toe Phalanx, Right R Toe Phalanx, Left	Ø Open 3 Percutaneous 4 Percutaneous Endoscopic	4 Internal Fixation Device 5 External Fixation Device Z No Device	Z No Qualifier
2 Pelvic Bone, Right 3 Pelvic Bone, Left D Patella, Right F Patella, Left L Tarsal, Right M Tarsal, Left N Metatarsal, Right P Metatarsal, Left Q Toe Phalanx, Right R Toe Phalanx, Left	X External	Z No Device	Z No Qualifier
6 Upper Femur, Right 7 Upper Femur, Left 8 Femoral Shaft, Right 9 Femoral Shaft, Left B Lower Femur, Right C Lower Femur, Left G Tibia, Right H Tibia, Left J Fibula, Right K Fibula, Left	Ø Open 3 Percutaneous 4 Percutaneous Endoscopic	4 Internal Fixation Device 5 External Fixation Device 6 Internal Fixation Device, Intramedullary B External Fixation Device, Monoplanar C External Fixation Device, Ring D External Fixation Device, Hybrid Z No Device	Z No Qualifier

SECTION: Ø MEDICAL AND SURGICAL
BODY SYSTEM: Q LOWER BONES
OPERATION: S REPOSITION: *(continued)*
Moving to its normal location, or other suitable location, all or a portion of a body part

Body Part	Approach	Device	Qualifier
6 Upper Femur, Right 7 Upper Femur, Left 8 Femoral Shaft, Right 9 Femoral Shaft, Left B Lower Femur, Right C Lower Femur, Left G Tibia, Right H Tibia, Left J Fibula, Right K Fibula, Left	X External	Z No Device	Z No Qualifier
N Metatarsal, Right P Metatarsal, Left	Ø Open 3 Percutaneous 4 Percutaneous Endoscopic	4 Internal Fixation Device 5 External Fixation Device Z No Device	2 Sesamoid Bone(s) 1st Toe Z No Qualifier
N Metatarsal, Right P Metatarsal, Left	X External	Z No Device	2 Sesamoid Bone(s) 1st Toe Z No Qualifier

SECTION: Ø MEDICAL AND SURGICAL
BODY SYSTEM: Q LOWER BONES
OPERATION: T RESECTION: Cutting out or off, without replacement, all of a body part

Body Part	Approach	Device	Qualifier
2 Pelvic Bone, Right 3 Pelvic Bone, Left 4 Acetabulum, Right 5 Acetabulum, Left 6 Upper Femur, Right 7 Upper Femur, Left 8 Femoral Shaft, Right 9 Femoral Shaft, Left B Lower Femur, Right C Lower Femur, Left D Patella, Right F Patella, Left G Tibia, Right H Tibia, Left J Fibula, Right K Fibula, Left L Tarsal, Right M Tarsal, Left N Metatarsal, Right P Metatarsal, Left Q Toe Phalanx, Right R Toe Phalanx, Left S Coccyx	Ø Open	Z No Device	Z No Qualifier

SECTION: Ø MEDICAL AND SURGICAL
BODY SYSTEM: Q LOWER BONES
OPERATION: U SUPPLEMENT: Putting in or on biological or synthetic material that physically reinforces and/or augments the function of a portion of a body part

Body Part	Approach	Device	Qualifier
Ø Lumbar Vertebra 1 Sacrum 2 Pelvic Bone, Right 3 Pelvic Bone, Left 4 Acetabulum, Right 5 Acetabulum, Left 6 Upper Femur, Right 7 Upper Femur, Left 8 Femoral Shaft, Right 9 Femoral Shaft, Left B Lower Femur, Right C Lower Femur, Left D Patella, Right F Patella, Left G Tibia, Right H Tibia, Left J Fibula, Right K Fibula, Left L Tarsal, Right M Tarsal, Left N Metatarsal, Right P Metatarsal, Left Q Toe Phalanx, Right R Toe Phalanx, Left S Coccyx	Ø Open 3 Percutaneous 4 Percutaneous Endoscopic	7 Autologous Tissue Substitute J Synthetic Substitute K Nonautologous Tissue Substitute	Z No Qualifier

SECTION: Ø MEDICAL AND SURGICAL
BODY SYSTEM: Q LOWER BONES
OPERATION: **W REVISION:** Correcting, to the extent possible, a portion of a malfunctioning device or the position of a displaced device

Body Part	Approach	Device	Qualifier
Ø Lumbar Vertebra 1 Sacrum 4 Acetabulum, Right 5 Acetabulum, Left S Coccyx	Ø Open 3 Percutaneous 4 Percutaneous Endoscopic X External	4 Internal Fixation Device 7 Autologous Tissue Substitute J Synthetic Substitute K Nonautologous Tissue Substitute	Z No Qualifier
2 Pelvic Bone, Right 3 Pelvic Bone, Left 6 Upper Femur, Right 7 Upper Femur, Left 8 Femoral Shaft, Right 9 Femoral Shaft, Left B Lower Femur, Right C Lower Femur, Left D Patella, Right F Patella, Left G Tibia, Right H Tibia, Left J Fibula, Right K Fibula, Left L Tarsal, Right M Tarsal, Left N Metatarsal, Right P Metatarsal, Left Q Toe Phalanx, Right R Toe Phalanx, Left	Ø Open 3 Percutaneous 4 Percutaneous Endoscopic X External	4 Internal Fixation Device 5 External Fixation Device 7 Autologous Tissue Substitute J Synthetic Substitute K Nonautologous Tissue Substitute	Z No Qualifier
Y Lower Bone	Ø Open 3 Percutaneous 4 Percutaneous Endoscopic X External	Ø Drainage Device M Bone Growth Stimulator	Z No Qualifier

New/Revised Text in Blue   ~~deleted~~   Deleted

W: REVISION

Q: LOWER BONES

Ø: M/S

ØR. Upper Joints...387
    ØR2. Change 388
    ØR5. Destruction...388
    ØR9. Drainage 389
    ØRB. Excision 391
    ØRC. Extirpation...392
    ØRG. Fusion 393
    ØRH. Insertion..394
    ØRJ. Inspection 395
    ØRN. Release 396
    ØRP. Removal 396
    ØRQ. Repair 398
    ØRR. Replacement 399
    ØRS. Reposition..400
    ØRT. Resection..401
    ØRU. Supplement 402
    ØRW. Revision...403

SECTION: Ø MEDICAL AND SURGICAL
BODY SYSTEM: R UPPER JOINTS
OPERATION: 2 CHANGE: Taking out or off a device from a body part and putting back an identical or similar device in or on the same body part without cutting or puncturing the skin or a mucous membrane

Body Part	Approach	Device	Qualifier
Y Upper Joint	X External	Ø Drainage Device Y Other Device	Z No Qualifier

SECTION: Ø MEDICAL AND SURGICAL
BODY SYSTEM: R UPPER JOINTS
OPERATION: 5 DESTRUCTION: Physical eradication of all or a portion of a body part by the direct use of energy, force, or destructive agent

Body Part	Approach	Device	Qualifier
Ø Occipital-cervical Joint 1 Cervical Vertebral Joint 3 Cervical Vertebral Disc 4 Cervicothoracic Vertebral Joint 5 Cervicothoracic Vertebral Disc 6 Thoracic Vertebral Joint 9 Thoracic Vertebral Disc A Thoracolumbar Vertebral Joint B Thoracolumbar Vertebral Disc C Temporomandibular Joint, Right D Temporomandibular Joint, Left E Sternoclavicular Joint, Right F Sternoclavicular Joint, Left G Acromioclavicular Joint, Right H Acromioclavicular Joint, Left J Shoulder Joint, Right K Shoulder Joint, Left L Elbow Joint, Right M Elbow Joint, Left N Wrist Joint, Right P Wrist Joint, Left Q Carpal Joint, Right R Carpal Joint, Left S Carpometacarpal Joint, Right T Carpometacarpal Joint, Left U Metacarpophalangeal Joint, Right V Metacarpophalangeal Joint, Left W Finger Phalangeal Joint, Right X Finger Phalangeal Joint, Left	Ø Open 3 Percutaneous 4 Percutaneous Endoscopic	Z No Device	Z No Qualifier

Ø: M/S   R: UPPER JOINTS   2: CHANGE   5: DESTRUCTION

SECTION: Ø MEDICAL AND SURGICAL
BODY SYSTEM: R UPPER JOINTS
OPERATION: 9 DRAINAGE: *(on multiple pages)*

Taking or letting out fluids and/or gases from a body part

Body Part	Approach	Device	Qualifier
Ø Occipital-cervical Joint	Ø Open	Ø Drainage Device	Z No Qualifier
1 Cervical Vertebral Joint	3 Percutaneous		
3 Cervical Vertebral Disc	4 Percutaneous Endoscopic		
4 Cervicothoracic Vertebral Joint			
5 Cervicothoracic Vertebral Disc			
6 Thoracic Vertebral Joint			
9 Thoracic Vertebral Disc			
A Thoracolumbar Vertebral Joint			
B Thoracolumbar Vertebral Disc			
C Temporomandibular Joint, Right			
D Temporomandibular Joint, Left			
E Sternoclavicular Joint, Right			
F Sternoclavicular Joint, Left			
G Acromioclavicular Joint, Right			
H Acromioclavicular Joint, Left			
J Shoulder Joint, Right			
K Shoulder Joint, Left			
L Elbow Joint, Right			
M Elbow Joint, Left			
N Wrist Joint, Right			
P Wrist Joint, Left			
Q Carpal Joint, Right			
R Carpal Joint, Left			
S Carpometacarpal Joint, Right			
T Carpometacarpal Joint, Left			
U Metacarpophalangeal Joint, Right			
V Metacarpophalangeal Joint, Left			
W Finger Phalangeal Joint, Right			
X Finger Phalangeal Joint, Left			

SECTION: Ø MEDICAL AND SURGICAL
BODY SYSTEM: R UPPER JOINTS
OPERATION: 9 DRAINAGE: *(continued)*
Taking or letting out fluids and/or gases from a body part

Body Part	Approach	Device	Qualifier
Ø Occipital-cervical Joint 1 Cervical Vertebral Joint 3 Cervical Vertebral Disc 4 Cervicothoracic Vertebral Joint 5 Cervicothoracic Vertebral Disc 6 Thoracic Vertebral Joint 9 Thoracic Vertebral Disc A Thoracolumbar Vertebral Joint B Thoracolumbar Vertebral Disc C Temporomandibular Joint, Right D Temporomandibular Joint, Left E Sternoclavicular Joint, Right F Sternoclavicular Joint, Left G Acromioclavicular Joint, Right H Acromioclavicular Joint, Left J Shoulder Joint, Right K Shoulder Joint, Left L Elbow Joint, Right M Elbow Joint, Left N Wrist Joint, Right P Wrist Joint, Left Q Carpal Joint, Right R Carpal Joint, Left S Carpometacarpal Joint, Right T Carpometacarpal Joint, Left U Metacarpophalangeal Joint, Right V Metacarpophalangeal Joint, Left W Finger Phalangeal Joint, Right X Finger Phalangeal Joint, Left	Ø Open 3 Percutaneous 4 Percutaneous Endoscopic	Z No Device	X Diagnostic Z No Qualifier

New/Revised Text in Blue   ~~deleted~~ Deleted

SECTION: Ø MEDICAL AND SURGICAL
BODY SYSTEM: R UPPER JOINTS
OPERATION: B EXCISION: Cutting out or off, without replacement, a portion of a body part

Body Part	Approach	Device	Qualifier
Ø Occipital-cervical Joint	Ø Open	Z No Device	X Diagnostic
1 Cervical Vertebral Joint	3 Percutaneous		Z No Qualifier
3 Cervical Vertebral Disc	4 Percutaneous Endoscopic		
4 Cervicothoracic Vertebral Joint			
5 Cervicothoracic Vertebral Disc			
6 Thoracic Vertebral Joint			
9 Thoracic Vertebral Disc			
A Thoracolumbar Vertebral Joint			
B Thoracolumbar Vertebral Disc			
C Temporomandibular Joint, Right			
D Temporomandibular Joint, Left			
E Sternoclavicular Joint, Right			
F Sternoclavicular Joint, Left			
G Acromioclavicular Joint, Right			
H Acromioclavicular Joint, Left			
J Shoulder Joint, Right			
K Shoulder Joint, Left			
L Elbow Joint, Right			
M Elbow Joint, Left			
N Wrist Joint, Right			
P Wrist Joint, Left			
Q Carpal Joint, Right			
R Carpal Joint, Left			
S Carpometacarpal Joint, Right			
T Carpometacarpal Joint, Left			
U Metacarpophalangeal Joint, Right			
V Metacarpophalangeal Joint, Left			
W Finger Phalangeal Joint, Right			
X Finger Phalangeal Joint, Left			

SECTION: Ø MEDICAL AND SURGICAL
BODY SYSTEM: R UPPER JOINTS
OPERATION: C EXTIRPATION: Taking or cutting out solid matter from a body part

Body Part	Approach	Device	Qualifier
Ø Occipital-cervical Joint 1 Cervical Vertebral Joint 3 Cervical Vertebral Disc 4 Cervicothoracic Vertebral Joint 5 Cervicothoracic Vertebral Disc 6 Thoracic Vertebral Joint 9 Thoracic Vertebral Disc A Thoracolumbar Vertebral Joint B Thoracolumbar Vertebral Disc C Temporomandibular Joint, Right D Temporomandibular Joint, Left E Sternoclavicular Joint, Right F Sternoclavicular Joint, Left G Acromioclavicular Joint, Right H Acromioclavicular Joint, Left J Shoulder Joint, Right K Shoulder Joint, Left L Elbow Joint, Right M Elbow Joint, Left N Wrist Joint, Right P Wrist Joint, Left Q Carpal Joint, Right R Carpal Joint, Left S Carpometacarpal Joint, Right T Carpometacarpal Joint, Left U Metacarpophalangeal Joint, Right V Metacarpophalangeal Joint, Left W Finger Phalangeal Joint, Right X Finger Phalangeal Joint, Left	Ø Open 3 Percutaneous 4 Percutaneous Endoscopic	Z No Device	Z No Qualifier

C: EXTIRPATION   R: UPPER JOINTS   Ø: M/S

New/Revised Text in Blue   ~~deleted~~ Deleted

SECTION: Ø MEDICAL AND SURGICAL
BODY SYSTEM: R UPPER JOINTS
OPERATION: G FUSION: Joining together portions of an articular body part, rendering the articular body part immobile

Body Part	Approach	Device	Qualifier
Ø Occipital-cervical Joint 1 Cervical Vertebral Joint 2 Cervical Vertebral Joints, 2 or more 4 Cervicothoracic Vertebral Joint 6 Thoracic Vertebral Joint 7 Thoracic Vertebral Joint, 2 to 7 8 Thoracic Vertebral Joint, 8 or more A Thoracolumbar Vertebral Joint	Ø Open 3 Percutaneous 4 Percutaneous Endoscopic	7 Autologous Tissue Substitute A Interbody Fusion Device J Synthetic Substitute K Nonautologous Tissue Substitute Z No Device	Ø Anterior Approach, Anterior Column 1 Posterior Approach, Posterior Column J Posterior Approach, Anterior Column
Ø Occipital-cervical Joint 1 Cervical Vertebral Joint 2 Cervical Vertebral Joints, 2 or more 4 Cervicothoracic Vertebral Joint 6 Thoracic Vertebral Joint 7 Thoracic Vertebral Joints, 2 to 7 8 Thoracic Vertebral Joints, 8 or more A Thoracolumbar Vertebral Joint	Ø Open 3 Percutaneous 4 Percutaneous Endoscopic	A Interbody Fusion Device	Ø Anterior Approach, Anterior Column J Posterior Approach, Anterior Column
C Temporomandibular Joint, Right D Temporomandibular Joint, Left E Sternoclavicular Joint, Right F Sternoclavicular Joint, Left G Acromioclavicular Joint, Right H Acromioclavicular Joint, Left J Shoulder Joint, Right K Shoulder Joint, Left	Ø Open 3 Percutaneous 4 Percutaneous Endoscopic	4 Internal Fixation Device 7 Autologous Tissue Substitute J Synthetic Substitute K Nonautologous Tissue Substitute Z No Device	Z No Qualifier
L Elbow Joint, Right M Elbow Joint, Left N Wrist Joint, Right P Wrist Joint, Left Q Carpal Joint, Right R Carpal Joint, Left S Carpometacarpal Joint, Right T Carpometacarpal Joint, Left U Metacarpophalangeal Joint, Right V Metacarpophalangeal Joint, Left W Finger Phalangeal Joint, Right X Finger Phalangeal Joint, Left	Ø Open 3 Percutaneous 4 Percutaneous Endoscopic	4 Internal Fixation Device 5 External Fixation Device 7 Autologous Tissue Substitute J Synthetic Substitute K Nonautologous Tissue Substitute Z No Device	Z No Qualifier

Ø: M/S

R: UPPER JOINTS

G: FUSION

SECTION: Ø MEDICAL AND SURGICAL
BODY SYSTEM: R UPPER JOINTS
OPERATION: H INSERTION: Putting in a nonbiological appliance that monitors, assists, performs, or prevents a physiological function but does not physically take the place of a body part

Body Part	Approach	Device	Qualifier
Ø Occipital-cervical Joint 1 Cervical Vertebral Joint 4 Cervicothoracic Vertebral Joint 6 Thoracic Vertebral Joint A Thoracolumbar Vertebral Joint	Ø Open 3 Percutaneous 4 Percutaneous Endoscopic	3 Infusion Device 4 Internal Fixation Device 8 Spacer B Spinal Stabilization Device, Interspinous Process C Spinal Stabilization Device, Pedicle-Based D Spinal Stabilization Device, Facet Replacement	Z No Qualifier
3 Cervical Vertebral Disc 5 Cervicothoracic Vertebral Disc 9 Thoracic Vertebral Disc B Thoracolumbar Vertebral Disc	Ø Open 3 Percutaneous 4 Percutaneous Endoscopic	3 Infusion Device	Z No Qualifier
C Temporomandibular Joint, Right D Temporomandibular Joint, Left E Sternoclavicular Joint, Right F Sternoclavicular Joint, Left G Acromioclavicular Joint, Right H Acromioclavicular Joint, Left J Shoulder Joint, Right K Shoulder Joint, Left	Ø Open 3 Percutaneous 4 Percutaneous Endoscopic	3 Infusion Device 4 Internal Fixation Device 8 Spacer	Z No Qualifier
L Elbow Joint, Right M Elbow Joint, Left N Wrist Joint, Right P Wrist Joint, Left Q Carpal Joint, Right R Carpal Joint, Left S Carpometacarpal Joint, Right T Carpometacarpal Joint, Left U Metacarpophalangeal Joint, Right V Metacarpophalangeal Joint, Left W Finger Phalangeal Joint, Right X Finger Phalangeal Joint, Left	Ø Open 3 Percutaneous 4 Percutaneous Endoscopic	3 Infusion Device 4 Internal Fixation Device 5 External Fixation Device 8 Spacer	Z No Qualifier

SECTION: Ø MEDICAL AND SURGICAL
BODY SYSTEM: R UPPER JOINTS
OPERATION: J INSPECTION: Visually and/or manually exploring a body part

Body Part	Approach	Device	Qualifier
Ø Occipital-cervical Joint	Ø Open	Z No Device	Z No Qualifier
1 Cervical Vertebral Joint	3 Percutaneous		
3 Cervical Vertebral Disc	4 Percutaneous Endoscopic		
4 Cervicothoracic Vertebral Joint	X External		
5 Cervicothoracic Vertebral Disc			
6 Thoracic Vertebral Joint			
9 Thoracic Vertebral Disc			
A Thoracolumbar Vertebral Joint			
B Thoracolumbar Vertebral Disc			
C Temporomandibular Joint, Right			
D Temporomandibular Joint, Left			
E Sternoclavicular Joint, Right			
F Sternoclavicular Joint, Left			
G Acromioclavicular Joint, Right			
H Acromioclavicular Joint, Left			
J Shoulder Joint, Right			
K Shoulder Joint, Left			
L Elbow Joint, Right			
M Elbow Joint, Left			
N Wrist Joint, Right			
P Wrist Joint, Left			
Q Carpal Joint, Right			
R Carpal Joint, Left			
S Carpometacarpal Joint, Right			
T Carpometacarpal Joint, Left			
U Metacarpophalangeal Joint, Right			
V Metacarpophalangeal Joint, Left			
W Finger Phalangeal Joint, Right			
X Finger Phalangeal Joint, Left			

SECTION: Ø MEDICAL AND SURGICAL
BODY SYSTEM: R UPPER JOINTS
OPERATION: N RELEASE: Freeing a body part from an abnormal physical constraint by cutting or by the use of force

Body Part	Approach	Device	Qualifier
Ø Occipital-cervical Joint	Ø Open	Z No Device	Z No Qualifier
1 Cervical Vertebral Joint	3 Percutaneous		
3 Cervical Vertebral Disc	4 Percutaneous Endoscopic		
4 Cervicothoracic Vertebral Joint	X External		
5 Cervicothoracic Vertebral Disc			
6 Thoracic Vertebral Joint			
9 Thoracic Vertebral Disc			
A Thoracolumbar Vertebral Joint			
B Thoracolumbar Vertebral Disc			
C Temporomandibular Joint, Right			
D Temporomandibular Joint, Left			
E Sternoclavicular Joint, Right			
F Sternoclavicular Joint, Left			
G Acromioclavicular Joint, Right			
H Acromioclavicular Joint, Left			
J Shoulder Joint, Right			
K Shoulder Joint, Left			
L Elbow Joint, Right			
M Elbow Joint, Left			
N Wrist Joint, Right			
P Wrist Joint, Left			
Q Carpal Joint, Right			
R Carpal Joint, Left			
S Carpometacarpal Joint, Right			
T Carpometacarpal Joint, Left			
U Metacarpophalangeal Joint, Right			
V Metacarpophalangeal Joint, Left			
W Finger Phalangeal Joint, Right			
X Finger Phalangeal Joint, Left			

SECTION: Ø MEDICAL AND SURGICAL
BODY SYSTEM: R UPPER JOINTS
OPERATION: P REMOVAL: (on multiple pages)
Taking out or off a device from a body part

Body Part	Approach	Device	Qualifier
Ø Occipital-cervical Joint	Ø Open	Ø Drainage Device	Z No Qualifier
1 Cervical Vertebral Joint	3 Percutaneous	3 Infusion Device	
4 Cervicothoracic Vertebral Joint	4 Percutaneous Endoscopic	4 Internal Fixation Device	
6 Thoracic Vertebral Joint		7 Autologous Tissue Substitute	
A Thoracolumbar Vertebral Joint		8 Spacer	
		A Interbody Fusion Device	
		J Synthetic Substitute	
		K Nonautologous Tissue Substitute	

New/Revised Text in Blue   ~~deleted~~ Deleted

SECTION: Ø MEDICAL AND SURGICAL
BODY SYSTEM: R UPPER JOINTS
OPERATION: P REMOVAL: *(continued)*
Taking out or off a device from a body part

Body Part	Approach	Device	Qualifier
Ø Occipital-cervical Joint 1 Cervical Vertebral Joint 4 Cervicothoracic Vertebral Joint 6 Thoracic Vertebral Joint A Thoracolumbar Vertebral Joint	X External	Ø Drainage Device 3 Infusion Device 4 Internal Fixation Device	Z No Qualifier
3 Cervical Vertebral Disc 5 Cervicothoracic Vertebral Disc 9 Thoracic Vertebral Disc B Thoracolumbar Vertebral Disc	Ø Open 3 Percutaneous 4 Percutaneous Endoscopic	Ø Drainage Device 3 Infusion Device 7 Autologous Tissue Substitute J Synthetic Substitute K Nonautologous Tissue Substitute	Z No Qualifier
3 Cervical Vertebral Disc 5 Cervicothoracic Vertebral Disc 9 Thoracic Vertebral Disc B Thoracolumbar Vertebral Disc	X External	Ø Drainage Device 3 Infusion Device	Z No Qualifier
C Temporomandibular Joint, Right D Temporomandibular Joint, Left E Sternoclavicular Joint, Right F Sternoclavicular Joint, Left G Acromioclavicular Joint, Right H Acromioclavicular Joint, Left J Shoulder Joint, Right K Shoulder Joint, Left	Ø Open 3 Percutaneous 4 Percutaneous Endoscopic	Ø Drainage Device 3 Infusion Device 4 Internal Fixation Device 7 Autologous Tissue Substitute 8 Spacer J Synthetic Substitute K Nonautologous Tissue Substitute	Z No Qualifier
C Temporomandibular Joint, Right D Temporomandibular Joint, Left E Sternoclavicular Joint, Right F Sternoclavicular Joint, Left G Acromioclavicular Joint, Right H Acromioclavicular Joint, Left J Shoulder Joint, Right K Shoulder Joint, Left	X External	Ø Drainage Device 3 Infusion Device 4 Internal Fixation Device	Z No Qualifier
L Elbow Joint, Right M Elbow Joint, Left N Wrist Joint, Right P Wrist Joint, Left Q Carpal Joint, Right R Carpal Joint, Left S Carpometacarpal Joint, Right T Carpometacarpal Joint, Left U Metacarpophalangeal Joint, Right V Metacarpophalangeal Joint, Left W Finger Phalangeal Joint, Right X Finger Phalangeal Joint, Left	Ø Open 3 Percutaneous 4 Percutaneous Endoscopic	Ø Drainage Device 3 Infusion Device 4 Internal Fixation Device 5 External Fixation Device 7 Autologous Tissue Substitute 8 Spacer J Synthetic Substitute K Nonautologous Tissue Substitute	Z No Qualifier

SECTION: Ø MEDICAL AND SURGICAL

BODY SYSTEM: R UPPER JOINTS

OPERATION: P REMOVAL: *(continued)*
Taking out or off a device from a body part

Body Part	Approach	Device	Qualifier
L Elbow Joint, Right M Elbow Joint, Left N Wrist Joint, Right P Wrist Joint, Left Q Carpal Joint, Right R Carpal Joint, Left S Carpometacarpal Joint, Right T Carpometacarpal Joint, Left U Metacarpophalangeal Joint, Right V Metacarpophalangeal Joint, Left W Finger Phalangeal Joint, Right X Finger Phalangeal Joint, Left	X External	Ø Drainage Device 3 Infusion Device 4 Internal Fixation Device 5 External Fixation Device	Z No Qualifier

SECTION: Ø MEDICAL AND SURGICAL

BODY SYSTEM: R UPPER JOINTS

OPERATION: Q REPAIR: Restoring, to the extent possible, a body part to its normal anatomic structure and function

Body Part	Approach	Device	Qualifier
Ø Occipital-cervical Joint 1 Cervical Vertebral Joint 3 Cervical Vertebral Disc 4 Cervicothoracic Vertebral Joint 5 Cervicothoracic Vertebral Disc 6 Thoracic Vertebral Joint 9 Thoracic Vertebral Disc A Thoracolumbar Vertebral Joint B Thoracolumbar Vertebral Disc C Temporomandibular Joint, Right D Temporomandibular Joint, Left E Sternoclavicular Joint, Right F Sternoclavicular Joint, Left G Acromioclavicular Joint, Right H Acromioclavicular Joint, Left J Shoulder Joint, Right K Shoulder Joint, Left L Elbow Joint, Right M Elbow Joint, Left N Wrist Joint, Right P Wrist Joint, Left Q Carpal Joint, Right R Carpal Joint, Left S Carpometacarpal Joint, Right T Carpometacarpal Joint, Left U Metacarpophalangeal Joint, Right V Metacarpophalangeal Joint, Left W Finger Phalangeal Joint, Right X Finger Phalangeal Joint, Left	Ø Open 3 Percutaneous 4 Percutaneous Endoscopic X External	Z No Device	Z No Qualifier

New/Revised Text in Blue   ~~deleted~~ Deleted

SECTION: Ø **MEDICAL AND SURGICAL**
BODY SYSTEM: R **UPPER JOINTS**
OPERATION: R **REPLACEMENT:** Putting in or on biological or synthetic material that physically takes the place and/or function of all or a portion of a body part

Body Part	Approach	Device	Qualifier
Ø Occipital-cervical Joint 1 Cervical Vertebral Joint 3 Cervical Vertebral Disc 4 Cervicothoracic Vertebral Joint 5 Cervicothoracic Vertebral Disc 6 Thoracic Vertebral Joint 9 Thoracic Vertebral Disc A Thoracolumbar Vertebral Joint B Thoracolumbar Vertebral Disc C Temporomandibular Joint, Right D Temporomandibular Joint, Left E Sternoclavicular Joint, Right F Sternoclavicular Joint, Left G Acromioclavicular Joint, Right H Acromioclavicular Joint, Left L Elbow Joint, Right M Elbow Joint, Left N Wrist Joint, Right P Wrist Joint, Left Q Carpal Joint, Right R Carpal Joint, Left S Carpometacarpal Joint, Right T Carpometacarpal Joint, Left U Metacarpophalangeal Joint, Right V Metacarpophalangeal Joint, Left W Finger Phalangeal Joint, Right X Finger Phalangeal Joint, Left	Ø Open	7 Autologous Tissue Substitute J Synthetic Substitute K Nonautologous Tissue Substitute	Z No Qualifier
J Shoulder Joint, Right K Shoulder Joint, Left	Ø Open	Ø Synthetic Substitute, Reverse Ball and Socket 7 Autologous Tissue Substitute K Nonautologous Tissue Substitute	Z No Qualifier
J Shoulder Joint, Right K Shoulder Joint, Left	Ø Open	J Synthetic Substitute	6 Humeral Surface 7 Glenoid Surface Z No Qualifier

SECTION: Ø MEDICAL AND SURGICAL
BODY SYSTEM: R UPPER JOINTS
OPERATION: S REPOSITION: Moving to its normal location, or other suitable location, all or a portion of a body part

Body Part	Approach	Device	Qualifier
Ø Occipital-cervical Joint 1 Cervical Vertebral Joint 4 Cervicothoracic Vertebral Joint 6 Thoracic Vertebral Joint A Thoracolumbar Vertebral Joint C Temporomandibular Joint, Right D Temporomandibular Joint, Left E Sternoclavicular Joint, Right F Sternoclavicular Joint, Left G Acromioclavicular Joint, Right H Acromioclavicular Joint, Left J Shoulder Joint, Right K Shoulder Joint, Left	Ø Open 3 Percutaneous 4 Percutaneous Endoscopic X External	4 Internal Fixation Device Z No Device	Z No Qualifier
L Elbow Joint, Right M Elbow Joint, Left N Wrist Joint, Right P Wrist Joint, Left Q Carpal Joint, Right R Carpal Joint, Left S Carpometacarpal Joint, Right T Carpometacarpal Joint, Left U Metacarpophalangeal Joint, Right V Metacarpophalangeal Joint, Left W Finger Phalangeal Joint, Right X Finger Phalangeal Joint, Left	Ø Open 3 Percutaneous 4 Percutaneous Endoscopic X External	4 Internal Fixation Device 5 External Fixation Device Z No Device	Z No Qualifier

New/Revised Text in Blue   ~~deleted~~ Deleted

SECTION: Ø MEDICAL AND SURGICAL
BODY SYSTEM: R UPPER JOINTS
OPERATION: T RESECTION: Cutting out or off, without replacement, all of a body part

Body Part	Approach	Device	Qualifier
3 Cervical Vertebral Disc	Ø Open	Z No Device	Z No Qualifier
4 Cervicothoracic Vertebral Joint			
5 Cervicothoracic Vertebral Disc			
9 Thoracic Vertebral Disc			
B Thoracolumbar Vertebral Disc			
C Temporomandibular Joint, Right			
D Temporomandibular Joint, Left			
E Sternoclavicular Joint, Right			
F Sternoclavicular Joint, Left			
G Acromioclavicular Joint, Right			
H Acromioclavicular Joint, Left			
J Shoulder Joint, Right			
K Shoulder Joint, Left			
L Elbow Joint, Right			
M Elbow Joint, Left			
N Wrist Joint, Right			
P Wrist Joint, Left			
Q Carpal Joint, Right			
R Carpal Joint, Left			
S Carpometacarpal Joint, Right			
T Carpometacarpal Joint, Left			
U Metacarpophalangeal Joint, Right			
V Metacarpophalangeal Joint, Left			
W Finger Phalangeal Joint, Right			
X Finger Phalangeal Joint, Left			

SECTION: Ø MEDICAL AND SURGICAL
BODY SYSTEM: R UPPER JOINTS
OPERATION: U SUPPLEMENT: Putting in or on biological or synthetic material that physically reinforces and/or augments the function of a portion of a body part

Body Part	Approach	Device	Qualifier
Ø Occipital-cervical Joint 1 Cervical Vertebral Joint 3 Cervical Vertebral Disc 4 Cervicothoracic Vertebral Joint 5 Cervicothoracic Vertebral Disc 6 Thoracic Vertebral Joint 9 Thoracic Vertebral Disc A Thoracolumbar Vertebral Joint B Thoracolumbar Vertebral Disc C Temporomandibular Joint, Right D Temporomandibular Joint, Left E Sternoclavicular Joint, Right F Sternoclavicular Joint, Left G Acromioclavicular Joint, Right H Acromioclavicular Joint, Left J Shoulder Joint, Right K Shoulder Joint, Left L Elbow Joint, Right M Elbow Joint, Left N Wrist Joint, Right P Wrist Joint, Left Q Carpal Joint, Right R Carpal Joint, Left S Carpometacarpal Joint, Right T Carpometacarpal Joint, Left U Metacarpophalangeal Joint, Right V Metacarpophalangeal Joint, Left W Finger Phalangeal Joint, Right X Finger Phalangeal Joint, Left	Ø Open 3 Percutaneous 4 Percutaneous Endoscopic	7 Autologous Tissue Substitute J Synthetic Substitute K Nonautologous Tissue Substitute	Z No Qualifier

SECTION: Ø MEDICAL AND SURGICAL
BODY SYSTEM: R UPPER JOINTS
OPERATION: W REVISION: Correcting, to the extent possible, a portion of a malfunctioning device or the position of a displaced device

Body Part	Approach	Device	Qualifier
Ø Occipital-cervical Joint 1 Cervical Vertebral Joint 4 Cervicothoracic Vertebral Joint 6 Thoracic Vertebral Joint A Thoracolumbar Vertebral Joint	Ø Open 3 Percutaneous 4 Percutaneous Endoscopic X External	Ø Drainage Device 3 Infusion Device 4 Internal Fixation Device 7 Autologous Tissue Substitute 8 Spacer A Interbody Fusion Device J Synthetic Substitute K Nonautologous Tissue Substitute	Z No Qualifier
3 Cervical Vertebral Disc 5 Cervicothoracic Vertebral Disc 9 Thoracic Vertebral Disc B Thoracolumbar Vertebral Disc	Ø Open 3 Percutaneous 4 Percutaneous Endoscopic X External	Ø Drainage Device 3 Infusion Device 7 Autologous Tissue Substitute J Synthetic Substitute K Nonautologous Tissue Substitute	Z No Qualifier
C Temporomandibular Joint, Right D Temporomandibular Joint, Left E Sternoclavicular Joint, Right F Sternoclavicular Joint, Left G Acromioclavicular Joint, Right H Acromioclavicular Joint, Left J Shoulder Joint, Right K Shoulder Joint, Left	Ø Open 3 Percutaneous 4 Percutaneous Endoscopic X External	Ø Drainage Device 3 Infusion Device 4 Internal Fixation Device 7 Autologous Tissue Substitute 8 Spacer J Synthetic Substitute K Nonautologous Tissue Substitute	Z No Qualifier
L Elbow Joint, Right M Elbow Joint, Left N Wrist Joint, Right P Wrist Joint, Left Q Carpal Joint, Right R Carpal Joint, Left S Carpometacarpal Joint, Right T Carpometacarpal Joint, Left U Metacarpophalangeal Joint, Right V Metacarpophalangeal Joint, Left W Finger Phalangeal Joint, Right X Finger Phalangeal Joint, Left	Ø Open 3 Percutaneous 4 Percutaneous Endoscopic X External	Ø Drainage Device 3 Infusion Device 4 Internal Fixation Device 5 External Fixation Device 7 Autologous Tissue Substitute 8 Spacer J Synthetic Substitute K Nonautologous Tissue Substitute	Z No Qualifier

ØS. Lower Joints.. 404
    ØS2. Change 405
    ØS5. Destruction 405
    ØS9. Drainage 406
    ØSB. Excision 407
    ØSC. Extirpation 407
    ØSG. Fusion 408
    ØSH. Insertion 409
    ØSJ. Inspection 410
    ØSN. Release 410
    ØSP. Removal 411
    ØSQ. Repair 414
    ØSR. Replacement 415
    ØSS. Reposition 417
    ØST. Resection 417
    ØSU. Supplement 418
    ØSW. Revision 419

SECTION: Ø MEDICAL AND SURGICAL

BODY SYSTEM: S LOWER JOINTS

OPERATION: 2 CHANGE: Taking out or off a device from a body part and putting back an identical or similar device in or on the same body part without cutting or puncturing the skin or a mucous membrane

Body Part	Approach	Device	Qualifier
Y Lower Joint	X External	Ø Drainage Device Y Other Device	Z No Qualifier

SECTION: Ø MEDICAL AND SURGICAL

BODY SYSTEM: S LOWER JOINTS

OPERATION: 5 DESTRUCTION: Physical eradication of all or a portion of a body part by the direct use of energy, force, or destructive agent

Body Part	Approach	Device	Qualifier
Ø Lumbar Vertebral Joint 2 Lumbar Vertebral Disc 3 Lumbosacral Joint 4 Lumbosacral Disc 5 Sacrococcygeal Joint 6 Coccygeal Joint 7 Sacroiliac Joint, Right 8 Sacroiliac Joint, Left 9 Hip Joint, Right B Hip Joint, Left C Knee Joint, Right D Knee Joint, Left F Ankle Joint, Right G Ankle Joint, Left H Tarsal Joint, Right J Tarsal Joint, Left K Tarsometatarsal Joint, Right L Tarsometatarsal Joint, Left M Metatarsal-Phalangeal Joint, Right N Metatarsal-Phalangeal Joint, Left P Toe Phalangeal Joint, Right Q Toe Phalangeal Joint, Left	Ø Open 3 Percutaneous 4 Percutaneous Endoscopic	Z No Device	Z No Qualifier

SECTION:　Ø MEDICAL AND SURGICAL
BODY SYSTEM: S LOWER JOINTS
OPERATION:　9 **DRAINAGE:** Taking or letting out fluids and/or gases from a body part

Body Part	Approach	Device	Qualifier
Ø Lumbar Vertebral Joint 2 Lumbar Vertebral Disc 3 Lumbosacral Joint 4 Lumbosacral Disc 5 Sacrococcygeal Joint 6 Coccygeal Joint 7 Sacroiliac Joint, Right 8 Sacroiliac Joint, Left 9 Hip Joint, Right B Hip Joint, Left C Knee Joint, Right D Knee Joint, Left F Ankle Joint, Right G Ankle Joint, Left H Tarsal Joint, Right J Tarsal Joint, Left K Tarsometatarsal Joint, Right L Tarsometatarsal Joint, Left M Metatarsal-Phalangeal Joint, Right N Metatarsal-Phalangeal Joint, Left P Toe Phalangeal Joint, Right Q Toe Phalangeal Joint, Left	Ø Open 3 Percutaneous 4 Percutaneous Endoscopic	Ø Drainage Device	Z No Qualifier
Ø Lumbar Vertebral Joint 2 Lumbar Vertebral Disc 3 Lumbosacral Joint 4 Lumbosacral Disc 5 Sacrococcygeal Joint 6 Coccygeal Joint 7 Sacroiliac Joint, Right 8 Sacroiliac Joint, Left 9 Hip Joint, Right B Hip Joint, Left C Knee Joint, Right D Knee Joint, Left F Ankle Joint, Right G Ankle Joint, Left H Tarsal Joint, Right J Tarsal Joint, Left K Tarsometatarsal Joint, Right L Tarsometatarsal Joint, Left M Metatarsal-Phalangeal Joint, Right N Metatarsal-Phalangeal Joint, Left P Toe Phalangeal Joint, Right Q Toe Phalangeal Joint, Left	Ø Open 3 Percutaneous 4 Percutaneous Endoscopic	Z No Device	X Diagnostic Z No Qualifier

9: DRAINAGE

S: LOWER JOINTS

Ø: M/S

SECTION: Ø MEDICAL AND SURGICAL
BODY SYSTEM: S LOWER JOINTS
OPERATION: **B EXCISION:** Cutting out or off, without replacement, a portion of a body part

Body Part	Approach	Device	Qualifier
Ø Lumbar Vertebral Joint 2 Lumbar Vertebral Disc 3 Lumbosacral Joint 4 Lumbosacral Disc 5 Sacrococcygeal Joint 6 Coccygeal Joint 7 Sacroiliac Joint, Right 8 Sacroiliac Joint, Left 9 Hip Joint, Right B Hip Joint, Left C Knee Joint, Right D Knee Joint, Left F Ankle Joint, Right G Ankle Joint, Left H Tarsal Joint, Right J Tarsal Joint, Left K Tarsometatarsal Joint, Right L Tarsometatarsal Joint, Left M Metatarsal-Phalangeal Joint, Right N Metatarsal-Phalangeal Joint, Left P Toe Phalangeal Joint, Right Q Toe Phalangeal Joint, Left	Ø Open 3 Percutaneous 4 Percutaneous Endoscopic	Z No Device	X Diagnostic Z No Qualifier

SECTION: Ø MEDICAL AND SURGICAL
BODY SYSTEM: S LOWER JOINTS
OPERATION: **C EXTIRPATION:** Taking or cutting out solid matter from a body part

Body Part	Approach	Device	Qualifier
Ø Lumbar Vertebral Joint 2 Lumbar Vertebral Disc 3 Lumbosacral Joint 4 Lumbosacral Disc 5 Sacrococcygeal Joint 6 Coccygeal Joint 7 Sacroiliac Joint, Right 8 Sacroiliac Joint, Left 9 Hip Joint, Right B Hip Joint, Left C Knee Joint, Right D Knee Joint, Left F Ankle Joint, Right G Ankle Joint, Left H Tarsal Joint, Right J Tarsal Joint, Left K Tarsometatarsal Joint, Right L Tarsometatarsal Joint, Left M Metatarsal-Phalangeal Joint, Right N Metatarsal-Phalangeal Joint, Left P Toe Phalangeal Joint, Right Q Toe Phalangeal Joint, Left	Ø Open 3 Percutaneous 4 Percutaneous Endoscopic	Z No Device	Z No Qualifier

SECTION: Ø MEDICAL AND SURGICAL
BODY SYSTEM: S LOWER JOINTS
OPERATION: **G FUSION:** Joining together portions of an articular body part, rendering the articular body part immobile

Body Part	Approach	Device	Qualifier
Ø Lumbar Vertebral Joint 1 Lumbar Vertebral Joints, 2 or more 3 Lumbosacral Joint	Ø Open 3 Percutaneous 4 Percutaneous Endoscopic	7 Autologous Tissue Substitute A Interbody Fusion Device J Synthetic Substitute K Nonautologous Tissue Substitute Z No Device	Ø Anterior Approach, Anterior Column 1 Posterior Approach, Posterior Column J Posterior Approach, Anterior Column
Ø Lumbar Vertebral Joint 1 Lumbar Vertebral Joints, 2 or more 3 Lumbosacral Joint	Ø Open 3 Percutaneous 4 Percutaneous Endoscopic	A Interbody Fusion Device	Ø Anterior Approach, Anterior Column J Posterior Approach, Anterior Column
5 Sacrococcygeal Joint 6 Coccygeal Joint 7 Sacroiliac Joint, Right 8 Sacroiliac Joint, Left	Ø Open 3 Percutaneous 4 Percutaneous Endoscopic	4 Internal Fixation Device 7 Autologous Tissue Substitute J Synthetic Substitute K Nonautologous Tissue Substitute Z No Device	Z No Qualifier
9 Hip Joint, Right B Hip Joint, Left C Knee Joint, Right D Knee Joint, Left F Ankle Joint, Right G Ankle Joint, Left H Tarsal Joint, Right J Tarsal Joint, Left K Tarsometatarsal Joint, Right L Tarsometatarsal Joint, Left M Metatarsal-Phalangeal Joint, Right N Metatarsal-Phalangeal Joint, Left P Toe Phalangeal Joint, Right Q Toe Phalangeal Joint, Left	Ø Open 3 Percutaneous 4 Percutaneous Endoscopic	4 Internal Fixation Device 5 External Fixation Device 7 Autologous Tissue Substitute J Synthetic Substitute K Nonautologous Tissue Substitute Z No Device	Z No Qualifier

SECTION: Ø MEDICAL AND SURGICAL
BODY SYSTEM: S LOWER JOINTS
OPERATION: H INSERTION: Putting in a nonbiological appliance that monitors, assists, performs, or prevents a physiological function but does not physically take the place of a body part

Body Part	Approach	Device	Qualifier
Ø Lumbar Vertebral Joint 3 Lumbosacral Joint	Ø Open 3 Percutaneous 4 Percutaneous Endoscopic	3 Infusion Device 4 Internal Fixation Device 8 Spacer B Spinal Stabilization Device, Interspinous Process C Spinal Stabilization Device, Pedicle-Based D Spinal Stabilization Device, Facet Replacement	Z No Qualifier
2 Lumbar Vertebral Disc 4 Lumbosacral Disc	Ø Open 3 Percutaneous 4 Percutaneous Endoscopic	3 Infusion Device 8 Spacer	Z No Qualifier
5 Sacrococcygeal Joint 6 Coccygeal Joint 7 Sacroiliac Joint, Right 8 Sacroiliac Joint, Left	Ø Open 3 Percutaneous 4 Percutaneous Endoscopic	3 Infusion Device 4 Internal Fixation Device 8 Spacer	Z No Qualifier
9 Hip Joint, Right B Hip Joint, Left C Knee Joint, Right D Knee Joint, Left F Ankle Joint, Right G Ankle Joint, Left H Tarsal Joint, Right J Tarsal Joint, Left K Tarsometatarsal Joint, Right L Tarsometatarsal Joint, Left M Metatarsal-Phalangeal Joint, Right N Metatarsal-Phalangeal Joint, Left P Toe Phalangeal Joint, Right Q Toe Phalangeal Joint, Left	Ø Open 3 Percutaneous 4 Percutaneous Endoscopic	3 Infusion Device 4 Internal Fixation Device 5 External Fixation Device 8 Spacer	Z No Qualifier

J: INSPECTION   N: RELEASE

S: LOWER JOINTS

Ø: M/S

SECTION: Ø MEDICAL AND SURGICAL
BODY SYSTEM: S LOWER JOINTS
OPERATION: J **INSPECTION:** Visually and/or manually exploring a body part

Body Part	Approach	Device	Qualifier
Ø Lumbar Vertebral Joint 2 Lumbar Vertebral Disc 3 Lumbosacral Joint 4 Lumbosacral Disc 5 Sacrococcygeal Joint 6 Coccygeal Joint 7 Sacroiliac Joint, Right 8 Sacroiliac Joint, Left 9 Hip Joint, Right B Hip Joint, Left C Knee Joint, Right D Knee Joint, Left F Ankle Joint, Right G Ankle Joint, Left H Tarsal Joint, Right J Tarsal Joint, Left K Tarsometatarsal Joint, Right L Tarsometatarsal Joint, Left M Metatarsal-Phalangeal Joint, Right N Metatarsal-Phalangeal Joint, Left P Toe Phalangeal Joint, Right Q Toe Phalangeal Joint, Left	Ø Open 3 Percutaneous 4 Percutaneous Endoscopic X External	Z No Device	Z No Qualifier

SECTION: Ø MEDICAL AND SURGICAL
BODY SYSTEM: S LOWER JOINTS
OPERATION: N **RELEASE:** Freeing a body part from an abnormal physical constraint by cutting or by the use of force

Body Part	Approach	Device	Qualifier
Ø Lumbar Vertebral Joint 2 Lumbar Vertebral Disc 3 Lumbosacral Joint 4 Lumbosacral Disc 5 Sacrococcygeal Joint 6 Coccygeal Joint 7 Sacroiliac Joint, Right 8 Sacroiliac Joint, Left 9 Hip Joint, Right B Hip Joint, Left C Knee Joint, Right D Knee Joint, Left F Ankle Joint, Right G Ankle Joint, Left H Tarsal Joint, Right J Tarsal Joint, Left K Tarsometatarsal Joint, Right L Tarsometatarsal Joint, Left M Metatarsal-Phalangeal Joint, Right N Metatarsal-Phalangeal Joint, Left P Toe Phalangeal Joint, Right Q Toe Phalangeal Joint, Left	Ø Open 3 Percutaneous 4 Percutaneous Endoscopic X External	Z No Device	Z No Qualifier

New/Revised Text in Blue   ~~deleted~~ Deleted

SECTION: Ø MEDICAL AND SURGICAL
BODY SYSTEM: S LOWER JOINTS
OPERATION: P REMOVAL: *(on multiple pages)*
Taking out or off a device from a body part

Body Part	Approach	Device	Qualifier
Ø Lumbar Vertebral Joint 3 Lumbosacral Joint	Ø Open 3 Percutaneous 4 Percutaneous Endoscopic	Ø Drainage Device 3 Infusion Device 4 Internal Fixation Device 7 Autologous Tissue Substitute 8 Spacer A Interbody Fusion Device J Synthetic Substitute K Nonautologous Tissue Substitute	Z No Qualifier
Ø Lumbar Vertebral Joint 3 Lumbosacral Joint	X External	Ø Drainage Device 3 Infusion Device 4 Internal Fixation Device	Z No Qualifier
2 Lumbar Vertebral Disc 4 Lumbosacral Disc	Ø Open 3 Percutaneous 4 Percutaneous Endoscopic	Ø Drainage Device 3 Infusion Device 7 Autologous Tissue Substitute J Synthetic Substitute K Nonautologous Tissue Substitute	Z No Qualifier
2 Lumbar Vertebral Disc 4 Lumbosacral Disc	X External	Ø Drainage Device 3 Infusion Device	Z No Qualifier
5 Sacrococcygeal Joint 6 Coccygeal Joint 7 Sacroiliac Joint, Right 8 Sacroiliac Joint, Left	Ø Open 3 Percutaneous 4 Percutaneous Endoscopic	Ø Drainage Device 3 Infusion Device 4 Internal Fixation Device 7 Autologous Tissue Substitute 8 Spacer J Synthetic Substitute K Nonautologous Tissue Substitute	Z No Qualifier
5 Sacrococcygeal Joint 6 Coccygeal Joint 7 Sacroiliac Joint, Right 8 Sacroiliac Joint, Left	X External	Ø Drainage Device 3 Infusion Device 4 Internal Fixation Device	Z No Qualifier
9 Hip Joint, Right B Hip Joint, Left	Ø Open	Ø Drainage Device 3 Infusion Device 4 Internal Fixation Device 5 External Fixation Device 7 Autologous Tissue Substitute 8 Spacer 9 Liner B Resurfacing Device J Synthetic Substitute K Nonautologous Tissue Substitute	Z No Qualifier
9 Hip Joint, Right B Hip Joint, Left	3 Percutaneous 4 Percutaneous Endoscopic	Ø Drainage Device 3 Infusion Device 4 Internal Fixation Device 5 External Fixation Device 7 Autologous Tissue Substitute 8 Spacer J Synthetic Substitute K Nonautologous Tissue Substitute	Z No Qualifier

SECTION: Ø MEDICAL AND SURGICAL
BODY SYSTEM: S LOWER JOINTS
OPERATION: P REMOVAL: *(continued)*
Taking out or off a device from a body part

Body Part	Approach	Device	Qualifier
9 Hip Joint, Right B Hip Joint, Left	X External	Ø Drainage Device 3 Infusion Device 4 Internal Fixation Device 5 External Fixation Device	Z No Qualifier
A Hip Joint, Acetabular Surface, Right E Hip Joint, Acetabular Surface, Left R Hip Joint, Femoral Surface, Right S Hip Joint, Femoral Surface, Left T Knee Joint, Femoral Surface, Right U Knee Joint, Femoral Surface, Left V Knee Joint, Tibial Surface, Right W Knee Joint, Tibial Surface, Left	Ø Open 3 Percutaneous 4 Percutaneous Endoscopic	J Synthetic Substitute	Z No Qualifier
C Knee Joint, Right D Knee Joint, Left	Ø Open	Ø Drainage Device 3 Infusion Device 4 Internal Fixation Device 5 External Fixation Device 7 Autologous Tissue Substitute 8 Spacer 9 Liner K Nonautologous Tissue Substitute	Z No Qualifier
C Knee Joint, Right D Knee Joint, Left	Ø Open	J Synthetic Substitute	C Patellar Surface Z No Qualifier
C Knee Joint, Right D Knee Joint, Left	3 Percutaneous 4 Percutaneous Endoscopic	Ø Drainage Device 3 Infusion Device 4 Internal Fixation Device 5 External Fixation Device 7 Autologous Tissue Substitute 8 Spacer K Nonautologous Tissue Substitute	Z No Qualifier
C Knee Joint, Right D Knee Joint, Left	3 Percutaneous 4 Percutaneous Endoscopic	J Synthetic Substitute	C Patellar Surface Z No Qualifier
C Knee Joint, Right D Knee Joint, Left	X External	Ø Drainage Device 3 Infusion Device 4 Internal Fixation Device 5 External Fixation Device	Z No Qualifier

SECTION: Ø MEDICAL AND SURGICAL
BODY SYSTEM: S LOWER JOINTS
OPERATION: P REMOVAL: *(continued)*
Taking out or off a device from a body part

Body Part	Approach	Device	Qualifier
F Ankle Joint, Right G Ankle Joint, Left H Tarsal Joint, Right J Tarsal Joint, Left K Tarsometatarsal Joint, Right L Tarsometatarsal Joint, Left M Metatarsal-Phalangeal Joint, Right N Metatarsal-Phalangeal Joint, Left P Toe Phalangeal Joint, Right Q Toe Phalangeal Joint, Left	Ø Open 3 Percutaneous 4 Percutaneous Endoscopic	Ø Drainage Device 3 Infusion Device 4 Internal Fixation Device 5 External Fixation Device 7 Autologous Tissue Substitute 8 Spacer J Synthetic Substitute K Nonautologous Tissue Substitute	Z No Qualifier
F Ankle Joint, Right G Ankle Joint, Left H Tarsal Joint, Right J Tarsal Joint, Left K Tarsometatarsal Joint, Right L Tarsometatarsal Joint, Left M Metatarsal-Phalangeal Joint, Right N Metatarsal-Phalangeal Joint, Left P Toe Phalangeal Joint, Right Q Toe Phalangeal Joint, Left	X External	Ø Drainage Device 3 Infusion Device 4 Internal Fixation Device 5 External Fixation Device	Z No Qualifier

SECTION: Ø MEDICAL AND SURGICAL
BODY SYSTEM: S LOWER JOINTS
OPERATION: Q **REPAIR:** Restoring, to the extent possible, a body part to its normal anatomic structure and function

Body Part	Approach	Device	Qualifier
Ø Lumbar Vertebral Joint 2 Lumbar Vertebral Disc 3 Lumbosacral Joint 4 Lumbosacral Disc 5 Sacrococcygeal Joint 6 Coccygeal Joint 7 Sacroiliac Joint, Right 8 Sacroiliac Joint, Left 9 Hip Joint, Right B Hip Joint, Left C Knee Joint, Right D Knee Joint, Left F Ankle Joint, Right G Ankle Joint, Left H Tarsal Joint, Right J Tarsal Joint, Left K Tarsometatarsal Joint, Right L Tarsometatarsal Joint, Left M Metatarsal-Phalangeal Joint, Right N Metatarsal-Phalangeal Joint, Left P Toe Phalangeal Joint, Right Q Toe Phalangeal Joint, Left	Ø Open 3 Percutaneous 4 Percutaneous Endoscopic X External	Z No Device	Z No Qualifier

SECTION: Ø MEDICAL AND SURGICAL
BODY SYSTEM: S LOWER JOINTS
OPERATION: R REPLACEMENT: *(on multiple pages)*

Putting in or on biological or synthetic material that physically takes the place and/or function of all or a portion of a body part

Body Part	Approach	Device	Qualifier
Ø Lumbar Vertebral Joint 2 Lumbar Vertebral Disc 3 Lumbosacral Joint 4 Lumbosacral Disc 5 Sacrococcygeal Joint 6 Coccygeal Joint 7 Sacroiliac Joint, Right 8 Sacroiliac Joint, Left H Tarsal Joint, Right J Tarsal Joint, Left K Tarsometatarsal Joint, Right L Tarsometatarsal Joint, Left M Metatarsal-Phalangeal Joint, Right N Metatarsal-Phalangeal Joint, Left P Toe Phalangeal Joint, Right Q Toe Phalangeal Joint, Left	Ø Open	7 Autologous Tissue Substitute J Synthetic Substitute K Nonautologous Tissue Substitute	Z No Qualifier
9 Hip Joint, Right B Hip Joint, Left	Ø Open	1 Synthetic Substitute, Metal 2 Synthetic Substitute, Metal on Polyethylene 3 Synthetic Substitute, Ceramic 4 Synthetic Substitute, Ceramic on Polyethylene 6 Synthetic Substitute, Oxidized Zirconium on Polyethylene J Synthetic Substitute	9 Cemented A Uncemented Z No Qualifier
9 Hip Joint, Right B Hip Joint, Left	Ø Open	7 Autologous Tissue Substitute K Nonautologous Tissue Substitute	Z No Qualifier
A Hip Joint, Acetabular Surface, Right E Hip Joint, Acetabular Surface, Left	Ø Open	Ø Synthetic Substitute, Polyethylene 1 Synthetic Substitute, Metal 3 Synthetic Substitute, Ceramic J Synthetic Substitute	9 Cemented A Uncemented Z No Qualifier
A Hip Joint, Acetabular Surface, Right E Hip Joint, Acetabular Surface, Left	Ø Open	7 Autologous Tissue Substitute K Nonautologous Tissue Substitute	Z No Qualifier

SECTION: Ø MEDICAL AND SURGICAL
BODY SYSTEM: S LOWER JOINTS
OPERATION: R REPLACEMENT: *(continued)*
Putting in or on biological or synthetic material that physically takes the place and/or function of all or a portion of a body part

Body Part	Approach	Device	Qualifier
C Knee Joint, Right D Knee Joint, Left	Ø Open	6 Synthetic Substitute, Oxidized Zirconium on Polyethylene J Synthetic Substitute L Synthetic Substitute, Unicondylar	9 Cemented A Uncemented Z No Qualifier
C Knee Joint, Right D Knee Joint, Left	Ø Open	7 Autologous Tissue Substitute K Nonautologous Tissue Substitute	Z No Qualifier
F Ankle Joint, Right G Ankle Joint, Left T Knee Joint, Femoral Surface, Right U Knee Joint, Femoral Surface, Left V Knee Joint, Tibial Surface, Right W Knee Joint, Tibial Surface, Left	Ø Open	7 Autologous Tissue Substitute K Nonautologous Tissue Substitute	Z No Qualifier
F Ankle Joint, Right G Ankle Joint, Left T Knee Joint, Femoral Surface, Right U Knee Joint, Femoral Surface, Left V Knee Joint, Tibial Surface, Right W Knee Joint, Tibial Surface, Left	Ø Open	J Synthetic Substitute	9 Cemented A Uncemented Z No Qualifier
R Hip Joint, Femoral Surface, Right S Hip Joint, Femoral Surface, Left	Ø Open	1 Synthetic Substitute, Metal 3 Synthetic Substitute, Ceramic J Synthetic Substitute	9 Cemented A Uncemented Z No Qualifier
R Hip Joint, Femoral Surface, Right S Hip Joint, Femoral Surface, Left	Ø Open	7 Autologous Tissue Substitute K Nonautologous Tissue Substitute	Z No Qualifier

SECTION: Ø MEDICAL AND SURGICAL
BODY SYSTEM: S LOWER JOINTS
OPERATION: S REPOSITION: Moving to its normal location, or other suitable location, all or a portion of a body part

Body Part	Approach	Device	Qualifier
Ø Lumbar Vertebral Joint 3 Lumbosacral Joint 5 Sacrococcygeal Joint 6 Coccygeal Joint 7 Sacroiliac Joint, Right 8 Sacroiliac Joint, Left	Ø Open 3 Percutaneous 4 Percutaneous Endoscopic X External	4 Internal Fixation Device Z No Device	Z No Qualifier
9 Hip Joint, Right B Hip Joint, Left C Knee Joint, Right D Knee Joint, Left F Ankle Joint, Right G Ankle Joint, Left H Tarsal Joint, Right J Tarsal Joint, Left K Tarsometatarsal Joint, Right L Tarsometatarsal Joint, Left M Metatarsal-Phalangeal Joint, Right N Metatarsal-Phalangeal Joint, Left P Toe Phalangeal Joint, Right Q Toe Phalangeal Joint, Left	Ø Open 3 Percutaneous 4 Percutaneous Endoscopic X External	4 Internal Fixation Device 5 External Fixation Device Z No Device	Z No Qualifier

SECTION: Ø MEDICAL AND SURGICAL
BODY SYSTEM: S LOWER JOINTS
OPERATION: T RESECTION: Cutting out or off, without replacement, all of a body part

Body Part	Approach	Device	Qualifier
2 Lumbar Vertebral Disc 4 Lumbosacral Disc 5 Sacrococcygeal Joint 6 Coccygeal Joint 7 Sacroiliac Joint, Right 8 Sacroiliac Joint, Left 9 Hip Joint, Right B Hip Joint, Left C Knee Joint, Right D Knee Joint, Left F Ankle Joint, Right G Ankle Joint, Left H Tarsal Joint, Right J Tarsal Joint, Left K Tarsometatarsal Joint, Right L Tarsometatarsal Joint, Left M Metatarsal-Phalangeal Joint, Right N Metatarsal-Phalangeal Joint, Left P Toe Phalangeal Joint, Right Q Toe Phalangeal Joint, Left	Ø Open	Z No Device	Z No Qualifier

SECTION: Ø MEDICAL AND SURGICAL
BODY SYSTEM: S LOWER JOINTS
OPERATION: U SUPPLEMENT: Putting in or on biological or synthetic material that physically reinforces and/or augments the function of a portion of a body part

Body Part	Approach	Device	Qualifier
Ø Lumbar Vertebral Joint 2 Lumbar Vertebral Disc 3 Lumbosacral Joint 4 Lumbosacral Disc 5 Sacrococcygeal Joint 6 Coccygeal Joint 7 Sacroiliac Joint, Right 8 Sacroiliac Joint, Left F Ankle Joint, Right G Ankle Joint, Left H Tarsal Joint, Right J Tarsal Joint, Left K Tarsometatarsal Joint, Right L Tarsometatarsal Joint, Left M Metatarsal-Phalangeal Joint, Right N Metatarsal-Phalangeal Joint, Left P Toe Phalangeal Joint, Right Q Toe Phalangeal Joint, Left	Ø Open 3 Percutaneous 4 Percutaneous Endoscopic	7 Autologous Tissue Substitute J Synthetic Substitute K Nonautologous Tissue Substitute	Z No Qualifier
9 Hip Joint, Right B Hip Joint, Left	Ø Open	7 Autologous Tissue Substitute 9 Liner B Resurfacing Device J Synthetic Substitute K Nonautologous Tissue Substitute	Z No Qualifier
9 Hip Joint, Right B Hip Joint, Left	3 Percutaneous 4 Percutaneous Endoscopic	7 Autologous Tissue Substitute J Synthetic Substitute K Nonautologous Tissue Substitute	Z No Qualifier
A Hip Joint, Acetabular Surface, Right E Hip Joint, Acetabular Surface, Left R Hip Joint, Femoral Surface, Right S Hip Joint, Femoral Surface, Left	Ø Open	9 Liner B Resurfacing Device	Z No Qualifier
C Knee Joint, Right D Knee Joint, Left	Ø Open	7 Autologous Tissue Substitute J Synthetic Substitute K Nonautologous Tissue Substitute	Z No Qualifier
C Knee Joint, Right D Knee Joint, Left	Ø Open	9 Liner	C Patellar Surface Z No Qualifier
C Knee Joint, Right D Knee Joint, Left	3 Percutaneous 4 Percutaneous Endoscopic	7 Autologous Tissue Substitute J Synthetic Substitute K Nonautologous Tissue Substitute	Z No Qualifier
T Knee Joint, Femoral Surface, Right U Knee Joint, Femoral Surface, Left V Knee Joint, Tibial Surface, Right W Knee Joint, Tibial Surface, Left	Ø Open	9 Liner	Z No Qualifier

SECTION: Ø MEDICAL AND SURGICAL
BODY SYSTEM: S LOWER JOINTS
OPERATION: W REVISION: *(on multiple pages)*
Correcting, to the extent possible, a portion of a malfunctioning device or the position of a displaced device

Body Part	Approach	Device	Qualifier
Ø Lumbar Vertebral Joint 3 Lumbosacral Joint	Ø Open 3 Percutaneous 4 Percutaneous Endoscopic X External	Ø Drainage Device 3 Infusion Device 4 Internal Fixation Device 7 Autologous Tissue Substitute 8 Spacer A Interbody Fusion Device J Synthetic Substitute K Nonautologous Tissue Substitute	Z No Qualifier
2 Lumbar Vertebral Disc 4 Lumbosacral Disc	Ø Open 3 Percutaneous 4 Percutaneous Endoscopic X External	Ø Drainage Device 3 Infusion Device 7 Autologous Tissue Substitute J Synthetic Substitute K Nonautologous Tissue Substitute	Z No Qualifier
5 Sacrococcygeal Joint 6 Coccygeal Joint 7 Sacroiliac Joint, Right 8 Sacroiliac Joint, Left	Ø Open 3 Percutaneous 4 Percutaneous Endoscopic X External	Ø Drainage Device 3 Infusion Device 4 Internal Fixation Device 7 Autologous Tissue Substitute 8 Spacer J Synthetic Substitute K Nonautologous Tissue Substitute	Z No Qualifier
9 Hip Joint, Right B Hip Joint, Left	Ø Open	Ø Drainage Device 3 Infusion Device 4 Internal Fixation Device 5 External Fixation Device 7 Autologous Tissue Substitute 8 Spacer 9 Liner B Resurfacing Device J Synthetic Substitute K Nonautologous Tissue Substitute	Z No Qualifier
9 Hip Joint, Right B Hip Joint, Left	3 Percutaneous 4 Percutaneous Endoscopic X External	Ø Drainage Device 3 Infusion Device 4 Internal Fixation Device 5 External Fixation Device 7 Autologous Tissue Substitute 8 Spacer J Synthetic Substitute K Nonautologous Tissue Substitute	Z No Qualifier

SECTION: Ø MEDICAL AND SURGICAL
BODY SYSTEM: S LOWER JOINTS
OPERATION: W REVISION: *(continued)*

Correcting, to the extent possible, a portion of a malfunctioning device or the position of a displaced device

Body Part	Approach	Device	Qualifier
A Hip Joint, Acetabular Surface, Right E Hip Joint, Acetabular Surface, Left R Hip Joint, Femoral Surface, Right S Hip Joint, Femoral Surface, Left T Knee Joint, Femoral Surface, Right U Knee Joint, Femoral Surface, Left V Knee Joint, Tibial Surface, Right W Knee Joint, Tibial Surface, Left	Ø Open 3 Percutaneous 4 Percutaneous Endoscopic X External	J Synthetic Substitute	Z No Qualifier
C Knee Joint, Right D Knee Joint, Left	Ø Open	Ø Drainage Device 3 Infusion Device 4 Internal Fixation Device 5 External Fixation Device 7 Autologous Tissue Substitute 8 Spacer 9 Liner K Nonautologous Tissue Substitute	Z No Qualifier
C Knee Joint, Right D Knee Joint, Left	Ø Open	J Synthetic Substitute	C Patellar Surface Z No Qualifier
C Knee Joint, Right D Knee Joint, Left	3 Percutaneous 4 Percutaneous Endoscopic X External	Ø Drainage Device 3 Infusion Device 4 Internal Fixation Device 5 External Fixation Device 7 Autologous Tissue Substitute 8 Spacer K Nonautologous Tissue Substitute	Z No Qualifier
C Knee Joint, Right D Knee Joint, Left	3 Percutaneous 4 Percutaneous Endoscopic X External	J Synthetic Substitute	C Patellar Surface Z No Qualifier
F Ankle Joint, Right G Ankle Joint, Left H Tarsal Joint, Right J Tarsal Joint, Left K Tarsometatarsal Joint, Right L Tarsometatarsal Joint, Left M Metatarsal-Phalangeal Joint, Right N Metatarsal-Phalangeal Joint, Left P Toe Phalangeal Joint, Right Q Toe Phalangeal Joint, Left	Ø Open 3 Percutaneous 4 Percutaneous Endoscopic X External	Ø Drainage Device 3 Infusion Device 4 Internal Fixation Device 5 External Fixation Device 7 Autologous Tissue Substitute 8 Spacer J Synthetic Substitute K Nonautologous Tissue Substitute	Z No Qualifier

ØT. Urinary System...421
    ØT1. Bypass...422
    ØT2. Change 422
    ØT5. Destruction...423
    ØT7. Dilation...423
    ØT8. Division...423
    ØT9. Drainage 424
    ØTB. Excision...425
    ØTC. Extirpation..425
    ØTD. Extraction...425
    ØTF. Fragmentation...426
    ØTH. Insertion...426
    ØTJ. Inspection...427
    ØTL. Occlusion..427
    ØTM. Reattachment...428
    ØTN. Release 428
    ØTP. Removal..429
    ØTQ. Repair 430
    ØTR. Replacement...431
    ØTS. Reposition..431
    ØTT. Resection...432
    ØTU. Supplement..432
    ØTV. Restriction...433
    ØTW. Revision...434
    ØTY. Transplantation...436

SECTION: Ø MEDICAL AND SURGICAL
BODY SYSTEM: T **URINARY SYSTEM**
OPERATION: 1 **BYPASS:** Altering the route of passage of the contents of a tubular body part

Body Part	Approach	Device	Qualifier
3 Kidney Pelvis, Right 4 Kidney Pelvis, Left	Ø Open 4 Percutaneous Endoscopic	7 Autologous Tissue Substitute J Synthetic Substitute K Nonautologous Tissue Substitute Z No Device	3 Kidney Pelvis, Right 4 Kidney Pelvis, Left 6 Ureter, Right 7 Ureter, Left 8 Colon 9 Colocutaneous A Ileum B Bladder C Ileocutaneous D Cutaneous
3 Kidney Pelvis, Right 4 Kidney Pelvis, Left	3 Percutaneous	J Synthetic Substitute	D Cutaneous
6 Ureter, Right 7 Ureter, Left 8 Ureters, Bilateral	Ø Open 4 Percutaneous Endoscopic	7 Autologous Tissue Substitute J Synthetic Substitute K Nonautologous Tissue Substitute Z No Device	6 Ureter, Right 7 Ureter, Left 8 Colon 9 Colocutaneous A Ileum B Bladder C Ileocutaneous D Cutaneous
6 Ureter, Right 7 Ureter, Left 8 Ureters, Bilateral	3 Percutaneous	J Synthetic Substitute	D Cutaneous
B Bladder	Ø Open 4 Percutaneous Endoscopic	7 Autologous Tissue Substitute J Synthetic Substitute K Nonautologous Tissue Substitute Z No Device	9 Colocutaneous C Ileocutaneous D Cutaneous
B Bladder	3 Percutaneous	J Synthetic Substitute	D Cutaneous

SECTION: Ø MEDICAL AND SURGICAL
BODY SYSTEM: T **URINARY SYSTEM**
OPERATION: 2 **CHANGE:** Taking out or off a device from a body part and putting back an identical or similar device in or on the same body part without cutting or puncturing the skin or a mucous membrane

Body Part	Approach	Device	Qualifier
5 Kidney 9 Ureter B Bladder D Urethra	X External	Ø Drainage Device Y Other Device	Z No Qualifier

1: BYPASS   2: CHANGE   T: URINARY SYSTEM   Ø: M/S

SECTION: Ø MEDICAL AND SURGICAL
BODY SYSTEM: T URINARY SYSTEM
OPERATION: 5 DESTRUCTION: Physical eradication of all or a portion of a body part by the direct use of energy, force, or a destructive agent

Body Part	Approach	Device	Qualifier
Ø Kidney, Right 1 Kidney, Left 3 Kidney Pelvis, Right 4 Kidney Pelvis, Left 6 Ureter, Right 7 Ureter, Left B Bladder C Bladder Neck	Ø Open 3 Percutaneous 4 Percutaneous Endoscopic 7 Via Natural or Artificial Opening 8 Via Natural or Artificial Opening Endoscopic	Z No Device	Z No Qualifier
D Urethra	Ø Open 3 Percutaneous 4 Percutaneous Endoscopic 7 Via Natural or Artificial Opening 8 Via Natural or Artificial Opening Endoscopic X External	Z No Device	Z No Qualifier

SECTION: Ø MEDICAL AND SURGICAL
BODY SYSTEM: T URINARY SYSTEM
OPERATION: 7 DILATION: Expanding an orifice or the lumen of a tubular body part

Body Part	Approach	Device	Qualifier
3 Kidney Pelvis, Right 4 Kidney Pelvis, Left 6 Ureter, Right 7 Ureter, Left 8 Ureters, Bilateral B Bladder C Bladder Neck D Urethra	Ø Open 3 Percutaneous 4 Percutaneous Endoscopic 7 Via Natural or Artificial Opening 8 Via Natural or Artificial Opening Endoscopic	D Intraluminal Device Z No Device	Z No Qualifier

SECTION: Ø MEDICAL AND SURGICAL
BODY SYSTEM: T URINARY SYSTEM
OPERATION: 8 DIVISION: Cutting into a body part, without draining fluids and/or gases from the body part, in order to separate or transect a body part

Body Part	Approach	Device	Qualifier
2 Kidneys, Bilateral C Bladder Neck	Ø Open 3 Percutaneous 4 Percutaneous Endoscopic	Z No Device	Z No Qualifier

SECTION: Ø MEDICAL AND SURGICAL
BODY SYSTEM: T URINARY SYSTEM
OPERATION: 9 DRAINAGE: Taking or letting out fluids and/or gases from a body part

Body Part	Approach	Device	Qualifier
Ø Kidney, Right 1 Kidney, Left 3 Kidney Pelvis, Right 4 Kidney Pelvis, Left 6 Ureter, Right 7 Ureter, Left 8 Ureters, Bilateral B Bladder C Bladder Neck	Ø Open 3 Percutaneous 4 Percutaneous Endoscopic 7 Via Natural or Artificial Opening 8 Via Natural or Artificial Opening Endoscopic	Ø Drainage Device	Z No Qualifier
Ø Kidney, Right 1 Kidney, Left 3 Kidney Pelvis, Right 4 Kidney Pelvis, Left 6 Ureter, Right 7 Ureter, Left 8 Ureters, Bilateral B Bladder C Bladder Neck	Ø Open 3 Percutaneous 4 Percutaneous Endoscopic 7 Via Natural or Artificial Opening 8 Via Natural or Artificial Opening Endoscopic	Z No Device	X Diagnostic Z No Qualifier
D Urethra	Ø Open 3 Percutaneous 4 Percutaneous Endoscopic 7 Via Natural or Artificial Opening 8 Via Natural or Artificial Opening Endoscopic X External	Ø Drainage Device	Z No Qualifier
D Urethrav	Ø Open 3 Percutaneous 4 Percutaneous Endoscopic 7 Via Natural or Artificial Opening 8 Via Natural or Artificial Opening Endoscopic X External	Z No Device	X Diagnostic Z No Qualifier

9: DRAINAGE

T: URINARY SYSTEM

Ø: M/S

New/Revised Text in Blue ~~deleted~~ Deleted

SECTION: Ø MEDICAL AND SURGICAL
BODY SYSTEM: T URINARY SYSTEM
OPERATION: B EXCISION: Cutting out or off, without replacement, a portion of a body part

Body Part	Approach	Device	Qualifier
Ø Kidney, Right 1 Kidney, Left 3 Kidney Pelvis, Right 4 Kidney Pelvis, Left 6 Ureter, Right 7 Ureter, Left B Bladder C Bladder Neck	Ø Open 3 Percutaneous 4 Percutaneous Endoscopic 7 Via Natural or Artificial Opening 8 Via Natural or Artificial Opening Endoscopic	Z No Device	X Diagnostic Z No Qualifier
D Urethra	Ø Open 3 Percutaneous 4 Percutaneous Endoscopic 7 Via Natural or Artificial Opening 8 Via Natural or Artificial Opening Endoscopic X External	Z No Device	X Diagnostic Z No Qualifier

SECTION: Ø MEDICAL AND SURGICAL
BODY SYSTEM: T URINARY SYSTEM
OPERATION: C EXTIRPATION: Taking or cutting out solid matter from a body part

Body Part	Approach	Device	Qualifier
Ø Kidney, Right 1 Kidney, Left 3 Kidney Pelvis, Right 4 Kidney Pelvis, Left 6 Ureter, Right 7 Ureter, Left B Bladder C Bladder Neck	Ø Open 3 Percutaneous 4 Percutaneous Endoscopic 7 Via Natural or Artificial Opening 8 Via Natural or Artificial Opening Endoscopic	Z No Device	Z No Qualifier
D Urethra	Ø Open 3 Percutaneous 4 Percutaneous Endoscopic 7 Via Natural or Artificial Opening 8 Via Natural or Artificial Opening Endoscopic X External	Z No Device	Z No Qualifier

SECTION: Ø MEDICAL AND SURGICAL
BODY SYSTEM: T URINARY SYSTEM
OPERATION: D EXTRACTION: Pulling or stripping out or off all or a portion of a body part by the use of force

Body Part	Approach	Device	Qualifier
Ø Kidney, Right 1 Kidney, Left	Ø Open 3 Percutaneous 4 Percutaneous Endoscopic	Z No Device	Z No Qualifier

SECTION: Ø MEDICAL AND SURGICAL
BODY SYSTEM: T URINARY SYSTEM
OPERATION: F FRAGMENTATION: Breaking solid matter in a body part into pieces

Body Part	Approach	Device	Qualifier
3 Kidney Pelvis, Right 4 Kidney Pelvis, Left 6 Ureter, Right 7 Ureter, Left B Bladder C Bladder Neck D Urethra	Ø Open 3 Percutaneous 4 Percutaneous Endoscopic 7 Via Natural or Artificial Opening 8 Via Natural or Artificial Opening Endoscopic X External	Z No Device	Z No Qualifier

SECTION: Ø MEDICAL AND SURGICAL
BODY SYSTEM: T URINARY SYSTEM
OPERATION: H INSERTION: Putting in a nonbiological appliance that monitors, assists, performs, or prevents a physiological function but does not physically take the place of a body part

Body Part	Approach	Device	Qualifier
5 Kidney	Ø Open 3 Percutaneous 4 Percutaneous Endoscopic 7 Via Natural or Artificial Opening 8 Via Natural or Artificial Opening Endoscopic	2 Monitoring Device 3 Infusion Device Y Other Device	Z No Qualifier
9 Ureter	Ø Open 3 Percutaneous 4 Percutaneous Endoscopic 7 Via Natural or Artificial Opening 8 Via Natural or Artificial Opening Endoscopic	2 Monitoring Device 3 Infusion Device M Stimulator Lead Y Other Device	Z No Qualifier
B Bladder	Ø Open 3 Percutaneous 4 Percutaneous Endoscopic 7 Via Natural or Artificial Opening 8 Via Natural or Artificial Opening Endoscopic	2 Monitoring Device 3 Infusion Device L Artificial Sphincter M Stimulator Lead Y Other Device	Z No Qualifier
C Bladder Neck	Ø Open 3 Percutaneous 4 Percutaneous Endoscopic 7 Via Natural or Artificial Opening 8 Via Natural or Artificial Opening Endoscopic	L Artificial Sphincter	Z No Qualifier
D Urethra	Ø Open 3 Percutaneous 4 Percutaneous Endoscopic 7 Via Natural or Artificial Opening 8 Via Natural or Artificial Opening Endoscopic X~~External~~	2 Monitoring Device 3 Infusion Device L Artificial Sphincter Y Other Device	Z No Qualifier
D Urethra	X External	2 Monitoring Device 3 Infusion Device L Artificial Sphincter	Z No Qualifier

Side tab: F: FRAGMENTATION H: INSERTION
Side tab: T: URINARY SYSTEM
Side tab: Ø: M/S

SECTION: Ø MEDICAL AND SURGICAL
BODY SYSTEM: T URINARY SYSTEM
OPERATION: J INSPECTION: Visually and/or manually exploring a body part

Body Part	Approach	Device	Qualifier
5 Kidney 9 Ureter B Bladder D Urethra	Ø Open 3 Percutaneous 4 Percutaneous Endoscopic 7 Via Natural or Artificial Opening 8 Via Natural or Artificial Opening Endoscopic X External	Z No Device	Z No Qualifier

SECTION: Ø MEDICAL AND SURGICAL
BODY SYSTEM: T URINARY SYSTEM
OPERATION: L OCCLUSION: Completely closing an orifice or the lumen of a tubular body part

Body Part	Approach	Device	Qualifier
3 Kidney Pelvis, Right 4 Kidney Pelvis, Left 6 Ureter, Right 7 Ureter, Left B Bladder C Bladder Neck	Ø Open 3 Percutaneous 4 Percutaneous Endoscopic	C Extraluminal Device D Intraluminal Device Z No Device	Z No Qualifier
3 Kidney Pelvis, Right 4 Kidney Pelvis, Left 6 Ureter, Right 7 Ureter, Left B Bladder C Bladder Neck	7 Via Natural or Artificial Opening 8 Via Natural or Artificial Opening Endoscopic	D Intraluminal Device Z No Device	Z No Qualifier
D Urethra	Ø Open 3 Percutaneous 4 Percutaneous Endoscopic X External	C Extraluminal Device D Intraluminal Device Z No Device	Z No Qualifier
D Urethra	7 Via Natural or Artificial Opening 8 Via Natural or Artificial Opening Endoscopic	D Intraluminal Device Z No Device	Z No Qualifier

SECTION: Ø MEDICAL AND SURGICAL
BODY SYSTEM: T URINARY SYSTEM
OPERATION: M REATTACHMENT: Putting back in or on all or a portion of a separated body part to its normal location or other suitable location

Body Part	Approach	Device	Qualifier
Ø Kidney, Right 1 Kidney, Left 2 Kidneys, Bilateral 3 Kidney Pelvis, Right 4 Kidney Pelvis, Left 6 Ureter, Right 7 Ureter, Left 8 Ureters, Bilateral B Bladder C Bladder Neck D Urethra	Ø Open 4 Percutaneous Endoscopic	Z No Device	Z No Qualifier

SECTION: Ø MEDICAL AND SURGICAL
BODY SYSTEM: T URINARY SYSTEM
OPERATION: N RELEASE: Freeing a body part from an abnormal physical constraint by cutting or by the use of force

Body Part	Approach	Device	Qualifier
Ø Kidney, Right 1 Kidney, Left 3 Kidney Pelvis, Right 4 Kidney Pelvis, Left 6 Ureter, Right 7 Ureter, Left B Bladder C Bladder Neck	Ø Open 3 Percutaneous 4 Percutaneous Endoscopic 7 Via Natural or Artificial Opening 8 Via Natural or Artificial Opening Endoscopic	Z No Device	Z No Qualifier
D Urethra	Ø Open 3 Percutaneous 4 Percutaneous Endoscopic 7 Via Natural or Artificial Opening 8 Via Natural or Artificial Opening Endoscopic X External	Z No Device	Z No Qualifier

New/Revised Text in Blue   ~~deleted~~ Deleted

SECTION: Ø MEDICAL AND SURGICAL
BODY SYSTEM: T URINARY SYSTEM
OPERATION: P REMOVAL: *(on multiple pages)*
Taking out or off a device from a body part

Body Part	Approach	Device	Qualifier
5 Kidney	Ø Open 3 Percutaneous 4 Percutaneous Endoscopic 7 Via Natural or Artificial Opening 8 Via Natural or Artificial Opening Endoscopic	Ø Drainage Device 2 Monitoring Device 3 Infusion Device 7 Autologous Tissue Substitute C Extraluminal Device D Intraluminal Device J Synthetic Substitute K Nonautologous Tissue Substitute Y Other Device	Z No Qualifier
5 Kidney	X External	Ø Drainage Device 2 Monitoring Device 3 Infusion Device D Intraluminal Device	Z No Qualifier
9 Ureter	Ø Open 3 Percutaneous 4 Percutaneous Endoscopic 7 Via Natural or Artificial Opening 8 Via Natural or Artificial Opening Endoscopic	Ø Drainage Device 2 Monitoring Device 3 Infusion Device 7 Autologous Tissue Substitute C Extraluminal Device D Intraluminal Device J Synthetic Substitute K Nonautologous Tissue Substitute M Stimulator Lead Y Other Device	Z No Qualifier
9 Ureter	X External	Ø Drainage Device 2 Monitoring Device 3 Infusion Device D Intraluminal Device M Stimulator Lead	Z No Qualifier
B Bladder	Ø Open 3 Percutaneous 4 Percutaneous Endoscopic 7 Via Natural or Artificial Opening 8 Via Natural or Artificial Opening Endoscopic	Ø Drainage Device 2 Monitoring Device 3 Infusion Device 7 Autologous Tissue Substitute C Extraluminal Device D Intraluminal Device J Synthetic Substitute K Nonautologous Tissue Substitute L Artificial Sphincter M Stimulator Lead Y Other Device	Z No Qualifier
B Bladder	X External	Ø Drainage Device 2 Monitoring Device 3 Infusion Device D Intraluminal Device L Artificial Sphincter M Stimulator Lead	Z No Qualifier

SECTION: Ø MEDICAL AND SURGICAL

BODY SYSTEM: T URINARY SYSTEM
OPERATION: P REMOVAL: *(continued)*
Taking out or off a device from a body part

Body Part	Approach	Device	Qualifier
D Urethra	Ø Open 3 Percutaneous 4 Percutaneous Endoscopic 7 Via Natural or Artificial Opening 8 Via Natural or Artificial Opening Endoscopic	Ø Drainage Device 2 Monitoring Device 3 Infusion Device 7 Autologous Tissue Substitute C Extraluminal Device D Intraluminal Device J Synthetic Substitute K Nonautologous Tissue Substitute L Artificial Sphincter Y Other Device	Z No Qualifier
D Urethra	X External	Ø Drainage Device 2 Monitoring Device 3 Infusion Device D Intraluminal Device L Artificial Sphincter	Z No Qualifier

SECTION: Ø MEDICAL AND SURGICAL

BODY SYSTEM: T URINARY SYSTEM
OPERATION: Q REPAIR: Restoring, to the extent possible, a body part to its normal anatomic structure and function

Body Part	Approach	Device	Qualifier
Ø Kidney, Right 1 Kidney, Left 3 Kidney Pelvis, Right 4 Kidney Pelvis, Left 6 Ureter, Right 7 Ureter, Left B Bladder C Bladder Neck	Ø Open 3 Percutaneous 4 Percutaneous Endoscopic 7 Via Natural or Artificial Opening 8 Via Natural or Artificial Opening Endoscopic	Z No Device	Z No Qualifier
D Urethra	Ø Open 3 Percutaneous 4 Percutaneous Endoscopic 7 Via Natural or Artificial Opening 8 Via Natural or Artificial Opening Endoscopic X External	Z No Device	Z No Qualifier

New/Revised Text in Blue   ~~deleted~~ Deleted

SECTION: Ø MEDICAL AND SURGICAL
BODY SYSTEM: T URINARY SYSTEM
OPERATION: R REPLACEMENT: Putting in or on biological or synthetic material that physically takes the place and/or function of all or a portion of a body part

Body Part	Approach	Device	Qualifier
3 Kidney Pelvis, Right 4 Kidney Pelvis, Left 6 Ureter, Right 7 Ureter, Left B Bladder C Bladder Neck	Ø Open 4 Percutaneous Endoscopic 7 Via Natural or Artificial Opening 8 Via Natural or Artificial Opening Endoscopic	7 Autologous Tissue Substitute J Synthetic Substitute K Nonautologous Tissue Substitute	Z No Qualifier
D Urethra	Ø Open 4 Percutaneous Endoscopic 7 Via Natural or Artificial Opening 8 Via Natural or Artificial Opening Endoscopic X External	7 Autologous Tissue Substitute J Synthetic Substitute K Nonautologous Tissue Substitute	Z No Qualifier

SECTION: Ø MEDICAL AND SURGICAL
BODY SYSTEM: T URINARY SYSTEM
OPERATION: S REPOSITION: Moving to its normal location, or other suitable location, all or a portion of a body part

Body Part	Approach	Device	Qualifier
Ø Kidney, Right 1 Kidney, Left 2 Kidneys, Bilateral 3 Kidney Pelvis, Right 4 Kidney Pelvis, Left 6 Ureter, Right 7 Ureter, Left 8 Ureters, Bilateral B Bladder C Bladder Neck D Urethra	Ø Open 4 Percutaneous Endoscopic	Z No Device	Z No Qualifier

Ø: M/S

T: URINARY SYSTEM

R: REPLACEMENT

S: REPOSITION

SECTION: Ø MEDICAL AND SURGICAL
BODY SYSTEM: T URINARY SYSTEM
OPERATION: T RESECTION: Cutting out or off, without replacement, all of a body part

Body Part	Approach	Device	Qualifier
Ø Kidney, Right 1 Kidney, Left 2 Kidneys, Bilateral	Ø Open 4 Percutaneous Endoscopic	Z No Device	Z No Qualifier
3 Kidney Pelvis, Right 4 Kidney Pelvis, Left 6 Ureter, Right 7 Ureter, Left B Bladder C Bladder Neck D Urethra	Ø Open 4 Percutaneous Endoscopic 7 Via Natural or Artificial Opening 8 Via Natural or Artificial Opening Endoscopic	Z No Device	Z No Qualifier

SECTION: Ø MEDICAL AND SURGICAL
BODY SYSTEM: T URINARY SYSTEM
OPERATION: U SUPPLEMENT: Putting in or on biological or synthetic material that physically reinforces and/or augments the function of a portion of a body part

Body Part	Approach	Device	Qualifier
3 Kidney Pelvis, Right 4 Kidney Pelvis, Left 6 Ureter, Right 7 Ureter, Left B Bladder C Bladder Neck	Ø Open 4 Percutaneous Endoscopic 7 Via Natural or Artificial Opening 8 Via Natural or Artificial Opening Endoscopic	7 Autologous Tissue Substitute J Synthetic Substitute K Nonautologous Tissue Substitute	Z No Qualifier
D Urethra	Ø Open 4 Percutaneous Endoscopic 7 Via Natural or Artificial Opening 8 Via Natural or Artificial Opening Endoscopic X External	7 Autologous Tissue Substitute J Synthetic Substitute K Nonautologous Tissue Substitute	Z No Qualifier

New/Revised Text in Blue   ~~deleted~~ Deleted

SECTION: Ø MEDICAL AND SURGICAL
BODY SYSTEM: T URINARY SYSTEM
OPERATION: V RESTRICTION: Partially closing an orifice or the lumen of a tubular body part

Body Part	Approach	Device	Qualifier
3 Kidney Pelvis, Right 4 Kidney Pelvis, Left 6 Ureter, Right 7 Ureter, Left B Bladder C Bladder Neck	Ø Open 3 Percutaneous 4 Percutaneous Endoscopic	C Extraluminal Device D Intraluminal Device Z No Device	Z No Qualifier
3 Kidney Pelvis, Right 4 Kidney Pelvis, Left 6 Ureter, Right 7 Ureter, Left B Bladder C Bladder Neck	7 Via Natural or Artificial Opening 8 Via Natural or Artificial Opening Endoscopic	D Intraluminal Device Z No Device	Z No Qualifier
D Urethra	Ø Open 3 Percutaneous 4 Percutaneous Endoscopic	C Extraluminal Device D Intraluminal Device Z No Device	Z No Qualifier
D Urethra	7 Via Natural or Artificial Opening 8 Via Natural or Artificial Opening Endoscopic	D Intraluminal Device Z No Device	Z No Qualifier
D Urethra	X External	Z No Device	Z No Qualifier

SECTION: Ø MEDICAL AND SURGICAL
BODY SYSTEM: T URINARY SYSTEM
OPERATION: W REVISION: *(on multiple pages)*
Correcting, to the extent possible, a portion of a malfunctioning device or the position of a displaced device

Body Part	Approach	Device	Qualifier
5 Kidney	Ø Open 3 Percutaneous 4 Percutaneous Endoscopic 7 Via Natural or Artificial Opening 8 Via Natural or Artificial Opening Endoscopic X External	Ø Drainage Device 2 Monitoring Device 3 Infusion Device 7 Autologous Tissue Substitute C Extraluminal Device D Intraluminal Device J Synthetic Substitute K Nonautologous Tissue Substitute Y Other Device	Z No Qualifier
5 Kidney	X External	Ø Drainage Device 2 Monitoring Device 3 Infusion Device 7 Autologous Tissue Substitute C Extraluminal Device D Intraluminal Device J Synthetic Substitute K Nonautologous Tissue Substitute	Z No Qualifier
9 Ureter	Ø Open 3 Percutaneous 4 Percutaneous Endoscopic 7 Via Natural or Artificial Opening 8 Via Natural or Artificial Opening Endoscopic X External	Ø Drainage Device 2 Monitoring Device 3 Infusion Device 7 Autologous Tissue Substitute C Extraluminal Device D Intraluminal Device J Synthetic Substitute K Nonautologous Tissue Substitute M Stimulator Lead Y Other Device	Z No Qualifier
9 Ureter	X External	Ø Drainage Device 2 Monitoring Device 3 Infusion Device 7 Autologous Tissue Substitute C Extraluminal Device D Intraluminal Device J Synthetic Substitute K Nonautologous Tissue Substitute M Stimulator Lead	Z No Qualifier

W: REVISION

T: URINARY SYSTEM

Ø: M/S

New/Revised Text in Blue   ~~deleted~~ Deleted

SECTION: Ø MEDICAL AND SURGICAL
BODY SYSTEM: T URINARY SYSTEM
OPERATION: W REVISION: *(continued)*

Correcting, to the extent possible, a portion of a malfunctioning device or the position of a displaced device

Body Part	Approach	Device	Qualifier
B Bladder	Ø Open 3 Percutaneous 4 Percutaneous Endoscopic 7 Via Natural or Artificial Opening 8 Via Natural or Artificial Opening Endoscopic ~~X External~~	Ø Drainage Device 2 Monitoring Device 3 Infusion Device 7 Autologous Tissue Substitute C Extraluminal Device D Intraluminal Device J Synthetic Substitute K Nonautologous Tissue Substitute L Artificial Sphincter M Stimulator Lead Y Other Device	Z No Qualifier
B Bladder	X External	Ø Drainage Device 2 Monitoring Device 3 Infusion Device 7 Autologous Tissue Substitute C Extraluminal Device D Intraluminal Device J Synthetic Substitute K Nonautologous Tissue Substitute L Artificial Sphincter M Stimulator Lead	Z No Qualifier
D Urethra	Ø Open 3 Percutaneous 4 Percutaneous Endoscopic 7 Via Natural or Artificial Opening 8 Via Natural or Artificial Opening Endoscopic ~~X External~~	Ø Drainage Device 2 Monitoring Device 3 Infusion Device 7 Autologous Tissue Substitute C Extraluminal Device D Intraluminal Device J Synthetic Substitute K Nonautologous Tissue Substitute L Artificial Sphincter Y Other Device	Z No Qualifier
D Urethra	X External	Ø Drainage Device 2 Monitoring Device 3 Infusion Device 7 Autologous Tissue Substitute C Extraluminal Device D Intraluminal Device J Synthetic Substitute K Nonautologous Tissue Substitute L Artificial Sphincter	Z No Qualifier

SECTION: Ø MEDICAL AND SURGICAL
BODY SYSTEM: T URINARY SYSTEM
OPERATION: Y TRANSPLANTATION: Putting in or on all or a portion of a living body part taken from another individual or animal to physically take the place and/or function of all or a portion of a similar body part

Body Part	Approach	Device	Qualifier
Ø Kidney, Right 1 Kidney, Left	Ø Open	Z No Device	Ø Allogeneic 1 Syngeneic 2 Zooplastic

New/Revised Text in Blue   ~~deleted~~ Deleted

ØU. Female Reproductive System...437
    ØU1. Bypass...438
    ØU2. Change...438
    ØU5. Destruction...439
    ØU7. Dilation...440
    ØU8. Division...440
    ØU9. Drainage..441
    ØUB. Excision...442
    ØUC. Extirpation..443
    ØUD. Extraction..444
    ØUF. Fragmentation...444
    ØUH. Insertion...445
    ØUJ. Inspection..446
    ØUL. Occlusion...446
    ØUM. Reattachment..447
    ØUN. Release...447
    ØUP. Removal...448
    ØUQ. Repair..449
    ØUS. Reposition..450
    ØUT. Resection...450
    ØUU. Supplement...451
    ØUV. Restriction...451
    ØUW. Revision...452
    ØUY. Transplantation...453

SECTION: Ø MEDICAL AND SURGICAL

BODY SYSTEM: U FEMALE REPRODUCTIVE SYSTEM
OPERATION: 1 BYPASS: Altering the route of passage of the contents of a tubular body part

Body Part	Approach	Device	Qualifier
5 Fallopian Tube, Right 6 Fallopian Tube, Left	Ø Open 4 Percutaneous Endoscopic	7 Autologous Tissue Substitute J Synthetic Substitute K Nonautologous Tissue Substitute Z No Device	5 Fallopian Tube, Right 6 Fallopian Tube, Left 9 Uterus

SECTION: Ø MEDICAL AND SURGICAL

BODY SYSTEM: U FEMALE REPRODUCTIVE SYSTEM
OPERATION: 2 CHANGE: Taking out or off a device from a body part and putting back an identical or similar device in or on the same body part without cutting or puncturing the skin or a mucous membrane

Body Part	Approach	Device	Qualifier
3 Ovary 8 Fallopian Tube M Vulva	X External	Ø Drainage Device Y Other Device	Z No Qualifier
D Uterus and Cervix	X External	Ø Drainage Device H Contraceptive Device Y Other Device	Z No Qualifier
H Vagina and Cul-de-sac	X External	Ø Drainage Device G Intraluminal Device, Pessary Y Other Device	Z No Qualifier

SECTION: Ø MEDICAL AND SURGICAL
BODY SYSTEM: U FEMALE REPRODUCTIVE SYSTEM
OPERATION: 5 DESTRUCTION: Physical eradication of all or a portion of a body part by the direct use of energy, force, or a destructive agent

Body Part	Approach	Device	Qualifier
Ø Ovary, Right 1 Ovary, Left 2 Ovaries, Bilateral 4 Uterine Supporting Structure	Ø Open 3 Percutaneous 4 Percutaneous Endoscopic 8 Via Natural or Artificial Opening Endoscopic	Z No Device	Z No Qualifier
5 Fallopian Tube, Right 6 Fallopian Tube, Left 7 Fallopian Tubes, Bilateral 9 Uterus B Endometrium C Cervix F Cul-de-sac	Ø Open 3 Percutaneous 4 Percutaneous Endoscopic 7 Via Natural or Artificial Opening 8 Via Natural or Artificial Opening Endoscopic	Z No Device	Z No Qualifier
G Vagina K Hymen	Ø Open 3 Percutaneous 4 Percutaneous Endoscopic 7 Via Natural or Artificial Opening 8 Via Natural or Artificial Opening Endoscopic X External	Z No Device	Z No Qualifier
J Clitoris L Vestibular Gland M Vulva	Ø Open X External	Z No Device	Z No Qualifier

SECTION: Ø MEDICAL AND SURGICAL
BODY SYSTEM: U FEMALE REPRODUCTIVE SYSTEM
OPERATION: 7 **DILATION:** Expanding an orifice or the lumen of a tubular body part

Body Part	Approach	Device	Qualifier
5 Fallopian Tube, Right 6 Fallopian Tube, Left 7 Fallopian Tubes, Bilateral 9 Uterus C Cervix G Vagina	Ø Open 3 Percutaneous 4 Percutaneous Endoscopic 7 Via Natural or Artificial Opening 8 Via Natural or Artificial Opening Endoscopic	D Intraluminal Device Z No Device	Z No Qualifier
K Hymen	Ø Open 3 Percutaneous 4 Percutaneous Endoscopic 7 Via Natural or Artificial Opening 8 Via Natural or Artificial Opening Endoscopic X External	D Intraluminal Device Z No Device	Z No Qualifier

SECTION: Ø MEDICAL AND SURGICAL
BODY SYSTEM: U FEMALE REPRODUCTIVE SYSTEM
OPERATION: 8 **DIVISION:** Cutting into a body part, without draining fluids and/or gases from the body part, in order to separate or transect a body part

Body Part	Approach	Device	Qualifier
Ø Ovary, Right 1 Ovary, Left 2 Ovaries, Bilateral 4 Uterine Supporting Structure	Ø Open 3 Percutaneous 4 Percutaneous Endoscopic	Z No Device	Z No Qualifier
K Hymen	7 Via Natural or Artificial Opening 8 Via Natural or Artificial Opening Endoscopic X External	Z No Device	Z No Qualifier

SECTION: 0 MEDICAL AND SURGICAL
BODY SYSTEM: U FEMALE REPRODUCTIVE SYSTEM
OPERATION: 9 DRAINAGE: *(on multiple pages)*
Taking or letting out fluids and/or gases from a body part

Body Part	Approach	Device	Qualifier
0 Ovary, Right 1 Ovary, Left 2 Ovaries, Bilateral	0 Open 3 Percutaneous 4 Percutaneous Endoscopic 8 Via Natural or Artificial Opening Endoscopic	0 Drainage Device	Z No Qualifier
0 Ovary, Right 1 Ovary, Left 2 Ovaries, Bilateral	0 Open 3 Percutaneous 4 Percutaneous Endoscopic 8 Via Natural or Artificial Opening Endoscopic	Z No Device	X Diagnostic Z No Qualifier
0 Ovary, Right 1 Ovary, Left 2 Ovaries, Bilateral	X External	Z No Device	Z No Qualifier
4 Uterine Supporting Structure	0 Open 3 Percutaneous 4 Percutaneous Endoscopic 8 Via Natural or Artificial Opening Endoscopic	0 Drainage Device	Z No Qualifier
4 Uterine Supporting Structure	0 Open 3 Percutaneous 4 Percutaneous Endoscopic 8 Via Natural or Artificial Opening Endoscopic	Z No Device	X Diagnostic Z No Qualifier
5 Fallopian Tube, Right 6 Fallopian Tube, Left 7 Fallopian Tubes, Bilateral 9 Uterus C Cervix F Cul-de-sac	0 Open 3 Percutaneous 4 Percutaneous Endoscopic 7 Via Natural or Artificial Opening 8 Via Natural or Artificial Opening Endoscopic	0 Drainage Device	Z No Qualifier
5 Fallopian Tube, Right 6 Fallopian Tube, Left 7 Fallopian Tubes, Bilateral 9 Uterus C Cervix F Cul-de-sac	0 Open 3 Percutaneous 4 Percutaneous Endoscopic 7 Via Natural or Artificial Opening 8 Via Natural or Artificial Opening Endoscopic	Z No Device	X Diagnostic Z No Qualifier
G Vagina K Hymen	0 Open 3 Percutaneous 4 Percutaneous Endoscopic 7 Via Natural or Artificial Opening 8 Via Natural or Artificial Opening Endoscopic X External	0 Drainage Device	Z No Qualifier

SECTION: Ø MEDICAL AND SURGICAL
BODY SYSTEM: U FEMALE REPRODUCTIVE SYSTEM
OPERATION: 9 DRAINAGE: *(continued)*
Taking or letting out fluids and/or gases from a body part

Body Part	Approach	Device	Qualifier
G Vagina K Hymen	Ø Open 3 Percutaneous 4 Percutaneous Endoscopic 7 Via Natural or Artificial Opening 8 Via Natural or Artificial Opening Endoscopic X External	Z No Device	X Diagnostic Z No Qualifier
J Clitoris L Vestibular Gland M Vulva	Ø Open X External	Ø Drainage Device	Z No Qualifier
J Clitoris L Vestibular Gland M Vulva	Ø Open X External	Z No Device	X Diagnostic Z No Qualifier

SECTION: Ø MEDICAL AND SURGICAL
BODY SYSTEM: U FEMALE REPRODUCTIVE SYSTEM
OPERATION: B EXCISION: Cutting out or off, without replacement, a portion of a body part

Body Part	Approach	Device	Qualifier
Ø Ovary, Right 1 Ovary, Left 2 Ovaries, Bilateral 4 Uterine Supporting Structure 5 Fallopian Tube, Right 6 Fallopian Tube, Left 7 Fallopian Tubes, Bilateral 9 Uterus C Cervix F Cul-de-sac	Ø Open 3 Percutaneous 4 Percutaneous Endoscopic 7 Via Natural or Artificial Opening 8 Via Natural or Artificial Opening Endoscopic	Z No Device	X Diagnostic Z No Qualifier
G Vagina K Hymen	Ø Open 3 Percutaneous 4 Percutaneous Endoscopic 7 Via Natural or Artificial Opening 8 Via Natural or Artificial Opening Endoscopic X External	Z No Device	X Diagnostic Z No Qualifier
J Clitoris L Vestibular Gland M Vulva	Ø Open X External	Z No Device	X Diagnostic Z No Qualifier

SECTION: Ø MEDICAL AND SURGICAL
BODY SYSTEM: U FEMALE REPRODUCTIVE SYSTEM
OPERATION: C EXTIRPATION: Taking or cutting out solid matter from a body part

Body Part	Approach	Device	Qualifier
Ø Ovary, Right 1 Ovary, Left 2 Ovaries, Bilateral 4 Uterine Supporting Structure	Ø Open 3 Percutaneous 4 Percutaneous Endoscopic 8 Via Natural or Artificial Opening Endoscopic	Z No Device	Z No Qualifier

5 Fallopian Tube, Right
6 Fallopian Tube, Left
7 Fallopian Tubes, Bilateral
9 Uterus
B Endometrium
C Cervix
F Cul-de-sac
	Ø Open
	3 Percutaneous
	4 Percutaneous Endoscopic
	7 Via Natural or Artificial
	   Opening
	8 Via Natural or Artificial
	   Opening Endoscopic
		Z No Device	Z No Qualifier

G Vagina
K Hymen
	Ø Open
	3 Percutaneous
	4 Percutaneous Endoscopic
	7 Via Natural or Artificial
	   Opening
	8 Via Natural or Artificial
	   Opening Endoscopic
	X External
		Z No Device	Z No Qualifier

J Clitoris L Vestibular Gland M Vulva	Ø Open X External	Z No Device	Z No Qualifier

SECTION: Ø MEDICAL AND SURGICAL
BODY SYSTEM: U FEMALE REPRODUCTIVE SYSTEM
OPERATION: D **EXTRACTION:** Pulling or stripping out or off all or a portion of a body part by the use of force

Body Part	Approach	Device	Qualifier
B Endometrium	7 Via Natural or Artificial Opening 8 Via Natural or Artificial Opening Endoscopic	Z No Device	X Diagnostic Z No Qualifier
N Ova	Ø Open 3 Percutaneous 4 Percutaneous Endoscopic	Z No Device	Z No Qualifier

SECTION: Ø MEDICAL AND SURGICAL
BODY SYSTEM: U FEMALE REPRODUCTIVE SYSTEM
OPERATION: F **FRAGMENTATION:** Breaking solid matter in a body part into pieces

Body Part	Approach	Device	Qualifier
5 Fallopian Tube, Right 6 Fallopian Tube, Left 7 Fallopian Tubes, Bilateral 9 Uterus	Ø Open 3 Percutaneous 4 Percutaneous Endoscopic 7 Via Natural or Artificial Opening 8 Via Natural or Artificial Opening Endoscopic X External	Z No Device	Z No Qualifier

Sidebar: F: FRAGMENTATION | D: EXTRACTION | U: FEMALE REPRODUCTIVE SYSTEM | Ø: M/S

SECTION: Ø MEDICAL AND SURGICAL
BODY SYSTEM: U FEMALE REPRODUCTIVE SYSTEM
OPERATION: H INSERTION: Putting in a nonbiological appliance that monitors, assists, performs, or prevents a physiological function but does not physically take the place of a body part

Body Part	Approach	Device	Qualifier
3 Ovary	Ø Open 3 Percutaneous 4 Percutaneous Endoscopic	3 Infusion Device Y Other Device	Z No Qualifier
3 Ovary	7 Via Natural or Artificial Opening 8 Via Natural or Artificial Opening Endoscopic	Y Other Device	Z No Qualifier
8 Fallopian Tube D Uterus and Cervix H Vagina and Cul-de-sac	Ø Open 3 Percutaneous 4 Percutaneous Endoscopic 7 Via Natural or Artificial Opening 8 Via Natural or Artificial Opening Endoscopic	3 Infusion Device Y Other Device	Z No Qualifier
9 Uterus	Ø Open 7 Via Natural or Artificial Opening 8 Via Natural or Artificial Opening Endoscopic	H Contraceptive Device	Z No Qualifier
C Cervix	Ø Open 3 Percutaneous 4 Percutaneous Endoscopic	1 Radioactive Element	Z No Qualifier
C Cervix	7 Via Natural or Artificial Opening 8 Via Natural or Artificial Opening Endoscopic	1 Radioactive Element H Contraceptive Device	Z No Qualifier
F Cul-de-sac	7 Via Natural or Artificial Opening 8 Via Natural or Artificial Opening Endoscopic	G Intraluminal Device, Pessary	Z No Qualifier
G Vagina	Ø Open 3 Percutaneous 4 Percutaneous Endoscopic X External	1 Radioactive Element	Z No Qualifier
G Vagina	7 Via Natural or Artificial Opening 8 Via Natural or Artificial Opening Endoscopic	1 Radioactive Element G Intraluminal Device, Pessary	Z No Qualifier

Ø: M/S

U: FEMALE REPRODUCTIVE SYSTEM

H: INSERTION

SECTION: Ø MEDICAL AND SURGICAL
BODY SYSTEM: U FEMALE REPRODUCTIVE SYSTEM
OPERATION: J INSPECTION: Visually and/or manually exploring a body part

Body Part	Approach	Device	Qualifier
3 Ovary	Ø Open 3 Percutaneous 4 Percutaneous Endoscopic 8 Via Natural or Artificial Opening Endoscopic X External	Z No Device	Z No Qualifier
8 Fallopian Tube D Uterus and Cervix H Vagina and Cul-de-sac	Ø Open 3 Percutaneous 4 Percutaneous Endoscopic 7 Via Natural or Artificial Opening 8 Via Natural or Artificial Opening Endoscopic X External	Z No Device	Z No Qualifier
M Vulva	Ø Open X External	Z No Device	Z No Qualifier

SECTION: Ø MEDICAL AND SURGICAL
BODY SYSTEM: U FEMALE REPRODUCTIVE SYSTEM
OPERATION: L OCCLUSION: Completely closing an orifice or the lumen of a tubular body part

Body Part	Approach	Device	Qualifier
5 Fallopian Tube, Right 6 Fallopian Tube, Left 7 Fallopian Tubes, Bilateral	Ø Open 3 Percutaneous 4 Percutaneous Endoscopic	C Extraluminal Device D Intraluminal Device Z No Device	Z No Qualifier
5 Fallopian Tube, Right 6 Fallopian Tube, Left 7 Fallopian Tubes, Bilateral	7 Via Natural or Artificial Opening 8 Via Natural or Artificial Opening Endoscopic	D Intraluminal Device Z No Device	Z No Qualifier
F Cul-de-sac G Vagina	7 Via Natural or Artificial Opening 8 Via Natural or Artificial Opening Endoscopic	D Intraluminal Device Z No Device	Z No Qualifier

SECTION: Ø MEDICAL AND SURGICAL
BODY SYSTEM: U FEMALE REPRODUCTIVE SYSTEM
OPERATION: M REATTACHMENT: Putting back in or on all or a portion of a separated body part to its normal location or other suitable location

Body Part	Approach	Device	Qualifier
Ø Ovary, Right 1 Ovary, Left 2 Ovaries, Bilateral 4 Uterine Supporting Structure 5 Fallopian Tube, Right 6 Fallopian Tube, Left 7 Fallopian Tubes, Bilateral 9 Uterus C Cervix F Cul-de-sac G Vagina	Ø Open 4 Percutaneous Endoscopic	Z No Device	Z No Qualifier
J Clitoris M Vulva	X External	Z No Device	Z No Qualifier
K Hymen	Ø Open 4 Percutaneous Endoscopic X External	Z No Device	Z No Qualifier

SECTION: Ø MEDICAL AND SURGICAL
BODY SYSTEM: U FEMALE REPRODUCTIVE SYSTEM
OPERATION: N RELEASE: Freeing a body part from an abnormal physical constraint by cutting or by the use of force

Body Part	Approach	Device	Qualifier
Ø Ovary, Right 1 Ovary, Left 2 Ovaries, Bilateral 4 Uterine Supporting Structure	Ø Open 3 Percutaneous 4 Percutaneous Endoscopic 8 Via Natural or Artificial Opening Endoscopic	Z No Device	Z No Qualifier
5 Fallopian Tube, Right 6 Fallopian Tube, Left 7 Fallopian Tubes, Bilateral 9 Uterus C Cervix F Cul-de-sac	Ø Open 3 Percutaneous 4 Percutaneous Endoscopic 7 Via Natural or Artificial Opening 8 Via Natural or Artificial Opening Endoscopic	Z No Device	Z No Qualifier
G Vagina K Hymen	Ø Open 3 Percutaneous 4 Percutaneous Endoscopic 7 Via Natural or Artificial Opening 8 Via Natural or Artificial Opening Endoscopic X External	Z No Device	Z No Qualifier
J Clitoris L Vestibular Gland M Vulva	Ø Open X External	Z No Device	Z No Qualifier

SECTION: Ø MEDICAL AND SURGICAL
BODY SYSTEM: U FEMALE REPRODUCTIVE SYSTEM
OPERATION: P REMOVAL: *(on multiple pages)*
Taking out or off a device from a body part

Body Part	Approach	Device	Qualifier
3 Ovary	Ø Open 3 Percutaneous 4 Percutaneous Endoscopic X External	Ø Drainage Device 3 Infusion Device Y Other Device	Z No Qualifier
3 Ovary	7 Via Natural or Artificial Opening 8 Via Natural or Artificial Opening Endoscopic	Y Other Device	Z No Qualifier
3 Ovary	X External	Ø Drainage Device 3 Infusion Device	Z No Qualifier
8 Fallopian Tube	Ø Open 3 Percutaneous 4 Percutaneous Endoscopic 7 Via Natural or Artificial Opening 8 Via Natural or Artificial Opening Endoscopic	Ø Drainage Device 3 Infusion Device 7 Autologous Tissue Substitute C Extraluminal Device D Intraluminal Device J Synthetic Substitute K Nonautologous Tissue Substitute Y Other Device	Z No Qualifier
8 Fallopian Tube	X External	Ø Drainage Device 3 Infusion Device D Intraluminal Device	Z No Qualifier
D Uterus and Cervix	Ø Open 3 Percutaneous 4 Percutaneous Endoscopic 7 Via Natural or Artificial Opening 8 Via Natural or Artificial Opening Endoscopic	Ø Drainage Device 1 Radioactive Element 3 Infusion Device 7 Autologous Tissue Substitute C Extraluminal Device D Intraluminal Device H Contraceptive Device J Synthetic Substitute K Nonautologous Tissue Substitute Y Other Device	Z No Qualifier
D Uterus and Cervix	X External	Ø Drainage Device 3 Infusion Device D Intraluminal Device H Contraceptive Device	Z No Qualifier
H Vagina and Cul-de-sac	Ø Open 3 Percutaneous 4 Percutaneous Endoscopic 7 Via Natural or Artificial Opening 8 Via Natural or Artificial Opening Endoscopic	Ø Drainage Device 1 Radioactive Element 3 Infusion Device 7 Autologous Tissue Substitute D Intraluminal Device J Synthetic Substitute K Nonautologous Tissue Substitute Y Other Device	Z No Qualifier

P: REMOVAL

U: FEMALE REPRODUCTIVE SYSTEM

Ø: M/S

SECTION: Ø MEDICAL AND SURGICAL
BODY SYSTEM: U FEMALE REPRODUCTIVE SYSTEM
OPERATION: P REMOVAL: *(continued)*
Taking out or off a device from a body part

Body Part	Approach	Device	Qualifier
H Vagina and Cul-de-sac	X External	Ø Drainage Device 1 Radioactive Element 3 Infusion Device D Intraluminal Device	Z No Qualifier
M Vulva	Ø Open	Ø Drainage Device 7 Autologous Tissue Substitute J Synthetic Substitute K Nonautologous Tissue Substitute	Z No Qualifier
M Vulva	X External	Ø Drainage Device	Z No Qualifier

SECTION: Ø MEDICAL AND SURGICAL
BODY SYSTEM: U FEMALE REPRODUCTIVE SYSTEM
OPERATION: Q REPAIR: Restoring, to the extent possible, a body part to its normal anatomic structure and function

Body Part	Approach	Device	Qualifier
Ø Ovary, Right 1 Ovary, Left 2 Ovaries, Bilateral 4 Uterine Supporting Structure	Ø Open 3 Percutaneous 4 Percutaneous Endoscopic 8 Via Natural or Artificial Opening Endoscopic	Z No Device	Z No Qualifier
5 Fallopian Tube, Right 6 Fallopian Tube, Left 7 Fallopian Tubes, Bilateral 9 Uterus C Cervix F Cul-de-sac	Ø Open 3 Percutaneous 4 Percutaneous Endoscopic 7 Via Natural or Artificial Opening 8 Via Natural or Artificial Opening Endoscopic	Z No Device	Z No Qualifier
G Vagina K Hymen	Ø Open 3 Percutaneous 4 Percutaneous Endoscopic 7 Via Natural or Artificial Opening 8 Via Natural or Artificial Opening Endoscopic X External	Z No Device	Z No Qualifier
J Clitoris L Vestibular Gland M Vulva	Ø Open X External	Z No Device	Z No Qualifier

SECTION: Ø MEDICAL AND SURGICAL
BODY SYSTEM: U FEMALE REPRODUCTIVE SYSTEM
OPERATION: S REPOSITION: Moving to its normal location, or other suitable location, all or a portion of a body part

Body Part	Approach	Device	Qualifier
Ø Ovary, Right 1 Ovary, Left 2 Ovaries, Bilateral 4 Uterine Supporting Structure 5 Fallopian Tube, Right 6 Fallopian Tube, Left 7 Fallopian Tubes, Bilateral C Cervix F Cul-de-sac	Ø Open 4 Percutaneous Endoscopic 8 Via Natural or Artificial Opening Endoscopic	Z No Device	Z No Qualifier
9 Uterus G Vagina	Ø Open 4 Percutaneous Endoscopic 7 Via Natural or Artificial Opening 8 Via Natural or Artificial Opening Endoscopic X External	Z No Device	Z No Qualifier

SECTION: Ø MEDICAL AND SURGICAL
BODY SYSTEM: U FEMALE REPRODUCTIVE SYSTEM
OPERATION: T RESECTION: Cutting out or off, without replacement, all of a body part

Body Part	Approach	Device	Qualifier
Ø Ovary, Right 1 Ovary, Left 2 Ovaries, Bilateral 5 Fallopian Tube, Right 6 Fallopian Tube, Left 7 Fallopian Tubes, Bilateral 9 Uterus	Ø Open 4 Percutaneous Endoscopic 7 Via Natural or Artificial Opening 8 Via Natural or Artificial Opening Endoscopic F Via Natural or Artificial Opening With Percutaneous Endoscopic Assistance	Z No Device	Z No Qualifier
4 Uterine Supporting Structure C Cervix F Cul-de-sac G Vagina	Ø Open 4 Percutaneous Endoscopic 7 Via Natural or Artificial Opening 8 Via Natural or Artificial Opening Endoscopic	Z No Device	Z No Qualifier
9 Uterus	Ø Open 4 Percutaneous Endoscopic 7 Via Natural or Artificial Opening 8 Via Natural or Artificial Opening Endoscopic F Via Natural or Artificial Opening With Percutaneous Endoscopic Assistance	Z No Device	L Supracervical Z No Qualifier
J Clitoris L Vestibular Gland M Vulva	Ø Open X External	Z No Device	Z No Qualifier
K Hymen	Ø Open 4 Percutaneous Endoscopic 7 Via Natural or Artificial Opening 8 Via Natural or Artificial Opening Endoscopic X External	Z No Device	Z No Qualifier

New/Revised Text in Blue ~~deleted~~ Deleted

SECTION: Ø MEDICAL AND SURGICAL
BODY SYSTEM: U FEMALE REPRODUCTIVE SYSTEM
OPERATION: U SUPPLEMENT: Putting in or on biological or synthetic material that physically reinforces and/or augments the function of a portion of a body part

Body Part	Approach	Device	Qualifier
4 Uterine Supporting Structure	Ø Open 4 Percutaneous Endoscopic	7 Autologous Tissue Substitute J Synthetic Substitute K Nonautologous Tissue Substitute	Z No Qualifier
5 Fallopian Tube Right 6 Fallopian Tube, Left 7 Fallopian Tubes, Bilateral F Cul-de-sac	Ø Open 4 Percutaneous Endoscopic 7 Via Natural or Artificial Opening 8 Via Natural or Artificial Opening Endoscopic	7 Autologous Tissue Substitute J Synthetic Substitute K Nonautologous Tissue Substitute	Z No Qualifier
G Vagina K Hymen	Ø Open 4 Percutaneous Endoscopic 7 Via Natural or Artificial Opening 8 Via Natural or Artificial Opening Endoscopic X External	7 Autologous Tissue Substitute J Synthetic Substitute K Nonautologous Tissue Substitute	Z No Qualifier
J Clitoris M Vulva	Ø Open X External	7 Autologous Tissue Substitute J Synthetic Substitute K Nonautologous Tissue Substitute	Z No Qualifier

SECTION: Ø MEDICAL AND SURGICAL
BODY SYSTEM: U FEMALE REPRODUCTIVE SYSTEM
OPERATION: V RESTRICTION: Partially closing an orifice or the lumen of a tubular body part

Body Part	Approach	Device	Qualifier
C Cervix	Ø Open 3 Percutaneous 4 Percutaneous Endoscopic	C Extraluminal Device D Intraluminal Device Z No Device	Z No Qualifier
C Cervix	7 Via Natural or Artificial Opening 8 Via Natural or Artificial Opening Endoscopic	D Intraluminal Device Z No Device	Z No Qualifier

SECTION: Ø MEDICAL AND SURGICAL
BODY SYSTEM: U FEMALE REPRODUCTIVE SYSTEM
OPERATION: W REVISION: *(on multiple pages)*
Correcting, to the extent possible, a portion of a malfunctioning device or the position of a displaced device

Body Part	Approach	Device	Qualifier
3 Ovary	Ø Open 3 Percutaneous 4 Percutaneous Endoscopic ~~X External~~	Ø Drainage Device 3 Infusion Device Y Other Device	Z No Qualifier
3 Ovary	7 Via Natural or Artificial Opening 8 Via Natural or Artificial Opening Endoscopic	Y Other Device	Z No Qualifier
3 Ovary	X External	Ø Drainage Device 3 Infusion Device	Z No Qualifier
8 Fallopian Tube	Ø Open 3 Percutaneous 4 Percutaneous Endoscopic 7 Via Natural or Artificial Opening 8 Via Natural or Artificial Opening Endoscopic ~~X External~~	Ø Drainage Device 3 Infusion Device 7 Autologous Tissue Substitute C Extraluminal Device D Intraluminal Device J Synthetic Substitute K Nonautologous Tissue Substitute Y Other Device	Z No Qualifier
8 Fallopian Tube	X External	Ø Drainage Device 3 Infusion Device 7 Autologous Tissue Substitute C Extraluminal Device D Intraluminal Device J Synthetic Substitute K Nonautologous Tissue Substitute	Z No Qualifier
D Uterus and Cervix	Ø Open 3 Percutaneous 4 Percutaneous Endoscopic 7 Via Natural or Artificial Opening 8 Via Natural or Artificial Opening Endoscopic	Ø Drainage Device 1 Radioactive Element 3 Infusion Device 7 Autologous Tissue Substitute C Extraluminal Device D Intraluminal Device H Contraceptive Device J Synthetic Substitute K Nonautologous Tissue Substitute Y Other Device	Z No Qualifier
D Uterus and Cervix	X External	Ø Drainage Device 3 Infusion Device 7 Autologous Tissue Substitute C Extraluminal Device D Intraluminal Device H Contraceptive Device J Synthetic Substitute K Nonautologous Tissue Substitute	Z No Qualifier
H Vagina and Cul-de-sac	Ø Open 3 Percutaneous 4 Percutaneous Endoscopic 7 Via Natural or Artificial Opening 8 Via Natural or Artificial Opening Endoscopic	Ø Drainage Device 1 Radioactive Element 3 Infusion Device 7 Autologous Tissue Substitute D Intraluminal Device J Synthetic Substitute K Nonautologous Tissue Substitute Y Other Device	Z No Qualifier

SECTION: Ø MEDICAL AND SURGICAL
BODY SYSTEM: U FEMALE REPRODUCTIVE SYSTEM
OPERATION: W REVISION: *(continued)*
Correcting, to the extent possible, a portion of a malfunctioning device or the position of a displaced device

Body Part	Approach	Device	Qualifier
H Vagina and Cul-de-sac	X External	Ø Drainage Device 3 Infusion Device 7 Autologous Tissue Substitute D Intraluminal Device J Synthetic Substitute K Nonautologous Tissue Substitute	Z No Qualifier
M Vulva	Ø Open X External	Ø Drainage Device 7 Autologous Tissue Substitute J Synthetic Substitute K Nonautologous Tissue Substitute	Z No Qualifier

SECTION: Ø MEDICAL AND SURGICAL
BODY SYSTEM: U FEMALE REPRODUCTIVE SYSTEM
OPERATION: Y TRANSPLANTATION: Putting in or on all or a portion of a living body part taken from another individual or animal to physically take the place and/or function of all or a portion of a similar body part

Body Part	Approach	Device	Qualifier
Ø Ovary, Right 1 Ovary, Left	Ø Open	Z No Device	Ø Allogeneic 1 Syngeneic 2 Zooplastic

ØV. Male Reproductive System 454
    ØV1. Bypass.. 455
    ØV2. Change 455
    ØV5. Destruction.. 456
    ØV7. Dilation.. 456
    ØV9. Drainage 457
    ØVB. Excision 458
    ØVC. Extirpation 459
    ØVH. Insertion 460
    ØVJ. Inspection 460
    ØVL. Occlusion 461
    ØVM. Reattachment.. 461
    ØVN. Release 462
    ØVP. Removal 463
    ØVQ. Repair 464
    ØVR. Replacement 465
    ØVS. Reposition.. 465
    ØVT. Resection.. 466
    ØVU. Supplement 467
    ØVW. Revision.. 468

SECTION: Ø MEDICAL AND SURGICAL

BODY SYSTEM: V MALE REPRODUCTIVE SYSTEM
OPERATION: 1 BYPASS: Altering the route of passage of the contents of a tubular body part

Body Part	Approach	Device	Qualifier
N Vas Deferens, Right P Vas Deferens, Left Q Vas Deferens, Bilateral	Ø Open 4 Percutaneous Endoscopic	7 Autologous Tissue Substitute J Synthetic Substitute K Nonautologous Tissue Substitute Z No Device	J Epididymis, Right K Epididymis, Left N Vas Deferens, Right P Vas Deferens, Left

SECTION: Ø MEDICAL AND SURGICAL

BODY SYSTEM: V MALE REPRODUCTIVE SYSTEM
OPERATION: 2 CHANGE: Taking out or off a device from a body part and putting back an identical or similar device in or on the same body part without cutting or puncturing the skin or a mucous membrane

Body Part	Approach	Device	Qualifier
4 Prostate and Seminal Vesicles 8 Scrotum and Tunica Vaginalis D Testis M Epididymis and Spermatic Cord R Vas Deferens S Penis	X External	Ø Drainage Device Y Other Device	Z No Qualifier

SECTION: Ø MEDICAL AND SURGICAL
BODY SYSTEM: V MALE REPRODUCTIVE SYSTEM
OPERATION: 5 DESTRUCTION: Physical eradication of all or a portion of a body part by the direct use of energy, force, or a destructive agent

Body Part	Approach	Device	Qualifier
Ø Prostate	Ø Open 3 Percutaneous 4 Percutaneous Endoscopic 7 Via Natural or Artificial Opening 8 Via Natural or Artificial Opening Endoscopic	Z No Device	Z No Qualifier
1 Seminal Vesicle, Right 2 Seminal Vesicle, Left 3 Seminal Vesicles, Bilateral 6 Tunica Vaginalis, Right 7 Tunica Vaginalis, Left 9 Testis, Right B Testis, Left C Testes, Bilateral ~~F Spermatic Cord, Right~~ ~~G Spermatic Cord, Left~~ ~~H Spermatic Cords, Bilateral~~ ~~J Epididymis, Right~~ ~~K Epididymis, Left~~ ~~L Epididymis, Bilateral~~ ~~N Vas Deferens, Right~~ ~~P Vas Deferens, Left A~~ ~~Q Vas Deferens, Bilateral A~~	Ø Open 3 Percutaneous 4 Percutaneous Endoscopic	Z No Device	Z No Qualifier
5 Scrotum S Penis T Prepuce	Ø Open 3 Percutaneous 4 Percutaneous Endoscopic X External	Z No Device	Z No Qualifier
F Spermatic Cord, Right G Spermatic Cord, Left H Spermatic Cords, Bilateral J Epididymis, Right K Epididymis, Left L Epididymis, Bilateral N Vas Deferens, Right P Vas Deferens, Left Q Vas Deferens, Bilateral	Ø Open 3 Percutaneous 4 Percutaneous Endoscopic 8 Via Natural or Artificial Opening Endoscopic	Z No Device	Z No Qualifier

SECTION: Ø MEDICAL AND SURGICAL
BODY SYSTEM: V MALE REPRODUCTIVE SYSTEM
OPERATION: 7 DILATION: Expanding an orifice or the lumen of a tubular body part

Body Part	Approach	Device	Qualifier
N Vas Deferens, Right P Vas Deferens, Left Q Vas Deferens, Bilateral	Ø Open 3 Percutaneous 4 Percutaneous Endoscopic	D Intraluminal Device Z No Device	Z No Qualifier

SECTION: Ø MEDICAL AND SURGICAL
BODY SYSTEM: V MALE REPRODUCTIVE SYSTEM
OPERATION: 9 DRAINAGE: *(on multiple pages)*
Taking or letting out fluids and/or gases from a body part

Body Part	Approach	Device	Qualifier
Ø Prostate	Ø Open 3 Percutaneous 4 Percutaneous Endoscopic 7 Via Natural or Artificial Opening 8 Via Natural or Artificial Opening Endoscopic	Ø Drainage Device	Z No Qualifier
Ø Prostate	Ø Open 3 Percutaneous 4 Percutaneous Endoscopic 7 Via Natural or Artificial Opening 8 Via Natural or Artificial Opening Endoscopic	Z No Device	X Diagnostic Z No Qualifier
1 Seminal Vesicle, Right 2 Seminal Vesicle, Left 3 Seminal Vesicles, Bilateral 6 Tunica Vaginalis, Right 7 Tunica Vaginalis, Left 9 Testis, Right B Testis, Left C Testes, Bilateral F Spermatic Cord, Right G Spermatic Cord, Left H Spermatic Cords, Bilateral J Epididymis, Right K Epididymis, Left L Epididymis, Bilateral N Vas Deferens, Right P Vas Deferens, Left Q Vas Deferens, Bilateral	Ø Open 3 Percutaneous 4 Percutaneous Endoscopic	Ø Drainage Device	Z No Qualifier
1 Seminal Vesicle, Right 2 Seminal Vesicle, Left 3 Seminal Vesicles, Bilateral 6 Tunica Vaginalis, Right 7 Tunica Vaginalis, Left 9 Testis, Right B Testis, Left C Testes, Bilateral F Spermatic Cord, Right G Spermatic Cord, Left H Spermatic Cords, Bilateral J Epididymis, Right K Epididymis, Left L Epididymis, Bilateral N Vas Deferens, Right P Vas Deferens, Left Q Vas Deferens, Bilateral	Ø Open 3 Percutaneous 4 Percutaneous Endoscopic	Z No Device	X Diagnostic Z No Qualifier

SECTION: Ø MEDICAL AND SURGICAL
BODY SYSTEM: V MALE REPRODUCTIVE SYSTEM
OPERATION: 9 DRAINAGE: *(continued)*
Taking or letting out fluids and/or gases from a body part

Body Part	Approach	Device	Qualifier
5 Scrotum S Penis T Prepuce	Ø Open 3 Percutaneous 4 Percutaneous Endoscopic X External	Ø Drainage Device	Z No Qualifier
5 Scrotum S Penis T Prepuce	Ø Open 3 Percutaneous 4 Percutaneous Endoscopic X External	Z No Device	X Diagnostic Z No Qualifier

SECTION: Ø MEDICAL AND SURGICAL
BODY SYSTEM: V MALE REPRODUCTIVE SYSTEM
OPERATION: B EXCISION: *(on multiple pages)*
Cutting out or off, without replacement, a portion of a body part

Body Part	Approach	Device	Qualifier
Ø Prostate	Ø Open 3 Percutaneous 4 Percutaneous Endoscopic 7 Via Natural or Artificial Opening 8 Via Natural or Artificial Opening Endoscopic	Z No Device	X Diagnostic Z No Qualifier
1 Seminal Vesicle, Right 2 Seminal Vesicle, Left 3 Seminal Vesicles, Bilateral 6 Tunica Vaginalis, Right 7 Tunica Vaginalis, Left 9 Testis, Right B Testis, Left C Testes, Bilateral ~~F Spermatic Cord, Right~~ ~~G Spermatic Cord, Left~~ ~~H Spermatic Cords, Bilateral~~ ~~J Epididymis, Right~~ ~~K Epididymis, Left~~ ~~L Epididymis, Bilateral~~ ~~N Vas Deferens, Right~~ ~~P Vas Deferens, Left~~ ~~Q Vas Deferens, Bilateral~~	Ø Open 3 Percutaneous 4 Percutaneous Endoscopic	Z No Device	X Diagnostic Z No Qualifier
5 Scrotum S Penis T Prepuce	Ø Open 3 Percutaneous 4 Percutaneous Endoscopic X External	Z No Device	X Diagnostic Z No Qualifier

SECTION: Ø MEDICAL AND SURGICAL
BODY SYSTEM: V MALE REPRODUCTIVE SYSTEM
OPERATION: B EXCISION: *(continued)*
Cutting out or off, without replacement, a portion of a body part

Body Part	Approach	Device	Qualifier
F Spermatic Cord, Right G Spermatic Cord, Left H Spermatic Cords, Bilateral J Epididymis, Right K Epididymis, Left L Epididymis, Bilateral N Vas Deferens, Right P Vas Deferens, Left Q Vas Deferens, Bilateral	Ø Open 3 Percutaneous 4 Percutaneous Endoscopic 8 Via Natural or Artificial Opening Endoscopic	Z No Device	X Diagnostic Z No Qualifier

SECTION: Ø MEDICAL AND SURGICAL
BODY SYSTEM: V MALE REPRODUCTIVE SYSTEM
OPERATION: C EXTIRPATION: Taking or cutting out solid matter from a body part

Body Part	Approach	Device	Qualifier
Ø Prostate	Ø Open 3 Percutaneous 4 Percutaneous Endoscopic 7 Via Natural or Artificial Opening 8 Via Natural or Artificial Opening Endoscopic	Z No Device	Z No Qualifier
1 Seminal Vesicle, Right 2 Seminal Vesicle, Left 3 Seminal Vesicles, Bilateral 6 Tunica Vaginalis, Right 7 Tunica Vaginalis, Left 9 Testis, Right B Testis, Left C Testes, Bilateral F Spermatic Cord, Right G Spermatic Cord, Left H Spermatic Cords, Bilateral J Epididymis, Right K Epididymis, Left L Epididymis, Bilateral N Vas Deferens, Right P Vas Deferens, Left Q Vas Deferens, Bilateral	Ø Open 3 Percutaneous 4 Percutaneous Endoscopic	Z No Device	Z No Qualifier
5 Scrotum S Penis T Prepuce	Ø Open 3 Percutaneous 4 Percutaneous Endoscopic X External	Z No Device	Z No Qualifier

SECTION: Ø MEDICAL AND SURGICAL
BODY SYSTEM: V MALE REPRODUCTIVE SYSTEM
OPERATION: H INSERTION: Putting in a nonbiological appliance that monitors, assists, performs, or prevents a physiological function but does not physically take the place of a body part

Body Part	Approach	Device	Qualifier
Ø Prostate	Ø Open 3 Percutaneous 4 Percutaneous Endoscopic 7 Via Natural or Artificial Opening 8 Via Natural or Artificial Opening Endoscopic	1 Radioactive Element	Z No Qualifier
4 Prostate and Seminal Vesicles 8 Scrotum and Tunica Vaginalis D Testis M Epididymis and Spermatic Cord R Vas Deferens	Ø Open 3 Percutaneous 4 Percutaneous Endoscopic 7 Via Natural or Artificial Opening 8 Via Natural or Artificial Opening Endoscopic	3 Infusion Device Y Other Device	Z No Qualifier
S Penis	Ø Open 3 Percutaneous 4 Percutaneous Endoscopic X External	3 Infusion Device Y Other Device	Z No Qualifier
S Penis	7 Via Natural or Artificial Opening 8 Via Natural or Artificial Opening Endoscopic	Y Other Device	Z No Qualifier
S Penis	X External	3 Infusion Device	Z No Qualifier

SECTION: Ø MEDICAL AND SURGICAL
BODY SYSTEM: V MALE REPRODUCTIVE SYSTEM
OPERATION: J INSPECTION: Visually and/or manually exploring a body part

Body Part	Approach	Device	Qualifier
4 Prostate and Seminal Vesicles 8 Scrotum and Tunica Vaginalis D Testis M Epididymis and Spermatic Cord R Vas Deferens S Penis	Ø Open 3 Percutaneous 4 Percutaneous Endoscopic X External	Z No Device	Z No Qualifier

SECTION: Ø MEDICAL AND SURGICAL

BODY SYSTEM: V MALE REPRODUCTIVE SYSTEM
OPERATION: L OCCLUSION: Completely closing an orifice or the lumen of a tubular body part

Body Part	Approach	Device	Qualifier
F Spermatic Cord, Right G Spermatic Cord, Left H Spermatic Cords, Bilateral N Vas Deferens, Right P Vas Deferens, Left Q Vas Deferens, Bilateral	Ø Open 3 Percutaneous 4 Percutaneous Endoscopic 8 Via Natural or Artificial Opening Endoscopic	C Extraluminal Device D Intraluminal Device Z No Device	Z No Qualifier

SECTION: Ø MEDICAL AND SURGICAL

BODY SYSTEM: V MALE REPRODUCTIVE SYSTEM
OPERATION: M REATTACHMENT: Putting back in or on all or a portion of a separated body part to its normal location or other suitable location

Body Part	Approach	Device	Qualifier
5 Scrotum S Penis	X External	Z No Device	Z No Qualifier
6 Tunica Vaginalis, Right 7 Tunica Vaginalis, Left 9 Testis, Right B Testis, Left C Testes, Bilateral F Spermatic Cord, Right G Spermatic Cord, Left H Spermatic Cords, Bilateral	Ø Open 4 Percutaneous Endoscopic	Z No Device	Z No Qualifier

SECTION: Ø MEDICAL AND SURGICAL
BODY SYSTEM: V MALE REPRODUCTIVE SYSTEM
OPERATION: N RELEASE: Freeing a body part from an abnormal physical restraint by cutting or by the use of force

Body Part	Approach	Device	Qualifier
Ø Prostate	Ø Open 3 Percutaneous 4 Percutaneous Endoscopic 7 Via Natural or Artificial Opening 8 Via Natural or Artificial Opening Endoscopic	Z No Device	Z No Qualifier
1 Seminal Vesicle, Right 2 Seminal Vesicle, Left 3 Seminal Vesicles, Bilateral 6 Tunica Vaginalis, Right 7 Tunica Vaginalis, Left 9 Testis, Right B Testis, Left C Testes, Bilateral ~~F Spermatic Cord, Right~~ ~~G Spermatic Cord, Left~~ ~~H Spermatic Cords, Bilateral~~ ~~J Epididymis, Right~~ ~~K Epididymis, Left~~ ~~L Epididymis, Bilateral~~ ~~N Vas Deferens, Right~~ ~~P Vas Deferens, Left~~ ~~Q Vas Deferens, Bilateral~~	Ø Open 3 Percutaneous 4 Percutaneous Endoscopic	Z No Device	Z No Qualifier
5 Scrotum S Penis T Prepuce	Ø Open 3 Percutaneous 4 Percutaneous Endoscopic X External	Z No Device	Z No Qualifier
F Spermatic Cord, Right G Spermatic Cord, Left H Spermatic Cords, Bilateral J Epididymis, Right K Epididymis, Left L Epididymis, Bilateral N Vas Deferens, Right P Vas Deferens, Left Q Vas Deferens, Bilateral	Ø Open 3 Percutaneous 4 Percutaneous Endoscopic 8 Via Natural or Artificial Opening Endoscopic	Z No Device	Z No Qualifier

New/Revised Text in Blue   ~~deleted~~ Deleted

SECTION: Ø MEDICAL AND SURGICAL
BODY SYSTEM: V MALE REPRODUCTIVE SYSTEM
OPERATION: P REMOVAL: Taking out or off a device from a body part

Body Part	Approach	Device	Qualifier
4 Prostate and Seminal Vesicles	Ø Open 3 Percutaneous 4 Percutaneous Endoscopic 7 Via Natural or Artificial Opening 8 Via Natural or Artificial Opening Endoscopic	Ø Drainage Device 1 Radioactive Element 3 Infusion Device 7 Autologous Tissue Substitute J Synthetic Substitute K Nonautologous Tissue Substitute Y Other Device	Z No Qualifier
4 Prostate and Seminal Vesicles	X External	Ø Drainage Device 1 Radioactive Element 3 Infusion Device	Z No Qualifier
8 Scrotum and Tunica Vaginalis D Testis S Penis	Ø Open 3 Percutaneous 4 Percutaneous Endoscopic 7 Via Natural or Artificial Opening 8 Via Natural or Artificial Opening Endoscopic	Ø Drainage Device 3 Infusion Device 7 Autologous Tissue Substitute J Synthetic Substitute K Nonautologous Tissue Substitute Y Other Device	Z No Qualifier
8 Scrotum and Tunica Vaginalis D Testis S Penis	X External	Ø Drainage Device 3 Infusion Device	Z No Qualifier
M Epididymis and Spermatic Cord	Ø Open 3 Percutaneous 4 Percutaneous Endoscopic 7 Via Natural or Artificial Opening 8 Via Natural or Artificial Opening Endoscopic	Ø Drainage Device 3 Infusion Device 7 Autologous Tissue Substitute C Extraluminal Device J Synthetic Substitute K Nonautologous Tissue Substitute Y Other Device	Z No Qualifier
M Epididymis and Spermatic Cord	X External	Ø Drainage Device 3 Infusion Device	Z No Qualifier
R Vas Deferens	Ø Open 3 Percutaneous 4 Percutaneous Endoscopic 7 Via Natural or Artificial Opening 8 Via Natural or Artificial Opening Endoscopic	Ø Drainage Device 3 Infusion Device 7 Autologous Tissue Substitute C Extraluminal Device D Intraluminal Device J Synthetic Substitute K Nonautologous Tissue Substitute Y Other Device	Z No Qualifier
R Vas Deferens	X External	Ø Drainage Device 3 Infusion Device D Intraluminal Device	Z No Qualifier

SECTION: Ø MEDICAL AND SURGICAL
BODY SYSTEM: V MALE REPRODUCTIVE SYSTEM
OPERATION: Q REPAIR: Restoring, to the extent possible, a body part to its normal anatomic structure and function

Body Part	Approach	Device	Qualifier
Ø Prostate	Ø Open 3 Percutaneous 4 Percutaneous Endoscopic 7 Via Natural or Artificial Opening 8 Via Natural or Artificial Opening Endoscopic	Z No Device	Z No Qualifier
1 Seminal Vesicle, Right 2 Seminal Vesicle, Left 3 Seminal Vesicles, Bilateral 6 Tunica Vaginalis, Right 7 Tunica Vaginalis, Left 9 Testis, Right B Testis, Left C Testes, Bilateral ~~F Spermatic Cord, Right~~ ~~G Spermatic Cord, Left~~ ~~H Spermatic Cords, Bilateral~~ ~~J Epididymis, Right~~ ~~K Epididymis, Left~~ ~~L Epididymis, Bilateral~~ ~~N Vas Deferens, Right~~ ~~P Vas Deferens, Left~~ ~~Q Vas Deferens, Bilateral~~	Ø Open 3 Percutaneous 4 Percutaneous Endoscopic	Z No Device	Z No Qualifier
5 Scrotum S Penis T Prepuce	Ø Open 3 Percutaneous 4 Percutaneous Endoscopic X External	Z No Device	Z No Qualifier
F Spermatic Cord, Right G Spermatic Cord, Left H Spermatic Cords, Bilateral J Epididymis, Right K Epididymis, Left L Epididymis, Bilateral N Vas Deferens, Right P Vas Deferens, Left Q Vas Deferens, Bilateral	Ø Open 3 Percutaneous 4 Percutaneous Endoscopic 8 Via Natural or Artificial Opening Endoscopic	Z No Device	Z No Qualifier

Q: REPAIR

V: MALE REPRODUCTIVE SYSTEM

Ø: M/S

       New/Revised Text in Blue   ~~deleted~~ Deleted

SECTION: Ø MEDICAL AND SURGICAL
BODY SYSTEM: V MALE REPRODUCTIVE SYSTEM
OPERATION: R REPLACEMENT: Putting in or on biological or synthetic material that physically takes the place and/or function of all or a portion of a body part

Body Part	Approach	Device	Qualifier
9 Testis, Right B Testis, Left C Testis, Bilateral	Ø Open	J Synthetic Substitute	Z No Qualifier

SECTION: Ø MEDICAL AND SURGICAL
BODY SYSTEM: V MALE REPRODUCTIVE SYSTEM
OPERATION: S REPOSITION: Moving to its normal location or other suitable location all or a portion of a body part

Body Part	Approach	Device	Qualifier
9 Testis, Right B Testis, Left C Testes, Bilateral F Spermatic Cord, Right G Spermatic Cord, Left H Spermatic Cords, Bilateral	Ø Open 3 Percutaneous 4 Percutaneous Endoscopic 8 Via Natural or Artificial Opening Endoscopic	Z No Device	Z No Qualifier

SECTION: Ø MEDICAL AND SURGICAL
BODY SYSTEM: V MALE REPRODUCTIVE SYSTEM
OPERATION: T RESECTION: Cutting out or off, without replacement, all of a body part

Body Part	Approach	Device	Qualifier
Ø Prostate	Ø Open 4 Percutaneous Endoscopic 7 Via Natural or Artificial Opening 8 Via Natural or Artificial Opening Endoscopic	Z No Device	Z No Qualifier
1 Seminal Vesicle, Right 2 Seminal Vesicle, Left 3 Seminal Vesicles, Bilateral 6 Tunica Vaginalis, Right 7 Tunica Vaginalis, Left 9 Testis, Right B Testis, Left C Testes, Bilateral F Spermatic Cord, Right G Spermatic Cord, Left H Spermatic Cords, Bilateral J Epididymis, Right K Epididymis, Left L Epididymis, Bilateral N Vas Deferens, Right P Vas Deferens, Left Q Vas Deferens, Bilateral	Ø Open 4 Percutaneous Endoscopic	Z No Device	Z No Qualifier
5 Scrotum S Penis T Prepuce	Ø Open 4 Percutaneous Endoscopic X External	Z No Device	Z No Qualifier

SECTION: Ø MEDICAL AND SURGICAL
BODY SYSTEM: V MALE REPRODUCTIVE SYSTEM
OPERATION: U SUPPLEMENT: Putting in or on biological or synthetic material that physically reinforces and/or augments the function of a portion of a body part

Body Part	Approach	Device	Qualifier
1 Seminal Vesicle, Right 2 Seminal Vesicle, Left 3 Seminal Vesicles, Bilateral 6 Tunica Vaginalis, Right 7 Tunica Vaginalis, Left F Spermatic Cord, Right G Spermatic Cord, Left H Spermatic Cords, Bilateral J Epididymis, Right K Epididymis, Left L Epididymis, Bilateral N Vas Deferens, Right P Vas Deferens, Left Q Vas Deferens, Bilateral	Ø Open 4 Percutaneous Endoscopic 8 Via Natural or Artificial Opening Endoscopic	7 Autologous Tissue Substitute J Synthetic Substitute K Nonautologous Tissue Substitute	Z No Qualifier
5 Scrotum S Penis T Prepuce	Ø Open 4 Percutaneous Endoscopic X External	7 Autologous Tissue Substitute J Synthetic Substitute K Nonautologous Tissue Substitute	Z No Qualifier
9 Testis, Right B Testis, Left C Testis, Bilateral	Ø Open	7 Autologous Tissue Substitute J Synthetic Substitute K Nonautologous Tissue Substitute	Z No Qualifier

SECTION: Ø MEDICAL AND SURGICAL
BODY SYSTEM: V MALE REPRODUCTIVE SYSTEM
OPERATION: W REVISION: Correcting, to the extent possible, a portion of a malfunctioning device or the position of a displaced device

Body Part	Approach	Device	Qualifier
4 Prostate and Seminal Vesicles 8 Scrotum and Tunica Vaginalis D Testis A S Penis A	Ø Open 3 Percutaneous 4 Percutaneous Endoscopic 7 Via Natural or Artificial Opening 8 Via Natural or Artificial Opening Endoscopic X̶ ̶E̶x̶t̶e̶r̶n̶a̶l̶	Ø Drainage Device 3 Infusion Device 7 Autologous Tissue Substitute J Synthetic Substitute K Nonautologous Tissue Substitute Y Other Device	Z No Qualifier
4 Prostate and Seminal Vesicles 8 Scrotum and Tunica Vaginalis D Testis S Penis	X External	Ø Drainage Device 3 Infusion Device 7 Autologous Tissue Substitute J Synthetic Substitute K Nonautologous Tissue Substitute	Z No Qualifier
M Epididymis and Spermatic Cord	Ø Open 3 Percutaneous 4 Percutaneous Endoscopic 7 Via Natural or Artificial Opening 8 Via Natural or Artificial Opening Endoscopic X̶ ̶E̶x̶t̶e̶r̶n̶a̶l̶	Ø Drainage Device 3 Infusion Device 7 Autologous Tissue Substitute C Extraluminal Device J Synthetic Substitute K Nonautologous Tissue Substitute Y Other Device	Z No Qualifier
M Epididymis and Spermatic Cord	X External	Ø Drainage Device 3 Infusion Device 7 Autologous Tissue Substitute C Extraluminal Device J Synthetic Substitute K Nonautologous Tissue Substitute	Z No Qualifier
R Vas Deferens	Ø Open 3 Percutaneous 4 Percutaneous Endoscopic 7 Via Natural or Artificial Opening 8 Via Natural or Artificial Opening Endoscopic X̶ ̶E̶x̶t̶e̶r̶n̶a̶l̶	Ø Drainage Device 3 Infusion Device 7 Autologous Tissue Substitute C Extraluminal Device D Intraluminal Device J Synthetic Substitute K Nonautologous Tissue Substitute Y Other Device	Z No Qualifier
R Vas Deferens	X External	Ø Drainage Device 3 Infusion Device 7 Autologous Tissue Substitute C Extraluminal Device D Intraluminal Device J Synthetic Substitute K Nonautologous Tissue Substitute	Z No Qualifier

New/Revised Text in Blue   ~~deleted~~ Deleted

ØW. Anatomical Regions, General 469
   ØWØ. Alteration 470
   ØW1. Bypass 470
   ØW2. Change 471
   ØW3. Control 471
   ØW4. Creation 472
   ØW8. Division 472
   ØW9. Drainage 473
   ØWB. Excision 474
   ØWC. Extirpation 474
   ØWF. Fragmentation 475
   ØWH. Insertion 476
   ØWJ. Inspection 477
   ØWM. Reattachment 477
   ØWP. Removal 478
   ØWQ. Repair 479
   ØWU. Supplement 479
   ØWW. Revision 480
   ØWY. Transplantation 480

SECTION: Ø MEDICAL AND SURGICAL
BODY SYSTEM: W ANATOMICAL REGIONS, GENERAL
OPERATION: Ø **ALTERATION:** Modifying the anatomic structure of a body part without affecting the function of the body part

Body Part	Approach	Device	Qualifier
Ø Head 2 Face 4 Upper Jaw 5 Lower Jaw 6 Neck 8 Chest Wall F Abdominal Wall K Upper Back L Lower Back M Perineum, Male N Perineum, Female	Ø Open 3 Percutaneous 4 Percutaneous Endoscopic	7 Autologous Tissue Substitute J Synthetic Substitute K Nonautologous Tissue Substitute Z No Device	Z No Qualifier

SECTION: Ø MEDICAL AND SURGICAL
BODY SYSTEM: W ANATOMICAL REGIONS, GENERAL
OPERATION: 1 **BYPASS:** Altering the route of passage of the contents of a tubular body part

Body Part	Approach	Device	Qualifier
1 Cranial Cavity	Ø Open	J Synthetic Substitute	9 Pleural Cavity, Right B Pleural Cavity, Left G Peritoneal Cavity J Pelvic Cavity
9 Pleural Cavity, Right B Pleural Cavity, Left G Peritoneal Cavity J Pelvic Cavity	Ø Open 4 Percutaneous Endoscopic	J Synthetic Substitute	4 Cutaneous 9 Pleural Cavity, Right B Pleural Cavity, Left G Peritoneal Cavity J Pelvic Cavity Y Lower Vein
9 Pleural Cavity, Right B Pleural Cavity, Left G Peritoneal Cavity J Pelvic Cavity	3 Percutaneous	J Synthetic Substitute	4 Cutaneous

SECTION: Ø MEDICAL AND SURGICAL
BODY SYSTEM: W ANATOMICAL REGIONS, GENERAL
OPERATION: 2 CHANGE: Taking out or off a device from a body part and putting back an identical or similar device in or on the same body part without cutting or puncturing the skin or a mucous membrane

Body Part	Approach	Device	Qualifier
Ø Head 1 Cranial Cavity 2 Face 4 Upper Jaw 5 Lower Jaw 6 Neck 8 Chest Wall 9 Pleural Cavity, Right B Pleural Cavity, Left C Mediastinum D Pericardial Cavity F Abdominal Wall G Peritoneal Cavity H Retroperitoneum J Pelvic Cavity K Upper Back L Lower Back M Perineum, Male N Perineum, Female	X External	Ø Drainage Device Y Other Device	Z No Qualifier

SECTION: Ø MEDICAL AND SURGICAL
BODY SYSTEM: W ANATOMICAL REGIONS, GENERAL
OPERATION: 3 CONTROL: *(on multiple pages)*
Stopping, or attempting to stop, postprocedure or other acute bleeding

Body Part	Approach	Device	Qualifier
Ø Head 1 Cranial Cavity 2 Face 3 Oral Cavity and Throat 4 Upper Jaw 5 Lower Jaw 6 Neck 8 Chest Wall 9 Pleural Cavity, Right B Pleural Cavity, Left C Mediastinum D Pericardial Cavity F Abdominal Wall G Peritoneal Cavity H Retroperitoneum J Pelvic Cavity K Upper Back L Lower Back M Perineum, Male N Perineum, Female	Ø Open 3 Percutaneous 4 Percutaneous Endoscopic	Z No Device	Z No Qualifier

SECTION: Ø MEDICAL AND SURGICAL
BODY SYSTEM: W ANATOMICAL REGIONS, GENERAL
OPERATION: 3 CONTROL: *(continued)*
Stopping, or attempting to stop, postprocedure or other acute bleeding

Body Part	Approach	Device	Qualifier
3 Oral Cavity and Throat	Ø Open 3 Percutaneous 4 Percutaneous Endoscopic 7 Via Natural or Artificial Opening 8 Via Natural or Artificial Opening Endoscopic X External	Z No Device	Z No Qualifier
P Gastrointestinal Tract Q Respiratory Tract R Genitourinary Tract	Ø Open 3 Percutaneous 4 Percutaneous Endoscopic 7 Via Natural or Artificial Opening 8 Via Natural or Artificial Opening Endoscopic	Z No Device	Z No Qualifier

SECTION: Ø MEDICAL AND SURGICAL
BODY SYSTEM: W ANATOMICAL REGIONS, GENERAL
OPERATION: 4 CREATION: Putting in or on biological or synthetic material to form a new body part that to the extent possible replicates the anatomic structure or function of an absent body part

Body Part	Approach	Device	Qualifier
M Perineum, Male	Ø Open	7 Autologous Tissue Substitute J Synthetic Substitute K Nonautologous Tissue Substitute Z No Device	Ø Vagina
N Perineum, Female	Ø Open	7 Autologous Tissue Substitute J Synthetic Substitute K Nonautologous Tissue Substitute Z No Device	1 Penis

SECTION: Ø MEDICAL AND SURGICAL
BODY SYSTEM: W ANATOMICAL REGIONS, GENERAL
OPERATION: 8 DIVISION: Cutting into a body part, without draining fluids and/or gases from the body part, in order to separate or transect a body part

Body Part	Approach	Device	Qualifier
N Perineum, Female	X External	Z No Device	Z No Qualifier

W: ANATOMICAL REGIONS, GENERAL · 3: CONTROL · 4: CREATION · 8: DIVISION · Ø: M/S

SECTION: Ø MEDICAL AND SURGICAL
BODY SYSTEM: W ANATOMICAL REGIONS, GENERAL
OPERATION: 9 DRAINAGE: Taking or letting out fluids and/or gases from a body part

Body Part	Approach	Device	Qualifier
Ø Head 1 Cranial Cavity 2 Face 3 Oral Cavity and Throat 4 Upper Jaw 5 Lower Jaw 6 Neck 8 Chest Wall 9 Pleural Cavity, Right B Pleural Cavity, Left C Mediastinum D Pericardial Cavity F Abdominal Wall G Peritoneal Cavity H Retroperitoneum J Pelvic Cavity K Upper Back L Lower Back M Perineum, Male N Perineum, Female	Ø Open 3 Percutaneous 4 Percutaneous Endoscopic	Ø Drainage Device	Z No Qualifier
Ø Head 1 Cranial Cavity 2 Face 3 Oral Cavity and Throat 4 Upper Jaw 5 Lower Jaw 6 Neck 8 Chest Wall 9 Pleural Cavity, Right B Pleural Cavity, Left C Mediastinum D Pericardial Cavity F Abdominal Wall G Peritoneal Cavity H Retroperitoneum J Pelvic Cavity K Upper Back L Lower Back M Perineum, Male N Perineum, Female	Ø Open 3 Percutaneous 4 Percutaneous Endoscopic	Z No Device	X Diagnostic Z No Qualifier

SECTION: Ø MEDICAL AND SURGICAL
BODY SYSTEM: W ANATOMICAL REGIONS, GENERAL
OPERATION: B EXCISION: Cutting out or off, without replacement, a portion of a body part

Body Part	Approach	Device	Qualifier
Ø Head 2 Face 3 Oral Cavity and Throat 4 Upper Jaw 5 Lower Jaw 8 Chest Wall K Upper Back L Lower Back M Perineum, Male N Perineum, Female	Ø Open 3 Percutaneous 4 Percutaneous Endoscopic X External	Z No Device	X Diagnostic Z No Qualifier
6 Neck F Abdominal Wall	Ø Open 3 Percutaneous 4 Percutaneous Endoscopic	Z No Device	X Diagnostic Z No Qualifier
6 Neck F Abdominal Wall	X External	Z No Device	2 Stoma X Diagnostic Z No Qualifier
C Mediastinum H Retroperitoneum	Ø Open 3 Percutaneous 4 Percutaneous Endoscopic	Z No Device	X Diagnostic Z No Qualifier

SECTION: Ø MEDICAL AND SURGICAL
BODY SYSTEM: W ANATOMICAL REGIONS, GENERAL
OPERATION: C EXTIRPATION: Taking or cutting out solid matter from a body part

Body Part	Approach	Device	Qualifier
1 Cranial Cavity 3 Oral Cavity and Throat 9 Pleural Cavity, Right B Pleural Cavity, Left C Mediastinum D Pericardial Cavity G Peritoneal Cavity H Retroperitoneum J Pelvic Cavity	Ø Open 3 Percutaneous 4 Percutaneous Endoscopic X External	Z No Device	Z No Qualifier
P Gastrointestinal Tract Q Respiratory Tract R Genitourinary Tract	Ø Open 3 Percutaneous 4 Percutaneous Endoscopic 7 Via Natural or Artificial Opening 8 Via Natural or Artificial Opening Endoscopic X External	Z No Device	Z No Qualifier

SECTION: Ø MEDICAL AND SURGICAL
BODY SYSTEM: W ANATOMICAL REGIONS, GENERAL
OPERATION: F FRAGMENTATION: Breaking solid matter in a body part into pieces

Body Part	Approach	Device	Qualifier
1 Cranial Cavity 3 Oral Cavity and Throat 9 Pleural Cavity, Right B Pleural Cavity, Left C Mediastinum D Pericardial Cavity G Peritoneal Cavity J Pelvic Cavity	Ø Open 3 Percutaneous 4 Percutaneous Endoscopic X External	Z No Device	Z No Qualifier
P Gastrointestinal Tract Q Respiratory Tract R Genitourinary Tract	Ø Open 3 Percutaneous 4 Percutaneous Endoscopic 7 Via Natural or Artificial Opening 8 Via Natural or Artificial Opening Endoscopic X External	Z No Device	Z No Qualifier

SECTION: Ø MEDICAL AND SURGICAL
BODY SYSTEM: W ANATOMICAL REGIONS, GENERAL
OPERATION: H INSERTION: Putting in a nonbiological appliance that monitors, assists, performs, or prevents a physiological function but does not physically take the place of a body part

Body Part	Approach	Device	Qualifier
Ø Head 1 Cranial Cavity 2 Face 3 Oral Cavity and Throat 4 Upper Jaw 5 Lower Jaw 6 Neck 8 Chest Wall 9 Pleural Cavity, Right B Pleural Cavity, Left C Mediastinum D Pericardial Cavity F Abdominal Wall G Peritoneal Cavity H Retroperitoneum J Pelvic Cavity K Upper Back L Lower Back M Perineum, Male N Perineum, Female	Ø Open 3 Percutaneous 4 Percutaneous Endoscopic	1 Radioactive Element 3 Infusion Device Y Other Device	Z No Qualifier
P Gastrointestinal Tract Q Respiratory Tract R Genitourinary Tract	Ø Open 3 Percutaneous 4 Percutaneous Endoscopic 7 Via Natural or Artificial Opening 8 Via Natural or Artificial Opening Endoscopic	1 Radioactive Element 3 Infusion Device Y Other Device	Z No Qualifier

SECTION: Ø MEDICAL AND SURGICAL
BODY SYSTEM: W ANATOMICAL REGIONS, GENERAL
OPERATION: J INSPECTION: Visually and/or manually exploring a body part

Body Part	Approach	Device	Qualifier
Ø Head 2 Face 3 Oral Cavity and Throat 4 Upper Jaw 5 Lower Jaw 6 Neck 8 Chest Wall F Abdominal Wall K Upper Back L Lower Back M Perineum, Male N Perineum, Female	Ø Open 3 Percutaneous 4 Percutaneous Endoscopic X External	Z No Device	Z No Qualifier
1 Cranial Cavity 9 Pleural Cavity, Right B Pleural Cavity, Left C Mediastinum D Pericardial Cavity G Peritoneal Cavity H Retroperitoneum J Pelvic Cavity	Ø Open 3 Percutaneous 4 Percutaneous Endoscopic	Z No Device	Z No Qualifier
P Gastrointestinal Tract Q Respiratory Tract R Genitourinary Tract	Ø Open 3 Percutaneous 4 Percutaneous Endoscopic 7 Via Natural or Artificial Opening 8 Via Natural or Artificial Opening Endoscopic	Z No Device	Z No Qualifier

SECTION: Ø MEDICAL AND SURGICAL
BODY SYSTEM: W ANATOMICAL REGIONS, GENERAL
OPERATION: M REATTACHMENT: Putting back in or on all or a portion of a separated body part to its normal location or other suitable location

Body Part	Approach	Device	Qualifier
2 Face 4 Upper Jaw 5 Lower Jaw 6 Neck 8 Chest Wall F Abdominal Wall K Upper Back L Lower Back M Perineum, Male N Perineum, Female	Ø Open	Z No Device	Z No Qualifier

SECTION: Ø MEDICAL AND SURGICAL
BODY SYSTEM: W ANATOMICAL REGIONS, GENERAL
OPERATION: P REMOVAL: Taking out or off a device from a body part

Body Part	Approach	Device	Qualifier
Ø Head 2 Face 4 Upper Jaw 5 Lower Jaw 6 Neck 8 Chest Wall C Mediastinum F Abdominal Wall K Upper Back L Lower Back M Perineum, Male N Perineum, Female	Ø Open 3 Percutaneous 4 Percutaneous Endoscopic X External	Ø Drainage Device 1 Radioactive Element 3 Infusion Device 7 Autologous Tissue Substitute J Synthetic Substitute K Nonautologous Tissue Substitute Y Other Device	Z No Qualifier
1 Cranial Cavity 9 Pleural Cavity, Right B Pleural Cavity, Left G Peritoneal Cavity J Pelvic Cavity	Ø Open 3 Percutaneous 4 Percutaneous Endoscopic	Ø Drainage Device 1 Radioactive Element 3 Infusion Device J Synthetic Substitute Y Other Device	Z No Qualifier
1 Cranial Cavity 9 Pleural Cavity, Right B Pleural Cavity, Left G Peritoneal Cavity J Pelvic Cavity	X External	Ø Drainage Device 1 Radioactive Element 3 Infusion Device	Z No Qualifier
D Pericardial Cavity H Retroperitoneum	Ø Open 3 Percutaneous 4 Percutaneous Endoscopic	Ø Drainage Device 1 Radioactive Element 3 Infusion Device Y Other Device	Z No Qualifier
D Pericardial Cavity H Retroperitoneum	X External	Ø Drainage Device 1 Radioactive Element 3 Infusion Device	Z No Qualifier
P Gastrointestinal Tract Q Respiratory Tract R Genitourinary Tract	Ø Open 3 Percutaneous 4 Percutaneous Endoscopic 7 Via Natural or Artificial Opening 8 Via Natural or Artificial Opening Endoscopic X External	1 Radioactive Element 3 Infusion Device Y Other Device	Z No Qualifier

New/Revised Text in Blue   ~~deleted~~ Deleted

SECTION: Ø MEDICAL AND SURGICAL

BODY SYSTEM: W ANATOMICAL REGIONS, GENERAL

OPERATION: Q REPAIR: Restoring, to the extent possible, a body part to its normal anatomic structure and function

Body Part	Approach	Device	Qualifier
Ø Head 2 Face 3 Oral Cavity and Throat 4 Upper Jaw 5 Lower Jaw 8 Chest Wall K Upper Back L Lower Back M Perineum, Male N Perineum, Female	Ø Open 3 Percutaneous 4 Percutaneous Endoscopic X External	Z No Device	Z No Qualifier
6 Neck F Abdominal Wall	Ø Open 3 Percutaneous 4 Percutaneous Endoscopic	Z No Device	Z No Qualifier
6 Neck F Abdominal Wall	X External	Z No Device	2 Stoma Z No Qualifier
C Mediastinum	Ø Open 3 Percutaneous 4 Percutaneous Endoscopic	Z No Device	Z No Qualifier

SECTION: Ø MEDICAL AND SURGICAL

BODY SYSTEM: W ANATOMICAL REGIONS, GENERAL

OPERATION: U SUPPLEMENT: Putting in or on biological or synthetic material that physically reinforces and/or augments the function of a portion of a body part

Body Part	Approach	Device	Qualifier
Ø Head 2 Face 4 Upper Jaw 5 Lower Jaw 6 Neck 8 Chest Wall C Mediastinum F Abdominal Wall K Upper Back L Lower Back M Perineum, Male N Perineum, Female	Ø Open 4 Percutaneous Endoscopic	7 Autologous Tissue Substitute J Synthetic Substitute K Nonautologous Tissue Substitute	Z No Qualifier

SECTION: Ø MEDICAL AND SURGICAL
BODY SYSTEM: W ANATOMICAL REGIONS, GENERAL
OPERATION: W REVISION: Correcting, to the extent possible, a portion of a malfunctioning device or the position of a displaced device

Body Part	Approach	Device	Qualifier
Ø Head 2 Face 4 Upper Jaw 5 Lower Jaw 6 Neck 8 Chest Wall C Mediastinum F Abdominal Wall K Upper Back L Lower Back M Perineum, Male N Perineum, Female	Ø Open 3 Percutaneous 4 Percutaneous Endoscopic X External	Ø Drainage Device 1 Radioactive Element 3 Infusion Device 7 Autologous Tissue Substitute J Synthetic Substitute K Nonautologous Tissue Substitute Y Other Device	Z No Qualifier
1 Cranial Cavity 9 Pleural Cavity, Right B Pleural Cavity, Left G Peritoneal Cavity J Pelvic Cavity	Ø Open 3 Percutaneous 4 Percutaneous Endoscopic X External	Ø Drainage Device 1 Radioactive Element 3 Infusion Device J Synthetic Substitute Y Other Device	Z No Qualifier
D Pericardial Cavity H Retroperitoneum	Ø Open 3 Percutaneous 4 Percutaneous Endoscopic X External	Ø Drainage Device 1 Radioactive Element 3 Infusion Device Y Other Device	Z No Qualifier
P Gastrointestinal Tract Q Respiratory Tract R Genitourinary Tract	Ø Open 3 Percutaneous 4 Percutaneous Endoscopic 7 Via Natural or Artificial Opening 8 Via Natural or Artificial Opening Endoscopic X External	1 Radioactive Element 3 Infusion Device Y Other Device	Z No Qualifier

SECTION: Ø MEDICAL AND SURGICAL
BODY SYSTEM: W ANATOMICAL REGIONS, GENERAL
OPERATION: Y TRANSPLANTATION: Putting in or on all or a portion of a living body part taken from another individual or animal to physically take the place and/or function of all or a portion of a similar body part

Body Part	Approach	Device	Qualifier
2 Face	Ø Open	Z No Device	Ø Allogeneic 1 Syngeneic

ØX. Anatomical Regions, Upper Extremities..481
   ØXØ. Alteration...482
   ØX2. Change 482
   ØX3. Control 482
   ØX6. Detachment 483
   ØX9. Drainage 484
   ØXB. Excision 485
   ØXH. Insertion 485
   ØXJ. Inspection 486
   ØXM. Reattachment 486
   ØXP. Removal 487
   ØXQ. Repair 487
   ØXR. Replacement 488
   ØXU. Supplement 488
   ØXW. Revision 489
   ØXX. Transfer 489
   ØXY. Transplantation..489

SECTION: Ø MEDICAL AND SURGICAL
BODY SYSTEM: X ANATOMICAL REGIONS, UPPER EXTREMITIES
OPERATION: Ø ALTERATION: Modifying the anatomic structure of a body part without affecting the function of the body part

Body Part	Approach	Device	Qualifier
2 Shoulder Region, Right 3 Shoulder Region, Left 4 Axilla, Right 5 Axilla, Left 6 Upper Extremity, Right 7 Upper Extremity, Left 8 Upper Arm, Right 9 Upper Arm, Left B Elbow Region, Right C Elbow Region, Left D Lower Arm, Right F Lower Arm, Left G Wrist Region, Right H Wrist Region, Left	Ø Open 3 Percutaneous 4 Percutaneous Endoscopic	7 Autologous Tissue Substitute J Synthetic Substitute K Nonautologous Tissue Substitute Z No Device	Z No Qualifier

SECTION: Ø MEDICAL AND SURGICAL
BODY SYSTEM: X ANATOMICAL REGIONS, UPPER EXTREMITIES
OPERATION: 2 CHANGE: Taking out or off a device from a body part and putting back an identical or similar device in or on the same body part without cutting or puncturing the skin or a mucous membrane

Body Part	Approach	Device	Qualifier
6 Upper Extremity, Right 7 Upper Extremity, Left	X External	Ø Drainage Device Y Other Device	Z No Qualifier

SECTION: Ø MEDICAL AND SURGICAL
BODY SYSTEM: X ANATOMICAL REGIONS, UPPER EXTREMITIES
OPERATION: 3 CONTROL: Stopping, or attempting to stop, postprocedure or other acute bleeding

Body Part	Approach	Device	Qualifier
2 Shoulder Region, Right 3 Shoulder Region, Left 4 Axilla, Right 5 Axilla, Left 6 Upper Extremity, Right 7 Upper Extremity, Left 8 Upper Arm, Right 9 Upper Arm, Left B Elbow Region, Right C Elbow Region, Left D Lower Arm, Right F Lower Arm, Left G Wrist Region, Right H Wrist Region, Left J Hand, Right K Hand, Left	Ø Open 3 Percutaneous 4 Percutaneous Endoscopic	Z No Device	Z No Qualifier

SECTION: Ø MEDICAL AND SURGICAL
BODY SYSTEM: X ANATOMICAL REGIONS, UPPER EXTREMITIES
OPERATION: 6 DETACHMENT: Cutting off all or a portion of the upper or lower extremities

Body Part	Approach	Device	Qualifier
Ø Forequarter, Right 1 Forequarter, Left 2 Shoulder Region, Right 3 Shoulder Region, Left B Elbow Region, Right C Elbow Region, Left	Ø Open	Z No Device	Z No Qualifier
8 Upper Arm, Right 9 Upper Arm, Left D Lower Arm, Right F Lower Arm, Left	Ø Open	Z No Device	1 High 2 Mid 3 Low
J Hand, Right K Hand, Left	Ø Open	Z No Device	Ø Complete 4 Complete 1st Ray 5 Complete 2nd Ray 6 Complete 3rd Ray 7 Complete 4th Ray 8 Complete 5th Ray 9 Partial 1st Ray B Partial 2nd Ray C Partial 3rd Ray D Partial 4th Ray F Partial 5th Ray
L Thumb, Right M Thumb, Left N Index Finger, Right P Index Finger, Left Q Middle Finger, Right R Middle Finger, Left S Ring Finger, Right T Ring Finger, Left V Little Finger, Right W Little Finger, Left	Ø Open	Z No Device	Ø Complete 1 High 2 Mid 3 Low

SECTION: Ø MEDICAL AND SURGICAL
BODY SYSTEM: X ANATOMICAL REGIONS, UPPER EXTREMITIES
OPERATION: 9 DRAINAGE: Taking or letting out fluids and/or gases from a body part

Body Part	Approach	Device	Qualifier
2 Shoulder Region, Right 3 Shoulder Region, Left 4 Axilla, Right 5 Axilla, Left 6 Upper Extremity, Right 7 Upper Extremity, Left 8 Upper Arm, Right 9 Upper Arm, Left B Elbow Region, Right C Elbow Region, Left D Lower Arm, Right F Lower Arm, Left G Wrist Region, Right H Wrist Region, Left J Hand, Right K Hand, Left	Ø Open 3 Percutaneous 4 Percutaneous Endoscopic	Ø Drainage Device	Z No Qualifier
2 Shoulder Region, Right 3 Shoulder Region, Left 4 Axilla, Right 5 Axilla, Left 6 Upper Extremity, Right 7 Upper Extremity, Left 8 Upper Arm, Right 9 Upper Arm, Left B Elbow Region, Right C Elbow Region, Left D Lower Arm, Right F Lower Arm, Left G Wrist Region, Right H Wrist Region, Left J Hand, Right K Hand, Left	Ø Open 3 Percutaneous 4 Percutaneous Endoscopic	Z No Device	X Diagnostic Z No Qualifier

SECTION: Ø MEDICAL AND SURGICAL
BODY SYSTEM: X ANATOMICAL REGIONS, UPPER EXTREMITIES
OPERATION: B EXCISION: Cutting out or off, without replacement, a portion of a body part

Body Part	Approach	Device	Qualifier
2 Shoulder Region, Right 3 Shoulder Region, Left 4 Axilla, Right 5 Axilla, Left 6 Upper Extremity, Right 7 Upper Extremity, Left 8 Upper Arm, Right 9 Upper Arm, Left B Elbow Region, Right C Elbow Region, Left D Lower Arm, Right F Lower Arm, Left G Wrist Region, Right H Wrist Region, Left J Hand, Right K Hand, Left	Ø Open 3 Percutaneous 4 Percutaneous Endoscopic	Z No Device	X Diagnostic Z No Qualifier

SECTION: Ø MEDICAL AND SURGICAL
BODY SYSTEM: X ANATOMICAL REGIONS, UPPER EXTREMITIES
OPERATION: H INSERTION: Putting in a nonbiological appliance that monitors, assists, performs, or prevents a physiological function but does not physically take the place of a body part

Body Part	Approach	Device	Qualifier
2 Shoulder Region, Right 3 Shoulder Region, Left 4 Axilla, Right 5 Axilla, Left 6 Upper Extremity, Right 7 Upper Extremity, Left 8 Upper Arm, Right 9 Upper Arm, Left B Elbow Region, Right C Elbow Region, Left D Lower Arm, Right F Lower Arm, Left G Wrist Region, Right H Wrist Region, Left J Hand, Right K Hand, Left	Ø Open 3 Percutaneous 4 Percutaneous Endoscopic	1 Radioactive Element 3 Infusion Device Y Other Device	Z No Qualifier

SECTION: Ø MEDICAL AND SURGICAL
BODY SYSTEM: X ANATOMICAL REGIONS, UPPER EXTREMITIES
OPERATION: J INSPECTION: Visually and/or manually exploring a body part

Body Part	Approach	Device	Qualifier
2 Shoulder Region, Right 3 Shoulder Region, Left 4 Axilla, Right 5 Axilla, Left 6 Upper Extremity, Right 7 Upper Extremity, Left 8 Upper Arm, Right 9 Upper Arm, Left B Elbow Region, Right C Elbow Region, Left D Lower Arm, Right F Lower Arm, Left G Wrist Region, Right H Wrist Region, Left J Hand, Right K Hand, Left	Ø Open 3 Percutaneous 4 Percutaneous Endoscopic X External	Z No Device	Z No Qualifier

SECTION: Ø MEDICAL AND SURGICAL
BODY SYSTEM: X ANATOMICAL REGIONS, UPPER EXTREMITIES
OPERATION: M REATTACHMENT: Putting back in or on all or a portion of a separated body part to its normal location or other suitable location

Body Part	Approach	Device	Qualifier
Ø Forequarter, Right 1 Forequarter, Left 2 Shoulder Region, Right 3 Shoulder Region, Left 4 Axilla, Right 5 Axilla, Left 6 Upper Extremity, Right 7 Upper Extremity, Left 8 Upper Arm, Right 9 Upper Arm, Left B Elbow Region, Right C Elbow Region, Left D Lower Arm, Right F Lower Arm, Left G Wrist Region, Right H Wrist Region, Left J Hand, Right K Hand, Left L Thumb, Right M Thumb, Left N Index Finger, Right P Index Finger, Left Q Middle Finger, Right R Middle Finger, Left S Ring Finger, Right T Ring Finger, Left V Little Finger, Right W Little Finger, Left	Ø Open	Z No Device	Z No Qualifier

SECTION: Ø MEDICAL AND SURGICAL
BODY SYSTEM: X ANATOMICAL REGIONS, UPPER EXTREMITIES
OPERATION: P REMOVAL: Taking out or off a device from a body part

Body Part	Approach	Device	Qualifier
6 Upper Extremity, Right 7 Upper Extremity, Left	Ø Open 3 Percutaneous 4 Percutaneous Endoscopic X External	Ø Drainage Device 1 Radioactive Element 3 Infusion Device 7 Autologous Tissue Substitute J Synthetic Substitute K Nonautologous Tissue Substitute Y Other Device	Z No Qualifier

SECTION: Ø MEDICAL AND SURGICAL
BODY SYSTEM: X ANATOMICAL REGIONS, UPPER EXTREMITIES
OPERATION: Q REPAIR: Restoring, to the extent possible, a body part to its normal anatomic structure and function

Body Part	Approach	Device	Qualifier
2 Shoulder Region, Right 3 Shoulder Region, Left 4 Axilla, Right 5 Axilla, Left 6 Upper Extremity, Right 7 Upper Extremity, Left 8 Upper Arm, Right 9 Upper Arm, Left B Elbow Region, Right C Elbow Region, Left D Lower Arm, Right F Lower Arm, Left G Wrist Region, Right H Wrist Region, Left J Hand, Right K Hand, Left L Thumb, Right M Thumb, Left N Index Finger, Right P Index Finger, Left Q Middle Finger, Right R Middle Finger, Left S Ring Finger, Right T Ring Finger, Left V Little Finger, Right W Little Finger, Left	Ø Open 3 Percutaneous 4 Percutaneous Endoscopic X External	Z No Device	Z No Qualifier

SECTION: Ø MEDICAL AND SURGICAL
BODY SYSTEM: X ANATOMICAL REGIONS, UPPER EXTREMITIES
OPERATION: R REPLACEMENT: Putting in or on biological or synthetic material that physically takes the place and/or function of all or a portion of a body part

Body Part	Approach	Device	Qualifier
L Thumb, Right M Thumb, Left	Ø Open 4 Percutaneous Endoscopic	7 Autologous Tissue Substitute	N Toe, Right P Toe, Left

SECTION: Ø MEDICAL AND SURGICAL
BODY SYSTEM: X ANATOMICAL REGIONS, UPPER EXTREMITIES
OPERATION: U SUPPLEMENT: Putting in or on biological or synthetic material that physically reinforces and/or augments the function of a portion of a body part

Body Part	Approach	Device	Qualifier
2 Shoulder Region, Right 3 Shoulder Region, Left 4 Axilla, Right 5 Axilla, Left 6 Upper Extremity, Right 7 Upper Extremity, Left 8 Upper Arm, Right 9 Upper Arm, Left B Elbow Region, Right C Elbow Region, Left D Lower Arm, Right F Lower Arm, Left G Wrist Region, Right H Wrist Region, Left J Hand, Right K Hand, Left L Thumb, Right M Thumb, Left N Index Finger, Right P Index Finger, Left Q Middle Finger, Right R Middle Finger, Left S Ring Finger, Right T Ring Finger, Left V Little Finger, Right W Little Finger, Left	Ø Open 4 Percutaneous Endoscopic	7 Autologous Tissue Substitute J Synthetic Substitute K Nonautologous Tissue Substitute	Z No Qualifier

New/Revised Text in Blue   ~~deleted~~ Deleted

SECTION: Ø MEDICAL AND SURGICAL
BODY SYSTEM: X ANATOMICAL REGIONS, UPPER EXTREMITIES
OPERATION: W REVISION: Correcting, to the extent possible, a portion of a malfunctioning device or the position of displaced device

Body Part	Approach	Device	Qualifier
6 Upper Extremity, Right 7 Upper Extremity, Left	Ø Open 3 Percutaneous 4 Percutaneous Endoscopic X External	Ø Drainage Device 3 Infusion Device 7 Autologous Tissue Substitute J Synthetic Substitute K Nonautologous Tissue Substitute Y Other Device	Z No Qualifier

SECTION: Ø MEDICAL AND SURGICAL
BODY SYSTEM: X ANATOMICAL REGIONS, UPPER EXTREMITIES
OPERATION: X TRANSFER: Moving, without taking out, all or a portion of a body part to another location to take over the function of all or a portion of a body part

Body Part	Approach	Device	Qualifier
N Index Finger, Right	Ø Open	Z No Device	L Thumb, Right
P Index Finger, Left	Ø Open	Z No Device	M Thumb, Left

SECTION: Ø MEDICAL AND SURGICAL
BODY SYSTEM: X ANATOMICAL REGIONS, UPPER EXTREMITIES
OPERATION: Y TRANSPLANTATION: Putting in or on all or a portion of a living body part taken from another individual or animal to physically take the place and/or function of all or a portion of a similar body part

Body Part	Approach	Device	Qualifier
J Hand, Right K Hand, Left	Ø Open	Z No Device	Ø Allogeneic 1 Syngeneic

ØY. Anatomical Regions, Lower Extremities 490
   ØYØ. Alteration 491
   ØY2. Change 491
   ØY3. Control 491
   ØY6. Detachment 492
   ØY9. Drainage 493
   ØYB. Excision 494
   ØYH. Insertion 494
   ØYJ. Inspection 495
   ØYM. Reattachment 496
   ØYP. Removal 496
   ØYQ. Repair 497
   ØYU. Supplement 498
   ØYW. Revision..498

SECTION: Ø MEDICAL AND SURGICAL
BODY SYSTEM: Y ANATOMICAL REGIONS, LOWER EXTREMITIES
OPERATION: Ø **ALTERATION:** Modifying the anatomic structure of a body part without affecting the function of the body part

Body Part	Approach	Device	Qualifier
Ø Buttock, Right 1 Buttock, Left 9 Lower Extremity, Right B Lower Extremity, Left C Upper Leg, Right D Upper Leg, Left F Knee Region, Right G Knee Region, Left H Lower Leg, Right J Lower Leg, Left K Ankle Region, Right L Ankle Region, Left	Ø Open 3 Percutaneous 4 Percutaneous Endoscopic	7 Autologous Tissue Substitute J Synthetic Substitute K Nonautologous Tissue Substitute Z No Device	Z No Qualifier

SECTION: Ø MEDICAL AND SURGICAL
BODY SYSTEM: Y ANATOMICAL REGIONS, LOWER EXTREMITIES
OPERATION: 2 **CHANGE:** Taking out or off a device from a body part and putting back an identical or similar device in or on the same body part without cutting or puncturing the skin or a mucous membrane

Body Part	Approach	Device	Qualifier
9 Lower Extremity, Right B Lower Extremity, Left	X External	Ø Drainage Device Y Other Device	Z No Qualifier

SECTION: Ø MEDICAL AND SURGICAL
BODY SYSTEM: Y ANATOMICAL REGIONS, LOWER EXTREMITIES
OPERATION: 3 **CONTROL:** Stopping, or attempting to stop, postprocedure or other acute bleeding

Body Part	Approach	Device	Qualifier
Ø Buttock, Right 1 Buttock, Left 5 Inguinal Region, Right 6 Inguinal Region, Left 7 Femoral Region, Right 8 Femoral Region, Left 9 Lower Extremity, Right B Lower Extremity, Left C Upper Leg, Right D Upper Leg, Left F Knee Region, Right G Knee Region, Left H Lower Leg, Right J Lower Leg, Left K Ankle Region, Right L Ankle Region, Left M Foot, Right N Foot, Left	Ø Open 3 Percutaneous 4 Percutaneous Endoscopic	Z No Device	Z No Qualifier

SECTION: Ø MEDICAL AND SURGICAL
BODY SYSTEM: Y ANATOMICAL REGIONS, LOWER EXTREMITIES
OPERATION: 6 DETACHMENT: Cutting off all or a portion of the upper or lower extremities

Body Part	Approach	Device	Qualifier
2 Hindquarter, Right 3 Hindquarter, Left 4 Hindquarter, Bilateral 7 Femoral Region, Right 8 Femoral Region, Left F Knee Region, Right G Knee Region, Left	Ø Open	Z No Device	Z No Qualifier
C Upper Leg, Right D Upper Leg, Left H Lower Leg, Right J Lower Leg, Left	Ø Open	Z No Device	1 High 2 Mid 3 Low
M Foot, Right N Foot, Left	Ø Open	Z No Device	Ø Complete 4 Complete 1st Ray 5 Complete 2nd Ray 6 Complete 3rd Ray 7 Complete 4th Ray 8 Complete 5th Ray 9 Partial 1st Ray B Partial 2nd Ray C Partial 3rd Ray D Partial 4th Ray F Partial 5th Ray
P 1st Toe, Right Q 1st Toe, Left R 2nd Toe, Right S 2nd Toe, Left T 3rd Toe, Right U 3rd Toe, Left V 4th Toe, Right W 4th Toe, Left X 5th Toe, Right Y 5th Toe, Left	Ø Open	Z No Device	Ø Complete 1 High 2 Mid 3 Low

SECTION: Ø MEDICAL AND SURGICAL

BODY SYSTEM: Y ANATOMICAL REGIONS, LOWER EXTREMITIES
OPERATION: 9 DRAINAGE: Taking or letting out fluids and/or gases from a body part

Body Part	Approach	Device	Qualifier
Ø Buttock, Right 1 Buttock, Left 5 Inguinal Region, Right 6 Inguinal Region, Left 7 Femoral Region, Right 8 Femoral Region, Left 9 Lower Extremity, Right B Lower Extremity, Left C Upper Leg, Right D Upper Leg, Left F Knee Region, Right G Knee Region, Left H Lower Leg, Right J Lower Leg, Left K Ankle Region, Right L Ankle Region, Left M Foot, Right N Foot, Left	Ø Open 3 Percutaneous 4 Percutaneous Endoscopic	Ø Drainage Device	Z No Qualifier
Ø Buttock, Right 1 Buttock, Left 5 Inguinal Region, Right 6 Inguinal Region, Left 7 Femoral Region, Right 8 Femoral Region, Left 9 Lower Extremity, Right B Lower Extremity, Left C Upper Leg, Right D Upper Leg, Left F Knee Region, Right G Knee Region, Left H Lower Leg, Right J Lower Leg, Left K Ankle Region, Right L Ankle Region, Left M Foot, Right N Foot, Left	Ø Open 3 Percutaneous 4 Percutaneous Endoscopic	Z No Device	X Diagnostic Z No Qualifier

SECTION: Ø MEDICAL AND SURGICAL
BODY SYSTEM: Y ANATOMICAL REGIONS, LOWER EXTREMITIES
OPERATION: B EXCISION: Cutting out or off, without replacement, a portion of a body part

Body Part	Approach	Device	Qualifier
Ø Buttock, Right 1 Buttock, Left 5 Inguinal Region, Right 6 Inguinal Region, Left 7 Femoral Region, Right 8 Femoral Region, Left 9 Lower Extremity, Right B Lower Extremity, Left C Upper Leg, Right D Upper Leg, Left F Knee Region, Right G Knee Region, Left H Lower Leg, Right J Lower Leg, Left K Ankle Region, Right L Ankle Region, Left M Foot, Right N Foot, Left	Ø Open 3 Percutaneous 4 Percutaneous Endoscopic	Z No Device	X Diagnostic Z No Qualifier

SECTION: Ø MEDICAL AND SURGICAL
BODY SYSTEM: Y ANATOMICAL REGIONS, LOWER EXTREMITIES
OPERATION: H INSERTION: Putting in a nonbiological appliance that monitors, assists, performs, or prevents a physiological function but does not physically take the place of a body part

Body Part	Approach	Device	Qualifier
Ø Buttock, Right 1 Buttock, Left 5 Inguinal Region, Right 6 Inguinal Region, Left 7 Femoral Region, Right 8 Femoral Region, Left 9 Lower Extremity, Right B Lower Extremity, Left C Upper Leg, Right D Upper Leg, Left F Knee Region, Right G Knee Region, Left H Lower Leg, Right J Lower Leg, Left K Ankle Region, Right L Ankle Region, Left M Foot, Right N Foot, Left	Ø Open 3 Percutaneous 4 Percutaneous Endoscopic	1 Radioactive Element 3 Infusion Device Y Other Device	Z No Qualifier

SECTION: Ø MEDICAL AND SURGICAL
BODY SYSTEM: Y ANATOMICAL REGIONS, LOWER EXTREMITIES
OPERATION: J INSPECTION: Visually and/or manually exploring a body part

Body Part	Approach	Device	Qualifier
Ø Buttock, Right	Ø Open	Z No Device	Z No Qualifier
1 Buttock, Left	3 Percutaneous		
5 Inguinal Region, Right	4 Percutaneous Endoscopic		
6 Inguinal Region, Left	X External		
7 Femoral Region, Right			
8 Femoral Region, Left			
9 Lower Extremity, Right			
A Inguinal Region, Bilateral			
B Lower Extremity, Left			
C Upper Leg, Right			
D Upper Leg, Left			
E Femoral Region, Bilateral			
F Knee Region, Right			
G Knee Region, Left			
H Lower Leg, Right			
J Lower Leg, Left			
K Ankle Region, Right			
L Ankle Region, Left			
M Foot, Right			
N Foot, Left			

SECTION: Ø MEDICAL AND SURGICAL
BODY SYSTEM: Y ANATOMICAL REGIONS, LOWER EXTREMITIES
OPERATION: M REATTACHMENT: Putting back in or on all or a portion of a separated body part to its normal location or other suitable location

Body Part	Approach	Device	Qualifier
Ø Buttock, Right	Ø Open	Z No Device	Z No Qualifier
1 Buttock, Left			
2 Hindquarter, Right			
3 Hindquarter, Left			
4 Hindquarter, Bilateral			
5 Inguinal Region, Right			
6 Inguinal Region, Left			
7 Femoral Region, Right			
8 Femoral Region, Left			
9 Lower Extremity, Right			
B Lower Extremity, Left			
C Upper Leg, Right			
D Upper Leg, Left			
F Knee Region, Right			
G Knee Region, Left			
H Lower Leg, Right			
J Lower Leg, Left			
K Ankle Region, Right			
L Ankle Region, Left			
M Foot, Right			
N Foot, Left			
P 1st Toe, Right			
Q 1st Toe, Left			
R 2nd Toe, Right			
S 2nd Toe, Left			
T 3rd Toe, Right			
U 3rd Toe, Left			
V 4th Toe, Right			
W 4th Toe, Left			
X 5th Toe, Right			
Y 5th Toe, Left			

SECTION: Ø MEDICAL AND SURGICAL
BODY SYSTEM: Y ANATOMICAL REGIONS, LOWER EXTREMITIES
OPERATION: P REMOVAL: Taking out or off a device from a body part

Body Part	Approach	Device	Qualifier
9 Lower Extremity, Right	Ø Open	Ø Drainage Device	Z No Qualifier
B Lower Extremity, Left	3 Percutaneous	1 Radioactive Element	
	4 Percutaneous Endoscopic	3 Infusion Device	
	X External	7 Autologous Tissue Substitute	
		J Synthetic Substitute	
		K Nonautologous Tissue Substitute	
		Y Other Device	

New/Revised Text in Blue ~~deleted~~ Deleted

SECTION: Ø MEDICAL AND SURGICAL
BODY SYSTEM: Y ANATOMICAL REGIONS, LOWER EXTREMITIES
OPERATION: Q **REPAIR:** Restoring, to the extent possible, a body part to its normal anatomic structure and function

Body Part	Approach	Device	Qualifier
Ø Buttock, Right	Ø Open	Z No Device	Z No Qualifier
1 Buttock, Left	3 Percutaneous		
5 Inguinal Region, Right	4 Percutaneous Endoscopic		
6 Inguinal Region, Left	X External		
7 Femoral Region, Right			
8 Femoral Region, Left			
9 Lower Extremity, Right			
A Inguinal Region, Bilateral			
B Lower Extremity, Left			
C Upper Leg, Right			
D Upper Leg, Left			
E Femoral Region, Bilateral			
F Knee Region, Right			
G Knee Region, Left			
H Lower Leg, Right			
J Lower Leg, Left			
K Ankle Region, Right			
L Ankle Region, Left			
M Foot, Right			
N Foot, Left			
P 1st Toe, Right			
Q 1st Toe, Left			
R 2nd Toe, Right			
S 2nd Toe, Left			
T 3rd Toe, Right			
U 3rd Toe, Left			
V 4th Toe, Right			
W 4th Toe, Left			
X 5th Toe, Right			
Y 5th Toe, Left			

SECTION: Ø MEDICAL AND SURGICAL
BODY SYSTEM: Y ANATOMICAL REGIONS, LOWER EXTREMITIES
OPERATION: U SUPPLEMENT: Putting in or on biological or synthetic material that physically reinforces and/or augments the function of a portion of a body part

Body Part	Approach	Device	Qualifier
Ø Buttock, Right 1 Buttock, Left 5 Inguinal Region, Right 6 Inguinal Region, Left 7 Femoral Region, Right 8 Femoral Region, Left 9 Lower Extremity, Right A Inguinal Region, Bilateral B Lower Extremity, Left C Upper Leg, Right D Upper Leg, Left E Femoral Region, Bilateral F Knee Region, Right G Knee Region, Left H Lower Leg, Right J Lower Leg, Left K Ankle Region, Right L Ankle Region, Left M Foot, Right N Foot, Left P 1st Toe, Right Q 1st Toe, Left R 2nd Toe, Right S 2nd Toe, Left T 3rd Toe, Right U 3rd Toe, Left V 4th Toe, Right W 4th Toe, Left X 5th Toe, Right Y 5th Toe, Left	Ø Open 4 Percutaneous Endoscopic	7 Autologous Tissue Substitute J Synthetic Substitute K Nonautologous Tissue Substitute	Z No Qualifier

SECTION: Ø MEDICAL AND SURGICAL
BODY SYSTEM: Y ANATOMICAL REGIONS, LOWER EXTREMITIES
OPERATION: W REVISION: Correcting, to the extent possible, a portion of a malfunctioning device or the position of a displaced device

Body Part	Approach	Device	Qualifier
9 Lower Extremity, Right B Lower Extremity, Left	Ø Open 3 Percutaneous 4 Percutaneous Endoscopic X External	Ø Drainage Device 3 Infusion Device 7 Autologous Tissue Substitute J Synthetic Substitute K Nonautologous Tissue Substitute Y Other Device	Z No Qualifier

1   Obstetrics...**499**
    1Ø2. Pregnancy, Change 500
    1Ø9. Pregnancy, Drainage...500
    1ØA. Pregnancy, Abortion 500
    1ØD. Pregnancy, Extraction 501
    1ØE. Pregnancy, Delivery 501
    1ØH. Pregnancy, Insertion 501
    1ØJ. Pregnancy, Inspection 502
    1ØP. Pregnancy, Removal...502
    1ØQ. Pregnancy, Repair 502
    1ØS. Pregnancy, Reposition 503
    1ØT. Pregnancy, Resection...503
    1ØY. Pregnancy, Transplantation 503

ICD-10-PCS Coding Guidelines

Obstetric Section Guidelines (section 1)

C. Obstetrics Section

Products of conception

C1

Procedures performed on the products of conception are coded to the Obstetrics section. Procedures performed on the pregnant female other than the products of conception are coded to the appropriate root operation in the Medical and Surgical section.

Example: Amniocentesis is coded to the products of conception body part in the Obstetrics section. Repair of obstetric urethral laceration is coded to the urethra body part in the Medical and Surgical section.

Procedures following delivery or abortion

C2

Procedures performed following a delivery or abortion for curettage of the endometrium or evacuation of retained products of conception are all coded in the Obstetrics section, to the root operation Extraction and the body part Products of Conception, Retained. Diagnostic or therapeutic dilation and curettage performed during times other than the postpartum or post-abortion period are all coded in the Medical and Surgical section, to the root operation Extraction and the body part Endometrium.

SECTION: 1 OBSTETRICS
BODY SYSTEM: Ø PREGNANCY
OPERATION: 2 CHANGE: Taking out or off a device from a body part and putting back an identical or similar device in or on the same body part without cutting or puncturing the skin or a mucous membrane

Body Part	Approach	Device	Qualifier
Ø Products of Conception	7 Via Natural or Artificial Opening	3 Monitoring Electrode Y Other Device	Z No Qualifier

SECTION: 1 OBSTETRICS
BODY SYSTEM: Ø PREGNANCY
OPERATION: 9 DRAINAGE: Taking or letting out fluids and/or gases from a body part

Body Part	Approach	Device	Qualifier
Ø Products of Conception	Ø Open 3 Percutaneous 4 Percutaneous Endoscopic 7 Via Natural or Artificial Opening 8 Via Natural or Artificial Opening Endoscopic	Z No Device	9 Fetal Blood A Fetal Cerebrospinal Fluid B Fetal Fluid, Other C Amniotic Fluid, Therapeutic D Fluid, Other U Amniotic Fluid, Diagnostic

SECTION: 1 OBSTETRICS
BODY SYSTEM: Ø PREGNANCY
OPERATION: A ABORTION: Artificially terminating a pregnancy

Body Part	Approach	Device	Qualifier
Ø Products of Conception	Ø Open 3 Percutaneous 4 Percutaneous Endoscopic 8 Via Natural or Artificial Opening Endoscopic	Z No Device	Z No Qualifier
Ø Products of Conception	7 Via Natural or Artificial Opening	Z No Device	6 Vacuum W Laminaria X Abortifacient Z No Qualifier

SECTION: 1 OBSTETRICS
BODY SYSTEM: Ø PREGNANCY
OPERATION: D EXTRACTION: Pulling or stripping out or off all or a portion of a body part by the use of force

Body Part	Approach	Device	Qualifier
Ø Products of Conception	Ø Open	Z No Device	Ø Classical 1 Low Cervical 2 Extraperitoneal
Ø Products of Conception	7 Via Natural or Artificial Opening	Z No Device	3 Low Forceps 4 Mid Forceps 5 High Forceps 6 Vacuum 7 Internal Version 8 Other
1 Products of Conception, Retained 2 Products of Conception, Ectopic	7 Via Natural or Artificial Opening 8 Via Natural or Artificial Opening Endoscopic	Z No Device	9 Manual Z No Qualifier
2 Products of Conception, Ectopic	7 Via Natural or Artificial Opening 8 Via Natural or Artificial Opening Endoscopic	Z No Device	Z No Qualifier

SECTION: 1 OBSTETRICS
BODY SYSTEM: Ø PREGNANCY
OPERATION: E DELIVERY: Assisting the passage of the products of conception from the genital canal

Body Part	Approach	Device	Qualifier
Ø Products of Conception	X External	Z No Device	Z No Qualifier

SECTION: 1 OBSTETRICS
BODY SYSTEM: Ø PREGNANCY
OPERATION: H INSERTION: Putting in a nonbiological appliance that monitors, assists, performs, or prevents a physiological function but does not physically take the place of a body part

Body Part	Approach	Device	Qualifier
Ø Products of Conception	Ø Open 7 Via Natural or Artificial Opening	3 Monitoring Electrode Y Other Device	Z No Qualifier

SECTION: 1 OBSTETRICS

BODY SYSTEM: Ø PREGNANCY
OPERATION: J INSPECTION: Visually and/or manually exploring a body part

Body Part	Approach	Device	Qualifier
Ø Products of Conception 1 Products of Conception, Retained 2 Products of Conception, Ectopic	Ø Open 3 Percutaneous 4 Percutaneous Endoscopic 7 Via Natural or Artificial Opening 8 Via Natural or Artificial Opening Endoscopic X External	Z No Device	Z No Qualifier

SECTION: 1 OBSTETRICS

BODY SYSTEM: Ø PREGNANCY
OPERATION: P REMOVAL: Taking out or off a device from a body part, region or orifice

Body Part	Approach	Device	Qualifier
Ø Products of Conception	Ø Open 7 Via Natural or Artificial Opening	3 Monitoring Electrode Y Other Device	Z No Qualifier

SECTION: 1 OBSTETRICS

BODY SYSTEM: Ø PREGNANCY
OPERATION: Q REPAIR: Restoring, to the extent possible, a body part to its normal anatomic structure and function

Body Part	Approach	Device	Qualifier
Ø Products of Conception	Ø Open 3 Percutaneous 4 Percutaneous Endoscopic 7 Via Natural or Artificial Opening 8 Via Natural or Artificial Opening Endoscopic	Y Other Device Z No Device	E Nervous System F Cardiovascular System G Lymphatics and Hemic H Eye J Ear, Nose, and Sinus K Respiratory System L Mouth and Throat M Gastrointestinal System N Hepatobiliary and Pancreas P Endocrine System Q Skin R Musculoskeletal System S Urinary System T Female Reproductive System V Male Reproductive System Y Other Body System

SECTION: 1 OBSTETRICS

BODY SYSTEM: Ø **PREGNANCY**

OPERATION: S **REPOSITION:** Moving to its normal location or other suitable location all or a portion of a body part

Body Part	Approach	Device	Qualifier
Ø Products of Conception	7 Via Natural or Artificial Opening X External	Z No Device	Z No Qualifier
2 Products of Conception, Ectopic	Ø Open 3 Percutaneous 4 Percutaneous Endoscopic 7 Via Natural or Artificial Opening 8 Via Natural or Artificial Opening Endoscopic	Z No Device	Z No Qualifier

SECTION: 1 OBSTETRICS

BODY SYSTEM: Ø **PREGNANCY**

OPERATION: T **RESECTION:** Cutting out or off, without replacement, all of a body part

Body Part	Approach	Device	Qualifier
2 Products of Conception, Ectopic	Ø Open 3 Percutaneous 4 Percutaneous Endoscopic 7 Via Natural or Artificial Opening 8 Via Natural or Artificial Opening Endoscopic	Z No Device	Z No Qualifier

SECTION: 1 OBSTETRICS

BODY SYSTEM: Ø **PREGNANCY**

OPERATION: Y **TRANSPLANTATION:** Putting in or on all or a portion of a living body part taken from another individual or animal to physically take the place and/or function of all or a portion of a similar body part

Body Part	Approach	Device	Qualifier
Ø Products of Conception	3 Percutaneous 4 Percutaneous Endoscopic 7 Via Natural or Artificial Opening	Z No Device	E Nervous System F Cardiovascular System G Lymphatics and Hemic H Eye J Ear, Nose, and Sinus K Respiratory System L Mouth and Throat M Gastrointestinal System N Hepatobiliary and Pancreas P Endocrine System Q Skin R Musculoskeletal System S Urinary System T Female Reproductive System V Male Reproductive System Y Other Body System

2   Placement..**504**

   2W. Anatomical Regions...505

       2W0. Change 505

       2W1. Compression 506

       2W2. Dressing 507

       2W3. Immobilization 508

       2W4. Packing 509

       2W5. Removal 510

       2W6. Traction 511

   2Y.   Anatomical Orifices 512

       2Y0. Change 512

       2Y4. Packing 512

       2Y5. Removal 512

SECTION: 2 PLACEMENT
BODY SYSTEM: W ANATOMICAL REGIONS
OPERATION: Ø CHANGE: Taking out or off a device from a body part and putting back an identical or similar device in or on the same body part without cutting or puncturing the skin or a mucous membrane

Body Region	Approach	Device	Qualifier
Ø Head 2 Neck 3 Abdominal Wall 4 Chest Wall 5 Back 6 Inguinal Region, Right 7 Inguinal Region, Left 8 Upper Extremity, Right 9 Upper Extremity, Left A Upper Arm, Right B Upper Arm, Left C Lower Arm, Right D Lower Arm, Left E Hand, Right F Hand, Left G Thumb, Right H Thumb, Left J Finger, Right K Finger, Left L Lower Extremity, Right M Lower Extremity, Left N Upper Leg, Right P Upper Leg, Left Q Lower Leg, Right R Lower Leg, Left S Foot, Right T Foot, Left U Toe, Right V Toe, Left	X External	Ø Traction Apparatus 1 Splint 2 Cast 3 Brace 4 Bandage 5 Packing Material 6 Pressure Dressing 7 Intermittent Pressure Device Y Other Device	Z No Qualifier
1 Face	X External	Ø Traction Apparatus 1 Splint 2 Cast 3 Brace 4 Bandage 5 Packing Material 6 Pressure Dressing 7 Intermittent Pressure Device 9 Wire Y Other Device	Z No Qualifier

SECTION: 2 PLACEMENT
BODY SYSTEM: W ANATOMICAL REGIONS
OPERATION: 1 COMPRESSION: Putting pressure on a body region

Body Region	Approach	Device	Qualifier
Ø Head	X External	6 Pressure Dressing	Z No Qualifier
1 Face		7 Intermittent Pressure Device	
2 Neck			
3 Abdominal Wall			
4 Chest Wall			
5 Back			
6 Inguinal Region, Right			
7 Inguinal Region, Left			
8 Upper Extremity, Right			
9 Upper Extremity, Left			
A Upper Arm, Right			
B Upper Arm, Left			
C Lower Arm, Right			
D Lower Arm, Left			
E Hand, Right			
F Hand, Left			
G Thumb, Right			
H Thumb, Left			
J Finger, Right			
K Finger, Left			
L Lower Extremity, Right			
M Lower Extremity, Left			
N Upper Leg, Right			
P Upper Leg, Left			
Q Lower Leg, Right			
R Lower Leg, Left			
S Foot, Right			
T Foot, Left			
U Toe, Right			
V Toe, Left			

1: COMPRESSION

W: ANATOMICAL REGIONS

2: PLACEMENT

SECTION: 2 PLACEMENT
BODY SYSTEM: W ANATOMICAL REGIONS
OPERATION: 2 DRESSING: Putting material on a body region for protection

Body Region	Approach	Device	Qualifier
Ø Head	X External	4 Bandage	Z No Qualifier
1 Face			
2 Neck			
3 Abdominal Wall			
4 Chest Wall			
5 Back			
6 Inguinal Region, Right			
7 Inguinal Region, Left			
8 Upper Extremity, Right			
9 Upper Extremity, Left			
A Upper Arm, Right			
B Upper Arm, Left			
C Lower Arm, Right			
D Lower Arm, Left			
E Hand, Right			
F Hand, Left			
G Thumb, Right			
H Thumb, Left			
J Finger, Right			
K Finger, Left			
L Lower Extremity, Right			
M Lower Extremity, Left			
N Upper Leg, Right			
P Upper Leg, Left			
Q Lower Leg, Right			
R Lower Leg, Left			
S Foot, Right			
T Foot, Left			
U Toe, Right			
V Toe, Left			

SECTION: 2 PLACEMENT
BODY SYSTEM: W ANATOMICAL REGIONS
OPERATION: 3 IMMOBILIZATION: Limiting or preventing motion of a body region

3: IMMOBILIZATION

W: ANATOMICAL REGIONS

2: PLACEMENT

Body Region	Approach	Device	Qualifier
Ø Head 2 Neck 3 Abdominal Wall 4 Chest Wall 5 Back 6 Inguinal Region, Right 7 Inguinal Region, Left 8 Upper Extremity, Right 9 Upper Extremity, Left A Upper Arm, Right B Upper Arm, Left C Lower Arm, Right D Lower Arm, Left E Hand, Right F Hand, Left G Thumb, Right H Thumb, Left J Finger, Right K Finger, Left L Lower Extremity, Right M Lower Extremity, Left N Upper Leg, Right P Upper Leg, Left Q Lower Leg, Right R Lower Leg, Left S Foot, Right T Foot, Left U Toe, Right V Toe, Left	X External	1 Splint 2 Cast 3 Brace Y Other Device	Z No Qualifier
1 Face	X External	1 Splint 2 Cast 3 Brace 9 Wire Y Other Device	Z No Qualifier

SECTION: 2 PLACEMENT
BODY SYSTEM: W ANATOMICAL REGIONS
OPERATION: 4 PACKING: Putting material in a body region or orifice

Body Region	Approach	Device	Qualifier
Ø Head	X External	5 Packing Material	Z No Qualifier
1 Face			
2 Neck			
3 Abdominal Wall			
4 Chest Wall			
5 Back			
6 Inguinal Region, Right			
7 Inguinal Region, Left			
8 Upper Extremity, Right			
9 Upper Extremity, Left			
A Upper Arm, Right			
B Upper Arm, Left			
C Lower Arm, Right			
D Lower Arm, Left			
E Hand, Right			
F Hand, Left			
G Thumb, Right			
H Thumb, Left			
J Finger, Right			
K Finger, Left			
L Lower Extremity, Right			
M Lower Extremity, Left			
N Upper Leg, Right			
P Upper Leg, Left			
Q Lower Leg, Right			
R Lower Leg, Left			
S Foot, Right			
T Foot, Left			
U Toe, Right			
V Toe, Left			

SECTION: 2 PLACEMENT
BODY SYSTEM: W ANATOMICAL REGIONS
OPERATION: 5 REMOVAL: Taking out or off a device from a body part

5: REMOVAL

W: ANATOMICAL REGIONS

2: PLACEMENT

Body Region	Approach	Device	Qualifier
Ø Head 2 Neck 3 Abdominal Wall 4 Chest Wall 5 Back 6 Inguinal Region, Right 7 Inguinal Region, Left 8 Upper Extremity, Right 9 Upper Extremity, Left A Upper Arm, Right B Upper Arm, Left C Lower Arm, Right D Lower Arm, Left E Hand, Right F Hand, Left G Thumb, Right H Thumb, Left J Finger, Right K Finger, Left L Lower Extremity, Right M Lower Extremity, Left N Upper Leg, Right P Upper Leg, Left Q Lower Leg, Right R Lower Leg, Left S Foot, Right T Foot, Left U Toe, Right V Toe, Left	X External	Ø Traction Apparatus 1 Splint 2 Cast 3 Brace 4 Bandage 5 Packing Material 6 Pressure Dressing 7 Intermittent Pressure Device Y Other Device	Z No Qualifier
1 Face	X External	Ø Traction Apparatus 1 Splint 2 Cast 3 Brace 4 Bandage 5 Packing Material 6 Pressure Dressing 7 Intermittent Pressure Device 9 Wire Y Other Device	Z No Qualifier

SECTION: 2 PLACEMENT
BODY SYSTEM: W ANATOMICAL REGIONS
OPERATION: 6 TRACTION: Exerting a pulling force on a body region in a distal direction

Body Region	Approach	Device	Qualifier
Ø Head	X External	Ø Traction Apparatus	Z No Qualifier
1 Face		Z No Device	
2 Neck			
3 Abdominal Wall			
4 Chest Wall			
5 Back			
6 Inguinal Region, Right			
7 Inguinal Region, Left			
8 Upper Extremity, Right			
9 Upper Extremity, Left			
A Upper Arm, Right			
B Upper Arm, Left			
C Lower Arm, Right			
D Lower Arm, Left			
E Hand, Right			
F Hand, Left			
G Thumb, Right			
H Thumb, Left			
J Finger, Right			
K Finger, Left			
L Lower Extremity, Right			
M Lower Extremity, Left			
N Upper Leg, Right			
P Upper Leg, Left			
Q Lower Leg, Right			
R Lower Leg, Left			
S Foot, Right			
T Foot, Left			
U Toe, Right			
V Toe, Left			

SECTION: 2 PLACEMENT
BODY SYSTEM: Y ANATOMICAL ORIFICES
OPERATION: 0 CHANGE: Taking out or off a device from a body part and putting back an identical or similar device in or on the same body part without cutting or puncturing the skin or a mucous membrane

Body Region	Approach	Device	Qualifier
0 Mouth and Pharynx 1 Nasal 2 Ear 3 Anorectal 4 Female Genital Tract 5 Urethra	X External	5 Packing Material	Z No Qualifier

SECTION: 2 PLACEMENT
BODY SYSTEM: Y ANATOMICAL ORIFICES
OPERATION: 4 PACKING: Putting material in a body region or orifice

Body Region	Approach	Device	Qualifier
0 Mouth and Pharynx 1 Nasal 2 Ear 3 Anorectal 4 Female Genital Tract 5 Urethra	X External	5 Packing Material	Z No Qualifier

SECTION: 2 PLACEMENT
BODY SYSTEM: Y ANATOMICAL ORIFICES
OPERATION: 5 REMOVAL: Taking out or off a device from a body part

Body Region	Approach	Device	Qualifier
0 Mouth and Pharynx 1 Nasal 2 Ear 3 Anorectal 4 Female Genital Tract 5 Urethra	X External	5 Packing Material	Z No Qualifier

3 Administration **513**
    3Ø. Circulatory 514
        3Ø2. Transfusion 514
    3C. Indwelling Device 516
        3C1. Irrigation 516
    3E. Physiological Systems and Anatomical Regions 516
        3EØ. Introduction 516
        3E1. Irrigation 53Ø

SECTION: 3 ADMINISTRATION
BODY SYSTEM: 0 CIRCULATORY
OPERATION: 2 **TRANSFUSION:** *(on multiple pages)*
Putting in blood or blood products

Body System / Region	Approach	Substance	Qualifier
3 Peripheral Vein 4 Central Vein	Ø Open 3 Percutaneous	A Stem Cells, Embryonic	Z No Qualifier
3 Peripheral Vein 4 Central Vein	Ø Open 3 Percutaneous	G Bone Marrow X Stem Cells, Cord Blood Y Stem Cells, Hematopoietic	Ø Autologous 2 Allogeneic, Related 3 Allogeneic, Unrelated 4 Allogeneic, Unspecified
3 Peripheral Vein 4 Central Vein	Ø Open 3 Percutaneous	H Whole Blood J Serum Albumin K Frozen Plasma L Fresh Plasma M Plasma Cryoprecipitate N Red Blood Cells P Frozen Red Cells Q White Cells R Platelets S Globulin T Fibrinogen V Antihemophilic Factors W Factor IX	Ø Autologous 1 Nonautologous
5 Peripheral Artery 6 Central Artery	Ø Open 3 Percutaneous	G Bone Marrow H Whole Blood J Serum Albumin K Frozen Plasma L Fresh Plasma M Plasma Cryoprecipitate N Red Blood Cells P Frozen Red Cells Q White Cells R Platelets S Globulin T Fibrinogen V Antihemophilic Factors W Factor IX X Stem Cells, Cord Blood Y Stem Cells, Hematopoietic	Ø Autologous 1 Nonautologous

SECTION: 3 ADMINISTRATION
BODY SYSTEM: 0 CIRCULATORY
OPERATION: 2 TRANSFUSION: *(continued)*
Putting in blood or blood products

Body System / Region	Approach	Substance	Qualifier
7 Products of Conception, Circulatory	3 Percutaneous 7 Via Natural or Artificial Opening	H Whole Blood J Serum Albumin K Frozen Plasma L Fresh Plasma M Plasma Cryoprecipitate N Red Blood Cells P Frozen Red Cells Q White Cells R Platelets S Globulin T Fibrinogen V Antihemophilic Factors W Factor IX	1 Nonautologous
8 Vein	Ø Open 3 Percutaneous	B 4-Factor Prothrombin Complex Concentrate	1 Nonautologous

SECTION: 3 ADMINISTRATION
BODY SYSTEM: C INDWELLING DEVICE
OPERATION: 1 IRRIGATION: Putting in or on a cleansing substance

Body System / Region	Approach	Substance	Qualifier
Z None	X External	8 Irrigating Substance	Z No Qualifier

SECTION: 3 ADMINISTRATION
BODY SYSTEM: E PHYSIOLOGICAL SYSTEMS AND ANATOMICAL REGIONS
OPERATION: 0 INTRODUCTION: *(on multiple pages)*
Putting in or on a therapeutic, diagnostic, nutritional, physiological, or prophylactic substance except blood or blood products

Body System / Region	Approach	Substance	Qualifier
0 Skin and Mucous Membranes	X External	0 Antineoplastic	5 Other Antineoplastic M Monoclonal Antibody
0 Skin and Mucous Membranes	X External	2 Anti-infective	8 Oxazolidinones 9 Other Anti-infective
0 Skin and Mucous Membranes	X External	3 Anti-inflammatory 4 Serum, Toxoid and Vaccine B Anesthetic Agent K Other Diagnostic Substance M Pigment N Analgesics, Hypnotics, Sedatives T Destructive Agent	Z No Qualifier
0 Skin and Mucous Membranes	X External	G Other Therapeutic Substance	C Other Substance
1 Subcutaneous Tissue	0 Open	2 Anti-infective	A Anti-Infective Envelope
1 Subcutaneous Tissue	3 Percutaneous	0 Antineoplastic	5 Other Antineoplastic M Monoclonal Antibody
1 Subcutaneous Tissue	3 Percutaneous	2 Anti-infective	8 Oxazolidinones 9 Other Anti-infective A Anti-Infective Envelope
1 Subcutaneous Tissue	3 Percutaneous	3 Anti-inflammatory 4 Serum, Toxoid, and Vaccine 6 Nutritional Substance 7 Electrolytic and Water Balance Substance B Anesthetic Agent H Radioactive Substance K Other Diagnostic Substance N Analgesics, Hypnotics, Sedatives T Destructive Agent	Z No Qualifier
1 Subcutaneous Tissue	3 Percutaneous	4 Serum, Toxoid and Vaccine	0 Influenza Vaccine Z No Qualifier
1 Subcutaneous Tissue	3 Percutaneous	G Other Therapeutic Substance	C Other Substance
1 Subcutaneous Tissue	3 Percutaneous	V Hormone	G Insulin J Other Hormone
2 Muscle	3 Percutaneous	0 Antineoplastic	5 Other Antineoplastic M Monoclonal Antibody

SECTION: 3 ADMINISTRATION
BODY SYSTEM: E PHYSIOLOGICAL SYSTEMS AND ANATOMICAL REGIONS
OPERATION: 0 INTRODUCTION: *(continued)*

Putting in or on a therapeutic, diagnostic, nutritional, physiological, or prophylactic substance except blood or blood products

Body System / Region	Approach	Substance	Qualifier
2 Muscle	3 Percutaneous	2 Anti-infective	8 Oxazolidinones 9 Other Anti-infective
2 Muscle	3 Percutaneous	3 Anti-inflammatory 4 Serum, Toxoid and Vaccine 6 Nutritional Substance 7 Electrolytic and Water Balance Substance B Anesthetic Agent H Radioactive Substance K Other Diagnostic Substance N Analgesics, Hypnotics, Sedatives T Destructive Agent	Z No Qualifier
2 Muscle	3 Percutaneous	G Other Therapeutic Substance	C Other Substance
3 Peripheral Vein	0 Open	0 Antineoplastic	2 High-dose Interleukin-2 3 Low-dose Interleukin-2 5 Other Antineoplastic M Monoclonal Antibody P Clofarabine
3 Peripheral Vein	0 Open	1 Thrombolytic	6 Recombinant Human-activated Protein C 7 Other Thrombolytic
3 Peripheral Vein	0 Open	2 Anti-infective	8 Oxazolidinones 9 Other Anti-infective
3 Peripheral Vein	0 Open	3 Anti-inflammatory 4 Serum, Toxoid and Vaccine 6 Nutritional Substance 7 Electrolytic and Water Balance Substance F Intracirculatory Anesthetic H Radioactive Substance K Other Diagnostic Substance N Analgesics, Hypnotics, Sedatives P Platelet Inhibitor R Antiarrhythmic T Destructive Agent X Vasopressor	Z No Qualifier
3 Peripheral Vein	0 Open	G Other Therapeutic Substance	C Other Substance N Blood Brain Barrier Disruption
3 Peripheral Vein	0 Open	U Pancreatic Islet Cells	0 Autologous 1 Nonautologous
3 Peripheral Vein	0 Open	V Hormone	G Insulin H Human B-type Natriuretic Peptide J Other Hormone
3 Peripheral Vein	0 Open	W Immunotherapeutic	K Immunostimulator L Immunosuppressive

SECTION: 3 ADMINISTRATION
BODY SYSTEM: E PHYSIOLOGICAL SYSTEMS AND ANATOMICAL REGIONS
OPERATION: Ø INTRODUCTION: *(continued)*
Putting in or on a therapeutic, diagnostic, nutritional, physiological, or prophylactic substance except blood or blood products

Body System / Region	Approach	Substance	Qualifier
3 Peripheral Vein	3 Percutaneous	Ø Antineoplastic	2 High-dose Interleukin-2 3 Low-dose Interleukin-2 5 Other Antineoplastic M Monoclonal Antibody P Clofarabine
3 Peripheral Vein	3 Percutaneous	1 Thrombolytic	6 Recombinant Human-activated Protein C 7 Other Thrombolytic
3 Peripheral Vein	3 Percutaneous	2 Anti-infective	8 Oxazolidinones 9 Other Anti-infective
3 Peripheral Vein	3 Percutaneous	3 Anti-inflammatory 4 Serum, Toxoid and Vaccine 6 Nutritional Substance 7 Electrolytic and Water Balance Substance F Intracirculatory Anesthetic H Radioactive Substance K Other Diagnostic Substance N Analgesics, Hypnotics, Sedatives P Platelet Inhibitor R Antiarrhythmic T Destructive Agent X Vasopressor	Z No Qualifier
3 Peripheral Vein	3 Percutaneous	G Other Therapeutic Substance	C Other Substance N Blood Brain Barrier Disruption Q Glucarpidase
3 Peripheral Vein	3 Percutaneous	U Pancreatic Islet Cells	Ø Autologous 1 Nonautologous
3 Peripheral Vein	3 Percutaneous	V Hormone	G Insulin H Human B-type Natriuretic Peptide J Other Hormone
3 Peripheral Vein	3 Percutaneous	W Immunotherapeutic	K Immunostimulator L Immunosuppressive
4 Central Vein	Ø Open	Ø Antineoplastic	2 High-dose Interleukin-2 3 Low-dose Interleukin-2 5 Other Antineoplastic M Monoclonal Antibody P Clofarabine
4 Central Vein	Ø Open	1 Thrombolytic	6 Recombinant Human-activated Protein C 7 Other Thrombolytic
4 Central Vein	Ø Open	2 Anti-infective	8 Oxazolidinones 9 Other Anti-infective

New/Revised Text in Blue   ~~deleted~~ Deleted

SECTION: 3 ADMINISTRATION
BODY SYSTEM: E PHYSIOLOGICAL SYSTEMS AND ANATOMICAL REGIONS
OPERATION: Ø INTRODUCTION: *(continued)*

Putting in or on a therapeutic, diagnostic, nutritional, physiological, or prophylactic substance except blood or blood products

Body System / Region	Approach	Substance	Qualifier
4 Central Vein	Ø Open	3 Anti-inflammatory 4 Serum, Toxoid and Vaccine 6 Nutritional Substance 7 Electrolytic and Water Balance Substance F Intracirculatory Anesthetic H Radioactive Substance K Other Diagnostic Substance N Analgesics, Hypnotics, Sedatives P Platelet Inhibitor R Antiarrhythmic T Destructive Agent X Vasopressor	Z No Qualifier
4 Central Vein	Ø Open	G Other Therapeutic Substance	C Other Substance N Blood Brain Barrier Disruption
4 Central Vein	Ø Open	V Hormone	G Insulin H Human B-type Natriuretic Peptide J Other Hormone
4 Central Vein	Ø Open	W Immunotherapeutic	K Immunostimulator L Immunosuppressive
4 Central Vein	3 Percutaneous	Ø Antineoplastic	2 High-dose Interleukin-2 3 Low-dose Interleukin-2 5 Other Antineoplastic M Monoclonal Antibody P Clofarabine
4 Central Vein	3 Percutaneous	1 Thrombolytic	6 Recombinant Human-activated Protein C 7 Other Thrombolytic
4 Central Vein	3 Percutaneous	2 Anti-infective	8 Oxazolidinones 9 Other Anti-infective
4 Central Vein	3 Percutaneous	3 Anti-inflammatory 4 Serum, Toxoid and Vaccine 6 Nutritional Substance 7 Electrolytic and Water Balance Substance F Intracirculatory Anesthetic H Radioactive Substance K Other Diagnostic Substance N Analgesics, Hypnotics, Sedatives P Platelet Inhibitor R Antiarrhythmic T Destructive Agent X Vasopressor	Z No Qualifier
4 Central Vein	3 Percutaneous	G Other Therapeutic Substance	C Other Substance N Blood Brain Barrier Disruption Q Glucarpidase
4 Central Vein	3 Percutaneous	V Hormone	G Insulin H Human B-type Natriuretic Peptide J Other Hormone

SECTION: 3 ADMINISTRATION

BODY SYSTEM: E PHYSIOLOGICAL SYSTEMS AND ANATOMICAL REGIONS
OPERATION: Ø INTRODUCTION: *(continued)*
Putting in or on a therapeutic, diagnostic, nutritional, physiological, or prophylactic substance except blood or blood products

Body System / Region	Approach	Substance	Qualifier
4 Central Vein	3 Percutaneous	W Immunotherapeutic	K Immunostimulator L Immunosuppressive
5 Peripheral Artery 6 Central Artery	Ø Open 3 Percutaneous	Ø Antineoplastic	2 High-dose Interleukin-2 3 Low-dose Interleukin-2 5 Other Antineoplastic M Monoclonal Antibody P Clofarabine
5 Peripheral Artery 6 Central Artery	Ø Open 3 Percutaneous	1 Thrombolytic	6 Recombinant Human-activated Protein C 7 Other Thrombolytic
5 Peripheral Artery 6 Central Artery	Ø Open 3 Percutaneous	2 Anti-infective	8 Oxazolidinones 9 Other Anti-infective
5 Peripheral Artery 6 Central Artery	Ø Open 3 Percutaneous	3 Anti-inflammatory 4 Serum, Toxoid and Vaccine 6 Nutritional Substance 7 Electrolytic and Water Balance Substance F Intracirculatory Anesthetic H Radioactive Substance K Other Diagnostic Substance N Analgesics, Hypnotics, Sedatives P Platelet Inhibitor R Antiarrhythmic T Destructive Agent X Vasopressor	Z No Qualifier
5 Peripheral Artery 6 Central Artery	Ø Open 3 Percutaneous	G Other Therapeutic Substance	C Other Substance N Blood Brain Barrier Disruption
5 Peripheral Artery 6 Central Artery	Ø Open 3 Percutaneous	V Hormone	G Insulin H Human B-type Natriuretic Peptide J Other Hormone
5 Peripheral Artery 6 Central Artery	Ø Open 3 Percutaneous	W Immunotherapeutic	K Immunostimulator L Immunosuppressive
7 Coronary Artery 8 Heart	Ø Open 3 Percutaneous	1 Thrombolytic	6 Recombinant Human-activated Protein C 7 Other Thrombolytic
7 Coronary Artery 8 Heart	Ø Open 3 Percutaneous	G Other Therapeutic Substance	C Other Substance
7 Coronary Artery 8 Heart	Ø Open 3 Percutaneous	K Other Diagnostic Substance P Platelet Inhibitor	Z No Qualifier
7 Coronary Artery 8 Heart	4 Percutaneous Endoscopic	G Other Therapeutic Substance	C Other Substance
9 Nose	3 Percutaneous 7 Via Natural or Artificial Opening X External	Ø Antineoplastic	5 Other Antineoplastic M Monoclonal Antibody
9 Nose	3 Percutaneous 7 Via Natural or Artificial Opening X External	2 Anti-infective	8 Oxazolidinones 9 Other Anti-infective

New/Revised Text in Blue ~~deleted~~ Deleted

SECTION: 3 ADMINISTRATION

BODY SYSTEM: E PHYSIOLOGICAL SYSTEMS AND ANATOMICAL REGIONS
OPERATION: Ø INTRODUCTION: *(continued)*

Putting in or on a therapeutic, diagnostic, nutritional, physiological, or prophylactic substance except blood or blood products

Body System / Region	Approach	Substance	Qualifier
9 Nose	3 Percutaneous 7 Via Natural or Artificial Opening X External	3 Anti-inflammatory 4 Serum, Toxoid and Vaccine B Anesthetic Agent H Radioactive Substance K Other Diagnostic Substance N Analgesics, Hypnotics, Sedatives T Destructive Agent	Z No Qualifier
9 Nose	3 Percutaneous 7 Via Natural or Artificial Opening X External	G Other Therapeutic Substance	C Other Substance
A Bone Marrow	3 Percutaneous	Ø Antineoplastic	5 Other Antineoplastic M Monoclonal Antibody
A Bone Marrow	3 Percutaneous	G Other Therapeutic Substance	C Other Substance
B Ear	3 Percutaneous 7 Via Natural or Artificial Opening X External	Ø Antineoplastic	4 Liquid Brachytherapy Radioisotope 5 Other Antineoplastic M Monoclonal Antibody
B Ear	3 Percutaneous 7 Via Natural or Artificial Opening X External	2 Anti-infective	8 Oxazolidinones 9 Other Anti-infective
B Ear	3 Percutaneous 7 Via Natural or Artificial Opening X External	3 Anti-inflammatory B Anesthetic Agent H Radioactive Substance K Other Diagnostic Substance N Analgesics, Hypnotics, Sedatives T Destructive Agent	Z No Qualifier
B Ear	3 Percutaneous 7 Via Natural or Artificial Opening X External	G Other Therapeutic Substance	C Other Substance
C Eye	3 Percutaneous 7 Via Natural or Artificial Opening X External	Ø Antineoplastic	4 Liquid Brachytherapy Radioisotope 5 Other Antineoplastic M Monoclonal Antibody
C Eye	3 Percutaneous 7 Via Natural or Artificial Opening X External	2 Anti-infective	8 Oxazolidinones 9 Other Anti-infective
C Eye	3 Percutaneous 7 Via Natural or Artificial Opening X External	3 Anti-inflammatory B Anesthetic Agent H Radioactive Substance K Other Diagnostic Substance M Pigment N Analgesics, Hypnotics, Sedatives T Destructive Agent	Z No Qualifier
C Eye	3 Percutaneous 7 Via Natural or Artificial Opening X External	G Other Therapeutic Substance	C Other Substance

New/Revised Text in Blue   ~~deleted~~   Deleted

SECTION: 3 ADMINISTRATION
BODY SYSTEM: E PHYSIOLOGICAL SYSTEMS AND ANATOMICAL REGIONS
OPERATION: Ø INTRODUCTION: *(continued)*
Putting in or on a therapeutic, diagnostic, nutritional, physiological, or prophylactic substance except blood or blood products

Body System / Region	Approach	Substance	Qualifier
C Eye	3 Percutaneous 7 Via Natural or Artificial Opening X External	S Gas	F Other Gas
D Mouth and Pharynx	3 Percutaneous 7 Via Natural or Artificial Opening X External	Ø Antineoplastic	4 Liquid Brachytherapy Radioisotope 5 Other Antineoplastic M Monoclonal Antibody
D Mouth and Pharynx	3 Percutaneous 7 Via Natural or Artificial Opening X External	2 Anti-infective	8 Oxazolidinones 9 Other Anti-infective
D Mouth and Pharynx	3 Percutaneous 7 Via Natural or Artificial Opening X External	3 Anti-inflammatory 4 Serum, Toxoid and Vaccine 6 Nutritional Substance 7 Electrolytic and Water Balance Substance B Anesthetic Agent H Radioactive Substance K Other Diagnostic Substance N Analgesics, Hypnotics, Sedatives R Antiarrhythmic T Destructive Agent	Z No Qualifier
D Mouth and Pharynx	3 Percutaneous 7 Via Natural or Artificial Opening X External	G Other Therapeutic Substance	C Other Substance
E Products of Conception G Upper GI H Lower GI K Genitourinary Tract N Male Reproductive	3 Percutaneous 7 Via Natural or Artificial Opening 8 Via Natural or Artificial Opening Endoscopic	Ø Antineoplastic	4 Liquid Brachytherapy Radioisotope 5 Other Antineoplastic M Monoclonal Antibody
E Products of Conception G Upper GI H Lower GI K Genitourinary Tract N Male Reproductive	3 Percutaneous 7 Via Natural or Artificial Opening 8 Via Natural or Artificial Opening Endoscopic	2 Anti-infective	8 Oxazolidinones 9 Other Anti-infective
E Products of Conception G Upper GI H Lower GI K Genitourinary Tract N Male Reproductive	3 Percutaneous 7 Via Natural or Artificial Opening 8 Via Natural or Artificial Opening Endoscopic	3 Anti-inflammatory 6 Nutritional Substance 7 Electrolytic and Water Balance Substance B Anesthetic Agent H Radioactive Substance K Other Diagnostic Substance N Analgesics, Hypnotics, Sedatives T Destructive Agent	Z No Qualifier
E Products of Conception G Upper GI H Lower GI K Genitourinary Tract N Male Reproductive	3 Percutaneous 7 Via Natural or Artificial Opening 8 Via Natural or Artificial Opening Endoscopic	G Other Therapeutic Substance	C Other Substance
E Products of Conception G Upper GI H Lower GI K Genitourinary Tract N Male Reproductive	3 Percutaneous 7 Via Natural or Artificial Opening 8 Via Natural or Artificial Opening Endoscopic	S Gas	F Other Gas

SECTION: 3 ADMINISTRATION
BODY SYSTEM: E PHYSIOLOGICAL SYSTEMS AND ANATOMICAL REGIONS
OPERATION: Ø INTRODUCTION: *(continued)*

Putting in or on a therapeutic, diagnostic, nutritional, physiological, or prophylactic substance except blood or blood products

Body System / Region	Approach	Substance	Qualifier
E Products of Conception G Upper GI H Lower GI K Genitourinary Tract N Male Reproductive	4 Percutaneous Endoscopic	G Other Therapeutic Substance	C Other Substance
F Respiratory Tract	3 Percutaneous 7 Via Natural or Artificial Opening 8 Via Natural or Artificial Opening Endoscopic	Ø Antineoplastic	4 Liquid Brachytherapy Radioisotope 5 Other Antineoplastic M Monoclonal Antibody
F Respiratory Tract	3 Percutaneous 7 Via Natural or Artificial Opening 8 Via Natural or Artificial Opening Endoscopic	2 Anti-infective	8 Oxazolidinones 9 Other Anti-infective
F Respiratory Tract	3 Percutaneous 7 Via Natural or Artificial Opening 8 Via Natural or Artificial Opening Endoscopic	3 Anti-inflammatory 6 Nutritional Substance 7 Electrolytic and Water Balance Substance B Anesthetic Agent H Radioactive Substance K Other Diagnostic Substance N Analgesics, Hypnotics, Sedatives T Destructive Agent	Z No Qualifier
F Respiratory Tract	3 Percutaneous 7 Via Natural or Artificial Opening 8 Via Natural or Artificial Opening Endoscopic	G Other Therapeutic Substance	C Other Substance
F Respiratory Tract	3 Percutaneous 7 Via Natural or Artificial Opening 8 Via Natural or Artificial Opening Endoscopic	S Gas	D Nitric Oxide F Other Gas
F Respiratory Tract	4 Percutaneous Endoscopic	G Other Therapeutic Substance	C Other Substance
~~F Respiratory Tract~~	~~7 Via Natural or Artificial Opening~~ ~~8 Via Natural or Artificial Opening Endoscopic~~	~~Ø Antineoplastic~~	~~4 Liquid Brachytherapy Radioisotope~~ ~~5 Other Antineoplastic~~ ~~M Monoclonal Antibody~~
~~F Respiratory Tract~~	~~7 Via Natural or Artificial Opening~~ ~~8 Via Natural or Artificial Opening Endoscopic~~	~~2 Anti-infective~~	~~8 Oxazolidinones~~ ~~9 Other Anti-infective~~
~~F Respiratory Tract~~	~~7 Via Natural or Artificial Opening~~ ~~8 Via Natural or Artificial Opening Endoscopic~~	~~3 Anti-inflammatory~~ ~~6 Nutritional Substance~~ ~~7 Electrolytic and Water Balance Substance~~ ~~B Local Anesthetic~~ ~~D Inhalation Anesthetic~~ ~~H Radioactive Substance~~ ~~K Other Diagnostic Substance~~ ~~N Analgesics, Hypnotics, Sedatives~~ ~~T Destructive Agent~~	~~Z No Qualifier~~
~~F Respiratory Tract~~	~~7 Via Natural or Artificial Opening~~ ~~8 Via Natural or Artificial Opening Endoscopic~~	~~G Other Therapeutic Substance~~	~~C Other Substance~~
~~F Respiratory Tract~~	~~7 Via Natural or Artificial Opening~~ ~~8 Via Natural or Artificial Opening Endoscopic~~	~~S Gas~~	~~D Nitric Oxide~~ ~~F Other Gas~~

New/Revised Text in Blue   ~~deleted~~ Deleted

SECTION: 3 ADMINISTRATION
BODY SYSTEM: E PHYSIOLOGICAL SYSTEMS AND ANATOMICAL REGIONS
OPERATION: Ø INTRODUCTION: *(continued)*
Putting in or on a therapeutic, diagnostic, nutritional, physiological, or prophylactic substance except blood or blood products

Body System / Region	Approach	Substance	Qualifier
J Biliary and Pancreatic Tract	3 Percutaneous 7 Via Natural or Artificial Opening 8 Via Natural or Artificial Opening Endoscopic	Ø Antineoplastic	4 Liquid Brachytherapy Radioisotope 5 Other Antineoplastic M Monoclonal Antibody
J Biliary and Pancreatic Tract	3 Percutaneous 7 Via Natural or Artificial Opening 8 Via Natural or Artificial Opening Endoscopic	2 Anti-infective	8 Oxazolidinones 9 Other Anti-infective
J Biliary and Pancreatic Tract	3 Percutaneous 7 Via Natural or Artificial Opening 8 Via Natural or Artificial Opening Endoscopic	3 Anti-inflammatory 6 Nutritional Substance 7 Electrolytic and Water Balance Substance B Anesthetic Agent H Radioactive Substance K Other Diagnostic Substance N Analgesics, Hypnotics, Sedatives T Destructive Agent	Z No Qualifier
J Biliary and Pancreatic Tract	3 Percutaneous 7 Via Natural or Artificial Opening 8 Via Natural or Artificial Opening Endoscopic	G Other Therapeutic Substance	C Other Substance
J Biliary and Pancreatic Tract	3 Percutaneous 7 Via Natural or Artificial Opening 8 Via Natural or Artificial Opening Endoscopic	S Gas	F Other Gas
J Biliary and Pancreatic Tract	3 Percutaneous 7 Via Natural or Artificial Opening 8 Via Natural or Artificial Opening Endoscopic	U Pancreatic Islet Cells	Ø Autologous 1 Nonautologous
J Biliary and Pancreatic Tract	4 Percutaneous Endoscopic	G Other Therapeutic Substance	C Other Substance
L Pleural Cavity M Peritoneal Cavity	Ø Open	5 Adhesion Barrier	Z No Qualifier
L Pleural Cavity M Peritoneal Cavity	3 Percutaneous	Ø Antineoplastic	4 Liquid Brachytherapy Radioisotope 5 Other Antineoplastic M Monoclonal Antibody
L Pleural Cavity M Peritoneal Cavity	3 Percutaneous	2 Anti-infective	8 Oxazolidinones 9 Other Anti-infective
L Pleural Cavity M Peritoneal Cavity	3 Percutaneous	3 Anti-inflammatory 5 Adhesion Barrier 6 Nutritional Substance 7 Electrolytic and Water Balance Substance B Anesthetic Agent H Radioactive Substance K Other Diagnostic Substance N Analgesics, Hypnotics, Sedatives T Destructive Agent	Z No Qualifier

SECTION: 3 ADMINISTRATION
BODY SYSTEM: E PHYSIOLOGICAL SYSTEMS AND ANATOMICAL REGIONS
OPERATION: Ø INTRODUCTION: *(continued)*

Putting in or on a therapeutic, diagnostic, nutritional, physiological, or prophylactic substance except blood or blood products

Body System / Region	Approach	Substance	Qualifier
L Pleural Cavity M Peritoneal Cavity	3 Percutaneous	G Other Therapeutic Substance	C Other Substance
L Pleural Cavity M Peritoneal Cavity	3 Percutaneous	S Gas	F Other Gas
L Pleural Cavity M Peritoneal Cavity	4 Percutaneous Endoscopic	5 Adhesion Barrier	Z No Qualifier
L Pleural Cavity M Peritoneal Cavity	4 Percutaneous Endoscopic	G Other Therapeutic Substance	C Other Substance
L Pleural Cavity M Peritoneal Cavity	7 Via Natural or Artificial Opening	Ø Antineoplastic	4 Liquid Brachytherapy Radioisotope 5 Other Antineoplastic M Monoclonal Antibody
L Pleural Cavity M Peritoneal Cavity	7 Via Natural or Artificial Opening	S Gas	F Other Gas
P Female Reproductive	Ø Open	5 Adhesion Barrier	Z No Qualifier
P Female Reproductive	3 Percutaneous 7 Via Natural or Artificial Opening	Ø Antineoplastic	4 Liquid Brachytherapy Radioisotope 5 Other Antineoplastic M Monoclonal Antibody
P Female Reproductive	3 Percutaneous 7 Via Natural or Artificial Opening	2 Anti-infective	8 Oxazolidinones 9 Other Anti-infective
P Female Reproductive	3 Percutaneous 7 Via Natural or Artificial Opening	3 Anti-inflammatory 5 Adhesion Barrier 6 Nutritional Substance 7 Electrolytic and Water Balance Substance B Anesthetic Agent H Radioactive Substance K Other Diagnostic Substance L Sperm N Analgesics, Hypnotics, Sedatives T Destructive Agent V Hormone	Z No Qualifier
P Female Reproductive	3 Percutaneous 7 Via Natural or Artificial Opening	G Other Therapeutic Substance	C Other Substance
P Female Reproductive	3 Percutaneous 7 Via Natural or Artificial Opening	Q Fertilized Ovum	Ø Autologous 1 Nonautologous
P Female Reproductive	3 Percutaneous 7 Via Natural or Artificial Opening	S Gas	F Other Gas
P Female Reproductive	4 Percutaneous Endoscopic	5 Adhesion Barrier	Z No Qualifier
P Female Reproductive	4 Percutaneous Endoscopic	G Other Therapeutic Substance	C Other Substance
P Female Reproductive	7 Via Natural or Artificial Opening	Ø Antineoplastic	4 Liquid Brachytherapy Radioisotope 5 Other Antineoplastic M Monoclonal Antibody
P Female Reproductive	7 Via Natural or Artificial Opening	2 Anti-infective	8 Oxazolidinones 9 Other Anti-infective

SECTION: 3 ADMINISTRATION
BODY SYSTEM: E PHYSIOLOGICAL SYSTEMS AND ANATOMICAL REGIONS
OPERATION: Ø INTRODUCTION: *(continued)*

Putting in or on a therapeutic, diagnostic, nutritional, physiological, or prophylactic substance except blood or blood products

Body System / Region	Approach	Substance	Qualifier
P Female Reproductive	7 Via Natural or Artificial Opening	3 Anti-inflammatory 6 Nutritional Substance 7 Electrolytic and Water Balance Substance B Anesthetic Agent H Radioactive Substance K Other Diagnostic Substance L Sperm N Analgesics, Hypnotics, Sedatives T Destructive Agent V Hormone	Z No Qualifier
P Female Reproductive	7 Via Natural or Artificial Opening	G Other Therapeutic Substance	C Other Substance
P Female Reproductive	7 Via Natural or Artificial Opening	Q Fertilized Ovum	Ø Autologous 1 Nonautologous
P Female Reproductive	7 Via Natural or Artificial Opening	S Gas	F Other Gas
P Female Reproductive	8 Via Natural or Artificial Opening Endoscopic	Ø Antineoplastic	4 Liquid Brachytherapy Radioisotope 5 Other Antineoplastic M Monoclonal Antibody
P Female Reproductive	8 Via Natural or Artificial Opening Endoscopic	2 Anti-infective	8 Oxazolidinones 9 Other Anti-infective
P Female Reproductive	8 Via Natural or Artificial Opening Endoscopic	3 Anti-inflammatory 6 Nutritional Substance 7 Electrolytic and Water Balance Substance B Anesthetic Agent H Radioactive Substance K Other Diagnostic Substance N Analgesics, Hypnotics, Sedatives T Destructive Agent	Z No Qualifier
P Female Reproductive	8 Via Natural or Artificial Opening Endoscopic	G Other Therapeutic Substance	C Other Substance
P Female Reproductive	8 Via Natural or Artificial Opening Endoscopic	S Gas	F Other Gas
Q Cranial Cavity and Brain	Ø Open 3 Percutaneous	Ø Antineoplastic	4 Liquid Brachytherapy Radioisotope 5 Other Antineoplastic M Monoclonal Antibody
Q Cranial Cavity and Brain	Ø Open 3 Percutaneous	2 Anti-infective	8 Oxazolidinones 9 Other Anti-infective
Q Cranial Cavity and Brain	Ø Open 3 Percutaneous	3 Anti-inflammatory 6 Nutritional Substance 7 Electrolytic and Water Balance Substance A Stem Cells, Embryonic B Anesthetic Agent H Radioactive Substance K Other Diagnostic Substance N Analgesics, Hypnotics, Sedatives T Destructive Agent	Z No Qualifier

SECTION: 3 ADMINISTRATION

BODY SYSTEM: E PHYSIOLOGICAL SYSTEMS AND ANATOMICAL REGIONS
OPERATION: Ø INTRODUCTION: *(continued)*

Putting in or on a therapeutic, diagnostic, nutritional, physiological, or prophylactic substance except blood or blood products

Body System / Region	Approach	Substance	Qualifier
Q Cranial Cavity and Brain	Ø Open 3 Percutaneous	E Stem Cells, Somatic	Ø Autologous 1 Nonautologous
Q Cranial Cavity and Brain	Ø Open 3 Percutaneous	G Other Therapeutic Substance	C Other Substance
Q Cranial Cavity and Brain	Ø Open 3 Percutaneous	S Gas	F Other Gas
Q Cranial Cavity and Brain	7 Via Natural or Artificial Opening	Ø Antineoplastic	4 Liquid Brachytherapy Radioisotope 5 Other Antineoplastic M Monoclonal Antibody
Q Cranial Cavity and Brain	7 Via Natural or Artificial Opening	S Gas	F Other Gas
R Spinal Canal	Ø Open	A Stem Cells, Embryonic	Z No Qualifier
R Spinal Canal	Ø Open	A Stem Cells, Somatic	Ø Autologous 1 Nonautologous
R Spinal Canal	3 Percutaneous	Ø Antineoplastic	2 High-dose Interleukin-2 3 Low-dose Interleukin-2 4 Liquid Brachytherapy Radioisotope 5 Other Antineoplastic M Monoclonal Antibody
R Spinal Canal	3 Percutaneous	2 Anti-infective	8 Oxazolidinones 9 Other Anti-infective
R Spinal Canal	3 Percutaneous	3 Anti-inflammatory 6 Nutritional Substance 7 Electrolytic and Water Balance Substance A Stem Cells, Embryonic B Anesthetic Agent C Regional Anesthetic H Radioactive Substance K Other Diagnostic Substance N Analgesics, Hypnotics, Sedatives T Destructive Agent	Z No Qualifier
R Spinal Canal	3 Percutaneous	E Stem Cells, Somatic	Ø Autologous 1 Nonautologous
R Spinal Canal	3 Percutaneous	G Other Therapeutic Substance	C Other Substance
R Spinal Canal	3 Percutaneous	S Gas	F Other Gas
R Spinal Canal	7 Via Natural or Artificial Opening	S Gas	F Other Gas
S Epidural Space	3 Percutaneous	Ø Antineoplastic	2 High-dose Interleukin-2 3 Low-dose Interleukin-2 4 Liquid Brachytherapy Radioisotope 5 Other Antineoplastic M Monoclonal Antibody
S Epidural Space	3 Percutaneous	2 Anti-infective	8 Oxazolidinones 9 Other Anti-infective

SECTION: 3 ADMINISTRATION
BODY SYSTEM: E PHYSIOLOGICAL SYSTEMS AND ANATOMICAL REGIONS
OPERATION: Ø INTRODUCTION: *(continued)*
Putting in or on a therapeutic, diagnostic, nutritional, physiological, or prophylactic substance except blood or blood products

Body System / Region	Approach	Substance	Qualifier
S Epidural Space	3 Percutaneous	3 Anti-inflammatory 6 Nutritional Substance 7 Electrolytic and Water Balance Substance B Anesthetic Agent C Regional Anesthetic H Radioactive Substance K Other Diagnostic Substance N Analgesics, Hypnotics, Sedatives T Destructive Agent	Z No Qualifier
S Epidural Space	3 Percutaneous	G Other Therapeutic Substance	C Other Substance
S Epidural Space	3 Percutaneous	S Gas	F Other Gas
S Epidural Space	7 Via Natural or Artificial Opening	S Gas	F Other Gas
T Peripheral Nerves and Plexi X Cranial Nerves	3 Percutaneous	3 Anti-inflammatory B Anesthetic Agent C Regional Anesthetic T Destructive Agent	Z No Qualifier
T Peripheral Nerves and Plexi X Cranial Nerves	3 Percutaneous	G Other Therapeutic Substance	C Other Substance
U Joints	Ø Open	2 Anti-infective	8 Oxazolidinones 9 Other Anti-infective
U Joints	Ø Open	G Other Therapeutic Substance	B Recombinant Bone Morphogenetic Protein
U Joints	3 Percutaneous	Ø Antineoplastic	4 Liquid Brachytherapy Radioisotope 5 Other Antineoplastic M Monoclonal Antibody
U Joints	3 Percutaneous	2 Anti-infective	8 Oxazolidinones 9 Other Anti-infective
U Joints	3 Percutaneous	3 Anti-inflammatory 6 Nutritional Substance 7 Electrolytic and Water Balance Substance B Anesthetic Agent H Radioactive Substance K Other Diagnostic Substance N Analgesics, Hypnotics, Sedatives T Destructive Agent	Z No Qualifier
U Joints	3 Percutaneous	G Other Therapeutic Substance	B Recombinant Bone Morphogenetic Protein C Other Substance
U Joints	3 Percutaneous	S Gas	F Other Gas
U Joints	3 Percutaneous Endoscopic	G Other Therapeutic Substance	C Other Substance

SECTION: 3 ADMINISTRATION
BODY SYSTEM: E PHYSIOLOGICAL SYSTEMS AND ANATOMICAL REGIONS
OPERATION: Ø INTRODUCTION: *(continued)*
Putting in or on a therapeutic, diagnostic, nutritional, physiological, or prophylactic substance except blood or blood products

Body System / Region	Approach	Substance	Qualifier
V Bones	Ø Open	G Other Therapeutic Substance	B Recombinant Bone Morphogenetic Protein
V Bones	3 Percutaneous	Ø Antineoplastic	5 Other Antineoplastic M Monoclonal Antibody
V Bones	3 Percutaneous	2 Anti-infective	8 Oxazolidinones 9 Other Anti-infective
V Bones	3 Percutaneous	3 Anti-inflammatory 6 Nutritional Substance 7 Electrolytic and Water Balance Substance B Anesthetic Agent H Radioactive Substance K Other Diagnostic Substance N Analgesics, Hypnotics, Sedatives T Destructive Agent	Z No Qualifier
V Bones	3 Percutaneous	G Other Therapeutic Substance	B Recombinant Bone Morphogenetic Protein C Other Substance
W Lymphatics	3 Percutaneous	Ø Antineoplastic	5 Other Antineoplastic M Monoclonal Antibody
W Lymphatics	3 Percutaneous	2 Anti-infective	8 Oxazolidinones 9 Other Anti-infective
W Lymphatics	3 Percutaneous	3 Anti-inflammatory 6 Nutritional Substance 7 Electrolytic and Water Balance Substance B Anesthetic Agent H Radioactive Substance K Other Diagnostic Substance N Analgesics, Hypnotics, Sedatives T Destructive Agent	Z No Qualifier
W Lymphatics	3 Percutaneous	G Other Therapeutic Substance	C Other Substance
Y Pericardial Cavity	3 Percutaneous	Ø Antineoplastic	4 Liquid Brachytherapy Radioisotope 5 Other Antineoplastic M Monoclonal Antibody
Y Pericardial Cavity	3 Percutaneous	2 Anti-infective	8 Oxazolidinones 9 Other Anti-infective
Y Pericardial Cavity	3 Percutaneous	3 Anti-inflammatory 6 Nutritional Substance 7 Electrolytic and Water Balance Substance B Anesthetic Agent H Radioactive Substance K Other Diagnostic Substance N Analgesics, Hypnotics, Sedatives T Destructive Agent	Z No Qualifier

SECTION: 3 ADMINISTRATION
BODY SYSTEM: E PHYSIOLOGICAL SYSTEMS AND ANATOMICAL REGIONS
OPERATION: 0 INTRODUCTION: *(continued)*
Putting in or on a therapeutic, diagnostic, nutritional, physiological, or prophylactic substance except blood or blood products

Body System / Region	Approach	Substance	Qualifier
Y Pericardial Cavity	3 Percutaneous	G Other Therapeutic Substance	C Other Substance
Y Pericardial Cavity	3 Percutaneous	S Gas	F Other Gas
Y Pericardial Cavity	3 Percutaneous Endoscopic	G Other Therapeutic Substance	C Other Substance
Y Pericardial Cavity	7 Via Natural or Artificial Opening	0 Antineoplastic	4 Liquid Brachytherapy Radioisotope 5 Other Antineoplastic M Monoclonal Antibody
Y Pericardial Cavity	7 Via Natural or Artificial Opening	S Gas	F Other Gas

SECTION: 3 ADMINISTRATION
BODY SYSTEM: E PHYSIOLOGICAL SYSTEMS AND ANATOMICAL REGIONS
OPERATION: 1 IRRIGATION: Putting in or on a cleansing substance

Body System / Region	Approach	Substance	Qualifier
0 Skin and Mucous Membranes C Eye	3 Percutaneous X External	8 Irrigating Substance	X Diagnostic Z No Qualifier
9 Nose B Ear F Respiratory Tract G Upper GI H Lower GI J Biliary and Pancreatic Tract K Genitourinary Tract N Male Reproductive P Female Reproductive	3 Percutaneous 7 Via Natural or Artificial Opening 8 Via Natural or Artificial Opening Endoscopic	8 Irrigating Substance	X Diagnostic Z No Qualifier
L Pleural Cavity Q Cranial Cavity and Brain R Spinal Canal S Epidural Space U Joints Y Pericardial Cavity	3 Percutaneous	8 Irrigating Substance	X Diagnostic Z No Qualifier
M Peritoneal Cavity	3 Percutaneous	8 Irrigating Substance	X Diagnostic Z No Qualifier
M Peritoneal Cavity	3 Percutaneous	9 Dialysate	Z No Qualifier

0; 1

E: PHYSIOLOGICAL SYSTEMS AND ANATOMICAL REGIONS

3: ADMINISTRATION

4   Measurement and Monitoring **531**
  4A. Physiological Systems 532
    4AØ. Measurement 532
    4A1. Monitoring 534
  4B. Physiological Devices 536
    4BØ. Measurement 536

SECTION: 4 MEASUREMENT AND MONITORING
BODY SYSTEM: A **PHYSIOLOGICAL SYSTEMS**
OPERATION: Ø **MEASUREMENT:** *(on multiple pages)*
Determining the level of a physiological or physical function at a point in time

Body System	Approach	Function / Device	Qualifier
Ø Central Nervous	Ø Open	2 Conductivity 4 Electrical Activity B Pressure	Z No Qualifier
Ø Central Nervous	3 Percutaneous 7 Via Natural or Artificial Opening 8 Via Natural or Artificial Opening Endoscopic	4 Electrical Activity	Z No Qualifier
Ø Central Nervous	3 Percutaneous 7 Via Natural or Artificial Opening 8 Via Natural or Artificial Opening Endoscopic	B Pressure K Temperature R Saturation	D Intracranial
~~Ø Central Nervous~~	~~7 Via Natural or Artificial Opening~~	~~B Pressure~~ ~~K Temperature~~ ~~R Saturation~~	~~D Intracranial~~
Ø Central Nervous	X External	2 Conductivity 4 Electrical Activity	Z No Qualifier
1 Peripheral Nervous	Ø Open 3 Percutaneous 7 Via Natural or Artificial Opening 8 Via Natural or Artificial Opening Endoscopic X External	2 Conductivity	9 Sensory B Motor
1 Peripheral Nervous	Ø Open 3 Percutaneous 7 Via Natural or Artificial Opening 8 Via Natural or Artificial Opening Endoscopic X External	4 Electrical Activity	Z No Qualifier
2 Cardiac	Ø Open 3 Percutaneous 7 Via Natural or Artificial Opening 8 Via Natural or Artificial Opening Endoscopic	4 Electrical Activity 9 Output C Rate F Rhythm H Sound P Action Currents	Z No Qualifier
2 Cardiac	Ø Open 3 Percutaneous 7 Via Natural or Artificial Opening 8 Via Natural or Artificial Opening Endoscopic	N Sampling and Pressure	6 Right Heart 7 Left Heart 8 Bilateral
2 Cardiac	X External	4 Electrical Activity	A Guidance Z No Qualifier
2 Cardiac	X External	9 Output C Rate F Rhythm H Sound P Action Currents	Z No Qualifier
2 Cardiac	X External	M Total Activity	4 Stress
3 Arterial	Ø Open 3 Percutaneous	5 Flow J Pulse	1 Peripheral 3 Pulmonary C Coronary
3 Arterial	Ø Open 3 Percutaneous	B Pressure	1 Peripheral 3 Pulmonary C Coronary F Other Thoracic

SECTION: 4 MEASUREMENT AND MONITORING
BODY SYSTEM: A PHYSIOLOGICAL SYSTEMS
OPERATION: 0 MEASUREMENT: *(continued)*
Determining the level of a physiological or physical function at a point in time

Body System	Approach	Function / Device	Qualifier
3 Arterial	0 Open 3 Percutaneous	H Sound R Saturation	1 Peripheral
3 Arterial	X External	5 Flow B Pressure H Sound J Pulse R Saturation	1 Peripheral
4 Venous	0 Open 3 Percutaneous	5 Flow B Pressure J Pulse	0 Central 1 Peripheral 2 Portal 3 Pulmonary
4 Venous	0 Open 3 Percutaneous	R Saturation	1 Peripheral
4 Venous	X External	5 Flow B Pressure J Pulse R Saturation	1 Peripheral
5 Circulatory	X External	L Volume	Z No Qualifier
6 Lymphatic	0 Open 3 Percutaneous 7 Via Natural or Artificial Opening 8 Via Natural or Artificial Opening Endoscopic	5 Flow B Pressure	Z No Qualifier
7 Visual	X External	0 Acuity 7 Mobility B Pressure	Z No Qualifier
8 Olfactory	X External	0 Acuity	Z No Qualifier
9 Respiratory	7 Via Natural or Artificial Opening 8 Via Natural or Artificial Opening Endoscopic X External	1 Capacity 5 Flow C Rate D Resistance L Volume M Total Activity	Z No Qualifier
B Gastrointestinal	7 Via Natural or Artificial Opening 8 Via Natural or Artificial Opening Endoscopic	8 Motility B Pressure G Secretion	Z No Qualifier
C Biliary	3 Percutaneous 4 Percutaneous Endoscopic 7 Via Natural or Artificial Opening 8 Via Natural or Artificial Opening Endoscopic	5 Flow B Pressure	Z No Qualifier
D Urinary	7 Via Natural or Artificial Opening 8 Via Natural or Artificial Opening Endoscopic	3 Contractility 5 Flow B Pressure D Resistance L Volume	Z No Qualifier
F Musculoskeletal	3 Percutaneous X External	3 Contractility	Z No Qualifier
H Products of Conception, Cardiac	7 Via Natural or Artificial Opening 8 Via Natural or Artificial Opening Endoscopic X External	4 Electrical Activity C Rate F Rhythm H Sound	Z No Qualifier

SECTION: **4 MEASUREMENT AND MONITORING**
BODY SYSTEM: **A PHYSIOLOGICAL SYSTEMS**
OPERATION: **Ø MEASUREMENT:** *(continued)*
     Determining the level of a physiological or physical function at a point in time

Body System	Approach	Function / Device	Qualifier
J Products of Conception, Nervous	7 Via Natural or Artificial Opening 8 Via Natural or Artificial Opening Endoscopic X External	2 Conductivity 4 Electrical Activity B Pressure	Z No Qualifier
Z None	7 Via Natural or Artificial Opening	6 Metabolism K Temperature	Z No Qualifier
Z None	X External	6 Metabolism K Temperature Q Sleep	Z No Qualifier

SECTION: **4 MEASUREMENT AND MONITORING**
BODY SYSTEM: **A PHYSIOLOGICAL SYSTEMS**
OPERATION: **1 MONITORING:** *(on multiple pages)*
     Determining the level of a physiological or physical function repetitively over a period of time

Body System	Approach	Function / Device	Qualifier
Ø Central Nervous	Ø Open	2 Conductivity B Pressure	Z No Qualifier
Ø Central Nervous	Ø Open	4 Electrical Activity	G Intraoperative Z No Qualifier
Ø Central Nervous	3 Percutaneous 7 Via Natural or Artificial Opening 8 Via Natural or Artificial Opening Endoscopic	4 Electrical Activity	G Intraoperative Z No Qualifier
~~Ø Central Nervous~~	~~3 Percutaneous~~	~~B Pressure~~ ~~K Temperature~~ ~~R Saturation~~	~~D Intracranial~~
Ø Central Nervous	3 Percutaneous 7 Via Natural or Artificial Opening 8 Via Natural or Artificial Opening Endoscopic	B Pressure K Temperature R Saturation	D Intracranial
Ø Central Nervous	X External	2 Conductivity	Z No Qualifier
Ø Central Nervous	X External	4 Electrical Activity	G Intraoperative Z No Qualifier
1 Peripheral Nervous	Ø Open 3 Percutaneous 7 Via Natural or Artificial Opening 8 Via Natural or Artificial Opening Endoscopic X External	2 Conductivity	9 Sensory B Motor
1 Peripheral Nervous	Ø Open 3 Percutaneous 7 Via Natural or Artificial Opening 8 Via Natural or Artificial Opening Endoscopic X External	4 Electrical Activity	G Intraoperative Z No Qualifier

(Side tab: 4: MEASUREMENT AND MONITORING   A: PHYSIOLOGICAL SYSTEMS   Ø: MEASUREMENT   1: MONITORING)

SECTION: 4 MEASUREMENT AND MONITORING
BODY SYSTEM: A PHYSIOLOGICAL SYSTEMS
OPERATION: 1 MONITORING: *(continued)*

Determining the level of a physiological or physical function repetitively over a period of time

Body System	Approach	Function / Device	Qualifier
2 Cardiac	0 Open 3 Percutaneous 7 Via Natural or Artificial Opening 8 Via Natural or Artificial Opening Endoscopic	4 Electrical Activity 9 Output C Rate F Rhythm H Sound	Z No Qualifier
2 Cardiac	X External	4 Electrical Activity	5 Ambulatory Z No Qualifier
2 Cardiac	X External	9 Output C Rate F Rhythm H Sound	Z No Qualifier
2 Cardiac	X External	M Total Activity	4 Stress
2 Cardiac	X External	S Vascular Perfusion	H Indocyanine Green Dye
3 Arterial	0 Open 3 Percutaneous	5 Flow B Pressure J Pulse	1 Peripheral 3 Pulmonary C Coronary
3 Arterial	0 Open 3 Percutaneous	H Sound R Saturation	1 Peripheral
3 Arterial	X External	5 Flow B Pressure H Sound J Pulse R Saturation	1 Peripheral
4 Venous	0 Open 3 Percutaneous	5 Flow B Pressure J Pulse	0 Central 1 Peripheral 2 Portal 3 Pulmonary
4 Venous	0 Open 3 Percutaneous	R Saturation	0 Central 2 Portal 3 Pulmonary
4 Venous	X External	5 Flow B Pressure J Pulse	1 Peripheral
6 Lymphatic	0 Open 3 Percutaneous 7 Via Natural or Artificial Opening 8 Via Natural or Artificial Opening Endoscopic	5 Flow B Pressure	Z No Qualifier
9 Respiratory	7 Via Natural or Artificial Opening X External	1 Capacity 5 Flow C Rate D Resistance L Volume	Z No Qualifier
B Gastrointestinal	7 Via Natural or Artificial Opening 8 Via Natural or Artificial Opening Endoscopic	8 Motility B Pressure G Secretion	Z No Qualifier

SECTION: 4 MEASUREMENT AND MONITORING
BODY SYSTEM: A PHYSIOLOGICAL SYSTEMS
OPERATION: 1 MONITORING: *(continued)*
Determining the level of a physiological or physical function repetitively over a period of time

Body System	Approach	Function / Device	Qualifier
B Gastrointestinal	X External	S Vascular Perfusion	H Indocyanine Green Dye
D Urinary	7 Via Natural or Artificial Opening 8 Via Natural or Artificial Opening Endoscopic	3 Contractility 5 Flow B Pressure D Resistance L Volume	Z No Qualifier
G Skin and Breast	X External	S Vascular Perfusion	H Indocyanine Green Dye
H Products of Conception, Cardiac	7 Via Natural or Artificial Opening 8 Via Natural or Artificial Opening Endoscopic X External	4 Electrical Activity C Rate F Rhythm H Sound	Z No Qualifier
J Products of Conception, Nervous	7 Via Natural or Artificial Opening 8 Via Natural or Artificial Opening Endoscopic X External	2 Conductivity 4 Electrical Activity B Pressure	Z No Qualifier
Z None	7 Via Natural or Artificial Opening	K Temperature	Z No Qualifier
Z None	X External	K Temperature Q Sleep	Z No Qualifier

SECTION: 4 MEASUREMENT AND MONITORING
BODY SYSTEM: B PHYSIOLOGICAL DEVICES
OPERATION: Ø MEASUREMENT: Determining the level of a physiological or physical function at a point in time

Body System	Approach	Function / Device	Qualifier
Ø Central Nervous 1 Peripheral Nervous F Musculoskeletal	X External	V Stimulator	Z No Qualifier
2 Cardiac	X External	S Pacemaker T Defibrillator	Z No Qualifier
9 Respiratory	X External	S Pacemaker	Z No Qualifier

Side tabs: B: PHYSIOLOGICAL DEVICES · A: PHYSIOLOGICAL SYSTEMS · 4: MEASUREMENT AND MONITORING

5 Extracorporeal or Systemic **Assistance and Performance** **537**
   5A. Physiological Systems 538
      5A∅. Assistance 538
      5A1. Performance 539
      5A2. Restoration 539

SECTION: 5 EXTRACORPOREAL OR SYSTEMIC ASSISTANCE AND PERFORMANCE

BODY SYSTEM: A PHYSIOLOGICAL SYSTEMS

OPERATION: Ø ASSISTANCE: Taking over a portion of a physiological function by extracorporeal means

Body System	Duration	Function	Qualifier
2 Cardiac	1 Intermittent 2 Continuous	1 Output	Ø Balloon Pump 5 Pulsatile Compression 6 Pump D Impeller Pump
5 Circulatory	1 Intermittent 2 Continuous	2 Oxygenation	1 Hyperbaric C Supersaturated
9 Respiratory	2 Continuous	Ø Filtration	Z No Qualifier
9 Respiratory	3 Less than 24 Consecutive Hours 4 24-96 Consecutive Hours 5 Greater than 96 Consecutive Hours	5 Ventilation	7 Continuous Positive Airway Pressure 8 Intermittent Positive Airway Pressure 9 Continuous Negative Airway Pressure B Intermittent Negative Airway Pressure Z No Qualifier

A: PHYSIOLOGICAL SYSTEMS

5: EXTRACORPOREAL OR SYSTEMIC ASSISTANCE AND PERFORMANCE

SECTION: **5 EXTRACORPOREAL OR SYSTEMIC ASSISTANCE AND PERFORMANCE**

BODY SYSTEM: **A PHYSIOLOGICAL SYSTEMS**

OPERATION: **1 PERFORMANCE:** Completely taking over a physiological function by extracorporeal means

Body System	Duration	Function	Qualifier
2 Cardiac	Ø Single	1 Output	2 Manual
2 Cardiac	1 Intermittent	3 Pacing	Z No Qualifier
2 Cardiac	2 Continuous	1 Output 3 Pacing	Z No Qualifier
5 Circulatory	2 Continuous	2 Oxygenation	3 Membrane
9 Respiratory	Ø Single	5 Ventilation	4 Nonmechanical
9 Respiratory	3 Less than 24 Consecutive Hours 4 24-96 Consecutive Hours 5 Greater than 96 Consecutive Hours	5 Ventilation	Z No Qualifier
C Biliary ~~D Urinary~~	Ø Single 6 Multiple	Ø Filtration	Z No Qualifier
D Urinary	7 Intermittent, Less than 6 Hours Per Day 8 Prolonged Intermittent, 6-18 Hours Per Day 9 Continuous, Greater than 18 Hours Per Day	Ø Filtration	Z No Qualifier

SECTION: **5 EXTRACORPOREAL OR SYSTEMIC ASSISTANCE AND PERFORMANCE**

BODY SYSTEM: **A PHYSIOLOGICAL SYSTEMS**

OPERATION: **2 RESTORATION:** Returning, or attempting to return, a physiological function to its original state by extracorporeal means

Body System	Duration	Function	Qualifier
2 Cardiac	Ø Single	4 Rhythm	Z No Qualifier

6 Extracorporeal Or Systemic Therapies..**540**

   6A. Physiological Systems 541

       6AØ. Atmospheric Control 541

       6A1. Decompression 541

       6A2. Electromagnetic Therapy 541

       6A3. Hyperthermia 541

       6A4. Hypothermia 541

       6A5. Pheresis 542

       6A6. Phototherapy 542

       6A7. Ultrasound Therapy 542

       6A8. Ultraviolet Light Therapy 542

       6A9. Shock Wave Therapy 543

       6AB. Perfusion 543

SECTION: 6 EXTRACORPOREAL OR SYSTEMIC THERAPIES
BODY SYSTEM: A PHYSIOLOGICAL SYSTEMS
OPERATION: Ø ATMOSPHERIC CONTROL: Extracorporeal control of atmospheric pressure and composition

Body System	Duration	Qualifier	Qualifier
Z None	Ø Single 1 Multiple	Z No Qualifier	Z No Qualifier

SECTION: 6 EXTRACORPOREAL OR SYSTEMIC THERAPIES
BODY SYSTEM: A PHYSIOLOGICAL SYSTEMS
OPERATION: 1 DECOMPRESSION: Extracorporeal elimination of undissolved gas from body fluids

Body System	Duration	Qualifier	Qualifier
5 Circulatory	Ø Single 1 Multiple	Z No Qualifier	Z No Qualifier

SECTION: 6 EXTRACORPOREAL OR SYSTEMIC THERAPIES
BODY SYSTEM: A PHYSIOLOGICAL SYSTEMS
OPERATION: 2 ELECTROMAGNETIC THERAPY: Extracorporeal treatment by electromagnetic rays

Body System	Duration	Qualifier	Qualifier
1 Urinary 2 Central Nervous	Ø Single 1 Multiple	Z No Qualifier	Z No Qualifier

SECTION: 6 EXTRACORPOREAL OR SYSTEMIC THERAPIES
BODY SYSTEM: A PHYSIOLOGICAL SYSTEMS
OPERATION: 3 HYPERTHERMIA: Extracorporeal raising of body temperature

Body System	Duration	Qualifier	Qualifier
Z None	Ø Single 1 Multiple	Z No Qualifier	Z No Qualifier

SECTION: 6 EXTRACORPOREAL OR SYSTEMIC THERAPIES
BODY SYSTEM: A PHYSIOLOGICAL SYSTEMS
OPERATION: 4 HYPOTHERMIA: Extracorporeal lowering of body temperature

Body System	Duration	Qualifier	Qualifier
Z None	Ø Single 1 Multiple	Z No Qualifier	Z No Qualifier

6: EXTRACORPOREAL OR SYSTEMIC THERAPIES   A: PHYSIOLOGICAL SYSTEMS   Ø; 1; 2; 3; 4

SECTION: 6 EXTRACORPOREAL OR SYSTEMIC THERAPIES
BODY SYSTEM: A PHYSIOLOGICAL SYSTEMS
OPERATION: 5 PHERESIS: Extracorporeal separation of blood products

Body System	Duration	Qualifier	Qualifier
5 Circulatory	Ø Single 1 Multiple	Z No Qualifier	Ø Erythrocytes 1 Leukocytes 2 Platelets 3 Plasma T Stem Cells, Cord Blood V Stem Cells, Hematopoietic

SECTION: 6 EXTRACORPOREAL OR SYSTEMIC THERAPIES
BODY SYSTEM: A PHYSIOLOGICAL SYSTEMS
OPERATION: 6 PHOTOTHERAPY: Extracorporeal treatment by light rays

Body System	Duration	Qualifier	Qualifier
Ø Skin 5 Circulatory	Ø Single 1 Multiple	Z No Qualifier	Z No Qualifier

SECTION: 6 EXTRACORPOREAL OR SYSTEMIC THERAPIES
BODY SYSTEM: A PHYSIOLOGICAL SYSTEMS
OPERATION: 7 ULTRASOUND THERAPY: Extracorporeal treatment by ultrasound

Body System	Duration	Qualifier	Qualifier
5 Circulatory	Ø Single 1 Multiple	Z No Qualifier	4 Head and Neck Vessels 5 Heart 6 Peripheral Vessels 7 Other Vessels Z No Qualifier

SECTION: 6 EXTRACORPOREAL OR SYSTEMIC THERAPIES
BODY SYSTEM: A PHYSIOLOGICAL SYSTEMS
OPERATION: 8 ULTRAVIOLET LIGHT THERAPY: Extracorporeal treatment by ultraviolet light

Body System	Duration	Qualifier	Qualifier
Ø Skin	Ø Single 1 Multiple	Z No Qualifier	Z No Qualifier

SECTION: 6 EXTRACORPOREAL OR SYSTEMIC THERAPIES
BODY SYSTEM: A PHYSIOLOGICAL SYSTEMS
OPERATION: 9 SHOCK WAVE THERAPY: Extracorporeal treatment by shock waves

Body System	Duration	Qualifier	Qualifier
3 Musculoskeletal	Ø Single 1 Multiple	Z No Qualifier	Z No Qualifier

SECTION: 6 EXTRACORPOREAL OR SYSTEMIC THERAPIES
BODY SYSTEM: A PHYSIOLOGICAL SYSTEMS
OPERATION: B PERFUSION: Extracorporeal treatment by diffusion of therapeutic fluid

Body System	Duration	Qualifier	Qualifier
5 Circulatory B Respiratory System F Hepatobiliary System and Pancreas T Urinary System	Ø Single	B Donor Organ	Z No Qualifier

6: EXTRACORPOREAL OR SYSTEMIC THERAPIES

A: PHYSIOLOGICAL SYSTEMS

9; B

7 Osteopathic...**544**

   7W. Anatomical Regions..545

       7WØ. Treatment...545

SECTION: 7 OSTEOPATHIC
BODY SYSTEM: W ANATOMICAL REGIONS
OPERATION: **Ø TREATMENT:** Manual treatment to eliminate or alleviate somatic dysfunction and related disorders

Body Region	Approach	Method	Qualifier
Ø Head	X External	Ø Articulatory-Raising	Z None
1 Cervical		1 Fascial Release	
2 Thoracic		2 General Mobilization	
3 Lumbar		3 High Velocity-Low Amplitude	
4 Sacrum		4 Indirect	
5 Pelvis		5 Low Velocity-High Amplitude	
6 Lower Extremities		6 Lymphatic Pump	
7 Upper Extremities		7 Muscle Energy-Isometric	
8 Rib Cage		8 Muscle Energy-Isotonic	
9 Abdomen		9 Other Method	

8   Other Procedures..**546**
   8C. Indwelling Device 547
      8CØ. Other Procedures 547
   8E. Physiological Systems and Anatomical Regions...548
      8EØ. Other Procedures..548

SECTION: 8 OTHER PROCEDURES
BODY SYSTEM: C INDWELLING DEVICE
OPERATION: Ø OTHER PROCEDURES: Methodologies which attempt to remediate or cure a disorder or disease

Body Region	Approach	Method	Qualifier
1 Nervous System	X External	6 Collection	J Cerebrospinal Fluid L Other Fluid
2 Circulatory System	X External	6 Collection	K Blood L Other Fluid

SECTION: 8 OTHER PROCEDURES
BODY SYSTEM: E PHYSIOLOGICAL SYSTEMS AND ANATOMICAL REGIONS
OPERATION: Ø OTHER PROCEDURES: Methodologies which attempt to remediate
or cure a disorder or disease

0: OTHER PROCEDURES

E: PHYSIOLOGICAL SYSTEMS AND ANATOMICAL REGIONS

8: OTHER PROCEDURES

Body Region	Approach	Method	Qualifier
1 Nervous System U Female Reproductive System	X External	Y Other Method	7 Examination
2 Circulatory System	3 Percutaneous	D Near Infrared Spectroscopy	Z No Qualifier
9 Head and Neck Region W Trunk Region	Ø Open 3 Percutaneous 4 Percutaneous Endoscopic 7 Via Natural or Artificial Opening 8 Via Natural or Artificial Opening Endoscopic	C Robotic Assisted Procedure	Z No Qualifier
9 Head and Neck Region W Trunk Region	X External	B Computer Assisted Procedure	F With Fluoroscopy G With Computerized Tomography H With Magnetic Resonance Imaging Z No Qualifier
9 Head and Neck Region W Trunk Region	X External	C Robotic Assisted Procedure	Z No Qualifier
9 Head and Neck Region W Trunk Region	X External	Y Other Method	8 Suture Removal
H Integumentary System and Breast	3 Percutaneous	Ø Acupuncture	Ø Anesthesia Z No Qualifier
H Integumentary System and Breast	X External	6 Collection	2 Breast Milk
H Integumentary System and Breast	X External	Y Other Method	9 Piercing
K Musculoskeletal System	X External	1 Therapeutic Massage	Z No Qualifier
K Musculoskeletal System	X External	Y Other Method	7 Examination
V Male Reproductive System	X External	1 Therapeutic Massage	C Prostate D Rectum
V Male Reproductive System	X External	6 Collection	3 Sperm
X Upper Extremity Y Lower Extremity	Ø Open 3 Percutaneous 4 Percutaneous Endoscopic	C Robotic Assisted Procedure	Z No Qualifier
X Upper Extremity Y Lower Extremity	X External	B Computer Assisted Procedure	F With Fluoroscopy G With Computerized Tomography H With Magnetic Resonance Imaging Z No Qualifier
X Upper Extremity Y Lower Extremity	X External	C Robotic Assisted Procedure	Z No Qualifier
X Upper Extremity Y Lower Extremity	X External	Y Other Method	8 Suture Removal
Z None	X External	Y Other Method	1 In Vitro Fertilization 4 Yoga Therapy 5 Meditation 6 Isolation

New/Revised Text in Blue   ~~deleted~~ Deleted

9 Chiropractic..**549**

9W. Anatomical Regions...550

9WB. Manipulation...550

SECTION: 9 CHIROPRACTIC
BODY SYSTEM: W ANATOMICAL REGIONS
OPERATION: B **MANIPULATION:** Manual procedure that involves a directed thrust to move a joint past the physiological range of motion, without exceeding the anatomical limit

Body Region	Approach	Method	Qualifier
Ø Head	X External	B Non-Manual	Z None
1 Cervical		C Indirect Visceral	
2 Thoracic		D Extra-Articular	
3 Lumbar		F Direct Visceral	
4 Sacrum		G Long Lever Specific Contact	
5 Pelvis		H Short Lever Specific Contact	
6 Lower Extremities		J Long and Short Lever Specific Contact	
7 Upper Extremities		K Mechanically Assisted	
8 Rib Cage		L Other Method	
9 Abdomen			

B: MANIPULATION

W: ANATOMICAL REGIONS

9: CHIROPRACTIC

New/Revised Text in Blue   ~~deleted~~ Deleted

B Imaging..**551**

    BØ. Central Nervous System...553

        BØØ. Plain Radiography...553

        BØ1. Fluoroscopy...553

        BØ2. Computerized Tomography (CT SCAN)..............553

        BØ3. Magnetic Resonance Imaging (MRI)...................554

        BØ4. Ultrasonography..554

    B2. Heart...555

        B2Ø. Plain Radiography...555

        B21. Fluoroscopy...555

        B22. Computerized Tomography (CT SCAN)..............556

        B23. Magnetic Resonance Imaging (MRI)...................556

        B24. Ultrasonography..557

    B3. Upper Arteries...558

        B3Ø. Plain Radiography...558

        B31. Fluoroscopy...559

        B32. Computerized Tomography (CT SCAN)..............561

        B33. Magnetic Resonance Imaging (MRI)...................562

        B34. Ultrasonography..562

    B4. Lower Arteries...563

        B4Ø. Plain Radiography...563

        B41. Fluoroscopy...564

        B42. Computerized Tomography (CT SCAN)..............565

        B43. Magnetic Resonance Imaging (MRI)...................565

        B44. Ultrasonography..566

    B5. Veins...567

        B5Ø. Plain Radiography...567

        B51. Fluoroscopy...568

        B52. Computerized Tomography (CT SCAN)..............569

        B53. Magnetic Resonance Imaging (MRI)...................570

        B54. Ultrasonography..571

    B7. Lymphatic System..572

        B7Ø. Plain Radiography...572

    B8. Eye..573

        B8Ø. Plain Radiography...573

        B82. Computerized Tomography (CT SCAN)..............573

        B83. Magnetic Resonance Imaging (MRI)...................574

        B84. Ultrasonography..574

    B9. Ear, Nose, Mouth, and Throat...575

        B9Ø. Plain Radiography...575

        B91. Fluoroscopy...575

        B92. Computerized Tomography (CT SCAN)..............576

        B93. Magnetic Resonance Imaging (MRI)...................576

    BB. Respiratory System..577

        BBØ. Plain Radiography...577

        BB1. Fluoroscopy...577

        BB2. Computerized Tomography (CT SCAN)..............577

        BB3. Magnetic Resonance Imaging (MRI)...................578

        BB4. Ultrasonography..578

    BD. Gastrointestinal System...579

        BD1. Fluoroscopy...579

        BD2. Computerized Tomography (CT SCAN)..............579

        BD4. Ultrasonography..579

    BF. Hepatobiliary System and Pancreas.................................58Ø

        BFØ. Plain Radiography...58Ø

        BF1. Fluoroscopy...58Ø

        BF2. Computerized Tomography (CT SCAN)..............581

        BF3. Magnetic Resonance Imaging (MRI)...................581

        BF4. Ultrasonography..581

BG. Endocrine System 582
   BG2. Computerized Tomography (CT SCAN) 582
   BG3. Magnetic Resonance Imaging (MRI) 582
   BG4. Ultrasonography 582
BH. Skin, Subcutaneous Tissue and Breast 583
   BHØ. Plain Radiography 583
   BH3. Magnetic Resonance Imaging (MRI) 583
   BH4. Ultrasonography 584
BL. Connective Tissue 585
   BL3. Magnetic Resonance Imaging (MRI) 585
   BL4. Ultrasonography 585
BN. Skull and Facial Bones 586
   BNØ. Plain Radiography 586
   BN1. Fluoroscopy 586
   BN2. Computerized Tomography (CT SCAN) 587
   BN3. Magnetic Resonance Imaging (MRI) 587
BP. Non-Axial Upper Bones 588
   BPØ. Plain Radiography 588
   BP1. Fluoroscopy 589
   BP2. Computerized Tomography (CT SCAN) 590
   BP3. Magnetic Resonance Imaging (MRI) 591
   BP4. Ultrasonography 591
BQ. Non-Axial Lower Bones 592
   BQØ. Plain Radiography 592
   BQ1. Fluoroscopy 593
   BQ2. Computerized Tomography (CT SCAN) 594
   BQ3. Magnetic Resonance Imaging (MRI) 595
   BQ4. Ultrasonography 596
BR. Axial Skeleton, Except Skull and Facial Bones 597
   BRØ. Plain Radiography 597
   BR1. Fluoroscopy 597
   BR2. Computerized Tomography (CT SCAN) 598
   BR3. Magnetic Resonance Imaging (MRI) 598
   BR4. Ultrasonography 598
BT. Urinary System 599
   BTØ. Plain Radiography 599
   BT1. Fluoroscopy 599
   BT2. Computerized Tomography (CT SCAN) 600
   BT3. Magnetic Resonance Imaging (MRI) 600
   BT4. Ultrasonography 601
BU. Female Reproductive System 602
   BUØ. Plain Radiography 602
   BU1. Fluoroscopy 602
   BU3. Magnetic Resonance Imaging (MRI) 603
   BU4. Ultrasonography 603
BV. Male Reproductive System 604
   BVØ. Plain Radiography 604
   BV1. Fluoroscopy 604
   BV2. Computerized Tomography (CT SCAN) 605
   BV3. Magnetic Resonance Imaging (MRI) 605
   BV4. Ultrasonography 605
BW. Anatomical Regions 606
   BWØ. Plain Radiography 606
   BW1. Fluoroscopy 606
   BW2. Computerized Tomography (CT SCAN) 606
   BW3. Magnetic Resonance Imaging (MRI) 607
   BW4. Ultrasonography 607
BY. Fetus and Obstetrical 608
   BY3. Magnetic Resonance Imaging (MRI) 608
   BY4. Ultrasonography 608

New/Revised Text in Blue   ~~deleted~~ Deleted

SECTION: B IMAGING
BODY SYSTEM: 0 CENTRAL NERVOUS SYSTEM
TYPE: 0 **PLAIN RADIOGRAPHY:** Planar display of an image developed from the capture of external ionizing radiation on photographic or photoconductive plate

Body Part	Contrast	Qualifier	Qualifier
B Spinal Cord	0 High Osmolar 1 Low Osmolar Y Other Contrast Z None	Z None	Z None

SECTION: B IMAGING
BODY SYSTEM: 0 CENTRAL NERVOUS SYSTEM
TYPE: 1 **FLUOROSCOPY:** Single plane or bi-plane real time display of an image developed from the capture of external ionizing radiation on a fluorescent screen. The image may also be stored by either digital or analog means

Body Part	Contrast	Qualifier	Qualifier
B Spinal Cord	0 High Osmolar 1 Low Osmolar Y Other Contrast Z None	Z None	Z None

SECTION: B IMAGING
BODY SYSTEM: 0 CENTRAL NERVOUS SYSTEM
TYPE: 2 **COMPUTERIZED TOMOGRAPHY (CT SCAN):** Computer reformatted digital display of multiplanar images developed from the capture of multiple exposures of external ionizing radiation

Body Part	Contrast	Qualifier	Qualifier
0 Brain 7 Cisterna 8 Cerebral Ventricle(s) 9 Sella Turcica/Pituitary Gland B Spinal Cord	0 High Osmolar 1 Low Osmolar Y Other Contrast	0 Unenhanced and Enhanced Z None	Z None
0 Brain 7 Cisterna 8 Cerebral Ventricle(s) 9 Sella Turcica/Pituitary Gland B Spinal Cord	Z None	Z None	Z None

SECTION: B IMAGING
BODY SYSTEM: 0 CENTRAL NERVOUS SYSTEM
TYPE: 3 MAGNETIC RESONANCE IMAGING (MRI): Computer reformatted digital display of multiplanar images developed from the capture of radiofrequency signals emitted by nuclei in a body site excited within a magnetic field

Body Part	Contrast	Qualifier	Qualifier
Ø Brain 9 Sella Turcica/Pituitary Gland B Spinal Cord C Acoustic Nerves	Y Other Contrast	Ø Unenhanced and Enhanced Z None	Z None
Ø Brain 9 Sella Turcica/Pituitary Gland B Spinal Cord C Acoustic Nerves	Z None	Z None	Z None

SECTION: B IMAGING
BODY SYSTEM: 0 CENTRAL NERVOUS SYSTEM
TYPE: 4 ULTRASONOGRAPHY: Real time display of images of anatomy or flow information developed from the capture of reflected and attenuated high frequency sound waves

Body Part	Contrast	Qualifier	Qualifier
Ø Brain B Spinal Cord	Z None	Z None	Z None

3; 4

Ø: CENTRAL NERVOUS SYSTEM

B: IMAGING

SECTION: B IMAGING
BODY SYSTEM: 2 HEART
TYPE: Ø **PLAIN RADIOGRAPHY:** Planar display of an image developed from the capture of external ionizing radiation on photographic or photoconductive plate

Body Part	Contrast	Qualifier	Qualifier
Ø Coronary Artery, Single 1 Coronary Arteries, Multiple 2 Coronary Artery Bypass Graft, Single 3 Coronary Artery Bypass Grafts, Multiple 4 Heart, Right 5 Heart, Left 6 Heart, Right and Left 7 Internal Mammary Bypass Graft, Right 8 Internal Mammary Bypass Graft, Left F Bypass Graft, Other	Ø High Osmolar 1 Low Osmolar Y Other Contrast	Z None	Z None

SECTION: B IMAGING
BODY SYSTEM: 2 HEART
TYPE: 1 **FLUOROSCOPY:** Single plane or bi-plane real time display of an image developed from the capture of external ionizing radiation on a fluorescent screen. The image may also be stored by either digital or analog means

Body Part	Contrast	Qualifier	Qualifier
Ø Coronary Artery, Single 1 Coronary Arteries, Multiple 2 Coronary Artery Bypass Graft, Single 3 Coronary Artery Bypass Grafts, Multiple	Ø High Osmolar 1 Low Osmolar Y Other Contrast	1 Laser	Ø Intraoperative
Ø Coronary Artery, Single 1 Coronary Arteries, Multiple 2 Coronary Artery Bypass Graft, Single 3 Coronary Artery Bypass Grafts, Multiple	Ø High Osmolar 1 Low Osmolar Y Other Contrast	Z None	Z None
4 Heart, Right 5 Heart, Left 6 Heart, Right and Left 7 Internal Mammary Bypass Graft, Right 8 Internal Mammary Bypass Graft, Left F Bypass Graft, Other	Ø High Osmolar 1 Low Osmolar Y Other Contrast	Z None	Z None

B: IMAGING 2: HEART Ø: PLAIN RADIOGRAPHY 1: FLUOROSCOPY

3: MAGNETIC RESONANCE IMAGING (MRI)   2: COMPUTERIZED TOMOGRAPHY (CT SCAN)   2: HEART   B: IMAGING

SECTION: B IMAGING

BODY SYSTEM: 2 HEART

TYPE: 2 **COMPUTERIZED TOMOGRAPHY (CT SCAN):** Computer reformatted digital display of multiplanar images developed from the capture of multiple exposures of external ionizing radiation

Body Part	Contrast	Qualifier	Qualifier
1 Coronary Arteries, Multiple 3 Coronary Artery Bypass Grafts, Multiple 6 Heart, Right and Left	Ø High Osmolar 1 Low Osmolar Y Other Contrast	Ø Unenhanced and Enhanced Z None	Z None
1 Coronary Arteries, Multiple 3 Coronary Artery Bypass Grafts, Multiple 6 Heart, Right and Left	Z None	2 Intravascular Optical Coherence Z None	Z None

SECTION: B IMAGING

BODY SYSTEM: 2 HEART

TYPE: 3 **MAGNETIC RESONANCE IMAGING (MRI):** Computer reformatted digital display of multiplanar images developed from the capture of radiofrequency signals emitted by nuclei in a body site excited within a magnetic field

Body Part	Contrast	Qualifier	Qualifier
1 Coronary Arteries, Multiple 3 Coronary Artery Bypass Grafts, Multiple 6 Heart, Right and Left	Y Other Contrast	Ø Unenhanced and Enhanced Z None	Z None
1 Coronary Arteries, Multiple 3 Coronary Artery Bypass Grafts, Multiple 6 Heart, Right and Left	Z None	Z None	Z None

SECTION: B IMAGING
BODY SYSTEM: 2 HEART
TYPE: 4 **ULTRASONOGRAPHY:** Real time display of images of anatomy or flow information developed from the capture of reflected and attenuated high frequency sound waves

Body Part	Contrast	Qualifier	Qualifier
Ø Coronary Artery, Single 1 Coronary Arteries, Multiple 4 Heart, Right 5 Heart, Left 6 Heart, Right and Left B Heart with Aorta C Pericardium D Pediatric Heart	Y Other Contrast	Z None	Z None
Ø Coronary Artery, Single 1 Coronary Arteries, Multiple 4 Heart, Right 5 Heart, Left 6 Heart, Right and Left B Heart with Aorta C Pericardium D Pediatric Heart	Z None	Z None	3 Intravascular 4 Transesophageal Z None

SECTION: B IMAGING
BODY SYSTEM: 3 UPPER ARTERIES
TYPE: Ø **PLAIN RADIOGRAPHY:** Planar display of an image developed from the capture of external ionizing radiation on photographic or photoconductive plate

Body Part	Contrast	Qualifier	Qualifier
Ø Thoracic Aorta	Ø High Osmolar	Z None	Z None
1 Brachiocephalic-Subclavian Artery, Right	1 Low Osmolar		
2 Subclavian Artery, Left	Y Other Contrast		
3 Common Carotid Artery, Right	Z None		
4 Common Carotid Artery, Left			
5 Common Carotid Arteries, Bilateral			
6 Internal Carotid Artery, Right			
7 Internal Carotid Artery, Left			
8 Internal Carotid Arteries, Bilateral			
9 External Carotid Artery, Right			
B External Carotid Artery, Left			
C External Carotid Arteries, Bilateral			
D Vertebral Artery, Right			
F Vertebral Artery, Left			
G Vertebral Arteries, Bilateral			
H Upper Extremity Arteries, Right			
J Upper Extremity Arteries, Left			
K Upper Extremity Arteries, Bilateral			
L Intercostal and Bronchial Arteries			
M Spinal Arteries			
N Upper Arteries, Other			
P Thoraco-Abdominal Aorta			
Q Cervico-Cerebral Arch			
R Intracranial Arteries			
S Pulmonary Artery, Right			
T Pulmonary Artery, Left			

Ø: PLAIN RADIOGRAPHY

3: UPPER ARTERIES

B: IMAGING

SECTION: **B IMAGING**
BODY SYSTEM: **3   UPPER ARTERIES**
TYPE: **1   FLUOROSCOPY:** *(on multiple pages)*
Single plane or bi-plane real time display of an image developed from the capture of external ionizing radiation on a fluorescent screen. The image may also be stored by either digital or analog means

Body Part	Contrast	Qualifier	Qualifier
Ø Thoracic Aorta	Ø High Osmolar	1 Laser	Ø Intraoperative
1 Brachiocephalic-Subclavian Artery, Right	1 Low Osmolar		
2 Subclavian Artery, Left	Y Other Contrast		
3 Common Carotid Artery, Right			
4 Common Carotid Artery, Left			
5 Common Carotid Arteries, Bilateral			
6 Internal Carotid Artery, Right			
7 Internal Carotid Artery, Left			
8 Internal Carotid Arteries, Bilateral			
9 External Carotid Artery, Right			
B External Carotid Artery, Left			
C External Carotid Arteries, Bilateral			
D Vertebral Artery, Right			
F Vertebral Artery, Left			
G Vertebral Arteries, Bilateral			
H Upper Extremity Arteries, Right			
J Upper Extremity Arteries, Left			
K Upper Extremity Arteries, Bilateral			
L Intercostal and Bronchial Arteries			
M Spinal Arteries			
N Upper Arteries, Other			
P Thoraco-Abdominal Aorta			
Q Cervico-Cerebral Arch			
R Intracranial Arteries			
S Pulmonary Artery, Right			
T Pulmonary Artery, Left			
U Pulmonary Trunk			

B: IMAGING   3: UPPER ARTERIES   1: FLUOROSCOPY

SECTION: B IMAGING
BODY SYSTEM: 3 UPPER ARTERIES
TYPE: 1 FLUOROSCOPY: *(continued)*

Single plane or bi-plane real time display of an image developed from the capture of external ionizing radiation on a fluorescent screen. The image may also be stored by either digital or analog means

Body Part	Contrast	Qualifier	Qualifier
Ø Thoracic Aorta	Ø High Osmolar	Z None	Z None
1 Brachiocephalic-Subclavian Artery, Right	1 Low Osmolar		
2 Subclavian Artery, Left	Y Other Contrast		
3 Common Carotid Artery, Right			
4 Common Carotid Artery, Left			
5 Common Carotid Arteries, Bilateral			
6 Internal Carotid Artery, Right			
7 Internal Carotid Artery, Left			
8 Internal Carotid Arteries, Bilateral			
9 External Carotid Artery, Right			
B External Carotid Artery, Left			
C External Carotid Arteries, Bilateral			
D Vertebral Artery, Right			
F Vertebral Artery, Left			
G Vertebral Arteries, Bilateral			
H Upper Extremity Arteries, Right			
J Upper Extremity Arteries, Left			
K Upper Extremity Arteries, Bilateral			
L Intercostal and Bronchial Arteries			
M Spinal Arteries			
N Upper Arteries, Other			
P Thoraco-Abdominal Aorta			
Q Cervico-Cerebral Arch			
R Intracranial Arteries			
S Pulmonary Artery, Right			
T Pulmonary Artery, Left			
U Pulmonary Trunk			

1: FLUOROSCOPY

3: UPPER ARTERIES

B: IMAGING

New/Revised Text in Blue   ~~deleted~~ Deleted

SECTION: **B IMAGING**
BODY SYSTEM: **3 UPPER ARTERIES**
TYPE: **1 FLUOROSCOPY:** *(continued)*

Single plane or bi-plane real time display of an image developed from the capture of external ionizing radiation on a fluorescent screen. The image may also be stored by either digital or analog means

Body Part	Contrast	Qualifier	Qualifier
Ø Thoracic Aorta	Z None	Z None	Z None
1 Brachiocephalic-Subclavian Artery, Right			
2 Subclavian Artery, Left			
3 Common Carotid Artery, Right			
4 Common Carotid Artery, Left			
5 Common Carotid Arteries, Bilateral			
6 Internal Carotid Artery, Right			
7 Internal Carotid Artery, Left			
8 Internal Carotid Arteries, Bilateral			
9 External Carotid Artery, Right			
B External Carotid Artery, Left			
C External Carotid Arteries, Bilateral			
D Vertebral Artery, Right			
F Vertebral Artery, Left			
G Vertebral Arteries, Bilateral			
H Upper Extremity Arteries, Right			
J Upper Extremity Arteries, Left			
K Upper Extremity Arteries, Bilateral			
L Intercostal and Bronchial Arteries			
M Spinal Arteries			
N Upper Arteries, Other			
P Thoraco-Abdominal Aorta			
Q Cervico-Cerebral Arch			
R Intracranial Arteries			
S Pulmonary Artery, Right			
T Pulmonary Artery, Left			
U Pulmonary Trunk			

SECTION: **B IMAGING**
BODY SYSTEM: **3 UPPER ARTERIES**
TYPE: **2 COMPUTERIZED TOMOGRAPHY (CT SCAN):** Computer reformatted digital display of multiplanar images developed from the capture of multiple exposures of external ionizing radiation

Body Part	Contrast	Qualifier	Qualifier
Ø Thoracic Aorta	Ø High Osmolar	Z None	Z None
5 Common Carotid Arteries, Bilateral	1 Low Osmolar		
8 Internal Carotid Arteries, Bilateral	Y Other Contrast		
G Vertebral Arteries, Bilateral			
R Intracranial Arteries			
S Pulmonary Artery, Right			
T Pulmonary Artery, Left			
Ø Thoracic Aorta	Z None	2 Intravascular Optical Coherence	Z None
5 Common Carotid Arteries, Bilateral		Z None	
8 Internal Carotid Arteries, Bilateral			
G Vertebral Arteries, Bilateral			
R Intracranial Arteries			
S Pulmonary Artery, Right			
T Pulmonary Artery, Left			

SECTION: B IMAGING
BODY SYSTEM: 3 UPPER ARTERIES
TYPE: 3 **MAGNETIC RESONANCE IMAGING (MRI):** Computer reformatted digital display of multiplanar images developed from the capture of radiofrequency signals emitted by nuclei in a body site excited within a magnetic field

Body Part	Contrast	Qualifier	Qualifier
Ø Thoracic Aorta 5 Common Carotid Arteries, Bilateral 8 Internal Carotid Arteries, Bilateral G Vertebral Arteries, Bilateral H Upper Extremity Arteries, Right J Upper Extremity Arteries, Left K Upper Extremity Arteries, Bilateral M Spinal Arteries Q Cervico-Cerebral Arch R Intracranial Arteries	Y Other Contrast	Ø Unenhanced and Enhanced Z None	Z None
Ø Thoracic Aorta 5 Common Carotid Arteries, Bilateral 8 Internal Carotid Arteries, Bilateral G Vertebral Arteries, Bilateral H Upper Extremity Arteries, Right J Upper Extremity Arteries, Left K Upper Extremity Arteries, Bilateral M Spinal Arteries Q Cervico-Cerebral Arch R Intracranial Arteries	Z None	Z None	Z None

SECTION: B IMAGING
BODY SYSTEM: 3 UPPER ARTERIES
TYPE: 4 **ULTRASONOGRAPHY:** Real time display of images of anatomy or flow information developed from the capture of reflected and attenuated high frequency sound waves

Body Part	Contrast	Qualifier	Qualifier
Ø Thoracic Aorta 1 Brachiocephalic-Subclavian Artery, Right 2 Subclavian Artery, Left 3 Common Carotid Artery, Right 4 Common Carotid Artery, Left 5 Common Carotid Arteries, Bilateral 6 Internal Carotid Artery, Right 7 Internal Carotid Artery, Left 8 Internal Carotid Arteries, Bilateral H Upper Extremity Arteries, Right J Upper Extremity Arteries, Left K Upper Extremity Arteries, Bilateral R Intracranial Arteries S Pulmonary Artery, Right T Pulmonary Artery, Left V Ophthalmic Arteries	Z None	Z None	3 Intravascular Z None

New/Revised Text in Blue   ~~deleted~~ Deleted

SECTION: B IMAGING
BODY SYSTEM: 4 LOWER ARTERIES
TYPE: Ø PLAIN RADIOGRAPHY: Planar display of an image developed from the capture of external ionizing radiation on photographic or photoconductive plate

Body Part	Contrast	Qualifier	Qualifier
Ø Abdominal Aorta	Ø High Osmolar	Z None	Z None
2 Hepatic Artery	1 Low Osmolar		
3 Splenic Arteries	Y Other Contrast		
4 Superior Mesenteric Artery			
5 Inferior Mesenteric Artery			
6 Renal Artery, Right			
7 Renal Artery, Left			
8 Renal Arteries, Bilateral			
9 Lumbar Arteries			
B Intra-Abdominal Arteries, Other			
C Pelvic Arteries			
D Aorta and Bilateral Lower Extremity Arteries			
F Lower Extremity Arteries, Right			
G Lower Extremity Arteries, Left			
J Lower Arteries, Other			
M Renal Artery Transplant			

SECTION: B IMAGING
BODY SYSTEM: 4 LOWER ARTERIES
TYPE: 1 **FLUOROSCOPY:** Single plane or bi-plane real time display of an image developed from the capture of external ionizing radiation on a fluorescent screen. The image may also be stored by either digital or analog means

Body Part	Contrast	Qualifier	Qualifier
Ø Abdominal Aorta 2 Hepatic Artery 3 Splenic Arteries 4 Superior Mesenteric Artery 5 Inferior Mesenteric Artery 6 Renal Artery, Right 7 Renal Artery, Left 8 Renal Arteries, Bilateral 9 Lumbar Arteries B Intra-Abdominal Arteries, Other C Pelvic Arteries D Aorta and Bilateral Lower Extremity Arteries F Lower Extremity Arteries, Right G Lower Extremity Arteries, Left J Lower Arteries, Other	Ø High Osmolar 1 Low Osmolar Y Other Contrast	1 Laser	Ø Intraoperative
Ø Abdominal Aorta 2 Hepatic Artery 3 Splenic Arteries 4 Superior Mesenteric Artery 5 Inferior Mesenteric Artery 6 Renal Artery, Right 7 Renal Artery, Left 8 Renal Arteries, Bilateral 9 Lumbar Arteries B Intra-Abdominal Arteries, Other C Pelvic Arteries D Aorta and Bilateral Lower Extremity Arteries F Lower Extremity Arteries, Right G Lower Extremity Arteries, Left J Lower Arteries, Other	Ø High Osmolar 1 Low Osmolar Y Other Contrast	Z None	Z None
Ø Abdominal Aorta 2 Hepatic Artery 3 Splenic Arteries 4 Superior Mesenteric Artery 5 Inferior Mesenteric Artery 6 Renal Artery, Right 7 Renal Artery, Left 8 Renal Arteries, Bilateral 9 Lumbar Arteries B Intra-Abdominal Arteries, Other C Pelvic Arteries D Aorta and Bilateral Lower Extremity Arteries F Lower Extremity Arteries, Right G Lower Extremity Arteries, Left J Lower Arteries, Other	Z None	Z None	Z None

1: FLUOROSCOPY

4: LOWER ARTERIES

B: IMAGING

New/Revised Text in Blue ~~deleted~~ Deleted

SECTION: B IMAGING
BODY SYSTEM: 4 LOWER ARTERIES
TYPE: 2 COMPUTERIZED TOMOGRAPHY (CT SCAN): Computer reformatted digital display of multiplanar images developed from the capture of multiple exposures of external ionizing radiation

Body Part	Contrast	Qualifier	Qualifier
Ø Abdominal Aorta 1 Celiac Artery 4 Superior Mesenteric Artery 8 Renal Arteries, Bilateral C Pelvic Arteries F Lower Extremity Arteries, Right G Lower Extremity Arteries, Left H Lower Extremity Arteries, Bilateral M Renal Artery Transplant	Ø High Osmolar 1 Low Osmolar Y Other Contrast	Z None	Z None
Ø Abdominal Aorta 1 Celiac Artery 4 Superior Mesenteric Artery 8 Renal Arteries, Bilateral C Pelvic Arteries F Lower Extremity Arteries, Right G Lower Extremity Arteries, Left H Lower Extremity Arteries, Bilateral M Renal Artery Transplant	Z None	2 Intravascular Optical Coherence Z None	Z None

SECTION: B IMAGING
BODY SYSTEM: 4 LOWER ARTERIES
TYPE: 3 MAGNETIC RESONANCE IMAGING (MRI): Computer reformatted digital display of multiplanar images developed from the capture of radiofrequency signals emitted by nuclei in a body site excited within a magnetic field

Body Part	Contrast	Qualifier	Qualifier
Ø Abdominal Aorta 1 Celiac Artery 4 Superior Mesenteric Artery 8 Renal Arteries, Bilateral C Pelvic Arteries F Lower Extremity Arteries, Right G Lower Extremity Arteries, Left H Lower Extremity Arteries, Bilateral	Y Other Contrast	Ø Unenhanced and Enhanced Z None	Z None
Ø Abdominal Aorta 1 Celiac Artery 4 Superior Mesenteric Artery 8 Renal Arteries, Bilateral C Pelvic Arteries F Lower Extremity Arteries, Right G Lower Extremity Arteries, Left H Lower Extremity Arteries, Bilateral	Z None	Z None	Z None

B: IMAGING

4: LOWER ARTERIES

2: COMPUTERIZED TOMOGRAPHY

3: MAGNETIC RESONANCE IMAGING

SECTION: B IMAGING
BODY SYSTEM: 4 **LOWER ARTERIES**
TYPE: 4 **ULTRASONOGRAPHY:** Real time display of images of anatomy or flow information developed from the capture of reflected and attenuated high frequency sound waves

Body Part	Contrast	Qualifier	Qualifier
Ø Abdominal Aorta 4 Superior Mesenteric Artery 5 Inferior Mesenteric Artery 6 Renal Artery, Right 7 Renal Artery, Left 8 Renal Arteries, Bilateral B Intra-Abdominal Arteries, Other F Lower Extremity Arteries, Right G Lower Extremity Arteries, Left H Lower Extremity Arteries, Bilateral K Celiac and Mesenteric Arteries L Femoral Artery N Penile Arteries	Z None	Z None	3 Intravascular Z None

SECTION: B IMAGING
BODY SYSTEM: 5 VEINS
TYPE: Ø PLAIN RADIOGRAPHY: Planar display of an image developed from the capture of external ionizing radiation on photographic or photoconductive plate

Body Part	Contrast	Qualifier	Qualifier
Ø Epidural Veins	Ø High Osmolar	Z None	Z None
1 Cerebral and Cerebellar Veins	1 Low Osmolar		
2 Intracranial Sinuses	Y Other Contrast		
3 Jugular Veins, Right			
4 Jugular Veins, Left			
5 Jugular Veins, Bilateral			
6 Subclavian Vein, Right			
7 Subclavian Vein, Left			
8 Superior Vena Cava			
9 Inferior Vena Cava			
B Lower Extremity Veins, Right			
C Lower Extremity Veins, Left			
D Lower Extremity Veins, Bilateral			
F Pelvic (Iliac) Veins, Right			
G Pelvic (Iliac) Veins, Left			
H Pelvic (Iliac) Veins, Bilateral			
J Renal Vein, Right			
K Renal Vein, Left			
L Renal Veins, Bilateral			
M Upper Extremity Veins, Right			
N Upper Extremity Veins, Left			
P Upper Extremity Veins, Bilateral			
Q Pulmonary Vein, Right			
R Pulmonary Vein, Left			
S Pulmonary Veins, Bilateral			
T Portal and Splanchnic Veins			
V Veins, Other			
W Dialysis Shunt/Fistula			

B: IMAGING

5: VEINS

Ø: PLAIN RADIOGRAPHY

SECTION: B IMAGING
BODY SYSTEM: 5   VEINS
TYPE: 1   FLUOROSCOPY: Single plane or bi-plane real time display of an image developed from the capture of external ionizing radiation on a fluorescent screen. The image may also be stored by either digital or analog means

Body Part	Contrast	Qualifier	Qualifier
Ø Epidural Veins	Ø High Osmolar	Z None	A Guidance
1 Cerebral and Cerebellar Veins	1 Low Osmolar		Z None
2 Intracranial Sinuses	Y Other Contrast		
3 Jugular Veins, Right	Z None		
4 Jugular Veins, Left			
5 Jugular Veins, Bilateral			
6 Subclavian Vein, Right			
7 Subclavian Vein, Left			
8 Superior Vena Cava			
9 Inferior Vena Cava			
B Lower Extremity Veins, Right			
C Lower Extremity Veins, Left			
D Lower Extremity Veins, Bilateral			
F Pelvic (Iliac) Veins, Right			
G Pelvic (Iliac) Veins, Left			
H Pelvic (Iliac) Veins, Bilateral			
J Renal Vein, Right			
K Renal Vein, Left			
L Renal Veins, Bilateral			
M Upper Extremity Veins, Right			
N Upper Extremity Veins, Left			
P Upper Extremity Veins, Bilateral			
Q Pulmonary Vein, Right			
R Pulmonary Vein, Left			
S Pulmonary Veins, Bilateral			
T Portal and Splanchnic Veins			
V Veins, Other			
W Dialysis Shunt/Fistula			

1: FLUOROSCOPY

5: VEINS

B: IMAGING

SECTION: B IMAGING
BODY SYSTEM: 5 **VEINS**
TYPE: 2 **COMPUTERIZED TOMOGRAPHY (CT SCAN):** Computer reformatted digital display of multiplanar images developed from the capture of multiple exposures of external ionizing radiation

Body Part	Contrast	Qualifier	Qualifier
2 Intracranial Sinuses 8 Superior Vena Cava 9 Inferior Vena Cava F Pelvic (Iliac) Veins, Right G Pelvic (Iliac) Veins, Left H Pelvic (Iliac) Veins, Bilateral J Renal Vein, Right K Renal Vein, Left L Renal Veins, Bilateral Q Pulmonary Vein, Right R Pulmonary Vein, Left S Pulmonary Veins, Bilateral T Portal and Splanchnic Veins	Ø High Osmolar 1 Low Osmolar Y Other Contrast	Ø Unenhanced and Enhanced Z None	Z None
2 Intracranial Sinuses 8 Superior Vena Cava 9 Inferior Vena Cava F Pelvic (Iliac) Veins, Right G Pelvic (Iliac) Veins, Left H Pelvic (Iliac) Veins, Bilateral J Renal Vein, Right K Renal Vein, Left L Renal Veins, Bilateral Q Pulmonary Vein, Right R Pulmonary Vein, Left S Pulmonary Veins, Bilateral T Portal and Splanchnic Veins	Z None	2 Intravascular Optical Coherence Z None	Z None

SECTION: B IMAGING
BODY SYSTEM: 5 **VEINS**
TYPE: 3 **MAGNETIC RESONANCE IMAGING (MRI):** Computer reformatted digital display of multiplanar images developed from the capture of radiofrequency signals emitted by nuclei in a body site excited within a magnetic field

Body Part	Contrast	Qualifier	Qualifier
1 Cerebral and Cerebellar Veins 2 Intracranial Sinuses 5 Jugular Veins, Bilateral 8 Superior Vena Cava 9 Inferior Vena Cava B Lower Extremity Veins, Right C Lower Extremity Veins, Left D Lower Extremity Veins, Bilateral H Pelvic (Iliac) Veins, Bilateral L Renal Veins, Bilateral M Upper Extremity Veins, Right N Upper Extremity Veins, Left P Upper Extremity Veins, Bilateral S Pulmonary Veins, Bilateral T Portal and Splanchnic Veins V Veins, Other	Y Other Contrast	Ø Unenhanced and Enhanced Z None	Z None
1 Cerebral and Cerebellar Veins 2 Intracranial Sinuses 5 Jugular Veins, Bilateral 8 Superior Vena Cava 9 Inferior Vena Cava B Lower Extremity Veins, Right C Lower Extremity Veins, Left D Lower Extremity Veins, Bilateral H Pelvic (Iliac) Veins, Bilateral L Renal Veins, Bilateral M Upper Extremity Veins, Right N Upper Extremity Veins, Left P Upper Extremity Veins, Bilateral S Pulmonary Veins, Bilateral T Portal and Splanchnic Veins V Veins, Other	Z None	Z None	Z None

3: MAGNETIC RESONANCE IMAGING (MRI)   5: VEINS   B: IMAGING

New/Revised Text in Blue   ~~deleted~~ Deleted

SECTION: B IMAGING
BODY SYSTEM: 5 VEINS
TYPE: 4 ULTRASONOGRAPHY: Real time display of images of anatomy or flow information developed from the capture of reflected and attenuated high frequency sound waves

Body Part	Contrast	Qualifier	Qualifier
3 Jugular Veins, Right	Z None	Z None	3 Intravascular
4 Jugular Veins, Left			A Guidance
6 Subclavian Vein, Right			Z None
7 Subclavian Vein, Left			
9 Inferior Vena Cava			
B Lower Extremity Veins, Right			
C Lower Extremity Veins, Left			
D Lower Extremity Veins, Bilateral			
J Renal Vein, Right			
K Renal Vein, Left			
L Renal Veins, Bilateral			
M Upper Extremity Veins, Right			
N Upper Extremity Veins, Left			
P Upper Extremity Veins, Bilateral			
T Portal and Splanchnic Veins			

B: IMAGING

5: VEINS

4: ULTRASONOGRAPHY

SECTION: B IMAGING
BODY SYSTEM: 7 **LYMPHATIC SYSTEM**
TYPE: Ø **PLAIN RADIOGRAPHY:** Planar display of an image developed from the capture of external ionizing radiation on photographic or photoconductive plate

Body Part	Contrast	Qualifier	Qualifier
Ø Abdominal/Retroperitoneal Lymphatics, Unilateral 1 Abdominal/Retroperitoneal Lymphatics, Bilateral 4 Lymphatics, Head and Neck 5 Upper Extremity Lymphatics, Right 6 Upper Extremity Lymphatics, Left 7 Upper Extremity Lymphatics, Bilateral 8 Lower Extremity Lymphatics, Right 9 Lower Extremity Lymphatics, Left B Lower Extremity Lymphatics, Bilateral C Lymphatics, Pelvic	Ø High Osmolar 1 Low Osmolar Y Other Contrast	Z None	Z None

New/Revised Text in Blue   ~~deleted~~ Deleted

SECTION: B IMAGING
BODY SYSTEM: 8 EYE
TYPE: Ø **PLAIN RADIOGRAPHY:** Planar display of an image developed from the capture of external ionizing radiation on photographic or photoconductive plate

Body Part	Contrast	Qualifier	Qualifier
Ø Lacrimal Duct, Right 1 Lacrimal Duct, Left 2 Lacrimal Ducts, Bilateral	Ø High Osmolar 1 Low Osmolar Y Other Contrast	Z None	Z None
3 Optic Foramina, Right 4 Optic Foramina, Left 5 Eye, Right 6 Eye, Left 7 Eyes, Bilateral	Z None	Z None	Z None

SECTION: B IMAGING
BODY SYSTEM: 8 EYE
TYPE: 2 **COMPUTERIZED TOMOGRAPHY (CT SCAN):** Computer reformatted digital display of multiplanar images developed from the capture of multiple exposures of external ionizing radiation

Body Part	Contrast	Qualifier	Qualifier
5 Eye, Right 6 Eye, Left 7 Eyes, Bilateral	Ø High Osmolar 1 Low Osmolar Y Other Contrast	Ø Unenhanced and Enhanced Z None	Z None
5 Eye, Right 6 Eye, Left 7 Eyes, Bilateral	Z None	Z None	Z None

SECTION: B IMAGING
BODY SYSTEM: 8 EYE
TYPE: 3 **MAGNETIC RESONANCE IMAGING (MRI):** Computer reformatted digital display of multiplanar images developed from the capture of radiofrequency signals emitted by nuclei in a body site excited within a magnetic field

Body Part	Contrast	Qualifier	Qualifier
5 Eye, Right 6 Eye, Left 7 Eyes, Bilateral	Y Other Contrast	Ø Unenhanced and Enhanced Z None	Z None
5 Eye, Right 6 Eye, Left 7 Eyes, Bilateral	Z None	Z None	Z None

SECTION: B IMAGING
BODY SYSTEM: 8 EYE
TYPE: 4 **ULTRASONOGRAPHY:** Real time display of images of anatomy or flow information developed from the capture of reflected and attenuated high frequency sound waves

Body Part	Contrast	Qualifier	Qualifier
5 Eye, Right 6 Eye, Left 7 Eyes, Bilateral	Z None	Z None	Z None

SECTION: B IMAGING
BODY SYSTEM: 9 **EAR, NOSE, MOUTH, AND THROAT**
TYPE: Ø **PLAIN RADIOGRAPHY:** Planar display of an image developed from the capture of external ionizing radiation on photographic or photoconductive plate

Body Part	Contrast	Qualifier	Qualifier
2 Paranasal Sinuses F Nasopharynx/Oropharynx H Mastoids	Z None	Z None	Z None
4 Parotid Gland, Right 5 Parotid Gland, Left 6 Parotid Glands, Bilateral 7 Submandibular Gland, Right 8 Submandibular Gland, Left 9 Submandibular Glands, Bilateral B Salivary Gland, Right C Salivary Gland, Left D Salivary Glands, Bilateral	Ø High Osmolar 1 Low Osmolar Y Other Contrast	Z None	Z None

SECTION: B IMAGING
BODY SYSTEM: 9 **EAR, NOSE, MOUTH, AND THROAT**
TYPE: 1 **FLUOROSCOPY:** Single plane or bi-plane real time display of an image developed from the capture of external ionizing radiation on a fluorescent screen. The image may also be stored by either digital or analog means

Body Part	Contrast	Qualifier	Qualifier
G Pharynx and Epiglottis J Larynx	Y Other Contrast Z None	Z None	Z None

SECTION: B IMAGING
BODY SYSTEM: 9 EAR, NOSE, MOUTH, AND THROAT
TYPE: 2 COMPUTERIZED TOMOGRAPHY (CT SCAN): Computer reformatted digital display of multiplanar images developed from the capture of multiple exposures of external ionizing radiation

Body Part	Contrast	Qualifier	Qualifier
Ø Ear 2 Paranasal Sinuses 6 Parotid Glands, Bilateral 9 Submandibular Glands, Bilateral D Salivary Glands, Bilateral F Nasopharynx/Oropharynx J Larynx	Ø High Osmolar 1 Low Osmolar Y Other Contrast	Ø Unenhanced and Enhanced Z None	Z None
Ø Ear 2 Paranasal Sinuses 6 Parotid Glands, Bilateral 9 Submandibular Glands, Bilateral D Salivary Glands, Bilateral F Nasopharynx/Oropharynx J Larynx	Z None	Z None	Z None

SECTION: B IMAGING
BODY SYSTEM: 9 EAR, NOSE, MOUTH, AND THROAT
TYPE: 3 MAGNETIC RESONANCE IMAGING (MRI): Computer reformatted digital display of multiplanar images developed from the capture of radiofrequency signals emitted by nuclei in a body site excited within a magnetic field

Body Part	Contrast	Qualifier	Qualifier
Ø Ear 2 Paranasal Sinuses 6 Parotid Glands, Bilateral 9 Submandibular Glands, Bilateral D Salivary Glands, Bilateral F Nasopharynx/Oropharynx J Larynx	Y Other Contrast	Ø Unenhanced and Enhanced Z None	Z None
Ø Ear 2 Paranasal Sinuses 6 Parotid Glands, Bilateral 9 Submandibular Glands, Bilateral D Salivary Glands, Bilateral F Nasopharynx/Oropharynx J Larynx	Z None	Z None	Z None

SECTION: B IMAGING
BODY SYSTEM: B RESPIRATORY SYSTEM
TYPE: Ø PLAIN RADIOGRAPHY: Planar display of an image developed from the capture of external ionizing radiation on photographic or photoconductive plate

Body Part	Contrast	Qualifier	Qualifier
7 Tracheobronchial Tree, Right 8 Tracheobronchial Tree, Left 9 Tracheobronchial Trees, Bilateral	Y Other Contrast	Z None	Z None
D Upper Airways	Z None	Z None	Z None

SECTION: B IMAGING
BODY SYSTEM: B RESPIRATORY SYSTEM
TYPE: 1 FLUOROSCOPY: Single plane or bi-plane real time display of an image developed from the capture of external ionizing radiation on a fluorescent screen. The image may also be stored by either digital or analog means

Body Part	Contrast	Qualifier	Qualifier
2 Lung, Right 3 Lung, Left 4 Lungs, Bilateral 6 Diaphragm C Mediastinum D Upper Airways	Z None	Z None	Z None
7 Tracheobronchial Tree, Right 8 Tracheobronchial Tree, Left 9 Tracheobronchial Trees, Bilateral	Y Other Contrast	Z None	Z None

SECTION: B IMAGING
BODY SYSTEM: B RESPIRATORY SYSTEM
TYPE: 2 COMPUTERIZED TOMOGRAPHY (CT SCAN): Computer reformatted digital display of multiplanar images developed from the capture of multiple exposures of external ionizing radiation

Body Part	Contrast	Qualifier	Qualifier
4 Lungs, Bilateral 7 Tracheobronchial Tree, Right 8 Tracheobronchial Tree, Left 9 Tracheobronchial Trees, Bilateral F Trachea/Airways	Ø High Osmolar 1 Low Osmolar Y Other Contrast	Ø Unenhanced and Enhanced Z None	Z None
4 Lungs, Bilateral 7 Tracheobronchial Tree, Right 8 Tracheobronchial Tree, Left 9 Tracheobronchial Trees, Bilateral F Trachea/Airways	Z None	Z None	Z None

SECTION: B IMAGING
BODY SYSTEM: B RESPIRATORY SYSTEM
TYPE: 3 MAGNETIC RESONANCE IMAGING (MRI): Computer reformatted digital display of multiplanar images developed from the capture of radiofrequency signals emitted by nuclei in a body site excited within a magnetic field

Body Part	Contrast	Qualifier	Qualifier
G Lung Apices	Y Other Contrast	Ø Unenhanced and Enhanced Z None	Z None
G Lung Apices	Z None	Z None	Z None

SECTION: B IMAGING
BODY SYSTEM: B RESPIRATORY SYSTEM
TYPE: 4 ULTRASONOGRAPHY: Real time display of images of anatomy or flow information developed from the capture of reflected and attenuated high frequency sound waves

Body Part	Contrast	Qualifier	Qualifier
B Pleura C Mediastinum	Z None	Z None	Z None

SECTION: B IMAGING
BODY SYSTEM: D GASTROINTESTINAL SYSTEM
TYPE: 1 **FLUOROSCOPY:** Single plane or bi-plane real time display of an image developed from the capture of external ionizing radiation on a fluorescent screen. The image may also be stored by either digital or analog means

Body Part	Contrast	Qualifier	Qualifier
1 Esophagus 2 Stomach 3 Small Bowel 4 Colon 5 Upper GI 6 Upper GI and Small Bowel 9 Duodenum B Mouth/Oropharynx	Y Other Contrast Z None	Z None	Z None

SECTION: B IMAGING
BODY SYSTEM: D GASTROINTESTINAL SYSTEM
TYPE: 2 **COMPUTERIZED TOMOGRAPHY (CT SCAN):** Computer reformatted digital display of multiplanar images developed from the capture of multiple exposures of external ionizing radiation

Body Part	Contrast	Qualifier	Qualifier
4 Colon	Ø High Osmolar 1 Low Osmolar Y Other Contrast	Ø Unenhanced and Enhanced Z None	Z None
4 Colon	Z None	Z None	Z None

SECTION: B IMAGING
BODY SYSTEM: D GASTROINTESTINAL SYSTEM
TYPE: 4 **ULTRASONOGRAPHY:** Real time display of images of anatomy or flow information developed from the capture of reflected and attenuated high frequency sound waves

Body Part	Contrast	Qualifier	Qualifier
1 Esophagus 2 Stomach 7 Gastrointestinal Tract 8 Appendix 9 Duodenum C Rectum	Z None	Z None	Z None

B: IMAGING   D: GASTROINTESTINAL SYSTEM   1: FLUOROSCOPY   2: CT SCAN   4: ULTRASONOGRAPHY

SECTION: B IMAGING
BODY SYSTEM: F HEPATOBILIARY SYSTEM AND PANCREAS
TYPE: Ø PLAIN RADIOGRAPHY: Planar display of an image developed from the capture of external ionizing radiation on photographic or photoconductive plate

Body Part	Contrast	Qualifier	Qualifier
Ø Bile Ducts 3 Gallbladder and Bile Ducts C Hepatobiliary System, All	Ø High Osmolar 1 Low Osmolar Y Other Contrast	Z None	Z None

SECTION: B IMAGING
BODY SYSTEM: F HEPATOBILIARY SYSTEM AND PANCREAS
TYPE: 1 FLUOROSCOPY: Single plane or bi-plane real time display of an image developed from the capture of external ionizing radiation on a fluorescent screen. The image may also be stored by either digital or analog means

Body Part	Contrast	Qualifier	Qualifier
Ø Bile Ducts 1 Biliary and Pancreatic Ducts 2 Gallbladder 3 Gallbladder and Bile Ducts 4 Gallbladder, Bile Ducts, and Pancreatic Ducts 8 Pancreatic Ducts	Ø High Osmolar 1 Low Osmolar Y Other Contrast	Z None	Z None

SECTION: B IMAGING
BODY SYSTEM: F HEPATOBILIARY SYSTEM AND PANCREAS
TYPE: 2 **COMPUTERIZED TOMOGRAPHY (CT SCAN):** Computer reformatted digital display of multiplanar images developed from the capture of multiple exposures of external ionizing radiation

Body Part	Contrast	Qualifier	Qualifier
5 Liver 6 Liver and Spleen 7 Pancreas C Hepatobiliary System, All	Ø High Osmolar 1 Low Osmolar Y Other Contrast	Ø Unenhanced and Enhanced Z None	Z None
5 Liver 6 Liver and Spleen 7 Pancreas C Hepatobiliary System, All	Z None	Z None	Z None

SECTION: B IMAGING
BODY SYSTEM: F HEPATOBILIARY SYSTEM AND PANCREAS
TYPE: 3 **MAGNETIC RESONANCE IMAGING (MRI):** Computer reformatted digital display of multiplanar images developed from the capture of radiofrequency signals emitted by nuclei in a body site excited within a magnetic field

Body Part	Contrast	Qualifier	Qualifier
5 Liver 6 Liver and Spleen 7 Pancreas	Y Other Contrast	Ø Unenhanced and Enhanced Z None	Z None
5 Liver 6 Liver and Spleen 7 Pancreas	Z None	Z None	Z None

SECTION: B IMAGING
BODY SYSTEM: F HEPATOBILIARY SYSTEM AND PANCREAS
TYPE: 4 **ULTRASONOGRAPHY:** Real time display of images of anatomy or flow information developed from the capture of reflected and attenuated high frequency sound waves

Body Part	Contrast	Qualifier	Qualifier
Ø Bile Ducts 2 Gallbladder 3 Gallbladder and Bile Ducts 5 Liver 6 Liver and Spleen 7 Pancreas C Hepatobiliary System, All	Z None	Z None	Z None

SECTION: B IMAGING
BODY SYSTEM: G ENDOCRINE SYSTEM
TYPE: 2 **COMPUTERIZED TOMOGRAPHY (CT SCAN):** Computer reformatted digital display of multiplanar images developed from the capture of multiple exposures of external ionizing radiation

Body Part	Contrast	Qualifier	Qualifier
2 Adrenal Glands, Bilateral 3 Parathyroid Glands 4 Thyroid Gland	Ø High Osmolar 1 Low Osmolar Y Other Contrast	Ø Unenhanced and Enhanced Z None	Z None
2 Adrenal Glands, Bilateral 3 Parathyroid Glands 4 Thyroid Gland	Z None	Z None	Z None

SECTION: B IMAGING
BODY SYSTEM: G ENDOCRINE SYSTEM
TYPE: 3 **MAGNETIC RESONANCE IMAGING (MRI):** Computer reformatted digital display of multiplanar images developed from the capture of radiofrequency signals emitted by nuclei in a body site excited within a magnetic field

Body Part	Contrast	Qualifier	Qualifier
2 Adrenal Glands, Bilateral 3 Parathyroid Glands 4 Thyroid Gland	Y Other Contrast	Ø Unenhanced and Enhanced Z None	Z None
2 Adrenal Glands, Bilateral 3 Parathyroid Glands 4 Thyroid Gland	Z None	Z None	Z None

SECTION: B IMAGING
BODY SYSTEM: G ENDOCRINE SYSTEM
TYPE: 4 **ULTRASONOGRAPHY:** Real time display of images of anatomy or flow information developed from the capture of reflected and attenuated high frequency sound waves

Body Part	Contrast	Qualifier	Qualifier
Ø Adrenal Gland, Right 1 Adrenal Gland, Left 2 Adrenal Glands, Bilateral 3 Parathyroid Glands 4 Thyroid Gland	Z None	Z None	Z None

SECTION: B IMAGING
BODY SYSTEM: H SKIN, SUBCUTANEOUS TISSUE AND BREAST
TYPE: Ø **PLAIN RADIOGRAPHY:** Planar display of an image developed from the capture of external ionizing radiation on photographic or photoconductive plate

Body Part	Contrast	Qualifier	Qualifier
Ø Breast, Right 1 Breast, Left 2 Breasts, Bilateral	Z None	Z None	Z None
3 Single Mammary Duct, Right 4 Single Mammary Duct, Left 5 Multiple Mammary Ducts, Right 6 Multiple Mammary Ducts, Left	Ø High Osmolar 1 Low Osmolar Y Other Contrast Z None	Z None	Z None

SECTION: B IMAGING
BODY SYSTEM: H SKIN, SUBCUTANEOUS TISSUE AND BREAST
TYPE: 3 **MAGNETIC RESONANCE IMAGING (MRI):** Computer reformatted digital display of multiplanar images developed from the capture of radiofrequency signals emitted by nuclei in a body site excited within a magnetic field

Body Part	Contrast	Qualifier	Qualifier
Ø Breast, Right 1 Breast, Left 2 Breasts, Bilateral D Subcutaneous Tissue, Head/Neck F Subcutaneous Tissue, Upper Extremity G Subcutaneous Tissue, Thorax H Subcutaneous Tissue, Abdomen and Pelvis J Subcutaneous Tissue, Lower Extremity	Y Other Contrast	Ø Unenhanced and Enhanced Z None	Z None
Ø Breast, Right 1 Breast, Left 2 Breasts, Bilateral D Subcutaneous Tissue, Head/Neck F Subcutaneous Tissue, Upper Extremity G Subcutaneous Tissue, Thorax H Subcutaneous Tissue, Abdomen and Pelvis J Subcutaneous Tissue, Lower Extremity	Z None	Z None	Z None

SECTION: B IMAGING
BODY SYSTEM: H SKIN, SUBCUTANEOUS TISSUE AND BREAST
TYPE: 4 ULTRASONOGRAPHY: Real time display of images of anatomy or flow information developed from the capture of reflected and attenuated high frequency sound waves

Body Part	Contrast	Qualifier	Qualifier
Ø Breast, Right 1 Breast, Left 2 Breasts, Bilateral 7 Extremity, Upper 8 Extremity, Lower 9 Abdominal Wall B Chest Wall C Head and Neck	Z None	Z None	Z None

SECTION: B IMAGING
BODY SYSTEM: L CONNECTIVE TISSUE
TYPE: 3 **MAGNETIC RESONANCE IMAGING (MRI):** Computer reformatted digital display of multiplanar images developed from the capture of radiofrequency signals emitted by nuclei in a body site excited within a magnetic field

Body Part	Contrast	Qualifier	Qualifier
Ø Connective Tissue, Upper Extremity 1 Connective Tissue, Lower Extremity 2 Tendons, Upper Extremity 3 Tendons, Lower Extremity	Y Other Contrast	Ø Unenhanced and Enhanced Z None	Z None
Ø Connective Tissue, Upper Extremity 1 Connective Tissue, Lower Extremity 2 Tendons, Upper Extremity 3 Tendons, Lower Extremity	Z None	Z None	Z None

SECTION: B IMAGING
BODY SYSTEM: L CONNECTIVE TISSUE
TYPE: 4 **ULTRASONOGRAPHY:** Real time display of images of anatomy or flow information developed from the capture of reflected and attenuated high frequency sound waves

Body Part	Contrast	Qualifier	Qualifier
Ø Connective Tissue, Upper Extremity 1 Connective Tissue, Lower Extremity 2 Tendons, Upper Extremity 3 Tendons, Lower Extremity	Z None	Z None	Z None

SECTION: B IMAGING

BODY SYSTEM: N **SKULL AND FACIAL BONES**

TYPE: Ø **PLAIN RADIOGRAPHY:** Planar display of an image developed from the capture of external ionizing radiation on photographic or photoconductive plate

Body Part	Contrast	Qualifier	Qualifier
Ø Skull 1 Orbit, Right 2 Orbit, Left 3 Orbits, Bilateral 4 Nasal Bones 5 Facial Bones 6 Mandible B Zygomatic Arch, Right C Zygomatic Arch, Left D Zygomatic Arches, Bilateral G Tooth, Single H Teeth, Multiple J Teeth, All	Z None	Z None	Z None
7 Temporomandibular Joint, Right 8 Temporomandibular Joint, Left 9 Temporomandibular Joints, Bilateral	Ø High Osmolar 1 Low Osmolar Y Other Contrast Z None	Z None	Z None

SECTION: B IMAGING

BODY SYSTEM: N **SKULL AND FACIAL BONES**

TYPE: 1 **FLUOROSCOPY:** Single plane or bi-plane real time display of an image developed from the capture of external ionizing radiation on a fluorescent screen. The image may also be stored by either digital or analog means

Body Part	Contrast	Qualifier	Qualifier
7 Temporomandibular Joint, Right 8 Temporomandibular Joint, Left 9 Temporomandibular Joints, Bilateral	Ø High Osmolar 1 Low Osmolar Y Other Contrast Z None	Z None	Z None

SECTION: B IMAGING
BODY SYSTEM: N SKULL AND FACIAL BONES
TYPE: 2 **COMPUTERIZED TOMOGRAPHY (CT SCAN):** Computer reformatted digital display of multiplanar images developed from the capture of multiple exposures of external ionizing radiation

Body Part	Contrast	Qualifier	Qualifier
Ø Skull 3 Orbits, Bilateral 5 Facial Bones 6 Mandible 9 Temporomandibular Joints, Bilateral F Temporal Bones	Ø High Osmolar 1 Low Osmolar Y Other Contrast Z None	Z None	Z None

SECTION: B IMAGING
BODY SYSTEM: N SKULL AND FACIAL BONES
TYPE: 3 **MAGNETIC RESONANCE IMAGING (MRI):** Computer reformatted digital display of multiplanar images developed from the capture of radiofrequency signals emitted by nuclei in a body site excited within a magnetic field

Body Part	Contrast	Qualifier	Qualifier
9 Temporomandibular Joints, Bilateral	Y Other Contrast Z None	Z None	Z None

B: IMAGING

N: SKULL AND FACIAL BONES

2: CT SCAN   3: MRI

SECTION: B IMAGING
BODY SYSTEM: P NON-AXIAL UPPER BONES
TYPE: Ø **PLAIN RADIOGRAPHY:** Planar display of an image developed from the capture of external ionizing radiation on photographic or photoconductive plate

Body Part	Contrast	Qualifier	Qualifier
Ø Sternoclavicular Joint, Right 1 Sternoclavicular Joint, Left 2 Sternoclavicular Joints, Bilateral 3 Acromioclavicular Joints, Bilateral 4 Clavicle, Right 5 Clavicle, Left 6 Scapula, Right 7 Scapula, Left A Humerus, Right B Humerus, Left E Upper Arm, Right F Upper Arm, Left J Forearm, Right K Forearm, Left N Hand, Right P Hand, Left R Finger(s), Right S Finger(s), Left X Ribs, Right Y Ribs, Left	Z None	Z None	Z None
8 Shoulder, Right 9 Shoulder, Left C Hand/Finger Joint, Right D Hand/Finger Joint, Left G Elbow, Right H Elbow, Left L Wrist, Right M Wrist, Left	Ø High Osmolar 1 Low Osmolar Y Other Contrast Z None	Z None	Z None

SECTION: B IMAGING
BODY SYSTEM: P NON-AXIAL UPPER BONES
TYPE: 1 **FLUOROSCOPY:** Single plane or bi-plane real time display of an image developed from the capture of external ionizing radiation on a fluorescent screen. The image may also be stored by either digital or analog means

Body Part	Contrast	Qualifier	Qualifier
Ø Sternoclavicular Joint, Right 1 Sternoclavicular Joint, Left 2 Sternoclavicular Joints, Bilateral 3 Acromioclavicular Joints, Bilateral 4 Clavicle, Right 5 Clavicle, Left 6 Scapula, Right 7 Scapula, Left A Humerus, Right B Humerus, Left E Upper Arm, Right F Upper Arm, Left J Forearm, Right K Forearm, Left N Hand, Right P Hand, Left R Finger(s), Right S Finger(s), Left X Ribs, Right Y Ribs, Left	Z None	Z None	Z None
8 Shoulder, Right 9 Shoulder, Left L Wrist, Right M Wrist, Left	Ø High Osmolar 1 Low Osmolar Y Other Contrast Z None	Z None	Z None
C Hand/Finger Joint, Right D Hand/Finger Joint, Left G Elbow, Right H Elbow, Left	Ø High Osmolar 1 Low Osmolar Y Other Contrast	Z None	Z None

SECTION: B IMAGING
BODY SYSTEM: P NON-AXIAL UPPER BONES
TYPE: 2 COMPUTERIZED TOMOGRAPHY (CT SCAN): Computer reformatted digital display of multiplanar images developed from the capture of multiple exposures of external ionizing radiation

Body Part	Contrast	Qualifier	Qualifier
Ø Sternoclavicular Joint, Right 1 Sternoclavicular Joint, Left W Thorax	Ø High Osmolar 1 Low Osmolar Y Other Contrast	Z None	Z None
2 Sternoclavicular Joints, Bilateral 3 Acromioclavicular Joints, Bilateral 4 Clavicle, Right 5 Clavicle, Left 6 Scapula, Right 7 Scapula, Left 8 Shoulder, Right 9 Shoulder, Left A Humerus, Right B Humerus, Left E Upper Arm, Right F Upper Arm, Left G Elbow, Right H Elbow, Left J Forearm, Right K Forearm, Left L Wrist, Right M Wrist, Left N Hand, Right P Hand, Left Q Hands and Wrists, Bilateral R Finger(s), Right S Finger(s), Left T Upper Extremity, Right U Upper Extremity, Left V Upper Extremities, Bilateral X Ribs, Right Y Ribs, Left	Ø High Osmolar 1 Low Osmolar Y Other Contrast Z None	Z None	Z None
C Hand/Finger Joint, Right D Hand/Finger Joint, Left	Z None	Z None	Z None

P: NON-AXIAL UPPER BONES   2: COMPUTERIZED TOMOGRAPHY (CT SCAN)

B: IMAGING

SECTION: B IMAGING
BODY SYSTEM: P NON-AXIAL UPPER BONES
TYPE: 3 **MAGNETIC RESONANCE IMAGING (MRI):** Computer reformatted digital display of multiplanar images developed from the capture of radiofrequency signals emitted by nuclei in a body site excited within a magnetic field

Body Part	Contrast	Qualifier	Qualifier
8 Shoulder, Right 9 Shoulder, Left C Hand/Finger Joint, Right D Hand/Finger Joint, Left E Upper Arm, Right F Upper Arm, Left G Elbow, Right H Elbow, Left J Forearm, Right K Forearm, Left L Wrist, Right M Wrist, Left	Y Other Contrast	Ø Unenhanced and Enhanced Z None	Z None
8 Shoulder, Right 9 Shoulder, Left C Hand/Finger Joint, Right D Hand/Finger Joint, Left E Upper Arm, Right F Upper Arm, Left G Elbow, Right H Elbow, Left J Forearm, Right K Forearm, Left L Wrist, Right M Wrist, Left	Z None	Z None	Z None

SECTION: B IMAGING
BODY SYSTEM: P NON-AXIAL UPPER BONES
TYPE: 4 **ULTRASONOGRAPHY:** Real time display of images of anatomy or flow information developed from the capture of reflected and attenuated high frequency sound waves

Body Part	Contrast	Qualifier	Qualifier
8 Shoulder, Right 9 Shoulder, Left G Elbow, Right H Elbow, Left L Wrist, Right M Wrist, Left N Hand, Right P Hand, Left	Z None	Z None	1 Densitometry Z None

SECTION: B IMAGING
BODY SYSTEM: Q NON-AXIAL LOWER BONES
TYPE: 0 **PLAIN RADIOGRAPHY:** Planar display of an image developed from the capture of external ionizing radiation on photographic or photoconductive plate

Body Part	Contrast	Qualifier	Qualifier
0 Hip, Right 1 Hip, Left	0 High Osmolar 1 Low Osmolar Y Other Contrast	Z None	Z None
0 Hip, Right 1 Hip, Left	Z None	Z None	1 Densitometry Z None
3 Femur, Right 4 Femur, Left	Z None	Z None	1 Densitometry Z None
7 Knee, Right 8 Knee, Left G Ankle, Right H Ankle, Left	0 High Osmolar 1 Low Osmolar Y Other Contrast Z None	Z None	Z None
D Lower Leg, Right F Lower Leg, Left J Calcaneus, Right K Calcaneus, Left L Foot, Right M Foot, Left P Toe(s), Right Q Toe(s), Left V Patella, Right W Patella, Left	Z None	Z None	Z None
X Foot/Toe Joint, Right Y Foot/Toe Joint, Left	0 High Osmolar 1 Low Osmolar Y Other Contrast	Z None	Z None

SECTION: B IMAGING
BODY SYSTEM: Q NON-AXIAL LOWER BONES
TYPE: 1 FLUOROSCOPY: Single plane or bi-plane real time display of an image developed from the capture of external ionizing radiation on a fluorescent screen. The image may also be stored by either digital or analog means

Body Part	Contrast	Qualifier	Qualifier
Ø Hip, Right 1 Hip, Left 7 Knee, Right 8 Knee, Left G Ankle, Right H Ankle, Left X Foot/Toe Joint, Right Y Foot/Toe Joint, Left	Ø High Osmolar 1 Low Osmolar Y Other Contrast Z None	Z None	Z None
3 Femur, Right 4 Femur, Left D Lower Leg, Right F Lower Leg, Left J Calcaneus, Right K Calcaneus, Left L Foot, Right M Foot, Left P Toe(s), Right Q Toe(s), Left V Patella, Right W Patella, Left	Z None	Z None	Z None

B: IMAGING

Q: NON-AXIAL LOWER BONES

1: FLUOROSCOPY

SECTION: B IMAGING
BODY SYSTEM: Q **NON-AXIAL LOWER BONES**
TYPE: 2 **COMPUTERIZED TOMOGRAPHY (CT SCAN):** Computer reformatted digital display of multiplanar images developed from the capture of multiple exposures of external ionizing radiation

Body Part	Contrast	Qualifier	Qualifier
Ø Hip, Right 1 Hip, Left 3 Femur, Right 4 Femur, Left 7 Knee, Right 8 Knee, Left D Lower Leg, Right F Lower Leg, Left G Ankle, Right H Ankle, Left J Calcaneus, Right K Calcaneus, Left L Foot, Right M Foot, Left P Toe(s), Right Q Toe(s), Left R Lower Extremity, Right S Lower Extremity, Left V Patella, Right W Patella, Left X Foot/Toe Joint, Right Y Foot/Toe Joint, Left	Ø High Osmolar 1 Low Osmolar Y Other Contrast Z None	Z None	Z None
B Tibia/Fibula, Right C Tibia/Fibula, Left	Ø High Osmolar 1 Low Osmolar Y Other Contrast	Z None	Z None

SECTION: B IMAGING
BODY SYSTEM: Q NON-AXIAL LOWER BONES
TYPE: 3 MAGNETIC RESONANCE IMAGING (MRI): Computer reformatted digital display of multiplanar images developed from the capture of radiofrequency signals emitted by nuclei in a body site excited within a magnetic field

Body Part	Contrast	Qualifier	Qualifier
Ø Hip, Right 1 Hip, Left 3 Femur, Right 4 Femur, Left 7 Knee, Right 8 Knee, Left D Lower Leg, Right F Lower Leg, Left G Ankle, Right H Ankle, Left J Calcaneus, Right K Calcaneus, Left L Foot, Right M Foot, Left P Toe(s), Right Q Toe(s), Left V Patella, Right W Patella, Left	Y Other Contrast	Ø Unenhanced and Enhanced Z None	Z None
Ø Hip, Right 1 Hip, Left 3 Femur, Right 4 Femur, Left 7 Knee, Right 8 Knee, Left D Lower Leg, Right F Lower Leg, Left G Ankle, Right H Ankle, Left J Calcaneus, Right K Calcaneus, Left L Foot, Right M Foot, Left P Toe(s), Right Q Toe(s), Left V Patella, Right W Patella, Left	Z None	Z None	Z None

SECTION: B IMAGING
BODY SYSTEM: Q NON-AXIAL LOWER BONES
TYPE: 4 **ULTRASONOGRAPHY:** Real time display of images of anatomy or flow information developed from the capture of reflected and attenuated high frequency sound waves

Body Part	Contrast	Qualifier	Qualifier
Ø Hip, Right 1 Hip, Left 2 Hips, Bilateral 7 Knee, Right 8 Knee, Left 9 Knees, Bilateral	Z None	Z None	Z None

SECTION: B IMAGING

BODY SYSTEM: R AXIAL SKELETON, EXCEPT SKULL AND FACIAL BONES
TYPE: Ø PLAIN RADIOGRAPHY: Planar display of an image developed from the capture of external ionizing radiation on photographic or photoconductive plate

Body Part	Contrast	Qualifier	Qualifier
Ø Cervical Spine 7 Thoracic Spine 9 Lumbar Spine G Whole Spine	Z None	Z None	1 Densitometry Z None
1 Cervical Disc(s) 2 Thoracic Disc(s) 3 Lumbar Disc(s) 4 Cervical Facet Joint(s) 5 Thoracic Facet Joint(s) 6 Lumbar Facet Joint(s) D Sacroiliac Joints	Ø High Osmolar 1 Low Osmolar Y Other Contrast Z None	Z None	Z None
8 Thoracolumbar Joint B Lumbosacral Joint C Pelvis F Sacrum and Coccyx H Sternum	Z None	Z None	Z None

SECTION: B IMAGING

BODY SYSTEM: R AXIAL SKELETON, EXCEPT SKULL AND FACIAL BONES
TYPE: 1 FLUOROSCOPY: Single plane or bi-plane real time display of an image developed from the capture of external ionizing radiation on a fluorescent screen. The image may also be stored by either digital or analog means

Body Part	Contrast	Qualifier	Qualifier
Ø Cervical Spine 1 Cervical Disc(s) 2 Thoracic Disc(s) 3 Lumbar Disc(s) 4 Cervical Facet Joint(s) 5 Thoracic Facet Joint(s) 6 Lumbar Facet Joint(s) 7 Thoracic Spine 8 Thoracolumbar Joint 9 Lumbar Spine B Lumbosacral Joint C Pelvis D Sacroiliac Joints F Sacrum and Coccyx G Whole Spine H Sternum	Ø High Osmolar 1 Low Osmolar Y Other Contrast Z None	Z None	Z None

SECTION: B IMAGING

BODY SYSTEM: R AXIAL SKELETON, EXCEPT SKULL AND FACIAL BONES

TYPE: 2 COMPUTERIZED TOMOGRAPHY (CT SCAN): Computer reformatted digital display of multiplanar images developed from the capture of multiple exposures of external ionizing radiation

Body Part	Contrast	Qualifier	Qualifier
Ø Cervical Spine 7 Thoracic Spine 9 Lumbar Spine C Pelvis D Sacroiliac Joints F Sacrum and Coccyx	Ø High Osmolar 1 Low Osmolar Y Other Contrast Z None	Z None	Z None

SECTION: B IMAGING

BODY SYSTEM: R AXIAL SKELETON, EXCEPT SKULL AND FACIAL BONES

TYPE: 3 MAGNETIC RESONANCE IMAGING (MRI): Computer reformatted digital display of multiplanar images developed from the capture of radiofrequency signals emitted by nuclei in a body site excited within a magnetic field

Body Part	Contrast	Qualifier	Qualifier
Ø Cervical Spine 1 Cervical Disc(s) 2 Thoracic Disc(s) 3 Lumbar Disc(s) 7 Thoracic Spine 9 Lumbar Spine C Pelvis F Sacrum and Coccyx	Y Other Contrast	Ø Unenhanced and Enhanced Z None	Z None
Ø Cervical Spine 1 Cervical Disc(s) 2 Thoracic Disc(s) 3 Lumbar Disc(s) 7 Thoracic Spine 9 Lumbar Spine C Pelvis F Sacrum and Coccyx	Z None	Z None	Z None

SECTION: B IMAGING

BODY SYSTEM: R AXIAL SKELETON, EXCEPT SKULL AND FACIAL BONES

TYPE: 4 ULTRASONOGRAPHY: Real time display of images of anatomy or flow information developed from the capture of reflected and attenuated high frequency sound waves

Body Part	Contrast	Qualifier	Qualifier
Ø Cervical Spine 7 Thoracic Spine 9 Lumbar Spine F Sacrum and Coccyx	Z None	Z None	Z None

New/Revised Text in Blue   ~~deleted~~ Deleted

SECTION: B IMAGING
BODY SYSTEM: T URINARY SYSTEM
TYPE: **0 PLAIN RADIOGRAPHY:** Planar display of an image developed from the capture of external ionizing radiation on photographic or photoconductive plate

Body Part	Contrast	Qualifier	Qualifier
0 Bladder 1 Kidney, Right 2 Kidney, Left 3 Kidneys, Bilateral 4 Kidneys, Ureters, and Bladder 5 Urethra 6 Ureter, Right 7 Ureter, Left 8 Ureters, Bilateral B Bladder and Urethra C Ileal Diversion Loop	0 High Osmolar 1 Low Osmolar Y Other Contrast Z None	Z None	Z None

SECTION: B IMAGING
BODY SYSTEM: T URINARY SYSTEM
TYPE: **1 FLUOROSCOPY:** Single plane or bi-plane real time display of an image developed from the capture of external ionizing radiation on a fluorescent screen. The image may also be stored by either digital or analog means

Body Part	Contrast	Qualifier	Qualifier
0 Bladder 1 Kidney, Right 2 Kidney, Left 3 Kidneys, Bilateral 4 Kidneys, Ureters, and Bladder 5 Urethra 6 Ureter, Right 7 Ureter, Left B Bladder and Urethra C Ileal Diversion Loop D Kidney, Ureter, and Bladder, Right F Kidney, Ureter, and Bladder, Left G Ileal Loop, Ureters, and Kidneys	0 High Osmolar 1 Low Osmolar Y Other Contrast Z None	Z None	Z None

SECTION: B IMAGING
BODY SYSTEM: T URINARY SYSTEM
TYPE: 2 **COMPUTERIZED TOMOGRAPHY (CT SCAN):** Computer reformatted digital display of multiplanar images developed from the capture of multiple exposures of external ionizing radiation

Body Part	Contrast	Qualifier	Qualifier
Ø Bladder 1 Kidney, Right 2 Kidney, Left 3 Kidneys, Bilateral 9 Kidney Transplant	Ø High Osmolar 1 Low Osmolar Y Other Contrast	Ø Unenhanced and Enhanced Z None	Z None
Ø Bladder 1 Kidney, Right 2 Kidney, Left 3 Kidneys, Bilateral 9 Kidney Transplant	Z None	Z None	Z None

SECTION: B IMAGING
BODY SYSTEM: T URINARY SYSTEM
TYPE: 3 **MAGNETIC RESONANCE IMAGING (MRI):** Computer reformatted digital display of multiplanar images developed from the capture of radiofrequency signals emitted by nuclei in a body site excited within a magnetic field

Body Part	Contrast	Qualifier	Qualifier
Ø Bladder 1 Kidney, Right 2 Kidney, Left 3 Kidneys, Bilateral 9 Kidney Transplant	Y Other Contrast	Ø Unenhanced and Enhanced Z None	Z None
Ø Bladder 1 Kidney, Right 2 Kidney, Left 3 Kidneys, Bilateral 9 Kidney Transplant	Z None	Z None	Z None

2: CT SCAN   3: MRI

T: URINARY SYSTEM

B: IMAGING

New/Revised Text in Blue   ~~deleted~~ Deleted

SECTION: B IMAGING
BODY SYSTEM: T URINARY SYSTEM
TYPE: 4 ULTRASONOGRAPHY: Real time display of images of anatomy or flow information developed from the capture of reflected and attenuated high frequency sound waves

Body Part	Contrast	Qualifier	Qualifier
Ø Bladder 1 Kidney, Right 2 Kidney, Left 3 Kidneys, Bilateral 5 Urethra 6 Ureter, Right 7 Ureter, Left 8 Ureters, Bilateral 9 Kidney Transplant J Kidneys and Bladder	Z None	Z None	Z None

Ø: PLAIN RADIOGRAPHY   1: FLUOROSCOPY

SECTION: B IMAGING

BODY SYSTEM: U FEMALE REPRODUCTIVE SYSTEM

TYPE: Ø **PLAIN RADIOGRAPHY:** Planar display of an image developed from the capture of external ionizing radiation on photographic or photoconductive plate

Body Part	Contrast	Qualifier	Qualifier
Ø Fallopian Tube, Right 1 Fallopian Tube, Left 2 Fallopian Tubes, Bilateral 6 Uterus 8 Uterus and Fallopian Tubes 9 Vagina	Ø High Osmolar 1 Low Osmolar Y Other Contrast	Z None	Z None

SECTION: B IMAGING

BODY SYSTEM: U FEMALE REPRODUCTIVE SYSTEM

TYPE: 1 **FLUOROSCOPY:** Single plane or bi-plane real time display of an image developed from the capture of external ionizing radiation on a fluorescent screen. The image may also be stored by either digital or analog means

Body Part	Contrast	Qualifier	Qualifier
Ø Fallopian Tube, Right 1 Fallopian Tube, Left 2 Fallopian Tubes, Bilateral 6 Uterus 8 Uterus and Fallopian Tubes 9 Vagina	Ø High Osmolar 1 Low Osmolar Y Other Contrast Z None	Z None	Z None

U: FEMALE REPRODUCTIVE SYSTEM

B: IMAGING

SECTION: B IMAGING
BODY SYSTEM: U FEMALE REPRODUCTIVE SYSTEM
TYPE: 3 MAGNETIC RESONANCE IMAGING (MRI): Computer reformatted digital display of multiplanar images developed from the capture of radiofrequency signals emitted by nuclei in a body site excited within a magnetic field

Body Part	Contrast	Qualifier	Qualifier
3 Ovary, Right 4 Ovary, Left 5 Ovaries, Bilateral 6 Uterus 9 Vagina B Pregnant Uterus C Uterus and Ovaries	Y Other Contrast	Ø Unenhanced and Enhanced Z None	Z None
3 Ovary, Right 4 Ovary, Left 5 Ovaries, Bilateral 6 Uterus 9 Vagina B Pregnant Uterus C Uterus and Ovaries	Z None	Z None	Z None

SECTION: B IMAGING
BODY SYSTEM: U FEMALE REPRODUCTIVE SYSTEM
TYPE: 4 ULTRASONOGRAPHY: Real time display of images of anatomy or flow information developed from the capture of reflected and attenuated high frequency sound waves

Body Part	Contrast	Qualifier	Qualifier
Ø Fallopian Tube, Right 1 Fallopian Tube, Left 2 Fallopian Tubes, Bilateral 3 Ovary, Right 4 Ovary, Left 5 Ovaries, Bilateral 6 Uterus C Uterus and Ovaries	Y Other Contrast Z None	Z None	Z None

SECTION: B IMAGING
BODY SYSTEM: V MALE REPRODUCTIVE SYSTEM
TYPE: Ø PLAIN RADIOGRAPHY: Planar display of an image developed from the capture of external ionizing radiation on photographic or photoconductive plate

Body Part	Contrast	Qualifier	Qualifier
Ø Corpora Cavernosa 1 Epididymis, Right 2 Epididymis, Left 3 Prostate 5 Testicle, Right 6 Testicle, Left 8 Vasa Vasorum	Ø High Osmolar 1 Low Osmolar Y Other Contrast	Z None	Z None

SECTION: B IMAGING
BODY SYSTEM: V MALE REPRODUCTIVE SYSTEM
TYPE: 1 FLUOROSCOPY: Single plane or bi-plane real time display of an image developed from the capture of external ionizing radiation on a fluorescent screen. The image may also be stored by either digital or analog means

Body Part	Contrast	Qualifier	Qualifier
Ø Corpora Cavernosa 8 Vasa Vasorum	Ø High Osmolar 1 Low Osmolar Y Other Contrast Z None	Z None	Z None

SECTION:　B IMAGING
BODY SYSTEM: V MALE REPRODUCTIVE SYSTEM
TYPE:　2 **COMPUTERIZED TOMOGRAPHY (CT SCAN):** Computer reformatted digital display of multiplanar images developed from the capture of multiple exposures of external ionizing radiation

Body Part	Contrast	Qualifier	Qualifier
3　Prostate	Ø　High Osmolar 1　Low Osmolar Y　Other Contrast	Ø　Unenhanced and Enhanced Z　None	Z　None
3　Prostate	Z　None	Z　None	Z　None

SECTION:　B IMAGING
BODY SYSTEM: V MALE REPRODUCTIVE SYSTEM
TYPE:　3 **MAGNETIC RESONANCE IMAGING (MRI):** Computer reformatted digital display of multiplanar images developed from the capture of radiofrequency signals emitted by nuclei in a body site excited within a magnetic field

Body Part	Contrast	Qualifier	Qualifier
Ø　Corpora Cavernosa 3　Prostate 4　Scrotum 5　Testicle, Right 6　Testicle, Left 7　Testicles, Bilateral	Y　Other Contrast	Ø　Unenhanced and Enhanced Z　None	Z　None
Ø　Corpora Cavernosa 3　Prostate 4　Scrotum 5　Testicle, Right 6　Testicle, Left 7　Testicles, Bilateral	Z　None	Z　None	Z　None

SECTION:　B IMAGING
BODY SYSTEM: V MALE REPRODUCTIVE SYSTEM
TYPE:　4 **ULTRASONOGRAPHY:** Real time display of images of anatomy or flow information developed from the capture of reflected and attenuated high frequency sound waves

Body Part	Contrast	Qualifier	Qualifier
4　Scrotum 9　Prostate and Seminal Vesicles B　Penis	Z　None	Z　None	Z　None

2: CT SCAN

1: FLUOROSCOPY

Ø: PLAIN RADIOGRAPHY

W: ANATOMICAL REGIONS

B: IMAGING

SECTION: B IMAGING
BODY SYSTEM: W ANATOMICAL REGIONS
TYPE: Ø **PLAIN RADIOGRAPHY:** Planar display of an image developed from the capture of external ionizing radiation on photographic or photoconductive plate

Body Part	Contrast	Qualifier	Qualifier
Ø Abdomen 1 Abdomen and Pelvis 3 Chest B Long Bones, All C Lower Extremity J Upper Extremity K Whole Body L Whole Skeleton M Whole Body, Infant	Z None	Z None	Z None

SECTION: B IMAGING
BODY SYSTEM: W ANATOMICAL REGIONS
TYPE: 1 **FLUOROSCOPY:** Single plane or bi-plane real time display of an image developed from the capture of external ionizing radiation on a fluorescent screen. The image may also be stored by either digital or analog means

Body Part	Contrast	Qualifier	Qualifier
1 Abdomen and Pelvis 9 Head and Neck C Lower Extremity J Upper Extremity	Ø High Osmolar 1 Low Osmolar Y Other Contrast Z None	Z None	Z None

SECTION: B IMAGING
BODY SYSTEM: W ANATOMICAL REGIONS
TYPE: 2 **COMPUTERIZED TOMOGRAPHY (CT SCAN):** Computer reformatted digital display of multiplanar images developed from the capture of multiple exposures of external ionizing radiation

Body Part	Contrast	Qualifier	Qualifier
Ø Abdomen 1 Abdomen and Pelvis 4 Chest and Abdomen 5 Chest, Abdomen, and Pelvis 8 Head 9 Head and Neck F Neck G Pelvic Region	Ø High Osmolar 1 Low Osmolar Y Other Contrast	Ø Unenhanced and Enhanced Z None	Z None
Ø Abdomen 1 Abdomen and Pelvis 4 Chest and Abdomen 5 Chest, Abdomen, and Pelvis 8 Head 9 Head and Neck F Neck G Pelvic Region	Z None	Z None	Z None

New/Revised Text in Blue   ~~deleted~~ Deleted

SECTION: **B IMAGING**
BODY SYSTEM: **W ANATOMICAL REGIONS**
TYPE: **3 MAGNETIC RESONANCE IMAGING (MRI):** Computer reformatted digital display of multiplanar images developed from the capture of radiofrequency signals emitted by nuclei in a body site excited within a magnetic field

Body Part	Contrast	Qualifier	Qualifier
Ø Abdomen 8 Head F Neck G Pelvic Region H Retroperitoneum P Brachial Plexus	Y Other Contrast	Ø Unenhanced and Enhanced Z None	Z None
Ø Abdomen 8 Head F Neck G Pelvic Region H Retroperitoneum P Brachial Plexus	Z None	Z None	Z None
3 Chest	Y Other Contrast	Ø Unenhanced and Enhanced Z None	Z None

SECTION: **B IMAGING**
BODY SYSTEM: **W ANATOMICAL REGIONS**
TYPE: **4 ULTRASONOGRAPHY:** Real time display of images of anatomy or flow information developed from the capture of reflected and attenuated high frequency sound waves

Body Part	Contrast	Qualifier	Qualifier
Ø Abdomen 1 Abdomen and Pelvis F Neck G Pelvic Region	Z None	Z None	Z None

SECTION: B IMAGING

BODY SYSTEM: Y FETUS AND OBSTETRICAL

TYPE: 3 MAGNETIC RESONANCE IMAGING (MRI): Computer reformatted digital display of multiplanar images developed from the capture of radiofrequency signals emitted by nuclei in a body site excited within a magnetic field

Body Part	Contrast	Qualifier	Qualifier
Ø Fetal Head 1 Fetal Heart 2 Fetal Thorax 3 Fetal Abdomen 4 Fetal Spine 5 Fetal Extremities 6 Whole Fetus	Y Other Contrast	Ø Unenhanced and Enhanced Z None	Z None
Ø Fetal Head 1 Fetal Heart 2 Fetal Thorax 3 Fetal Abdomen 4 Fetal Spine 5 Fetal Extremities 6 Whole Fetus	Z None	Z None	Z None

SECTION: B IMAGING

BODY SYSTEM: Y FETUS AND OBSTETRICAL

TYPE: 4 ULTRASONOGRAPHY: Real time display of images of anatomy or flow information developed from the capture of reflected and attenuated high frequency sound waves

Body Part	Contrast	Qualifier	Qualifier
7 Fetal Umbilical Cord 8 Placenta 9 First Trimester, Single Fetus B First Trimester, Multiple Gestation C Second Trimester, Single Fetus D Second Trimester, Multiple Gestation F Third Trimester, Single Fetus G Third Trimester, Multiple Gestation	Z None	Z None	Z None

C   Nuclear Medicine..609
    CØ. Central Nervous System..610
        CØ1. Planar Nuclear Medicine Imaging...610
        CØ2. Tomographic (TOMO) Nuclear Medicine Imaging..................................610
        CØ3. Positron Emission Tomographic (PET) Imaging.......................................611
        CØ5. Nonimaging Nuclear Medicine Probe...611
    C2. Heart..612
        C21. Planar Nuclear Medicine Imaging...612
        C22. Tomographic (TOMO) Nuclear Medicine Imaging..................................612
        C23. Positron Emission Tomographic (PET) Imaging.......................................613
        C25. Nonimaging Nuclear Medicine Probe...613
    C5. Veins..614
        C51. Planar Nuclear Medicine Imaging...614
    C7. Lymphatic and Hematologic System...615
        C71. Planar Nuclear Medicine Imaging...615
        C72. Tomographic (TOMO) Nuclear Medicine Imaging..................................615
        C75. Nonimaging Nuclear Medicine Probe...616
        C76. Nonimaging Nuclear Medicine Assay..616
    C8. Eye...617
        C81. Planar Nuclear Medicine Imaging...617
    C9. Ear, Nose, Mouth, and Throat...618
        C91. Planar Nuclear Medicine Imaging...618
    CB. Respiratory System...619
        CB1. Planar Nuclear Medicine Imaging...619
        CB2. Tomographic (TOMO) Nuclear Medicine Imaging..................................619
        CB3. Positron Emission Tomographic (PET) Imaging.......................................619
    CD. Gastrointestinal System...620
        CD1. Planar Nuclear Medicine Imaging...620
        CD2. Tomographic (TOMO) Nuclear Medicine Imaging..................................620
    CF. Hepatobiliary System and Pancreas...621
        CF1. Planar Nuclear Medicine Imaging...621
        CF2. Tomographic (TOMO) Nuclear Medicine Imaging..................................621
    CG. Endocrine System...622
        CG1. Planar Nuclear Medicine Imaging...622
        CG2. Tomographic (TOMO) Nuclear Medicine Imaging..................................622
        CG4. Nonimaging Nuclear Medicine Uptake...622
    CH. Skin, Subcutaneous Tissue and Breast...623
        CH1. Planar Nuclear Medicine Imaging...623
        CH2. Tomographic (TOMO) Nuclear Medicine Imaging..................................623
    CP. Musculoskeletal System..624
        CP1. Planar Nuclear Medicine Imaging...624
        CP2. Tomographic (TOMO) Nuclear Medicine Imaging..................................624
        CP5. Nonimaging Nuclear Medicine Probe...625
    CT. Urinary System...626
        CT1. Planar Nuclear Medicine Imaging...626
        CT2. Tomographic (TOMO) Nuclear Medicine Imaging..................................626
        CT6. Nonimaging Nuclear Medicine Assay..626
    CV. Male Reproductive System..627
        CV1. Planar Nuclear Medicine Imaging...627
    CW. Anatomical Regions...628
        CW1. Planar Nuclear Medicine Imaging...628
        CW2. Tomographic (TOMO) Nuclear Medicine Imaging..................................628
        CW3. Positron Emission Tomographic (PET) Imaging.......................................629
        CW5. Nonimaging Nuclear Medicine Probe...629
        CW7. Systemic Nuclear Medicine Therapy...629

SECTION: C NUCLEAR MEDICINE
BODY SYSTEM: Ø CENTRAL NERVOUS SYSTEM
TYPE: 1 PLANAR NUCLEAR MEDICINE IMAGING: Introduction of radioactive materials into the body for single plane display of images developed from the capture of radioactive emissions

Body Part	Radionuclide	Qualifier	Qualifier
Ø Brain	1 Technetium 99m (Tc-99m) Y Other Radionuclide	Z None	Z None
5 Cerebrospinal Fluid	D Indium 111 (In-111) Y Other Radionuclide	Z None	Z None
Y Central Nervous System	Y Other Radionuclide	Z None	Z None

SECTION: C NUCLEAR MEDICINE
BODY SYSTEM: Ø CENTRAL NERVOUS SYSTEM
TYPE: 2 TOMOGRAPHIC (TOMO) NUCLEAR MEDICINE IMAGING: Introduction of radioactive materials into the body for three dimensional display of images developed from the capture of radioactive emissions

Body Part	Radionuclide	Qualifier	Qualifier
Ø Brain	1 Technetium 99m (Tc-99m) F Iodine 123 (I-123) S Thallium 2Ø1 (Tl-2Ø1) Y Other Radionuclide	Z None	Z None
5 Cerebrospinal Fluid	D Indium 111 (In-111) Y Other Radionuclide	Z None	Z None
Y Central Nervous System	Y Other Radionuclide	Z None	Z None

SECTION: C NUCLEAR MEDICINE
BODY SYSTEM: Ø **CENTRAL NERVOUS SYSTEM**
TYPE: 3 **POSITRON EMISSION TOMOGRAPHIC (PET) IMAGING:** Introduction of radioactive materials into the body for three dimensional display of images developed from the simultaneous capture, 18Ø degrees apart, of radioactive emissions

Body Part	Radionuclide	Qualifier	Qualifier
Ø Brain	B Carbon 11 (C-11) K Fluorine 18 (F-18) M Oxygen 15 (O-15) Y Other Radionuclide	Z None	Z None
Y Central Nervous System	Y Other Radionuclide	Z None	Z None

SECTION: C NUCLEAR MEDICINE
BODY SYSTEM: Ø **CENTRAL NERVOUS SYSTEM**
TYPE: 5 **NONIMAGING NUCLEAR MEDICINE PROBE:** Introduction of radioactive materials into the body for the study of distribution and fate of certain substances by the detection of radioactive emissions; or, alternatively, measurement of absorption of radioactive emissions from an external source

Body Part	Radionuclide	Qualifier	Qualifier
Ø Brain	V Xenon 133 (Xe-133) Y Other Radionuclide	Z None	Z None
Y Central Nervous System	Y Other Radionuclide	Z None	Z None

C: NUCLEAR MEDICINE

Ø: CENTRAL NERVOUS SYSTEM

3; 5

SECTION: C NUCLEAR MEDICINE

BODY SYSTEM: 2 HEART
TYPE: 1 **PLANAR NUCLEAR MEDICINE IMAGING:** Introduction of radioactive materials into the body for single plane display of images developed from the capture of radioactive emissions

Body Part	Radionuclide	Qualifier	Qualifier
6 Heart, Right and Left	1 Technetium 99m (Tc-99m) Y Other Radionuclide	Z None	Z None
G Myocardium	1 Technetium 99m (Tc-99m) D Indium 111 (In-111) S Thallium 201 (Tl-201) Y Other Radionuclide Z None	Z None	Z None
Y Heart	Y Other Radionuclide	Z None	Z None

SECTION: C NUCLEAR MEDICINE

BODY SYSTEM: 2 HEART
TYPE: 2 **TOMOGRAPHIC (TOMO) NUCLEAR MEDICINE IMAGING:** Introduction of radioactive materials into the body for three dimensional display of images developed from the capture of radioactive emissions

Body Part	Radionuclide	Qualifier	Qualifier
6 Heart, Right and Left	1 Technetium 99m (Tc-99m) Y Other Radionuclide	Z None	Z None
G Myocardium	1 Technetium 99m (Tc-99m) D Indium 111 (In-111) K Fluorine 18 (F-18) S Thallium 201 (Tl-201) Y Other Radionuclide Z None	Z None	Z None
Y Heart	Y Other Radionuclide	Z None	Z None

New/Revised Text in Blue   deleted Deleted

SECTION: C NUCLEAR MEDICINE
BODY SYSTEM: 2 HEART
TYPE: 3 **POSITRON EMISSION TOMOGRAPHIC (PET) IMAGING:** Introduction of radioactive materials into the body for three dimensional display of images developed from the simultaneous capture, 18Ø degrees apart, of radioactive emissions

Body Part	Radionuclide	Qualifier	Qualifier
G Myocardium	K Fluorine 18 (F-18) M Oxygen 15 (O-15) Q Rubidium 82 (Rb-82) R Nitrogen 13 (N-13) Y Other Radionuclide	Z None	Z None
Y Heart	Y Other Radionuclide	Z None	Z None

SECTION: C NUCLEAR MEDICINE
BODY SYSTEM: 2 HEART
TYPE: 5 **NONIMAGING NUCLEAR MEDICINE PROBE:** Introduction of radioactive materials into the body for the study of distribution and fate of certain substances by the detection of radioactive emissions; or, alternatively, measurement of absorption of radioactive emissions from an external source

Body Part	Radionuclide	Qualifier	Qualifier
6 Heart, Right and Left	1 Technetium 99m (Tc-99m) Y Other Radionuclide	Z None	Z None
Y Heart	Y Other Radionuclide	Z None	Z None

1: PLANAR NUCLEAR MEDICINE IMAGING

5: VEINS

C: NUCLEAR MEDICINE

SECTION: C NUCLEAR MEDICINE
BODY SYSTEM: 5 VEINS
TYPE: 1 PLANAR NUCLEAR MEDICINE IMAGING: Introduction of radioactive materials into the body for single plane display of images developed from the capture of radioactive emissions

Body Part	Radionuclide	Qualifier	Qualifier
B Lower Extremity Veins, Right C Lower Extremity Veins, Left D Lower Extremity Veins, Bilateral N Upper Extremity Veins, Right P Upper Extremity Veins, Left Q Upper Extremity Veins, Bilateral R Central Veins	1 Technetium 99m (Tc-99m) Y Other Radionuclide	Z None	Z None
Y Veins	Y Other Radionuclide	Z None	Z None

SECTION: **C NUCLEAR MEDICINE**
BODY SYSTEM: **7 LYMPHATIC AND HEMATOLOGIC SYSTEM**
TYPE: **1 PLANAR NUCLEAR MEDICINE IMAGING:** Introduction of radioactive materials into the body for single plane display of images developed from the capture of radioactive emissions

Body Part	Radionuclide	Qualifier	Qualifier
Ø Bone Marrow	1 Technetium 99m (Tc-99m) D Indium 111 (In-111) Y Other Radionuclide	Z None	Z None
2 Spleen 5 Lymphatics, Head and Neck D Lymphatics, Pelvic J Lymphatics, Head K Lymphatics, Neck L Lymphatics, Upper Chest M Lymphatics, Trunk N Lymphatics, Upper Extremity P Lymphatics, Lower Extremity	1 Technetium 99m (Tc-99m) Y Other Radionuclide	Z None	Z None
3 Blood	D Indium 111 (In-111) Y Other Radionuclide	Z None	Z None
Y Lymphatic and Hematologic System	Y Other Radionuclide	Z None	Z None

SECTION: **C NUCLEAR MEDICINE**
BODY SYSTEM: **7 LYMPHATIC AND HEMATOLOGIC SYSTEM**
TYPE: **2 TOMOGRAPHIC (TOMO) NUCLEAR MEDICINE IMAGING:** Introduction of radioactive materials into the body for three dimensional display of images developed from the capture of radioactive emissions

Body Part	Radionuclide	Qualifier	Qualifier
2 Spleen	1 Technetium 99m (Tc-99m) Y Other Radionuclide	Z None	Z None
Y Lymphatic and Hematologic System	Y Other Radionuclide	Z None	Z None

SECTION: C NUCLEAR MEDICINE
BODY SYSTEM: 7 LYMPHATIC AND HEMATOLOGIC SYSTEM
TYPE: 5 NONIMAGING NUCLEAR MEDICINE PROBE: Introduction of radioactive materials into the body for the study of distribution and fate of certain substances by the detection of radioactive emissions; or, alternatively, measurement of absorption of radioactive emissions from an external source

Body Part	Radionuclide	Qualifier	Qualifier
5 Lymphatics, Head and Neck D Lymphatics, Pelvic J Lymphatics, Head K Lymphatics, Neck L Lymphatics, Upper Chest M Lymphatics, Trunk N Lymphatics, Upper Extremity P Lymphatics, Lower Extremity	1 Technetium 99m (Tc-99m) Y Other Radionuclide	Z None	Z None
Y Lymphatic and Hematologic System	Y Other Radionuclide	Z None	Z None

SECTION: C NUCLEAR MEDICINE
BODY SYSTEM: 7 LYMPHATIC AND HEMATOLOGIC SYSTEM
TYPE: 6 NONIMAGING NUCLEAR MEDICINE ASSAY: Introduction of radioactive materials into the body for the study of body fluids and blood elements, by the detection of radioactive emissions

Body Part	Radionuclide	Qualifier	Qualifier
3 Blood	1 Technetium 99m (Tc-99m) 7 Cobalt 58 (Co-58) C Cobalt 57 (Co-57) D Indium 111 (In-111) H Iodine 125 (I-125) W Chromium (Cr-51) Y Other Radionuclide	Z None	Z None
Y Lymphatic and Hematologic System	Y Other Radionuclide	Z None	Z None

SECTION: C NUCLEAR MEDICINE
BODY SYSTEM: 8 EYE
TYPE: 1 **PLANAR NUCLEAR MEDICINE IMAGING:** Introduction of radioactive materials into the body for single plane display of images developed from the capture of radioactive emissions

Body Part	Radionuclide	Qualifier	Qualifier
9 Lacrimal Ducts, Bilateral	1 Technetium 99m (Tc-99m) Y Other Radionuclide	Z None	Z None
Y Eye	Y Other Radionuclide	Z None	Z None

SECTION: **C NUCLEAR MEDICINE**
BODY SYSTEM: 9 **EAR, NOSE, MOUTH, AND THROAT**
TYPE: 1 **PLANAR NUCLEAR MEDICINE IMAGING:** Introduction of radioactive materials into the body for single plane display of images developed from the capture of radioactive emissions

Body Part	Radionuclide	Qualifier	Qualifier
B Salivary Glands, Bilateral	1 Technetium 99m (Tc-99m) Y Other Radionuclide	Z None	Z None
Y Ear, Nose, Mouth and Throat	Y Other Radionuclide	Z None	Z None

SECTION: C NUCLEAR MEDICINE
BODY SYSTEM: B RESPIRATORY SYSTEM
TYPE: 1 **PLANAR NUCLEAR MEDICINE IMAGING:** Introduction of radioactive materials into the body for single plane display of images developed from the capture of radioactive emissions

Body Part	Radionuclide	Qualifier	Qualifier
2 Lungs and Bronchi	1 Technetium 99m (Tc-99m) 9 Krypton (Kr-81m) T Xenon 127 (Xe-127) V Xenon 133 (Xe-133) Y Other Radionuclide	Z None	Z None
Y Respiratory System	Y Other Radionuclide	Z None	Z None

SECTION: C NUCLEAR MEDICINE
BODY SYSTEM: B RESPIRATORY SYSTEM
TYPE: 2 **TOMOGRAPHIC (TOMO) NUCLEAR MEDICINE IMAGING:** Introduction of radioactive materials into the body for three dimensional display of images developed from the capture of radioactive emissions

Body Part	Radionuclide	Qualifier	Qualifier
2 Lungs and Bronchi	1 Technetium 99m (Tc-99m) 9 Krypton (Kr-81m) Y Other Radionuclide	Z None	Z None
Y Respiratory System	Y Other Radionuclide	Z None	Z None

SECTION: C NUCLEAR MEDICINE
BODY SYSTEM: B RESPIRATORY SYSTEM
TYPE: 3 **POSITRON EMISSION TOMOGRAPHIC (PET) IMAGING:** Introduction of radioactive materials into the body for three dimensional display of images developed from the simultaneous capture, 18Ø degrees apart, of radioactive emissions

Body Part	Radionuclide	Qualifier	Qualifier
2 Lungs and Bronchi	K Fluorine 18 (F-18) Y Other Radionuclide	Z None	Z None
Y Respiratory System	Y Other Radionuclide	Z None	Z None

SECTION: **C NUCLEAR MEDICINE**
BODY SYSTEM: **D GASTROINTESTINAL SYSTEM**
TYPE: **1 PLANAR NUCLEAR MEDICINE IMAGING:** Introduction of radioactive materials into the body for single plane display of images developed from the capture of radioactive emissions

Body Part	Radionuclide	Qualifier	Qualifier
5 Upper Gastrointestinal Tract 7 Gastrointestinal Tract	1 Technetium 99m (Tc-99m) D Indium 111 (In-111) Y Other Radionuclide	Z None	Z None
Y Digestive System	Y Other Radionuclide	Z None	Z None

SECTION: **C NUCLEAR MEDICINE**
BODY SYSTEM: **D GASTROINTESTINAL SYSTEM**
TYPE: **2 TOMOGRAPHIC (TOMO) NUCLEAR MEDICINE IMAGING:** Introduction of radioactive materials into the body for three dimensional display of images developed from the capture of radioactive emissions

Body Part	Radionuclide	Qualifier	Qualifier
7 Gastrointestinal Tract	1 Technetium 99m (Tc-99m) D Indium 111 (In-111) Y Other Radionuclide	Z None	Z None
Y Digestive System	Y Other Radionuclide	Z None	Z None

C: NUCLEAR MEDICINE

D: GASTROINTESTINAL SYSTEM

1; 2

SECTION: C NUCLEAR MEDICINE
BODY SYSTEM: F HEPATOBILIARY SYSTEM AND PANCREAS
TYPE: **1 PLANAR NUCLEAR MEDICINE IMAGING:** Introduction of radioactive materials into the body for single plane display of images developed from the capture of radioactive emissions

Body Part	Radionuclide	Qualifier	Qualifier
4 Gallbladder 5 Liver 6 Liver and Spleen C Hepatobiliary System, All	1 Technetium 99m (Tc-99m) Y Other Radionuclide	Z None	Z None
Y Hepatobiliary System and Pancreas	Y Other Radionuclide	Z None	Z None

SECTION: C NUCLEAR MEDICINE
BODY SYSTEM: F HEPATOBILIARY SYSTEM AND PANCREAS
TYPE: **2 TOMOGRAPHIC (TOMO) NUCLEAR MEDICINE IMAGING:** Introduction of radioactive materials into the body for three dimensional display of images developed from the capture of radioactive emissions

Body Part	Radionuclide	Qualifier	Qualifier
4 Gallbladder 5 Liver 6 Liver and Spleen	1 Technetium 99m (Tc-99m) Y Other Radionuclide	Z None	Z None
Y Hepatobiliary System and Pancreas	Y Other Radionuclide	Z None	Z None

SECTION: C NUCLEAR MEDICINE
BODY SYSTEM: G ENDOCRINE SYSTEM
TYPE: 1 **PLANAR NUCLEAR MEDICINE IMAGING:** Introduction of radioactive materials into the body for single plane display of images developed from the capture of radioactive emissions

Body Part	Radionuclide	Qualifier	Qualifier
1 Parathyroid Glands	1 Technetium 99m (Tc-99m) S Thallium 201 (Tl-201) Y Other Radionuclide	Z None	Z None
2 Thyroid Gland	1 Technetium 99m (Tc-99m) F Iodine 123 (I-123) G Iodine 131 (I-131) Y Other Radionuclide	Z None	Z None
4 Adrenal Glands, Bilateral	G Iodine 131 (I-131) Y Other Radionuclide	Z None	Z None
Y Endocrine System	Y Other Radionuclide	Z None	Z None

SECTION: C NUCLEAR MEDICINE
BODY SYSTEM: G ENDOCRINE SYSTEM
TYPE: 2 **TOMOGRAPHIC (TOMO) NUCLEAR MEDICINE IMAGING:** Introduction of radioactive materials into the body for three dimensional display of images developed from the capture of radioactive emissions

Body Part	Radionuclide	Qualifier	Qualifier
1 Parathyroid Glands	1 Technetium 99m (Tc-99m) S Thallium 201 (Tl-201) Y Other Radionuclide	Z None	Z None
Y Endocrine System	Y Other Radionuclide	Z None	Z None

SECTION: C NUCLEAR MEDICINE
BODY SYSTEM: G ENDOCRINE SYSTEM
TYPE: 4 **NONIMAGING NUCLEAR MEDICINE UPTAKE:** Introduction of radioactive materials into the body for measurements of organ function, from the detection of radioactive emissions

Body Part	Radionuclide	Qualifier	Qualifier
2 Thyroid Gland	1 Technetium 99m (Tc-99m) F Iodine 123 (I-123) G Iodine 131 (I-131) Y Other Radionuclide	Z None	Z None
Y Endocrine System	Y Other Radionuclide	Z None	Z None

SECTION: C NUCLEAR MEDICINE
BODY SYSTEM: H SKIN, SUBCUTANEOUS TISSUE AND BREAST
TYPE: 1 **PLANAR NUCLEAR MEDICINE IMAGING:** Introduction of radioactive materials into the body for single plane display of images developed from the capture of radioactive emissions

Body Part	Radionuclide	Qualifier	Qualifier
Ø Breast, Right 1 Breast, Left 2 Breasts, Bilateral	1 Technetium 99m (Tc-99m) S Thallium 201 (Tl-201) Y Other Radionuclide	Z None	Z None
Y Skin, Subcutaneous Tissue, and Breast	Y Other Radionuclide	Z None	Z None

SECTION: C NUCLEAR MEDICINE
BODY SYSTEM: H SKIN, SUBCUTANEOUS TISSUE AND BREAST
TYPE: 2 **TOMOGRAPHIC (TOMO) NUCLEAR MEDICINE IMAGING:** Introduction of radioactive materials into the body for three dimensional display of images developed from the capture of radioactive emissions

Body Part	Radionuclide	Qualifier	Qualifier
Ø Breast, Right 1 Breast, Left 2 Breasts, Bilateral	1 Technetium 99m (Tc-99m) S Thallium 201 (Tl-201) Y Other Radionuclide	Z None	Z None
Y Skin, Subcutaneous Tissue, and Breast	Y Other Radionuclide	Z None	Z None

SECTION: C NUCLEAR MEDICINE
BODY SYSTEM: P MUSCULOSKELETAL SYSTEM
TYPE: 1 **PLANAR NUCLEAR MEDICINE IMAGING:** Introduction of radioactive materials into the body for single plane display of images developed from the capture of radioactive emissions

Body Part	Radionuclide	Qualifier	Qualifier
1 Skull 4 Thorax 5 Spine 6 Pelvis 7 Spine and Pelvis 8 Upper Extremity, Right 9 Upper Extremity, Left B Upper Extremities, Bilateral C Lower Extremity, Right D Lower Extremity, Left F Lower Extremities, Bilateral Z Musculoskeletal System, All	1 Technetium 99m (Tc-99m) Y Other Radionuclide	Z None	Z None
Y Musculoskeletal System, Other	Y Other Radionuclide	Z None	Z None

SECTION: C NUCLEAR MEDICINE
BODY SYSTEM: P MUSCULOSKELETAL SYSTEM
TYPE: 2 **TOMOGRAPHIC (TOMO) NUCLEAR MEDICINE IMAGING:** Introduction of radioactive materials into the body for three dimensional display of images developed from the capture of radioactive emissions

Body Part	Radionuclide	Qualifier	Qualifier
1 Skull 2 Cervical Spine 3 Skull and Cervical Spine 4 Thorax 6 Pelvis 7 Spine and Pelvis 8 Upper Extremity, Right 9 Upper Extremity, Left B Upper Extremities, Bilateral C Lower Extremity, Right D Lower Extremity, Left F Lower Extremities, Bilateral G Thoracic Spine H Lumbar Spine J Thoracolumbar Spine	1 Technetium 99m (Tc-99m) Y Other Radionuclide	Z None	Z None
Y Musculoskeletal System, Other	Y Other Radionuclide	Z None	Z None

SECTION: **C NUCLEAR MEDICINE**
BODY SYSTEM: P **MUSCULOSKELETAL SYSTEM**
TYPE: **5 NONIMAGING NUCLEAR MEDICINE PROBE:** Introduction of radioactive materials into the body for the study of distribution and fate of certain substances by the detection of radioactive emissions; or, alternatively, measurement of absorption of radioactive emissions from an external source

Body Part	Radionuclide	Qualifier	Qualifier
5 Spine N Upper Extremities P Lower Extremities	Z None	Z None	Z None
Y Musculoskeletal System, Other	Y Other Radionuclide	Z None	Z None

SECTION: C NUCLEAR MEDICINE

BODY SYSTEM: T   URINARY SYSTEM

TYPE: 1   **PLANAR NUCLEAR MEDICINE IMAGING:** Introduction of radioactive materials into the body for single plane display of images developed from the capture of radioactive emissions

Body Part	Radionuclide	Qualifier	Qualifier
3 Kidneys, Ureters, and Bladder	1 Technetium 99m (Tc-99m) F Iodine 123 (I-123) G Iodine 131 (I-131) Y Other Radionuclide	Z None	Z None
H Bladder and Ureters	1 Technetium 99m (Tc-99m) Y Other Radionuclide	Z None	Z None
Y Urinary System	Y Other Radionuclide	Z None	Z None

SECTION: C NUCLEAR MEDICINE

BODY SYSTEM: T   URINARY SYSTEM

TYPE: 2   **TOMOGRAPHIC (TOMO) NUCLEAR MEDICINE IMAGING:** Introduction of radioactive materials into the body for three dimensional display of images developed from the capture of radioactive emissions

Body Part	Radionuclide	Qualifier	Qualifier
3 Kidneys, Ureters, and Bladder	1 Technetium 99m (Tc-99m) Y Other Radionuclide	Z None	Z None
Y Urinary System	Y Other Radionuclide	Z None	Z None

SECTION: C NUCLEAR MEDICINE

BODY SYSTEM: T   URINARY SYSTEM

TYPE: 6   **NONIMAGING NUCLEAR MEDICINE ASSAY:** Introduction of radioactive materials into the body for the study of body fluids and blood elements, by the detection of radioactive emissions

Body Part	Radionuclide	Qualifier	Qualifier
3 Kidneys, Ureters, and Bladder	1 Technetium 99m (Tc-99m) F Iodine 123 (I-123) G Iodine 131 (I-131) H Iodine 125 (I-125) Y Other Radionuclide	Z None	Z None
Y Urinary System	Y Other Radionuclide	Z None	Z None

SECTION: C NUCLEAR MEDICINE
BODY SYSTEM: V   MALE REPRODUCTIVE SYSTEM
TYPE: 1   **PLANAR NUCLEAR MEDICINE IMAGING:** Introduction of radioactive materials into the body for single plane display of images developed from the capture of radioactive emissions

Body Part	Radionuclide	Qualifier	Qualifier
9 Testicles, Bilateral	1 Technetium 99m (Tc-99m) Y Other Radionuclide	Z None	Z None
Y Male Reproductive System	Y Other Radionuclide	Z None	Z None

SECTION: C NUCLEAR MEDICINE
BODY SYSTEM: W ANATOMICAL REGIONS
TYPE: 1 **PLANAR NUCLEAR MEDICINE IMAGING:** Introduction of radioactive materials into the body for single plane display of images developed from the capture of radioactive emissions

Body Part	Radionuclide	Qualifier	Qualifier
Ø Abdomen 1 Abdomen and Pelvis 4 Chest and Abdomen 6 Chest and Neck B Head and Neck D Lower Extremity J Pelvic Region M Upper Extremity N Whole Body	1 Technetium 99m (Tc-99m) D Indium 111 (In-111) F Iodine 123 (I-123) G Iodine 131 (I-131) L Gallium 67 (Ga-67) S Thallium 201 (Tl-201) Y Other Radionuclide	Z None	Z None
3 Chest	1 Technetium 99m (Tc-99m) D Indium 111 (In-111) F Iodine 123 (I-123) G Iodine 131 (I-131) K Fluorine 18 (F-18) L Gallium 67 (Ga-67) S Thallium 201 (Tl-201) Y Other Radionuclide	Z None	Z None
Y Anatomical Regions, Multiple	Y Other Radionuclide	Z None	Z None
Z Anatomical Region, Other	Z None	Z None	Z None

SECTION: C NUCLEAR MEDICINE
BODY SYSTEM: W ANATOMICAL REGIONS
TYPE: 2 **TOMOGRAPHIC (TOMO) NUCLEAR MEDICINE IMAGING:** Introduction of radioactive materials into the body for three dimensional display of images developed from the capture of radioactive emissions

Body Part	Radionuclide	Qualifier	Qualifier
Ø Abdomen 1 Abdomen and Pelvis 3 Chest 4 Chest and Abdomen 6 Chest and Neck B Head and Neck D Lower Extremity J Pelvic Region M Upper Extremity	1 Technetium 99m (Tc-99m) D Indium 111 (In-111) F Iodine 123 (I-123) G Iodine 131 (I-131) K Fluorine 18 (F-18) L Gallium 67 (Ga-67) S Thallium 201 (Tl-201) Y Other Radionuclide	Z None	Z None
Y Anatomical Regions, Multiple	Y Other Radionuclide	Z None	Z None

W: ANATOMICAL REGIONS

C: NUCLEAR MEDICINE

1; 2

SECTION:　C NUCLEAR MEDICINE
BODY SYSTEM: W ANATOMICAL REGIONS
TYPE:　　　3 **POSITRON EMISSION TOMOGRAPHIC (PET) IMAGING:** Introduction of radioactive materials into the body for three dimensional display of images developed from the simultaneous capture, 18Ø degrees apart, of radioactive emissions

Body Part	Radionuclide	Qualifier	Qualifier
N Whole Body	Y Other Radionuclide	Z None	Z None

SECTION:　C NUCLEAR MEDICINE
BODY SYSTEM: W ANATOMICAL REGIONS
TYPE:　　　5 **NONIMAGING NUCLEAR MEDICINE PROBE:** Introduction of radioactive materials into the body for the study of distribution and fate of certain substances by the detection of radioactive emissions; or, alternatively, measurement of absorption of radioactive emissions from an external source

Body Part	Radionuclide	Qualifier	Qualifier
Ø Abdomen 1 Abdomen and Pelvis 3 Chest 4 Chest and Abdomen 6 Chest and Neck B Head and Neck D Lower Extremity J Pelvic Region M Upper Extremity	1 Technetium 99m (Tc-99m) D Indium 111 (In-111) Y Other Radionuclide	Z None	Z None

SECTION:　C NUCLEAR MEDICINE
BODY SYSTEM: W ANATOMICAL REGIONS
TYPE:　　　7 **SYSTEMIC NUCLEAR MEDICINE THERAPY:** Introduction of unsealed radioactive materials into the body for treatment

Body Part	Radionuclide	Qualifier	Qualifier
Ø Abdomen 3 Chest	N Phosphorus 32 (P-32) Y Other Radionuclide	Z None	Z None
G Thyroid	G Iodine 131 (I-131) Y Other Radionuclide	Z None	Z None
N Whole Body	8 Samarium 153 (Sm-153) G Iodine 131 (I-131) N Phosphorus 32 (P-32) P Strontium 89 (Sr-89) Y Other Radionuclide	Z None	Z None
Y Anatomical Regions, Multiple	Y Other Radionuclide	Z None	Z None

D   Radiation Therapy...**630**
    DØ. Central and Peripheral Nervous System...632
        DØØ. Beam Radiation 632
        DØ1. Brachytherapy 632
        DØ2. Stereotactic Radiosurgery 632
        DØY. Other Radiation 632
    D7. Lymphatic and Hematologic System 633
        D7Ø. Beam Radiation 633
        D71. Brachytherapy 633
        D72. Stereotactic Radiosurgery 634
        D7Y. Other Radiation 634
    D8. Eye..635
        D8Ø. Beam Radiation 635
        D81. Brachytherapy 635
        D82. Stereotactic Radiosurgery 635
        D8Y. Other Radiation 635
    D9. Ear, Nose, Mouth, and Throat 636
        D9Ø. Beam Radiation 636
        D91. Brachytherapy 636
        D92. Stereotactic Radiosurgery 637
        D9Y. Other Radiation 637
    DB. Respiratory System 638
        DBØ. Beam Radiation 638
        DB1. Brachytherapy 638
        DB2. Stereotactic Radiosurgery 639
        DBY. Other Radiation 639
    DD. Gastrointestinal System 640
        DDØ. Beam Radiation 640
        DD1. Brachytherapy 640
        DD2. Stereotactic Radiosurgery 641
        DDY. Other Radiation 641
    DF. Hepatobiliary System and Pancreas 642
        DFØ. Beam Radiation 642
        DF1. Brachytherapy 642
        DF2. Stereotactic Radiosurgery 642
        DFY. Other Radiation 642
    DG. Endocrine System 643
        DGØ. Beam Radiation 643
        DG1. Brachytherapy 643
        DG2. Stereotactic Radiosurgery 643
        DGY. Other Radiation 643
    DH. Skin 644
        DHØ. Beam Radiation 644
        DHY. Other Radiation 644
    DM. Breast 645
        DMØ. Beam Radiation 645
        DM1. Brachytherapy 645
        DM2. Stereotactic Radiosurgery 645
        DMY. Other Radiation 645
    DP. Musculoskeletal System 646
        DPØ. Beam Radiation 646
        DPY. Other Radiation 646
    DT. Urinary System 647
        DTØ. Beam Radiation 647
        DT1. Brachytherapy 647
        DT2. Stereotactic Radiosurgery 647
        DTY. Other Radiation 647

DU. Female Reproductive System 648
    DUØ. Beam Radiation 648
    DU1. Brachytherapy...648
    DU2. Stereotactic Radiosurgery 649
    DUY. Other Radiation 649
DV. Male Reproductive System 650
    DVØ. Beam Radiation 650
    DV1. Brachytherapy...650
    DV2. Stereotactic Radiosurgery 651
    DVY. Other Radiation 651
DW. Anatomical Regions...652
    DWØ. Beam Radiation 652
    DW1. Brachytherapy..652
    DW2. Stereotactic Radiosurgery 653
    DWY. Other Radiation 653

SECTION: D RADIATION THERAPY
BODY SYSTEM: 0 CENTRAL AND PERIPHERAL NERVOUS SYSTEM
MODALITY: 0 BEAM RADIATION

Treatment Site	Modality Qualifier	Isotope	Qualifier
0 Brain 1 Brain Stem 6 Spinal Cord 7 Peripheral Nerve	0 Photons <1 MeV 1 Photons 1 - 10 MeV 2 Photons >10 MeV 4 Heavy Particles (Protons,Ions) 5 Neutrons 6 Neutron Capture	Z None	Z None
0 Brain 1 Brain Stem 6 Spinal Cord 7 Peripheral Nerve	3 Electrons	Z None	0 Intraoperative Z None

SECTION: D RADIATION THERAPY
BODY SYSTEM: 0 CENTRAL AND PERIPHERAL NERVOUS SYSTEM
MODALITY: 1 BRACHYTHERAPY

Treatment Site	Modality Qualifier	Isotope	Qualifier
0 Brain 1 Brain Stem 6 Spinal Cord 7 Peripheral Nerve	9 High Dose Rate (HDR) B Low Dose Rate (LDR)	7 Cesium 137 (Cs-137) 8 Iridium 192 (Ir-192) 9 Iodine 125 (I-125) B Palladium 103 (Pd-103) C Californium 252 (Cf-252) Y Other Isotope	Z None

SECTION: D RADIATION THERAPY
BODY SYSTEM: 0 CENTRAL AND PERIPHERAL NERVOUS SYSTEM
MODALITY: 2 STEREOTACTIC RADIOSURGERY

Treatment Site	Modality Qualifier	Isotope	Qualifier
0 Brain 1 Brain Stem 6 Spinal Cord 7 Peripheral Nerve	D Stereotactic Other Photon Radiosurgery H Stereotactic Particulate Radiosurgery J Stereotactic Gamma Beam Radiosurgery	Z None	Z None

SECTION: D RADIATION THERAPY
BODY SYSTEM: 0 CENTRAL AND PERIPHERAL NERVOUS SYSTEM
MODALITY: Y OTHER RADIATION

Treatment Site	Modality Qualifier	Isotope	Qualifier
0 Brain 1 Brain Stem 6 Spinal Cord 7 Peripheral Nerve	7 Contact Radiation 8 Hyperthermia F Plaque Radiation K Laser Interstitial Thermal Therapy	Z None	Z None

SECTION: D RADIATION THERAPY
BODY SYSTEM: 7 LYMPHATIC AND HEMATOLOGIC SYSTEM
MODALITY: Ø BEAM RADIATION

Treatment Site	Modality Qualifier	Isotope	Qualifier
Ø Bone Marrow 1 Thymus 2 Spleen 3 Lymphatics, Neck 4 Lymphatics, Axillary 5 Lymphatics, Thorax 6 Lymphatics, Abdomen 7 Lymphatics, Pelvis 8 Lymphatics, Inguinal	Ø Photons <1 MeV 1 Photons 1 - 1Ø MeV 2 Photons >1Ø MeV 4 Heavy Particles (Protons, Ions) 5 Neutrons 6 Neutron Capture	Z None	Z None
Ø Bone Marrow 1 Thymus 2 Spleen 3 Lymphatics, Neck 4 Lymphatics, Axillary 5 Lymphatics, Thorax 6 Lymphatics, Abdomen 7 Lymphatics, Pelvis 8 Lymphatics, Inguinal	3 Electrons	Z None	Ø Intraoperative Z None

SECTION: D RADIATION THERAPY
BODY SYSTEM: 7 LYMPHATIC AND HEMATOLOGIC SYSTEM
MODALITY: 1 BRACHYTHERAPY

Treatment Site	Modality Qualifier	Isotope	Qualifier
Ø Bone Marrow 1 Thymus 2 Spleen 3 Lymphatics, Neck 4 Lymphatics, Axillary 5 Lymphatics, Thorax 6 Lymphatics, Abdomen 7 Lymphatics, Pelvis 8 Lymphatics, Inguinal	9 High Dose Rate (HDR) B Low Dose Rate (LDR)	7 Cesium 137 (Cs-137) 8 Iridium 192 (Ir-192) 9 Iodine 125 (I-125) B Palladium 1Ø3 (Pd-1Ø3) C Californium 252 (Cf-252) Y Other Isotope	Z None

SECTION: **D RADIATION THERAPY**
BODY SYSTEM: 7 **LYMPHATIC AND HEMATOLOGIC SYSTEM**
MODALITY: 2 **STEREOTACTIC RADIOSURGERY**

Treatment Site	Modality Qualifier	Isotope	Qualifier
Ø Bone Marrow 1 Thymus 2 Spleen 3 Lymphatics, Neck 4 Lymphatics, Axillary 5 Lymphatics, Thorax 6 Lymphatics, Abdomen 7 Lymphatics, Pelvis 8 Lymphatics, Inguinal	D Stereotactic Other Photon Radiosurgery H Stereotactic Particulate Radiosurgery J Stereotactic Gamma Beam Radiosurgery	Z None	Z None

SECTION: **D RADIATION THERAPY**
BODY SYSTEM: 7 **LYMPHATIC AND HEMATOLOGIC SYSTEM**
MODALITY: Y **OTHER RADIATION**

Treatment Site	Modality Qualifier	Isotope	Qualifier
Ø Bone Marrow 1 Thymus 2 Spleen 3 Lymphatics, Neck 4 Lymphatics, Axillary 5 Lymphatics, Thorax 6 Lymphatics, Abdomen 7 Lymphatics, Pelvis 8 Lymphatics, Inguinal	8 Hyperthermia F Plaque Radiation	Z None	Z None

New/Revised Text in Blue   ~~deleted~~ Deleted

SECTION: D RADIATION THERAPY
BODY SYSTEM: 8 EYE
MODALITY: Ø BEAM RADIATION

Treatment Site	Modality Qualifier	Isotope	Qualifier
Ø Eye	Ø Photons <1 MeV 1 Photons 1 - 1Ø MeV 2 Photons >1Ø MeV 4 Heavy Particles (Protons, Ions) 5 Neutrons 6 Neutron Capture	Z None	Z None
Ø Eye	3 Electrons	Z None	Ø Intraoperative Z None

SECTION: D RADIATION THERAPY
BODY SYSTEM: 8 EYE
MODALITY: 1 BRACHYTHERAPY

Treatment Site	Modality Qualifier	Isotope	Qualifier
Ø Eye	9 High Dose Rate (HDR) B Low Dose Rate (LDR)	7 Cesium 137 (Cs-137) 8 Iridium 192 (Ir-192) 9 Iodine 125 (I-125) B Palladium 1Ø3 (Pd-1Ø3) C Californium 252 (Cf-252) Y Other Isotope	Z None

SECTION: D RADIATION THERAPY
BODY SYSTEM: 8 EYE
MODALITY: 2 STEREOTACTIC RADIOSURGERY

Treatment Site	Modality Qualifier	Isotope	Qualifier
Ø Eye	D Stereotactic Other Photon Radiosurgery H Stereotactic Particulate Radiosurgery J Stereotactic Gamma Beam Radiosurgery	Z None	Z None

SECTION: D RADIATION THERAPY
BODY SYSTEM: 8 EYE
MODALITY: Y OTHER RADIATION

Treatment Site	Modality Qualifier	Isotope	Qualifier
Ø Eye	7 Contact Radiation 8 Hyperthermia F Plaque Radiation	Z None	Z None

SECTION: D RADIATION THERAPY
BODY SYSTEM: 9 EAR, NOSE, MOUTH, AND THROAT
MODALITY: Ø BEAM RADIATION

Treatment Site	Modality Qualifier	Isotope	Qualifier
Ø Ear 1 Nose 3 Hypopharynx 4 Mouth 5 Tongue 6 Salivary Glands 7 Sinuses 8 Hard Palate 9 Soft Palate B Larynx D Nasopharynx F Oropharynx	Ø Photons <1 MeV 1 Photons 1 - 1Ø MeV 2 Photons >1Ø MeV 4 Heavy Particles (Protons, Ions) 5 Neutrons 6 Neutron Capture	Z None	Z None
Ø Ear 1 Nose 3 Hypopharynx 4 Mouth 5 Tongue 6 Salivary Glands 7 Sinuses 8 Hard Palate 9 Soft Palate B Larynx D Nasopharynx F Oropharynx	3 Electrons	Z None	Ø Intraoperative Z None

SECTION: D RADIATION THERAPY
BODY SYSTEM: 9 EAR, NOSE, MOUTH, AND THROAT
MODALITY: 1 BRACHYTHERAPY

Treatment Site	Modality Qualifier	Isotope	Qualifier
Ø Ear 1 Nose 3 Hypopharynx 4 Mouth 5 Tongue 6 Salivary Glands 7 Sinuses 8 Hard Palate 9 Soft Palate B Larynx D Nasopharynx F Oropharynx	9 High Dose Rate (HDR) B Low Dose Rate (LDR)	7 Cesium 137 (Cs-137) 8 Iridium 192 (Ir-192) 9 Iodine 125 (I-125) B Palladium 1Ø3 (Pd-1Ø3) C Californium 252 (Cf-252) Y Other Isotope	Z None

SECTION: D RADIATION THERAPY
BODY SYSTEM: 9 EAR, NOSE, MOUTH, AND THROAT
MODALITY: 2 STEREOTACTIC RADIOSURGERY

Treatment Site	Modality Qualifier	Isotope	Qualifier
Ø Ear 1 Nose 4 Mouth 5 Tongue 6 Salivary Glands 7 Sinuses 8 Hard Palate 9 Soft Palate B Larynx C Pharynx D Nasopharynx	D Stereotactic Other Photon Radiosurgery H Stereotactic Particulate Radiosurgery J Stereotactic Gamma Beam Radiosurgery	Z None	Z None

SECTION: D RADIATION THERAPY
BODY SYSTEM: 9 EAR, NOSE, MOUTH, AND THROAT
MODALITY: Y OTHER RADIATION

Treatment Site	Modality Qualifier	Isotope	Qualifier
Ø Ear 1 Nose 5 Tongue 6 Salivary Glands 7 Sinuses 8 Hard Palate 9 Soft Palate	7 Contact Radiation 8 Hyperthermia F Plaque Radiation	Z None	Z None
3 Hypopharynx F Oropharynx	7 Contact Radiation 8 Hyperthermia	Z None	Z None
4 Mouth B Larynx D Nasopharynx	7 Contact Radiation 8 Hyperthermia C Intraoperative Radiation Therapy (IORT) F Plaque Radiation	Z None	Z None
C Pharynx	C Intraoperative Radiation Therapy (IORT) F Plaque Radiation	Z None	Z None

SECTION: D RADIATION THERAPY
BODY SYSTEM: B RESPIRATORY SYSTEM
MODALITY: Ø BEAM RADIATION

Treatment Site	Modality Qualifier	Isotope	Qualifier
Ø Trachea 1 Bronchus 2 Lung 5 Pleura 6 Mediastinum 7 Chest Wall 8 Diaphragm	Ø Photons <1 MeV 1 Photons 1 - 1Ø MeV 2 Photons >1Ø MeV 4 Heavy Particles (Protons, Ions) 5 Neutrons 6 Neutron Capture	Z None	Z None
Ø Trachea 1 Bronchus 2 Lung 5 Pleura 6 Mediastinum 7 Chest Wall 8 Diaphragm	3 Electrons	Z None	Ø Intraoperative Z None

SECTION: D RADIATION THERAPY
BODY SYSTEM: B RESPIRATORY SYSTEM
MODALITY: 1 BRACHYTHERAPY

Treatment Site	Modality Qualifier	Isotope	Qualifier
Ø Trachea 1 Bronchus 2 Lung 5 Pleura 6 Mediastinum 7 Chest Wall 8 Diaphragm	9 High Dose Rate (HDR) B Low Dose Rate (LDR)	7 Cesium 137 (Cs-137) 8 Iridium 192 (Ir-192) 9 Iodine 125 (I-125) B Palladium 1Ø3 (Pd-1Ø3) C Californium 252 (Cf-252) Y Other Isotope	Z None

SECTION: D RADIATION THERAPY
BODY SYSTEM: B RESPIRATORY SYSTEM
MODALITY: 2 STEREOTACTIC RADIOSURGERY

Treatment Site	Modality Qualifier	Isotope	Qualifier
Ø Trachea 1 Bronchus 2 Lung 5 Pleura 6 Mediastinum 7 Chest Wall 8 Diaphragm	D Stereotactic Other Photon Radiosurgery H Stereotactic Particulate Radiosurgery J Stereotactic Gamma Beam Radiosurgery	Z None	Z None

SECTION: D RADIATION THERAPY
BODY SYSTEM: B RESPIRATORY SYSTEM
MODALITY: Y OTHER RADIATION

Treatment Site	Modality Qualifier	Isotope	Qualifier
Ø Trachea 1 Bronchus 2 Lung 5 Pleura 6 Mediastinum 7 Chest Wall 8 Diaphragm	7 Contact Radiation 8 Hyperthermia F Plaque Radiation K Laser Interstitial Thermal Therapy	Z None	Z None

SECTION: D RADIATION THERAPY
BODY SYSTEM: D GASTROINTESTINAL SYSTEM
MODALITY: Ø BEAM RADIATION

Treatment Site	Modality Qualifier	Isotope	Qualifier
Ø Esophagus 1 Stomach 2 Duodenum 3 Jejunum 4 Ileum 5 Colon 7 Rectum	Ø Photons <1 MeV 1 Photons 1 - 1Ø MeV 2 Photons >1Ø MeV 4 Heavy Particles (Protons, Ions) 5 Neutrons 6 Neutron Capture	Z None	Z None
Ø Esophagus 1 Stomach 2 Duodenum 3 Jejunum 4 Ileum 5 Colon 7 Rectum	3 Electrons	Z None	Ø Intraoperative Z None

SECTION: D RADIATION THERAPY
BODY SYSTEM: D GASTROINTESTINAL SYSTEM
MODALITY: 1 BRACHYTHERAPY

Treatment Site	Modality Qualifier	Isotope	Qualifier
Ø Esophagus 1 Stomach 2 Duodenum 3 Jejunum 4 Ileum 5 Colon 7 Rectum	9 High Dose Rate (HDR) B Low Dose Rate (LDR)	7 Cesium 137 (Cs-137) 8 Iridium 192 (Ir-192) 9 Iodine 125 (I-125) B Palladium 1Ø3 (Pd-1Ø3) C Californium 252 (Cf-252) Y Other Isotope	Z None

SECTION: **D RADIATION THERAPY**
BODY SYSTEM: **D GASTROINTESTINAL SYSTEM**
MODALITY: **2 STEREOTACTIC RADIOSURGERY**

Treatment Site	Modality Qualifier	Isotope	Qualifier
Ø Esophagus 1 Stomach 2 Duodenum 3 Jejunum 4 Ileum 5 Colon 7 Rectum	D Stereotactic Other Photon Radiosurgery H Stereotactic Particulate Radiosurgery J Stereotactic Gamma Beam Radiosurgery	Z None	Z None

SECTION: **D RADIATION THERAPY**
BODY SYSTEM: **D GASTROINTESTINAL SYSTEM**
MODALITY: **Y OTHER RADIATION**

Treatment Site	Modality Qualifier	Isotope	Qualifier
Ø Esophagus	7 Contact Radiation 8 Hyperthermia F Plaque Radiation K Laser Interstitial Thermal Therapy	Z None	Z None
1 Stomach 2 Duodenum 3 Jejunum 4 Ileum 5 Colon 7 Rectum	7 Contact Radiation 8 Hyperthermia C Intraoperative Radiation Therapy (IORT) F Plaque Radiation K Laser Interstitial Thermal Therapy	Z None	Z None
8 Anus	C Intraoperative Radiation Therapy (IORT) F Plaque Radiation K Laser Interstitial Thermal Therapy	Z None	Z None

SECTION: D RADIATION THERAPY
BODY SYSTEM: F HEPATOBILIARY SYSTEM AND PANCREAS
MODALITY: Ø BEAM RADIATION

Treatment Site	Modality Qualifier	Isotope	Qualifier
Ø Liver 1 Gallbladder 2 Bile Ducts 3 Pancreas	Ø Photons <1 MeV 1 Photons 1 - 1Ø MeV 2 Photons >1Ø MeV 4 Heavy Particles (Protons, Ions) 5 Neutrons 6 Neutron Capture	Z None	Z None
Ø Liver 1 Gallbladder 2 Bile Ducts 3 Pancreas	3 Electrons	Z None	Ø Intraoperative Z None

SECTION: D RADIATION THERAPY
BODY SYSTEM: F HEPATOBILIARY SYSTEM AND PANCREAS
MODALITY: 1 BRACHYTHERAPY

Treatment Site	Modality Qualifier	Isotope	Qualifier
Ø Liver 1 Gallbladder 2 Bile Ducts 3 Pancreas	9 High Dose Rate (HDR) B Low Dose Rate (LDR)	7 Cesium 137 (Cs-137) 8 Iridium 192 (Ir-192) 9 Iodine 125 (I-125) B Palladium 1Ø3 (Pd-1Ø3) C Californium 252 (Cf-252) Y Other Isotope	Z None

SECTION: D RADIATION THERAPY
BODY SYSTEM: F HEPATOBILIARY SYSTEM AND PANCREAS
MODALITY: 2 STEREOTACTIC RADIOSURGERY

Treatment Site	Modality Qualifier	Isotope	Qualifier
Ø Liver 1 Gallbladder 2 Bile Ducts 3 Pancreas	D Stereotactic Other Photon Radiosurgery H Stereotactic Particulate Radiosurgery J Stereotactic Gamma Beam Radiosurgery	Z None	Z None

SECTION: D RADIATION THERAPY
BODY SYSTEM: F HEPATOBILIARY SYSTEM AND PANCREAS
MODALITY: Y OTHER RADIATION

Treatment Site	Modality Qualifier	Isotope	Qualifier
Ø Liver 1 Gallbladder 2 Bile Ducts 3 Pancreas	7 Contact Radiation 8 Hyperthermia C Intraoperative Radiation Therapy (IORT) F Plaque Radiation K Laser Interstitial Thermal Therapy	Z None	Z None

SECTION: D RADIATION THERAPY
BODY SYSTEM: G ENDOCRINE SYSTEM
MODALITY: Ø BEAM RADIATION

Treatment Site	Modality Qualifier	Isotope	Qualifier
Ø Pituitary Gland 1 Pineal Body 2 Adrenal Glands 4 Parathyroid Glands 5 Thyroid	Ø Photons <1 MeV 1 Photons 1 - 1Ø MeV 2 Photons >1Ø MeV 5 Neutrons 6 Neutron Capture	Z None	Z None
Ø Pituitary Gland 1 Pineal Body 2 Adrenal Glands 4 Parathyroid Glands 5 Thyroid	3 Electrons	Z None	Ø Intraoperative Z None

SECTION: D RADIATION THERAPY
BODY SYSTEM: G ENDOCRINE SYSTEM
MODALITY: 1 BRACHYTHERAPY

Treatment Site	Modality Qualifier	Isotope	Qualifier
Ø Pituitary Gland 1 Pineal Body 2 Adrenal Glands 4 Parathyroid Glands 5 Thyroid	9 High Dose Rate (HDR) B Low Dose Rate (LDR)	7 Cesium 137 (Cs-137) 8 Iridium 192 (Ir-192) 9 Iodine 125 (I-125) B Palladium 1Ø3 (Pd-1Ø3) C Californium 252 (Cf-252) Y Other Isotope	Z None

SECTION: D RADIATION THERAPY
BODY SYSTEM: G ENDOCRINE SYSTEM
MODALITY: 2 STEREOTACTIC RADIOSURGERY

Treatment Site	Modality Qualifier	Isotope	Qualifier
Ø Pituitary Gland 1 Pineal Body 2 Adrenal Glands 4 Parathyroid Glands 5 Thyroid	D Stereotactic Other Photon Radiosurgery H Stereotactic Particulate Radiosurgery J Stereotactic Gamma Beam Radiosurgery	Z None	Z None

SECTION: D RADIATION THERAPY
BODY SYSTEM: G ENDOCRINE SYSTEM
MODALITY: Y OTHER RADIATION

Treatment Site	Modality Qualifier	Isotope	Qualifier
Ø Pituitary Gland 1 Pineal Body 2 Adrenal Glands 4 Parathyroid Glands 5 Thyroid	7 Contact Radiation 8 Hyperthermia F Plaque Radiation K Laser Interstitial Thermal Therapy	Z None	Z None

SECTION: D RADIATION THERAPY
BODY SYSTEM: H SKIN
MODALITY: Ø BEAM RADIATION

Treatment Site	Modality Qualifier	Isotope	Qualifier
2 Skin, Face 3 Skin, Neck 4 Skin, Arm 6 Skin, Chest 7 Skin, Back 8 Skin, Abdomen 9 Skin, Buttock B Skin, Leg	Ø Photons <1 MeV 1 Photons 1 - 1Ø MeV 2 Photons >1Ø MeV 4 Heavy Particles (Protons, Ions) 5 Neutrons 6 Neutron Capture	Z None	Z None
2 Skin, Face 3 Skin, Neck 4 Skin, Arm 6 Skin, Chest 7 Skin, Back 8 Skin, Abdomen 9 Skin, Buttock B Skin, Leg	3 Electrons	Z None	Ø Intraoperative Z None

SECTION: D RADIATION THERAPY
BODY SYSTEM: H SKIN
MODALITY: Y OTHER RADIATION

Treatment Site	Modality Qualifier	Isotope	Qualifier
2 Skin, Face 3 Skin, Neck 4 Skin, Arm 6 Skin, Chest 7 Skin, Back 8 Skin, Abdomen 9 Skin, Buttock B Skin, Leg	7 Contact Radiation 8 Hyperthermia F Plaque Radiation	Z None	Z None
5 Skin, Hand C Skin, Foot	F Plaque Radiation	Z None	Z None

SECTION: D RADIATION THERAPY
BODY SYSTEM: M BREAST
MODALITY: Ø BEAM RADIATION

Treatment Site	Modality Qualifier	Isotope	Qualifier
Ø Breast, Left 1 Breast, Right	Ø Photons <1 MeV 1 Photons 1 - 1Ø MeV 2 Photons >1Ø MeV 4 Heavy Particles (Protons, Ions) 5 Neutrons 6 Neutron Capture	Z None	Z None
Ø Breast, Left 1 Breast, Right	3 Electrons	Z None	Ø Intraoperative Z None

SECTION: D RADIATION THERAPY
BODY SYSTEM: M BREAST
MODALITY: 1 BRACHYTHERAPY

Treatment Site	Modality Qualifier	Isotope	Qualifier
Ø Breast, Left 1 Breast, Right	9 High Dose Rate (HDR) B Low Dose Rate (LDR)	7 Cesium 137 (Cs-137) 8 Iridium 192 (Ir-192) 9 Iodine 125 (I-125) B Palladium 1Ø3 (Pd-1Ø3) C Californium 252 (Cf-252) Y Other Isotope	Z None

SECTION: D RADIATION THERAPY
BODY SYSTEM: M BREAST
MODALITY: 2 STEREOTACTIC RADIOSURGERY

Treatment Site	Modality Qualifier	Isotope	Qualifier
Ø Breast, Left 1 Breast, Right	D Stereotactic Other Photon Radiosurgery H Stereotactic Particulate Radiosurgery J Stereotactic Gamma Beam Radiosurgery	Z None	Z None

SECTION: D RADIATION THERAPY
BODY SYSTEM: M BREAST
MODALITY: Y OTHER RADIATION

Treatment Site	Modality Qualifier	Isotope	Qualifier
Ø Breast, Left 1 Breast, Right	7 Contact Radiation 8 Hyperthermia F Plaque Radiation K Laser Interstitial Thermal Therapy	Z None	Z None

SECTION: D RADIATION THERAPY
BODY SYSTEM: P MUSCULOSKELETAL SYSTEM
MODALITY: Ø BEAM RADIATION

Treatment Site	Modality Qualifier	Isotope	Qualifier
Ø Skull 2 Maxilla 3 Mandible 4 Sternum 5 Rib(s) 6 Humerus 7 Radius/Ulna 8 Pelvic Bones 9 Femur B Tibia/Fibula C Other Bone	Ø Photons <1 MeV 1 Photons 1 - 1Ø MeV 2 Photons >1Ø MeV 4 Heavy Particles (Protons, Ions) 5 Neutrons 6 Neutron Capture	Z None	Z None
Ø Skull 2 Maxilla 3 Mandible 4 Sternum 5 Rib(s) 6 Humerus 7 Radius/Ulna 8 Pelvic Bones 9 Femur B Tibia/Fibula C Other Bone	3 Electrons	Z None	Ø Intraoperative Z None

SECTION: D RADIATION THERAPY
BODY SYSTEM: P MUSCULOSKELETAL SYSTEM
MODALITY: Y OTHER RADIATION

Treatment Site	Modality Qualifier	Isotope	Qualifier
Ø Skull 2 Maxilla 3 Mandible 4 Sternum 5 Rib(s) 6 Humerus 7 Radius/Ulna 8 Pelvic Bones 9 Femur B Tibia/Fibula C Other Bone	7 Contact Radiation 8 Hyperthermia F Plaque Radiation	Z None	Z None

SECTION: D RADIATION THERAPY
BODY SYSTEM: T URINARY SYSTEM
MODALITY: Ø BEAM RADIATION

Treatment Site	Modality Qualifier	Isotope	Qualifier
Ø Kidney 1 Ureter 2 Bladder 3 Urethra	Ø Photons <1 MeV 1 Photons 1 - 1Ø MeV 2 Photons >1Ø MeV 4 Heavy Particles (Protons, Ions) 5 Neutrons 6 Neutron Capture	Z None	Z None
Ø Kidney 1 Ureter 2 Bladder 3 Urethra	3 Electrons	Z None	Ø Intraoperative Z None

SECTION: D RADIATION THERAPY
BODY SYSTEM: T URINARY SYSTEM
MODALITY: 1 BRACHYTHERAPY

Treatment Site	Modality Qualifier	Isotope	Qualifier
Ø Kidney 1 Ureter 2 Bladder 3 Urethra	9 High Dose Rate (HDR) B Low Dose Rate (LDR)	7 Cesium 137 (Cs-137) 8 Iridium 192 (Ir-192) 9 Iodine 125 (I-125) B Palladium 1Ø3 (Pd-1Ø3) C Californium 252 (Cf-252) Y Other Isotope	Z None

SECTION: D RADIATION THERAPY
BODY SYSTEM: T URINARY SYSTEM
MODALITY: 2 STEREOTACTIC RADIOSURGERY

Treatment Site	Modality Qualifier	Isotope	Qualifier
Ø Kidney 1 Ureter 2 Bladder 3 Urethra	D Stereotactic Other Photon Radiosurgery H Stereotactic Particulate Radiosurgery J Stereotactic Gamma Beam Radiosurgery	Z None	Z None

SECTION: D RADIATION THERAPY
BODY SYSTEM: T URINARY SYSTEM
MODALITY: Y OTHER RADIATION

Treatment Site	Modality Qualifier	Isotope	Qualifier
Ø Kidney 1 Ureter 2 Bladder 3 Urethra	7 Contact Radiation 8 Hyperthermia C Intraoperative Radiation Therapy (IORT) F Plaque Radiation	Z None	Z None

SECTION: **D RADIATION THERAPY**
BODY SYSTEM: U FEMALE REPRODUCTIVE SYSTEM
MODALITY: Ø BEAM RADIATION

Treatment Site	Modality Qualifier	Isotope	Qualifier
Ø Ovary 1 Cervix 2 Uterus	Ø Photons <1 MeV 1 Photons 1 - 1Ø MeV 2 Photons >1Ø MeV 4 Heavy Particles (Protons, Ions) 5 Neutrons 6 Neutron Capture	Z None	Z None
Ø Ovary 1 Cervix 2 Uterus	3 Electrons	Z None	Ø Intraoperative Z None

SECTION: **D RADIATION THERAPY**
BODY SYSTEM: U FEMALE REPRODUCTIVE SYSTEM
MODALITY: 1 BRACHYTHERAPY

Treatment Site	Modality Qualifier	Isotope	Qualifier
Ø Ovary 1 Cervix 2 Uterus	9 High Dose Rate (HDR) B Low Dose Rate (LDR)	7 Cesium 137 (Cs-137) 8 Iridium 192 (Ir-192) 9 Iodine 125 (I-125) B Palladium 1Ø3 (Pd-1Ø3) C Californium 252 (Cf-252) Y Other Isotope	Z None

Ø; 1

U: FEMALE REPRODUCTIVE SYSTEM

D: RADIATION THERAPY

SECTION: D RADIATION THERAPY
BODY SYSTEM: U FEMALE REPRODUCTIVE SYSTEM
MODALITY: 2 STEREOTACTIC RADIOSURGERY

Treatment Site	Modality Qualifier	Isotope	Qualifier
Ø Ovary 1 Cervix 2 Uterus	D Stereotactic Other Photon Radiosurgery H Stereotactic Particulate Radiosurgery J Stereotactic Gamma Beam Radiosurgery	Z None	Z None

SECTION: D RADIATION THERAPY
BODY SYSTEM: U FEMALE REPRODUCTIVE SYSTEM
MODALITY: Y OTHER RADIATION

Treatment Site	Modality Qualifier	Isotope	Qualifier
Ø Ovary 1 Cervix 2 Uterus	7 Contact Radiation 8 Hyperthermia C Intraoperative Radiation Therapy (IORT) F Plaque Radiation	Z None	Z None

SECTION: D RADIATION THERAPY
BODY SYSTEM: V MALE REPRODUCTIVE SYSTEM
MODALITY: Ø BEAM RADIATION

Treatment Site	Modality Qualifier	Isotope	Qualifier
Ø Prostate 1 Testis	Ø Photons <1 MeV 1 Photons 1 - 1Ø MeV 2 Photons >1Ø MeV 4 Heavy Particles (Protons, Ions) 5 Neutrons 6 Neutron Capture	Z None	Z None
Ø Prostate 1 Testis	3 Electrons	Z None	Ø Intraoperative Z None

SECTION: D RADIATION THERAPY
BODY SYSTEM: V MALE REPRODUCTIVE SYSTEM
MODALITY: 1 BRACHYTHERAPY

Treatment Site	Modality Qualifier	Isotope	Qualifier
Ø Prostate 1 Testis	9 High Dose Rate (HDR) B Low Dose Rate (LDR)	7 Cesium 137 (Cs-137) 8 Iridium 192 (Ir-192) 9 Iodine 125 (I-125) B Palladium 1Ø3 (Pd-1Ø3) C Californium 252 (Cf-252) Y Other Isotope	Z None

New/Revised Text in Blue   ~~deleted~~ Deleted

SECTION: D RADIATION THERAPY
BODY SYSTEM: V MALE REPRODUCTIVE SYSTEM
MODALITY: 2 STEREOTACTIC RADIOSURGERY

Treatment Site	Modality Qualifier	Isotope	Qualifier
Ø Prostate 1 Testis	D Stereotactic Other Photon Radiosurgery H Stereotactic Particulate Radiosurgery J Stereotactic Gamma Beam Radiosurgery	Z None	Z None

SECTION: D RADIATION THERAPY
BODY SYSTEM: V MALE REPRODUCTIVE SYSTEM
MODALITY: Y OTHER RADIATION

Treatment Site	Modality Qualifier	Isotope	Qualifier
Ø Prostate	7 Contact Radiation 8 Hyperthermia C Intraoperative Radiation Therapy (IORT) F Plaque Radiation K Laser Interstitial Thermal Therapy	Z None	Z None
1 Testis	7 Contact Radiation 8 Hyperthermia F Plaque Radiation	Z None	Z None

SECTION: **D RADIATION THERAPY**
BODY SYSTEM: **W ANATOMICAL REGIONS**
MODALITY: **Ø BEAM RADIATION**

Treatment Site	Modality Qualifier	Isotope	Qualifier
1 Head and Neck 2 Chest 3 Abdomen 4 Hemibody 5 Whole Body 6 Pelvic Region	Ø Photons <1 MeV 1 Photons 1 - 1Ø MeV 2 Photons >1Ø MeV 4 Heavy Particles (Protons, Ions) 5 Neutrons 6 Neutron Capture	Z None	Z None
1 Head and Neck 2 Chest 3 Abdomen 4 Hemibody 5 Whole Body 6 Pelvic Region	3 Electrons	Z None	Ø Intraoperative Z None

SECTION: **D RADIATION THERAPY**
BODY SYSTEM: **W ANATOMICAL REGIONS**
MODALITY: **1 BRACHYTHERAPY**

Treatment Site	Modality Qualifier	Isotope	Qualifier
1 Head and Neck 2 Chest 3 Abdomen 6 Pelvic Region	9 High Dose Rate (HDR) B Low Dose Rate (LDR)	7 Cesium 137 (Cs-137) 8 Iridium 192 (Ir-192) 9 Iodine 125 (I-125) B Palladium 1Ø3 (Pd-1Ø3) C Californium 252 (Cf-252) Y Other Isotope	Z None

W: ANATOMICAL REGIONS
Ø; 1
D: RADIATION THERAPY

New/Revised Text in Blue   ~~deleted~~ Deleted

SECTION: D RADIATION THERAPY
BODY SYSTEM: W ANATOMICAL REGIONS
MODALITY: 2 STEREOTACTIC RADIOSURGERY

Treatment Site	Modality Qualifier	Isotope	Qualifier
1 Head and Neck 2 Chest 3 Abdomen 6 Pelvic Region	D Stereotactic Other Photon Radiosurgery H Stereotactic Particulate Radiosurgery J Stereotactic Gamma Beam Radiosurgery	Z None	Z None

SECTION: D RADIATION THERAPY
BODY SYSTEM: W ANATOMICAL REGIONS
MODALITY: Y OTHER RADIATION

Treatment Site	Modality Qualifier	Isotope	Qualifier
1 Head and Neck 2 Chest 3 Abdomen 4 Hemibody 6 Pelvic Region	7 Contact Radiation 8 Hyperthermia F Plaque Radiation	Z None	Z None
5 Whole Body	7 Contact Radiation 8 Hyperthermia F Plaque Radiation	Z None	Z None
5 Whole Body	G Isotope Administration	D Iodine 131 (I-131) F Phosphorus 32 (P-32) G Strontium 89 (Sr-89) H Strontium 90 (Sr-90) Y Other Isotope	Z None

F   Physical Rehabilitation and Diagnostic Audiology **654**
    F0. Rehabilitation 655
        F00. Speech Assessment 655
        F01. Motor and/or Nerve Function Assessment.. 657
        F02. Activities of Daily Living Assessment.. 659
        F06. Speech Treatment.. 661
        F07. Motor Treatment.. 663
        F08. Activities of Daily Living Treatment.. 665
        F09. Hearing Treatment... 666
        F0B. Cochlear Implant Treatment... 666
        F0C. Vestibular Treatment... 667
        F0D. Device Fitting... 667
        F0F. Caregiver Training.. 668
    F1. Diagnostic Audiology 669
        F13. Hearing Assessment... 669
        F14. Hearing Aid Assessment.. 670
        F15. Vestibular Assessment... 671

New/Revised Text in Blue   ~~deleted~~ Deleted

SECTION:

F PHYSICAL REHABILITATION AND DIAGNOSTIC AUDIOLOGY

SECTION QUALIFIER: Ø REHABILITATION

TYPE: **Ø SPEECH ASSESSMENT:** *(on multiple pages)*

Measurement of speech and related functions

Body System – Body Region	Type Qualifier	Equipment	Qualifier
3 Neurological System - Whole Body	G Communicative/Cognitive Integration Skills	K Audiovisual M Augmentative/Alternative Communication P Computer Y Other Equipment Z None	Z None
Z None	Ø Filtered Speech 3 Staggered Spondaic Word Q Performance Intensity Phonetically Balanced Speech Discrimination R Brief Tone Stimuli S Distorted Speech T Dichotic Stimuli V Temporal Ordering of Stimuli W Masking Patterns	1 Audiometer 2 Sound Field/Booth K Audiovisual Z None	Z None
Z None	1 Speech Threshold 2 Speech/Word Recognition	1 Audiometer 2 Sound Field/Booth 9 Cochlear Implant K Audiovisual Z None	Z None
Z None	4 Sensorineural Acuity Level	1 Audiometer 2 Sound Field/Booth Z None	Z None
Z None	5 Synthetic Sentence Identification	1 Audiometer 2 Sound Field/Booth 9 Cochlear Implant K Audiovisual	Z None
Z None	6 Speech and/or Language Screening 7 Nonspoken Language 8 Receptive/Expressive Language C Aphasia G Communicative/Cognitive Integration Skills L Augmentative/Alternative Communication System	K Audiovisual M Augmentative/Alternative Communication P Computer Y Other Equipment Z None	Z None
Z None	9 Articulation/Phonology	K Audiovisual P Computer Q Speech Analysis Y Other Equipment Z None	Z None
Z None	B Motor Speech	K Audiovisual N Biosensory Feedback P Computer Q Speech Analysis T Aerodynamic Function Y Other Equipment Z None	Z None

SECTION: F PHYSICAL REHABILITATION AND DIAGNOSTIC AUDIOLOGY

SECTION QUALIFIER: Ø **REHABILITATION**

TYPE: Ø **SPEECH ASSESSMENT:** *(continued)*
Measurement of speech and related functions

Body System – Body Region	Type Qualifier	Equipment	Qualifier
Z None	D Fluency	K Audiovisual N Biosensory Feedback P Computer Q Speech Analysis S Voice Analysis T Aerodynamic Function Y Other Equipment Z None	Z None
Z None	F Voice	K Audiovisual N Biosensory Feedback P Computer S Voice Analysis T Aerodynamic Function Y Other Equipment Z None	Z None
Z None	H Bedside Swallowing and Oral Function P Oral Peripheral Mechanism	Y Other Equipment Z None	Z None
Z None	J Instrumental Swallowing and Oral Function	T Aerodynamic Function W Swallowing Y Other Equipment	Z None
Z None	K Orofacial Myofunctional	K Audiovisual P Computer Y Other Equipment Z None	Z None
Z None	M Voice Prosthetic	K Audiovisual P Computer S Voice Analysis V Speech Prosthesis Y Other Equipment Z None	Z None
Z None	N Non-invasive Instrumental Status	N Biosensory Feedback P Computer Q Speech Analysis S Voice Analysis T Aerodynamic Function Y Other Equipment	Z None
Z None	X Other Specified Central Auditory Processing	Z None	Z None

SECTION: F PHYSICAL REHABILITATION AND DIAGNOSTIC AUDIOLOGY

SECTION QUALIFIER: Ø REHABILITATION

TYPE: 1 MOTOR AND/OR NERVE FUNCTION ASSESSMENT: *(on multiple pages)*
Measurement of motor, nerve, and related functions

Body System – Body Region	Type Qualifier	Equipment	Qualifier
Ø Neurological System - Head and Neck 1 Neurological System - Upper Back/Upper Extremity 2 Neurological System - Lower Back/Lower Extremity 3 Neurological System - Whole Body	Ø Muscle Performance	E Orthosis F Assistive, Adaptive, Supportive or Protective U Prosthesis Y Other Equipment Z None	Z None
Ø Neurological System - Head and Neck 1 Neurological System - Upper Back/Upper Extremity 2 Neurological System - Lower Back/Lower Extremity 3 Neurological System - Whole Body	1 Integumentary Integrity 3 Coordination/Dexterity 4 Motor Function G Reflex Integrity	Z None	Z None
Ø Neurological System - Head and Neck 1 Neurological System - Upper Back/Upper Extremity 2 Neurological System - Lower Back/Lower Extremity 3 Neurological System - Whole Body	5 Range of Motion and Joint Integrity 6 Sensory Awareness/ Processing/Integrity	Y Other Equipment Z None	Z None
D Integumentary System - Head and Neck F Integumentary System - Upper Back/Upper Extremity G Integumentary System - Lower Back/Lower Extremity H Integumentary System - Whole Body J Musculoskeletal System - Head and Neck K Musculoskeletal System - Upper Back/Upper Extremity L Musculoskeletal System - Lower Back/Lower Extremity M Musculoskeletal System - Whole Body	Ø Muscle Performance	E Orthosis F Assistive, Adaptive, Supportive or Protective U Prosthesis Y Other Equipment Z None	Z None
D Integumentary System - Head and Neck F Integumentary System - Upper Back/Upper Extremity G Integumentary System - Lower Back/Lower Extremity H Integumentary System - Whole Body J Musculoskeletal System - Head and Neck K Musculoskeletal System - Upper Back/Upper Extremity L Musculoskeletal System - Lower Back/Lower Extremity M Musculoskeletal System - Whole Body	1 Integumentary Integrity	Z None	Z None
D Integumentary System - Head and Neck F Integumentary System - Upper Back/Upper Extremity G Integumentary System - Lower Back/Lower Extremity H Integumentary System - Whole Body J Musculoskeletal System - Head and Neck K Musculoskeletal System - Upper Back/Upper Extremity L Musculoskeletal System - Lower Back/Lower Extremity M Musculoskeletal System - Whole Body	5 Range of Motion and Joint Integrity 6 Sensory Awareness/ Processing/Integrity	Y Other Equipment Z None	Z None

SECTION: F PHYSICAL REHABILITATION AND DIAGNOSTIC AUDIOLOGY

SECTION QUALIFIER: Ø REHABILITATION
TYPE: 1 MOTOR AND/OR NERVE FUNCTION
ASSESSMENT: *(continued)*
Measurement of motor, nerve, and related functions

Body System – Body Region	Type Qualifier	Equipment	Qualifier
N Genitourinary System	Ø Muscle Performance	E Orthosis F Assistive, Adaptive, Supportive or Protective U Prosthesis Y Other Equipment Z None	Z None
Z None	2 Visual Motor Integration	K Audiovisual M Augmentative/Alternative Communication N Biosensory Feedback P Computer Q Speech Analysis S Voice Analysis Y Other Equipment Z None	Z None
Z None	7 Facial Nerve Function	7 Electrophysiologic	Z None
Z None	9 Somatosensory Evoked Potentials	J Somatosensory	Z None
Z None	B Bed Mobility C Transfer F Wheelchair Mobility	E Orthosis F Assistive, Adaptive, Supportive or Protective U Prosthesis Z None	Z None
Z None	D Gait and/or Balance	E Orthosis F Assistive, Adaptive, Supportive or Protective U Prosthesis Y Other Equipment Z None	Z None

SECTION: F PHYSICAL REHABILITATION AND DIAGNOSTIC AUDIOLOGY

SECTION QUALIFIER: Ø REHABILITATION
TYPE: 2 ACTIVITIES OF DAILY LIVING ASSESSMENT: *(on multiple pages)*
Measurement of functional level for activities of daily living

Body System – Body Region	Type Qualifier	Equipment	Qualifier
Ø Neurological System - Head and Neck	9 Cranial Nerve Integrity D Neuromotor Development	Y Other Equipment Z None	Z None
1 Neurological System - Upper Back/Upper Extremity 2 Neurological System - Lower Back/Lower Extremity 3 Neurological System - Whole Body	D Neuromotor Development	Y Other Equipment Z None	Z None
4 Circulatory System - Head and Neck 5 Circulatory System - Upper Back/Upper Extremity 6 Circulatory System - Lower Back/Lower Extremity 8 Respiratory System - Head and Neck 9 Respiratory System - Upper Back/Upper Extremity B Respiratory System - Lower Back/Lower Extremity	G Ventilation, Respiration and Circulation	C Mechanical G Aerobic Endurance and Conditioning Y Other Equipment Z None	Z None
7 Circulatory System - Whole Body C Respiratory System - Whole Body	7 Aerobic Capacity and Endurance	E Orthosis G Aerobic Endurance and Conditioning U Prosthesis Y Other Equipment Z None	Z None
7 Circulatory System - Whole Body C Respiratory System - Whole Body	G Ventilation, Respiration and Circulation	C Mechanical G Aerobic Endurance and Conditioning Y Other Equipment Z None	Z None

SECTION: F PHYSICAL REHABILITATION AND DIAGNOSTIC AUDIOLOGY

SECTION QUALIFIER: Ø REHABILITATION

TYPE: 2 ACTIVITIES OF DAILY LIVING ASSESSMENT: *(continued)*
Measurement of functional level for activities of daily living

Body System – Body Region	Type Qualifier	Equipment	Qualifier
Z None	Ø Bathing/Showering 1 Dressing 3 Grooming/Personal Hygiene 4 Home Management	E Orthosis F Assistive, Adaptive, Supportive or Protective U Prosthesis Z None	Z None
Z None	2 Feeding/Eating 8 Anthropometric Characteristics F Pain	Y Other Equipment Z None	Z None
Z None	5 Perceptual Processing	K Audiovisual M Augmentative/Alternative Communication N Biosensory Feedback P Computer Q Speech Analysis S Voice Analysis Y Other Equipment Z None	Z None
Z None	6 Psychosocial Skills	Z None	Z None
Z None	B Environmental, Home and Work Barriers C Ergonomics and Body Mechanics	E Orthosis F Assistive, Adaptive, Supportive or Protective U Prosthesis Y Other Equipment Z None	Z None
Z None	H Vocational Activities and Functional Community or Work Reintegration Skills	E Orthosis F Assistive, Adaptive, Supportive or Protective G Aerobic Endurance and Conditioning U Prosthesis Y Other Equipment Z None	Z None

SECTION: **F PHYSICAL REHABILITATION AND DIAGNOSTIC AUDIOLOGY**

SECTION QUALIFIER: Ø   REHABILITATION

TYPE: 6   **SPEECH TREATMENT:** *(on multiple pages)*
Application of techniques to improve, augment, or compensate for speech and related functional impairment

Body System – Body Region	Type Qualifier	Equipment	Qualifier
3 Neurological System - Whole Body	6 Communicative/Cognitive Integration Skills	K Audiovisual M Augmentative/Alternative Communication P Computer Y Other Equipment Z None	Z None
Z None	Ø Nonspoken Language 3 Aphasia 6 Communicative/Cognitive Integration Skills	K Audiovisual M Augmentative/Alternative Communication P Computer Y Other Equipment Z None	Z None
Z None	1 Speech-Language Pathology and Related Disorders Counseling 2 Speech-Language Pathology and Related Disorders Prevention	K Audiovisual Z None	Z None
Z None	4 Articulation/Phonology	K Audiovisual P Computer Q Speech Analysis T Aerodynamic Function Y Other Equipment Z None	Z None
Z None	5 Aural Rehabilitation	K Audiovisual L Assistive Listening M Augmentative/Alternative Communication N Biosensory Feedback P Computer Q Speech Analysis S Voice Analysis Y Other Equipment Z None	Z None
Z None	7 Fluency	4 Electroacoustic Immitance/ Acoustic Reflex K Audiovisual N Biosensory Feedback Q Speech Analysis S Voice Analysis T Aerodynamic Function Y Other Equipment Z None	Z None

SECTION: F PHYSICAL REHABILITATION AND DIAGNOSTIC AUDIOLOGY

SECTION QUALIFIER: Ø REHABILITATION

TYPE: 6 SPEECH TREATMENT: *(continued)*

Application of techniques to improve, augment, or compensate for speech and related functional impairment

Body System – Body Region	Type Qualifier	Equipment	Qualifier
Z None	8 Motor Speech	K Audiovisual N Biosensory Feedback P Computer Q Speech Analysis S Voice Analysis T Aerodynamic Function Y Other Equipment Z None	Z None
Z None	9 Orofacial Myofunctional	K Audiovisual P Computer Y Other Equipment Z None	Z None
Z None	B Receptive/Expressive Language	K Audiovisual L Assistive Listening M Augmentative/Alternative Communication P Computer Y Other Equipment Z None	Z None
Z None	C Voice	K Audiovisual N Biosensory Feedback P Computer S Voice Analysis T Aerodynamic Function V Speech Prosthesis Y Other Equipment Z None	Z None
Z None	D Swallowing Dysfunction	M Augmentative/Alternative Communication T Aerodynamic Function V Speech Prosthesis Y Other Equipment Z None	Z None

F: PHYSICAL REHABILITATION AND DIAGNOSTIC AUDIOLOGY   Ø: REHABILITATION   6: SPEECH TREATMENT

SECTION: F PHYSICAL REHABILITATION AND DIAGNOSTIC AUDIOLOGY

SECTION QUALIFIER: Ø REHABILITATION

TYPE: 7 MOTOR TREATMENT: *(on multiple pages)*
Exercise or activities to increase or facilitate motor function

Body System – Body Region	Type Qualifier	Equipment	Qualifier
Ø Neurological System - Head and Neck 1 Neurological System - Upper Back/Upper Extremity 2 Neurological System - Lower Back/Lower Extremity 3 Neurological System - Whole Body D Integumentary System - Head and Neck F Integumentary System - Upper Back/Upper Extremity G Integumentary System - Lower Back/Lower Extremity H Integumentary System - Whole Body J Musculoskeletal System - Head and Neck K Musculoskeletal System - Upper Back/Upper Extremity L Musculoskeletal System - Lower Back/Lower Extremity M Musculoskeletal System - Whole Body	Ø Range of Motion and Joint Mobility 1 Muscle Performance 2 Coordination/Dexterity 3 Motor Function	E Orthosis F Assistive, Adaptive, Supportive or Protective U Prosthesis Y Other Equipment Z None	Z None
Ø Neurological System - Head and Neck 1 Neurological System - Upper Back/Upper Extremity 2 Neurological System - Lower Back/Lower Extremity 3 Neurological System - Whole Body D Integumentary System - Head and Neck F Integumentary System - Upper Back/Upper Extremity G Integumentary System - Lower Back/Lower Extremity H Integumentary System - Whole Body J Musculoskeletal System - Head and Neck K Musculoskeletal System - Upper Back/Upper Extremity L Musculoskeletal System - Lower Back/Lower Extremity M Musculoskeletal System - Whole Body	6 Therapeutic Exercise	B Physical Agents C Mechanical D Electrotherapeutic E Orthosis F Assistive, Adaptive, Supportive or Protective G Aerobic Endurance and Conditioning H Mechanical or Electromechanical U Prosthesis Y Other Equipment Z None	Z None
Ø Neurological System - Head and Neck 1 Neurological System - Upper Back/Upper Extremity 2 Neurological System - Lower Back/Lower Extremity 3 Neurological System - Whole Body D Integumentary System - Head and Neck F Integumentary System - Upper Back/Upper Extremity G Integumentary System - Lower Back/Lower Extremity H Integumentary System - Whole Body J Musculoskeletal System - Head and Neck K Musculoskeletal System - Upper Back/Upper Extremity L Musculoskeletal System - Lower Back/Lower Extremity M Musculoskeletal System - Whole Body	7 Manual Therapy Techniques	Z None	Z None

SECTION: F PHYSICAL REHABILITATION AND DIAGNOSTIC AUDIOLOGY

SECTION QUALIFIER: Ø REHABILITATION

TYPE: 7 MOTOR TREATMENT: *(continued)*

Exercise or activities to increase or facilitate motor function

Body System – Body Region	Type Qualifier	Equipment	Qualifier
4 Circulatory System - Head and Neck 5 Circulatory System - Upper Back/Upper Extremity 6 Circulatory System - Lower Back/Lower Extremity 7 Circulatory System - Whole Body 8 Respiratory System - Head and Neck 9 Respiratory System - Upper Back/Upper Extremity B Respiratory System - Lower Back/Lower Extremity C Respiratory System - Whole Body	6 Therapeutic Exercise	B Physical Agents C Mechanical D Electrotherapeutic E Orthosis F Assistive, Adaptive, Supportive or Protective G Aerobic Endurance and Conditioning H Mechanical or Electromechanical U Prosthesis Y Other Equipment Z None	Z None
N Genitourinary System	1 Muscle Performance	E Orthosis F Assistive, Adaptive, Supportive or Protective U Prosthesis Y Other Equipment Z None	Z None
N Genitourinary System	6 Therapeutic Exercise	B Physical Agents C Mechanical D Electrotherapeutic E Orthosis F Assistive, Adaptive, Supportive or Protective G Aerobic Endurance and Conditioning H Mechanical or Electromechanical U Prosthesis Y Other Equipment Z None	Z None
Z None	4 Wheelchair Mobility	D Electrotherapeutic E Orthosis F Assistive, Adaptive, Supportive or Protective U Prosthesis Y Other Equipment Z None	Z None
Z None	5 Bed Mobility	C Mechanical E Orthosis F Assistive, Adaptive, Supportive or Protective U Prosthesis Y Other Equipment Z None	Z None
Z None	8 Transfer Training	C Mechanical D Electrotherapeutic E Orthosis F Assistive, Adaptive, Supportive or Protective U Prosthesis Y Other Equipment Z None	Z None
Z None	9 Gait Training/Functional Ambulation	C Mechanical D Electrotherapeutic E Orthosis F Assistive, Adaptive, Supportive or Protective G Aerobic Endurance and Conditioning U Prosthesis Y Other Equipment Z None	Z None

New/Revised Text in Blue   ~~deleted~~ Deleted

SECTION: F PHYSICAL REHABILITATION AND DIAGNOSTIC AUDIOLOGY

SECTION QUALIFIER: Ø REHABILITATION

TYPE: 8 ACTIVITIES OF DAILY LIVING TREATMENT: Exercise or activities to facilitate functional competence for activities of daily living

Body System – Body Region	Type Qualifier	Equipment	Qualifier
D Integumentary System - Head and Neck F Integumentary System - Upper Back/Upper Extremity G Integumentary System - Lower Back/Lower Extremity H Integumentary System - Whole Body J Musculoskeletal System - Head and Neck K Musculoskeletal System - Upper Back/Upper Extremity L Musculoskeletal System - Lower Back/Lower Extremity M Musculoskeletal System - Whole Body	5 Wound Management	B Physical Agents C Mechanical D Electrotherapeutic E Orthosis F Assistive, Adaptive, Supportive or Protective U Prosthesis Y Other Equipment Z None	Z None
Z None	Ø Bathing/Showering Techniques 1 Dressing Techniques 2 Grooming/Personal Hygiene	E Orthosis F Assistive, Adaptive, Supportive or Protective U Prosthesis Y Other Equipment Z None	Z None
Z None	3 Feeding/Eating	C Mechanical D Electrotherapeutic E Orthosis F Assistive, Adaptive, Supportive or Protective U Prosthesis Y Other Equipment Z None	Z None
Z None	4 Home Management	D Electrotherapeutic E Orthosis F Assistive, Adaptive, Supportive or Protective U Prosthesis Y Other Equipment Z None	Z None
Z None	6 Psychosocial Skills	Z None	Z None
Z None	7 Vocational Activities and Functional Community or Work Reintegration Skills	B Physical Agents C Mechanical D Electrotherapeutic E Orthosis F Assistive, Adaptive, Supportive or Protective G Aerobic Endurance and Conditioning U Prosthesis Y Other Equipment Z None	Z None

SECTION: F PHYSICAL REHABILITATION AND DIAGNOSTIC AUDIOLOGY

SECTION QUALIFIER: Ø REHABILITATION

TYPE: 9 HEARING TREATMENT: Application of techniques to improve, augment, or compensate for hearing and related functional impairment

Body System – Body Region	Type Qualifier	Equipment	Qualifier
Z None	Ø Hearing and Related Disorders Counseling 1 Hearing and Related Disorders Prevention	K Audiovisual Z None	Z None
Z None	2 Auditory Processing	K Audiovisual L Assistive Listening P Computer Y Other Equipment Z None	Z None
Z None	3 Cerumen Management	X Cerumen Management Z None	Z None

SECTION: F PHYSICAL REHABILITATION AND DIAGNOSTIC AUDIOLOGY

SECTION QUALIFIER: Ø REHABILITATION

TYPE: B COCHLEAR IMPLANT TREATMENT: Application of techniques to improve the communication abilities of individuals with cochlear implant

Body System – Body Region	Type Qualifier	Equipment	Qualifier
Z None	Ø Cochlear Implant Rehabilitation	1 Audiometer 2 Sound Field/Booth 9 Cochlear Implant K Audiovisual P Computer Y Other Equipment	Z None

SECTION: F PHYSICAL REHABILITATION AND DIAGNOSTIC AUDIOLOGY

SECTION QUALIFIER: 0 REHABILITATION

TYPE: C VESTIBULAR TREATMENT: Application of techniques to improve, augment, or compensate for vestibular and related functional impairment

Body System – Body Region	Type Qualifier	Equipment	Qualifier
3 Neurological System - Whole Body H Integumentary System - Whole Body M Musculoskeletal System - Whole Body	3 Postural Control	E Orthosis F Assistive, Adaptive, Supportive or Protective U Prosthesis Y Other Equipment Z None	Z None
Z None	0 Vestibular	8 Vestibular/Balance Z None	Z None
Z None	1 Perceptual Processing 2 Visual Motor Integration	K Audiovisual L Assistive Listening N Biosensory Feedback P Computer Q Speech Analysis S Voice Analysis T Aerodynamic Function Y Other Equipment Z None	Z None

SECTION: F PHYSICAL REHABILITATION AND DIAGNOSTIC AUDIOLOGY

SECTION QUALIFIER: 0 REHABILITATION

TYPE: D DEVICE FITTING: Fitting of a device designed to facilitate or support achievement of a higher level of function

Body System – Body Region	Type Qualifier	Equipment	Qualifier
Z None	0 Tinnitus Masker	5 Hearing Aid Selection/Fitting/Test Z None	Z None
Z None	1 Monaural Hearing Aid 2 Binaural Hearing Aid 5 Assistive Listening Device	1 Audiometer 2 Sound Field/Booth 5 Hearing Aid Selection/Fitting/Test K Audiovisual L Assistive Listening Z None	Z None
Z None	3 Augmentative/Alternative Communication System	M Augmentative/Alternative Communication	Z None
Z None	4 Voice Prosthetic	S Voice Analysis V Speech Prosthesis	Z None
Z None	6 Dynamic Orthosis 7 Static Orthosis 8 Prosthesis 9 Assistive, Adaptive, Supportive or Protective Devices	E Orthosis F Assistive, Adaptive, Supportive or Protective U Prosthesis Z None	Z None

SECTION: F PHYSICAL REHABILITATION AND DIAGNOSTIC AUDIOLOGY

SECTION QUALIFIER: Ø **REHABILITATION**

TYPE: F **CAREGIVER TRAINING:** Training in activities to support patient's optimal level of function

Body System – Body Region	Type Qualifier	Equipment	Qualifier
Z None	Ø Bathing/Showering Technique 1 Dressing 2 Feeding and Eating 3 Grooming/Personal Hygiene 4 Bed Mobility 5 Transfer 6 Wheelchair Mobility 7 Therapeutic Exercise 8 Airway Clearance Techniques 9 Wound Management B Vocational Activities and Functional Community or Work Reintegration Skills C Gait Training/Functional Ambulation D Application, Proper Use and Care Devices F Application, Proper Use and Care of Orthoses G Application, Proper Use and Care of Prosthesis H Home Management	E Orthosis F Assistive, Adaptive, Supportive or Protective U Prosthesis Z None	Z None
Z None	J Communication Skills	K Audiovisual L Assistive Listening M Augmentative/Alternative Communication P Computer Z None	Z None

SECTION: F PHYSICAL REHABILITATION AND DIAGNOSTIC AUDIOLOGY

SECTION QUALIFIER: 1 DIAGNOSTIC AUDIOLOGY
TYPE: 3 HEARING ASSESSMENT: Measurement of hearing and related functions

Body System – Body Region	Type Qualifier	Equipment	Qualifier
Z None	Ø Hearing Screening	Ø Occupational Hearing 1 Audiometer 2 Sound Field/Booth 3 Tympanometer 8 Vestibular/Balance 9 Cochlear Implant Z None	Z None
Z None	1 Pure Tone Audiometry, Air 2 Pure Tone Audiometry, Air and Bone	Ø Occupational Hearing 1 Audiometer 2 Sound Field/Booth Z None	Z None
Z None	3 Bekesy Audiometry 6 Visual Reinforcement Audiometry 9 Short Increment Sensitivity Index B Stenger C Pure Tone Stenger	1 Audiometer 2 Sound Field/Booth Z None	Z None
Z None	4 Conditioned Play Audiometry 5 Select Picture Audiometry	1 Audiometer 2 Sound Field/Booth K Audiovisual Z None	Z None
Z None	7 Alternate Binaural or Monaural Loudness Balance	1 Audiometer K Audiovisual Z None	Z None
Z None	8 Tone Decay D Tympanometry F Eustachian Tube Function G Acoustic Reflex Patterns H Acoustic Reflex Threshold J Acoustic Reflex Decay	3 Tympanometer 4 Electroacoustic Immitance/Acoustic Reflex Z None	Z None
Z None	K Electrocochleography L Auditory Evoked Potentials	7 Electrophysiologic Z None	Z None
Z None	M Evoked Otoacoustic Emissions, Screening N Evoked Otoacoustic Emissions, Diagnostic	6 Otoacoustic Emission (OAE) Z None	Z None
Z None	P Aural Rehabilitation Status	1 Audiometer 2 Sound Field/Booth 4 Electroacoustic Immitance/Acoustic Reflex 9 Cochlear Implant K Audiovisual L Assistive Listening P Computer Z None	Z None
Z None	Q Auditory Processing	K Audiovisual P Computer Y Other Equipment Z None	Z None

SECTION:　　　F PHYSICAL REHABILITATION AND DIAGNOSTIC AUDIOLOGY

SECTION QUALIFIER: 1 DIAGNOSTIC AUDIOLOGY
TYPE:　　　　　**4** HEARING AID ASSESSMENT: Measurement of the appropriateness and/or effectiveness of a hearing device

Body System – Body Region	Type Qualifier	Equipment	Qualifier
Z None	Ø Cochlear Implant	1 Audiometer 2 Sound Field/Booth 3 Tympanometer 4 Electroacoustic Immitance/ Acoustic Reflex 5 Hearing Aid Selection/ Fitting/Test 7 Electrophysiologic 9 Cochlear Implant K Audiovisual L Assistive Listening P Computer Y Other Equipment Z None	Z None
Z None	1 Ear Canal Probe Microphone 6 Binaural Electroacoustic Hearing Aid Check 8 Monaural Electroacoustic Hearing Aid Check	5 Hearing Aid Selection/ Fitting/Test Z None	Z None
Z None	2 Monaural Hearing Aid 3 Binaural Hearing Aid	1 Audiometer 2 Sound Field/Booth 3 Tympanometer 4 Electroacoustic Immitance/ Acoustic Reflex 5 Hearing Aid Selection/ Fitting/Test K Audiovisual L Assistive Listening P Computer Z None	Z None
Z None	4 Assistive Listening System/ Device Selection	1 Audiometer 2 Sound Field/Booth 3 Tympanometer 4 Electroacoustic Immitance/ Acoustic Reflex K Audiovisual L Assistive Listening Z None	Z None
Z None	5 Sensory Aids	1 Audiometer 2 Sound Field/Booth 3 Tympanometer 4 Electroacoustic Immitance/ Acoustic Reflex 5 Hearing Aid Selection/ Fitting/Test K Audiovisual L Assistive Listening Z None	Z None
Z None	7 Ear Protector Attentuation	Ø Occupational Hearing Z None	Z None

New/Revised Text in Blue　~~deleted~~ Deleted

SECTION: F PHYSICAL REHABILITATION AND DIAGNOSTIC AUDIOLOGY
SECTION QUALIFIER: 1 DIAGNOSTIC AUDIOLOGY
TYPE: 5 **VESTIBULAR ASSESSMENT:** Measurement of the vestibular system and related functions

Body System – Body Region	Type Qualifier	Equipment	Qualifier
Z None	Ø Bithermal, Binaural Caloric Irrigation 1 Bithermal, Monaural Caloric Irrigation 2 Unithermal Binaural Screen 3 Oscillating Tracking 4 Sinusoidal Vertical Axis Rotational 5 Dix-Hallpike Dynamic 6 Computerized Dynamic Posturography	8 Vestibular/Balance Z None	Z None
Z None	7 Tinnitus Masker	5 Hearing Aid Selection/Fitting/Test Z None	Z None

G Mental Health...**672**
   GZ1. Psychological Tests 673
   GZ2. Crisis Intervention 673
   GZ3. Medication Management 673
   GZ5. Individual Psychotherapy...673
   GZ6. Counseling 674
   GZ7. Family Psychotherapy 674
   GZB. Electroconvulsive Therapy 674
   GZC. Biofeedback 674
   GZF. Hypnosis 675
   GZG. Narcosynthesis 675
   GZH. Group Psychotherapy...675
   GZJ. Light Therapy 675

New/Revised Text in Blue   ~~deleted~~ Deleted

SECTION: **G MENTAL HEALTH**
SECTION QUALIFIER: **Z NONE**
TYPE: **1 PSYCHOLOGICAL TESTS:** The administration and interpretation of standardized psychological tests and measurement instruments for the assessment of psychological function

Qualifier	Qualifier	Qualifier	Qualifier
Ø Developmental 1 Personality and Behavioral 2 Intellectual and Psychoeducational 3 Neuropsychological 4 Neurobehavioral and Cognitive Status	Z None	Z None	Z None

SECTION: **G MENTAL HEALTH**
SECTION QUALIFIER: **Z NONE**
TYPE: **2 CRISIS INTERVENTION:** Treatment of a traumatized, acutely disturbed or distressed individual for the purpose of short-term stabilization

Qualifier	Qualifier	Qualifier	Qualifier
Z None	Z None	Z None	Z None

SECTION: **G MENTAL HEALTH**
SECTION QUALIFIER: **Z NONE**
TYPE: **3 MEDICATION MANAGEMENT:** Monitoring and adjusting the use of medications for the treatment of a mental health disorder

Qualifier	Qualifier	Qualifier	Qualifier
Z None	Z None	Z None	Z None

SECTION: **G MENTAL HEALTH**
SECTION QUALIFIER: **Z NONE**
TYPE: **5 INDIVIDUAL PSYCHOTHERAPY:** Treatment of an individual with a mental health disorder by behavioral, cognitive, psychoanalytic, psychodynamic or psychophysiological means to improve functioning or well-being

Qualifier	Qualifier	Qualifier	Qualifier
Ø Interactive 1 Behavioral 2 Cognitive 3 Interpersonal 4 Psychoanalysis 5 Psychodynamic 6 Supportive 8 Cognitive-Behavioral 9 Psychophysiological	Z None	Z None	Z None

6; 7; B; C

Z: NONE

G: MENTAL HEALTH

SECTION: G MENTAL HEALTH
SECTION QUALIFIER: Z NONE
TYPE: 6 **COUNSELING:** The application of psychological methods to treat an individual with normal developmental issues and psychological problems in order to increase function, improve well-being, alleviate distress, maladjustment or resolve crises

Qualifier	Qualifier	Qualifier	Qualifier
Ø Educational 1 Vocational 3 Other Counseling	Z None	Z None	Z None

SECTION: G MENTAL HEALTH
SECTION QUALIFIER: Z NONE
TYPE: 7 **FAMILY PSYCHOTHERAPY:** Treatment that includes one or more family members of an individual with a mental health disorder by behavioral, cognitive, psychoanalytic, psychodynamic or psychophysiological means to improve functioning or well-being

Qualifier	Qualifier	Qualifier	Qualifier
2 Other Family Psychotherapy	Z None	Z None	Z None

SECTION: G MENTAL HEALTH
SECTION QUALIFIER: Z NONE
TYPE: B **ELECTROCONVULSIVE THERAPY:** The application of controlled electrical voltages to treat a mental health disorder

Qualifier	Qualifier	Qualifier	Qualifier
Ø Unilateral-Single Seizure 1 Unilateral-Multiple Seizure 2 Bilateral-Single Seizure 3 Bilateral-Multiple Seizure 4 Other Electroconvulsive Therapy	Z None	Z None	Z None

SECTION: G MENTAL HEALTH
SECTION QUALIFIER: Z NONE
TYPE: C **BIOFEEDBACK:** Provision of information from the monitoring and regulating of physiological processes in conjunction with cognitive-behavioral techniques to improve patient functioning or well-being

Qualifier	Qualifier	Qualifier	Qualifier
9 Other Biofeedback	Z None	Z None	Z None

SECTION: **G MENTAL HEALTH**
SECTION QUALIFIER: **Z** **NONE**
TYPE: **F** **HYPNOSIS:** Induction of a state of heightened suggestibility by auditory, visual, and tactile techniques to elicit an emotional or behavioral response

Qualifier	Qualifier	Qualifier	Qualifier
Z None	Z None	Z None	Z None

SECTION: **G MENTAL HEALTH**
SECTION QUALIFIER: **Z** **NONE**
TYPE: **G** **NARCOSYNTHESIS:** Administration of intravenous barbiturates in order to release suppressed or repressed thoughts

Qualifier	Qualifier	Qualifier	Qualifier
Z None	Z None	Z None	Z None

SECTION: **G MENTAL HEALTH**
SECTION QUALIFIER: **Z** **NONE**
TYPE: **H** **GROUP PSYCHOTHERAPY:** Treatment of two or more individuals with a mental health disorder by behavioral, cognitive, psychoanalytic, psychodynamic, or psychophysiological means to improve functioning or well-being

Qualifier	Qualifier	Qualifier	Qualifier
Z None	Z None	Z None	Z None

SECTION: **G MENTAL HEALTH**
SECTION QUALIFIER: **Z** **NONE**
TYPE: **J** **LIGHT THERAPY:** Application of specialized light treatments to improve functioning or well-being

Qualifier	Qualifier	Qualifier	Qualifier
Z None	Z None	Z None	Z None

H Substance Abuse Treatment 676
    HZ2. Detoxification Services 677
    HZ3. Individual Counseling 677
    HZ4. Group Counseling 677
    HZ5. Individual Psychotherapy 678
    HZ6. Family Counseling 678
    HZ8. Medication Management 678
    HZ9. Pharmacotherapy... 679

SECTION: **H SUBSTANCE ABUSE TREATMENT**
SECTION QUALIFIER: **Z NONE**
TYPE: **2 DETOXIFICATION SERVICES:** Detoxification from alcohol and/or drugs

Qualifier	Qualifier	Qualifier	Qualifier
Z None	Z None	Z None	Z None

SECTION: **H SUBSTANCE ABUSE TREATMENT**
SECTION QUALIFIER: **Z NONE**
TYPE: **3 INDIVIDUAL COUNSELING:** The application of psychological methods to treat an individual with addictive behavior

Qualifier	Qualifier	Qualifier	Qualifier
Ø Cognitive	Z None	Z None	Z None
1 Behavioral			
2 Cognitive-Behavioral			
3 12-Step			
4 Interpersonal			
5 Vocational			
6 Psychoeducation			
7 Motivational Enhancement			
8 Confrontational			
9 Continuing Care			
B Spiritual			
C Pre/Post-Test Infectious Disease			

SECTION: **H SUBSTANCE ABUSE TREATMENT**
SECTION QUALIFIER: **Z NONE**
TYPE: **4 GROUP COUNSELING:** The application of psychological methods to treat two or more individuals with addictive behavior

Qualifier	Qualifier	Qualifier	Qualifier
Ø Cognitive	Z None	Z None	Z None
1 Behavioral			
2 Cognitive-Behavioral			
3 12-Step			
4 Interpersonal			
5 Vocational			
6 Psychoeducation			
7 Motivational Enhancement			
8 Confrontational			
9 Continuing Care			
B Spiritual			
C Pre/Post-Test Infectious Disease			

5; 6; 8

Z: NONE

H: SUBSTANCE ABUSE TREATMENT

SECTION: **H SUBSTANCE ABUSE TREATMENT**
SECTION QUALIFIER: **Z NONE**
TYPE: **5 INDIVIDUAL PSYCHOTHERAPY:** Treatment of an individual with addictive behavior by behavioral, cognitive, psychoanalytic, psychodynamic, or psychophysiological means

Qualifier	Qualifier	Qualifier	Qualifier
0 Cognitive	Z None	Z None	Z None
1 Behavioral			
2 Cognitive-Behavioral			
3 12-Step			
4 Interpersonal			
5 Interactive			
6 Psychoeducation			
7 Motivational Enhancement			
8 Confrontational			
9 Supportive			
B Psychoanalysis			
C Psychodynamic			
D Psychophysiological			

SECTION: **H SUBSTANCE ABUSE TREATMENT**
SECTION QUALIFIER: **Z NONE**
TYPE: **6 FAMILY COUNSELING:** The application of psychological methods that includes one or more family members to treat an individual with addictive behavior

Qualifier	Qualifier	Qualifier	Qualifier
3 Other Family Counseling	Z None	Z None	Z None

SECTION: **H SUBSTANCE ABUSE TREATMENT**
SECTION QUALIFIER: **Z NONE**
TYPE: **8 MEDICATION MANAGEMENT:** Monitoring and adjusting the use of replacement medications for the treatment of addiction

Qualifier	Qualifier	Qualifier	Qualifier
0 Nicotine Replacement	Z None	Z None	Z None
1 Methadone Maintenance			
2 Levo-alpha-acetyl-methadol (LAAM)			
3 Antabuse			
4 Naltrexone			
5 Naloxone			
6 Clonidine			
7 Bupropion			
8 Psychiatric Medication			
9 Other Replacement Medication			

SECTION:
H SUBSTANCE ABUSE TREATMENT

SECTION QUALIFIER: Z NONE

TYPE: 9 **PHARMACOTHERAPY:** The use of replacement medications for the treatment of addiction

Qualifier	Qualifier	Qualifier	Qualifier
Ø Nicotine Replacement	Z None	Z None	Z None
1 Methadone Maintenance			
2 Levo-alpha-acetyl-methadol (LAAM)			
3 Antabuse			
4 Naltrexone			
5 Naloxone			
6 Clonidine			
7 Bupropion			
8 Psychiatric Medication			
9 Other Replacement Medication			

H: SUBSTANCE ABUSE TREATMENT Z: NONE 9: PHARMACOTHERAPY

X New Technology **68Ø**

    X2. Cardiovascular System.. 681
        X2A. Assistance 681
        X2C. Extirpation 681
        X2R. Replacement 681
    XH. Skin, Subcutaneous Tissue, Fascia and Breast.. 682
        XHR. Replacement... 682
    XK. Muscles, Tendons, Bursae and Ligaments.. 682
        XKØ. Introduction.. 682
    XN. Bones 683
        XNS. Reposition 683
    XR. Joints 683
        XR2. Monitoring 683
        XRG. Fusion 684
    XW. Anatomical Regions... 685
        XWØ. Introduction.. 685
    XY. Extracorporeal 686
        XYØ. Introduction... 686

ICD-10-PCS Coding Guidelines

New Technology Section Guidelines (section X)

D. New Technology Section

General guidelines

D1

Section X codes are standalone codes. They are not supplemental codes. Section X codes fully represent the specific procedure described in the code title, and do not require any additional codes from other sections of ICD-10-PCS. When section X contains a code title which describes a specific new technology procedure, only that X code is reported for the procedure. There is no need to report a broader, non-specific code in another section of ICD-10-PCS.

Example: XW04321 Introduction of Ceftazidime-Avibactam Anti-infective into Central Vein, Percutaneous Approach, New Technology Group 1, can be coded to indicate that Ceftazidime-Avibactam Anti-infective was administered via a central vein. A separate code from table 3E0 in the Administration section of ICD-10-PCS is not coded in addition to this code.

Selection of Principal Procedure

The following instructions should be applied in the selection of principal procedure and clarification on the importance of the relation to the principal diagnosis when more than one procedure is performed:

1. Procedure performed for definitive treatment of both principal diagnosis and secondary diagnosis

    a. Sequence procedure performed for definitive treatment most related to principal diagnosis as principal procedure.

2. Procedure performed for definitive treatment and diagnostic procedures performed for both principal diagnosis and secondary diagnosis

    a. Sequence procedure performed for definitive treatment most related to principal diagnosis as principal procedure

3. A diagnostic procedure was performed for the principal diagnosis and a procedure is performed for definitive treatment of a secondary diagnosis.

    a. Sequence diagnostic procedure as principal procedure, since the procedure most related to the principal diagnosis takes precedence.

4. No procedures performed that are related to principal diagnosis; procedures performed for definitive treatment and diagnostic procedures were performed for secondary diagnosis

    a. Sequence procedure performed for definitive treatment of secondary diagnosis as principal procedure, since there are no procedures (definitive or nondefinitive treatment) related to principal diagnosis.

SECTION: X NEW TECHNOLOGY
BODY SYSTEM: 2 CARDIOVASCULAR SYSTEM
OPERATION: A ASSISTANCE: Taking over a portion of a physiological function by extracorporeal means

Body Part	Approach	Device / Substance / Technology	Qualifier
5 Innominate Artery and Left Common Carotid Artery	3 Percutaneous	1 Cerebral Embolic Filtration, Dual Filter	2 New Technology Group 2

SECTION: X NEW TECHNOLOGY
BODY SYSTEM: 2 CARDIOVASCULAR SYSTEM
OPERATION: C EXTIRPATION: Taking or cutting out solid matter from a body part

Body Part	Approach	Device / Substance / Technology	Qualifier
Ø Coronary Artery, One Artery 1 Coronary Artery, Two Arteries 2 Coronary Artery, Three Arteries 3 Coronary Artery, Four or More Arteries	3 Percutaneous	6 Orbital Atherectomy Technology	1 New Technology Group 1

SECTION: X NEW TECHNOLOGY
BODY SYSTEM: 2 CARDIOVASCULAR SYSTEM
OPERATION: R REPLACEMENT: Putting in or on biological or synthetic material that physically takes the place and/or function of all or a portion of a body part

Body Part	Approach	Device / Substance / Technology	Qualifier
F Aortic Valve	Ø Open 3 Percutaneous 4 Percutaneous Endoscopic	3 Zooplastic Tissue, Rapid Deployment Technique	2 New Technology Group 2

SECTION: **X NEW TECHNOLOGY**
BODY SYSTEM: **H SKIN, SUBCUTANEOUS TISSUE, FASCIA AND BREAST**
OPERATION: **R REPLACEMENT:** Putting in or on biological or synthetic material that physically takes the place and/or function of all or a portion of a body part

Body Part	Approach	Device / Substance / Technology	Qualifier
P Skin	X External	L Skin Substitute, Porcine Liver Derived	2 New Technology Group 2

SECTION: **X NEW TECHNOLOGY**
BODY SYSTEM: **K MUSCLES, TENDONS, BURSAE AND LIGAMENTS**
OPERATION: **Ø INTRODUCTION:** Putting in or on a therapeutic, diagnostic, nutritional, physiological, or prophylactic substance except blood or blood products

Body Part	Approach	Device / Substance / Technology	Qualifier
2 Muscle	3 Percutaneous	Ø Concentrated Bone Marrow Aspirate	3 New Technology Group 3

SECTION: X NEW TECHNOLOGY
BODY SYSTEM: N BONES
OPERATION: S **REPOSITION:** Moving to its normal location, or other suitable location, all or a portion of a body part

Body Part	Approach	Device / Substance / Technology	Qualifier
Ø Lumbar Vertebra 3 Cervical Vertebra 4 Thoracic Vertebra	Ø Open 3 Percutaneous	3 Magnetically Controlled Growth Rod(s)	2 New Technology Group 2

SECTION: X NEW TECHNOLOGY
BODY SYSTEM: R JOINTS
OPERATION: 2 **MONITORING:** Determining the level of a physiological or physical function repetitively over a period of time

Body Part	Approach	Device / Substance / Technology	Qualifier
G Knee Joint, Right H Knee Joint, Left	Ø Open	2 Intraoperative Knee Replacement Sensor	1 New Technology Group 1

SECTION: X NEW TECHNOLOGY
BODY SYSTEM: R JOINTS *(on multiple pages)*
OPERATION: G FUSION: Joining together portions of an articular body part rendering the articular body part immobile

Body Part	Approach	Device / Substance / Technology	Qualifier
Ø Occipital-cervical Joint ~~1 Cervical Vertebral Joint~~ ~~2 Cervical Vertebral Joints, 2 or more~~ ~~4 Cervicothoracic Vertebral Joint~~ ~~6 Thoracic Vertebral Joint~~ ~~7 Thoracic Vertebral Joints, 2 to 7~~ ~~8 Thoracic Vertebral Joints, 8 or more~~ ~~A Thoracolumbar Vertebral Joint~~ ~~B Lumbar Vertebral Joint~~ ~~C Lumbar Vertebral Joints, 2 or more~~ ~~D Lumbosacral Joint~~	Ø Open	9 Interbody Fusion Device, Nanotextured Surface	2 New Technology Group 2
Ø Occipital-cervical Joint	Ø Open	F Interbody Fusion Device, Radiolucent Porous	3 New Technology Group 3
1 Cervical Vertebral Joint	Ø Open	9 Interbody Fusion Device, Nanotextured Surface	2 New Technology Group 2
1 Cervical Vertebral Joint	Ø Open	F Interbody Fusion Device, Radiolucent Porous	3 New Technology Group 3
2 Cervical Vertebral Joints, 2 or more	Ø Open	9 Interbody Fusion Device, Nanotextured Surface	2 New Technology Group 2
2 Cervical Vertebral Joints, 2 or more	Ø Open	F Interbody Fusion Device, Radiolucent Porous	3 New Technology Group 3
4 Cervicothoracic Vertebral Joint	Ø Open	9 Interbody Fusion Device, Nanotextured Surface	2 New Technology Group 2
4 Cervicothoracic Vertebral Joint	Ø Open	F Interbody Fusion Device, Radiolucent Porous	3 New Technology Group 3
6 Thoracic Vertebral Joint	Ø Open	9 Interbody Fusion Device, Nanotextured Surface	2 New Technology Group 2
6 Thoracic Vertebral Joint	Ø Open	F Interbody Fusion Device, Radiolucent Porous	3 New Technology Group 3
7 Thoracic Vertebral Joints, 2 to 7	Ø Open	9 Interbody Fusion Device, Nanotextured Surface	2 New Technology Group 2
7 Thoracic Vertebral Joints, 2 to 7	Ø Open	F Interbody Fusion Device, Radiolucent Porous	3 New Technology Group 3
8 Thoracic Vertebral Joints, 8 or more	Ø Open	9 Interbody Fusion Device, Nanotextured Surface	2 New Technology Group 2
8 Thoracic Vertebral Joints, 8 or more	Ø Open	F Interbody Fusion Device, Radiolucent Porous	3 New Technology Group 3
A Thoracolumbar Vertebral Joint	Ø Open	9 Interbody Fusion Device, Nanotextured Surface	2 New Technology Group 2

G: FUSION

R: JOINTS

X: NEW TECHNOLOGY

New/Revised Text in Blue   ~~deleted~~ Deleted

SECTION: X NEW TECHNOLOGY
BODY SYSTEM: R JOINTS *(continued)*
OPERATION: G FUSION: Joining together portions of an articular body part rendering the articular body part immobile

Body Part	Approach	Device / Substance / Technology	Qualifier
A Thoracolumbar Vertebral Joint	Ø Open	F Interbody Fusion Device, Radiolucent Porous	3 New Technology Group 3
B Lumbar Vertebral Joint	Ø Open	9 Interbody Fusion Device, Nanotextured Surface	2 New Technology Group 2
B Lumbar Vertebral Joint	Ø Open	F Interbody Fusion Device, Radiolucent Porous	3 New Technology Group 3
C Lumbar Vertebral, Joints, 2 or more	Ø Open	9 Interbody Fusion Device, Nanotextured Surface	2 New Technology Group 2
C Lumbar Vertebral Joints, 2 or more	Ø Open	F Interbody Fusion Device, Radiolucent Porous	3 New Technology Group 3
D Lumbosacral Joint	Ø Open	9 Interbody Fusion Device, Nanotextured Surface	2 New Technology Group 2
D Lumbosacral Joint	Ø Open	F Interbody Fusion Device, Radiolucent Porous	3 New Technology Group 3

SECTION: X NEW TECHNOLOGY
BODY SYSTEM: W ANATOMICAL REGIONS *(on multiple pages)*
OPERATION: Ø INTRODUCTION: Putting in or on a therapeutic, diagnostic, nutritional, physiological, or prophylactic substance except blood or blood products

Body Part	Approach	Device / Substance / Technology	Qualifier
3 Peripheral Vein	3 Percutaneous	2 Ceftazidime-Avibactam Anti-infective 3 Idarucizumab, Dabigatran Reversal Agent 4 Isavuconazole Anti-infective 5 Blinatumomab Antineoplastic Immunotherapy	1 New Technology Group 1
3 Peripheral Vein	3 Percutaneous	7 Andexanet Alfa, Factor Xa Inhibitor Reversal Agent 9 Defibrotide Sodium Anticoagulant	2 New Technology Group 2
3 Peripheral Vein	3 Percutaneous	A Bezlotoxumab Monoclonal Antibody B Cytarabine and Daunorubicin Liposome Antineoplastic C Engineered Autologous Chimeric Antigen Receptor T-cell Immunotherapy F Other New Technology Therapeutic Substance	3 New Technology Group 3

SECTION: X NEW TECHNOLOGY
BODY SYSTEM: W ANATOMICAL REGIONS *(continued)*
OPERATION: 0 INTRODUCTION: Putting in or on a therapeutic, diagnostic, nutritional, physiological, or prophylactic substance except blood or blood products

Body Part	Approach	Device / Substance / Technology	Qualifier
4 Central Vein	3 Percutaneous	2 Ceftazidime-Avibactam Anti-infective 3 Idarucizumab, Dabigatran Reversal Agent 4 Isavuconazole Antiinfective 5 Blinatumomab Antineoplastic Immunotherapy	1 New Technology Group 1
4 Central Vein	3 Percutaneous	7 Andexanet Alfa, Factor Xa Inhibitor Reversal Agent 9 Defibrotide Sodium Anticoagulant	2 New Technology Group 2
4 Central Vein	3 Percutaneous	A Bezlotoxumab Monoclonal Antibody B Cytarabine and Daunorubicin Liposome Antineoplastic C Engineered Autologous Chimeric Antigen Receptor T-cell Immunotherapy F Other New Technology Therapeutic Substance	3 New Technology Group 3
D Mouth and Pharynx	X External	8 Uridine Triacetate	2 New Technology Group 2

SECTION: X NEW TECHNOLOGY
BODY SYSTEM: Y EXTRACORPOREAL
OPERATION: 0 INTRODUCTION: Putting in or on a therapeutic, diagnostic, nutritional, physiological, or prophylactic substance except blood or blood products

Body Part	Approach	Device / Substance / Technology	Qualifier
V Vein Graft	X External	8 Endothelial Damage Inhibitor	3 New Technology Group 3

INDEX

3

3f (Aortic) Bioprosthesis valve *use* Zooplastic Tissue in Heart and Great Vessels

A

Abdominal aortic plexus *use* Abdominal Sympathetic Nerve
Abdominal esophagus *use* Esophagus, Lower
Abdominohysterectomy
  see Resection, Cervix 0UTC
  see Resection, Uterus 0UT9
Abdominoplasty
  see Alteration, Abdominal Wall, 0W0F
  see Repair, Abdominal Wall, 0WQF
  see Supplement, Abdominal Wall, 0WUF
Abductor hallucis muscle
  use Foot Muscle, Right
  use Foot Muscle, Left
AbioCor® Total Replacement Heart *use* Synthetic Substitute
Ablation *see* Destruction
Abortion
  Products of Conception 10A0
  Abortifacient 10A07ZX
  Laminaria 10A07ZW
  Vacuum 10A07Z6
Abrasion *see* Extraction
Absolute Pro Vascular (OTW) Self-Expanding Stent System *use* Intraluminal Device
Accessory cephalic vein
  use Cephalic Vein, Right
  use Cephalic Vein, Left
Accessory obturator nerve *use* Lumbar Plexus
Accessory phrenic nerve *use* Phrenic Nerve
Accessory spleen *use* Spleen
Acculink (RX) Carotid Stent System *use* Intraluminal Device
Acellular Hydrated Dermis *use* Nonautologous Tissue Substitute
Acetabular cup *use* Liner in Lower Joints
Acetabulectomy
  see Excision, Lower Bones 0QB
  see Resection, Lower Bones 0QT
Acetabulofemoral joint
  use Hip Joint, Right
  use Hip Joint, Left
Acetabuloplasty
  see Repair, Lower Bones 0QQ
  see Replacement, Lower Bones 0QR
  see Supplement, Lower Bones 0QU
Achilles tendon
  use Lower Leg Tendon, Right
  use Lower Leg Tendon, Left
Achillorrhaphy *use* Repair, Tendons 0LQ
Achillotenotomy, achillotomy
  see Division, Tendons 0L8
  see Drainage, Tendons 0L9
Acromioclavicular ligament
  use Shoulder Bursa and Ligament, Right
  use Shoulder Bursa and Ligament, Left
Acromion (process)
  use Scapula, Right
  use Scapula, Left
Acromionectomy
  see Excision, Upper Joints 0RB
  see Resection, Upper Joints 0RT
Acromioplasty
  see Repair, Upper Joints 0RQ
  see Replacement, Upper Joints 0RR
  see Supplement, Upper Joints 0RU
Activa PC neurostimulator *use* Stimulator Generator, Multiple Array in 0JH
Activa RC neurostimulator *use* Stimulator Generator, Multiple Array Rechargeable in 0JH
Activa SC neurostimulator *use* Stimulator Generator, Single Array in 0JH
Activities of Daily Living Assessment F02
Activities of Daily Living Treatment F08

ACUITY™ Steerable Lead
  use Cardiac Lead, Pacemaker in 02H
  use Cardiac Lead, Defibrillator in O2H
Acupuncture
  Breast
    Anesthesia 8E0H300
    No Qualifier 8E0H30Z
  Integumentary System
    Anesthesia 8E0H300
    No Qualifier 8E0H30Z
Adductor brevis muscle
  use Upper Leg Muscle, Right
  use Upper Leg Muscle, Left
Adductor hallucis muscle
  use Foot Muscle, Right
  use Foot Muscle, Left
Adductor longus muscle
  use Upper Leg Muscle, Right
  use Upper Leg Muscle, Left
Adductor magnus muscle
  use Upper Leg Muscle, Right
  use Upper Leg Muscle, Left
Adenohypophysis *use* Pituitary Gland
Adenoidectomy
  see Excision, Adenoids 0CBQ
  see Resection, Adenoids 0CTQ
Adenoidotomy *see* Drainage, Adenoids 0C9Q
Adhesiolysis *see* Release
Administration
  Blood products *see* Transfusion
  Other substance *see* Introduction of substance in or on
Adrenalectomy
  see Excision, Endocrine System 0GB
  see Resection, Endocrine System 0GT
Adrenalorrhaphy *see* Repair, Endocrine System 0GQ
Adrenalotomy *see* Drainage, Endocrine System 0G9
Advancement
  see Reposition
  see Transfer
Advisa (MRI) *use* Pacemaker, Dual Chamber in 0JH
AFX® Endovascular AAA System *use* Intraluminal Device
AIGISRx Antibacterial Envelope *use* Anti-Infective Envelope
Alar ligament of axis *use* Head and Neck Bursa and Ligament
Alimentation *see* Introduction of substance in or on
Alteration
  Abdominal Wall 0W0F
  Ankle Region
    Left 0Y0L
    Right 0Y0K
  Arm
    Lower
      Left 0X0F
      Right 0X0D
    Upper
      Left 0X09
      Right 0X08
  Axilla
    Left 0X05
    Right 0X04
  Back
    Lower 0W0L
    Upper 0W0K
  Breast
    Bilateral 0H0V
    Left 0H0U
    Right 0H0T
  Buttock
    Left 0Y01
    Right 0Y00
  Chest Wall 0W08
  Ear
    Bilateral 0902
    Left 0901
    Right 0900

Alteration *(Continued)*
  Elbow Region
    Left 0X0C
    Right 0X0B
  Extremity
    Lower
      Left 0Y0B
      Right 0Y09
    Upper
      Left 0X07
      Right 0X06
  Eyelid
    Lower
      Left 080R
      Right 080Q
    Upper
      Left 080P
      Right 080N
  Face 0W02
  Head 0W00
  Jaw
    Lower 0W05
    Upper 0W04
  Knee Region
    Left 0Y0G
    Right 0Y0F
  Leg
    Lower
      Left 0Y0J
      Right 0Y0H
    Upper
      Left 0Y0D
      Right 0Y0C
  Lip
    Lower 0C01X
    Upper 0C00X
  ▶Nasal Mucosa and Soft Tissue 090K
  Neck 0W06
  ~~Nose 090K~~
  Perineum
    Female 0W0N
    Male 0W0M
  Shoulder Region
    Left 0X03
    Right 0X02
  Subcutaneous Tissue and Fascia
    Abdomen 0J08
    Back 0J07
    Buttock 0J09
    Chest 0J06
    Face 0J01
    Lower Arm
      Left 0J0H
      Right 0J0G
    Lower Leg
      Left 0J0P
      Right 0J0N
    Neck
      ~~Anterior 0J04~~
      ~~Posterior 0J05~~
      ▶Left 0J05
      ▶Right 0J04
    Upper Arm
      Left 0J0F
      Right 0J0D
    Upper Leg
      Left 0J0M
      Right 0J0L
  Wrist Region
    Left 0X0H
    Right 0X0G
⟹**Alveolar process of mandible** *use* Maxilla
  ~~*use* Mandible, Right~~
  ~~*use* Mandible, Left~~
Alveolar process of maxilla
  use Maxilla, Right
  use Maxilla, Left
Alveolectomy
  see Excision, Head and Facial Bones 0NB
  see Resection, Head and Facial Bones 0NT

▶ New　⟹ Revised　~~deleted~~ Deleted

Alveoloplasty
  see Repair, Head and Facial Bones ØNQ
  see Replacement, Head and Facial Bones ØNR
  see Supplement, Head and Facial Bones ØNU
Alveolotomy
  see Division, Head and Facial Bones ØN8
  see Drainage, Head and Facial Bones ØN9
Ambulatory cardiac monitoring 4A12X45
Amniocentesis *see* Drainage, Products of
  Conception 1Ø9Ø
Amnioinfusion *see* Introduction of substance in
  or on, Products of Conception 3EØE
Amnioscopy 1ØJØ8ZZ
Amniotomy *see* Drainage, Products of
  Conception 1Ø9Ø
AMPLATZER® Muscular VSD Occluder *use*
  Synthetic Substitute
Amputation *see* Detachment
AMS 800® Urinary Control System *use*
  Artificial Sphincter in Urinary System
Anal orifice *use* Anus
Analog radiography *see* Plain Radiography
Analog radiology *see* Plain Radiography
Anastomosis *see* Bypass
Anatomical snuffbox
  use Lower Arm and Wrist Muscle, Right
  use Lower Arm and Wrist Muscle, Left
Andexanet Alfa, Factor Xa Inhibitor Reversal
  Agent XWØ
AneuRx® AAA Advantage® *use* Intraluminal
  Device
Angiectomy
  see Excision, Heart and Great Vessels Ø2B
  see Excision, Upper Arteries Ø3B
  see Excision, Lower Arteries Ø4B
  see Excision, Upper Veins Ø5B
  see Excision, Lower Veins Ø6B
Angiocardiography
  Combined right and left heart *see*
    Fluoroscopy, Heart, Right and Left B216
  Left Heart *see* Fluoroscopy, Heart, Left B215
  Right Heart *see* Fluoroscopy, Heart, Right B214
  SPY system intravascular fluorescence *see*
    Monitoring, Physiological Systems 4A1
Angiography
  see Plain Radiography, Heart B2Ø
  see Fluoroscopy, Heart B21
Angioplasty
  see Dilation, Heart and Great Vessels Ø27
  see Repair, Heart and Great Vessels Ø2Q
  see Replacement, Heart and Great Vessels Ø2R
  see Supplement, Heart and Great Vessels Ø2U
  see Dilation, Upper Arteries Ø37
  see Repair, Upper Arteries Ø3Q
  see Replacement, Upper Arteries Ø3R
  see Supplement, Upper Arteries Ø3U
  see Dilation, Lower Arteries Ø47
  see Repair, Lower Arteries Ø4Q
  see Replacement, Lower Arteries Ø4R
  see Supplement, Lower Arteries Ø4U
Angiorrhaphy
  see Repair, Heart and Great Vessels Ø2Q
  see Repair, Upper Arteries Ø3Q
  see Repair, Lower Arteries Ø4Q
Angioscopy
  Ø2JY4ZZ
  Ø3JY4ZZ
  Ø4JY4ZZ
Angiotripsy
  see Occlusion, Upper Arteries Ø3L
  see Occlusion, Lower Arteries Ø4L
Angular artery *use* Face Artery
Angular vein
  use Face Vein, Right
  use Face Vein, Left
Annular ligament
  use Elbow Bursa and Ligament, Right
  use Elbow Bursa and Ligament, Left
Annuloplasty
  see Repair, Heart and Great Vessels Ø2Q
  see Supplement, Heart and Great Vessels Ø2U
Annuloplasty ring *use* Synthetic Substitute

Anoplasty
  see Repair, Anus ØDQQ
  see Supplement, Anus ØDUQ
Anorectal junction *use* Rectum
Anoscopy ØDJD8ZZ
Ansa cervicalis *use* Cervical Plexus
Antabuse therapy HZ93ZZZ
Antebrachial fascia
  use Subcutaneous Tissue and Fascia, Right
    Lower Arm
  use Subcutaneous Tissue and Fascia, Left
    Lower Arm
Anterior (pectoral) lymph node
  use Lymphatic, Right Axillary
  use Lymphatic, Left Axillary
Anterior cerebral artery *use* Intracranial Artery
Anterior cerebral vein *use* Intracranial Vein
Anterior choroidal artery *use* Intracranial
  Artery
Anterior circumflex humeral artery
  use Axillary Artery, Right
  use Axillary Artery, Left
Anterior communicating artery *use* Intracranial
  Artery
Anterior cruciate ligament (ACL)
  use Knee Bursa and Ligament, Right
  use Knee Bursa and Ligament, Left
Anterior crural nerve *use* Femoral Nerve
Anterior facial vein
  use Face Vein, Right
  use Face Vein, Left
Anterior intercostal artery
  use Internal Mammary Artery, Right
  use Internal Mammary Artery, Left
Anterior interosseous nerve *use* Median Nerve
Anterior lateral malleolar artery
  use Anterior Tibial Artery, Right
  use Anterior Tibial Artery, Left
Anterior lingual gland *use* Minor Salivary
  Gland
Anterior medial malleolar artery
  use Anterior Tibial Artery, Right
  use Anterior Tibial Artery, Left
Anterior spinal artery
  use Vertebral Artery, Right
  use Vertebral Artery, Left
Anterior tibial recurrent artery
  use Anterior Tibial Artery, Right
  use Anterior Tibial Artery, Left
Anterior ulnar recurrent artery
  use Ulnar Artery, Right
  use Ulnar Artery, Left
Anterior vagal trunk *use* Vagus Nerve
Anterior vertebral muscle
  use Neck Muscle, Right
  use Neck Muscle, Left
▶**Antigen-free air conditioning** *see* Atmospheric
  Control, Physiological Systems 6AØ
Antihelix
  use External Ear, Right
  use External Ear, Left
  use External Ear, Bilateral
Antimicrobial envelope *use* Anti-Infective
  Envelope
Antitragus
  use External Ear, Right
  use External Ear, Left
  use External Ear, Bilateral
Antrostomy *see* Drainage, Ear, Nose, Sinus Ø99
Antrotomy *see* Drainage, Ear, Nose, Sinus Ø99
Antrum of Highmore
  use Maxillary Sinus, Right
  use Maxillary Sinus, Left
Aortic annulus *use* Aortic Valve
Aortic arch *use* Thoracic Aorta, Ascending/Arch
Aortic intercostal artery *use* Upper Artery
Aortography
  see Plain Radiography, Upper Arteries B3Ø
  see Fluoroscopy, Upper Arteries B31
  see Plain Radiography, Lower Arteries B4Ø
  see Fluoroscopy, Lower Arteries B41

Aortoplasty
  see Repair, Aorta, Thoracic, Descending
    Ø2QW
  see Repair, Aorta, Thoracic, Ascending/Arch
    Ø2QX
  see Replacement, Aorta, Thoracic, Descending
    Ø2RW
  see Replacement, Aorta, Thoracic, Ascending/
    Arch Ø2RX
  see Supplement, Aorta, Thoracic, Descending
    Ø2UW
  see Supplement, Aorta, Thoracic, Ascending/
    Arch Ø2UX
  see Repair, Aorta, Abdominal Ø4QØ
  see Replacement, Aorta, Abdominal Ø4RØ
  see Supplement, Aorta, Abdominal Ø4UØ
Apical (subclavicular) lymph node
  use Lymphatic, Axillary, Right
  use Lymphatic, Axillary, Left
Apneustic center *use* Pons
Appendectomy
  see Excision, Appendix ØDBJ
  see Resection, Appendix ØDTJ
Appendicolysis *see* Release, Appendix ØDNJ
Appendicotomy *see* Drainage, Appendix ØD9J
Application *see* Introduction of substance in
  or on
Aquapheresis 6A55ØZ3
Aqueduct of Sylvius *use* Cerebral Ventricle
Aqueous humour
  use Anterior Chamber, Right
  use Anterior Chamber, Left
Arachnoid mater, intracranial *use* Cerebral
  Meninges
Arachnoid mater, spinal *use* Spinal Meninges
Arcuate artery
  use Foot Artery, Right
  use Foot Artery, Left
Areola
  use Nipple, Right
  use Nipple, Left
AROM (artificial rupture of membranes)
  1Ø9Ø7ZC
Arterial canal (duct) *use* Pulmonary Artery,
  Left
Arterial pulse tracing *see* Measurement,
  Arterial 4AØ3
Arteriectomy
  see Excision, Heart and Great Vessels Ø2B
  see Excision, Upper Arteries Ø3B
  see Excision, Lower Arteries Ø4B
Arteriography
  see Plain Radiography, Heart B2Ø
  see Fluoroscopy, Heart B21
  see Plain Radiography, Upper Arteries
    B3Ø
  see Fluoroscopy, Upper Arteries B31
  see Plain Radiography, Lower Arteries
    B4Ø
  see Fluoroscopy, Lower Arteries B41
Arterioplasty
  see Repair, Heart and Great Vessels Ø2Q
  see Replacement, Heart and Great Vessels
    Ø2R
  see Supplement, Heart and Great Vessels
    Ø2U
  see Repair, Upper Arteries Ø3Q
  see Replacement, Upper Arteries Ø3R
  see Supplement, Upper Arteries Ø3U
  see Repair, Lower Arteries Ø4Q
  see Replacement, Lower Arteries Ø4R
  see Supplement, Lower Arteries Ø4U
Arteriorrhaphy
  see Repair, Heart and Great Vessels
    Ø2Q
  see Repair, Upper Arteries Ø3Q
  see Repair, Lower Arteries Ø4Q
Arterioscopy
  see Inspection, Great Vessel Ø2JY
  see Inspection, Artery, Upper Ø3JY
  see Inspection, Artery, Lower Ø4JY

Arthrectomy
see Excision, Upper Joints ØRB
see Resection, Upper Joints ØRT
see Excision, Lower Joints ØSB
see Resection, Lower Joints ØST
Arthrocentesis
see Drainage, Upper Joints ØR9
see Drainage, Lower Joints ØS9
Arthrodesis
see Fusion, Upper Joints ØRG
see Fusion, Lower Joints ØSG
Arthrography
see Plain Radiography, Skull and Facial Bones BNØ
see Plain Radiography, Non-Axial Upper Bones BPØ
see Plain Radiography, Non-Axial Lower Bones BQØ
Arthrolysis
see Release, Upper Joints ØRN
see Release, Lower Joints ØSN
Arthropexy
see Repair, Upper Joints ØRQ
see Reposition, Upper Joints ØRS
see Repair, Lower Joints ØSQ
see Reposition, Lower Joints ØSS
Arthroplasty
see Repair, Upper Joints ØRQ
see Replacement, Upper Joints ØRR
see Supplement, Upper Joints ØRU
see Repair, Lower Joints ØSQ
see Replacement, Lower Joints ØSR
see Supplement, Lower Joints ØSU
Arthroscopy
see Inspection, Upper Joints ØRJ
see Inspection, Lower Joints ØSJ
Arthrotomy
see Drainage, Upper Joints ØR9
see Drainage, Lower Joints ØS9
Artificial anal sphincter (AAS) use Artificial Sphincter in Gastrointestinal System
Artificial bowel sphincter (neosphincter) use Artificial Sphincter in Gastrointestinal System
Artificial Sphincter
Insertion of device in
Anus ØDHQ
Bladder ØTHB
Bladder Neck ØTHC
Urethra ØTHD
Removal of device from
Anus ØDPQ
Bladder ØTPB
Urethra ØTPD
Revision of device in
Anus ØDWQ
Bladder ØTWB
Urethra ØTWD
Artificial urinary sphincter (AUS) use Artificial Sphincter in Urinary System
Aryepiglottic fold use Larynx
Arytenoid cartilage use Larynx
Arytenoid muscle
use Neck Muscle, Right
use Neck Muscle, Left
Arytenoidectomy see Excision, Larynx ØCBS
Arytenoidopexy see Repair, Larynx ØCQS
Ascenda Intrathecal Catheter use Infusion Device
Ascending aorta use Thoracic Aorta, Ascending/Arch
Ascending palatine artery use Face Artery
Ascending pharyngeal artery
use External Carotid Artery, Right
use External Carotid Artery, Left
Aspiration, fine needle
fluid or gas see Drainage
tissue see Excision

Assessment
Activities of daily living see Activities of Daily Living Assessment, Rehabilitation F02
Hearing see Hearing Assessment, Diagnostic Audiology F13
Hearing aid see Hearing Aid Assessment, Diagnostic Audiology F14
Intravascular perfusion, using indocyanine green (ICG) dye see Monitoring, Physiological Systems 4A1
Motor function see Motor Function Assessment, Rehabilitation F01
Nerve function see Motor Function Assessment, Rehabilitation F01
Speech see Speech Assessment, Rehabilitation F00
Vestibular see Vestibular Assessment, Diagnostic Audiology F15
Vocational see Activities of Daily Living Treatment, Rehabilitation F08
Assistance
Cardiac
Continuous
Balloon Pump 5A02210
Impeller Pump 5A0221D
Other Pump 5A02216
Pulsatile Compression 5A02215
Intermittent
Balloon Pump 5A02110
Impeller Pump 5A0211D
Other Pump 5A02116
Pulsatile Compression 5A02115
Circulatory
Continuous
Hyperbaric 5A05221
Supersaturated 5A0522C
Intermittent
Hyperbaric 5A05121
Supersaturated 5A0512C
Respiratory
24-96 Consecutive Hours
Continuous Negative Airway Pressure 5A09459
Continuous Positive Airway Pressure 5A09457
Intermittent Negative Airway Pressure 5A0945B
Intermittent Positive Airway Pressure 5A09458
No Qualifier 5A0945Z
▶Continuous, Filtration 5A0920Z
Greater than 96 Consecutive Hours
Continuous Negative Airway Pressure 5A09559
Continuous Positive Airway Pressure 5A09557
Intermittent Negative Airway Pressure 5A0955B
Intermittent Positive Airway Pressure 5A09558
No Qualifier 5A0955Z
Less than 24 Consecutive Hours
Continuous Negative Airway Pressure 5A09359
Continuous Positive Airway Pressure 5A09357
Intermittent Negative Airway Pressure 5A0935B
Intermittent Positive Airway Pressure 5A09358
No Qualifier 5A0935Z
Assurant (Cobalt) stent use Intraluminal Device
Atherectomy
see Extirpation, Heart and Great Vessels Ø2C
see Extirpation, Upper Arteries Ø3C
see Extirpation, Lower Arteries Ø4C
Atlantoaxial joint use Cervical Vertebral Joint
Atmospheric Control 6AØZ
▶**AtriClip LAA Exclusion System** use Extraluminal Device

Atrioseptoplasty
see Repair, Heart and Great Vessels Ø2Q
see Replacement, Heart and Great Vessels Ø2R
see Supplement, Heart and Great Vessels Ø2U
Atrioventricular node use Conduction Mechanism
Atrium dextrum cordis use Atrium, Right
Atrium pulmonale use Atrium, Left
Attain Ability® lead
use Cardiac Lead, Pacemaker in Ø2H
use Cardiac Lead, Defibrillator in Ø2H
Attain StarFix® (OTW) lead
use Cardiac Lead, Pacemaker in Ø2H
use Cardiac Lead, Defibrillator in O2H
Audiology, diagnostic
see Hearing Assessment, Diagnostic Audiology F13
see Hearing Aid Assessment, Diagnostic Audiology F14
see Vestibular Assessment, Diagnostic Audiology F15
Audiometry see Hearing Assessment, Diagnostic Audiology F13
Auditory tube
use Eustachian Tube, Right
use Eustachian Tube, Left
Auerbach's (myenteric) plexus use Nerve, Abdominal Sympathetic
Auricle
use External Ear, Right
use External Ear, Left
use External Ear, Bilateral
Auricularis muscle use Head Muscle
Autograft use Autologous Tissue Substitute
Autologous artery graft
use Autologous Arterial Tissue in Heart and Great Vessels
use Autologous Arterial Tissue in Upper Arteries
use Autologous Arterial Tissue in Lower Arteries
use Autologous Arterial Tissue in Upper Veins
use Autologous Arterial Tissue in Lower Veins
Autologous vein graft
use Autologous Venous Tissue in Heart and Great Vessels
use Autologous Venous Tissue in Upper Arteries
use Autologous Venous Tissue in Lower Arteries
use Autologous Venous Tissue in Upper Veins
use Autologous Venous Tissue in Lower Veins
Autotransfusion see Transfusion
Autotransplant
Adrenal tissue see Reposition, Endocrine System ØGS
Kidney
see Reposition, Urinary System ØTS
Pancreatic tissue see Reposition, Pancreas ØFSG
Parathyroid tissue see Reposition, Endocrine System ØGS
Thyroid tissue see Reposition, Endocrine System ØGS
Tooth see Reattachment, Mouth and Throat ØCM
Avulsion see Extraction
Axial Lumbar Interbody Fusion System use Interbody Fusion Device in Lower Joints
AxiaLIF® System use Interbody Fusion Device in Lower Joints
▶**Axicabtagene Ciloeucel** use Engineered Autologous Chimeric Antigen Receptor T-cell Immunotherapy
Axillary fascia
use Subcutaneous Tissue and Fascia, Right Upper Arm
use Subcutaneous Tissue and Fascia, Left Upper Arm
Axillary nerve use Brachial Plexus

B

BAK/C® Interbody Cervical Fusion System *use*
  Interbody Fusion Device in Upper Joints
BAL (bronchial alveolar lavage), diagnostic *see*
  Drainage, Respiratory System 0B9
Balanoplasty
  see Repair, Penis 0VQS
  see Supplement, Penis 0VUS
▶ Balloon atrial septostomy (BAS) 02163Z7
Balloon Pump
  Continuous, Output 5A02210
  Intermittent, Output 5A02110
Bandage, Elastic *see* Compression
Banding
  see Occlusion
  see Restriction
▶ Banding, esophageal varices *see* Occlusion,
  Vein, Esophageal 06L3
▶ Banding, laparoscopic (adjustable) gastric
  ▶ Adjustment/revision 0DW64CZ
  ▶ Initial procedure 0DV64CZ
Bard® Composix® (E/X) (LP) mesh *use* Synthetic
  Substitute
Bard® Composix® Kugel® patch *use* Synthetic
  Substitute
Bard® Dulex™ mesh *use* Synthetic Substitute
Bard® Ventralex™ hernia patch *use* Synthetic
  Substitute
Barium swallow *see* Fluoroscopy,
  Gastrointestinal System BD1
Baroreflex Activation Therapy® (BAT®)
  use Stimulator Generator in Subcutaneous
    Tissue and Fascia
  use Stimulator Lead in Upper Arteries
Bartholin's (greater vestibular) gland *use*
  Vestibular Gland
Basal (internal) cerebral vein *use* Intracranial Vein
Basal metabolic rate (BMR) *see* Measurement,
  Physiological Systems 4A0Z
Basal nuclei *use* Basal Ganglia
Base of Tongue *use* Pharynx
Basilar artery *use* Intracranial Artery
Basis pontis *use* Pons
Beam Radiation
  Abdomen DW03
    Intraoperative DW033Z0
  Adrenal Gland DG02
    Intraoperative DG023Z0
  Bile Ducts DF02
    Intraoperative DF023Z0
  Bladder DT02
    Intraoperative DT023Z0
  Bone
    Other DP0C
      Intraoperative DP0C3Z0
  Bone Marrow D700
    Intraoperative D7003Z0
  Brain D000
    Intraoperative D0003Z0
  Brain Stem D001
    Intraoperative D0013Z0
  Breast
    Left DM00
      Intraoperative DM003Z0
    Right DM01
      Intraoperative DM013Z0
  Bronchus DB01
    Intraoperative DB013Z0
  Cervix DU01
    Intraoperative DU013Z0
  Chest DW02
    Intraoperative DW023Z0
  Chest Wall DB07
    Intraoperative DB073Z0
  Colon DD05
    Intraoperative DD053Z0
  Diaphragm DB08
    Intraoperative DB083Z0
  Duodenum DD02
    Intraoperative DD023Z0
  Ear D900
    Intraoperative D9003Z0

Beam Radiation (*Continued*)
  Esophagus DD00
    Intraoperative DD003Z0
  Eye D800
    Intraoperative D8003Z0
  Femur DP09
    Intraoperative DP093Z0
  Fibula DP0B
    Intraoperative DP0B3Z0
  Gallbladder DF01
    Intraoperative DF013Z0
  Gland
    Adrenal DG02
      Intraoperative DG023Z0
    Parathyroid DG04
      Intraoperative DG043Z0
    Pituitary DG00
      Intraoperative DG003Z0
    Thyroid DG05
      Intraoperative DG053Z0
  Glands
    Salivary D906
      Intraoperative D9063Z0
  Head and Neck DW01
    Intraoperative DW013Z0
  Hemibody DW04
    Intraoperative DW043Z0
  Humerus DP06
    Intraoperative DP063Z0
  Hypopharynx D903
    Intraoperative D9033Z0
  Ileum DD04
    Intraoperative DD043Z0
  Jejunum DD03
    Intraoperative DD033Z0
  Kidney DT00
    Intraoperative DT003Z0
  Larynx D90B
    Intraoperative D90B3Z0
  Liver DF00
    Intraoperative DF003Z0
  Lung DB02
    Intraoperative DB023Z0
  Lymphatics
    Abdomen D706
      Intraoperative D7063Z0
    Axillary D704
      Intraoperative D7043Z0
    Inguinal D708
      Intraoperative D7083Z0
    Neck D703
      Intraoperative D7033Z0
    Pelvis D707
      Intraoperative D7073Z0
    Thorax D705
      Intraoperative D7053Z0
  Mandible DP03
    Intraoperative DP033Z0
  Maxilla DP02
    Intraoperative DP023Z0
  Mediastinum DB06
    Intraoperative DB063Z0
  Mouth D904
    Intraoperative D9043Z0
  Nasopharynx D90D
    Intraoperative D90D3Z0
  Neck and Head DW01
    Intraoperative DW013Z0
  Nerve
    Peripheral D007
      Intraoperative D0073Z0
  Nose D901
    Intraoperative D9013Z0
  Oropharynx D90F
    Intraoperative D90F3Z0
  Ovary DU00
    Intraoperative DU003Z0
  Palate
    Hard D908
      Intraoperative D9083Z0
    Soft D909
      Intraoperative D9093Z0

Beam Radiation (*Continued*)
  Pancreas DF03
    Intraoperative DF033Z0
  Parathyroid Gland DG04
    Intraoperative DG043Z0
  Pelvic Bones DP08
    Intraoperative DP083Z0
  Pelvic Region DW06
    Intraoperative DW063Z0
  Pineal Body DG01
    Intraoperative DG013Z0
  Pituitary Gland DG00
    Intraoperative DG003Z0
  Pleura DB05
    Intraoperative DB053Z0
  Prostate DV00
    Intraoperative DV003Z0
  Radius DP07
    Intraoperative DP073Z0
  Rectum DD07
    Intraoperative DD073Z0
  Rib DP05
    Intraoperative DP053Z0
  Sinuses D907
    Intraoperative D9073Z0
  Skin
    Abdomen DH08
      Intraoperative DH083Z0
    Arm DH04
      Intraoperative DH043Z0
    Back DH07
      Intraoperative DH073Z0
    Buttock DH09
      Intraoperative DH093Z0
    Chest DH06
      Intraoperative DH063Z0
    Face DH02
      Intraoperative DH023Z0
    Leg DH0B
      Intraoperative DH0B3Z0
    Neck DH03
      Intraoperative DH033Z0
  Skull DP00
    Intraoperative DP003Z0
  Spinal Cord D006
    Intraoperative D0063Z0
  Spleen D702
    Intraoperative D7023Z0
  Sternum DP04
    Intraoperative DP043Z0
  Stomach DD01
    Intraoperative DD013Z0
  Testis DV01
    Intraoperative DV013Z0
  Thymus D701
    Intraoperative D7013Z0
  Thyroid Gland DG05
    Intraoperative DG053Z0
  Tibia DP0B
    Intraoperative DP0B3Z0
  Tongue D905
    Intraoperative D9053Z0
  Trachea DB00
    Intraoperative DB003Z0
  Ulna DP07
    Intraoperative DP073Z0
  Ureter DT01
    Intraoperative DT013Z0
  Urethra DT03
    Intraoperative DT033Z0
  Uterus DU02
    Intraoperative DU023Z0
  Whole Body DW05
    Intraoperative DW053Z0
Bedside swallow F00ZJWZ
Berlin Heart Ventricular Assist Device *use*
  Implantable Heart Assist System in Heart
    and Great Vessels
▶ Bezlotoxumab Monoclonal Antibody XW0
Biceps brachii muscle
  use Upper Arm Muscle, Right
  use Upper Arm Muscle, Left
Biceps femoris muscle
  use Upper Leg Muscle, Right
  use Upper Leg Muscle, Left

Bicipital aponeurosis
  use Subcutaneous Tissue and Fascia, Right
    Lower Arm
  use Subcutaneous Tissue and Fascia, Left
    Lower Arm
Bicuspid valve *use* Mitral Valve
Bililite therapy *see* Ultraviolet Light Therapy,
  Skin 6A8Ø
Bioactive embolization coil(s) *use* Intraluminal
  Device, Bioactive in Upper Arteries
Biofeedback GZC9ZZZ
Biopsy
  see Drainage with qualifier Diagnostic
  see Excision with qualifier Diagnostic
  Bone Marrow *see* Extraction with qualifier
    Diagnostic
BiPAP *see* Assistance, Respiratory 5A09
Bisection *see* Division
➡ **Biventricular external heart assist system** *use*
    Short-term External Heart Assist System in
    Heart and Great Vessels
Blepharectomy
  see Excision, Eye Ø8B
  see Resection, Eye Ø8T
Blepharoplasty
  see Repair, Eye Ø8Q
  see Replacement, Eye Ø8R
  see Reposition, Eye Ø8S
  see Supplement, Eye Ø8U
Blepharorrhaphy *see* Repair, Eye Ø8Q
Blepharotomy *see* Drainage, Eye Ø89
Blinatumomab Antineoplastic
  Immunotherapy XWØ
Block, Nerve, anesthetic injection 3EØT3CZ
Blood glucose monitoring system *use*
  Monitoring Device
Blood pressure *see* Measurement, Arterial 4A03
BMR (basal metabolic rate) *see* Measurement,
  Physiological Systems 4AØZ
Body of femur
  use Femoral Shaft, Right
  use Femoral Shaft, Left
Body of fibula
  use Fibula, Right
  use Fibula, Left
Bone anchored hearing device
  use Hearing Device, Bone Conduction in Ø9H
  use Hearing Device, in Head and Facial Bones
Bone bank bone graft *use* Nonautologous
  Tissue Substitute
Bone Growth Stimulator
  Insertion of device in
    Bone
      Facial ØNHW
      Lower ØQHY
      Nasal ØNHB
      Upper ØPHY
    Skull ØNHØ
  Removal of device from
    Bone
      Facial ØNPW
      Lower ØQPY
      Nasal ØNPB
      Upper ØPPY
    Skull ØNPØ
  Revision of device in
    Bone
      Facial ØNWW
      Lower ØQWY
      Nasal ØNWB
      Upper ØPWY
    Skull ØNWØ
Bone marrow transplant *see* Transfusion,
  Circulatory 3Ø2
Bone morphogenetic protein 2 (BMP 2) *use*
  Recombinant Bone Morphogenetic
  Protein
Bone screw (interlocking) (lag) (pedicle)
  (recessed)
  use Internal Fixation Device in Head and
    Facial Bones
  use Internal Fixation Device in Upper Bones
  use Internal Fixation Device in Lower Bones

Bony labyrinth
  use Inner Ear, Right
  use Inner Ear, Left
Bony orbit
  use Orbit, Right
  use Orbit, Left
Bony vestibule
  use Inner Ear, Right
  use Inner Ear, Left
Botallo's duct *use* Pulmonary Artery, Left
Bovine pericardial valve *use* Zooplastic Tissue
  in Heart and Great Vessels
Bovine pericardium graft *use* Zooplastic Tissue
  in Heart and Great Vessels
BP (blood pressure) *see* Measurement, Arterial
  4A03
Brachial (lateral) lymph node
  use Lymphatic, Axillary Right
  use Lymphatic, Axillary Left
Brachialis muscle
  use Upper Arm Muscle, Right
  use Upper Arm Muscle, Left
Brachiocephalic artery *use* Innominate Artery
Brachiocephalic trunk *use* Innominate Artery
Brachiocephalic vein
  use Innominate Vein, Right
  use Innominate Vein, Left
Brachioradialis muscle
  use Lower Arm and Wrist Muscle, Right
  use Lower Arm and Wrist Muscle, Left
Brachytherapy
  Abdomen DW13
  Adrenal Gland DG12
  Bile Ducts DF12
  Bladder DT12
  Bone Marrow D71Ø
  Brain DØ1Ø
  Brain Stem DØ11
  Breast
    Left DM1Ø
    Right DM11
  Bronchus DB11
  Cervix DU11
  Chest DW12
  Chest Wall DB17
  Colon DD15
  Diaphragm DB18
  Duodenum DD12
  Ear D91Ø
  Esophagus DD1Ø
  Eye D81Ø
  Gallbladder DF11
  Gland
    Adrenal DG12
    Parathyroid DG14
    Pituitary DG1Ø
    Thyroid DG15
  Glands, Salivary D916
  Head and Neck DW11
  Hypopharynx D913
  Ileum DD14
  Jejunum DD13
  Kidney DT1Ø
  Larynx D91B
  Liver DF1Ø
  Lung DB12
  Lymphatics
    Abdomen D716
    Axillary D714
    Inguinal D718
    Neck D713
    Pelvis D717
    Thorax D715
  Mediastinum DB16
  Mouth D914
  Nasopharynx D91D
  Neck and Head DW11
  Nerve, Peripheral DØ17
  Nose D911
  Oropharynx D91F
  Ovary DU1Ø

Brachytherapy *(Continued)*
  Palate
    Hard D918
    Soft D919
  Pancreas DF13
  Parathyroid Gland DG14
  Pelvic Region DW16
  Pineal Body DG11
  Pituitary Gland DG1Ø
  Pleura DB15
  Prostate DV1Ø
  Rectum DD17
  Sinuses D917
  Spinal Cord DØ16
  Spleen D712
  Stomach DD11
  Testis DV11
  Thymus D711
  Thyroid Gland DG15
  Tongue D915
  Trachea DB1Ø
  Ureter DT11
  Urethra DT13
  Uterus DU12
Brachytherapy seeds *use* Radioactive Element
Broad ligament *use* Uterine Supporting
  Structure
Bronchial artery *use* Upper Artery
Bronchography
  see Plain Radiography, Respiratory System
    BBØ
  see Fluoroscopy, Respiratory System BB1
Bronchoplasty
  see Repair, Respiratory System ØBQ
  see Supplement, Respiratory System ØBU
Bronchorrhaphy *see* Repair, Respiratory System
  ØBQ
Bronchoscopy ØBJ08ZZ
Bronchotomy *see* Drainage, Respiratory System
  ØB9
Bronchus Intermedius *use* Main Bronchus,
  Right
BRYAN® Cervical Disc System *use* Synthetic
  Substitute
Buccal gland *use* Buccal Mucosa
Buccinator lymph node *use* Lymphatic, Head
Buccinator muscle *use* Facial Muscle
Buckling, scleral with implant *see* Supplement,
  Eye Ø8U
Bulbospongiosus muscle *use* Perineum
  Muscle
Bulbourethral (Cowper's) gland *use* Urethra
Bundle of His *use* Conduction Mechanism
Bundle of Kent *use* Conduction Mechanism
Bunionectomy *see* Excision, Lower Bones
  ØQB
Bursectomy
  see Excision, Bursae and Ligaments ØMB
  see Resection, Bursae and Ligaments ØMT
Bursocentesis *see* Drainage, Bursae and
  Ligaments ØM9
Bursography
  see Plain Radiography, Non-Axial Upper
    Bones BPØ
  see Plain Radiography, Non-Axial Lower
    Bones BQØ
Bursotomy
  see Division, Bursae and Ligaments ØM8
  see Drainage, Bursae and Ligaments ØM9
➡ **BVS 5000 Ventricular Assist Device** *use*
    Short-term External Heart Assist System
    in Heart and Great Vessels
Bypass
  Anterior Chamber
    Left Ø8133
    Right Ø8123
  Aorta
    Abdominal Ø41Ø
    Thoracic
      Ascending/Arch Ø21X
      Descending Ø21W

▶ New   ➡ Revised   ~~deleted~~ Deleted

Bypass (*Continued*)
  Artery
    Axillary
      Left 0316Ø
      Right 0315Ø
    Brachial
      Left 0318Ø
      Right 0317Ø
    Common Carotid
      Left 031JØ
      Right 031HØ
    Common Iliac
      Left 041D
      Right 041C
    Coronary
      Four or More Arteries 0213
      One Artery 0210
      Three Arteries 0212
      Two Arteries 0211
    External Carotid
      Left 031NØ
      Right 031MØ
    External Iliac
      Left 041J
      Right 041H
    Femoral
      Left 041L
      Right 041K
    ▶Foot
      ▶Left 041W
      ▶Right 041V
    ▶Hepatic 0413
    Innominate 0312Ø
    Internal Carotid
      Left 031LØ
      Right 031KØ
    Internal Iliac
      Left 041F
      Right 041E
    Intracranial 031GØ
    ▶Peroneal
      ▶Left 041U
      ▶Right 041T
    Popliteal
      Left 041N
      Right 041M
    Pulmonary
      Left 021R
      Right 021Q
    Pulmonary Trunk 021P
    Radial
      Left 031CØ
      Right 031BØ
    Splenic 0414
    Subclavian
      Left 0314Ø
      Right 0313Ø
    Temporal
      Left 031TØ
      Right 031SØ
    Ulnar
      Left 031AØ
      Right 0319Ø
  Atrium
    Left 0217
    Right 0216
  Bladder 0T1B
  Cavity, Cranial 0W110J

Bypass (*Continued*)
  Cecum 0D1H
  Cerebral Ventricle 0016
  Colon
    Ascending 0D1K
    Descending 0D1M
    Sigmoid 0D1N
    Transverse 0D1L
  Duct
    Common Bile 0F19
    Cystic 0F18
    Hepatic
      ▶Common 0F17
      Left 0F16
      Right 0F15
    Lacrimal
      Left 081Y
      Right 081X
    Pancreatic 0F1D
      Accessory 0F1F
  Duodenum 0D19
  Ear
    Left 091EØ
    Right 091DØ
  Esophagus 0D15
    Lower 0D13
    Middle 0D12
    Upper 0D11
  Fallopian Tube
    Left 0U16
    Right 0U15
  Gallbladder 0F14
  Ileum 0D1B
  Jejunum 0D1A
  Kidney Pelvis
    Left 0T14
    Right 0T13
  Pancreas 0F1G
  Pelvic Cavity 0W1J
  Peritoneal Cavity 0W1G
  Pleural Cavity
    Left 0W1B
    Right 0W19
  Spinal Canal 001U
  Stomach 0D16
  Trachea 0B11
  Ureter
    Left 0T17
    Right 0T16
  Ureters, Bilateral 0T18
  Vas Deferens
    Bilateral 0V1Q
    Left 0V1P
    Right 0V1N
  Vein
    Axillary
      Left 0518
      Right 0517
    Azygos 0510
    Basilic
      Left 051C
      Right 051B
    Brachial
      Left 051A
      Right 0519
    Cephalic
      Left 051F
      Right 051D

Bypass (*Continued*)
  Vein (*Continued*)
    Colic 0617
    Common Iliac
      Left 061D
      Right 061C
    Esophageal 0613
    External Iliac
      Left 061G
      Right 061F
    External Jugular
      Left 051Q
      Right 051P
    Face
      Left 051V
      Right 051T
    Femoral
      Left 061N
      Right 061M
    Foot
      Left 061V
      Right 061T
    Gastric 0612
    ~~Greater Saphenous~~
      ~~Left 061Q~~
      ~~Right 061P~~
    Hand
      Left 051H
      Right 051G
    Hemiazygos 0511
    Hepatic 0614
    Hypogastric
      Left 061J
      Right 061H
    Inferior Mesenteric 0616
    Innominate
      Left 0514
      Right 0513
    Internal Jugular
      Left 051N
      Right 051M
    Intracranial 051L
    ~~Lesser Saphenous~~
      ~~Left 061S~~
      ~~Right 061R~~
    Portal 0618
    Renal
      Left 061B
      Right 0619
    ▶Saphenous
      ▶Left 061Q
      ▶Right 061P
    Splenic 0611
    Subclavian
      Left 0516
      Right 0515
    Superior Mesenteric 0615
    Vertebral
      Left 051S
      Right 051R
  Vena Cava
    Inferior 0610
    Superior 021V
  Ventricle
    Left 021L
    Right 021K
Bypass, cardiopulmonary 5A1221Z

▶ New   ⇒ Revised   ~~deleted~~ Deleted

C

Caesarean section *see* Extraction, Products of Conception 10D0
Calcaneocuboid joint
  use Tarsal Joint, Right
  use Tarsal Joint, Left
Calcaneocuboid ligament
  use Foot Bursa and Ligament, Right
  use Foot Bursa and Ligament, Left
Calcaneofibular ligament
  use Ankle Bursa and Ligament, Right
  use Ankle Bursa and Ligament, Left
Calcaneus
  use Tarsal, Right
  use Tarsal, Left
Cannulation
  see Bypass
  see Dilation
  see Drainage
  see Irrigation
Canthorrhaphy *see* Repair, Eye 08Q
Canthotomy *see* Release, Eye 08N
Capitate bone
  use Carpal, Right
  use Carpal, Left
Capsulectomy, lens *see* Excision, Eye 08B
Capsulorrhaphy, joint
  see Repair, Upper Joints 0RQ
  see Repair, Lower Joints 0SQ
Cardia *use* Esophagogastric Junction
Cardiac contractility modulation lead *use* Cardiac Lead in Heart and Great Vessels
Cardiac event recorder *use* Monitoring Device
Cardiac Lead
  Defibrillator
    Atrium
      Left 02H7
      Right 02H6
    Pericardium 02HN
    Vein, Coronary 02H4
    Ventricle
      Left 02HL
      Right 02HK
  Insertion of device in
    Atrium
      Left 02H7
      Right 02H6
    Pericardium 02HN
    Vein, Coronary 02H4
    Ventricle
      Left 02HL
      Right 02HK
  Pacemaker
    Atrium
      Left 02H7
      Right 02H6
    Pericardium 02HN
    Vein, Coronary 02H4
    Ventricle
      Left 02HL
      Right 02HK
  Removal of device from, Heart 02PA
  Revision of device in, Heart 02WA
Cardiac plexus *use* Nerve, Thoracic Sympathetic
Cardiac Resynchronization Defibrillator Pulse Generator
  Abdomen 0JH8
  Chest 0JH6
Cardiac Resynchronization Pacemaker Pulse Generator
  Abdomen 0JH8
  Chest 0JH6
Cardiac resynchronization therapy (CRT) lead
  use Cardiac Lead, Pacemaker in 02H
  use Cardiac Lead, Defibrillator in 02H
Cardiac Rhythm Related Device
  Insertion of device in
    Abdomen 0JH8
    Chest 0JH6

Cardiac Rhythm Related Device *(Continued)*
  Removal of device from, Subcutaneous Tissue and Fascia, Trunk 0JPT
  Revision of device in, Subcutaneous Tissue and Fascia, Trunk 0JWT
Cardiocentesis *see* Drainage, Pericardial Cavity 0W9D
Cardioesophageal junction *use* Esophagogastric Junction
Cardiolysis *see* Release, Heart and Great Vessels 02N
CardioMEMS® pressure sensor *use* Monitoring Device, Pressure Sensor in 02H
Cardiomyotomy *see* Division, Esophagogastric Junction 0D84
Cardioplegia *see* Introduction of substance in or on, Heart 3E08
Cardiorrhaphy *see* Repair, Heart and Great Vessels 02Q
Cardioversion 5A2204Z
Caregiver Training F0FZ
Caroticotympanic artery
  use Internal Carotid Artery, Right
  use Internal Carotid Artery, Left
Carotid (artery) sinus (baroreceptor) lead *use* Stimulator Lead in Upper Arteries
Carotid glomus
  use Carotid Body, Left
  use Carotid Body, Right
  use Carotid Bodies, Bilateral
Carotid sinus
  use Internal Carotid Artery, Right
  use Internal Carotid Artery, Left
Carotid sinus nerve *use* Glossopharyngeal Nerve
Carotid WALLSTENT® Monorail® Endoprosthesis *use* Intraluminal Device
Carpectomy
  see Excision, Upper Bones 0PB
  see Resection, Upper Bones 0PT
~~Carpometacarpal (CMC) joint~~
  ~~use Metacarpocarpal Joint, Right~~
  ~~use Metacarpocarpal Joint, Left~~
Carpometacarpal ligament
  use Hand Bursa and Ligament, Right
  use Hand Bursa and Ligament, Left
Casting *see* Immobilization
CAT scan *see* Computerized Tomography (CT Scan)
Catheterization
  see Dilation
  see Drainage
  see Insertion of device in
  see Irrigation
  Heart *see* Measurement, Cardiac 4A02
  Umbilical vein, for infusion 06H033T
Cauda equina *use* Lumbar Spinal Cord
Cauterization
  see Destruction
  see Repair
Cavernous plexus *use* Head and Neck Sympathetic Nerve
▶**CBMA (Concentrated Bone Marrow Aspirate)**
  use Concentrated Bone Marrow Aspirate
▶**CBMA (Concentrated Bone Marrow Aspirate) injection, intramuscular** XK02303
Cecectomy
  see Excision, Cecum 0DBH
  see Resection, Cecum 0DTH
Cecocolostomy
  see Bypass, Gastrointestinal System 0D1
  see Drainage, Gastrointestinal System 0D9
Cecopexy
  see Repair, Cecum 0DQH
  see Reposition, Cecum 0DSH
Cecoplication *see* Restriction, Cecum 0DVH
Cecorrhaphy *see* Repair, Cecum 0DQH
Cecostomy
  see Bypass, Cecum 0D1H
  see Drainage, Cecum 0D9H
Cecotomy *see* Drainage, Cecum 0D9H
Ceftazidime-Avibactam Anti-infective XW0
Celiac (solar) plexus *use* Abdominal Sympathetic Nerve

Celiac ganglion *use* Abdominal Sympathetic Nerve
Celiac lymph node *use* Lymphatic, Aortic
Celiac trunk *use* Celiac Artery
Central axillary lymph node
  use Lymphatic, Right Axillary
  use Lymphatic, Left Axillary
Central venous pressure *see* Measurement, Venous 4A04
▶**Centrimag® Blood Pump** *use* Short-term External Heart Assist System in Heart and Great Vessels
Cephalogram BN00ZZZ
Ceramic on ceramic bearing surface *use* Synthetic Substitute, Ceramic in 0SR
Cerclage *see* Restriction
Cerebral aqueduct (Sylvius) *use* Cerebral Ventricle
Cerebral Embolic Filtration, Dual Filter X2A5312
Cerebrum *use* Brain
Cervical esophagus *use* Esophagus, Upper
Cervical facet joint
  use Cervical Vertebral Joint
  use Cervical Vertebral Joint, 2 or more
Cervical ganglion *use* Head and Neck Sympathetic Nerve
Cervical interspinous ligament *use* Head and Neck Bursa and Ligament
Cervical intertransverse ligament *use* Head and Neck Bursa and Ligament
Cervical ligamentum flavum *use* Head and Neck Bursa and Ligament
Cervical lymph node
  use Lymphatic, Right Neck
  use Lymphatic, Left Neck
Cervicectomy
  see Excision, Cervix 0UBC
  see Resection, Cervix 0UTC
Cervicothoracic facet joint *use* Cervicothoracic Vertebral Joint
Cesarean section *see* Extraction, Products of Conception 10D0
▶**Cesium-131 Collagen Implant** *use* Radioactive Element, Cesium-131 Collagen Implant in 00H
Change device in
  Abdominal Wall 0W2FX
  Back
    Lower 0W2LX
    Upper 0W2KX
  Bladder 0T2BX
  Bone
    Facial 0N2WX
    Lower 0Q2YX
    Nasal 0N2BX
    Upper 0P2YX
  Bone Marrow 072TX
  Brain 0020X
  Breast
    Left 0H2UX
    Right 0H2TX
  Bursa and Ligament
    Lower 0M2YX
    Upper 0M2XX
  Cavity, Cranial 0W21X
  Chest Wall 0W28X
  Cisterna Chyli 072LX
  Diaphragm 0B2TX
  Duct
    Hepatobiliary 0F2BX
    Pancreatic 0F2DX
  Ear
    Left 092JX
    Right 092HX
  Epididymis and Spermatic Cord 0V2MX
  Extremity
    Lower
      Left 0Y2BX
      Right 0Y29X
    Upper
      Left 0X27X
      Right 0X26X

▶ New   ⇒ Revised   ~~deleted~~ Deleted

Change device in (Continued)
Eye
Left 0821X
Right 0820X
Face 0W22X
Fallopian Tube 0U28X
Gallbladder 0F24X
Gland
Adrenal 0G25X
Endocrine 0G2SX
Pituitary 0G20X
Salivary 0C2AX
Head 0W20X
Intestinal Tract
Lower 0D2DXUZ
Upper 0D20XUZ
Jaw
Lower 0W25X
Upper 0W24X
Joint
Lower 0S2YX
Upper 0R2YX
Kidney 0T25X
Larynx 0C2SX
Liver 0F20X
Lung
Left 0B2LX
Right 0B2KX
Lymphatic 072NX
Thoracic Duct 072KX
Mediastinum 0W2CX
Mesentery 0D2VX
Mouth and Throat 0C2YX
Muscle
Lower 0K2YX
Upper 0K2XX
▶ Nasal Mucosa and Soft Tissue 092KX
Neck 0W26X
Nerve
Cranial 002EX
Peripheral 012YX
~~Nose 092KX~~
Omentum 0D2UX
Ovary 0U23X
Pancreas 0F2GX
Parathyroid Gland 0G2RX
Pelvic Cavity 0W2JX
Penis 0V2SX
Pericardial Cavity 0W2DX
Perineum
Female 0W2NX
Male 0W2MX
Peritoneal Cavity 0W2GX
Peritoneum 0D2WX
Pineal Body 0G21X
Pleura 0B2QX
Pleural Cavity
Left 0W2BX
Right 0W29X
Products of Conception 10207
Prostate and Seminal Vesicles 0V24X
Retroperitoneum 0W2HX
Scrotum and Tunica Vaginalis 0V28X
Sinus 092YX
Skin 0H2PX
Skull 0N20X
Spinal Canal 002UX
Spleen 072PX
Subcutaneous Tissue and Fascia
Head and Neck 0J2SX
Lower Extremity 0J2WX
Trunk 0J2TX
Upper Extremity 0J2VX
Tendon
Lower 0L2YX
Upper 0L2XX
Testis 0V2DX
Thymus 072MX
Thyroid Gland 0G2KX
Trachea 0B21
Tracheobronchial Tree 0B20X

Change device in (Continued)
Ureter 0T29X
Urethra 0T2DX
Uterus and Cervix 0U2DXHZ
Vagina and Cul-de-sac 0U2HXGZ
Vas Deferens 0V2RX
Vulva 0U2MX
Change device in or on
Abdominal Wall 2W03X
Anorectal 2Y03X5Z
Arm
Lower
Left 2W0DX
Right 2W0CX
Upper
Left 2W0BX
Right 2W0AX
Back 2W05X
Chest Wall 2W04X
Ear 2Y02X5Z
Extremity
Lower
Left 2W0MX
Right 2W0LX
Upper
Left 2W09X
Right 2W08X
Face 2W01X
Finger
Left 2W0KX
Right 2W0JX
Foot
Left 2W0TX
Right 2W0SX
Genital Tract, Female 2Y04X5Z
Hand
Left 2W0FX
Right 2W0EX
Head 2W00X
Inguinal Region
Left 2W07X
Right 2W06X
Leg
Lower
Left 2W0RX
Right 2W0QX
Upper
Left 2W0PX
Right 2W0NX
Mouth and Pharynx 2Y00X5Z
Nasal 2Y01X5Z
Neck 2W02X
Thumb
Left 2W0HX
Right 2W0GX
Toe
Left 2W0VX
Right 2W0UX
Urethra 2Y05X5Z
Chemoembolization see Introduction of substance in or on
Chemosurgery, Skin 3E00XTZ
Chemothalamectomy see Destruction, Thalamus 0059
Chemotherapy, Infusion for cancer see Introduction of substance in or on
Chest x-ray see Plain Radiography, Chest BW03
Chiropractic Manipulation
Abdomen 9WB9X
Cervical 9WB1X
Extremities
Lower 9WB6X
Upper 9WB7X
Head 9WB0X
Lumbar 9WB3X
Pelvis 9WB5X
Rib Cage 9WB8X
Sacrum 9WB4X
Thoracic 9WB2X
Choana use Nasopharynx

Cholangiogram
see Plain Radiography, Hepatobiliary System and Pancreas BF0
see Fluoroscopy, Hepatobiliary System and Pancreas BF1
Cholecystectomy
see Excision, Gallbladder 0FB4
see Resection, Gallbladder 0FT4
Cholecystojejunostomy
see Bypass, Hepatobiliary System and Pancreas 0F1
see Drainage, Hepatobiliary System and Pancreas 0F9
Cholecystopexy
see Repair, Gallbladder 0FQ4
see Reposition, Gallbladder 0FS4
Cholecystoscopy 0FJ44ZZ
Cholecystostomy
see Bypass, Gallbladder 0F14
see Drainage, Gallbladder 0F94
Cholecystotomy see Drainage, Gallbladder 0F94
Choledochectomy
see Excision, Hepatobiliary System and Pancreas 0FB
see Resection, Hepatobiliary System and Pancreas 0FT
Choledocholithotomy see Extirpation, Duct, Common Bile 0FC9
Choledochoplasty
see Repair, Hepatobiliary System and Pancreas 0FQ
see Replacement, Hepatobiliary System and Pancreas 0FR
see Supplement, Hepatobiliary System and Pancreas 0FU
Choledochoscopy 0FJB8ZZ
Choledochotomy see Drainage, Hepatobiliary System and Pancreas 0F9
Cholelithotomy see Extirpation, Hepatobiliary System and Pancreas 0FC
Chondrectomy
see Excision, Upper Joints 0RB
see Excision, Lower Joints 0SB
Knee see Excision, Lower Joints 0SB
Semilunar cartilage see Excision, Lower Joints 0SB
Chondroglossus muscle use Tongue, Palate, Pharynx Muscle
Chorda tympani use Facial Nerve
▶ **Chordotomy** see Division, Central Nervous System and Cranial Nerves 008
Choroid plexus use Cerebral Ventricle
Choroidectomy
see Excision, Eye 08B
see Resection, Eye 08T
Ciliary body
use Eye, Right
use Eye, Left
Ciliary ganglion use Head and Neck Sympathetic Nerve
Circle of Willis use Intracranial Artery
Circumcision 0VTTXZZ
Circumflex iliac artery
use Femoral Artery, Right
use Femoral Artery, Left
Clamp and rod internal fixation system (CRIF)
use Internal Fixation Device in Upper Bones
use Internal Fixation Device in Lower Bones
Clamping see Occlusion
Claustrum use Basal Ganglia
Claviculectomy
see Excision, Upper Bones 0PB
see Resection, Upper Bones 0PT
Claviculotomy
see Division, Upper Bones 0P8
see Drainage, Upper Bones 0P9
▶ **Clipping, aneurysm**
▶ see Occlusion using Extraluminal Device
▶ see Restriction using Extraluminal Device
Clitorectomy, clitoridectomy
see Excision, Clitoris 0UBJ
see Resection, Clitoris 0UTJ

Clolar *use* Clofarabine
Closure
  see Occlusion
  see Repair
Clysis *see* Introduction of substance in or on
Coagulation *see* Destruction
▶**COALESCE® radiolucent interbody fusion device** *use* Interbody Fusion Device, Radiolucent Porous in New Technology
CoAxia NeuroFlo catheter *use* Intraluminal Device
Cobalt/chromium head and polyethylene socket *use* Synthetic Substitute, Metal on Polyethylene in ØSR
Cobalt/chromium head and socket *use* Synthetic Substitute, Metal in ØSR
Coccygeal body *use* Coccygeal Glomus
Coccygeus muscle
  use Trunk Muscle, Right
  use Trunk Muscle, Left
Cochlea
  use Inner Ear, Right
  use Inner Ear, Left
Cochlear implant (CI), multiple channel (electrode) *use* Hearing Device, Multiple Channel Cochlear Prosthesis in 09H
Cochlear implant (CI), single channel (electrode) *use* Hearing Device, Single Channel Cochlear Prosthesis in 09H
Cochlear Implant Treatment FØBZØ
Cochlear nerve *use* Acoustic Nerve
COGNIS® CRT-D *use* Cardiac Resynchronization Defibrillator Pulse Generator in ØJH
▶**COHERE® radiolucent interbody fusion device** *use* Interbody Fusion Device, Radiolucent Porous in New Technology
Colectomy
  see Excision, Gastrointestinal System ØDB
  see Resection, Gastrointestinal System ØDT
Collapse *see* Occlusion
Collection from
  Breast, Breast Milk 8EØHX62
  Indwelling Device
    Circulatory System
      Blood 8CØ2X6K
      Other Fluid 8CØ2X6L
    Nervous System
      Cerebrospinal Fluid 8CØ1X6J
      Other Fluid 8CØ1X6L
  Integumentary System, Breast Milk 8EØHX62
  Reproductive System, Male, Sperm 8EØVX63
Colocentesis *see* Drainage, Gastrointestinal System ØD9
Colofixation
  see Repair, Gastrointestinal System ØDQ
  see Reposition, Gastrointestinal System ØDS
Cololysis *see* Release, Gastrointestinal System ØDN
Colonic Z-Stent® *use* Intraluminal Device
Colonoscopy ØDJD8ZZ
Colopexy
  see Repair, Gastrointestinal System ØDQ
  see Reposition, Gastrointestinal System ØDS
Coloplication *see* Restriction, Gastrointestinal System ØDV
Coloproctectomy
  see Excision, Gastrointestinal System ØDB
  see Resection, Gastrointestinal System ØDT
Coloproctostomy
  see Bypass, Gastrointestinal System ØD1
  see Drainage, Gastrointestinal System ØD9
Colopuncture *see* Drainage, Gastrointestinal System ØD9
Colorrhaphy *see* Repair, Gastrointestinal System ØDQ
Colostomy
  see Bypass, Gastrointestinal System ØD1
  see Drainage, Gastrointestinal System ØD9
Colpectomy
  see Excision, Vagina ØUBG
  see Resection, Vagina ØUTG

Colpocentesis *see* Drainage, Vagina ØU9G
Colpopexy
  see Repair, Vagina ØUQG
  see Reposition, Vagina ØUSG
Colpoplasty
  see Repair, Vagina ØUQG
  see Supplement, Vagina ØUUG
Colporrhaphy *see* Repair, Vagina ØUQG
Colposcopy ØUJH8ZZ
➡**Columella** *use* Nasal Mucosa and Soft Tissue
Common digital vein
  use Foot Vein, Right
  use Foot Vein, Left
Common facial vein
  use Face Vein, Right
  use Face Vein, Left
Common fibular nerve *use* Peroneal Nerve
Common hepatic artery *use* Hepatic Artery
Common iliac (subaortic) lymph node *use* Lymphatic, Pelvis
Common interosseous artery
  use Ulnar Artery, Right
  use Ulnar Artery, Left
Common peroneal nerve *use* Peroneal Nerve
Complete (SE) stent *use* Intraluminal Device
Compression *see* Restriction
  Abdominal Wall 2W13X
  Arm
    Lower
      Left 2W1DX
      Right 2W1CX
    Upper
      Left 2W1BX
      Right 2W1AX
  Back 2W15X
  Chest Wall 2W14X
  Extremity
    Lower
      Left 2W1MX
      Right 2W1LX
    Upper
      Left 2W19X
      Right 2W18X
  Face 2W11X
  Finger
    Left 2W1KX
    Right 2W1JX
  Foot
    Left 2W1TX
    Right 2W1SX
  Hand
    Left 2W1FX
    Right 2W1EX
  Head 2W10X
  Inguinal Region
    Left 2W17X
    Right 2W16X
  Leg
    Lower
      Left 2W1RX
      Right 2W1QX
    Upper
      Left 2W1PX
      Right 2W1NX
  Neck 2W12X
  Thumb
    Left 2W1HX
    Right 2W1GX
  Toe
    Left 2W1VX
    Right 2W1UX
Computer Assisted Procedure
  Extremity
    Lower
      No Qualifier 8EØYXBZ
      With Computerized Tomography 8EØYXBG
      With Fluoroscopy 8EØYXBF
      With Magnetic Resonance Imaging 8EØYXBH

Computer Assisted Procedure *(Continued)*
  Extremity *(Continued)*
    Upper
      No Qualifier 8EØXXBZ
      With Computerized Tomography 8EØXXBG
      With Fluoroscopy 8EØXXBF
      With Magnetic Resonance Imaging 8EØXXBH
  Head and Neck Region
    No Qualifier 8EØ9XBZ
    With Computerized Tomography 8EØ9XBG
    With Fluoroscopy 8EØ9XBF
    With Magnetic Resonance Imaging 8EØ9XBH
  Trunk Region
    No Qualifier 8EØWXBZ
    With Computerized Tomography 8EØWXBG
    With Fluoroscopy 8EØWXBF
    With Magnetic Resonance Imaging 8EØWXBH
Computerized Tomography (CT Scan)
  Abdomen BW20
    Chest and Pelvis BW25
  Abdomen and Chest BW24
  Abdomen and Pelvis BW21
  Airway, Trachea BB2F
  Ankle
    Left BQ2H
    Right BQ2G
  Aorta
    Abdominal B420
      Intravascular Optical Coherence B420Z2Z
    Thoracic B320
      Intravascular Optical Coherence B320Z2Z
  Arm
    Left BP2F
    Right BP2E
  Artery
    Celiac B421
      Intravascular Optical Coherence B421Z2Z
    Common Carotid
      Bilateral B325
      Intravascular Optical Coherence B325Z2Z
    Coronary
      Bypass Graft
        Multiple B223
          Intravascular Optical Coherence B223Z2Z
      Multiple B221
        Intravascular Optical Coherence B221Z2Z
    Internal Carotid
      Bilateral B328
      Intravascular Optical Coherence B328Z2Z
    Intracranial B32R
      Intravascular Optical Coherence B32RZ2Z
    Lower Extremity
      Bilateral B42H
        Intravascular Optical Coherence B42HZ2Z
      Left B42G
        Intravascular Optical Coherence B42GZ2Z
      Right B42F
        Intravascular Optical Coherence B42FZ2Z
    Pelvic B42C
      Intravascular Optical Coherence B42CZ2Z
    Pulmonary
      Left B32T
        Intravascular Optical Coherence B32TZ2Z
      Right B32S
        Intravascular Optical Coherence B32SZ2Z

Computerized Tomography *(Continued)*
  Artery *(Continued)*
    Renal
      Bilateral B428
        Intravascular Optical Coherence
          B428Z2Z
      Transplant B42M
        Intravascular Optical Coherence
          B42MZ2Z
      Superior Mesenteric B424
        Intravascular Optical Coherence
          B424Z2Z
      Vertebral
        Bilateral B32G
        Intravascular Optical Coherence
          B32GZ2Z
  Bladder BT2Ø
  Bone
    Facial BN25
    Temporal BN2F
  Brain BØ2Ø
  Calcaneus
    Left BQ2K
    Right BQ2J
  Cerebral Ventricle BØ28
  Chest, Abdomen and Pelvis BW25
  Chest and Abdomen BW24
  Cisterna BØ27
  Clavicle
    Left BP25
    Right BP24
  Coccyx BR2F
  Colon BD24
  Ear B92Ø
  Elbow
    Left BP2H
    Right BP2G
  Extremity
    Lower
      Left BQ2S
      Right BQ2R
    Upper
      Bilateral BP2V
      Left BP2U
      Right BP2T
  Eye
    Bilateral B827
    Left B826
    Right B825
  Femur
    Left BQ24
    Right BQ23
  Fibula
    Left BQ2C
    Right BQ2B
  Finger
    Left BP2S
    Right BP2R
  Foot
    Left BQ2M
    Right BQ2L
  Forearm
    Left BP2K
    Right BP2J
  Gland
    Adrenal, Bilateral BG22
    Parathyroid BG23
    Parotid, Bilateral B926
    Salivary, Bilateral B92D
    Submandibular, Bilateral B929
    Thyroid BG24
  Hand
    Left BP2P
    Right BP2N
  Hands and Wrists, Bilateral BP2Q
  Head BW28
  Head and Neck BW29
  Heart
    Right and Left B226
    Intravascular Optical Coherence B226Z2Z
  Hepatobiliary System, All BF2C

Computerized Tomography *(Continued)*
  Hip
    Left BQ21
    Right BQ2Ø
  Humerus
    Left BP2B
    Right BP2A
  Intracranial Sinus B522
    Intravascular Optical Coherence B522Z2Z
  Joint
    Acromioclavicular, Bilateral BP23
    Finger
      Left BP2DZZZ
      Right BP2CZZZ
    Foot
      Left BQ2Y
      Right BQ2X
    Hand
      Left BP2DZZZ
      Right BP2CZZZ
    Sacroiliac BR2D
    Sternoclavicular
      Bilateral BP22
      Left BP21
      Right BP2Ø
    Temporomandibular, Bilateral BN29
    Toe
      Left BQ2Y
      Right BQ2X
  Kidney
    Bilateral BT23
    Left BT22
    Right BT21
    Transplant BT29
  Knee
    Left BQ28
    Right BQ27
  Larynx B92J
  Leg
    Left BQ2F
    Right BQ2D
  Liver BF25
  Liver and Spleen BF26
  Lung, Bilateral BB24
  Mandible BN26
  Nasopharynx B92F
  Neck BW2F
  Neck and Head BW29
  Orbit, Bilateral BN23
  Oropharynx B92F
  Pancreas BF27
  Patella
    Left BQ2W
    Right BQ2V
  Pelvic Region BW2G
  Pelvis BR2C
    Chest and Abdomen BW25
  Pelvis and Abdomen BW21
  Pituitary Gland BØ29
  Prostate BV23
  Ribs
    Left BP2Y
    Right BP2X
  Sacrum BR2F
  Scapula
    Left BP27
    Right BP26
  Sella Turcica BØ29
  Shoulder
    Left BP29
    Right BP28
  Sinus
    Intracranial B522
      Intravascular Optical Coherence B522Z2Z
    Paranasal B922
  Skull BN2Ø
  Spinal Cord BØ2B
  Spine
    Cervical BR2Ø
    Lumbar BR29
    Thoracic BR27

Computerized Tomography *(Continued)*
  Spleen and Liver BF26
  Thorax BP2W
  Tibia
    Left BQ2C
    Right BQ2B
  Toe
    Left BQ2Q
    Right BQ2P
  Trachea BB2F
  Tracheobronchial Tree
    Bilateral BB29
    Left BB28
    Right BB27
  Vein
    Pelvic (Iliac)
      Left B52G
        Intravascular Optical Coherence
          B52GZ2Z
      Right B52F
        Intravascular Optical Coherence
          B52FZ2Z
    Pelvic (Iliac) Bilateral B52H
      Intravascular Optical Coherence
        B52HZ2Z
    Portal B52T
      Intravascular Optical Coherence
        B52TZ2Z
    Pulmonary
      Bilateral B52S
        Intravascular Optical Coherence
          B52SZ2Z
      Left B52R
        Intravascular Optical Coherence
          B52RZ2Z
      Right B52Q
        Intravascular Optical Coherence
          B52QZ2Z
    Renal
      Bilateral B52L
        Intravascular Optical Coherence
          B52LZ2Z
      Left B52K
        Intravascular Optical Coherence
          B52KZ2Z
      Right B52J
        Intravascular Optical Coherence
          B52JZ2Z
    Spanchnic B52T
      Intravascular Optical Coherence
        B52TZ2Z
    Vena Cava
      Inferior B529
        Intravascular Optical Coherence
          B529Z2Z
      Superior B528
        Intravascular Optical Coherence
          B528Z2Z
    Ventricle, Cerebral BØ28
    Wrist
      Left BP2M
      Right BP2L
▶**Concentrated Bone Marrow Aspirate (CBMA) injection, intramuscular XKØ23Ø3**
Concerto II CRT-D *use* Cardiac
    Resynchronization Defibrillator Pulse
    Generator in ØJH
Condylectomy
    see Excision, Head and Facial Bones ØNB
    see Excision, Upper Bones ØPB
    see Excision, Lower Bones ØQB
Condyloid process
    use Mandible, Left
    use Mandible, Right
Condylotomy
    see Division, Head and Facial Bones ØN8
    see Drainage, Head and Facial Bones ØN9
    see Division, Upper Bones ØP8
    see Drainage, Upper Bones ØP9
    see Division, Lower Bones ØQ8
    see Drainage, Lower Bones ØQ9

Condylysis
see Release, Head and Facial Bones ØNN
see Release, Upper Bones ØPN
see Release, Lower Bones ØQN
Conization, cervix see Excision, Cervix ØUBC
Conjunctivoplasty
see Repair, Eye Ø8Q
see Replacement, Eye Ø8R
CONSERVE® PLUS Total Resurfacing Hip
System use Resurfacing Device in Lower
Joints
Construction
Auricle, ear see Replacement, Ear, Nose, Sinus
Ø9R
Ileal conduit see Bypass, Urinary System ØT1
Consulta CRT-D use Cardiac Resynchronization
Defibrillator Pulse Generator in ØJH
Consulta CRT-P use Cardiac Resynchronization
Pacemaker Pulse Generator in ØJH
Contact Radiation
Abdomen DWY37ZZ
Adrenal Gland DGY27ZZ
Bile Ducts DFY27ZZ
Bladder DTY27ZZ
Bone, Other DPYC7ZZ
Brain DØY07ZZ
Brain Stem DØY17ZZ
Breast
Left DMY07ZZ
Right DMY17ZZ
Bronchus DBY17ZZ
Cervix DUY17ZZ
Chest DWY27ZZ
Chest Wall DBY77ZZ
Colon DDY57ZZ
Diaphragm DBY87ZZ
Duodenum DDY27ZZ
Ear D9Y07ZZ
Esophagus DDY07ZZ
Eye D8Y07ZZ
Femur DPY97ZZ
Fibula DPYB7ZZ
Gallbladder DFY17ZZ
Gland
Adrenal DGY27ZZ
Parathyroid DGY47ZZ
Pituitary DGY07ZZ
Thyroid DGY57ZZ
Glands, Salivary D9Y67ZZ
Head and Neck DWY17ZZ
Hemibody DWY47ZZ
Humerus DPY67ZZ
Hypopharynx D9Y37ZZ
Ileum DDY47ZZ
Jejunum DDY37ZZ
Kidney DTY07ZZ
Larynx D9YB7ZZ
Liver DFY07ZZ
Lung DBY27ZZ
Mandible DPY37ZZ
Maxilla DPY27ZZ
Mediastinum DBY67ZZ
Mouth D9Y47ZZ
Nasopharynx D9YD7ZZ
Neck and Head DWY17ZZ
Nerve, Peripheral DØY77ZZ
Nose D9Y17ZZ
Oropharynx D9YF7ZZ
Ovary DUY07ZZ
Palate
Hard D9Y87ZZ
Soft D9Y97ZZ
Pancreas DFY37ZZ
Parathyroid Gland DGY47ZZ
Pelvic Bones DPY87ZZ
Pelvic Region DWY67ZZ
Pineal Body DGY17ZZ
Pituitary Gland DGY07ZZ
Pleura DBY57ZZ
Prostate DVY07ZZ
Radius DPY77ZZ
Rectum DDY77ZZ

Contact Radiation (Continued)
Rib DPY57ZZ
Sinuses D9Y77ZZ
Skin
Abdomen DHY87ZZ
Arm DHY47ZZ
Back DHY77ZZ
Buttock DHY97ZZ
Chest DHY67ZZ
Face DHY27ZZ
Leg DHYB7ZZ
Neck DHY37ZZ
Skull DPY07ZZ
Spinal Cord DØY67ZZ
Sternum DPY47ZZ
Stomach DDY17ZZ
Testis DVY17ZZ
Thyroid Gland DGY57ZZ
Tibia DPYB7ZZ
Tongue D9Y57ZZ
Trachea DBY07ZZ
Ulna DPY77ZZ
Ureter DTY17ZZ
Urethra DTY37ZZ
Uterus DUY27ZZ
Whole Body DWY57ZZ
CONTAK RENEWAL® 3 RF (HE) CRT-D use
Cardiac Resynchronization Defibrillator
Pulse Generator in ØJH
Contegra Pulmonary Valved Conduit use
Zooplastic Tissue in Heart and Great Vessels
Continuous Glucose Monitoring (CGM)
device use Monitoring Device
Continuous Negative Airway Pressure
24-96 Consecutive Hours, Ventilation 5A09459
Greater than 96 Consecutive Hours,
Ventilation 5A09559
Less than 24 Consecutive Hours, Ventilation
5A09359
Continuous Positive Airway Pressure
24-96 Consecutive Hours, Ventilation 5A09457
Greater than 96 Consecutive Hours,
Ventilation 5A09557
Less than 24 Consecutive Hours, Ventilation
5A09357
▶**Continuous renal replacement therapy (CRRT)**
5A1D90Z
Contraceptive Device
Change device in, Uterus and Cervix
ØU2DXHZ
Insertion of device in
Cervix ØUHC
Subcutaneous Tissue and Fascia
Abdomen ØJH8
Chest ØJH6
Lower Arm
Left ØJHH
Right ØJHG
Lower Leg
Left ØJHP
Right ØJHN
Upper Arm
Left ØJHF
Right ØJHD
Upper Leg
Left ØJHM
Right ØJHL
Uterus ØUH9
Removal of device from
Subcutaneous Tissue and Fascia
Lower Extremity ØJPW
Trunk ØJPT
Upper Extremity ØJPV
Uterus and Cervix ØUPD
Revision of device in
Subcutaneous Tissue and Fascia
Lower Extremity ØJWW
Trunk ØJWT
Upper Extremity ØJWV
Uterus and Cervix ØUWD
Contractility Modulation Device
Abdomen ØJH8
Chest ØJH6

Control bleeding in
Abdominal Wall ØW3F
Ankle Region
Left ØY3L
Right ØY3K
Arm
Lower
Left ØX3F
Right ØX3D
Upper
Left ØX39
Right ØX38
Axilla
Left ØX35
Right ØX34
Back
Lower ØW3L
Upper ØW3K
Buttock
Left ØY31
Right ØY30
Cavity, Cranial ØW31
Chest Wall ØW38
Elbow Region
Left ØX3C
Right ØX3B
Extremity
Lower
Left ØY3B
Right ØY39
Upper
Left ØX37
Right ØX36
Face ØW32
Femoral Region
Left ØY38
Right ØY37
Foot
Left ØY3N
Right ØY3M
Gastrointestinal Tract ØW3P
Genitourinary Tract ØW3R
Hand
Left ØX3K
Right ØX3J
Head ØW30
Inguinal Region
Left ØY36
Right ØY35
Jaw
Lower ØW35
Upper ØW34
Knee Region
Left ØY3G
Right ØY3F
Leg
Lower
Left ØY3J
Right ØY3H
Upper
Left ØY3D
Right ØY3C
Mediastinum ØW3C
Neck ØW36
Oral Cavity and Throat ØW33
Pelvic Cavity ØW3J
Pericardial Cavity ØW3D
Perineum
Female ØW3N
Male ØW3M
Peritoneal Cavity ØW3G
Pleural Cavity
Left ØW3B
Right ØW39
Respiratory Tract ØW3Q
Retroperitoneum ØW3H
Shoulder Region
Left ØX33
Right ØX32
Wrist Region
Left ØX3H
Right ØX3G

▶ New   ➡ Revised   ~~deleted~~ Deleted

Conus arteriosus *use* Ventricle, Right

Conus medullaris *use* Spinal Cord, Lumbar

Conversion
Cardiac rhythm 5A2204Z
Gastrostomy to jejunostomy feeding device
see Insertion of device in, Jejunum 0DHA

Cook Biodesign® Fistula Plug(s) *use* Nonautologous Tissue Substitute

Cook Biodesign® Hernia Graft(s) *use* Nonautologous Tissue Substitute

Cook Biodesign® Layered Graft(s) *use* Nonautologous Tissue Substitute

Cook Zenapro™ Layered Graft(s) *use* Nonautologous Tissue Substitute

Cook Zenith AAA Endovascular Graft
use Intraluminal Device, Branched or Fenestrated, One or Two Arteries in 04V
use Intraluminal Device, Branched or Fenestrated, Three or More Arteries in 04V
use Intraluminal Device

Coracoacromial ligament
use Shoulder Bursa and Ligament, Right
use Shoulder Bursa and Ligament, Left

Coracobrachialis muscle
use Upper Arm Muscle, Right
use Upper Arm Muscle, Left

Coracoclavicular ligament
use Shoulder Bursa and Ligament, Right
use Shoulder Bursa and Ligament, Left

Coracohumeral ligament
use Shoulder Bursa and Ligament, Right
use Shoulder Bursa and Ligament, Left

Coracoid process
use Scapula, Right
use Scapula, Left

Cordotomy *see* Division, Central Nervous System and Cranial Nerves 008

Core needle biopsy *see* Excision with qualifier Diagnostic

CoreValve transcatheter aortic valve *use* Zooplastic Tissue in Heart and Great Vessels

Cormet Hip Resurfacing System *use* Resurfacing Device in Lower Joints

Corniculate cartilage *use* Larynx

CoRoent® XL *use* Interbody Fusion Device in Lower Joints

Coronary arteriography
see Plain Radiography, Heart B20
see Fluoroscopy, Heart B21

Corox (OTW) Bipolar Lead
use Cardiac Lead, Pacemaker in 02H
use Cardiac Lead, Defibrillator in 02H

Corpus callosum *use* Brain

Corpus cavernosum *use* Penis

Corpus spongiosum *use* Penis

Corpus striatum *use* Basal Ganglia

Corrugator supercilii muscle *use* Facial Muscle

Cortical strip neurostimulator lead *use* Neurostimulator Lead in Central Nervous System and Cranial Nerves

Costatectomy
see Excision, Upper Bones 0PB
see Resection, Upper Bones 0PT

Costectomy
see Excision, Upper Bones 0PB
see Resection, Upper Bones 0PT

Costocervical trunk
use Subclavian Artery, Right
use Subclavian Artery, Left

Costochondrectomy
see Excision, Upper Bones 0PB
see Resection, Upper Bones 0PT

Costoclavicular ligament
use Shoulder Bursa and Ligament, Right
use Shoulder Bursa and Ligament, Left

Costosternoplasty
see Repair, Upper Bones 0PQ
see Replacement, Upper Bones 0PR
see Supplement, Upper Bones 0PU

Costotomy
see Division, Upper Bones 0P8
see Drainage, Upper Bones 0P9

Costotransverse joint *use* Thoracic Vertebral Joint

Costotransverse ligament
use Thorax Bursa and Ligament, Right
use Thorax Bursa and Ligament, Left
▶*use* Sternum Bursa and Ligament
▶*use* Rib(s) Bursa and Ligament

Costovertebral joint *use* Thoracic Vertebral Joint

Costoxiphoid ligament
use Thorax Bursa and Ligament, Right
use Thorax Bursa and Ligament, Left
▶*use* Sternum Bursa and Ligament
▶*use* Rib(s) Bursa and Ligament

Counseling
Family, for substance abuse, Other Family Counseling HZ63ZZZ
Group
12-Step HZ43ZZZ
Behavioral HZ41ZZZ
Cognitive HZ40ZZZ
Cognitive-Behavioral HZ42ZZZ
Confrontational HZ48ZZZ
Continuing Care HZ49ZZZ
Infectious Disease
Post-Test HZ4CZZZ
Pre-Test HZ4CZZZ
Interpersonal HZ44ZZZ
Motivational Enhancement HZ47ZZZ
Psychoeducation HZ46ZZZ
Spiritual HZ4BZZZ
Vocational HZ45ZZZ
Individual
12-Step HZ33ZZZ
Behavioral HZ31ZZZ
Cognitive HZ30ZZZ
Cognitive-Behavioral HZ32ZZZ
Confrontational HZ38ZZZ
Continuing Care HZ39ZZZ
Infectious Disease
Post-Test HZ3CZZZ
Pre-Test HZ3CZZZ
Interpersonal HZ34ZZZ
Motivational Enhancement HZ37ZZZ
Psychoeducation HZ36ZZZ
Spiritual HZ3BZZZ
Vocational HZ35ZZZ
Mental Health Services
Educational GZ60ZZZ
Other Counseling GZ63ZZZ
Vocational GZ61ZZZ

Countershock, cardiac 5A2204Z

Cowper's (bulbourethral) gland *use* Urethra

CPAP (continuous positive airway pressure)
see Assistance, Respiratory 5A09

Craniectomy
see Excision, Head and Facial Bones 0NB
see Resection, Head and Facial Bones 0NT

Cranioplasty
see Repair, Head and Facial Bones 0NQ
see Replacement, Head and Facial Bones 0NR
see Supplement, Head and Facial Bones 0NU

Craniotomy
see Drainage, Central Nervous System 009
▶*see* Drainage, Central Nervous System and Cranial Nerves 009
see Division, Head and Facial Bones 0N8
see Drainage, Head and Facial Bones 0N9

Creation
Perineum
Female 0W4N0
Male 0W4M0

Creation *(Continued)*
Valve
Aortic 024F0
Mitral 024G0
Tricuspid 024J0

Cremaster muscle *use* Perineum Muscle

Cribriform plate
use Ethmoid Bone, Right
use Ethmoid Bone, Left

Cricoid cartilage *use* Trachea

Cricoidectomy *see* Excision, Larynx 0CBS

Cricothyroid artery
use Thyroid Artery, Right
use Thyroid Artery, Left

Cricothyroid muscle
use Neck Muscle, Right
use Neck Muscle, Left

Crisis Intervention GZ2ZZZZ

▶CRRT (Continuous renal replacement therapy) 5A1D90Z

Crural fascia
use Subcutaneous Tissue and Fascia, Right Upper Leg
use Subcutaneous Tissue and Fascia, Left Upper Leg

Crushing, nerve
▶Cranial *see* Destruction, Central Nervous System and Cranial Nerves 005
Peripheral *see* Destruction, Peripheral Nervous System 015

Cryoablation *see* Destruction

Cryotherapy *see* Destruction

Cryptorchidectomy
see Excision, Male Reproductive System 0VB
see Resection, Male Reproductive System 0VT

Cryptorchiectomy
see Excision, Male Reproductive System 0VB
see Resection, Male Reproductive System 0VT

Cryptotomy
see Division, Gastrointestinal System 0D8
see Drainage, Gastrointestinal System 0D9

CT scan *see* Computerized Tomography (CT Scan)

CT sialogram *see* Computerized Tomography (CT Scan), Ear, Nose, Mouth and Throat B92

Cubital lymph node
use Lymphatic, Right Upper Extremity
use Lymphatic, Left Upper Extremity

Cubital nerve *use* Ulnar Nerve

Cuboid bone
use Tarsal, Right
use Tarsal, Left

Cuboideonavicular joint
use Tarsal Joint, Right
use Tarsal Joint, Left

Culdocentesis *see* Drainage, Cul-de-sac 0U9F

Culdoplasty
see Repair, Cul-de-sac 0UQF
see Supplement, Cul-de-sac 0UUF

Culdoscopy 0UJH8ZZ

Culdotomy *see* Drainage, Cul-de-sac 0U9F

Culmen *use* Cerebellum

Cultured epidermal cell autograft *use* Autologous Tissue Substitute

Cuneiform cartilage *use* Larynx

Cuneonavicular joint
use Tarsal Joint, Right
use Tarsal Joint, Left

Cuneonavicular ligament
use Foot Bursa and Ligament, Right
use Foot Bursa and Ligament, Left

Curettage
see Excision
see Extraction

Cutaneous (transverse) cervical nerve *use* Nerve, Cervical Plexus

CVP (central venous pressure) *see* Measurement, Venous 4A04

Cyclodiathermy *see* Destruction, Eye 085

Cyclophotocoagulation *see* Destruction, Eye 085

CYPHER® Stent *use* Intraluminal Device, Drug-eluting in Heart and Great Vessels
Cystectomy
  see Excision, Bladder ØTBB
  see Resection, Bladder ØTTB
Cystocele repair *see* Repair, Subcutaneous Tissue and Fascia, Pelvic Region ØJQC
Cystography
  see Plain Radiography, Urinary System BTØ
  see Fluoroscopy, Urinary System BT1
Cystolithotomy *see* Extirpation, Bladder ØTCB

Cystopexy
  see Repair, Bladder ØTQB
  see Reposition, Bladder ØTSB
Cystoplasty
  see Repair, Bladder ØTQB
  see Replacement, Bladder ØTRB
  see Supplement, Bladder ØTUB
Cystorrhaphy *see* Repair, Bladder ØTQB
Cystoscopy ØTJB8ZZ
Cystostomy *see* Bypass, Bladder ØT1B
Cystostomy tube *use* Drainage Device

Cystotomy *see* Drainage, Bladder ØT9B
Cystourethrography
  see Plain Radiography, Urinary System BTØ
  see Fluoroscopy, Urinary System BT1
Cystourethroplasty
  see Repair, Urinary System ØTQ
  see Replacement, Urinary System ØTR
  see Supplement, Urinary System ØTU
▶**Cytarabine and Daunorubicin Liposome Antineoplastic** XWØ

▶ New   ⇒ Revised   ~~deleted~~ Deleted

D

⬛►DBS lead *use* Neurostimulator Lead in Central Nervous System and Cranial Nerves

DeBakey Left Ventricular Assist Device *use* Implantable Heart Assist System in Heart and Great Vessels

Debridement
Excisional *see* Excision
Non-excisional *see* Extraction

Decompression, Circulatory 6A15

⬛►**Decortication, lung**
►*see* Extirpation, Respiratory System ØBC
►*see* Release, Respiratory System ØBN

Deep brain neurostimulator lead *use*
⬛►Neurostimulator Lead in Central Nervous System and Cranial Nerves

⬛►**Deep cervical fascia**
►*use* Subcutaneous Tissue and Fascia, Right Neck
►*use* Subcutaneous Tissue and Fascia, Left Neck

Deep cervical vein
use Vertebral Vein, Right
use Vertebral Vein, Left

Deep circumflex iliac artery
use External Iliac Artery, Right
use External Iliac Artery, Left

Deep facial vein
use Face Vein, Right
use Face Vein, Left

Deep femoral (profunda femoris) vein
use Femoral Vein, Right
use Femoral Vein, Left

Deep femoral artery
use Femoral Artery, Right
use Femoral Artery, Left

Deep Inferior Epigastric Artery Perforator Flap
~~Bilateral ØHRVØ77~~
~~Left ØHRUØ77~~
~~Right ØHRTØ77~~
►Replacement
►Bilateral ØHRVØ77
►Left ØHRUØ77
►Right ØHRTØ77
►Transfer
►Left ØKXG
►Right ØKXF

Deep palmar arch
use Hand Artery, Right
use Hand Artery, Left

Deep transverse perineal muscle *use* Perineum Muscle

Deferential artery
use Internal Iliac Artery, Right
use Internal Iliac Artery, Left

Defibrillator Generator
Abdomen ØJH8
Chest ØJH6

Defibrotide Sodium Anticoagulant XWØ

Defitelio *use* Defibrotide Sodium Anticoagulant

Delivery
Cesarean *see* Extraction, Products of Conception 10DØ
Forceps *see* Extraction, Products of Conception 10DØ
Manually assisted 10EØXZZ
Products of Conception 10EØXZZ
Vacuum assisted *see* Extraction, Products of Conception 10DØ

Delta frame external fixator
use External Fixation Device, Hybrid in ØPH
use External Fixation Device, Hybrid in ØPS
use External Fixation Device, Hybrid in ØQH
use External Fixation Device, Hybrid in ØQS

Delta III Reverse shoulder prosthesis *use* Synthetic Substitute, Reverse Ball and Socket in ØRR

Deltoid fascia
use Subcutaneous Tissue and Fascia, Right Upper Arm
use Subcutaneous Tissue and Fascia, Left Upper Arm

Deltoid ligament
use Ankle Bursa and Ligament, Right
use Ankle Bursa and Ligament, Left

Deltoid muscle
use Shoulder Muscle, Right
use Shoulder Muscle, Left

Deltopectoral (infraclavicular) lymph node
use Lymphatic, Right Upper Extremity
use Lymphatic, Left Upper Extremity

Denervation
⬛►Cranial nerve *see* Destruction, Central Nervous System and Cranial Nerves 005
Peripheral nerve *see* Destruction, Peripheral Nervous System 015

►**Dens** *use* Cervical Vertebra

Densitometry
Plain Radiography
Femur
Left BQ04ZZ1
Right BQ03ZZ1
Hip
Left BQ01ZZ1
Right BQ00ZZ1
Spine
Cervical BR00ZZ1
Lumbar BR09ZZ1
Thoracic BR07ZZ1
Whole BR0GZZ1
Ultrasonography
Elbow
Left BP4HZZ1
Right BP4GZZ1
Hand
Left BP4PZZ1
Right BP4NZZ1
Shoulder
Left BP49ZZ1
Right BP48ZZ1
Wrist
Left BP4MZZ1
Right BP4LZZ1

Denticulate (dentate) ligament *use* Spinal Meninges

Depressor anguli oris muscle *use* Facial Muscle

Depressor labii inferioris muscle *use* Facial Muscle

Depressor septi nasi muscle *use* Facial Muscle

Depressor supercilii muscle *use* Facial Muscle

Dermabrasion *see* Extraction, Skin and Breast ØHD

Dermis *see* Skin

Descending genicular artery
use Femoral Artery, Right
use Femoral Artery, Left

Destruction
Acetabulum
Left ØQ55
Right ØQ54
Adenoids ØC5Q
Ampulla of Vater ØF5C
Anal Sphincter ØD5R
Anterior Chamber
Left 08533ZZ
Right 08523ZZ
Anus ØD5Q
Aorta
Abdominal 0450
Thoracic
Ascending/Arch 025X
Descending 025W
Aortic Body ØG5D
Appendix ØD5J
Artery
Anterior Tibial
Left 045Q
Right 045P

Destruction (Continued)
Artery (Continued)
Axillary
Left 0356
Right 0355
Brachial
Left 0358
Right 0357
Celiac 0451
Colic
Left 0457
Middle 0458
Right 0456
Common Carotid
Left 035J
Right 035H
Common Iliac
Left 045D
Right 045C
External Carotid
Left 035N
Right 035M
External Iliac
Left 045J
Right 045H
Face 035R
Femoral
Left 045L
Right 045K
Foot
Left 045W
Right 045V
Gastric 0452
Hand
Left 035F
Right 035D
Hepatic 0453
Inferior Mesenteric 045B
Innominate 0352
Internal Carotid
Left 035L
Right 035K
Internal Iliac
Left 045F
Right 045E
Internal Mammary
Left 0351
Right 0350
Intracranial 035G
Lower 045Y
Peroneal
Left 045U
Right 045T
Popliteal
Left 045N
Right 045M
Posterior Tibial
Left 045S
Right 045R
Pulmonary
Left 025R
Right 025Q
Pulmonary Trunk 025P
Radial
Left 035C
Right 035B
Renal
Left 045A
Right 0459
Splenic 0454
Subclavian
Left 0354
Right 0353
Superior Mesenteric 0455
Temporal
Left 035T
Right 035S
Thyroid
Left 035V
Right 035U

Destruction (Continued)

Artery (Continued)
Ulnar
Left 035A
Right 0359
Upper 035Y
Vertebral
Left 035Q
Right 035P
Atrium
Left 0257
Right 0256
Auditory Ossicle
➡ Left 095A
➡ Right 0959
Basal Ganglia 0058
Bladder 0T5B
Bladder Neck 0T5C
Bone
Ethmoid
Left 0N5G
Right 0N5F
➤ Frontal 0N51
~~Left 0N52~~
~~Right 0N51~~
Hyoid 0N5X
Lacrimal
Left 0N5J
Right 0N5H
Nasal 0N5B
➤ Occipital 0N57
~~Left 0N58~~
~~Right 0N57~~
Palatine
Left 0N5L
Right 0N5K
Parietal
Left 0N54
Right 0N53
Pelvic
Left 0Q53
Right 0Q52
➤ Sphenoid 0N5C
~~Left 0N5D~~
~~Right 0N5C~~
Temporal
Left 0N56
Right 0N55
Zygomatic
Left 0N5N
Right 0N5M
Brain 0050
Breast
Bilateral 0H5V
Left 0H5U
Right 0H5T
Bronchus
Lingula 0B59
Lower Lobe
Left 0B5B
Right 0B56
Main
Left 0B57
Right 0B53
Middle Lobe, Right 0B55
Upper Lobe
Left 0B58
Right 0B54
Buccal Mucosa 0C54
Bursa and Ligament
Abdomen
Left 0M5J
Right 0M5H
Ankle
Left 0M5R
Right 0M5Q
Elbow
Left 0M54
Right 0M53
Foot
Left 0M5T
Right 0M5S

Destruction (Continued)

Bursa and Ligament (Continued)
Hand
Left 0M58
Right 0M57
Head and Neck 0M50
Hip
Left 0M5M
Right 0M5L
Knee
Left 0M5P
Right 0M5N
Lower Extremity
Left 0M5W
Right 0M5V
Perineum 0M5K
➤ Rib(s) 0M5G
Shoulder
Left 0M52
Right 0M51
➤ Spine
➤ Lower 0M5D
➤ Upper 0M5C
➤ Sternum 0M5F
~~Thorax~~
~~Left 0M5G~~
~~Right 0M5F~~
~~Trunk~~
~~Left 0M5D~~
~~Right 0M5C~~
Upper Extremity
Left 0M5B
Right 0M59
Wrist
Left 0M56
Right 0M55
Carina 0B52
Carotid Bodies, Bilateral 0G58
Carotid Body
Left 0G56
Right 0G57
Carpal
Left 0P5N
Right 0P5M
Cecum 0D5H
Cerebellum 005C
Cerebral Hemisphere 0057
Cerebral Meninges 0051
Cerebral Ventricle 0056
Cervix 0U5C
Chordae Tendineae 0259
Choroid
Left 085B
Right 085A
Cisterna Chyli 075L
Clavicle
Left 0P5B
Right 0P59
Clitoris 0U5J
Coccygeal Glomus 0G5B
Coccyx 0Q5S
Colon
Ascending 0D5K
Descending 0D5M
Sigmoid 0D5N
Transverse 0D5L
Conduction Mechanism 0258
Conjunctiva
Left 085TXZZ
Right 085SXZZ
Cord
Bilateral 0V5H
Left 0V5G
Right 0V5F
Cornea
Left 0859XZZ
Right 0858XZZ
Cul-de-sac 0U5F
➤ Diaphragm 0B5T
~~Left 0B5S~~
~~Right 0B5R~~

Destruction (Continued)

Disc
Cervical Vertebral 0R53
Cervicothoracic Vertebral 0R55
Lumbar Vertebral 0S52
Lumbosacral 0S54
Thoracic Vertebral 0R59
Thoracolumbar Vertebral 0R5B
Duct
Common Bile 0F59
Cystic 0F58
Hepatic
➤ Common 0F57
Left 0F56
Right 0F55
Lacrimal
Left 085Y
Right 085X
Pancreatic 0F5D
Accessory 0F5F
Parotid
Left 0C5C
Right 0C5B
Thoracic 075K
Duodenum 0D59
Dura Mater 0052
Ear
External
Left 0951
Right 0950
External Auditory Canal
Left 0954
Right 0953
Inner
➡ Left 095E
➡ Right 095D
Middle
➡ Left 0956
➡ Right 0955
Endometrium 0U5B
Epididymis
Bilateral 0V5L
Left 0V5K
Right 0V5J
Epiglottis 0C5R
Esophagogastric Junction 0D54
Esophagus 0D55
Lower 0D53
Middle 0D52
Upper 0D51
Eustachian Tube
Left 095G
Right 095F
Eye
Left 0851XZZ
Right 0850XZZ
Eyelid
Lower
Left 085R
Right 085Q
Upper
Left 085P
Right 085N
Fallopian Tube
Left 0U56
Right 0U55
Fallopian Tubes, Bilateral 0U57
Femoral Shaft
Left 0Q59
Right 0Q58
Femur
Lower
Left 0Q5C
Right 0Q5B
Upper
Left 0Q57
Right 0Q56
Fibula
Left 0Q5K
Right 0Q5J
Finger Nail 0H5QXZZ

➤ New ➡ Revised ~~deleted~~ Deleted

Destruction (*Continued*)
Gallbladder 0F54
Gingiva
  Lower 0C56
  Upper 0C55
Gland
  Adrenal
    Bilateral 0G54
    Left 0G52
    Right 0G53
  Lacrimal
    Left 085W
    Right 085V
  Minor Salivary 0C5J
  Parotid
    Left 0C59
    Right 0C58
  Pituitary 0G50
  Sublingual
    Left 0C5F
    Right 0C5D
  Submaxillary
    Left 0C5H
    Right 0C5G
  Vestibular 0U5L
Glenoid Cavity
  Left 0P58
  Right 0P57
Glomus Jugulare 0G5C
Humeral Head
  Left 0P5D
  Right 0P5C
Humeral Shaft
  Left 0P5G
  Right 0P5F
Hymen 0U5K
Hypothalamus 005A
Ileocecal Valve 0D5C
Ileum 0D5B
Intestine
  Large 0D5E
    Left 0D5G
    Right 0D5F
  Small 0D58
Iris
  Left 085D3ZZ
  Right 085C3ZZ
Jejunum 0D5A
Joint
  Acromioclavicular
    Left 0R5H
    Right 0R5G
  Ankle
    Left 0S5G
    Right 0S5F
  Carpal
    Left 0R5R
    Right 0R5Q
  ▶ Carpometacarpal
    ▶ Left 0R5T
    ▶ Right 0R5S
  Cervical Vertebral 0R51
  Cervicothoracic Vertebral 0R54
  Coccygeal 0S56
  Elbow
    Left 0R5M
    Right 0R5L
  Finger Phalangeal
    Left 0R5X
    Right 0R5W
  Hip
    Left 0S5B
    Right 0S59
  Knee
    Left 0S5D
    Right 0S5C
  Lumbar Vertebral 0S50
  Lumbosacral 0S53
  ~~Metacarpocarpal~~
    ~~Left 0R5T~~
    ~~Right 0R5S~~

Destruction (*Continued*)
Joint (*Continued*)
  Metacarpophalangeal
    Left 0R5V
    Right 0R5U
  Metatarsal-Phalangeal
    Left 0S5N
    Right 0S5M
  ~~Metatarsal-Tarsal~~
    ~~Left 0S5L~~
    ~~Right 0S5K~~
  Occipital-cervical 0R50
  Sacrococcygeal 0S55
  Sacroiliac
    Left 0S58
    Right 0S57
  Shoulder
    Left 0R5K
    Right 0R5J
  Sternoclavicular
    Left 0R5F
    Right 0R5E
  Tarsal
    Left 0S5J
    Right 0S5H
  ▶ Tarsometatarsal
    ▶ Left 0S5L
    ▶ Right 0S5K
  Temporomandibular
    Left 0R5D
    Right 0R5C
  Thoracic Vertebral 0R56
  Thoracolumbar Vertebral 0R5A
  Toe Phalangeal
    Left 0S5Q
    Right 0S5P
  Wrist
    Left 0R5P
    Right 0R5N
Kidney
  Left 0T51
  Right 0T50
Kidney Pelvis
  Left 0T54
  Right 0T53
Larynx 0C5S
Lens
  Left 085K3ZZ
  Right 085J3ZZ
Lip
  Lower 0C51
  Upper 0C50
Liver 0F50
  Left Lobe 0F52
  Right Lobe 0F51
Lung
  Bilateral 0B5M
  Left 0B5L
  Lower Lobe
    Left 0B5J
    Right 0B5F
  Middle Lobe, Right 0B5D
  Right 0B5K
  Upper Lobe
    Left 0B5G
    Right 0B5C
Lung Lingula 0B5H
Lymphatic
  Aortic 075D
  Axillary
    Left 0756
    Right 0755
  Head 0750
  Inguinal
    Left 075J
    Right 075H
  Internal Mammary
    Left 0759
    Right 0758
  Lower Extremity
    Left 075G
    Right 075F

Destruction (*Continued*)
Lymphatic (*Continued*)
  Mesenteric 075B
  Neck
    Left 0752
    Right 0751
  Pelvis 075C
  Thorax 0757
  Upper Extremity
    Left 0754
    Right 0753
Mandible
  Left 0N5V
  Right 0N5T
⮞ Maxilla 0N5R
  ~~Left 0N5S~~
  ~~Right 0N5R~~
Medulla Oblongata 005D
Mesentery 0D5V
Metacarpal
  Left 0P5Q
  Right 0P5P
Metatarsal
  Left 0Q5P
  Right 0Q5N
Muscle
  Abdomen
    Left 0K5L
    Right 0K5K
  Extraocular
    Left 085M
    Right 085L
  Facial 0K51
  Foot
    Left 0K5W
    Right 0K5V
  Hand
    Left 0K5D
    Right 0K5C
  Head 0K50
  Hip
    Left 0K5P
    Right 0K5N
  Lower Arm and Wrist
    Left 0K5B
    Right 0K59
  Lower Leg
    Left 0K5T
    Right 0K5S
  Neck
    Left 0K53
    Right 0K52
  Papillary 025D
  Perineum 0K5M
  Shoulder
    Left 0K56
    Right 0K55
  Thorax
    Left 0K5J
    Right 0K5H
  Tongue, Palate, Pharynx 0K54
  Trunk
    Left 0K5G
    Right 0K5F
  Upper Arm
    Left 0K58
    Right 0K57
  Upper Leg
    Left 0K5R
    Right 0K5Q
▶ Nasal Mucosa and Soft Tissue 095K
Nasopharynx 095N
Nerve
  Abdominal Sympathetic 015M
  Abducens 005L
  Accessory 005R
  Acoustic 005N
  Brachial Plexus 0153
  Cervical 0151
  Cervical Plexus 0153
  Facial 005M

Destruction *(Continued)*
  Nerve *(Continued)*
    Femoral 015D
    Glossopharyngeal 005P
    Head and Neck Sympathetic 015K
    Hypoglossal 005S
    Lumbar 015B
    Lumbar Plexus 0159
    Lumbar Sympathetic 015N
    Lumbosacral Plexus 015A
    Median 0155
    Oculomotor 005H
    Olfactory 005F
    Optic 005G
    Peroneal 015H
    Phrenic 0152
    Pudendal 015C
    Radial 0156
    Sacral 015R
    Sacral Plexus 015Q
    Sacral Sympathetic 015P
    Sciatic 015F
    Thoracic 0158
    Thoracic Sympathetic 015L
    Tibial 015G
    Trigeminal 005K
    Trochlear 005J
    Ulnar 0154
    Vagus 005Q
  Nipple
    Left 0H5X
    Right 0H5W
  Nose 095K
  ➠Omentum 0D5U
    Greater 0D5S
    Lesser 0D5T
  Orbit
    Left 0N5Q
    Right 0N5P
  Ovary
    Bilateral 0U52
    Left 0U51
    Right 0U50
  Palate
    Hard 0C52
    Soft 0C53
  Pancreas 0F5G
  Para-aortic Body 0G59
  Paraganglion Extremity 0G5F
  Parathyroid Gland 0G5R
    Inferior
      Left 0G5P
      Right 0G5N
    Multiple 0G5Q
    Superior
      Left 0G5M
      Right 0G5L
  Patella
    Left 0Q5F
    Right 0Q5D
  Penis 0V5S
  Pericardium 025N
  Peritoneum 0D5W
  Phalanx
    Finger
      Left 0P5V
      Right 0P5T
    Thumb
      Left 0P5S
      Right 0P5R
    Toe
      Left 0Q5R
      Right 0Q5Q
  Pharynx 0C5M
  Pineal Body 0G51
  Pleura
    Left 0B5P
    Right 0B5N
  Pons 005B
  Prepuce 0V5T
  Prostate 0V50

Destruction *(Continued)*
  Radius
    Left 0P5J
    Right 0P5H
  Rectum 0D5P
  Retina
    Left 085F3ZZ
    Right 085E3ZZ
  Retinal Vessel
    Left 085H3ZZ
    Right 085G3ZZ
  Rib
    Left 0P52
    Right 0P51
  ▶Ribs
    ▶1 to 2 0P51
    ▶3 or More 0P52
  Sacrum 0Q51
  Scapula
    Left 0P56
    Right 0P55
  Sclera
    Left 0857XZZ
    Right 0856XZZ
  Scrotum 0V55
  Septum
    Atrial 0255
    Nasal 095M
    Ventricular 025M
  Sinus
    Accessory 095P
    Ethmoid
      Left 095V
      Right 095U
    Frontal
      Left 095T
      Right 095S
    Mastoid
      Left 095C
      Right 095B
    Maxillary
      Left 095R
      Right 095Q
    Sphenoid
      Left 095X
      Right 095W
  Skin
    Abdomen 0H57XZ
    Back 0H56XZ
    Buttock 0H58XZ
    Chest 0H55XZ
    Ear
      Left 0H53XZ
      Right 0H52XZ
    Face 0H51XZ
    Foot
      Left 0H5NXZ
      Right 0H5MXZ
    Genitalia 0H5AXZ
    Hand
      Left 0H5GXZ
      Right 0H5FXZ
    ▶Inguinal 0H5AXZ
    Lower Arm
      Left 0H5EXZ
      Right 0H5DXZ
    Lower Leg
      Left 0H5LXZ
      Right 0H5KXZ
    Neck 0H54XZ
    Perineum 0H59XZ
    Scalp 0H50XZ
    Upper Arm
      Left 0H5CXZ
      Right 0H5BXZ
    Upper Leg
      Left 0H5JXZ
      Right 0H5HXZ
  Skull 0N50
  Spinal Cord
    Cervical 005W
    Lumbar 005Y
    Thoracic 005X

Destruction *(Continued)*
  Spinal Meninges 005T
  Spleen 075P
  Sternum 0P50
  Stomach 0D56
    Pylorus 0D57
  Subcutaneous Tissue and Fascia
    Abdomen 0J58
    Back 0J57
    Buttock 0J59
    Chest 0J56
    Face 0J51
    Foot
      Left 0J5R
      Right 0J5Q
    Hand
      Left 0J5K
      Right 0J5J
    Lower Arm
      Left 0J5H
      Right 0J5G
    Lower Leg
      Left 0J5P
      Right 0J5N
    Neck
      Anterior 0J54
      Posterior 0J55
      ▶Left 0J55
      ▶Right 0J54
    Pelvic Region 0J5C
    Perineum 0J5B
    Scalp 0J50
    Upper Arm
      Left 0J5F
      Right 0J5D
    Upper Leg
      Left 0J5M
      Right 0J5L
  Tarsal
    Left 0Q5M
    Right 0Q5L
  Tendon
    Abdomen
      Left 0L5G
      Right 0L5F
    Ankle
      Left 0L5T
      Right 0L5S
    Foot
      Left 0L5W
      Right 0L5V
    Hand
      Left 0L58
      Right 0L57
    Head and Neck 0L50
    Hip
      Left 0L5K
      Right 0L5J
    Knee
      Left 0L5R
      Right 0L5Q
    Lower Arm and Wrist
      Left 0L56
      Right 0L55
    Lower Leg
      Left 0L5P
      Right 0L5N
    Perineum 0L5H
    Shoulder
      Left 0L52
      Right 0L51
    Thorax
      Left 0L5D
      Right 0L5C
    Trunk
      Left 0L5B
      Right 0L59
    Upper Arm
      Left 0L54
      Right 0L53

▶ New   ➠ Revised   ~~deleted~~ Deleted

Destruction (Continued)
  Tendon (Continued)
    Upper Leg
      Left 0L5M
      Right 0L5L
  Testis
    Bilateral 0V5C
    Left 0V5B
    Right 0V59
  Thalamus 0059
  Thymus 075M
  Thyroid Gland
    Left Lobe 0G5G
    Right Lobe 0G5H
  Tibia
    Left 0Q5H
    Right 0Q5G
  Toe Nail 0H5RXZZ
  Tongue 0C57
  Tonsils 0C5P
  Tooth
    Lower 0C5X
    Upper 0C5W
  Trachea 0B51
  Tunica Vaginalis
    Left 0V57
    Right 0V56
  Turbinate, Nasal 095L
  Tympanic Membrane
    Left 0958
    Right 0959
  Ulna
    Left 0P5L
    Right 0P5K
  Ureter
    Left 0T57
    Right 0T56
  Urethra 0T5D
  Uterine Supporting Structure 0U54
  Uterus 0U59
  Uvula 0C5N
  Vagina 0U5G
  Valve
    Aortic 025F
    Mitral 025G
    Pulmonary 025H
    Tricuspid 025J
  Vas Deferens
    Bilateral 0V5Q
    Left 0V5P
    Right 0V5N
  Vein
    Axillary
      Left 0558
      Right 0557
    Azygos 0550
    Basilic
      Left 055C
      Right 055B
    Brachial
      Left 055A
      Right 0559
    Cephalic
      Left 055F
      Right 055D
    Colic 0657
    Common Iliac
      Left 065D
      Right 065C
    Coronary 0254
    Esophageal 0653
    External Iliac
      Left 065G
      Right 065F
    External Jugular
      Left 055Q
      Right 055P
    Face
      Left 055V
      Right 055T

Destruction (Continued)
  Vein (Continued)
    Femoral
      Left 065N
      Right 065M
    Foot
      Left 065V
      Right 065T
    Gastric 0652
    ~~Greater Saphenous~~
      ~~Left 065Q~~
      ~~Right 065P~~
    Hand
      Left 055H
      Right 055G
    Hemiazygos 0551
    Hepatic 0654
    Hypogastric
      Left 065J
      Right 065H
    Inferior Mesenteric 0656
    Innominate
      Left 0554
      Right 0553
    Internal Jugular
      Left 055N
      Right 055M
    Intracranial 055L
    ~~Lesser Saphenous~~
      ~~Left 065S~~
      ~~Right 065R~~
    Lower 065Y
    Portal 0658
    Pulmonary
      Left 025T
      Right 025S
    Renal
      Left 065B
      Right 0659
    ▶Saphenous
      ▶Left 065Q
      ▶Right 065P
    Splenic 0651
    Subclavian
      Left 0556
      Right 0555
    Superior Mesenteric 0655
    Upper 055Y
    Vertebral
      Left 055S
      Right 055R
  Vena Cava
    Inferior 0650
    Superior 025V
  Ventricle
    Left 025L
    Right 025K
  Vertebra
    Cervical 0P53
    Lumbar 0Q50
    Thoracic 0P54
  Vesicle
    Bilateral 0V53
    Left 0V52
    Right 0V51
  Vitreous
    Left 08553ZZ
    Right 08543ZZ
  Vocal Cord
    Left 0C5V
    Right 0C5T
  Vulva 0U5M
Detachment
  Arm
    Lower
      Left 0X6F0Z
      Right 0X6D0Z
    Upper
      Left 0X690Z
      Right 0X680Z

Detachment (Continued)
  Elbow Region
    Left 0X6C0ZZ
    Right 0X6B0ZZ
  Femoral Region
    Left 0Y680ZZ
    Right 0Y670ZZ
  Finger
    Index
      Left 0X6P0Z
      Right 0X6N0Z
    Little
      Left 0X6W0Z
      Right 0X6V0Z
    Middle
      Left 0X6R0Z
      Right 0X6Q0Z
    Ring
      Left 0X6T0Z
      Right 0X6S0Z
  Foot
    Left 0Y6N0Z
    Right 0Y6M0Z
  Forequarter
    Left 0X610ZZ
    Right 0X600ZZ
  Hand
    Left 0X6K0Z
    Right 0X6J0Z
  Hindquarter
    Bilateral 0Y640ZZ
    Left 0Y630ZZ
    Right 0Y620ZZ
  Knee Region
    Left 0Y6G0ZZ
    Right 0Y6F0ZZ
  Leg
    Lower
      Left 0Y6J0Z
      Right 0Y6H0Z
    Upper
      Left 0Y6D0Z
      Right 0Y6C0Z
  Shoulder Region
    Left 0X630ZZ
    Right 0X620ZZ
  Thumb
    Left 0X6M0Z
    Right 0X6L0Z
  Toe
    1st
      Left 0Y6Q0Z
      Right 0Y6P0Z
    2nd
      Left 0Y6S0Z
      Right 0Y6R0Z
    3rd
      Left 0Y6U0Z
      Right 0Y6T0Z
    4th
      Left 0Y6W0Z
      Right 0Y6V0Z
    5th
      Left 0Y6Y0Z
      Right 0Y6X0Z
Determination, Mental status GZ14ZZZ
Detorsion
  see Release
  see Reposition
Detoxification Services, for substance abuse
  HZ2ZZZZ
Device Fitting F0DZ
Diagnostic Audiology see Audiology,
  Diagnostic
Diagnostic imaging see Imaging, Diagnostic
Diagnostic radiology see Imaging, Diagnostic
Dialysis
  ➡Hemodialysis see Performance, Urinary 5A1D
    Peritoneal 3E1M39Z
Diaphragma sellae use Dura Mater
Diaphragmatic pacemaker generator use
  Stimulator Generator in Subcutaneous
  Tissue and Fascia

Diaphragmatic Pacemaker Lead
~~Insertion of device in~~
~~Left 0BHS~~
~~Right 0BHR~~
▶ Insertion of device in, Diaphragm 0BHT
Removal of device from, Diaphragm 0BPT
Revision of device in, Diaphragm 0BWT
Digital radiography, plain *see* Plain Radiography
Dilation
Ampulla of Vater 0F7C
Anus 0D7Q
Aorta
  Abdominal 0470
  Thoracic
    Ascending/Arch 027X
    Descending 027W
Artery
  Anterior Tibial
    Left 047Q
    Right 047P
  Axillary
    Left 0376
    Right 0375
  Brachial
    Left 0378
    Right 0377
  Celiac 0471
  Colic
    Left 0477
    Middle 0478
    Right 0476
  Common Carotid
    Left 037J
    Right 037H
  Common Iliac
    Left 047D
    Right 047C
  Coronary
    Four or More Arteries 0273
    One Artery 0270
    Three Arteries 0272
    Two Arteries 0271
  External Carotid
    Left 037N
    Right 037M
  External Iliac
    Left 047J
    Right 047H
  Face 037R
  Femoral
    Left 047L
    Right 047K
  Foot
    Left 047W
    Right 047V
  Gastric 0472
  Hand
    Left 037F
    Right 037D
  Hepatic 0473
  Inferior Mesenteric 047B
  Innominate 0372
  Internal Carotid
    Left 037L
    Right 037K
  Internal Iliac
    Left 047F
    Right 047E
  Internal Mammary
    Left 0371
    Right 0370
  Intracranial 037G
  Lower 047Y
  Peroneal
    Left 047U
    Right 047T
  Popliteal
    Left 047N
    Right 047M
  Posterior Tibial
    Left 047S
    Right 047R

Dilation *(Continued)*
Artery *(Continued)*
  Pulmonary
    Left 027R
    Right 027Q
  Pulmonary Trunk 027P
  Radial
    Left 037C
    Right 037B
  Renal
    Left 047A
    Right 0479
  Splenic 0474
  Subclavian
    Left 0374
    Right 0373
  Superior Mesenteric 0475
  Temporal
    Left 037T
    Right 037S
  Thyroid
    Left 037V
    Right 037U
  Ulnar
    Left 037A
    Right 0379
  Upper 037Y
  Vertebral
    Left 037Q
    Right 037P
Bladder 0T7B
Bladder Neck 0T7C
Bronchus
  Lingula 0B79
  Lower Lobe
    Left 0B7B
    Right 0B76
  Main
    Left 0B77
    Right 0B73
  Middle Lobe, Right 0B75
  Upper Lobe
    Left 0B78
    Right 0B74
Carina 0B72
Cecum 0D7H
▶ Cerebral Ventricle 0076
Cervix 0U7C
Colon
  Ascending 0D7K
  Descending 0D7M
  Sigmoid 0D7N
  Transverse 0D7L
Duct
  Common Bile 0F79
  Cystic 0F78
  Hepatic
    ▶ Common 0F77
    Left 0F76
    Right 0F75
  Lacrimal
    Left 087Y
    Right 087X
  Pancreatic 0F7D
    Accessory 0F7F
  Parotid
    Left 0C7C
    Right 0C7B
Duodenum 0D79
Esophagogastric Junction 0D74
Esophagus 0D75
  Lower 0D73
  Middle 0D72
  Upper 0D71
Eustachian Tube
  Left 097G
  Right 097F
Fallopian Tube
  Left 0U76
  Right 0U75
Fallopian Tubes, Bilateral 0U77

Dilation *(Continued)*
Hymen 0U7K
Ileocecal Valve 0D7C
Ileum 0D7B
Intestine
  Large 0D7E
    Left 0D7G
    Right 0D7F
  Small 0D78
Jejunum 0D7A
Kidney Pelvis
  Left 0T74
  Right 0T73
Larynx 0C7S
Pharynx 0C7M
Rectum 0D7P
Stomach 0D76
  Pylorus 0D77
Trachea 0B71
Ureter
  Left 0T77
  Right 0T76
Ureters, Bilateral 0T78
Urethra 0T7D
Uterus 0U79
Vagina 0U7G
Valve
  Aortic 027F
  Ileocecal 0D7C
  Mitral 027G
  Pulmonary 027H
  Tricuspid 027J
Vas Deferens
  Bilateral 0V7Q
  Left 0V7P
  Right 0V7N
Vein
  Axillary
    Left 0578
    Right 0577
  Azygos 0570
  Basilic
    Left 057C
    Right 057B
  Brachial
    Left 057A
    Right 0579
  Cephalic
    Left 057F
    Right 057D
  Colic 0677
  Common Iliac
    Left 067D
    Right 067C
  Esophageal 0673
  External Iliac
    Left 067G
    Right 067F
  External Jugular
    Left 057Q
    Right 057P
  Face
    Left 057V
    Right 057T
  Femoral
    Left 067N
    Right 067M
  Foot
    Left 067V
    Right 067T
  Gastric 0672
  ~~Greater Saphenous~~
    ~~Left 067Q~~
    ~~Right 067P~~
  Hand
    Left 057H
    Right 057G
  Hemiazygos 0571
  Hepatic 0674
  Hypogastric
    Left 067J
    Right 067H

▶ New   ⇒ Revised   ~~deleted~~ Deleted

Dilation *(Continued)*
  Vein *(Continued)*
    Inferior Mesenteric 0676
    Innominate
      Left 0574
      Right 0573
    Internal Jugular
      Left 057N
      Right 057M
    Intracranial 057L
    ~~Lesser Saphenous~~
      ~~Left 067S~~
      ~~Right 067R~~
    Lower 067Y
    Portal 0678
    Pulmonary
      Left 027T
      Right 027S
    Renal
      Left 067B
      Right 0679
    ▶ Saphenous
      ▶ Left 067Q
      ▶ Right 067P
    Splenic 0671
    Subclavian
      Left 0576
      Right 0575
    Superior Mesenteric 0675
    Upper 057Y
    Vertebral
      Left 057S
      Right 057R
  Vena Cava
    Inferior 0670
    Superior 027V
  ~~Ventricle, Right 027K~~
  ▶ Ventricle
    ▶ Left 027L
    ▶ Right 027K
Direct Lateral Interbody Fusion (DLIF) device
  use Interbody Fusion Device in Lower
    Joints
Disarticulation *see* Detachment
Discectomy, diskectomy
  see Excision, Upper Joints 0RB
  see Resection, Upper Joints 0RT
  see Excision, Lower Joints 0SB
  see Resection, Lower Joints 0ST
Discography
  see Plain Radiography, Axial Skeleton,
    Except Skull and Facial Bones BR0
  see Fluoroscopy, Axial Skeleton, Except Skull
    and Facial Bones BR1
Distal humerus
  use Humeral Shaft, Right
  use Humeral Shaft, Left
Distal humerus, involving joint
  use Elbow Joint, Right
  use Elbow Joint, Left
Distal radioulnar joint
  use Wrist Joint, Right
  use Wrist Joint, Left
Diversion *see* Bypass
Diverticulectomy *see* Excision, Gastrointestinal
  System 0DB
Division
  Acetabulum
    Left 0Q85
    Right 0Q84
  Anal Sphincter 0D8R
  Basal Ganglia 0088
  Bladder Neck 0T8C
  Bone
    Ethmoid
      Left 0N8G
      Right 0N8F
    ➡ Frontal 0N81
      ~~Left 0N82~~
      ~~Right 0N81~~
    Hyoid 0N8X

Division *(Continued)*
  Bone *(Continued)*
    Lacrimal
      Left 0N8J
      Right 0N8H
    Nasal 0N8B
    ➡ Occipital 0N87
      ~~Left 0N88~~
      ~~Right 0N87~~
    Palatine
      Left 0N8L
      Right 0N8K
    Parietal
      Left 0N84
      Right 0N83
    Pelvic
      Left 0Q83
      Right 0Q82
    ➡ Sphenoid 0N8C
      ~~Left 0N8D~~
      ~~Right 0N8C~~
    Temporal
      Left 0N86
      Right 0N85
    Zygomatic
      Left 0N8N
      Right 0N8M
  Brain 0080
  Bursa and Ligament
    Abdomen
      Left 0M8J
      Right 0M8H
    Ankle
      Left 0M8R
      Right 0M8Q
    Elbow
      Left 0M84
      Right 0M83
    Foot
      Left 0M8T
      Right 0M8S
    Hand
      Left 0M88
      Right 0M87
    Head and Neck 0M80
    Hip
      Left 0M8M
      Right 0M8L
    Knee
      Left 0M8P
      Right 0M8N
    Lower Extremity
      Left 0M8W
      Right 0M8V
    Perineum 0M8K
    ▶ Rib(s) 0M8G
    Shoulder
      Left 0M82
      Right 0M81
    ▶ Spine
      ▶ Lower 0M8D
      ▶ Upper 0M8C
    ▶ Sternum 0M8F
    ~~Thorax~~
      ~~Left 0M8G~~
      ~~Right 0M8F~~
    ~~Trunk~~
      ~~Left 0M8D~~
      ~~Right 0M8C~~
    Upper Extremity
      Left 0M8B
      Right 0M89
    Wrist
      Left 0M86
      Right 0M85
  Carpal
    Left 0P8N
    Right 0P8M
  Cerebral Hemisphere 0087
  Chordae Tendineae 0289

Division *(Continued)*
  Clavicle
    Left 0P8B
    Right 0P89
  Coccyx 0Q8S
  Conduction Mechanism 0288
  Esophagogastric Junction
    0D84
  Femoral Shaft
    Left 0Q89
    Right 0Q88
  Femur
    Lower
      Left 0Q8C
      Right 0Q8B
    Upper
      Left 0Q87
      Right 0Q86
  Fibula
    Left 0Q8K
    Right 0Q8J
  Gland, Pituitary 0G80
  Glenoid Cavity
    Left 0P88
    Right 0P87
  Humeral Head
    Left 0P8D
    Right 0P8C
  Humeral Shaft
    Left 0P8G
    Right 0P8F
  Hymen 0U8K
  Kidneys, Bilateral 0T82
  Mandible
    Left 0N8V
    Right 0N8T
  ➡ Maxilla 0N8R
    ~~Left 0N8S~~
    ~~Right 0N8R~~
  Metacarpal
    Left 0P8Q
    Right 0P8P
  Metatarsal
    Left 0Q8P
    Right 0Q8N
  Muscle
    Abdomen
      Left 0K8L
      Right 0K8K
    Facial 0K81
    Foot
      Left 0K8W
      Right 0K8V
    Hand
      Left 0K8D
      Right 0K8C
    Head 0K80
    Hip
      Left 0K8P
      Right 0K8N
    Lower Arm and Wrist
      Left 0K8B
      Right 0K89
    Lower Leg
      Left 0K8T
      Right 0K8S
    Neck
      Left 0K83
      Right 0K82
    Papillary 028D
    Perineum 0K8M
    Shoulder
      Left 0K86
      Right 0K85
    Thorax
      Left 0K8J
      Right 0K8H
    Tongue, Palate, Pharynx 0K84
    Trunk
      Left 0K8G
      Right 0K8F

▶ New   ➡ Revised   ~~deleted~~ Deleted

Division *(Continued)*
  Muscle *(Continued)*
    Upper Arm
      Left 0K88
      Right 0K87
    Upper Leg
      Left 0K8R
      Right 0K8Q
  Nerve
    Abdominal Sympathetic 018M
    Abducens 008L
    Accessory 008R
    Acoustic 008N
    Brachial Plexus 0183
    Cervical 0181
    Cervical Plexus 0180
    Facial 008M
    Femoral 018D
    Glossopharyngeal 008P
    Head and Neck Sympathetic 018K
    Hypoglossal 008S
    Lumbar 018B
    Lumbar Plexus 0189
    Lumbar Sympathetic 018N
    Lumbosacral Plexus 018A
    Median 0185
    Oculomotor 008H
    Olfactory 008F
    Optic 008G
    Peroneal 018H
    Phrenic 0182
    Pudendal 018C
    Radial 0186
    Sacral 018R
    Sacral Plexus 018Q
    Sacral Sympathetic 018P
    Sciatic 018F
    Thoracic 0188
    Thoracic Sympathetic 018L
    Tibial 018G
    Trigeminal 008K
    Trochlear 008J
    Ulnar 0184
    Vagus 008Q
  Orbit
    Left 0N8Q
    Right 0N8P
  Ovary
    Bilateral 0U82
    Left 0U81
    Right 0U80
  Pancreas 0F8G
  Patella
    Left 0Q8F
    Right 0Q8D
  Perineum, Female 0W8NXZZ
  Phalanx
    Finger
      Left 0P8V
      Right 0P8T
    Thumb
      Left 0P8S
      Right 0P8R
    Toe
      Left 0Q8R
      Right 0Q8Q
  Radius
    Left 0P8J
    Right 0P8H
  ~~Rib~~
    ~~Left 0P82~~
    ~~Right 0P81~~
  ▶Ribs
    ▶1 to 2 0P81
    ▶3 or More 0P82
  Sacrum 0Q81
  Scapula
    Left 0P86
    Right 0P85
  Skin
    Abdomen 0H87XZZ
    Back 0H86XZZ

Division *(Continued)*
  Skin *(Continued)*
    Buttock 0H88XZZ
    Chest 0H85XZZ
    Ear
      Left 0H83XZZ
      Right 0H82XZZ
    Face 0H81XZZ
    Foot
      Left 0H8NXZZ
      Right 0H8MXZZ
    ~~Genitalia 0H8AXZZ~~
    Hand
      Left 0H8GXZZ
      Right 0H8FXZZ
    ▶Inguinal 0H8AXZZ
    Lower Arm
      Left 0H8EXZZ
      Right 0H8DXZZ
    Lower Leg
      Left 0H8LXZZ
      Right 0H8KXZZ
    Neck 0H84XZZ
    Perineum 0H89XZZ
    Scalp 0H80XZZ
    Upper Arm
      Left 0H8CXZZ
      Right 0H8BXZZ
    Upper Leg
      Left 0H8JXZZ
      Right 0H8HXZZ
  Skull 0N80
  Spinal Cord
    Cervical 008W
    Lumbar 008Y
    Thoracic 008X
  Sternum 0P80
  Stomach, Pylorus 0D87
  Subcutaneous Tissue and Fascia
    Abdomen 0J88
    Back 0J87
    Buttock 0J89
    Chest 0J86
    Face 0J81
    Foot
      Left 0J8R
      Right 0J8Q
    Hand
      Left 0J8K
      Right 0J8J
    Head and Neck 0J8S
    Lower Arm
      Left 0J8H
      Right 0J8G
    Lower Extremity 0J8W
    Lower Leg
      Left 0J8P
      Right 0J8N
    Neck
      ~~Anterior 0J84~~
      ~~Posterior 0J85~~
      ▶Left 0J85
      ▶Right 0J84
    Pelvic Region 0J8C
    Perineum 0J8B
    Scalp 0J80
    Trunk 0J8T
    Upper Arm
      Left 0J8F
      Right 0J8D
    Upper Extremity 0J8V
    Upper Leg
      Left 0J8M
      Right 0J8L
  Tarsal
    Left 0Q8M
    Right 0Q8L
  Tendon
    Abdomen
      Left 0L8G
      Right 0L8F

Division *(Continued)*
  Tendon *(Continued)*
    Ankle
      Left 0L8T
      Right 0L8S
    Foot
      Left 0L8W
      Right 0L8V
    Hand
      Left 0L88
      Right 0L87
    Head and Neck 0L80
    Hip
      Left 0L8K
      Right 0L8J
    Knee
      Left 0L8R
      Right 0L8Q
    Lower Arm and Wrist
      Left 0L86
      Right 0L85
    Lower Leg
      Left 0L8P
      Right 0L8N
    Perineum 0L8H
    Shoulder
      Left 0L82
      Right 0L81
    Thorax
      Left 0L8D
      Right 0L8C
    Trunk
      Left 0L8B
      Right 0L89
    Upper Arm
      Left 0L84
      Right 0L83
    Upper Leg
      Left 0L8M
      Right 0L8L
  Thyroid Gland Isthmus 0G8J
  Tibia
    Left 0Q8H
    Right 0Q8G
  Turbinate, Nasal 098L
  Ulna
    Left 0P8L
    Right 0P8K
  Uterine Supporting Structure 0U84
  Vertebra
    Cervical 0P83
    Lumbar 0Q80
    Thoracic 0P84
Doppler study *see* Ultrasonography
Dorsal digital nerve *use* Radial Nerve
Dorsal metacarpal vein
  use Hand Vein, Right
  use Hand Vein, Left
Dorsal metatarsal artery
  use Foot Artery, Right
  use Foot Artery, Left
Dorsal metatarsal vein
  use Foot Vein, Right
  use Foot Vein, Left
Dorsal scapular artery
  use Subclavian Artery, Right
  use Subclavian Artery, Left
Dorsal scapular nerve *use* Brachial Plexus
Dorsal venous arch
  use Foot Vein, Right
  use Foot Vein, Left
Dorsalis pedis artery
  use Anterior Tibial Artery, Right
  use Anterior Tibial Artery, Left
Drainage
  Abdominal Wall 0W9F
  Acetabulum
    Left 0Q95
    Right 0Q94
  Adenoids 0C9Q
  Ampulla of Vater 0F9C
  Anal Sphincter 0D9R

▶ New   ⇒ Revised   ~~deleted~~ Deleted

Drainage *(Continued)*
Ankle Region
Left 0Y9L
Right 0Y9K
Anterior Chamber
Left 0893
Right 0892
Anus 0D9Q
Aorta, Abdominal 0490
Aortic Body 0G9D
Appendix 0D9J
Arm
Lower
Left 0X9F
Right 0X9D
Upper
Left 0X99
Right 0X98
Artery
Anterior Tibial
Left 049Q
Right 049P
Axillary
Left 0396
Right 0395
Brachial
Left 0398
Right 0397
Celiac 0491
Colic
Left 0497
Middle 0498
Right 0496
Common Carotid
Left 039J
Right 039H
Common Iliac
Left 049D
Right 049C
External Carotid
Left 039N
Right 039M
External Iliac
Left 049J
Right 049H
Face 039R
Femoral
Left 049L
Right 049K
Foot
Left 049W
Right 049V
Gastric 0492
Hand
Left 039F
Right 039D
Hepatic 0493
Inferior Mesenteric 049B
Innominate 0392
Internal Carotid
Left 039L
Right 039K
Internal Iliac
Left 049F
Right 049E
Internal Mammary
Left 0391
Right 0390
Intracranial 039G
Lower 049Y
Peroneal
Left 049U
Right 049T
Popliteal
Left 049N
Right 049M
Posterior Tibial
Left 049S
Right 049R
Radial
Left 039C
Right 039B

Drainage *(Continued)*
Artery *(Continued)*
Renal
Left 049A
Right 0499
Splenic 0494
Subclavian
Left 0394
Right 0393
Superior Mesenteric 0495
Temporal
Left 039T
Right 039S
Thyroid
Left 039V
Right 039U
Ulnar
Left 039A
Right 0399
Upper 039Y
Vertebral
Left 039Q
Right 039P
Auditory Ossicle
Left 099A
Right 0999
Axilla
Left 0X95
Right 0X94
Back
Lower 0W9L
Upper 0W9K
Basal Ganglia 0098
Bladder 0T9B
Bladder Neck 0T9C
Bone
Ethmoid
Left 0N9G
Right 0N9F
➡Frontal 0N91
Left 0N92
Right 0N91
Hyoid 0N9X
Lacrimal
Left 0N9J
Right 0N9H
Nasal 0N9B
➡Occipital 0N97
Left 0N98
Right 0N97
Palatine
Left 0N9L
Right 0N9K
Parietal
Left 0N94
Right 0N93
Pelvic
Left 0Q93
Right 0Q92
➡Sphenoid 0N9C
Left 0N9D
Right 0N9C
Temporal
Left 0N96
Right 0N95
Zygomatic
Left 0N9N
Right 0N9M
Bone Marrow 079T
Brain 0090
Breast
Bilateral 0H9V
Left 0H9U
Right 0H9T
Bronchus
Lingula 0B99
Lower Lobe
Left 0B9B
Right 0B96
Main
Left 0B97
Right 0B93

Drainage *(Continued)*
Bronchus *(Continued)*
Middle Lobe, Right 0B95
Upper Lobe
Left 0B98
Right 0B94
Buccal Mucosa 0C94
Bursa and Ligament
Abdomen
Left 0M9J
Right 0M9H
Ankle
Left 0M9R
Right 0M9Q
Elbow
Left 0M94
Right 0M93
Foot
Left 0M9T
Right 0M9S
Hand
Left 0M98
Right 0M97
Head and Neck 0M90
Hip
Left 0M9M
Right 0M9L
Knee
Left 0M9P
Right 0M9N
Lower Extremity
Left 0M9W
Right 0M9V
Perineum 0M9K
▶Rib(s) 0M9G
Shoulder
Left 0M92
Right 0M91
▶Spine
▶Lower 0M9D
▶Upper 0M9C
▶Sternum 0M9F
Thorax
Left 0M9G
Right 0M9F
Trunk
Left 0M9D
Right 0M9C
Upper Extremity
Left 0M9B
Right 0M99
Wrist
Left 0M96
Right 0M95
Buttock
Left 0Y91
Right 0Y90
Carina 0B92
Carotid Bodies, Bilateral 0G98
Carotid Body
Left 0G96
Right 0G97
Carpal
Left 0P9N
Right 0P9M
Cavity, Cranial 0W91
Cecum 0D9H
Cerebellum 009C
Cerebral Hemisphere 0097
Cerebral Meninges 0091
Cerebral Ventricle 0096
Cervix 0U9C
Chest Wall 0W98
Choroid
Left 089B
Right 089A
Cisterna Chyli 079L
Clavicle
Left 0P9B
Right 0P99
Clitoris 0U9J

New ➡ Revised ~~deleted~~ Deleted

Drainage (Continued)
Coccygeal Glomus 0G9B
Coccyx 0Q9S
Colon
  Ascending 0D9K
  Descending 0D9M
  Sigmoid 0D9N
  Transverse 0D9L
Conjunctiva
  Left 089T
  Right 089S
Cord
  Bilateral 0V9H
  Left 0V9G
  Right 0V9F
Cornea
  Left 0899
  Right 0898
Cul-de-sac 0U9F
➡ Diaphragm 0B9T
  ~~Left 0B9S~~
  ~~Right 0B9R~~
Disc
  Cervical Vertebral 0R93
  Cervicothoracic Vertebral 0R95
  Lumbar Vertebral 0S92
  Lumbosacral 0S94
  Thoracic Vertebral 0R99
  Thoracolumbar Vertebral 0R9B
Duct
  Common Bile 0F99
  Cystic 0F98
  Hepatic
  ▶ Common 0F97
    Left 0F96
    Right 0F95
  Lacrimal
    Left 089Y
    Right 089X
  Pancreatic 0F9D
    Accessory 0F9F
  Parotid
    Left 0C9C
    Right 0C9B
Duodenum 0D99
Dura Mater 0092
Ear
  External
    Left 0991
    Right 0990
  External Auditory Canal
    Left 0994
    Right 0993
  Inner
    Left 099E
    Right 099D
  Middle
    Left 0996
    Right 0995
Elbow Region
  Left 0X9C
  Right 0X9B
Epididymis
  Bilateral 0V9L
  Left 0V9K
  Right 0V9J
~~Epidural Space 0093~~
▶ Epidural Space, Intracranial 0093
Epiglottis 0C9R
Esophagogastric Junction 0D94
Esophagus 0D95
  Lower 0D93
  Middle 0D92
  Upper 0D91
Eustachian Tube
  Left 099G
  Right 099F
Extremity
  Lower
    Left 0Y9B
    Right 0Y99

Drainage (Continued)
Extremity (Continued)
  Upper
    Left 0X97
    Right 0X96
Eye
  Left 0891
  Right 0890
Eyelid
  Lower
    Left 089R
    Right 089Q
  Upper
    Left 089P
    Right 089N
Face 0W92
Fallopian Tube
  Left 0U96
  Right 0U95
Fallopian Tubes, Bilateral 0U97
Femoral Region
  Left 0Y98
  Right 0Y97
Femoral Shaft
  Left 0Q99
  Right 0Q98
Femur
  Lower
    Left 0Q9C
    Right 0Q9B
  Upper
    Left 0Q97
    Right 0Q96
Fibula
  Left 0Q9K
  Right 0Q9J
Finger Nail 0H9Q
Foot
  Left 0Y9N
  Right 0Y9M
Gallbladder 0F94
Gingiva
  Lower 0C96
  Upper 0C95
Gland
  Adrenal
    Bilateral 0G94
    Left 0G92
    Right 0G93
  Lacrimal
    Left 089W
    Right 089V
  Minor Salivary 0C9J
  Parotid
    Left 0C99
    Right 0C98
  Pituitary 0G90
  Sublingual
    Left 0C9F
    Right 0C9D
  Submaxillary
    Left 0C9H
    Right 0C9G
  Vestibular 0U9L
Glenoid Cavity
  Left 0P98
  Right 0P97
Glomus Jugulare 0G9C
Hand
  Left 0X9K
  Right 0X9J
Head 0W90
Humeral Head
  Left 0P9D
  Right 0P9C
Humeral Shaft
  Left 0P9G
  Right 0P9F
Hymen 0U9K
Hypothalamus 009A
Ileocecal Valve 0D9C

Drainage (Continued)
Ileum 0D9B
Inguinal Region
  Left 0Y96
  Right 0Y95
Intestine
  Large 0D9E
    Left 0D9G
    Right 0D9F
  Small 0D98
Iris
  Left 089D
  Right 089C
Jaw
  Lower 0W95
  Upper 0W94
Jejunum 0D9A
Joint
  Acromioclavicular
    Left 0R9H
    Right 0R9G
  Ankle
    Left 0S9G
    Right 0S9F
  Carpal
    Left 0R9R
    Right 0R9Q
  ▶ Carpometacarpal
    ▶ Left 0R9T
    ▶ Right 0R9S
  Cervical Vertebral 0R91
  Cervicothoracic Vertebral 0R94
  Coccygeal 0S96
  Elbow
    Left 0R9M
    Right 0R9L
  Finger Phalangeal
    Left 0R9X
    Right 0R9W
  Hip
    Left 0S9B
    Right 0S99
  Knee
    Left 0S9D
    Right 0S9C
  Lumbar Vertebral 0S90
  Lumbosacral 0S93
  ~~Metacarpocarpal~~
    ~~Left 0R9T~~
    ~~Right 0R9S~~
  Metacarpophalangeal
    Left 0R9V
    Right 0R9U
  Metatarsal-Phalangeal
    Left 0S9N
    Right 0S9M
  ~~Metatarsal-Tarsal~~
    ~~Left 0S9L~~
    ~~Right 0S9K~~
  Occipital-cervical 0R90
  Sacrococcygeal 0S95
  Sacroiliac
    Left 0S98
    Right 0S97
  Shoulder
    Left 0R9K
    Right 0R9J
  Sternoclavicular
    Left 0R9F
    Right 0R9E
  Tarsal
    Left 0S9J
    Right 0S9H
  ▶ Tarsometatarsal
    ▶ Left 0S9L
    ▶ Right 0S9K
  Temporomandibular
    Left 0R9D
    Right 0R9C
  Thoracic Vertebral 0R96
  Thoracolumbar Vertebral 0R9A

▶ New   ➡ Revised   ~~deleted~~ Deleted

Drainage *(Continued)*
  Joint *(Continued)*
    Toe Phalangeal
      Left 0S9Q
      Right 0S9P
    Wrist
      Left 0R9P
      Right 0R9N
  Kidney
    Left 0T91
    Right 0T90
  Kidney Pelvis
    Left 0T94
    Right 0T93
  Knee Region
    Left 0Y9G
    Right 0Y9F
  Larynx 0C9S
  Leg
    Lower
      Left 0Y9J
      Right 0Y9H
    Upper
      Left 0Y9D
      Right 0Y9C
  Lens
    Left 089K
    Right 089J
  Lip
    Lower 0C91
    Upper 0C90
  Liver 0F90
    Left Lobe 0F92
    Right Lobe 0F91
  Lung
    Bilateral 0B9M
    Left 0B9L
    Lower Lobe
      Left 0B9J
      Right 0B9F
    Middle Lobe, Right 0B9D
    Right 0B9K
    Upper Lobe
      Left 0B9G
      Right 0B9C
  Lung Lingula 0B9H
  Lymphatic
    Aortic 079D
    Axillary
      Left 0796
      Right 0795
    Head 0790
    Inguinal
      Left 079J
      Right 079H
    Internal Mammary
      Left 0799
      Right 0798
    Lower Extremity
      Left 079G
      Right 079F
    Mesenteric 079B
    Neck
      Left 0792
      Right 0791
    Pelvis 079C
    Thoracic Duct 079K
    Thorax 0797
    Upper Extremity
      Left 0794
      Right 0793
  Mandible
    Left 0N9V
    Right 0N9T
  ⇒Maxilla 0N9R
    ~~Left 0N9S~~
    ~~Right 0N9R~~
  Mediastinum 0W9C
  Medulla Oblongata 009D
  Mesentery 0D9V

Drainage *(Continued)*
  Metacarpal
    Left 0P9Q
    Right 0P9P
  Metatarsal
    Left 0Q9P
    Right 0Q9N
  Muscle
    Abdomen
      Left 0K9L
      Right 0K9K
    Extraocular
      Left 089M
      Right 089L
    Facial 0K91
    Foot
      Left 0K9W
      Right 0K9V
    Hand
      Left 0K9D
      Right 0K9C
    Head 0K90
    Hip
      Left 0K9P
      Right 0K9N
    Lower Arm and Wrist
      Left 0K9B
      Right 0K99
    Lower Leg
      Left 0K9T
      Right 0K9S
    Neck
      Left 0K93
      Right 0K92
    Perineum 0K9M
    Shoulder
      Left 0K96
      Right 0K95
    Thorax
      Left 0K9J
      Right 0K9H
    Tongue, Palate, Pharynx 0K94
    Trunk
      Left 0K9G
      Right 0K9F
    Upper Arm
      Left 0K98
      Right 0K97
    Upper Leg
      Left 0K9R
      Right 0K9Q
  ▶Nasal Mucosa and Soft Tissue 099K
  Nasopharynx 099N
  Neck 0W96
  Nerve
    Abdominal Sympathetic 019M
    Abducens 009L
    Accessory 009R
    Acoustic 009N
    Brachial Plexus 0193
    Cervical 0191
    Cervical Plexus 0190
    Facial 009M
    Femoral 019D
    Glossopharyngeal 009P
    Head and Neck Sympathetic 019K
    Hypoglossal 009S
    Lumbar 019B
    Lumbar Plexus 0199
    Lumbar Sympathetic 019N
    Lumbosacral Plexus 019A
    Median 0195
    Oculomotor 009H
    Olfactory 009F
    Optic 009G
    Peroneal 019H
    Phrenic 0192
    Pudendal 019C
    Radial 0196
    Sacral 019R
    Sacral Sympathetic 019P

Drainage *(Continued)*
  Nerve *(Continued)*
    Sciatic 019F
    Thoracic 0198
    Thoracic Sympathetic 019L
    Tibial 019G
    Trigeminal 009K
    Trochlear 009J
    Ulnar 0194
    Vagus 009Q
  Nipple
    Left 0H9X
    Right 0H9W
  ~~Nose 099K~~
  ⇒Omentum 0D9U
    ~~Greater 0D9S~~
    ~~Lesser 0D9T~~
  Oral Cavity and Throat 0W93
  Orbit
    Left 0N9Q
    Right 0N9P
  Ovary
    Bilateral 0U92
    Left 0U91
    Right 0U90
  Palate
    Hard 0C92
    Soft 0C93
  Pancreas 0F9G
  Para-aortic Body 0G99
  Paraganglion Extremity 0G9F
  Parathyroid Gland 0G9R
    Inferior
      Left 0G9P
      Right 0G9N
    Multiple 0G9Q
    Superior
      Left 0G9P
      Right 0G9L
  Patella
    Left 0Q9F
    Right 0Q9D
  Pelvic Cavity 0W9J
  Penis 0V9S
  Pericardial Cavity 0W9D
  Perineum
    Female 0W9N
    Male 0W9M
  Peritoneal Cavity 0W9G
  Peritoneum 0D9W
  Phalanx
    Finger
      Left 0P9V
      Right 0P9T
    Thumb
      Left 0P9S
      Right 0P9R
    Toe
      Left 0Q9R
      Right 0Q9Q
  Pharynx 0C9M
  Pineal Body 0G91
  Pleura
    Left 0B9P
    Right 0B9N
  Pleural Cavity
    Left 0W9B
    Right 0W99
  Pons 009B
  Prepuce 0V9T
  Products of Conception
    Amniotic Fluid
      Diagnostic 1090
      Therapeutic 1090
    Fetal Blood 1090
    Fetal Cerebrospinal Fluid 1090
    Fetal Fluid, Other 1090
    Fluid, Other 1090
  Prostate 0V90
  Radius
    Left 0P9J
    Right 0P9H

▶ New   ⇒ Revised   ~~deleted~~ Deleted

Drainage (Continued)
Rectum ØD9P
Retina
  Left Ø89F
  Right Ø89E
Retinal Vessel
  Left Ø89H
  Right Ø89G
Retroperitoneum ØW9H
Rib
  Left ØP92
  Right ØP91
▶ Ribs
  ▶ 1 to 2 ØP91
  ▶ 3 or More ØP92
Sacrum ØQ91
Scapula
  Left ØP96
  Right ØP95
Sclera
  Left Ø897
  Right Ø896
Scrotum ØV95
Septum, Nasal Ø99M
Shoulder Region
  Left ØX93
  Right ØX92
Sinus
  Accessory Ø99P
  Ethmoid
    Left Ø99V
    Right Ø99U
  Frontal
    Left Ø99T
    Right Ø99S
  Mastoid
    Left Ø99C
    Right Ø99B
  Maxillary
    Left Ø99R
    Right Ø99Q
  Sphenoid
    Left Ø99X
    Right Ø99W
Skin
  Abdomen ØH97
  Back ØH96
  Buttock ØH98
  Chest ØH95
  Ear
    Left ØH93
    Right ØH92
  Face ØH91
  Foot
    Left ØH9N
    Right ØH9M
  Genitalia ØH9A
  Hand
    Left ØH9G
    Right ØH9F
  ▶ Inguinal ØH9A
  Lower Arm
    Left ØH9E
    Right ØH9D
  Lower Leg
    Left ØH9L
    Right ØH9K
  Neck ØH94
  Perineum ØH99
  Scalp ØH90
  Upper Arm
    Left ØH9C
    Right ØH9B
  Upper Leg
    Left ØH9J
    Right ØH9H
Skull ØN90
Spinal Canal ØØ9U
Spinal Cord
  Cervical ØØ9W
  Lumbar ØØ9Y
  Thoracic ØØ9X

Drainage (Continued)
Spinal Meninges ØØ9T
Spleen Ø79P
Sternum ØP90
Stomach ØD96
  Pylorus ØD97
Subarachnoid Space ØØ95
▶ Subarachnoid Space, Intracranial ØØ95
Subcutaneous Tissue and Fascia
  Abdomen ØJ98
  Back ØJ97
  Buttock ØJ99
  Chest ØJ96
  Face ØJ91
  Foot
    Left ØJ9R
    Right ØJ9Q
  Hand
    Left ØJ9K
    Right ØJ9J
  Lower Arm
    Left ØJ9H
    Right ØJ9G
  Lower Leg
    Left ØJ9P
    Right ØJ9N
  Neck
    Anterior ØJ94
    Posterior ØJ95
    ▶ Left ØJ95
    ▶ Right ØJ94
  Pelvic Region ØJ9C
  Perineum ØJ9B
  Scalp ØJ90
  Upper Arm
    Left ØJ9F
    Right ØJ9D
  Upper Leg
    Left ØJ9M
    Right ØJ9L
Subdural Space ØØ94
▶ Subdural Space, Intracranial ØØ94
Tarsal
  Left ØQ9M
  Right ØQ9L
Tendon
  Abdomen
    Left ØL9G
    Right ØL9F
  Ankle
    Left ØL9T
    Right ØL9S
  Foot
    Left ØL9W
    Right ØL9V
  Hand
    Left ØL98
    Right ØL97
  Head and Neck ØL90
  Hip
    Left ØL9K
    Right ØL9J
  Knee
    Left ØL9R
    Right ØL9Q
  Lower Arm and Wrist
    Left ØL96
    Right ØL95
  Lower Leg
    Left ØL9P
    Right ØL9N
  Perineum ØL9H
  Shoulder
    Left ØL92
    Right ØL91
  Thorax
    Left ØL9D
    Right ØL9C
  Trunk
    Left ØL9B
    Right ØL99

Drainage (Continued)
Tendon (Continued)
  Upper Arm
    Left ØL94
    Right ØL93
  Upper Leg
    Left ØL9M
    Right ØL9L
Testis
  Bilateral ØV9C
  Left ØV9B
  Right ØV99
Thalamus ØØ99
Thymus Ø79M
Thyroid Gland ØG9K
  Left Lobe ØG9G
  Right Lobe ØG9H
Tibia
  Left ØQ9H
  Right ØQ9G
Toe Nail ØH9R
Tongue ØC97
Tonsils ØC9P
Tooth
  Lower ØC9X
  Upper ØC9W
Trachea ØB91
Tunica Vaginalis
  Left ØV97
  Right ØV96
Turbinate, Nasal Ø99L
Tympanic Membrane
  Left Ø998
  Right Ø997
Ulna
  Left ØP9L
  Right ØP9K
Ureter
  Left ØT97
  Right ØT96
Ureters, Bilateral ØT98
Urethra ØT9D
Uterine Supporting Structure ØU94
Uterus ØU99
Uvula ØC9N
Vagina ØU9G
Vas Deferens
  Bilateral ØV9Q
  Left ØV9P
  Right ØV9N
Vein
  Axillary
    Left Ø598
    Right Ø597
  Azygos Ø590
  Basilic
    Left Ø59C
    Right Ø59B
  Brachial
    Left Ø59A
    Right Ø599
  Cephalic
    Left Ø59F
    Right Ø59D
  Colic Ø697
  Common Iliac
    Left Ø69D
    Right Ø69C
  Esophageal Ø693
  External Iliac
    Left Ø69G
    Right Ø69F
  External Jugular
    Left Ø59Q
    Right Ø59P
  Face
    Left Ø59V
    Right Ø59T
  Femoral
    Left Ø69N
    Right Ø69M

▶ New   ⇒ Revised   ~~deleted~~ Deleted

Drainage *(Continued)*
Vein *(Continued)*
Foot
Left 069V
Right 069T
Gastric 0692
Greater Saphenous
Left 069Q
Right 069P
Hand
Left 059H
Right 059G
Hemiazygos 0591
Hepatic 0694
Hypogastric
Left 069J
Right 069H
Inferior Mesenteric 0696
Innominate
Left 0594
Right 0593
Internal Jugular
Left 059N
Right 059M
Intracranial 059L
Lesser Saphenous
Left 069S
Right 069R
Lower 069Y
Portal 0698
Renal
Left 069B
Right 0699
▶Saphenous
▶Left 069Q
▶Right 069P
Splenic 0691
Subclavian
Left 0596
Right 0595
Superior Mesenteric 0695
Upper 059Y
Vertebral
Left 059S
Right 059R
Vena Cava, Inferior 0690
Vertebra
Cervical 0P93
Lumbar 0Q90
Thoracic 0P94
Vesicle
Bilateral 0V93
Left 0V92
Right 0V91

Drainage *(Continued)*
Vitreous
Left 0895
Right 0894
Vocal Cord
Left 0C9V
Right 0C9T
Vulva 0U9M
Wrist Region
Left 0X9H
Right 0X9G
Dressing
Abdominal Wall 2W23X4Z
Arm
Lower
Left 2W2DX4Z
Right 2W2CX4Z
Upper
Left 2W2BX4Z
Right 2W2AX4Z
Back 2W25X4Z
Chest Wall 2W24X4Z
Extremity
Lower
Left 2W2MX4Z
Right 2W2LX4Z
Upper
Left 2W29X4Z
Right 2W28X4Z
Face 2W21X4Z
Finger
Left 2W2KX4Z
Right 2W2JX4Z
Foot
Left 2W2TX4Z
Right 2W2SX4Z
Hand
Left 2W2FX4Z
Right 2W2EX4Z
Head 2W20X4Z
Inguinal Region
Left 2W27X4Z
Right 2W26X4Z
Leg
Lower
Left 2W2RX4Z
Right 2W2QX4Z
Upper
Left 2W2PX4Z
Right 2W2NX4Z
Neck 2W22X4Z
Thumb
Left 2W2HX4Z
Right 2W2GX4Z

Dressing *(Continued)*
Toe
Left 2W2VX4Z
Right 2W2UX4Z
Driver stent (RX) (OTW) *use* Intraluminal
Device
Drotrecogin alfa *see* Introduction of
Recombinant Human-activated Protein C
Duct of Santorini *use* Duct, Pancreatic,
Accessory
Duct of Wirsung *use* Duct, Pancreatic
Ductogram, mammary *see* Plain Radiography,
Skin, Subcutaneous Tissue and Breast BH0
Ductography, mammary *see* Plain Radiography,
Skin, Subcutaneous Tissue and Breast BH0
Ductus deferens
use Vas Deferens, Right
use Vas Deferens, Left
use Vas Deferens, Bilateral
use Vas Deferens
Duodenal ampulla *use* Ampulla of Vater
Duodenectomy
see Excision, Duodenum 0DB9
see Resection, Duodenum 0DT9
Duodenocholedochotomy *see* Drainage,
Gallbladder 0F94
Duodenocystostomy
see Bypass, Gallbladder 0F14
see Drainage, Gallbladder 0F94
Duodenoenterostomy
see Bypass, Gastrointestinal System 0D1
see Drainage, Gastrointestinal System 0D9
Duodenojejunal flexure *use* Jejunum
Duodenolysis *see* Release, Duodenum 0DN9
Duodenorrhaphy *see* Repair, Duodenum 0DQ9
Duodenostomy
see Bypass, Duodenum 0D19
see Drainage, Duodenum 0D99
Duodenotomy *see* Drainage, Duodenum 0D99
▶**DuraGraft® Endothelial Damage Inhibitor** *use*
Endothelial Damage Inhibitor
DuraHeart Left Ventricular Assist System *use*
Implantable Heart Assist System in Heart
and Great Vessels
Dural venous sinus *use* Vein, Intracranial
Dura mater, intracranial *use* Dura Mater
Dura mater, spinal *use* Spinal Meninges
Durata® Defibrillation Lead *use* Cardiac Lead,
Defibrillator in 02H
Dynesys® Dynamic Stabilization System
use Spinal Stabilization Device, Pedicle-Based
in 0RH
use Spinal Stabilization Device, Pedicle-Based
in 0SH

E

E-Luminexx™ (Biliary) (Vascular) Stent *use*
Intraluminal Device
Earlobe
use External Ear, Right
use External Ear, Left
use External Ear, Bilateral
▶**ECCO2R (Extracorporeal Carbon Dioxide
Removal)** 5A0920Z
Echocardiogram *see* Ultrasonography, Heart
B24
Echography *see* Ultrasonography
ECMO *see* Performance, Circulatory 5A15
EDWARDS INTUITY Elite valve system *use*
Zooplastic Tissue, Rapid Deployment
Technique in New Technology
EEG (electroencephalogram) *see* Measurement,
Central Nervous 4A00
EGD (esophagogastroduodenoscopy)
0DJ08ZZ
Eighth cranial nerve *use* Acoustic Nerve
Ejaculatory duct
use Vas Deferens, Right
use Vas Deferens, Left
use Vas Deferens, Bilateral
use Vas Deferens
EKG (electrocardiogram) *see* Measurement,
Cardiac 4A02
Electrical bone growth stimulator (EBGS)
use Bone Growth Stimulator in Head and
Facial Bones
use Bone Growth Stimulator in Upper Bones
use Bone Growth Stimulator in Lower Bones
Electrical muscle stimulation (EMS) lead *use*
Stimulator Lead in Muscles
Electrocautery
Destruction *see* Destruction
Repair *see* Repair
Electroconvulsive Therapy
Bilateral-Multiple Seizure GZB3ZZZ
Bilateral-Single Seizure GZB2ZZZ
Electroconvulsive Therapy, Other GZB4ZZZ
Unilateral-Multiple Seizure GZB1ZZZ
Unilateral-Single Seizure GZB0ZZZ
Electroencephalogram (EEG) *see* Measurement,
Central Nervous 4A00
Electromagnetic Therapy
Central Nervous 6A22
Urinary 6A21
Electronic muscle stimulator lead *use*
Stimulator Lead in Muscles
Electrophysiologic stimulation (EPS) *see*
Measurement, Cardiac 4A02
Electroshock therapy *see* Electroconvulsive
Therapy
Elevation, bone fragments, skull *see*
Reposition, Head and Facial Bones 0NS
Eleventh cranial nerve *use* Accessory Nerve
Embolectomy *see* Extirpation
Embolization
see Occlusion
see Restriction
Embolization coil(s) *use* Intraluminal Device
EMG (electromyogram) *see* Measurement,
Musculoskeletal 4A0F
Encephalon *use* Brain
Endarterectomy
see Extirpation, Upper Arteries 03C
see Extirpation, Lower Arteries 04C
**Endeavor® (III) (IV) (Sprint) Zotarolimus-
eluting Coronary Stent System** *use*
Intraluminal Device, Drug-eluting in Heart
and Great Vessels
Endologix AFX® Endovascular AAA System
use Intraluminal Device
EndoSure® sensor *use* Monitoring Device,
Pressure Sensor in 02H
**ENDOTAK RELIANCE® (G) Defibrillation
Lead** *use* Cardiac Lead, Defibrillator in
02H

▶**Endothelial damage inhibitor, applied to vein
graft** XY0VX83
Endotracheal tube (cuffed) (double-lumen)
use Intraluminal Device, Endotracheal
Airway in Respiratory System
Endurant® Endovascular Stent Graft *use*
Intraluminal Device
Endurant® II AAA stent graft system *use*
Intraluminal Device
▶**Engineered Autologous Chimeric Antigen
Receptor T-cell Immunotherapy** XW0
Enlargement
see Dilation
see Repair
EnRhythm *use* Pacemaker, Dual Chamber in 0JH
Enterorrhaphy *see* Repair, Gastrointestinal
System 0DQ
Enterra gastric neurostimulator *use* Stimulator
Generator, Multiple Array in 0JH
Enucleation
Eyeball *see* Resection, Eye 08T
Eyeball with prosthetic implant *see*
Replacement, Eye 08R
Ependyma *use* Cerebral Ventricle
Epic™ Stented Tissue Valve (aortic) *use*
Zooplastic Tissue in Heart and Great Vessels
Epicel® cultured epidermal autograft *use*
Autologous Tissue Substitute
Epidermis *use* Skin
Epididymectomy
see Excision, Male Reproductive System 0VB
see Resection, Male Reproductive System
0VT
Epididymoplasty
see Repair, Male Reproductive System 0VQ
see Supplement, Male Reproductive System
0VU
Epididymorrhaphy *see* Repair, Male
Reproductive System 0VQ
Epididymotomy *see* Drainage, Male
Reproductive System 0V9
Epidural space, intracranial use Epidural Space
Epidural space, spinal *use* **Spinal Canal**
Epiphysiodesis
see Fusion, Upper Joints 0RG
see Fusion, Lower Joints 0SG
▶*see* Insertion of device in, Upper Bones 0PH
▶*see* Repair, Upper Bones 0PQ
▶*see* Insertion of device in, Lower Bones 0QH
▶*see* Repair, Lower Bones 0QQ
Epiploic foramen *use* Peritoneum
Epiretinal Visual Prosthesis
Left 08H105Z
Right 08H005Z
Episiorrhaphy *see* Repair, Perineum, Female
0WQN
Episiotomy *see* Division, Perineum, Female
0W8N
Epithalamus *use* Thalamus
Epitroclear lymph node
use Lymphatic, Right Upper Extremity
use Lymphatic, Left Upper Extremity
EPS (electrophysiologic stimulation) *see*
Measurement, Cardiac 4A02
Eptifibatide, infusion *see* Introduction of
Platelet Inhibitor
**ERCP (endoscopic retrograde
cholangiopancreatography)** *see* Fluoroscopy,
Hepatobiliary System and Pancreas BF1
Erector spinae muscle
use Trunk Muscle, Right
use Trunk Muscle, Left
Esophageal artery *use* Upper Artery
Esophageal obturator airway (EOA)
use Intraluminal Device, Airway in
Gastrointestinal System
Esophageal plexus *use* Thoracic Sympathetic
Nerve
Esophagectomy
see Excision, Gastrointestinal System 0DB
see Resection, Gastrointestinal System 0DT

Esophagocoloplasty
see Repair, Gastrointestinal System 0DQ
see Supplement, Gastrointestinal System 0DU
Esophagoenterostomy
see Bypass, Gastrointestinal System 0D1
see Drainage, Gastrointestinal System 0D9
Esophagoesophagostomy
see Bypass, Gastrointestinal System 0D1
see Drainage, Gastrointestinal System 0D9
Esophagogastrectomy
see Excision, Gastrointestinal System 0DB
see Resection, Gastrointestinal System 0DT
Esophagogastroduodenoscopy (EGD)
0DJ08ZZ
Esophagogastroplasty
see Repair, Gastrointestinal System 0DQ
see Supplement, Gastrointestinal System 0DU
Esophagogastroscopy 0DJ68ZZ
Esophagogastrostomy
see Bypass, Gastrointestinal System 0D1
see Drainage, Gastrointestinal System 0D9
Esophagojejunoplasty *see* Supplement,
Gastrointestinal System 0DU
Esophagojejunostomy
see Bypass, Gastrointestinal System 0D1
see Drainage, Gastrointestinal System 0D9
Esophagomyotomy *see* Division,
Esophagogastric Junction 0D84
Esophagoplasty
see Repair, Gastrointestinal System 0DQ
see Replacement, Esophagus 0DR5
see Supplement, Gastrointestinal System
0DU
Esophagoplication *see* Restriction,
Gastrointestinal System 0DV
Esophagorrhaphy *see* Repair, Gastrointestinal
System 0DQ
Esophagoscopy 0DJ08ZZ
Esophagotomy *see* Drainage, Gastrointestinal
System 0D9
Esteem® implantable hearing system *use*
Hearing Device in Ear, Nose, Sinus
ESWL (extracorporeal shock wave lithotripsy)
see Fragmentation
Ethmoidal air cell
use Ethmoid Sinus, Right
use Ethmoid Sinus, Left
Ethmoidectomy
see Excision, Ear, Nose, Sinus 09B
see Resection, Ear, Nose, Sinus 09T
see Excision, Head and Facial Bones 0NB
see Resection, Head and Facial Bones 0NT
Ethmoidotomy *see* Drainage, Ear, Nose, Sinus
099
Evacuation
Hematoma *see* Extirpation
Other Fluid *see* Drainage
Evera (XT)(S)(DR/VR) *use* Defibrillator
Generator in 0JH
Everolimus-eluting coronary stent *use*
Intraluminal Device, Drug-eluting in Heart
and Great Vessels
Evisceration
Eyeball *see* Resection, Eye 08T
Eyeball with prosthetic implant *see*
Replacement, Eye 08R
Ex-PRESS™ mini glaucoma shunt *use* Synthetic
Substitute
Examination *see* Inspection
Exchange *see* Change device in
Excision
Abdominal Wall 0WBF
Acetabulum
Left 0QB5
Right 0QB4
Adenoids 0CBQ
Ampulla of Vater 0FBC
Anal Sphincter 0DBR
Ankle Region
Left 0YBL
Right 0YBK

▶ New   ➡ Revised   ~~deleted~~ Deleted

Excision (*Continued*)
Anus 0DBQ
Aorta
  Abdominal 04B0
  Thoracic
    Ascending/Arch 02BX
    Descending 02BW
Aortic Body 0GBD
Appendix 0DBJ
Arm
  Lower
    Left 0XBF
    Right 0XBD
  Upper
    Left 0XB9
    Right 0XB8
Artery
  Anterior Tibial
    Left 04BQ
    Right 04BP
  Axillary
    Left 03B6
    Right 03B5
  Brachial
    Left 03B8
    Right 03B7
  Celiac 04B1
  Colic
    Left 04B7
    Middle 04B8
    Right 04B6
  Common Carotid
    Left 03BJ
    Right 03BH
  Common Iliac
    Left 04BD
    Right 04BC
  External Carotid
    Left 03BN
    Right 03BM
  External Iliac
    Left 04BJ
    Right 04BH
  Face 03BR
  Femoral
    Left 04BL
    Right 04BK
  Foot
    Left 04BW
    Right 04BV
  Gastric 04B2
  Hand
    Left 03BF
    Right 03BD
  Hepatic 04B3
  Inferior Mesenteric 04BB
  Innominate 03B2
  Internal Carotid
    Left 03BL
    Right 03BK
  Internal Iliac
    Left 04BF
    Right 04BE
  Internal Mammary
    Left 03B1
    Right 03B0
  Intracranial 03BG
  Lower 04BY
  Peroneal
    Left 04BU
    Right 04BT
  Popliteal
    Left 04BN
    Right 04BM
  Posterior Tibial
    Left 04BS
    Right 04BR
  Pulmonary
    Left 02BR
    Right 02BQ
  Pulmonary Trunk 02BP

Excision (*Continued*)
Artery (*Continued*)
  Radial
    Left 03BC
    Right 03BB
  Renal
    Left 04BA
    Right 04B9
  Splenic 04B4
  Subclavian
    Left 03B4
    Right 03B3
  Superior Mesenteric 04B5
  Temporal
    Left 03BT
    Right 03BS
  Thyroid
    Left 03BV
    Right 03BU
  Ulnar
    Left 03BA
    Right 03B9
  Upper 03BY
  Vertebral
    Left 03BQ
    Right 03BP
Atrium
  Left 02B7
  Right 02B6
Auditory Ossicle
  ➠Left 09BA
  ➠Right 09B9
Axilla
  Left 0XB5
  Right 0XB4
Back
  Lower 0WBL
  Upper 0WBK
Basal Ganglia 00B8
Bladder 0TBB
Bladder Neck 0TBC
Bone
  Ethmoid
    Left 0NBG
    Right 0NBF
  ➠Frontal 0NB1
    ~~Left 0NB2~~
    ~~Right 0NB1~~
  Hyoid 0NBX
  Lacrimal
    Left 0NBJ
    Right 0NBH
  Nasal 0NBB
  ➠Occipital 0NB7
    ~~Left 0NB8~~
    ~~Right 0NB7~~
  Palatine
    Left 0NBL
    Right 0NBK
  Parietal
    Left 0NB4
    Right 0NB3
  Pelvic
    Left 0QB3
    Right 0QB2
  ➠Sphenoid 0NBC
    ~~Left 0NBD~~
    ~~Right 0NBC~~
  Temporal
    Left 0NB6
    Right 0NB5
  Zygomatic
    Left 0NBN
    Right 0NBM
Brain 00B0
Breast
  Bilateral 0HBV
  Left 0HBU
  Right 0HBT
  Supernumerary 0HBY

Excision (*Continued*)
Bronchus
  Lingula 0BB9
  Lower Lobe
    Left 0BBB
    Right 0BB6
  Main
    Left 0BB7
    Right 0BB3
  Middle Lobe, Right 0BB5
  Upper Lobe
    Left 0BB8
    Right 0BB4
Buccal Mucosa 0CB4
Bursa and Ligament
  Abdomen
    Left 0MBJ
    Right 0MBH
  Ankle
    Left 0MBR
    Right 0MBQ
  Elbow
    Left 0MB4
    Right 0MB3
  Foot
    Left 0MBT
    Right 0MBS
  Hand
    Left 0MB8
    Right 0MB7
  Head and Neck 0MB0
  Hip
    Left 0MBM
    Right 0MBL
  Knee
    Left 0MBP
    Right 0MBN
  Lower Extremity
    Left 0MBW
    Right 0MBV
  Perineum 0MBK
  ▶Rib(s) 0MBG
  Shoulder
    Left 0MB2
    Right 0MB1
  ▶Spine
    ▶Lower 0MBD
    ▶Upper 0MBC
  ▶Sternum 0MBF
  ~~Thorax~~
    ~~Left 0MBG~~
    ~~Right 0MBF~~
  ~~Trunk~~
    ~~Left 0MBD~~
    ~~Right 0MBC~~
  Upper Extremity
    Left 0MBB
    Right 0MB9
  Wrist
    Left 0MB6
    Right 0MB5
Buttock
  Left 0YB1
  Right 0YB0
Carina 0BB2
Carotid Bodies, Bilateral 0GB8
Carotid Body
  Left 0GB6
  Right 0GB7
Carpal
  Left 0PBN
  Right 0PBM
Cecum 0DBH
Cerebellum 00BC
Cerebral Hemisphere 00B7
Cerebral Meninges 00B1
Cerebral Ventricle 00B6
Cervix 0UBC
Chest Wall 0WB8
Chordae Tendineae 02B9

Excision (*Continued*)
Choroid
    Left 08BB
    Right 08BA
Cisterna Chyli 07BL
Clavicle
    Left 0PBB
    Right 0PB9
Clitoris 0UBJ
Coccygeal Glomus 0GBB
Coccyx 0QBS
Colon
    Ascending 0DBK
    Descending 0DBM
    Sigmoid 0DBN
    Transverse 0DBL
Conduction Mechanism 02B8
Conjunctiva
    Left 08BTXZ
    Right 08BSXZ
Cord
    Bilateral 0VBH
    Left 0VBG
    Right 0VBF
Cornea
    Left 08B9XZ
    Right 08B8XZ
Cul-de-sac 0UBF
➡ Diaphragm 0BBT
    ~~Left 0BBS~~
    ~~Right 0BBR~~
Disc
    Cervical Vertebral 0RB3
    Cervicothoracic Vertebral 0RB5
    Lumbar Vertebral 0SB2
    Lumbosacral 0SB4
    Thoracic Vertebral 0RB9
    Thoracolumbar Vertebral 0RBB
Duct
    Common Bile 0FB9
    Cystic 0FB8
    Hepatic
    ▶ Common 0FB7
        Left 0FB6
        Right 0FB5
    Lacrimal
        Left 08BY
        Right 08BX
    Pancreatic 0FBD
        Accessory 0FBF
    Parotid
        Left 0CBC
        Right 0CBB
Duodenum 0DB9
Dura Mater 00B2
Ear
    External
        Left 09B1
        Right 09B0
    External Auditory Canal
        Left 09B4
        Right 09B3
    Inner
    ➡ Left 09BE
    ➡ Right 09BD
    Middle
    ➡ Left 09B6
    ➡ Right 09B5
Elbow Region
    Left 0XBC
    Right 0XBB
Epididymis
    Bilateral 0VBL
    Left 0VBK
    Right 0VBJ
Epiglottis 0CBR
Esophagogastric Junction 0DB4
Esophagus 0DB5
    Lower 0DB3
    Middle 0DB2
    Upper 0DB1

Excision (*Continued*)
Eustachian Tube
    Left 09BG
    Right 09BF
Extremity
    Lower
        Left 0YBB
        Right 0YB9
    Upper
        Left 0XB7
        Right 0XB6
Eye
    Left 08B1
    Right 08B0
Eyelid
    Lower
        Left 08BR
        Right 08BQ
    Upper
        Left 08BP
        Right 08BN
Face 0WB2
Fallopian Tube
    Left 0UB6
    Right 0UB5
Fallopian Tubes, Bilateral 0UB7
Femoral Region
    Left 0YB8
    Right 0YB7
Femoral Shaft
    Left 0QB9
    Right 0QB8
Femur
    Lower
        Left 0QBC
        Right 0QBB
    Upper
        Left 0QB7
        Right 0QB6
Fibula
    Left 0QBK
    Right 0QBJ
Finger Nail 0HBQXZ
▶ Floor of mouth *see* Excision, Oral Cavity and
        Throat 0WB3
Foot
    Left 0YBN
    Right 0YBM
Gallbladder 0FB4
Gingiva
    Lower 0CB6
    Upper 0CB5
Gland
    Adrenal
        Bilateral 0GB4
        Left 0GB2
        Right 0GB3
    Lacrimal
        Left 08BW
        Right 08BV
    Minor Salivary 0CBJ
    Parotid
        Left 0CB9
        Right 0CB8
    Pituitary 0GB0
    Sublingual
        Left 0CBF
        Right 0CBD
    Submaxillary
        Left 0CBH
        Right 0CBG
    Vestibular 0UBL
Glenoid Cavity
    Left 0PB8
    Right 0PB7
Glomus Jugulare 0GBC
Hand
    Left 0XBK
    Right 0XBJ
Head 0WB0
Humeral Head
    Left 0PBD
    Right 0PBC

Excision (*Continued*)
Humeral Shaft
    Left 0PBG
    Right 0PBF
Hymen 0UBK
Hypothalamus 00BA
Ileocecal Valve 0DBC
Ileum 0DBB
Inguinal Region
    Left 0YB6
    Right 0YB5
Intestine
    Large 0DBE
        Left 0DBG
        Right 0DBF
    Small 0DB8
Iris
    Left 08BD3Z
    Right 08BC3Z
Jaw
    Lower 0WB5
    Upper 0WB4
Jejunum 0DBA
Joint
    Acromioclavicular
        Left 0RBH
        Right 0RBG
    Ankle
        Left 0SBG
        Right 0SBF
    Carpal
        Left 0RBR
        Right 0RBQ
    ▶ Carpometacarpal
        ▶ Left 0RBT
        ▶ Right 0RBS
    Cervical Vertebral 0RB1
    Cervicothoracic Vertebral 0RB4
    Coccygeal 0SB6
    Elbow
        Left 0RBM
        Right 0RBL
    Finger Phalangeal
        Left 0RBX
        Right 0RBW
    Hip
        Left 0SBB
        Right 0SB9
    Knee
        Left 0SBD
        Right 0SBC
    Lumbar Vertebral 0SB0
    Lumbosacral 0SB3
    ~~Metacarpocarpal~~
        ~~Left 0RBT~~
        ~~Right 0RBS~~
    Metacarpophalangeal
        Left 0RBV
        Right 0RBU
    Metatarsal-Phalangeal
        Left 0SBN
        Right 0SBM
    ~~Metatarsal-Tarsal~~
        ~~Left 0SBL~~
        ~~Right 0SBK~~
    Occipital-cervical 0RB0
    Sacrococcygeal 0SB5
    Sacroiliac
        Left 0SB8
        Right 0SB7
    Shoulder
        Left 0RBK
        Right 0RBJ
    Sternoclavicular
        Left 0RBF
        Right 0RBE
    Tarsal
        Left 0SBJ
        Right 0SBH
    ▶ Tarsometatarsal
        ▶ Left 0SBL
        ▶ Right 0SBK

▶ New   ➡ Revised   ~~deleted~~ Deleted

Excision (*Continued*)
Joint (*Continued*)
 Temporomandibular
  Left 0RBD
  Right 0RBC
 Thoracic Vertebral 0RB6
 Thoracolumbar Vertebral 0RBA
 Toe Phalangeal
  Left 0SBQ
  Right 0SBP
 Wrist
  Left 0RBP
  Right 0RBN
Kidney
 Left 0TB1
 Right 0TB0
Kidney Pelvis
 Left 0TB4
 Right 0TB3
Knee Region
 Left 0YBG
 Right 0YBF
Larynx 0CBS
Leg
 Lower
  Left 0YBJ
  Right 0YBH
 Upper
  Left 0YBD
  Right 0YBC
Lens
 Left 08BK3Z
 Right 08BJ3Z
Lip
 Lower 0CB1
 Upper 0CB0
Liver 0FB0
 Left Lobe 0FB2
 Right Lobe 0FB1
Lung
 Bilateral 0BBM
 Left 0BBL
 Lower Lobe
  Left 0BBJ
  Right 0BBF
 Middle Lobe, Right 0BBD
 Right 0BBK
 Upper Lobe
  Left 0BBG
  Right 0BBC
Lung Lingula 0BBH
Lymphatic
 Aortic 07BD
 Axillary
  Left 07B6
  Right 07B5
 Head 07B0
 Inguinal
  Left 07BJ
  Right 07BH
 Internal Mammary
  Left 07B9
  Right 07B8
 Lower Extremity
  Left 07BG
  Right 07BF
 Mesenteric 07BB
 Neck
  Left 07B2
  Right 07B1
 Pelvis 07BC
 Thoracic Duct 07BK
 Thorax 07B7
 Upper Extremity
  Left 07B4
  Right 07B3
Mandible
 Left 0NBV
 Right 0NBT
➡Maxilla 0NBR
 ~~Left 0NBS~~
 ~~Right 0NBR~~

Excision (*Continued*)
Mediastinum 0WBC
Medulla Oblongata 00BD
Mesentery 0DBV
Metacarpal
 Left 0PBQ
 Right 0PBP
Metatarsal
 Left 0QBP
 Right 0QBN
Muscle
 Abdomen
  Left 0KBL
  Right 0KBK
 Extraocular
  Left 08BM
  Right 08BL
 Facial 0KB1
 Foot
  Left 0KBW
  Right 0KBV
 Hand
  Left 0KBD
  Right 0KBC
 Head 0KB0
 Hip
  Left 0KBP
  Right 0KBN
 Lower Arm and Wrist
  Left 0KBB
  Right 0KB9
 Lower Leg
  Left 0KBT
  Right 0KBS
 Neck
  Left 0KB3
  Right 0KB2
 Papillary 02BD
 Perineum 0KBM
 Shoulder
  Left 0KB6
  Right 0KB5
 Thorax
  Left 0KBJ
  Right 0KBH
 Tongue, Palate, Pharynx 0KB4
 Trunk
  Left 0KBG
  Right 0KBF
 Upper Arm
  Left 0KB8
  Right 0KB7
 Upper Leg
  Left 0KBR
  Right 0KBQ
▶Nasal Mucosa and Soft Tissue 09BK
Nasopharynx 09BN
Neck 0WB6
Nerve
 Abdominal Sympathetic 01BM
 Abducens 00BL
 Accessory 00BR
 Acoustic 00BN
 Brachial Plexus 01B3
 Cervical 01B1
 Cervical Plexus 01B0
 Facial 00BM
 Femoral 01BD
 Glossopharyngeal 00BP
 Head and Neck Sympathetic 01BK
 Hypoglossal 00BS
 Lumbar 01BB
 Lumbar Plexus 01B9
 Lumbar Sympathetic 01BN
 Lumbosacral Plexus 01BA
 Median 01B5
 Oculomotor 00BH
 Olfactory 00BF
 Optic 00BG
 Peroneal 01BH
 Phrenic 01B2

Excision (*Continued*)
Nerve (*Continued*)
 Pudendal 01BC
 Radial 01B6
 Sacral 01BR
 Sacral Plexus 01BQ
 Sacral Sympathetic 01BP
 Sciatic 01BF
 Thoracic 01B8
 Thoracic Sympathetic 01BL
 Tibial 01BG
 Trigeminal 00BK
 Trochlear 00BJ
 Ulnar 01B4
 Vagus 00BQ
Nipple
 Left 0HBX
 Right 0HBW
~~Nose 09BK~~
➡Omentum 0DBU
 ~~Greater 0DBS~~
 ~~Lesser 0DBT~~
▶Oral Cavity and Throat 0WB3
Orbit
 Left 0NBQ
 Right 0NBP
Ovary
 Bilateral 0UB2
 Left 0UB1
 Right 0UB0
Palate
 Hard 0CB2
 Soft 0CB3
Pancreas 0FBG
Para-aortic Body 0GB9
Paraganglion Extremity 0GBF
Parathyroid Gland 0GBR
 Inferior
  Left 0GBP
  Right 0GBN
 Multiple 0GBQ
 Superior
  Left 0GBM
  Right 0GBL
Patella
 Left 0QBF
 Right 0QBD
Penis 0VBS
Pericardium 02BN
Perineum
 Female 0WBN
 Male 0WBM
Peritoneum 0DBW
Phalanx
 Finger
  Left 0PBV
  Right 0PBT
 Thumb
  Left 0PBS
  Right 0PBR
 Toe
  Left 0QBR
  Right 0QBQ
Pharynx 0CBM
Pineal Body 0GB1
Pleura
 Left 0BBP
 Right 0BBN
Pons 00BB
Prepuce 0VBT
Prostate 0VB0
Radius
 Left 0PBJ
 Right 0PBH
Rectum 0DBP
Retina
 Left 08BF3Z
 Right 08BE3Z
Retroperitoneum 0WBH
~~Rib~~
 ~~Left 0PB2~~
 ~~Right 0PB1~~

Excision *(Continued)*
▶ Ribs
  ▶ 1 to 2 0PB1
  ▶ 3 or More 0PB2
Sacrum 0QB1
Scapula
  Left 0PB6
  Right 0PB5
Sclera
  Left 08B7XZ
  Right 08B6XZ
Scrotum 0VB5
Septum
  Atrial 02B5
  Nasal 09BM
  Ventricular 02BM
Shoulder Region
  Left 0XB3
  Right 0XB2
Sinus
  Accessory 09BP
  Ethmoid
    Left 09BV
    Right 09BU
  Frontal
    Left 09BT
    Right 09BS
  Mastoid
    Left 09BC
    Right 09BB
  Maxillary
    Left 09BR
    Right 09BQ
  Sphenoid
    Left 09BX
    Right 09BW
Skin
  Abdomen 0HB7XZ
  Back 0HB6XZ
  Buttock 0HB8XZ
  Chest 0HB5XZ
  Ear
    Left 0HB3XZ
    Right 0HB2XZ
  Face 0HB1XZ
  Foot
    Left 0HBNXZ
    Right 0HBMXZ
  ~~Genitalia 0HBAXZ~~
  Hand
    Left 0HBGXZ
    Right 0HBFXZ
  ▶ Inguinal 0HBAXZ
  Lower Arm
    Left 0HBEXZ
    Right 0HBDXZ
  Lower Leg
    Left 0HBLXZ
    Right 0HBKXZ
  Neck 0HB4XZ
  Perineum 0HB9XZ
  Scalp 0HB0XZ
  Upper Arm
    Left 0HBCXZ
    Right 0HBBXZ
  Upper Leg
    Left 0HBJXZ
    Right 0HBHXZ
Skull 0NB0
Spinal Cord
  Cervical 00BW
  Lumbar 00BY
  Thoracic 00BX
Spinal Meninges 00BT
Spleen 07BP
Sternum 0PB0
Stomach 0DB6
  Pylorus 0DB7
Subcutaneous Tissue and Fascia
  Abdomen 0JB8
  Back 0JB7

Excision *(Continued)*
Subcutaneous Tissue and Fascia *(Continued)*
  Buttock 0JB9
  Chest 0JB6
  Face 0JB1
  Foot
    Left 0JBR
    Right 0JBQ
  Hand
    Left 0JBK
    Right 0JBJ
  Lower Arm
    Left 0JBH
    Right 0JBG
  Lower Leg
    Left 0JBP
    Right 0JBN
  Neck
    ~~Anterior 0JB4~~
    ~~Posterior 0JB5~~
  ▶ Left 06B5
  ▶ Right 06B4
  Pelvic Region 0JBC
  Perineum 0JBB
  Scalp 0JB0
  Upper Arm
    Left 0JBF
    Right 0JBD
  Upper Leg
    Left 0JBM
    Right 0JBL
Tarsal
  Left 0QBM
  Right 0QBL
Tendon
  Abdomen
    Left 0LBG
    Right 0LBF
  Ankle
    Left 0LBT
    Right 0LBS
  Foot
    Left 0LBW
    Right 0LBV
  Hand
    Left 0LB8
    Right 0LB7
  Head and Neck 0LB0
  Hip
    Left 0LBK
    Right 0LBJ
  Knee
    Left 0LBR
    Right 0LBQ
  Lower Arm and Wrist
    Left 0LB6
    Right 0LB5
  Lower Leg
    Left 0LBP
    Right 0LBN
  Perineum 0LBH
  Shoulder
    Left 0LB2
    Right 0LB1
  Thorax
    Left 0LBD
    Right 0LBC
  Trunk
    Left 0LBB
    Right 0LB9
  Upper Arm
    Left 0LB4
    Right 0LB3
  Upper Leg
    Left 0LBM
    Right 0LBL
Testis
  Bilateral 0VBC
  Left 0VBB
  Right 0VB9
Thalamus 00B9
Thymus 07BM

Excision *(Continued)*
Thyroid Gland
  Left Lobe 0GBG
  Right Lobe 0GBH
▶ Thyroid Gland Isthmus 0GBJ
Tibia
  Left 0QBH
  Right 0QBG
Toe Nail 0HBRXZ
Tongue 0CB7
Tonsils 0CBP
Tooth
  Lower 0CBX
  Upper 0CBW
Trachea 0BB1
Tunica Vaginalis
  Left 0VB7
  Right 0VB6
Turbinate, Nasal 09BL
Tympanic Membrane
  Left 09B8
  Right 09B7
Ulna
  Left 0PBL
  Right 0PBK
Ureter
  Left 0TB7
  Right 0TB6
Urethra 0TBD
Uterine Supporting Structure 0UB4
Uterus 0UB9
Uvula 0CBN
Vagina 0UBG
Valve
  Aortic 02BF
  Mitral 02BG
  Pulmonary 02BH
  Tricuspid 02BJ
Vas Deferens
  Bilateral 0VBQ
  Left 0VBP
  Right 0VBN
Vein
  Axillary
    Left 05B8
    Right 05B7
  Azygos 05B0
  Basilic
    Left 05BC
    Right 05BB
  Brachial
    Left 05BA
    Right 05B9
  Cephalic
    Left 05BF
    Right 05BD
  Colic 06B7
  Common Iliac
    Left 06BD
    Right 06BC
  Coronary 02B4
  Esophageal 06B3
  External Iliac
    Left 06BG
    Right 06BF
  External Jugular
    Left 05BQ
    Right 05BP
  Face
    Left 05BV
    Right 05BT
  Femoral
    Left 06BN
    Right 06BM
  Foot
    Left 06BV
    Right 06BT
  Gastric 06B2
  ~~Greater Saphenous~~
    ~~Left 06BQ~~
    ~~Right 06BP~~

Excision *(Continued)*
Vein *(Continued)*
Hand
Left 05BH
Right 05BG
Hemiazygos 05B1
Hepatic 06B4
Hypogastric
Left 06BJ
Right 06BH
Inferior Mesenteric 06B6
Innominate
Left 05B4
Right 05B3
Internal Jugular
Left 05BN
Right 05BM
Intracranial 05BL
~~Lesser Saphenous~~
~~Left 06BS~~
~~Right 06BR~~
Lower 06BY
Portal 06B8
Pulmonary
Left 02BT
Right 02BS
Renal
Left 06BB
Right 06B9
▶Saphenous
▶Left 06BQ
▶Right 06BP
Splenic 06B1
Subclavian
Left 05B6
Right 05B5
Superior Mesenteric 06B5
Upper 05BY
Vertebral
Left 05BS
Right 05BR
Vena Cava
Inferior 06B0
Superior 02BV
Ventricle
Left 02BL
Right 02BK
Vertebra
Cervical 0PB3
Lumbar 0QB0
Thoracic 0PB4
Vesicle
Bilateral 0VB3
Left 0VB2
Right 0VB1
Vitreous
Left 08B53Z
Right 08B43Z
Vocal Cord
Left 0CBV
Right 0CBT
Vulva 0UBM
Wrist Region
Left 0XBH
Right 0XBG
EXCLUDER® AAA Endoprosthesis
use Intraluminal Device, Branched or
Fenestrated, One or Two Arteries in
04V
use Intraluminal Device, Branched or
Fenestrated, Three or More Arteries in
04V
use Intraluminal Device
EXCLUDER® IBE Endoprosthesis *use*
Intraluminal Device, Branched or
Fenestrated, One or Two Arteries in 04V
Exclusion, Left atrial appendage (LAA) *see*
Occlusion, Atrium, Left 02L7
Exercise, rehabilitation *see* Motor Treatment,
Rehabilitation F07
Exploration *see* Inspection

Express® (LD) Premounted Stent System *use*
Intraluminal Device
**Express® Biliary SD Monorail® Premounted
Stent System** *use* Intraluminal Device
**Express® SD Renal Monorail® Premounted
Stent System** *use* Intraluminal Device
Extensor carpi radialis muscle
use Lower Arm and Wrist Muscle, Right
use Lower Arm and Wrist Muscle, Left
Extensor carpi ulnaris muscle
use Lower Arm and Wrist Muscle, Right
use Lower Arm and Wrist Muscle, Left
Extensor digitorum brevis muscle
use Foot Muscle, Right
use Foot Muscle, Left
Extensor digitorum longus muscle
use Lower Leg Muscle, Right
use Lower Leg Muscle, Left
Extensor hallucis brevis muscle
use Foot Muscle, Right
use Foot Muscle, Left
Extensor hallucis longus muscle
use Lower Leg Muscle, Right
use Lower Leg Muscle, Left
External anal sphincter *use* Anal Sphincter
External auditory meatus
use External Auditory Canal, Right
use External Auditory Canal, Left
External fixator
use External Fixation Device in Head and
Facial Bones
use External Fixation Device in Upper Bones
use External Fixation Device in Lower Bones
use External Fixation Device in Upper Joints
use External Fixation Device in Lower Joints
External maxillary artery *use* Face Artery
➡**External naris** *use* Nasal Mucosa and Soft Tissue
External oblique aponeurosis *use*
Subcutaneous Tissue and Fascia, Trunk
External oblique muscle
use Abdomen Muscle, Right
use Abdomen Muscle, Left
External popliteal nerve *use* Peroneal
Nerve
External pudendal artery
use Femoral Artery, Right
use Femoral Artery, Left
External pudendal vein
~~use Greater Saphenous Vein, Right~~
~~use Greater Saphenous Vein, Left~~
▶*use* Saphenous Vein, Right
▶*use* Saphenous Vein, Left
External urethral sphincter *use* Urethra
Extirpation
Acetabulum
Left 0QC5
Right 0QC4
Adenoids 0CCQ
Ampulla of Vater 0FCC
Anal Sphincter 0DCR
Anterior Chamber
Left 08C3
Right 08C2
Anus 0DCQ
Aorta
Abdominal 04C0
Thoracic
Ascending/Arch 02CX
Descending 02CW
Aortic Body 0GCD
Appendix 0DCJ
Artery
Anterior Tibial
Left 04CQ
Right 04CP
Axillary
Left 03C6
Right 03C5
Brachial
Left 03C8
Right 03C7

Extirpation *(Continued)*
Artery *(Continued)*
Celiac 04C1
Colic
Left 04C7
Middle 04C8
Right 04C6
Common Carotid
Left 03CJ
Right 03CH
Common Iliac
Left 04CD
Right 04CC
Coronary
Four or More Arteries 02C3
One Artery 02C0
Three Arteries 02C2
Two Arteries 02C1
External Carotid
Left 03CN
Right 03CM
External Iliac
Left 04CJ
Right 04CH
Face 03CR
Femoral
Left 04CL
Right 04CK
Foot
Left 04CW
Right 04CV
Gastric 04C2
Hand
Left 03CF
Right 03CD
Hepatic 04C3
Inferior Mesenteric 04CB
Innominate 03C2
Internal Carotid
Left 03CL
Right 03CK
Internal Iliac
Left 04CF
Right 04CE
Internal Mammary
Left 03C1
Right 03C0
Intracranial 03CG
Lower 04CY
Peroneal
Left 04CU
Right 04CT
Popliteal
Left 04CN
Right 04CM
Posterior Tibial
Left 04CS
Right 04CR
Pulmonary
Left 02CR
Right 02CQ
Pulmonary Trunk 02CP
Radial
Left 03CC
Right 03CB
Renal
Left 04CA
Right 04C9
Splenic 04C4
Subclavian
Left 03C4
Right 03C3
Superior Mesenteric
04C5
Temporal
Left 03CT
Right 03CS
Thyroid
Left 03CV
Right 03CU

▶ New ➡ Revised ~~deleted~~ Deleted

Extirpation (Continued)
Artery (Continued)
Ulnar
Left 03CA
Right 03C9
Upper 03CY
Vertebral
Left 03CQ
Right 03CP
Atrium
Left 02C7
Right 02C6
Auditory Ossicle
➠Left 09CA
➠Right 09C9
Basal Ganglia 00C8
Bladder 0TCB
Bladder Neck 0TCC
Bone
Ethmoid
Left 0NCG
Right 0NCF
➠Frontal 0NC1
Left 0NC2
Right 0NC1
Hyoid 0NCX
Lacrimal
Left 0NCJ
Right 0NCH
Nasal 0NCB
➠Occipital 0NC7
Left 0NC8
Right 0NC7
Palatine
Left 0NCL
Right 0NCK
Parietal
Left 0NC4
Right 0NC3
Pelvic
Left 0QC3
Right 0QC2
➠Sphenoid 0NCC
Left 0NCD
Right 0NCC
Temporal
Left 0NC6
Right 0NC5
Zygomatic
Left 0NCN
Right 0NCM
Brain 00C0
Breast
Bilateral 0HCV
Left 0HCU
Right 0HCT
Bronchus
Lingula 0BC9
Lower Lobe
Left 0BCB
Right 0BC6
Main
Left 0BC7
Right 0BC3
Middle Lobe, Right 0BC5
Upper Lobe
Left 0BC8
Right 0BC4
Buccal Mucosa 0CC4
Bursa and Ligament
Abdomen
Left 0MCJ
Right 0MCH
Ankle
Left 0MCR
Right 0MCQ
Elbow
Left 0MC4
Right 0MC3
Foot
Left 0MCT
Right 0MCS

Extirpation (Continued)
Bursa and Ligament (Continued)
Hand
Left 0MC8
Right 0MC7
Head and Neck 0MC0
Hip
Left 0MCM
Right 0MCL
Knee
Left 0MCP
Right 0MCN
Lower Extremity
Left 0MCW
Right 0MCV
Perineum 0MCK
▶Rib(s) 0MCG
Shoulder
Left 0MC2
Right 0MC1
▶Spine
▶Lower 0MCD
▶Upper 0MCC
▶Sternum 0MCF
Thorax
Left 0MCG
Right 0MCF
Trunk
Left 0MCD
Right 0MCC
Upper Extremity
Left 0MCB
Right 0MC9
Wrist
Left 0MC6
Right 0MC5
Carina 0BC2
Carotid Bodies, Bilateral 0GC8
Carotid Body
Left 0GC6
Right 0GC7
Carpal
Left 0PCN
Right 0PCM
Cavity, Cranial 0WC1
Cecum 0DCH
Cerebellum 00CC
Cerebral Hemisphere 00C7
Cerebral Meninges 00C1
Cerebral Ventricle 00C6
Cervix 0UCC
Chordae Tendineae 02C9
Choroid
Left 08CB
Right 08CA
Cisterna Chyli 07CL
Clavicle
Left 0PCB
Right 0PC9
Clitoris 0UCJ
Coccygeal Glomus 0GCB
Coccyx 0QCS
Colon
Ascending 0DCK
Descending 0DCM
Sigmoid 0DCN
Transverse 0DCL
Conduction Mechanism 02C8
Conjunctiva
Left 08CTXZZ
Right 08CSXZZ
Cord
Bilateral 0VCH
Left 0VCG
Right 0VCF
Cornea
Left 08C9XZZ
Right 08C8XZZ
Cul-de-sac 0UCF
➠Diaphragm 0BCT
Left 0BCS
Right 0BCR

Extirpation (Continued)
Disc
Cervical Vertebral 0RC3
Cervicothoracic Vertebral 0RC5
Lumbar Vertebral 0SC2
Lumbosacral 0SC4
Thoracic Vertebral 0RC9
Thoracolumbar Vertebral 0RCB
Duct
Common Bile 0FC9
Cystic 0FC8
Hepatic
▶Common 0FC7
Left 0FC6
Right 0FC5
Lacrimal
Left 08CY
Right 08CX
Pancreatic 0FCD
Accessory 0FCF
Parotid
Left 0CCC
Right 0CCB
Duodenum 0DC9
Dura Mater 00C2
Ear
External
Left 09C1
Right 09C0
External Auditory Canal
Left 09C4
Right 09C3
Inner
➠Left 09CE
➠Right 09CD
Middle
➠Left 09C6
➠Right 09C5
Endometrium 0UCB
Epididymis
Bilateral 0VCL
Left 0VCK
Right 0VCJ
Epidural Space 00C3
▶Epidural Space, Intracranial 00C3
Epiglottis 0CCR
Esophagogastric Junction 0DC4
Esophagus 0DC5
Lower 0DC3
Middle 0DC2
Upper 0DC1
Eustachian Tube
Left 09CG
Right 09CF
Eye
Left 08C1XZZ
Right 08C0XZZ
Eyelid
Lower
Left 08CR
Right 08CQ
Upper
Left 08CP
Right 08CN
Fallopian Tube
Left 0UC6
Right 0UC5
Fallopian Tubes, Bilateral 0UC7
Femoral Shaft
Left 0QC9
Right 0QC8
Femur
Lower
Left 0QCC
Right 0QCB
Upper
Left 0QC7
Right 0QC6
Fibula
Left 0QCK
Right 0QCJ

▶ New   ➠ Revised   ~~deleted~~ Deleted

Extirpation *(Continued)*
Finger Nail ØHCQXZZ
Gallbladder ØFC4
Gastrointestinal Tract ØWCP
Genitourinary Tract ØWCR
Gingiva
  Lower ØCC6
  Upper ØCC5
Gland
  Adrenal
    Bilateral ØGC4
    Left ØGC2
    Right ØGC3
  Lacrimal
    Left Ø8CW
    Right Ø8CV
  Minor Salivary ØCCJ
  Parotid
    Left ØCC9
    Right ØCC8
  Pituitary ØGCØ
  Sublingual
    Left ØCCF
    Right ØCCD
  Submaxillary
    Left ØCCH
    Right ØCCG
  Vestibular ØUCL
Glenoid Cavity
  Left ØPC8
  Right ØPC7
Glomus Jugulare ØGCC
Humeral Head
  Left ØPCD
  Right ØPCC
Humeral Shaft
  Left ØPCG
  Right ØPCF
Hymen ØUCK
Hypothalamus ØØCA
Ileocecal Valve ØDCC
Ileum ØDCB
Intestine
  Large ØDCE
    Left ØDCG
    Right ØDCF
  Small ØDC8
Iris
  Left Ø8CD
  Right Ø8CC
Jejunum ØDCA
Joint
  Acromioclavicular
    Left ØRCH
    Right ØRCG
  Ankle
    Left ØSCG
    Right ØSCF
  Carpal
    Left ØRCR
    Right ØRCQ
  ▶Carpometacarpal
    ▶Left ØRCT
    ▶Right ØRCS
  Cervical Vertebral ØRC1
  Cervicothoracic Vertebral ØRC4
  Coccygeal ØSC6
  Elbow
    Left ØRCM
    Right ØRCL
  Finger Phalangeal
    Left ØRCX
    Right ØRCW
  Hip
    Left ØSCB
    Right ØSC9
  Knee
    Left ØSCD
    Right ØSCC
  Lumbar Vertebral ØSCØ
  Lumbosacral ØSC3

Extirpation *(Continued)*
Joint *(Continued)*
  ~~Metacarpocarpal~~
    ~~Left ØRCT~~
    ~~Right ØRCS~~
  Metacarpophalangeal
    Left ØRCV
    Right ØRCU
  Metatarsal-Phalangeal
    Left ØSCN
    Right ØSCM
  ~~Metatarsal-Tarsal~~
    ~~Left ØSCL~~
    ~~Right ØSCK~~
  Occipital-cervical ØRCØ
  Sacrococcygeal ØSC5
  Sacroiliac
    Left ØSC8
    Right ØSC7
  Shoulder
    Left ØRCK
    Right ØRCJ
  Sternoclavicular
    Left ØRCF
    Right ØRCE
  Tarsal
    Left ØSCJ
    Right ØSCH
  ▶Tarsometatarsal
    ▶Left ØSCL
    ▶Right ØSCK
  Temporomandibular
    Left ØRCD
    Right ØRCC
  Thoracic Vertebral ØRC6
  Thoracolumbar Vertebral ØRCA
  Toe Phalangeal
    Left ØSCQ
    Right ØSCP
  Wrist
    Left ØRCP
    Right ØRCN
Kidney
  Left ØTC1
  Right ØTCØ
Kidney Pelvis
  Left ØTC4
  Right ØTC3
Larynx ØCCS
Lens
  Left Ø8CK
  Right Ø8CJ
Lip
  Lower ØCC1
  Upper ØCCØ
Liver ØFCØ
  Left Lobe ØFC2
  Right Lobe ØFC1
Lung
  Bilateral ØBCM
  Left ØBCL
  Lower Lobe
    Left ØBCJ
    Right ØBCF
  Middle Lobe, Right ØBCD
  Right ØBCK
  Upper Lobe
    Left ØBCG
    Right ØBCC
Lung Lingula ØBCH
Lymphatic
  Aortic Ø7CD
  Axillary
    Left Ø7C6
    Right Ø7C5
  Head Ø7CØ
  Inguinal
    Left Ø7CJ
    Right Ø7CH
  Internal Mammary
    Left Ø7C9
    Right Ø7C8

Extirpation *(Continued)*
Lymphatic *(Continued)*
  Lower Extremity
    Left Ø7CG
    Right Ø7CF
  Mesenteric Ø7CB
  Neck
    Left Ø7C2
    Right Ø7C1
  Pelvis Ø7CC
  Thoracic Duct Ø7CK
  Thorax Ø7C7
  Upper Extremity
    Left Ø7C4
    Right Ø7C3
Mandible
  Left ØNCV
  Right ØNCT
➡Maxilla ØNCR
  ~~Left ØNCS~~
  ~~Right ØNCR~~
Mediastinum ØWCC
Medulla Oblongata ØØCD
Mesentery ØDCV
Metacarpal
  Left ØPCQ
  Right ØPCP
Metatarsal
  Left ØQCP
  Right ØQCN
Muscle
  Abdomen
    Left ØKCL
    Right ØKCK
  Extraocular
    Left Ø8CM
    Right Ø8CL
  Facial ØKC1
  Foot
    Left ØKCW
    Right ØKCV
  Hand
    Left ØKCD
    Right ØKCC
  Head ØKCØ
  Hip
    Left ØKCP
    Right ØKCN
  Lower Arm and Wrist
    Left ØKCB
    Right ØKC9
  Lower Leg
    Left ØKCT
    Right ØKCS
  Neck
    Left ØKC3
    Right ØKC2
  Papillary Ø2CD
  Perineum ØKCM
  Shoulder
    Left ØKC6
    Right ØKC5
  Thorax
    Left ØKCJ
    Right ØKCH
  Tongue, Palate, Pharynx ØKC4
  Trunk
    Left ØKCG
    Right ØKCF
  Upper Arm
    Left ØKC8
    Right ØKC7
  Upper Leg
    Left ØKCR
    Right ØKCQ
▶Nasal Mucosa and Soft Tissue Ø9CK
Nasopharynx Ø9CN
Nerve
  Abdominal Sympathetic Ø1CM
  Abducens ØØCL
  Accessory ØØCR

Extirpation *(Continued)*
Nerve *(Continued)*
- Acoustic 00CN
- Brachial Plexus 01C3
- Cervical 01C1
- Cervical Plexus 01C0
- Facial 00CM
- Femoral 01CD
- Glossopharyngeal 00CP
- Head and Neck Sympathetic 01CK
- Hypoglossal 00CS
- Lumbar 01CB
- Lumbar Plexus 01C9
- Lumbar Sympathetic 01CN
- Lumbosacral Plexus 01CA
- Median 01C5
- Oculomotor 00CH
- Olfactory 00CF
- Optic 00CG
- Peroneal 01CH
- Phrenic 01C2
- Pudendal 01CC
- Radial 01C6
- Sacral 01CR
- Sacral Plexus 01CQ
- Sacral Sympathetic 01CP
- Sciatic 01CF
- Thoracic 01C8
- Thoracic Sympathetic 01CL
- Tibial 01CG
- Trigeminal 00CK
- Trochlear 00CJ
- Ulnar 01C4
- Vagus 00CQ
Nipple
- Left 0HCX
- Right 0HCW
- ~~Nose 09CK~~
➡ Omentum 0DCU
- ~~Greater 0DCS~~
- ~~Lesser 0DCT~~
- Oral Cavity and Throat 0WC3
Orbit
- Left 0NCQ
- Right 0NCP
- Orbital Atherectomy Technology X2C
Ovary
- Bilateral 0UC2
- Left 0UC1
- Right 0UC0
Palate
- Hard 0CC2
- Soft 0CC3
- Pancreas 0FCG
- Para-aortic Body 0GC9
- Paraganglion Extremity 0GCF
- Parathyroid Gland 0GCR
Inferior
- Left 0GCP
- Right 0GCN
- Multiple 0GCQ
Superior
- Left 0GCM
- Right 0GCL
Patella
- Left 0QCF
- Right 0QCD
- Pelvic Cavity 0WCJ
- Penis 0VCS
- Pericardial Cavity 0WCD
- Pericardium 02CN
- Peritoneal Cavity 0WCG
- Peritoneum 0DCW
Phalanx
Finger
- Left 0PCV
- Right 0PCT
Thumb
- Left 0PCS
- Right 0PCR

Extirpation *(Continued)*
Phalanx *(Continued)*
Toe
- Left 0QCR
- Right 0QCQ
- Pharynx 0CCM
- Pineal Body 0GC1
Pleura
- Left 0BCP
- Right 0BCN
Pleural Cavity
- Left 0WCB
- Right 0WC9
- Pons 00CB
- Prepuce 0VCT
- Prostate 0VC0
Radius
- Left 0PCJ
- Right 0PCH
- Rectum 0DCP
- Respiratory Tract 0WCQ
Retina
- Left 08CF
- Right 08CE
Retinal Vessel
- Left 08CH
- Right 08CG
- ~~Rib~~
- ~~Left 0PC2~~
- ~~Right 0PC1~~
▶ Retroperitoneum 0WCH
▶ Ribs
- ▶ 1 to 2 0PC1
- ▶ 3 or More 0PC2
- Sacrum 0QC1
Scapula
- Left 0PC6
- Right 0PC5
Sclera
- Left 08C7XZZ
- Right 08C6XZZ
- Scrotum 0VC5
Septum
- Atrial 02C5
- Nasal 09CM
- Ventricular 02CM
Sinus
- Accessory 09CP
Ethmoid
- Left 09CV
- Right 09CU
Frontal
- Left 09CT
- Right 09CS
Mastoid
- Left 09CC
- Right 09CB
Maxillary
- Left 09CR
- Right 09CQ
Sphenoid
- Left 09CX
- Right 09CW
Skin
- Abdomen 0HC7XZZ
- Back 0HC6XZZ
- Buttock 0HC8XZZ
- Chest 0HC5XZZ
Ear
- Left 0HC3XZZ
- Right 0HC2XZZ
- Face 0HC1XZZ
Foot
- Left 0HCNXZZ
- Right 0HCMXZZ
- ~~Genitalia 0HCAXZZ~~
Hand
- Left 0HCGXZZ
- Right 0HCFXZZ
▶ Inguinal 0HCAXZZ

Extirpation *(Continued)*
Skin *(Continued)*
Lower Arm
- Left 0HCEXZZ
- Right 0HCDXZZ
Lower Leg
- Left 0HCLXZZ
- Right 0HCKXZZ
- Neck 0HC4XZZ
- Perineum 0HC9XZZ
- Scalp 0HC0XZZ
Upper Arm
- Left 0HCCXZZ
- Right 0HCBXZZ
Upper Leg
- Left 0HCJXZZ
- Right 0HCHXZZ
▶ Spinal Canal 00CU
Spinal Cord
- Cervical 00CW
- Lumbar 00CY
- Thoracic 00CX
- Spinal Meninges 00CT
- Spleen 07CP
- Sternum 0PC0
- Stomach 0DC6
- Pylorus 0DC7
- ~~Subarachnoid Space 00C5~~
▶ Subarachnoid Space, Intracranial 00C5
Subcutaneous Tissue and Fascia
- Abdomen 0JC8
- Back 0JC7
- Buttock 0JC9
- Chest 0JC6
- Face 0JC1
Foot
- Left 0JCR
- Right 0JCQ
Hand
- Left 0JCK
- Right 0JCJ
Lower Arm
- Left 0JCH
- Right 0JCG
Lower Leg
- Left 0JCP
- Right 0JCN
Neck
- ~~Anterior 0JC4~~
- ~~Posterior 0JC5~~
- ▶ Left 0JC5
- ▶ Right 0JC4
- Pelvic Region 0JCC
- Perineum 0JCB
- Scalp 0JC0
Upper Arm
- Left 0JCF
- Right 0JCD
Upper Leg
- Left 0JCM
- Right 0JCL
- ~~Subdural Space 00C4~~
▶ Subdural Space, Intracranial 00C4
Tarsal
- Left 0QCM
- Right 0QCL
Tendon
Abdomen
- Left 0LCG
- Right 0LCF
Ankle
- Left 0LCT
- Right 0LCS
Foot
- Left 0LCW
- Right 0LCV
Hand
- Left 0LC8
- Right 0LC7
- Head and Neck 0LC0

▶ New   ➡ Revised   ~~deleted~~ Deleted

Extirpation *(Continued)*
  Tendon *(Continued)*
    Hip
      Left 0LCK
      Right 0LCJ
    Knee
      Left 0LCR
      Right 0LCQ
    Lower Arm and Wrist
      Left 0LC6
      Right 0LC5
    Lower Leg
      Left 0LCP
      Right 0LCN
    Perineum 0LCH
    Shoulder
      Left 0LC2
      Right 0LC1
    Thorax
      Left 0LCD
      Right 0LCC
    Trunk
      Left 0LCB
      Right 0LC9
    Upper Arm
      Left 0LC4
      Right 0LC3
    Upper Leg
      Left 0LCM
      Right 0LCL
  Testis
    Bilateral 0VCC
    Left 0VCB
    Right 0VC9
  Thalamus 00C9
  Thymus 07CM
  Thyroid Gland 0GCK
    Left Lobe 0GCG
    Right Lobe 0GCH
  Tibia
    Left 0QCH
    Right 0QCG
  Toe Nail 0HCRXZZ
  Tongue 0CC7
  Tonsils 0CCP
  Tooth
    Lower 0CCX
    Upper 0CCW
  Trachea 0BC1
  Tunica Vaginalis
    Left 0VC7
    Right 0VC6
  Turbinate, Nasal 09CL
  Tympanic Membrane
    Left 09C8
    Right 09C7
  Ulna
    Left 0PCL
    Right 0PCK
  Ureter
    Left 0TC7
    Right 0TC6
  Urethra 0TCD
  Uterine Supporting Structure 0UC4
  Uterus 0UC9
  Uvula 0CCN
  Vagina 0UCG
  Valve
    Aortic 02CF
    Mitral 02CG
    Pulmonary 02CH
    Tricuspid 02CJ
  Vas Deferens
    Bilateral 0VCQ
    Left 0VCP
    Right 0VCN
  Vein
    Axillary
      Left 05C8
      Right 05C7
    Azygos 05C0

Extirpation *(Continued)*
  Vein *(Continued)*
    Basilic
      Left 05CC
      Right 05CB
    Brachial
      Left 05CA
      Right 05C9
    Cephalic
      Left 05CF
      Right 05CD
    Colic 06C7
    Common Iliac
      Left 06CD
      Right 06CC
    Coronary 02C4
    Esophageal 06C3
    External Iliac
      Left 06CG
      Right 06CF
    External Jugular
      Left 05CQ
      Right 05CP
    Face
      Left 05CV
      Right 05CT
    Femoral
      Left 06CN
      Right 06CM
    Foot
      Left 06CV
      Right 06CT
    Gastric 06C2
    ~~Greater Saphenous~~
      ~~Left 06CQ~~
      ~~Right 06CP~~
    Hand
      Left 05CH
      Right 05CG
    Hemiazygos 05C1
    Hepatic 06C4
    Hypogastric
      Left 06CJ
      Right 06CH
    Inferior Mesenteric 06C6
    Innominate
      Left 05C4
      Right 05C3
    Internal Jugular
      Left 05CN
      Right 05CM
    Intracranial 05CL
    ~~Lesser Saphenous~~
      ~~Left 06CS~~
      ~~Right 06CR~~
    Lower 06CY
    Portal 06C8
    Pulmonary
      Left 02CT
      Right 02CS
    Renal
      Left 06CB
      Right 06C9
    ► Saphenous
      ► Left 06CQ
      ► Right 06CP
    Splenic 06C1
    Subclavian
      Left 05C6
      Right 05C5
    Superior Mesenteric 06C5
    Upper 05CY
    Vertebral
      Left 05CS
      Right 05CR
    Vena Cava
      Inferior 06C0
      Superior 02CV
    Ventricle
      Left 02CL
      Right 02CK

Extirpation *(Continued)*
  Vertebra
    Cervical 0PC3
    Lumbar 0QC0
    Thoracic 0PC4
  Vesicle
    Bilateral 0VC3
    Left 0VC2
    Right 0VC1
  Vitreous
    Left 08C5
    Right 08C4
  Vocal Cord
    Left 0CCV
    Right 0CCT
  Vulva 0UCM
► **Extracorporeal Carbon Dioxide Removal (ECCO2R)** 5A0920Z
Extracorporeal shock wave lithotripsy *see*
  Fragmentation
Extracranial-intracranial bypass (EC-IC) *see*
  Bypass, Upper Arteries 031
Extraction
  ► Acetabulum
    ► Left 0QD50ZZ
    ► Right 0QD40ZZ
  ► Anus 0DDQ
  ► Appendix 0DDJ
  Auditory Ossicle
    Left 09DA0ZZ
    Right 09D90ZZ
  ► Bone
    ► Ethmoid
      ► Left 0NDG0ZZ
      ► Right 0NDF0ZZ
    ► Frontal 0ND10ZZ
    ► Hyoid 0NDX0ZZ
    ► Lacrimal
      ► Left 0NDJ0ZZ
      ► Right 0NDH0ZZ
    ► Nasal 0NDB0ZZ
    ► Occipital 0ND70ZZ
    ► Palatine
      ► Left 0NDL0ZZ
      ► Right 0NDK0ZZ
    ► Parietal
      ► Left 0ND40ZZ
      ► Right 0ND30ZZ
    ► Pelvic
      ► Left 0QD30ZZ
      ► Right 0QD20ZZ
    ► Sphenoid 0NDC0ZZ
    ► Temporal
      ► Left 0ND60ZZ
      ► Right 0ND50ZZ
    ► Zygomatic
      ► Left 0NDN0ZZ
      ► Right 0NDM0ZZ
  Bone Marrow
    Iliac 07DR
    Sternum 07DQ
    Vertebral 07DS
  ► Bronchus
    ► Lingula 0BD9
    ► Lower Lobe
      ► Left 0BDB
      ► Right 0BD6
    ► Main
      ► Left 0BD7
      ► Right 0BD3
    ► Middle Lobe, Right 0BD5
    ► Upper Lobe
      ► Left 0BD8
      ► Right 0BD4
  Bursa and Ligament
    Abdomen
      Left 0MDJ
      Right 0MDH
    Ankle
      Left 0MDR
      Right 0MDQ

Extraction (*Continued*)
Bursa and Ligament (*Continued*)
Elbow
Left 0MD4
Right 0MD3
Foot
Left 0MDT
Right 0MDS
Hand
Left 0MD8
Right 0MD7
Head and Neck 0MD0
Hip
Left 0MDM
Right 0MDL
Knee
Left 0MDP
Right 0MDN
Lower Extremity
Left 0MDW
Right 0MDV
Perineum 0MDK
▶ Rib(s) 0MDG
Shoulder
Left 0MD2
Right 0MD1
▶ Spine
▶ Lower 0MDD
▶ Upper 0MDC
▶ Sternum 0MDF
~~Thorax~~
~~Left 0MDG~~
~~Right 0MDF~~
~~Trunk~~
~~Left 0MDD~~
~~Right 0MDC~~
Upper Extremity
Left 0MDB
Right 0MD9
Wrist
Left 0MD6
Right 0MD5
▶ Carina 0BD2
▶ Carpal
▶ Left 0PDN0ZZ
▶ Right 0PDM0ZZ
▶ Cecum 0DDH
Cerebral Meninges 00D1
▶ Cisterna Chyli 07DL
▶ Clavicle
▶ Left 0PDB0ZZ
▶ Right 0PD90ZZ
▶ Coccyx 0QDS0ZZ
▶ Colon
▶ Ascending 0DDK
▶ Descending 0DDM
▶ Sigmoid 0DDN
▶ Transverse 0DDL
Cornea
Left 08D9XZ
Right 08D8XZ
▶ Duodenum 0DD9
Dura Mater 00D2
Endometrium 0UDB
▶ Esophagogastric Junction 0DD4
▶ Esophagus 0DD5
▶ Lower 0DD3
▶ Middle 0DD2
▶ Upper 0DD1
▶ Femoral Shaft
▶ Left 0QD90ZZ
▶ Right 0QD80ZZ
▶ Femur
▶ Lower
▶ Left 0QDC0ZZ
▶ Right 0QDB0ZZ
▶ Upper
▶ Left 0QD70ZZ
▶ Right 0QD60ZZ

Extraction (*Continued*)
▶ Fibula
▶ Left 0QDK0ZZ
▶ Right 0QDJ0ZZ
Finger Nail 0HDQXZZ
▶ Glenoid Cavity
▶ Left 0PD80ZZ
▶ Right 0PD70ZZ
Hair 0HDSXZZ
▶ Humeral Head
▶ Left 0PDD0ZZ
▶ Right 0PDC0ZZ
▶ Humeral Shaft
▶ Left 0PDG0ZZ
▶ Right 0PDF0ZZ
▶ Ileocecal Valve 0DDC
▶ Ileum 0DDB
▶ Intestine
▶ Large 0DDE
▶ Left 0DDG
▶ Right 0DDF
▶ Small 0DD8
▶ Jejunum 0DDA
Kidney
Left 0TD1
Right 0TD0
Lens
Left 08DK3ZZ
Right 08DJ3ZZ
▶ Lung
▶ Bilateral 0BDM
▶ Left 0BDL
▶ Lower Lobe
▶ Left 0BDJ
▶ Right 0BDF
▶ Middle Lobe, Right 0BDD
▶ Right 0BDK
▶ Upper Lobe
▶ Left 0BDG
▶ Right 0BDC
▶ Lung Lingula 0BDH
▶ Lymphatic
▶ Aortic 07DD
▶ Axillary
▶ Left 07D6
▶ Right 07D5
▶ Head 07D0
▶ Inguinal
▶ Left 07DJ
▶ Right 07DH
▶ Internal Mammary
▶ Left 07D9
▶ Right 07D8
▶ Lower Extremity
▶ Left 07DG
▶ Right 07DF
▶ Mesenteric 07DB
▶ Neck
▶ Left 07D2
▶ Right 07D1
▶ Pelvis 07DC
▶ Thoracic Duct 07DK
▶ Thorax 07D7
▶ Upper Extremity
▶ Left 07D4
▶ Right 07D3
▶ Mandible
▶ Left 0NDV0ZZ
▶ Right 0NDT0ZZ
▶ Maxilla 0NDR0ZZ
▶ Metacarpal
▶ Left 0PDQ0ZZ
▶ Right 0PDP0ZZ
▶ Metatarsal
▶ Left 0QDP0ZZ
▶ Right 0QDN0ZZ
▶ Muscle
▶ Abdomen
▶ Left 0KDL0ZZ
▶ Right 0KDK0ZZ
▶ Facial 0KD10ZZ

Extraction (*Continued*)
Muscle (*Continued*)
▶ Foot
▶ Left 0KDW0ZZ
▶ Right 0KDV0ZZ
▶ Hand
▶ Left 0KDD0ZZ
▶ Right 0KDC0ZZ
▶ Head 0KD00ZZ
▶ Hip
▶ Left 0KDP0ZZ
▶ Right 0KDN0ZZ
▶ Lower Arm and Wrist
▶ Left 0KDB0ZZ
▶ Right 0KD90ZZ
▶ Lower Leg
▶ Left 0KDT0ZZ
▶ Right 0KDS0ZZ
▶ Neck
▶ Left 0KD30ZZ
▶ Right 0KD20ZZ
▶ Perineum 0KDM0ZZ
▶ Shoulder
▶ Left 0KD60ZZ
▶ Right 0KD50ZZ
▶ Thorax
▶ Left 0KDJ0ZZ
▶ Right 0KDH0ZZ
▶ Tongue, Palate, Pharynx 0KD40ZZ
▶ Trunk
▶ Left 0KDG0ZZ
▶ Right 0KDF0ZZ
▶ Upper Arm
▶ Left 0KD80ZZ
▶ Right 0KD70ZZ
▶ Upper Leg
▶ Left 0KDR0ZZ
▶ Right 0KDQ0ZZ
Nerve
Abdominal Sympathetic 01DM
Abducens 00DL
Accessory 00DR
Acoustic 00DN
Brachial Plexus 01D3
Cervical 01D1
Cervical Plexus 01D0
Facial 00DM
Femoral 01DD
Glossopharyngeal 00DP
Head and Neck Sympathetic 01DK
Hypoglossal 00DS
Lumbar 01DB
Lumbar Plexus 01D9
Lumbar Sympathetic 01DN
Lumbosacral Plexus 01DA
Median 01D5
Oculomotor 00DH
Olfactory 00DF
Optic 00DG
Peroneal 01DH
Phrenic 01D2
Pudendal 01DC
Radial 01D6
Sacral 01DR
Sacral Plexus 01DQ
Sacral Sympathetic 01DP
Sciatic 01DF
Thoracic 01D8
Thoracic Sympathetic 01DL
Tibial 01DG
Trigeminal 00DK
Trochlear 00DJ
Ulnar 01D4
Vagus 00DQ
▶ Orbit
▶ Left 0NDQ0ZZ
▶ Right 0NDP0ZZ
▶ Patella
▶ Left 0QDF0ZZ
▶ Right 0QDD0ZZ

▶ New   ⇒ Revised   ~~deleted~~ Deleted

Extraction *(Continued)*
▶Phalanx
  ▶Finger
    ▶Left 0PDV0ZZ
    ▶Right 0PDT0ZZ
  ▶Thumb
    ▶Left 0PDS0ZZ
    ▶Right 0PDR0ZZ
  ▶Toe
    ▶Left 0QDR0ZZ
    ▶Right 0QDQ0ZZ
Ova 0UDN
Pleura
  Left 0BDP
  Right 0BDN
Products of Conception
  Classical 10D00Z0
  Ectopic 10D2
  Extraperitoneal 10D00Z2
  High Forceps 10D07Z5
  Internal Version 10D07Z7
  Low Cervical 10D00Z1
  Low Forceps 10D07Z3
  Mid Forceps 10D07Z4
  Other 10D07Z8
  Retained 10D1
  Vacuum 10D07Z6
▶Radius
  ▶Left 0PDJ0ZZ
  ▶Right 0PDH0ZZ
▶Rectum 0DDP
▶Ribs
  ▶1 to 2 0PD10ZZ
  ▶3 or More 0PD20ZZ
▶Sacrum 0QD10ZZ
▶Scapula
  ▶Left 0PD60ZZ
  ▶Right 0PD50ZZ
Septum, Nasal 09DM
Sinus
  Accessory 09DP
  Ethmoid
    Left 09DV
    Right 09DU
  Frontal
    Left 09DT
    Right 09DS
  Mastoid
    Left 09DC
    Right 09DB
  Maxillary
    Left 09DR
    Right 09DQ
  Sphenoid
    Left 09DX
    Right 09DW
Skin
  Abdomen 0HD7XZZ
  Back 0HD6XZZ
  Buttock 0HD8XZZ
  Chest 0HD5XZZ
  Ear
    Left 0HD3XZZ
    Right 0HD2XZZ
  Face 0HD1XZZ
  Foot
    Left 0HDNXZZ
    Right 0HDMXZZ
  ~~Genitalia 0HDAXZZ~~
  Hand
    Left 0HDGXZZ
    Right 0HDFXZZ
  ▶Inguinal 0HDAXZZ
  Lower Arm
    Left 0HDEXZZ
    Right 0HDDXZZ
  Lower Leg
    Left 0HDLXZZ
    Right 0HDKXZZ

Extraction *(Continued)*
  Skin *(Continued)*
    Neck 0HD4XZZ
    Perineum 0HD9XZZ
    Scalp 0HD0XZZ
    Upper Arm
      Left 0HDCXZZ
      Right 0HDBXZZ
    Upper Leg
      Left 0HDJXZZ
      Right 0HDHXZZ
▶Skull 0ND00ZZ
Spinal Meninges 00DT
▶Spleen 07DP
▶Sternum 0PD00ZZ
▶Stomach 0DD6
  ▶Pylorus 0DD7
Subcutaneous Tissue and Fascia
  Abdomen 0JD8
  Back 0JD7
  Buttock 0JD9
  Chest 0JD6
  Face 0JD1
  Foot
    Left 0JDR
    Right 0JDQ
  Hand
    Left 0JDK
    Right 0JDJ
  Lower Arm
    Left 0JDH
    Right 0JDG
  Lower Leg
    Left 0JDP
    Right 0JDN
  Neck
    ~~Anterior 0JD4~~
    ~~Posterior 0JD5~~
    ▶Left 0JD5
    ▶Right 0JD4
  Pelvic Region 0JDC
  Perineum 0JDB
  Scalp 0JD0
  Upper Arm
    Left 0JDF
    Right 0JDD
  Upper Leg
    Left 0JDM
    Right 0JDL
▶Tarsal
  ▶Left 0QDM0ZZ
  ▶Right 0QDL0ZZ
▶Tendon
  Abdomen
    ▶Left 0LDG0ZZ
    ▶Right 0LDF0ZZ
  ▶Ankle
    ▶Left 0LDT0ZZ
    ▶Right 0LDS0ZZ
  ▶Foot
    ▶Left 0LDW0ZZ
    ▶Right 0LDV0ZZ
  ▶Hand
    ▶Left 0LD80ZZ
    ▶Right 0LD70ZZ
  ▶Head and Neck 0LD00ZZ
  ▶Hip
    ▶Left 0LDK0ZZ
    ▶Right 0LDJ0ZZ
  ▶Knee
    ▶Left 0LDR0ZZ
    ▶Right 0LDQ0ZZ
  ▶Lower Arm and Wrist
    ▶Left 0LD60ZZ
    ▶Right 0LD50ZZ
  ▶Lower Leg
    ▶Left 0LDP0ZZ
    ▶Right 0LDN0ZZ

Extraction *(Continued)*
  Tendon *(Continued)*
    ▶Perineum 0LDH0ZZ
    ▶Shoulder
      ▶Left 0LD20ZZ
      ▶Right 0LD10ZZ
    ▶Thorax
      ▶Left 0LDD0ZZ
      ▶Right 0LDC0ZZ
    ▶Trunk
      ▶Left 0LDB0ZZ
      ▶Right 0LD90ZZ
    ▶Upper Arm
      ▶Left 0LD40ZZ
      ▶Right 0LD30ZZ
    ▶Upper Leg
      ▶Left 0LDM0ZZ
      ▶Right 0LDL0ZZ
  ▶Thymus 07DM
  ▶Tibia
    ▶Left 0QDH0ZZ
    ▶Right 0QDG0ZZ
  Toe Nail 0HDRXZZ
  Tooth
    Lower 0CDXXZ
    Upper 0CDWXZ
  ▶Trachea 0BD1
  Turbinate, Nasal 09DL
  Tympanic Membrane
    Left 09D8
    Right 09D7
  ▶Ulna
    ▶Left 0PDL0ZZ
    ▶Right 0PDK0ZZ
  Vein
    Basilic
      Left 05DC
      Right 05DB
    Brachial
      Left 05DA
      Right 05D9
    Cephalic
      Left 05DF
      Right 05DD
    Femoral
      Left 06DN
      Right 06DM
    Foot
      Left 06DV
      Right 06DT
    ~~Greater Saphenous~~
      ~~Left 06DQ~~
      ~~Right 06DP~~
    Hand
      Left 05DH
      Right 05DG
    ~~Lesser Saphenous~~
      ~~Left 06DS~~
      ~~Right 06DR~~
    Lower 06DY
    ▶Saphenous
      ▶Left 06DQ
      ▶Right 06DP
    Upper 05DY
  ▶Vertebra
    ▶Cervical 0PD30ZZ
    ▶Lumbar 0QD00ZZ
    ▶Thoracic 0PD40ZZ
  Vocal Cord
    Left 0CDV
    Right 0CDT
➡**Extradural space, intracranial** *use* Epidural Space, Intracranial
Extradural space, spinal *use* Spinal Canal
EXtreme Lateral Interbody Fusion (XLIF) device *use* Interbody Fusion Device in Lower Joints

▶ New   ➡ Revised   ~~deleted~~ Deleted

F

Face lift *see* Alteration, Face 0W02
Facet replacement spinal stabilization device
  use Spinal Stabilization Device, Facet
    Replacement in 0RH
  use Spinal Stabilization Device, Facet
    Replacement in 0SH
Facial artery *use* Face Artery
Factor Xa Inhibitor Reversal Agent, Andexanet
  Alfa *use* Andexanet Alfa, Factor Xa
    Inhibitor Reversal Agent
False vocal cord *use* Larynx
Falx cerebri *use* Dura Mater
Fascia lata
  use Subcutaneous Tissue and Fascia, Right
    Upper Leg
  use Subcutaneous Tissue and Fascia, Left
    Upper Leg
Fasciaplasty, fascioplasty
  see Repair, Subcutaneous Tissue and Fascia 0JQ
  see Replacement, Subcutaneous Tissue and
    Fascia 0JR
Fasciectomy
  see Excision, Subcutaneous Tissue and Fascia
    0JB
Fasciorrhaphy *see* Repair, Subcutaneous Tissue
  and Fascia 0JQ
Fasciotomy
  see Division, Subcutaneous Tissue and Fascia
    0J8
  see Drainage, Subcutaneous Tissue and Fascia
    0J9
  see Release
Feeding Device
  Change device in
    Lower 0D2DXUZ
    Upper 0D20XUZ
  Insertion of device in
    Duodenum 0DH9
    Esophagus 0DH5
    Ileum 0DHB
    Intestine, Small 0DH8
    Jejunum 0DHA
    Stomach 0DH6
  Removal of device from
    Esophagus 0DP5
    Intestinal Tract
      Lower 0DPD
      Upper 0DP0
    Stomach 0DP6
  Revision of device in
    Intestinal Tract
      Lower 0DWD
      Upper 0DW0
    Stomach 0DW6
Femoral head
  use Upper Femur, Right
  use Upper Femur, Left
Femoral lymph node
  use Lymphatic, Right Lower Extremity
  use Lymphatic, Left Lower Extremity
Femoropatellar joint
  use Knee Joint, Right
  use Knee Joint, Left
  use Knee Joint, Femoral Surface, Right
  use Knee Joint, Femoral Surface, Left
Femorotibial joint
  use Knee Joint, Right
  use Knee Joint, Left
  use Knee Joint, Tibial Surface, Right
  use Knee Joint, Tibial Surface, Left
Fibular artery
  use Peroneal Artery, Right
  use Peroneal Artery, Left
Fibularis brevis muscle
  use Lower Leg Muscle, Right
  use Lower Leg Muscle, Left
Fibularis longus muscle
  use Lower Leg Muscle, Right
  use Lower Leg Muscle, Left

Fifth cranial nerve *use* Trigeminal Nerve
Filum terminale *use* Spinal Meninges
Fimbriectomy
  see Excision, Female Reproductive System
    0UB
  see Resection, Female Reproductive System
    0UT
Fine needle aspiration
  fluid or gas *see* Drainage
  tissue *see* Excision
First cranial nerve *use* Olfactory Nerve
First intercostal nerve *use* Brachial
  Plexus
Fistulization
  see Bypass
  see Drainage
  see Repair
Fitting
  Arch bars, for fracture reduction *see*
    Reposition, Mouth and Throat 0CS
  Arch bars, for immobilization *see*
    Immobilization, Face 2W31
  Artificial limb *see* Device Fitting,
    Rehabilitation F0D
  Hearing aid *see* Device Fitting, Rehabilitation
    F0D
  Ocular prosthesis F0DZ8UZ
  Prosthesis, limb *see* Device Fitting,
    Rehabilitation F0D
  Prosthesis, ocular F0DZ8UZ
Fixation, bone
  External, with fracture reduction *see* Reposition
  External, without fracture reduction *see*
    Insertion
  Internal, with fracture reduction *see* Reposition
  Internal, without fracture reduction *see*
    Insertion
FLAIR® Endovascular Stent Graft *use*
  Intraluminal Device
Flexible Composite Mesh *use* Synthetic
  Substitute
Flexor carpi radialis muscle
  use Lower Arm and Wrist Muscle, Right
  use Lower Arm and Wrist Muscle, Left
Flexor carpi ulnaris muscle
  use Lower Arm and Wrist Muscle, Right
  use Lower Arm and Wrist Muscle, Left
Flexor digitorum brevis muscle
  use Foot Muscle, Right
  use Foot Muscle, Left
Flexor digitorum longus muscle
  use Lower Leg Muscle, Right
  use Lower Leg Muscle, Left
Flexor hallucis brevis muscle
  use Foot Muscle, Right
  use Foot Muscle, Left
Flexor hallucis longus muscle
  use Lower Leg Muscle, Right
  use Lower Leg Muscle, Left
Flexor pollicis longus muscle
  use Lower Arm and Wrist Muscle, Right
  use Lower Arm and Wrist Muscle, Left
Fluoroscopy
  Abdomen and Pelvis BW11
  Airway, Upper BB1DZZZ
  Ankle
    Left BQ1H
    Right BQ1G
  Aorta
    Abdominal B410
      Laser, Intraoperative B410
    Thoracic B310
      Laser, Intraoperative B310
    Thoraco-Abdominal B31P
      Laser, Intraoperative B31P
  Aorta and Bilateral Lower Extremity Arteries
    B41D
    Laser, Intraoperative B41D
  Arm
    Left BP1FZZZ
    Right BP1EZZZ

Fluoroscopy *(Continued)*
  Artery
    Brachiocephalic-Subclavian
      Right B311
        Laser, Intraoperative B311
    Bronchial B31L
      Laser, Intraoperative B31L
    Bypass Graft, Other B21F
    Cervico-Cerebral Arch B31Q
      Laser, Intraoperative B31Q
    Common Carotid
      Bilateral B315
        Laser, Intraoperative B315
      Left B314
        Laser, Intraoperative B314
      Right B313
        Laser, Intraoperative B313
    Coronary
      Bypass Graft
        Multiple B213
          Laser, Intraoperative B213
        Single B212
          Laser, Intraoperative B212
      Multiple B211
        Laser, Intraoperative B211
      Single B210
        Laser, Intraoperative B210
    External Carotid
      Bilateral B31C
        Laser, Intraoperative B31C
      Left B31B
        Laser, Intraoperative B31B
      Right B319
        Laser, Intraoperative B319
    Hepatic B412
      Laser, Intraoperative B412
    Inferior Mesenteric B415
      Laser, Intraoperative B415
    Intercostal B31L
      Laser, Intraoperative B31L
    Internal Carotid
      Bilateral B318
        Laser, Intraoperative B318
      Left B317
        Laser, Intraoperative B317
      Right B316
        Laser, Intraoperative B316
    Internal Mammary Bypass Graft
      Left B218
      Right B217
    Intra-Abdominal
      Other B41B
        Laser, Intraoperative B41B
    Intracranial B31R
      Laser, Intraoperative B31R
    Lower
      Other B41J
        Laser, Intraoperative B41J
    Lower Extremity
      Bilateral and Aorta B41D
        Laser, Intraoperative B41D
      Left B41G
        Laser, Intraoperative B41G
      Right B41F
        Laser, Intraoperative B41F
    Lumbar B419
      Laser, Intraoperative B419
    Pelvic B41C
      Laser, Intraoperative B41C
    Pulmonary
      Left B31T
        Laser, Intraoperative B31T
      Right B31S
        Laser, Intraoperative B31S
    ▶Pulmonary Trunk B31U
      ▶Laser, Intraoperative B31U
    Renal
      Bilateral B418
        Laser, Intraoperative B418
      Left B417
        Laser, Intraoperative B417
      Right B416
        Laser, Intraoperative B416

▶ New   ➡ Revised   ~~deleted~~ Deleted

Fluoroscopy *(Continued)*
  Artery *(Continued)*
    Spinal B31M
      Laser, Intraoperative B31M
    Splenic B413
      Laser, Intraoperative B413
    Subclavian, Left B312
      Left B312
      Laser, Intraoperative B312
    Superior Mesenteric B414
      Laser, Intraoperative B414
    Upper
      Other B31N
      Laser, Intraoperative B31N
    Upper Extremity
      Bilateral B31K
        Laser, Intraoperative B31K
      Left B31J
        Laser, Intraoperative B31J
      Right B31H
        Laser, Intraoperative B31H
    Vertebral
      Bilateral B31G
        Laser, Intraoperative B31G
      Left B31F
        Laser, Intraoperative B31F
      Right B31D
        Laser, Intraoperative B31D
  Bile Duct BF10
    Pancreatic Duct and Gallbladder BF14
  Bile Duct and Gallbladder BF13
  Biliary Duct BF11
  Bladder BT10
    Kidney and Ureter BT14
      Left BT1F
      Right BT1D
  Bladder and Urethra BT1B
  Bowel, Small BD1
  Calcaneus
    Left BQ1KZZZ
    Right BQ1JZZZ
  Clavicle
    Left BP15ZZZ
    Right BP14ZZZ
  Coccyx BR1F
  Colon BD14
  Corpora Cavernosa BV10
  Dialysis Fistula B51W
  Dialysis Shunt B51W
  Diaphragm BB16ZZZ
  Disc
    Cervical BR11
    Lumbar BR13
    Thoracic BR12
  Duodenum BD19
  Elbow
    Left BP1H
    Right BP1G
  Epiglottis B91G
  Esophagus BD11
  Extremity
    Lower BW1C
    Upper BW1J
  Facet Joint
    Cervical BR14
    Lumbar BR16
    Thoracic BR15
  Fallopian Tube
    Bilateral BU12
    Left BU11
    Right BU10
  Fallopian Tube and Uterus BU18
  Femur
    Left BQ14ZZZ
    Right BQ13ZZZ
  Finger
    Left BP1SZZZ
    Right BP1RZZZ
  Foot
    Left BQ1MZZZ
    Right BQ1LZZZ

Fluoroscopy *(Continued)*
  Forearm
    Left BP1KZZZ
    Right BP1JZZZ
  Gallbladder BF12
    Bile Duct and Pancreatic Duct BF14
  Gallbladder and Bile Duct BF13
  Gastrointestinal, Upper BD1
  Hand
    Left BP1PZZZ
    Right BP1NZZZ
  Head and Neck BW19
  Heart
    Left B215
    Right B214
    Right and Left B216
  Hip
    Left BQ11
    Right BQ10
  Humerus
    Left BP1BZZZ
    Right BP1AZZZ
  Ileal Diversion Loop BT1C
  Ileal Loop, Ureters and Kidney BT1G
  Intracranial Sinus B512
  Joint
    Acromioclavicular, Bilateral BP13ZZZ
    Finger
      Left BP1D
      Right BP1C
    Foot
      Left BQ1Y
      Right BQ1X
    Hand
      Left BP1D
      Right BP1C
    Lumbosacral BR1B
    Sacroiliac BR1D
    Sternoclavicular
      Bilateral BP12ZZZ
      Left BP11ZZZ
      Right BP10ZZZ
    Temporomandibular
      Bilateral BN19
      Left BN18
      Right BN17
    Thoracolumbar BR18
    Toe
      Left BQ1Y
      Right BQ1X
  Kidney
    Bilateral BT13
    Ileal Loop and Ureter BT1G
    Left BT12
    Right BT11
    Ureter and Bladder BT14
      Left BT1F
      Right BT1D
  Knee
    Left BQ18
    Right BQ17
  Larynx B91J
  Leg
    Left BQ1FZZZ
    Right BQ1DZZZ
  Lung
    Bilateral BB14ZZZ
    Left BB13ZZZ
    Right BB12ZZZ
  Mediastinum BB1CZZZ
  Mouth BD1B
  Neck and Head BW19
  Oropharynx BD1B
  Pancreatic Duct BF1
    Gallbladder and Bile Buct BF14
  Patella
    Left BQ1WZZZ
    Right BQ1VZZZ
  Pelvis BR1C
  Pelvis and Abdomen BW11
  Pharynix B91G

Fluoroscopy *(Continued)*
  Ribs
    Left BP1YZZZ
    Right BP1XZZZ
  Sacrum BR1F
  Scapula
    Left BP17ZZZ
    Right BP16ZZZ
  Shoulder
    Left BP19
    Right BP18
  Sinus, Intracranial B512
  Spinal Cord B01B
  Spine
    Cervical BR10
    Lumbar BR19
    Thoracic BR17
    Whole BR1G
  Sternum BR1H
  Stomach BD12
  Toe
    Left BQ1QZZZ
    Right BQ1PZZZ
  Tracheobronchial Tree
    Bilateral BB19YZZ
    Left BB18YZZ
    Right BB17YZZ
  Ureter
    Ileal Loop and Kidney BT1G
    Kidney and Bladder BT14
      Left BT1F
      Right BT1D
    Left BT17
    Right BT16
  Urethra BT15
  Urethra and Bladder BT1B
  Uterus BU16
  Uterus and Fallopian Tube BU18
  Vagina BU19
  Vasa Vasorum BV18
  Vein
    Cerebellar B511
    Cerebral B511
    Epidural B510
    Jugular
      Bilateral B515
      Left B514
      Right B513
    Lower Extremity
      Bilateral B51D
      Left B51C
      Right B51B
    Other B51V
    Pelvic (Iliac)
      Left B51G
      Right B51F
    Pelvic (Iliac) Bilateral B51H
    Portal B51T
    Pulmonary
      Bilateral B51S
      Left B51R
      Right B51Q
    Renal
      Bilateral B51L
      Left B51K
      Right B51J
    Spanchnic B51T
    Subclavian
      Left B517
      Right B516
    Upper Extremity
      Bilateral B51P
      Left B51N
      Right B51M
  Vena Cava
    Inferior B519
    Superior B518
  Wrist
    Left BP1M
    Right BP1L

Fluoroscopy, laser intraoperative
  see Fluoroscopy, Heart B21
  see Fluoroscopy, Upper Arteries B31
  see Fluoroscopy, Lower Arteries B41
Flushing *see* Irrigation
Foley catheter *use* Drainage Device
▶**Fontan completion procedure Stage II** *see*
    Bypass, Vena Cava, Inferior 0610
➠**Foramen magnum** *use* Occipital Bone
  use Bone, Occipital, Right
  use Bone, Occipital, Left
Foramen of Monro (intraventricular) *use*
    Cerebral Ventricle
Foreskin *use* Prepuce
Formula™ Balloon-Expandable Renal
    Stent System *use* Intraluminal
    Device
Fossa of Rosenmuller *use* Nasopharynx
Fourth cranial nerve *use* Nerve, Trochlear
Fourth ventricle *use* Cerebral Ventricle
Fovea
  use Retina, Right
  use Retina, Left
Fragmentation
  Ampulla of Vater 0FFC
  Anus 0DFQ
  Appendix 0DFJ
  Bladder 0TFB
  Bladder Neck 0TFC
  Bronchus
    Lingula 0BF9
    Lower Lobe
      Left 0BFB
      Right 0BF6
    Main
      Left 0BF7
      Right 0BF3
    Middle Lobe, Right 0BF5
    Upper Lobe
      Left 0BF8
      Right 0BF4
  Carina 0BF2
  Cavity, Cranial 0WF1
  Cecum 0DFH
  Cerebral Ventricle 00F6
  Colon
    Ascending 0DFK
    Descending 0DFM
    Sigmoid 0DFN
    Transverse 0DFL
  Duct
    Common Bile 0FF9
    Cystic 0FF8
    Hepatic
    ▶Common 0FF7
      Left 0FF6
      Right 0FF5
    Pancreatic 0FFD
      Accessory 0FFF
    Parotid
      Left 0CFC
      Right 0CFB
  Duodenum 0DF9
  Epidural Space 00F3
▶**Epidural Space, Intracranial** 00F3
  Esophagus 0DF5
  Fallopian Tube
    Left 0UF6
    Right 0UF5
  Fallopian Tubes, Bilateral 0UF7
  Gallbladder 0FF4
  Gastrointestinal Tract 0WFP
  Genitourinary Tract 0WFR
  Ileum 0DFB
  Intestine
    Large 0DFE
      Left 0DFG
      Right 0DFF
    Small 0DF8

Fragmentation *(Continued)*
  Jejunum 0DFA
  Kidney Pelvis
    Left 0TF4
    Right 0TF3
  Mediastinum 0WFC
  Oral Cavity and Throat 0WF3
  Pelvic Cavity 0WFJ
  Pericardial Cavity 0WFD
  Pericardium 02FN
  Peritoneal Cavity 0WFG
  Pleural Cavity
    Left 0WFB
    Right 0WF9
  Rectum 0DFP
  Respiratory Tract 0WFQ
  Spinal Canal 00FU
  Stomach 0DF6
  Subarachnoid Space 00F5
  Subdural Space 00F4
▶**Subarachnoid Space, Intracranial** 00F5
▶**Subdural Space, Intracranial** 00F4
  Trachea 0BF1
  Ureter
    Left 0TF7
    Right 0TF6
  Urethra 0TFD
  Uterus 0UF9
  Vitreous
    Left 08F5
    Right 08F4
Freestyle (Stentless) Aortic Root Bioprosthesis
    use Zooplastic Tissue in Heart and Great
    Vessels
Frenectomy
  see Excision, Mouth and Throat 0CB
  see Resection, Mouth and Throat 0CT
Frenoplasty, frenuloplasty
  see Repair, Mouth and Throat 0CQ
  see Replacement, Mouth and Throat 0CR
  see Supplement, Mouth and Throat 0CU
Frenotomy
  see Drainage, Mouth and Throat 0C9
  see Release, Mouth and Throat 0CN
Frenulotomy
  see Drainage, Mouth and Throat 0C9
  see Release, Mouth and Throat 0CN
Frenulum labii inferioris *use* Lower Lip
Frenulum labii superioris *use* Upper Lip
Frenulum linguae *use* Tongue
Frenulumectomy
  see Excision, Mouth and Throat 0CB
  see Resection, Mouth and Throat 0CT
Frontal lobe *use* Cerebral Hemisphere
Frontal vein
  use Face Vein, Right
  use Face Vein, Left
Fulguration *see* Destruction
Fundoplication, gastroesophageal *see*
    Restriction, Esophagogastric Junction
    0DV4
Fundus uteri *use* Uterus
Fusion
  Acromioclavicular
    Left 0RGH
    Right 0RGG
  Ankle
    Left 0SGG
    Right 0SGF
  Carpal
    Left 0RGR
    Right 0RGQ
▶Carpometacarpal
  ▶Left 0RGT
  ▶Right 0RGS
  Cervical Vertebral 0RG1
    2 or more 0RG2
      Interbody Fusion Device, Nanotextured
        Surface XRG2092

Fusion *(Continued)*
  Cervical Vertebral *(Continued)*
    ▶Interbody Fusion Device
      ▶Nanotextured Surface XRG2092
      ▶Radiolucent Porous XRG20F3
    Interbody Fusion Device, Nanotextured
      Surface XRG1092
    ▶Interbody Fusion Device
      ▶Nanotextured Surface XRG1092
      ▶Radiolucent Porous XRG10F3
  Cervicothoracic Vertebral 0RG4
    Interbody Fusion Device, Nanotextured
      Surface XRG4092
    ▶Interbody Fusion Device
      ▶Nanotextured Surface XRG4092
      ▶Radiolucent Porous XRG40F3
  Coccygeal 0SG6
  Elbow
    Left 0RGM
    Right 0RGL
  Finger Phalangeal
    Left 0RGX
    Right 0RGW
  Hip
    Left 0SGB
    Right 0SG9
  Knee
    Left 0SGD
    Right 0SGC
  Lumbar Vertebral 0SG0
    2 or more 0SG1
      Interbody Fusion Device, Nanotextured
        Surface XRGC092
    ▶Interbody Fusion Device
      ▶Nanotextured Surface XRGC092
      ▶Radiolucent Porous XRGC0F3
    Interbody Fusion Device, Nanotextured
      Surface XRGB092
    ▶Interbody Fusion Device
      ▶Nanotextured Surface XRGB092
      ▶Radiolucent Porous XRGB0F3
  Lumbosacral 0SG3
    Interbody Fusion Device, Nanotextured
      Surface XRGD092
    ▶Interbody Fusion Device
      ▶Nanotextured Surface XRGD092
      ▶Radiolucent Porous XRGD0F3
  Metacarpocarpal
    Left 0RGT
    Right 0RGS
  Metacarpophalangeal
    Left 0RGV
    Right 0RGU
  Metatarsal-Phalangeal
    Left 0SGN
    Right 0SGM
  Metatarsal-Tarsal
    Left 0SGL
    Right 0SGK
  Occipital-cervical 0RG0
    Interbody Fusion Device, Nanotextured
      Surface XRG0092
    ▶Interbody Fusion Device
      ▶Nanotextured Surface XRG0092
      ▶Radiolucent Porous XRG00F3
  Sacrococcygeal 0SG5
  Sacroiliac
    Left 0SG8
    Right 0SG7
  Shoulder
    Left 0RGK
    Right 0RGJ
  Sternoclavicular
    Left 0RGF
    Right 0RGE
  Tarsal
    Left 0SGJ
    Right 0SGH

▶ New   ➠ Revised   ~~deleted~~ Deleted

Fusion *(Continued)*
▶ Tarsometatarsal
  ▶ Left 0SGL
  ▶ Right 0SGK
 Temporomandibular
  Left 0RGD
  Right 0RGC
 Thoracic Vertebral 0RG6
  2 to 7 0RG7
   ~~Interbody Fusion Device, Nanotextured Surface XRG7092~~
   ▶ Interbody Fusion Device
    ▶ Nanotextured Surface XRG7092
    ▶ Radiolucent Porous XRG70F3
  8 or more 0RG8
   ~~Interbody Fusion Device, Nanotextured Surface XRG8092~~

Fusion *(Continued)*
 Thoracic Vertebral *(Continued)*
  ▶ Interbody Fusion Device
   ▶ Nanotextured Surface XRG8092
   ▶ Radiolucent Porous XRG80F3
  ~~Interbody Fusion Device, Nanotextured Surface XRG6092~~
  ▶ Interbody Fusion Device
   ▶ Nanotextured Surface XRG6092
   ▶ Radiolucent Porous XRG60F3
 Thoracolumbar Vertebral 0RGA
  ~~Interbody Fusion Device, Nanotextured Surface XRGA092~~

Fusion *(Continued)*
 Thoracolumbar Vertebral *(Continued)*
  ▶ Interbody Fusion Device
   ▶ Nanotextured Surface XRGA092
   ▶ Radiolucent Porous XRGA0F3
 Toe Phalangeal
  Left 0SGQ
  Right 0SGP
 Wrist
  Left 0RGP
  Right 0RGN
Fusion screw (compression) (lag) (locking)
 use Internal Fixation Device in Upper Joints
 use Internal Fixation Device in Lower Joints

G

Gait training *see* Motor Treatment,
  Rehabilitation F07
Galea aponeurotica *use* Subcutaneous Tissue
  and Fascia, Scalp
▶**GammaTile™** *use* Radioactive Element,
  Cesium-131 Collagen Implant in 00H
Ganglion impar (ganglion of Walther) *use*
  Sacral Sympathetic Nerve
Ganglionectomy
  Destruction of lesion *see* Destruction
  Excision of lesion *see* Excision
Gasserian ganglion *use* Trigeminal Nerve
Gastrectomy
  Partial *see* Excision, Stomach 0DB6
  Total *see* Resection, Stomach 0DT6
  Vertical (sleeve) *see* Excision, Stomach 0DB6
Gastric electrical stimulation (GES) lead *use*
  Stimulator Lead in Gastrointestinal System
Gastric lymph node *use* Lymphatic, Aortic
Gastric pacemaker lead *use* Stimulator Lead in
  Gastrointestinal System
Gastric plexus *see* Abdominal Sympathetic
  Nerve
Gastrocnemius muscle
  use Lower Leg Muscle, Right
  use Lower Leg Muscle, Left
➡**Gastrocolic ligament** *use* Omentum
➡**Gastrocolic omentum** *use* Omentum
Gastrocolostomy
  see Bypass, Gastrointestinal System 0D1
  see Drainage, Gastrointestinal System 0D9
Gastroduodenal artery *use* Hepatic Artery
Gastroduodenectomy
  see Excision, Gastrointestinal System 0DB
  see Resection, Gastrointestinal System 0DT
Gastroduodenoscopy 0DJ08ZZ
Gastroenteroplasty
  see Repair, Gastrointestinal System 0DQ
  see Supplement, Gastrointestinal System 0DU
Gastroenterostomy
  see Bypass, Gastrointestinal System 0D1
  see Drainage, Gastrointestinal System 0D9
Gastroesophageal (GE) junction *use*
  Esophagogastric Junction
Gastrogastrostomy
  see Bypass, Stomach 0D16
  see Drainage, Stomach 0D96
➡**Gastrohepatic omentum** *use* Omentum
Gastrojejunostomy
  see Bypass, Stomach 0D16
  see Drainage, Stomach 0D96
Gastrolysis *see* Release, Stomach 0DN6
Gastropexy
  see Repair, Stomach 0DQ6
  see Reposition, Stomach 0DS6
➡**Gastrophrenic ligament** *use* Omentum
Gastroplasty
  see Repair, Stomach 0DQ6
  see Supplement, Stomach 0DU6
Gastroplication *see* Restriction, Stomach 0DV6
Gastropylorectomy *see* Excision,
  Gastrointestinal System 0DB
Gastrorrhaphy *see* Repair, Stomach 0DQ6
Gastroscopy 0DJ68ZZ

➡**Gastrosplenic ligament** *use* Omentum
Gastrostomy
  see Bypass, Stomach 0D16
  see Drainage, Stomach 0D96
Gastrotomy *see* Drainage, Stomach 0D96
Gemellus muscle
  use Hip Muscle, Right
  use Hip Muscle, Left
Geniculate ganglion *use* Facial Nerve
Geniculate nucleus *use* Thalamus
Genioglossus muscle *use* Tongue, Palate,
  Pharynx Muscle
Genioplasty *see* Alteration, Jaw, Lower 0W05
Genitofemoral nerve *use* Lumbar Plexus
Gingivectomy *see* Excision, Mouth and Throat
  0CB
Gingivoplasty
  see Repair, Mouth and Throat 0CQ
  see Replacement, Mouth and Throat 0CR
  see Supplement, Mouth and Throat 0CU
Glans penis *use* Prepuce
Glenohumeral joint
  use Shoulder Joint, Right
  use Shoulder Joint, Left
Glenohumeral ligament
  use Shoulder Bursa and Ligament, Right
  use Shoulder Bursa and Ligament, Left
Glenoid fossa (of scapula)
  use Glenoid Cavity, Right
  use Glenoid Cavity, Left
Glenoid ligament (labrum)
  use Shoulder Joint, Right
  use Shoulder Joint, Left
Globus pallidus *use* Basal Ganglia
Glomectomy
  see Excision, Endocrine System 0GB
  see Resection, Endocrine System 0GT
Glossectomy
  see Excision, Tongue 0CB7
  see Resection, Tongue 0CT7
Glossoepiglottic fold *use* Epiglottis
Glossopexy
  see Repair, Tongue 0CQ7
  see Reposition, Tongue 0CS7
Glossoplasty
  see Repair, Tongue 0CQ7
  see Replacement, Tongue 0CR7
  see Supplement, Tongue 0CU7
Glossorrhaphy *see* Repair, Tongue 0CQ7
Glossotomy *see* Drainage, Tongue 0C97
Glottis *use* Larynx
Gluteal Artery Perforator Flap
  ~~Bilateral 0HRV079~~
  ~~Left 0HRU079~~
  ~~Right 0HRT079~~
  ▶Replacement
    ▶Bilateral 0HRV079
    ▶Left 0HRU079
    ▶Right 0HRT079
  ▶Transfer
    ▶Left 0KXG
    ▶Right 0KXF
Gluteal lymph node *use* Lymphatic, Pelvis
Gluteal vein
  use Hypogastric Vein, Right
  use Hypogastric Vein, Left

Gluteus maximus muscle
  use Hip Muscle, Right
  use Hip Muscle, Left
Gluteus medius muscle
  use Hip Muscle, Right
  use Hip Muscle, Left
Gluteus minimus muscle
  use Hip Muscle, Right
  use Hip Muscle, Left
GORE EXCLUDER® AAA Endoprosthesis
  use Intraluminal Device, Branched or
    Fenestrated, One or Two Arteries in
    04V
  use Intraluminal Device, Branched or
    Fenestrated, Three or More Arteries in
    04V
  use Intraluminal Device
GORE EXCLUDER® IBE Endoprosthesis *use*
  Intraluminal Device, Branched or
  Fenestrated, One or Two Arteries in
  04V
GORE TAG® Thoracic Endoprosthesis *use*
  Intraluminal Device
GORE® DUALMESH® *use* Synthetic
  Substitute
Gracilis muscle
  use Upper Leg Muscle, Right
  use Upper Leg Muscle, Left
Graft
  see Replacement
  see Supplement
Great auricular nerve *use* Lumbar Plexus
Great cerebral vein *use* Intracranial Vein
~~Great saphenous vein~~
  ~~use Greater Saphenous Vein, Right~~
  ~~use Greater Saphenous Vein, Left~~
▶**Great(er) saphenous vein**
  ▶*use* Saphenous Vein, Right
  ▶*use* Saphenous Vein, Left
➡**Greater alar cartilage** *use* Nasal Mucosa and
  Soft Tissue
Greater occipital nerve *use* Cervical Nerve
▶**Greater Omentum** *use* Omentum
Greater splanchnic nerve *use* Thoracic
  Sympathetic Nerve
Greater superficial petrosal nerve *use* Facial
  Nerve
Greater trochanter
  use Upper Femur, Right
  use Upper Femur, Left
Greater tuberosity
  use Humeral Head, Right
  use Humeral Head, Left
Greater vestibular (Bartholin's) gland
  use Vestibular Gland
➡**Greater wing** *use* Sphenoid Bone
  ~~use Sphenoid Bone, Right~~
  ~~use Sphenoid Bone, Left~~
Guedel airway *use* Intraluminal Device, Airway
  in Mouth and Throat
Guidance, catheter placement
  EKG *see* Measurement, Physiological Systems
    4A0
  Fluoroscopy *see* Fluoroscopy, Veins B51
  Ultrasound *see* Ultrasonography, Veins B54

H

Hallux
 use Toe, 1st, Right
 use Toe, 1st, Left
Hamate bone
 use Carpal, Right
 use Carpal, Left
Hancock Bioprosthesis (aortic) (mitral) valve
 use Zooplastic Tissue in Heart and Great Vessels
Hancock Bioprosthetic Valved Conduit *use* Zooplastic Tissue in Heart and Great Vessels
Harvesting, stem cells *see* Pheresis, Circulatory 6A55
Head of fibula
 use Fibula, Right
 use Fibula, Left
Hearing Aid Assessment F14Z
Hearing Assessment F13Z
Hearing Device
 Bone Conduction
  Left 09HE
  Right 09HD
 Insertion of device in
  Left 0NH6[034]SZ
  Right 0NH5[034]SZ
 Multiple Channel Cochlear Prosthesis
  Left 09HE
  Right 09HD
 Removal of device from, Skull 0NP0
 Revision of device in, Skull 0NW0
 Single Channel Cochlear Prosthesis
  Left 09HE
  Right 09HD
Hearing Treatment F09Z
Heart Assist System
 ~~External~~
  ~~Insertion of device in, Heart 02HA~~
  ~~Removal of device from, Heart 02PA~~
  ~~Revision of device in, Heart 02WA~~
 Implantable
  Insertion of device in, Heart 02HA
  Removal of device from, Heart 02PA
  Revision of device in, Heart 02WA
 ▶Short-term External
  ▶Insertion of device in, Heart 02HA
  ▶Removal of device from, Heart 02PA
  ▶Revision of device in, Heart 02WA
▶**HeartMate 3™ LVAS** *use* Implantable Heart Assist System in Heart and Great Vessels
HeartMate II® Left Ventricular Assist Device (LVAD) *use* Implantable Heart Assist System in Heart and Great Vessels
HeartMate XVE® Left Ventricular Assist Device (LVAD) *use* Implantable Heart Assist System in Heart and Great Vessels
HeartMate® implantable heart assist system *see* Insertion of device in, Heart 02HA
Helix
 use External Ear, Right
 use External Ear, Left
 use External Ear, Bilateral
Hematopoietic cell transplant (HCT) *see* Transfusion, Circulatory 302
Hemicolectomy *see* Resection, Gastrointestinal System 0DT
Hemicystectomy *see* Excision, Urinary System 0TB
Hemigastrectomy *see* Excision, Gastrointestinal System 0DB
Hemiglossectomy *see* Excision, Mouth and Throat 0CB
Hemilaminectomy
 see Excision, Upper Bones 0PB
 see Excision, Lower Bones 0QB
Hemilaminotomy
 see Release, Central Nervous System 00N
 see Release, Peripheral Nervous System 01N
 see Drainage, Upper Bones 0P9
 see Excision, Upper Bones 0PB

Hemilaminotomy *(Continued)*
 see Release, Upper Bones 0PN
 see Drainage, Lower Bones 0Q9
 see Excision, Lower Bones 0QB
 see Release, Lower Bones 0QN
Hemilaryngectomy *see* Excision, Larynx 0CBS
Hemimandibulectomy *see* Excision, Head and Facial Bones 0NB
Hemimaxillectomy *see* Excision, Head and Facial Bones 0NB
Hemipylorectomy *see* Excision, Gastrointestinal System 0DB
Hemispherectomy
 ~~see Excision, Central Nervous System 00B~~
 ~~see Resection, Central Nervous System 00T~~
 ▶*see* Excision, Central Nervous System and Cranial Nerves 00B
 ▶*see* Resection, Central Nervous System and Cranial Nerves 00T
Hemithyroidectomy
 see Excision, Endocrine System 0GB
 see Resection, Endocrine System 0GT
➠**Hemodialysis** *see* Performance, Urinary 5A1D
▶**Hemolung® Respiratory Assist System (RAS)** 5A0920Z
Hepatectomy
 see Excision, Hepatobiliary System and Pancreas 0FB
 see Resection, Hepatobiliary System and Pancreas 0FT
Hepatic artery proper *use* Hepatic Artery
➠**Hepatic flexure** *use* Transverse Colon
Hepatic lymph node *use* Aortic Lymphatic
Hepatic plexus *use* Abdominal Sympathetic Nerve
Hepatic portal vein *use* Portal Vein
Hepaticoduodenostomy
 see Bypass, Hepatobiliary System and Pancreas 0F1
 see Drainage, Hepatobiliary System and Pancreas 0F9
Hepaticotomy *see* Drainage, Hepatobiliary System and Pancreas 0F9
Hepatocholedochostomy *see* Drainage, Duct, Common Bile 0F99
➠**Hepatogastric ligament** *use* Omentum
Hepatopancreatic ampulla *use* Ampulla of Vater
Hepatopexy
 see Repair, Hepatobiliary System and Pancreas 0FQ
 see Reposition, Hepatobiliary System and Pancreas 0FS
Hepatorrhaphy *see* Repair, Hepatobiliary System and Pancreas 0FQ
Hepatotomy *see* Drainage, Hepatobiliary System and Pancreas 0F9
Herculink (RX) Elite Renal Stent System *use* Intraluminal Device
Herniorrhaphy
 see Repair, Anatomical Regions, General 0WQ
 see Repair, Anatomical Regions, Lower Extremities 0YQ
 with synthetic substitute
  see Supplement, Anatomical Regions, General 0WU
  see Supplement, Anatomical Regions, Lower Extremities 0YU
Hip (joint) liner *use* Liner in Lower Joints
Holter monitoring 4A12X45
Holter valve ventricular shunt *use* Synthetic Substitute
Humeroradial joint
 use Elbow Joint, Right
 use Elbow Joint, Left
Humeroulnar joint
 use Elbow Joint, Right
 use Elbow Joint, Left
Humerus, distal
 use Humeral Shaft, Right
 use Humeral Shaft, Left

Hydrocelectomy *see* Excision, Male Reproductive System 0VB
Hydrotherapy
 Assisted exercise in pool *see* Motor Treatment, Rehabilitation F07
 Whirlpool *see* Activities of Daily Living Treatment, Rehabilitation F08
Hymenectomy
 see Excision, Hymen 0UBK
 see Resection, Hymen 0UTK
Hymenoplasty
 see Repair, Hymen 0UQK
 see Supplement, Hymen 0UUK
Hymenorrhaphy *see* Repair, Hymen 0UQK
Hymenotomy
 see Division, Hymen 0U8K
 see Drainage, Hymen 0U9K
Hyoglossus muscle *use* Tongue, Palate, Pharynx Muscle
Hyoid artery
 use Thyroid Artery, Right
 use Thyroid Artery, Left
Hyperalimentation *see* Introduction of substance in or on
Hyperbaric oxygenation
 Decompression sickness treatment *see* Decompression, Circulatory 6A15
 Wound treatment *see* Assistance, Circulatory 5A05
Hyperthermia
 Radiation Therapy
  Abdomen DWY38ZZ
  Adrenal Gland DGY28ZZ
  Bile Ducts DFY28ZZ
  Bladder DTY28ZZ
  Bone, Other DPYC8ZZ
  Bone Marrow D7Y08ZZ
  Brain D0Y08ZZ
  Brain Stem D0Y18ZZ
  Breast
   Left DMY08ZZ
   Right DMY18ZZ
  Bronchus DBY18ZZ
  Cervix DUY18ZZ
  Chest DWY28ZZ
  Chest Wall DBY78ZZ
  Colon DDY58ZZ
  Diaphragm DBY88ZZ
  Duodenum DDY28ZZ
  Ear D9Y08ZZ
  Esophagus DDY08ZZ
  Eye D8Y08ZZ
  Femur DPY98ZZ
  Fibula DPYB8ZZ
  Gallbladder DFY18ZZ
  Gland
   Adrenal DGY28ZZ
   Parathyroid DGY48ZZ
   Pituitary DGY08ZZ
   Thyroid DGY58ZZ
  Glands, Salivary D9Y68ZZ
  Head and Neck DWY18ZZ
  Hemibody DWY48ZZ
  Humerus DPY68ZZ
  Hypopharynx D9Y38ZZ
  Ileum DDY48ZZ
  Jejunum DDY38ZZ
  Kidney DTY08ZZ
  Larynx D9YB8ZZ
  Liver DFY08ZZ
  Lung DBY28ZZ
  Lymphatics
   Abdomen D7Y68ZZ
   Axillary D7Y48ZZ
   Inguinal D7Y88ZZ
   Neck D7Y38ZZ
   Pelvis D7Y78ZZ
   Thorax D7Y58ZZ
  Mandible DPY38ZZ
  Maxilla DPY28ZZ
  Mediastinum DBY68ZZ

Hyperthermia *(Continued)*
  Radiation Therapy *(Continued)*
    Mouth D9Y48ZZ
    Nasopharynx D9YD8ZZ
    Neck and Head DWY18ZZ
    Nerve, Peripheral D0Y78ZZ
    Nose D9Y18ZZ
    Oropharynx D9YF8ZZ
    Ovary DUY08ZZ
    Palate
      Hard D9Y88ZZ
      Soft D9Y98ZZ
    Pancreas DFY38ZZ
    Parathyroid Gland DGY48ZZ
    Pelvic Bones DPY88ZZ
    Pelvic Region DWY68ZZ
    Pineal Body DGY18ZZ
    Pituitary Gland DGY08ZZ
    Pleura DBY58ZZ
    Prostate DVY08ZZ
    Radius DPY78ZZ
    Rectum DDY78ZZ
    Rib DPY58ZZ
    Sinuses D9Y78ZZ
    Skin
      Abdomen DHY88ZZ
      Arm DHY48ZZ
      Back DHY78ZZ
      Buttock DHY98ZZ
      Chest DHY68ZZ
      Face DHY28ZZ

Hyperthermia *(Continued)*
  Radiation Therapy *(Continued)*
    Skin *(Continued)*
      Leg DHYB8ZZ
      Neck DHY38ZZ
    Skull DPY08ZZ
    Spinal Cord D0Y68ZZ
    Spleen D7Y28ZZ
    Sternum DPY48ZZ
    Stomach DDY18ZZ
    Testis DVY18ZZ
    Thymus D7Y18ZZ
    Thyroid Gland DGY58ZZ
    Tibia DPYB8ZZ
    Tongue D9Y58ZZ
    Trachea DBY08ZZ
    Ulna DPY78ZZ
    Ureter DTY18ZZ
    Urethra DTY38ZZ
    Uterus DUY28ZZ
    Whole Body DWY58ZZ
  Whole Body 6A3Z
Hypnosis GZFZZZZZ
Hypogastric artery
  use Internal Iliac Artery, Right
  use Internal Iliac Artery, Left
Hypopharynx *use* Pharynx
Hypophysectomy
  see Excision, Gland, Pituitary 0GB0
  see Resection, Gland, Pituitary 0GT0

Hypophysis *use* Gland, Pituitary
Hypothalamotomy *see* Destruction, Thalamus 0059
Hypothenar muscle
  use Hand Muscle, Right
  use Hand Muscle, Left
Hypothermia, Whole Body 6A4Z
Hysterectomy
  supracervical *see* Resection, Uterus 0UT9
  ➡ total *see* Resection, Uterus 0UT9
    ~~see Resection, Uterus 0UT9~~
    ~~see Resection, Cervix 0UTC~~
Hysterolysis *see* Release, Uterus 0UN9
Hysteropexy
  see Repair, Uterus 0UQ9
  see Reposition, Uterus 0US9
Hysteroplasty
  see Repair, Uterus 0UQ9
Hysterorrhaphy *see* Repair, Uterus 0UQ9
Hysteroscopy 0UJD8ZZ
Hysterotomy
  see Drainage, Uterus 0U99
Hysterotrachelectomy
  see Resection, Uterus 0UT9
  see Resection, Cervix 0UTC
Hysterotracheloplasty
  see Repair, Uterus 0UQ9
Hysterotrachelorrhaphy *see* Repair, Uterus 0UQ9

▶ New   ➡ Revised   ~~deleted~~ Deleted

I

IABP (Intra-aortic balloon pump) *see* Assistance, Cardiac 5A02
IAEMT (Intraoperative anesthetic effect monitoring and titration) *see* Monitoring, Central Nervous 4A10
Idarucizumab, Dabigatran Reversal Agent XW0
▶**IHD (Intermittent hemodialysis)** 5A1D70Z
Ileal artery *use* Superior Mesenteric Artery
Ileectomy
  see Excision, Ileum 0DBB
  see Resection, Ileum 0DTB
Ileocolic artery *use* Superior Mesenteric Artery
Ileocolic vein *use* Colic Vein
Ileopexy
  see Repair, Ileum 0DQB
  see Reposition, Ileum 0DSB
Ileorrhaphy *see* Repair, Ileum 0DQB
Ileoscopy 0DJD8ZZ
Ileostomy
  see Bypass, Ileum 0D1B
  see Drainage, Ileum 0D9B
Ileotomy *see* Drainage, Ileum 0D9B
Ileoureterostomy *see* Bypass, Bladder 0T1B
Iliac crest
  use Pelvic Bone, Right
  use Pelvic Bone, Left
Iliac fascia
  use Subcutaneous Tissue and Fascia, Right Upper Leg
  use Subcutaneous Tissue and Fascia, Left Upper Leg
Iliac lymph node *use* Lymphatic, Pelvis
Iliacus muscle
  use Hip Muscle, Right
  use Hip Muscle, Left
Iliofemoral ligament
  use Hip Bursa and Ligament, Right
  use Hip Bursa and Ligament, Left
Iliohypogastric nerve *use* Lumbar Plexus
Ilioinguinal nerve *use* Lumbar Plexus
Iliolumbar artery
  use Internal Iliac Artery, Right
  use Internal Iliac Artery, Left
➡**Iliolumbar ligament** *use* Lower Spine Bursa and Ligament
  ~~use Trunk Bursa and Ligament, Right~~
  ~~use Trunk Bursa and Ligament, Left~~
Iliotibial tract (band)
  use Subcutaneous Tissue and Fascia, Right Upper Leg
  use Subcutaneous Tissue and Fascia, Left Upper Leg
Ilium
  use Pelvic Bone, Right
  use Pelvic Bone, Left
Ilizarov external fixator
  use External Fixation Device, Ring in 0PH
  use External Fixation Device, Ring in 0PS
  use External Fixation Device, Ring in 0QH
  use External Fixation Device, Ring in 0QS
Ilizarov-Vecklich device
  use External Fixation Device, Limb Lengthening in 0PH
  use External Fixation Device, Limb Lengthening in 0QH
Imaging, diagnostic
  see Plain Radiography
  see Fluoroscopy
  see Computerized Tomography (CT Scan)
  see Magnetic Resonance Imaging (MRI)
  see Ultrasonography
Immobilization
  Abdominal Wall 2W33X
  Arm
    Lower
      Left 2W3DX
      Right 2W3CX

Immobilization *(Continued)*
  Arm *(Continued)*
    Upper
      Left 2W3BX
      Right 2W3AX
  Back 2W35X
  Chest Wall 2W34X
  Extremity
    Lower
      Left 2W3MX
      Right 2W3LX
    Upper
      Left 2W39X
      Right 2W38X
  Face 2W31X
  Finger
    Left 2W3KX
    Right 2W3JX
  Foot
    Left 2W3TX
    Right 2W3SX
  Hand
    Left 2W3FX
    Right 2W3EX
  Head 2W30X
  Inguinal Region
    Left 2W37X
    Right 2W36X
  Leg
    Lower
      Left 2W3RX
      Right 2W3QX
    Upper
      Left 2W3PX
      Right 2W3NX
  Neck 2W32X
  Thumb
    Left 2W3HX
    Right 2W3GX
  Toe
    Left 2W3VX
    Right 2W3UX
Immunization *see* Introduction of Serum, Toxoid, and Vaccine
Immunotherapy *see* Introduction of Immunotherapeutic Substance
Immunotherapy, antineoplastic
  Interferon *see* Introduction of Low-dose Interleukin-2
  Interleukin-2 of high-dose *see* Introduction, High-dose Interleukin-2
  Interleukin-2, low-dose *see* Introduction of Low-dose Interleukin-2
  Monoclonal antibody *see* Introduction of Monoclonal Antibody
  Proleukin, high-dose *see* Introduction of High-dose Interleukin-2
  Proleukin, low-dose *see* Introduction of Low-dose Interleukin-2
▶**Impella® heart pump** *use* Short-term External Heart Assist System in Heart and Great Vessels
Impeller Pump
  Continuous, Output 5A0221D
  Intermittent, Output 5A0211D
Implantable cardioverter-defibrillator (ICD) *use* Defibrillator Generator in 0JH
Implantable drug infusion pump (anti-spasmodic) (chemotherapy) (pain) *use* Infusion Device, Pump in Subcutaneous Tissue and Fascia
Implantable glucose monitoring device *use* Monitoring Device
Implantable hemodynamic monitor (IHM) *use* Monitoring Device, Hemodynamic in 0JH
Implantable hemodynamic monitoring system (IHMS) *use* Monitoring Device, Hemodynamic in 0JH
Implantable Miniature Telescope™ (IMT) *use* Synthetic Substitute, Intraocular Telescope in 08R

Implantation
  see Replacement
  see Insertion
➡**Implanted (venous) (access) port** *use* Vascular Access Device, Totally Implantable in Subcutaneous Tissue and Fascia
IMV (intermittent mandatory ventilation) *see* Assistance, Respiratory 5A09
In Vitro Fertilization 8E0ZXY1
Incision, abscess *see* Drainage
Incudectomy
  see Excision, Ear, Nose, Sinus 09B
  see Resection, Ear, Nose, Sinus 09T
Incudopexy
  see Repair, Ear, Nose, Sinus 09Q
  see Reposition, Ear, Nose, Sinus 09S
Incus
  use Ossicle, Auditory, Right
  use Ossicle, Auditory, Left
Induction of labor
  Artificial rupture of membranes *see* Drainage, Pregnancy 109
  Oxytocin *see* Introduction of Hormone
InDura, intrathecal catheter (1P) (spinal) *use* Infusion Device
Inferior cardiac nerve *use* Thoracic Sympathetic Nerve
Inferior cerebellar vein *use* Intracranial Vein
Inferior cerebral vein *use* Intracranial Vein
Inferior epigastric artery
  use External Iliac Artery, Right
  use External Iliac Artery, Left
Inferior epigastric lymph node *use* Lymphatic, Pelvis
Inferior genicular artery
  use Popliteal Artery, Right
  use Popliteal Artery, Left
Inferior gluteal artery
  use Internal Iliac Artery, Right
  use Internal Iliac Artery, Left
Inferior gluteal nerve *use* Sacral Plexus Nerve
Inferior hypogastric plexus *use* Abdominal Sympathetic Nerve
Inferior labial artery *use* Face Artery
Inferior longitudinal muscle *use* Tongue, Palate, Pharynx Muscle
Inferior mesenteric ganglion *use* Abdominal Sympathetic Nerve
Inferior mesenteric lymph node *use* Mesenteric Lymphatic
Inferior mesenteric plexus *use* Abdominal Sympathetic Nerve
Inferior oblique muscle
  use Extraocular Muscle, Right
  use Extraocular Muscle, Left
Inferior pancreaticoduodenal artery *use* Superior Mesenteric Artery
Inferior phrenic artery *use* Abdominal Aorta
Inferior rectus muscle
  use Extraocular Muscle, Right
  use Extraocular Muscle, Left
Inferior suprarenal artery
  use Renal Artery, Right
  use Renal Artery, Left
Inferior tarsal plate
  use Lower Eyelid, Right
  use Lower Eyelid, Left
Inferior thyroid vein
  use Innominate Vein, Right
  use Innominate Vein, Left
Inferior tibiofibular joint
  use Ankle Joint, Right
  use Ankle Joint, Left
Inferior turbinate *use* Nasal Turbinate
Inferior ulnar collateral artery
  use Brachial Artery, Right
  use Brachial Artery, Left
Inferior vesical artery
  use Internal Iliac Artery, Right
  use Internal Iliac Artery, Left

Infraauricular lymph node use Lymphatic, Head
Infraclavicular (deltopectoral) lymph node
    use Lymphatic, Right Upper Extremity
    use Lymphatic, Left Upper Extremity
Infrahyoid muscle
    use Neck Muscle, Right
    use Neck Muscle, Left
Infraparotid lymph node use Lymphatic, Head
Infraspinatus fascia
    use Subcutaneous Tissue and Fascia, Right
        Upper Arm
    use Subcutaneous Tissue and Fascia, Left
        Upper Arm
Infraspinatus muscle
    use Shoulder Muscle, Right
    use Shoulder Muscle, Left
Infundibulopelvic ligament use Uterine
    Supporting Structure
Infusion see Introduction of substance in or on
Infusion Device, Pump
    Insertion of device in
        Abdomen 0JH8
        Back 0JH7
        Chest 0JH6
        Lower Arm
            Left 0JHH
            Right 0JHG
        Lower Leg
            Left 0JHP
            Right 0JHN
        Trunk 0JHT
        Upper Arm
            Left 0JHF
            Right 0JHD
        Upper Leg
            Left 0JHM
            Right 0JHL
    Removal of device from
        Lower Extremity 0JPW
        Trunk 0JPT
        Upper Extremity 0JPV
    Revision of device in
        Lower Extremity 0JWW
        Trunk 0JWT
        Upper Extremity 0JWV
Infusion, glucarpidase
    Central vein 3E043GQ
    Peripheral vein 3E033GQ
Inguinal canal
    use Inguinal Region, Right
    use Inguinal Region, Left
    use Inguinal Region, Bilateral
Inguinal triangle
    see Inguinal Region, Right
    see Inguinal Region, Left
    see Inguinal Region, Bilateral
Injection see Introduction of substance in or on
Injection reservoir, port use Vascular Access
    Device, Reservoir in Subcutaneous Tissue
    and Fascia
Injection reservoir, pump use Infusion Device,
    Pump in Subcutaneous Tissue and Fascia
▶**Injection, Concentrated Bone Marrow Aspirate**
    (CBMA), intramuscular XK02303
Insemination, artificial 3E0P7LZ
Insertion
    Antimicrobial envelope see Introduction of
        Anti-infective
    Aqueous drainage shunt
        see Bypass, Eye 081
        see Drainage, Eye 089
    Products of Conception 10H0
    Spinal Stabilization Device
        see Insertion of device in, Upper Joints 0RH
        see Insertion of device in, Lower Joints 0SH
Insertion of device in
    Abdominal Wall 0WHF
    Acetabulum
        Left 0QH5
        Right 0QH4
    Anal Sphincter 0DHR

Insertion of device in (Continued)
    Ankle Region
        Left 0YHL
        Right 0YHK
    Anus 0DHQ
    Aorta
        Abdominal 04H0
        Thoracic
            Ascending/Arch 02HX
            Descending 02HW
    Arm
        Lower
            Left 0XHF
            Right 0XHD
        Upper
            Left 0XH9
            Right 0XH8
    Artery
        Anterior Tibial
            Left 04HQ
            Right 04HP
        Axillary
            Left 03H6
            Right 03H5
        Brachial
            Left 03H8
            Right 03H7
        Celiac 04H1
        Colic
            Left 04H7
            Middle 04H8
            Right 04H6
        Common Carotid
            Left 03HJ
            Right 03HH
        Common Iliac
            Left 04HD
            Right 04HC
        External Carotid
            Left 03HN
            Right 03HM
        External Iliac
            Left 04HJ
            Right 04HH
        Face 03HR
        Femoral
            Left 04HL
            Right 04HK
        Foot
            Left 04HW
            Right 04HV
        Gastric 04H2
        Hand
            Left 03HF
            Right 03HD
        Hepatic 04H3
        Inferior Mesenteric 04HB
        Innominate 03H2
        Internal Carotid
            Left 03HL
            Right 03HK
        Internal Iliac
            Left 04HF
            Right 04HE
        Internal Mammary
            Left 03H1
            Right 03H0
        Intracranial 03HG
        Lower 04HY
        Peroneal
            Left 04HU
            Right 04HT
        Popliteal
            Left 04HN
            Right 04HM
        Posterior Tibial
            Left 04HS
            Right 04HR
        Pulmonary
            Left 02HR
            Right 02HQ
        Pulmonary Trunk 02HP

Insertion of device in (Continued)
    Artery (Continued)
        Radial
            Left 03HC
            Right 03HB
        Renal
            Left 04HA
            Right 04H9
        Splenic 04H4
        Subclavian
            Left 03H4
            Right 03H3
        Superior Mesenteric 04H5
        Temporal
            Left 03HT
            Right 03HS
        Thyroid
            Left 03HV
            Right 03HU
        Ulnar
            Left 03HA
            Right 03H9
        Upper 03HY
        Vertebral
            Left 03HQ
            Right 03HP
    Atrium
        Left 02H7
        Right 02H6
    Axilla
        Left 0XH5
        Right 0XH4
    Back
        Lower 0WHL
        Upper 0WHK
    Bladder 0THB
    Bladder Neck 0THC
    Bone
        Ethmoid
            Left 0NHG
            Right 0NHF
        Facial 0NHW
        ➥Frontal 0NH1
            ~~Left 0NH2~~
            ~~Right 0NH1~~
        Hyoid 0NHX
        Lacrimal
            Left 0NHJ
            Right 0NHH
        Lower 0QHY
        Nasal 0NHB
        ➥Occipital 0NH7
            ~~Left 0NH8~~
            ~~Right 0NH7~~
        Palatine
            Left 0NHL
            Right 0NHK
        Parietal
            Left 0NH4
            Right 0NH3
        Pelvic
            Left 0QH3
            Right 0QH2
        ➥Sphenoid 0NHC
            ~~Left 0NHD~~
            ~~Right 0NHC~~
        Temporal
            Left 0NH6
            Right 0NH5
        Upper 0PHY
        Zygomatic
            Left 0NHN
            Right 0NHM
    Brain 00H0
    Breast
        Bilateral 0HHV
        Left 0HHU
        Right 0HHT
    Bronchus
        Lingula 0BH9
        Lower Lobe
            Left 0BHB
            Right 0BH6

▶ New   ➥ Revised   ~~deleted~~ Deleted

Insertion of device in (Continued)
  Bronchus (Continued)
    Main
      Left 0BH7
      Right 0BH3
    Middle Lobe, Right 0BH5
    Upper Lobe
      Left 0BH8
      Right 0BH4
▶ Bursa and Ligament
  ▶ Lower 0MHY
  ▶ Upper 0MHX
  Buttock
    Left 0YH1
    Right 0YH0
  Carpal
    Left 0PHN
    Right 0PHM
  Cavity, Cranial 0WH1
  Cerebral Ventricle 00H6
  Cervix 0UHC
  Chest Wall 0WH8
  Cisterna Chyli 07HL
  Clavicle
    Left 0PHB
    Right 0PH9
  Coccyx 0QHS
  Cul-de-sac 0UHF
➡ Diaphragm 0BHT
    ~~Left 0BHS~~
    ~~Right 0BHR~~
  Disc
    Cervical Vertebral 0RH3
    Cervicothoracic Vertebral 0RH5
    Lumbar Vertebral 0SH2
    Lumbosacral 0SH4
    Thoracic Vertebral 0RH9
    Thoracolumbar Vertebral 0RHB
  Duct
    Hepatobiliary 0FHB
    Pancreatic 0FHD
  Duodenum 0DH9
  Ear
  ▶ Inner
    ▶ Left 09HE
    ▶ Right 09HD
  ➡ Left 09HJ
  ➡ Right 09HH
  Elbow Region
    Left 0XHC
    Right 0XHB
  Epididymis and Spermatic Cord 0VHM
  Esophagus 0DH5
  Extremity
    Lower
      Left 0YHB
      Right 0YH9
    Upper
      Left 0XH7
      Right 0XH6
  Eye
    Left 08H1
    Right 08H0
  Face 0WH2
  Fallopian Tube 0UH8
  Femoral Region
    Left 0YH8
    Right 0YH7
  Femoral Shaft
    Left 0QH9
    Right 0QH8
  Femur
    Lower
      Left 0QHC
      Right 0QHB
    Upper
      Left 0QH7
      Right 0QH6
  Fibula
    Left 0QHK
    Right 0QHJ

Insertion of device in (Continued)
  Foot
    Left 0YHN
    Right 0YHM
  Gallbladder 0FH4
  Gastrointestinal Tract 0WHP
  Genitourinary Tract 0WHR
  ~~Gland, Endocrine 0GHS~~
▶ Gland
  ▶ Endocrine 0GHS
  ▶ Salivary 0CHA
  Glenoid Cavity
    Left 0PH8
    Right 0PH7
  Hand
    Left 0XHK
    Right 0XHJ
  Head 0WH0
  Heart 02HA
  Humeral Head
    Left 0PHD
    Right 0PHC
  Humeral Shaft
    Left 0PHG
    Right 0PHF
  Ileum 0DHB
  Inguinal Region
    Left 0YH6
    Right 0YH5
▶ Intestinal Tract
  ▶ Lower 0DHD
  ▶ Upper 0DH0
  Intestine
    Large 0DHE
    Small 0DH8
  Jaw
    Lower 0WH5
    Upper 0WH4
  Jejunum 0DHA
  Joint
    Acromioclavicular
      Left 0RHH
      Right 0RHG
    Ankle
      Left 0SHG
      Right 0SHF
    Carpal
      Left 0RHR
      Right 0RHQ
  ▶ Carpometacarpal
    ▶ Left 0RHT
    ▶ Right 0RHS
    Cervical Vertebral 0RH1
    Cervicothoracic Vertebral 0RH4
    Coccygeal 0SH6
    Elbow
      Left 0RHM
      Right 0RHL
    Finger Phalangeal
      Left 0RHX
      Right 0RHW
    Hip
      Left 0SHB
      Right 0SH9
    Knee
      Left 0SHD
      Right 0SHC
    Lumbar Vertebral 0SH0
    Lumbosacral 0SH3
    ~~Metacarpocarpal~~
      ~~Left 0RHT~~
      ~~Right 0RHS~~
    Metacarpophalangeal
      Left 0RHV
      Right 0RHU
    Metatarsal-Phalangeal
      Left 0SHN
      Right 0SHM
    ~~Metatarsal-Tarsal~~
      ~~Left 0SHL~~
      ~~Right 0SHK~~

Insertion of device in (Continued)
  Joint (Continued)
    Occipital-cervical 0RH0
    Sacrococcygeal 0SH5
    Sacroiliac
      Left 0SH8
      Right 0SH7
    Shoulder
      Left 0RHK
      Right 0RHJ
    Sternoclavicular
      Left 0RHF
      Right 0RHE
    Tarsal
      Left 0SHJ
      Right 0SHH
    ▶ Tarsometatarsal
      ▶ Left 0SHL
      ▶ Right 0SHK
    Temporomandibular
      Left 0RHD
      Right 0RHC
    Thoracic Vertebral 0RH6
    Thoracolumbar Vertebral 0RHA
    Toe Phalangeal
      Left 0SHQ
      Right 0SHP
    Wrist
      Left 0RHP
      Right 0RHN
  Kidney 0TH5
  Knee Region
    Left 0YHG
    Right 0YHF
▶ Larynx 0CHS
  Leg
    Lower
      Left 0YHJ
      Right 0YHH
    Upper
      Left 0YHD
      Right 0YHC
  Liver 0FH0
    Left Lobe 0FH2
    Right Lobe 0FH1
  Lung
    Left 0BHL
    Right 0BHK
  Lymphatic 07HN
    Thoracic Duct 07HK
  Mandible
    Left 0NHV
    Right 0NHT
➡ Maxilla 0NHR
    ~~Left 0NHS~~
    ~~Right 0NHR~~
  Mediastinum 0WHC
  Metacarpal
    Left 0PHQ
    Right 0PHP
  Metatarsal
    Left 0QHP
    Right 0QHN
  Mouth and Throat 0CHY
  Muscle
    Lower 0KHY
    Upper 0KHX
▶ Nasal Mucosa and Soft Tissue 09HK
  Nasopharynx 09HN
  Neck 0WH6
  Nerve
    Cranial 00HE
    Peripheral 01HY
  Nipple
    Left 0HHX
    Right 0HHW
  Oral Cavity and Throat 0WH3
  Orbit
    Left 0NHQ
    Right 0NHP
  Ovary 0UH3

▶ New   ➡ Revised   ~~deleted~~ Deleted

Insertion of device in (*Continued*)
  Pancreas 0FHG
  Patella
    Left 0QHF
    Right 0QHD
  Pelvic Cavity 0WHJ
  Penis 0VHS
  Pericardial Cavity 0WHD
  Pericardium 02HN
  Perineum
    Female 0WHN
    Male 0WHM
  Peritoneal Cavity 0WHG
  Phalanx
    Finger
      Left 0PHV
      Right 0PHT
    Thumb
      Left 0PHS
      Right 0PHR
    Toe
      Left 0QHR
      Right 0QHQ
  ▶Pleura 0BHQ
  Pleural Cavity
    Left 0WHB
    Right 0WH9
  Prostate 0VH0
  Prostate and Seminal Vesicles 0VH4
  Radius
    Left 0PHJ
    Right 0PHH
  Rectum 0DHP
  Respiratory Tract 0WHQ
  Retroperitoneum 0WHH
  ~~Rib~~
    ~~Left 0PH2~~
    ~~Right 0PH1~~
  ▶Ribs
    ▶1 to 2 0PH1
    ▶3 or More 0PH2
  Sacrum 0QH1
  Scapula
    Left 0PH6
    Right 0PH5
  Scrotum and Tunica Vaginalis 0VH8
  Shoulder Region
    Left 0XH3
    Right 0XH2
  ▶Sinus 09HY
  ▶Skin 0HHPXYZ
  Skull 0NH0
  Spinal Canal 00HU
  Spinal Cord 00HV
  Spleen 07HP
  Sternum 0PH0
  Stomach 0DH6
  Subcutaneous Tissue and Fascia
    Abdomen 0JH8
    Back 0JH7
    Buttock 0JH9
    Chest 0JH6
    Face 0JH1
    Foot
      Left 0JHR
      Right 0JHQ
    Hand
      Left 0JHK
      Right 0JHJ
    Head and Neck 0JHS
    Lower Arm
      Left 0JHH
      Right 0JHG
    Lower Extremity 0JHW
    Lower Leg
      Left 0JHP
      Right 0JHN
    Neck
      ~~Anterior 0JH4~~
      ~~Posterior 0JH5~~
      ▶Left 0JH5
      ▶Right 0JH4

Insertion of device in (*Continued*)
  Subcutaneous Tissue and Fascia (*Continued*)
    Pelvic Region 0JHC
    Perineum 0JHB
    Scalp 0JH0
    Trunk 0JHT
    Upper Arm
      Left 0JHF
      Right 0JHD
    Upper Extremity 0JHV
    Upper Leg
      Left 0JHM
      Right 0JHL
  Tarsal
    Left 0QHM
    Right 0QHL
  ▶Tendon
    ▶Lower 0LHY
    ▶Upper 0LHX
  Testis 0VHD
  Thymus 07HM
  Tibia
    Left 0QHH
    Right 0QHG
  Tongue 0CH7
  Trachea 0BH1
  Tracheobronchial Tree 0BH0
  Ulna
    Left 0PHL
    Right 0PHK
  Ureter 0TH9
  Urethra 0THD
  Uterus 0UH9
  Uterus and Cervix 0UHD
  Vagina 0UHG
  Vagina and Cul-de-sac 0UHH
  Vas Deferens 0VHR
  Vein
    Axillary
      Left 05H8
      Right 05H7
    Azygos 05H0
    Basilic
      Left 05HC
      Right 05HB
    Brachial
      Left 05HA
      Right 05H9
    Cephalic
      Left 05HF
      Right 05HD
    Colic 06H7
    Common Iliac
      Left 06HD
      Right 06HC
    Coronary 02H4
    Esophageal 06H3
    External Iliac
      Left 06HG
      Right 06HF
    External Jugular
      Left 05HQ
      Right 05HP
    Face
      Left 05HV
      Right 05HT
    Femoral
      Left 06HN
      Right 06HM
    Foot
      Left 06HV
      Right 06HT
    Gastric 06H2
    ~~Greater Saphenous~~
      ~~Left 06HQ~~
      ~~Right 06HP~~
    Hand
      Left 05HH
      Right 05HG
    Hemiazygos 05H1
    Hepatic 06H4

Insertion of device in (*Continued*)
  Vein (*Continued*)
    Hypogastric
      Left 06HJ
      Right 06HH
    Inferior Mesenteric 06H6
    Innominate
      Left 05H4
      Right 05H3
    Internal Jugular
      Left 05HN
      Right 05HM
    Intracranial 05HL
    ~~Lesser Saphenous~~
      ~~Left 06HS~~
      ~~Right 06HR~~
    Lower 06HY
    Portal 06H8
    Pulmonary
      Left 02HT
      Right 02HS
    Renal
      Left 06HB
      Right 06H9
    ▶Saphenous
      ▶Left 06HQ
      ▶Right 06HP
    Splenic 06H1
    Subclavian
      Left 05H6
      Right 05H5
    Superior Mesenteric 06H5
    Upper 05HY
    Vertebral
      Left 05HS
      Right 05HR
    Vena Cava
      Inferior 06H0
      Superior 02HV
  Ventricle
    Left 02HL
    Right 02HK
  Vertebra
    Cervical 0PH3
    Lumbar 0QH0
    Thoracic 0PH4
  Wrist Region
    Left 0XHH
    Right 0XHG

Inspection
  Abdominal Wall 0WJF
  Ankle Region
    Left 0YJL
    Right 0YJK
  Arm
    Lower
      Left 0XJF
      Right 0XJD
    Upper
      Left 0XJ9
      Right 0XJ8
  Artery
    Lower 04JY
    Upper 03JY
  Axilla
    Left 0XJ5
    Right 0XJ4
  Back
    Lower 0WJL
    Upper 0WJK
  Bladder 0TJB
  Bone
    Facial 0NJW
    Lower 0QJY
    Nasal 0NJB
    Upper 0PJY
  Bone Marrow 07JT
  Brain 00J0
  Breast
    Left 0HJU
    Right 0HJT

Inspection (Continued)
Bursa and Ligament
  Lower 0MJY
  Upper 0MJX
Buttock
  Left 0YJ1
  Right 0YJ0
Cavity, Cranial 0WJ1
Chest Wall 0WJ8
Cisterna Chyli 07JL
Diaphragm 0BJT
Disc
  Cervical Vertebral 0RJ3
  Cervicothoracic Vertebral 0RJ5
  Lumbar Vertebral 0SJ2
  Lumbosacral 0SJ4
  Thoracic Vertebral 0RJ9
  Thoracolumbar Vertebral 0RJB
Duct
  Hepatobiliary 0FJB
  Pancreatic 0FJD
Ear
  Inner
    Left 09JE
    Right 09JD
  Left 09JJ
  Right 09JH
Elbow Region
  Left 0XJC
  Right 0XJB
Epididymis and Spermatic Cord 0VJM
Extremity
  Lower
    Left 0YJB
    Right 0YJ9
  Upper
    Left 0XJ7
    Right 0XJ6
Eye
  Left 08J1XZZ
  Right 08J0XZZ
Face 0WJ2
Fallopian Tube 0UJ8
Femoral Region
  Bilateral 0YJE
  Left 0YJ8
  Right 0YJ7
Finger Nail 0HJQXZZ
Foot
  Left 0YJN
  Right 0YJM
Gallbladder 0FJ4
Gastrointestinal Tract 0WJP
Genitourinary Tract 0WJR
Gland
  Adrenal 0GJ5
  Endocrine 0GJS
  Pituitary 0GJ0
  Salivary 0CJA
Great Vessel 02JY
Hand
  Left 0XJK
  Right 0XJJ
Head 0WJ0
Heart 02JA
Inguinal Region
  Bilateral 0YJA
  Left 0YJ6
  Right 0YJ5
Intestinal Tract
  Lower 0DJD
  Upper 0DJ0
Jaw
  Lower 0WJ5
  Upper 0WJ4
Joint
  Acromioclavicular
    Left 0RJH
    Right 0RJG
  Ankle
    Left 0SJG
    Right 0SJF

Inspection (Continued)
Joint (Continued)
  Carpal
    Left 0RJR
    Right 0RJQ
  ▶Carpometacarpal
    ▶Left 0RJT
    ▶Right 0RJS
  Cervical Vertebral 0RJ1
  Cervicothoracic Vertebral 0RJ4
  Coccygeal 0SJ6
  Elbow
    Left 0RJM
    Right 0RJL
  Finger Phalangeal
    Left 0RJX
    Right 0RJW
  Hip
    Left 0SJB
    Right 0SJ9
  Knee
    Left 0SJD
    Right 0SJC
  Lumbar Vertebral 0SJ0
  Lumbosacral 0SJ3
  ~~Metacarpocarpal~~
    ~~Left 0RJT~~
    ~~Right 0RJS~~
  Metacarpophalangeal
    Left 0RJV
    Right 0RJU
  Metatarsal-Phalangeal
    Left 0SJN
    Right 0SJM
  ~~Metatarsal-Tarsal~~
    ~~Left 0SJL~~
    ~~Right 0SJK~~
  Occipital-cervical 0RJ0
  Sacrococcygeal 0SJ5
  Sacroiliac
    Left 0SJ8
    Right 0SJ7
  Shoulder
    Left 0RJK
    Right 0RJJ
  Sternoclavicular
    Left 0RJF
    Right 0RJE
  Tarsal
    Left 0SJJ
    Right 0SJH
  ▶Tarsometatarsal
    ▶Left 0SJL
    ▶Right 0SJK
  Temporomandibular
    Left 0RJD
    Right 0RJC
  Thoracic Vertebral 0RJ6
  Thoracolumbar Vertebral 0RJA
  Toe Phalangeal
    Left 0SJQ
    Right 0SJP
  Wrist
    Left 0RJP
    Right 0RJN
Kidney 0TJ5
Knee Region
  Left 0YJG
  Right 0YJF
Larynx 0CJS
Leg
  Lower
    Left 0YJJ
    Right 0YJH
  Upper
    Left 0YJD
    Right 0YJC
Lens
  Left 08JKXZZ
  Right 08JJXZZ
Liver 0FJ0

Inspection (Continued)
Lung
  Left 0BJL
  Right 0BJK
Lymphatic 07JN
  Thoracic Duct 07JK
Mediastinum 0WJC
Mesentery 0DJV
Mouth and Throat 0CJY
Muscle
  Extraocular
    Left 08JM
    Right 08JL
  Lower 0KJY
  Upper 0KJX
▶Nasal Mucosa and Soft Tissue 09JK
Neck 0WJ6
Nerve
  Cranial 00JE
  Peripheral 01JY
~~Nose 09JK~~
Omentum 0DJU
Oral Cavity and Throat 0WJ3
Ovary 0UJ3
Pancreas 0FJG
Parathyroid Gland 0GJR
Pelvic Cavity 0WJD
Penis 0VJS
Pericardial Cavity 0WJD
Perineum
  Female 0WJN
  Male 0WJM
Peritoneal Cavity 0WJG
Peritoneum 0DJW
Pineal Body 0GJ1
Pleura 0BJQ
Pleural Cavity
  Left 0WJB
  Right 0WJ9
Products of Conception 10J0
  Ectopic 10J2
  Retained 10J1
Prostate and Seminal Vesicles 0VJ4
Respiratory Tract 0WJQ
Retroperitoneum 0WJH
Scrotum and Tunica Vaginalis 0VJ8
Shoulder Region
  Left 0XJ3
  Right 0XJ2
Sinus 09JY
Skin 0HJPXZZ
Skull 0NJ0
Spinal Canal 00JU
Spinal Cord 00JV
Spleen 07JP
Stomach 0DJ6
Subcutaneous Tissue and Fascia
  Head and Neck 0JJS
  Lower Extremity 0JJW
  Trunk 0JJT
  Upper Extremity 0JJV
Tendon
  Lower 0LJY
  Upper 0LJX
Testis 0VJD
Thymus 07JM
Thyroid Gland 0GJK
Toe Nail 0HJRXZZ
Trachea 0BJ1
Tracheobronchial Tree 0BJ0
Tympanic Membrane
  Left 09J8
  Right 09J7
Ureter 0TJ9
Urethra 0TJD
Uterus and Cervix 0UJD
Vagina and Cul-de-sac 0UJH
Vas Deferens 0VJR
Vein
  Lower 06JY
  Upper 05JY

▶ New   ⇒ Revised   ~~deleted~~ Deleted

Inspection *(Continued)*
  Vulva 0UJM
  Wall
    Abdominal 0WJF
    Chest 0WJ8
    Wrist Region
      Left 0XJH
      Right 0XJG
Instillation *see* Introduction of substance in
  or on
Insufflation *see* Introduction of substance in
  or on
Interatrial septum *use* Atrial Septum
Interbody fusion (spine) cage
  use Interbody Fusion Device in Upper Joints
  use Interbody Fusion Device in Lower Joints
~~Interbody Fusion Device, Nanotextured Surface~~
  ~~Cervical Vertebral XRG1092~~
    ~~2 or more XRG2092~~
  ~~Cervicothoracic Vertebral XRG4092~~
  ~~Lumbar Vertebral XRGB092~~
    ~~2 or more XRGC092~~
  ~~Lumbosacral XRGD092~~
  ~~Occipital-cervical XRG0092~~
  ~~Thoracic Vertebral XRG6092~~
    ~~2 to 7 XRG7092~~
    ~~8 or more XRG8092~~
  ~~Thoracolumbar Vertebral XRGA092~~
▶ **Interbody Fusion Device**
  ▶ Nanotextured Surface
    ▶ Cervical Vertebral XRG1092
      ▶ 2 or more XRG2092
    ▶ Cervicothoracic Vertebral XRG4092
    ▶ Lumbar Vertebral XRGB092
      ▶ 2 or more XRGC092
    ▶ Lumbosacral XRGD092
    ▶ Occipital-cervical XRG0092
    ▶ Thoracic Vertebral XRG6092
      ▶ 2 to 7 XRG7092
      ▶ 8 or more XRG8092
    ▶ Thoracolumbar Vertebral XRGA092
  ▶ Radiolucent Porous
    ▶ Cervical Vertebral XRG10F3
      ▶ 2 or more XRG20F3
    ▶ Cervicothoracic Vertebral XRG40F3
    ▶ Lumbar Vertebral XRGB0F3
      ▶ 2 or more XRGC0F3
    ▶ Lumbosacral XRGD0F3
    ▶ Occipital-cervical XRG00F3
    ▶ Thoracic Vertebral XRG60F3
      ▶ 2 to 7 XRG70F3
      ▶ 8 or more XRG80F3
    ▶ Thoracolumbar Vertebral XRGA0F3
Intercarpal joint
  use Carpal Joint, Right
  use Carpal Joint, Left
Intercarpal ligament
  use Hand Bursa and Ligament, Right
  use Hand Bursa and Ligament, Left
Interclavicular ligament
  use Shoulder Bursa and Ligament, Right
  use Shoulder Bursa and Ligament, Left
Intercostal lymph node *use* Lymphatic, Thorax
Intercostal muscle
  use Thorax Muscle, Right
  use Thorax Muscle, Left
Intercostal nerve *use* Thoracic Nerve
Intercostobrachial nerve *use* Thoracic Nerve
Intercuneiform joint
  use Tarsal Joint, Right
  use Tarsal Joint, Left
Intercuneiform ligament
  use Foot Bursa and Ligament, Right
  use Foot Bursa and Ligament, Left
Intermediate bronchus *use* Main Bronchus, Right
Intermediate cuneiform bone
  use Tarsal, Right
  use Tarsal, Left
▶ **Intermittent hemodialysis (IHD)** 5A1D70Z

Intermittent mandatory ventilation *see* Assistance, Respiratory 5A09
Intermittent Negative Airway Pressure
  24-96 Consecutive Hours, Ventilation 5A0945B
  Greater than 96 Consecutive Hours, Ventilation 5A0955B
  Less than 24 Consecutive Hours, Ventilation 5A0935B
Intermittent Positive Airway Pressure
  24-96 Consecutive Hours, Ventilation 5A09458
  Greater than 96 Consecutive Hours, Ventilation 5A09558
  Less than 24 Consecutive Hours, Ventilation 5A09358
Intermittent positive pressure breathing *see* Assistance, Respiratory 5A09
Internal (basal) cerebral vein *use* Intracranial Vein
Internal anal sphincter *use* Anal Sphincter
Internal carotid artery, intracranial portion *use* Intracranial Artery
Internal carotid plexus *use* Head and Neck Sympathetic Nerve
Internal iliac vein
  use Hypogastric Vein, Right
  use Hypogastric Vein, Left
Internal maxillary artery
  use External Carotid Artery, Right
  use External Carotid Artery, Left
➡ **Internal naris** *use* Nasal Mucosa and Soft Tissue
Internal oblique muscle
  use Abdomen Muscle, Right
  use Abdomen Muscle, Left
Internal pudendal artery
  use Internal Iliac Artery, Right
  use Internal Iliac Artery, Left
Internal pudendal vein
  use Hypogastric Vein, Right
  use Hypogastric Vein, Left
Internal thoracic artery
  use Internal Mammary Artery, Right
  use Internal Mammary Artery, Left
  use Subclavian Artery, Right
  use Subclavian Artery, Left
Internal urethral sphincter *use* Urethra
Interphalangeal (IP) joint
  use Finger Phalangeal Joint, Right
  use Finger Phalangeal Joint, Left
  use Toe Phalangeal Joint, Right
  use Toe Phalangeal Joint, Left
Interphalangeal ligament
  use Hand Bursa and Ligament, Right
  use Hand Bursa and Ligament, Left
  use Foot Bursa and Ligament, Right
  use Foot Bursa and Ligament, Left
Interrogation, cardiac rhythm related device
  Interrogation only *see* Measurement, Cardiac 4B02
  With cardiac function testing *see* Measurement, Cardiac 4A02
Interruption *see* Occlusion
Interspinalis muscle
  use Trunk Muscle, Right
  use Trunk Muscle, Left
Interspinous ligament
  use Head and Neck Bursa and Ligament
  ~~use Trunk Bursa and Ligament, Right~~
  ~~use Trunk Bursa and Ligament, Left~~
  ▶ *use* Upper Spine Bursa and Ligament
  ▶ *use* Lower Spine Bursa and Ligament
Interspinous process spinal stabilization device
  use Spinal Stabilization Device, Interspinous Process in 0RH
  use Spinal Stabilization Device, Interspinous Process in 0SH
InterStim® Therapy lead *use* Neurostimulator Lead in Peripheral Nervous System
InterStim® Therapy neurostimulator, *use* Stimulator Generator, Single Array in 0JH

Intertransversarius muscle
  use Trunk Muscle, Right
  use Trunk Muscle, Left
Intertransverse ligament
  ~~use Trunk Bursa and Ligament, Right~~
  ~~use Trunk Bursa and Ligament, Left~~
  ▶ *use* Upper Spine Bursa and Ligament
  ▶ *use* Lower Spine Bursa and Ligament
Interventricular foramen (Monro) *use* Cerebral Ventricle
Interventricular septum *use* Ventricular Septum
Intestinal lymphatic trunk *use* Cisterna Chyli
Intraluminal Device
  Airway
    Esophagus 0DH5
    Mouth and Throat 0CHY
    Nasopharynx 09HN
  Bioactive
    Occlusion
      Common Carotid
        Left 03LJ
        Right 03LH
      External Carotid
        Left 03LN
        Right 03LM
      Internal Carotid
        Left 03LL
        Right 03LK
      Intracranial 03LG
      Vertebral
        Left 03LQ
        Right 03LP
    Restriction
      Common Carotid
        Left 03VJ
        Right 03VH
      External Carotid
        Left 03VN
        Right 03VM
      Internal Carotid
        Left 03VL
        Right 03VK
      Intracranial 03VG
      Vertebral
        Left 03VQ
        Right 03VP
  Endobronchial Valve
    Lingula 0BH9
    Lower Lobe
      Left 0BHB
      Right 0BH6
    Main
      Left 0BH7
      Right 0BH3
    Middle Lobe, Right 0BH5
    Upper Lobe
      Left 0BH8
      Right 0BH4
  Endotracheal Airway
    Change device in, Trachea 0B21XEZ
    Insertion of device in, Trachea 0BH1
  Pessary
    Change device in, Vagina and Cul-de-sac 0U2HXGZ
    Insertion of device in
      Cul-de-sac 0UHF
      Vagina 0UHG
Intramedullary (IM) rod (nail)
  use Internal Fixation Device, Intramedullary in Upper Bones
  use Internal Fixation Device, Intramedullary in Lower Bones
Intramedullary skeletal kinetic distractor (ISKD)
  use Internal Fixation Device, Intramedullary in Upper Bones
  use Internal Fixation Device, Intramedullary in Lower Bones
Intraocular Telescope
  Left 08RK30Z
  Right 08RJ30Z

Intraoperative Knee Replacement Sensor
  XR2
Intraoperative Radiation Therapy (IORT)
  Anus DDY8CZZ
  Bile Ducts DFY2CZZ
  Bladder DTY2CZZ
  Cervix DUY1CZZ
  Colon DDY5CZZ
  Duodenum DDY2CZZ
  Gallbladder DFY1CZZ
  Ileum DDY4CZZ
  Jejunum DDY3CZZ
  Kidney DTY0CZZ
  Larynx D9YBCZZ
  Liver DFY0CZZ
  Mouth D9Y4CZZ
  Nasopharynx D9YDCZZ
  Ovary DUY0CZZ
  Pancreas DFY3CZZ
  Pharynx D9YCCZZ
  Prostate DVY0CZZ
  Rectum DDY7CZZ
  Stomach DDY1CZZ
  Ureter DTY1CZZ
  Urethra DTY3CZZ
  Uterus DUY2CZZ
Intrauterine device (IUD) *use* Contraceptive
  Device in Female Reproductive System
Intravascular fluorescence angiography (IFA)
  see Monitoring, Physiological Systems
  4A1
Introduction of substance in or on
  Artery
    Central 3E06
      Analgesics 3E06
      Anesthetic, Intracirculatory 3E06
      Anti-infective 3E06
      Anti-inflammatory 3E06
      Antiarrhythmic 3E06
      Antineoplastic 3E06
      Destructive Agent 3E06
      Diagnostic Substance, Other 3E06
      Electrolytic Substance 3E06
      Hormone 3E06
      Hypnotics 3E06
      Immunotherapeutic 3E06
      Nutritional Substance 3E06
      Platelet Inhibitor 3E06
      Radioactive Substance 3E06
      Sedatives 3E06
      Serum 3E06
      Thrombolytic 3E06
      Toxoid 3E06
      Vaccine 3E06
      Vasopressor 3E06
      Water Balance Substance 3E06
    Coronary 3E07
      Diagnostic Substance, Other 3E07
      Platelet Inhibitor 3E07
      Thrombolytic 3E07
    Peripheral 3E05
      Analgesics 3E05
      Anesthetic, Intracirculatory 3E05
      Anti-infective 3E05
      Anti-inflammatory 3E05
      Antiarrhythmic 3E05
      Antineoplastic 3E05
      Destructive Agent 3E05
      Diagnostic Substance, Other 3E05
      Electrolytic Substance 3E05
      Hormone 3E05
      Hypnotics 3E05
      Immunotherapeutic 3E05
      Nutritional Substance 3E05
      Platelet Inhibitor 3E05
      Radioactive Substance 3E05
      Sedatives 3E05
      Serum 3E05
      Thrombolytic 3E05
      Toxoid 3E05
      Vaccine 3E05

Introduction of substance in or on *(Continued)*
  Artery *(Continued)*
    Peripheral *(Continued)*
      Vasopressor 3E05
      Water Balance Substance 3E05
  Biliary Tract 3E0J
    Analgesics 3E0J
    ~~Anesthetic, Local 3E0J~~
    ▶ Anesthetic Agent 3E0J
    Anti-infective 3E0J
    Anti-inflammatory 3E0J
    Antineoplastic 3E0J
    Destructive Agent 3E0J
    Diagnostic Substance, Other 3E0J
    Electrolytic Substance 3E0J
    Gas 3E0J
    Hypnotics 3E0J
    Islet Cells, Pancreatic 3E0J
    Nutritional Substance 3E0J
    Radioactive Substance 3E0J
    Sedatives 3E0J
    Water Balance Substance 3E0J
  Bone 3E0V3G
    Analgesics 3E0V3NZ
    ~~Anesthetic, Local 3E0V3BZ~~
    ▶ Anesthetic Agent 3E0V3BZ
    Anti-infective 3E0V32
    Anti-inflammatory 3E0V33Z
    Antineoplastic 3E0V30
    Destructive Agent 3E0V3TZ
    Diagnostic Substance, Other 3E0V3KZ
    Electrolytic Substance 3E0V37Z
    Hypnotics 3E0V3NZ
    Nutritional Substance 3E0V36Z
    Radioactive Substance 3E0V3HZ
    Sedatives 3E0V3NZ
    Water Balance Substance 3E0V37Z
  Bone Marrow 3E0A3GC
    Antineoplastic 3E0A30
  Brain 3E0Q
    Analgesics 3E0Q
    ~~Anesthetic, Local 3E0Q~~
    ▶ Anesthetic Agent 3E0Q
    Anti-infective 3E0Q
    Anti-inflammatory 3E0Q
    Antineoplastic 3E0Q
    Destructive Agent 3E0Q
    Diagnostic Substance, Other 3E0Q
    Electrolytic Substance 3E0Q
    Gas 3E0Q
    Hypnotics 3E0Q
    Nutritional Substance 3E0Q
    Radioactive Substance 3E0Q
    Sedatives 3E0Q
    Stem Cells
      Embryonic 3E0Q
      Somatic 3E0Q
    Water Balance Substance 3E0Q
  Cranial Cavity 3E0Q
    Analgesics 3E0Q
    ~~Anesthetic, Local 3E0Q~~
    ▶ Anesthetic Agent 3E0Q
    Anti-infective 3E0Q
    Anti-inflammatory 3E0Q
    Antineoplastic 3E0Q
    Destructive Agent 3E0Q
    Diagnostic Substance, Other 3E0Q
    Electrolytic Substance 3E0Q
    Gas 3E0Q
    Hypnotics 3E0Q
    Nutritional Substance 3E0Q
    Radioactive Substance 3E0Q
    Sedatives 3E0Q
    Stem Cells
      Embryonic 3E0Q
      Somatic 3E0Q
    Water Balance Substance 3E0Q
  Ear 3E0B
    Analgesics 3E0B
    ~~Anesthetic, Local 3E0B~~
    ▶ Anesthetic Agent 3E0B
    Anti-infective 3E0B

Introduction of substance in or on *(Continued)*
  Ear *(Continued)*
    Anti-inflammatory 3E0B
    Antineoplastic 3E0B
    Destructive Agent 3E0B
    Diagnostic Substance, Other 3E0B
    Hypnotics 3E0B
    Radioactive Substance 3E0B
    Sedatives 3E0B
  Epidural Space 3E0S3GC
    Analgesics 3E0S3NZ
    ~~Anesthetic~~
      ~~Local 3E0S3BZ~~
      ~~Regional 3E0S3CZ~~
    ▶ Anesthetic Agent 3E0S3BZ
    Anti-infective 3E0S32
    Anti-inflammatory 3E0S33Z
    Antineoplastic 3E0S30
    Destructive Agent 3E0S3TZ
    Diagnostic Substance, Other 3E0S3KZ
    Electrolytic Substance 3E0S37Z
    Gas 3E0S
    Hypnotics 3E0S3NZ
    Nutritional Substance 3E0S36Z
    Radioactive Substance 3E0S3HZ
    Sedatives 3E0S3NZ
    Water Balance Substance 3E0S37Z
  Eye 3E0C
    Analgesics 3E0C
    ~~Anesthetic, Local 3E0C~~
    ▶ Anesthetic Agent 3E0C
    Anti-infective 3E0C
    Anti-inflammatory 3E0C
    Antineoplastic 3E0C
    Destructive Agent 3E0C
    Diagnostic Substance, Other 3E0C
    Gas 3E0C
    Hypnotics 3E0C
    Pigment 3E0C
    Radioactive Substance 3E0C
    Sedatives 3E0C
  Gastrointestinal Tract
    Lower 3E0H
      Analgesics 3E0H
      ~~Anesthetic, Local 3E0H~~
      ▶ Anesthetic Agent 3E0H
      Anti-infective 3E0H
      Anti-inflammatory 3E0H
      Antineoplastic 3E0H
      Destructive Agent 3E0H
      Diagnostic Substance, Other 3E0H
      Electrolytic Substance 3E0H
      Gas 3E0H
      Hypnotics 3E0H
      Nutritional Substance 3E0H
      Radioactive Substance 3E0H
      Sedatives 3E0H
      Water Balance Substance 3E0H
    Upper 3E0G
      Analgesics 3E0G
      ~~Anesthetic, Local 3E0G~~
      ▶ Anesthetic Agent 3E0G
      Anti-infective 3E0G
      Anti-inflammatory 3E0G
      Antineoplastic 3E0G
      Destructive Agent 3E0G
      Diagnostic Substance, Other 3E0G
      Electrolytic Substance 3E0G
      Gas 3E0G
      Hypnotics 3E0G
      Nutritional Substance 3E0G
      Radioactive Substance 3E0G
      Sedatives 3E0G
      Water Balance Substance 3E0G
  Genitourinary Tract 3E0K
    Analgesics 3E0K
    ~~Anesthetic, Local 3E0K~~
    ▶ Anesthetic Agent 3E0K
    Anti-infective 3E0K
    Anti-inflammatory 3E0K
    Antineoplastic 3E0K

▶ New   ⇒ Revised   ~~deleted~~ Deleted

Introduction of substance in or on (Continued)
  Genitourinary Tract (Continued)
    Destructive Agent 3E0K
    Diagnostic Substance, Other 3E0K
    Electrolytic Substance 3E0K
    Gas 3E0K
    Hypnotics 3E0K
    Nutritional Substance 3E0K
    Radioactive Substance 3E0K
    Sedatives 3E0K
    Water Balance Substance 3E0K
  Heart 3E08
    Diagnostic Substance, Other 3E08
    Platelet Inhibitor 3E08
    Thrombolytic 3E08
  Joint 3E0U
    Analgesics 3E0U3NZ
    Anesthetic, Local 3E0U3BZ
  ▶Anesthetic Agent 3E0U3BZ
    Anti-infective 3E0U
    Anti-inflammatory 3E0U33Z
    Antineoplastic 3E0U30
    Destructive Agent 3E0U3TZ
    Diagnostic Substance, Other 3E0U3KZ
    Electrolytic Substance 3E0U37Z
    Gas 3E0U3SF
    Hypnotics 3E0U3NZ
    Nutritional Substance 3E0U36Z
    Radioactive Substance 3E0U3HZ
    Sedatives 3E0U3NZ
    Water Balance Substance 3E0U37Z
  Lymphatic 3E0W3GC
    Analgesics 3E0W3NZ
    Anesthetic, Local 3E0W3BZ
  ▶Anesthetic Agent 3E0W3BZ
    Anti-infective 3E0W32
    Anti-inflammatory 3E0W33Z
    Antineoplastic 3E0W30
    Destructive Agent 3E0W3TZ
    Diagnostic Substance, Other 3E0W3KZ
    Electrolytic Substance 3E0W37Z
    Hypnotics 3E0W3NZ
    Nutritional Substance 3E0W36Z
    Radioactive Substance 3E0W3HZ
    Sedatives 3E0W3NZ
    Water Balance Substance 3E0W37Z
  Mouth 3E0D
    Analgesics 3E0D
    Anesthetic, Local 3E0D
  ▶Anesthetic Agent 3E0D
    Anti-infective 3E0D
    Anti-inflammatory 3E0D
    Antiarrhythmic 3E0D
    Antineoplastic 3E0D
    Destructive Agent 3E0D
    Diagnostic Substance, Other 3E0D
    Electrolytic Substance 3E0D
    Hypnotics 3E0D
    Nutritional Substance 3E0D
    Radioactive Substance 3E0D
    Sedatives 3E0D
    Serum 3E0D
    Toxoid 3E0D
    Vaccine 3E0D
    Water Balance Substance 3E0D
  Mucous Membrane 3E00XGC
    Analgesics 3E00XNZ
    Anesthetic, Local 3E00XBZ
  ▶Anesthetic Agent 3E00XBZ
    Anti-infective 3E00X2
    Anti-inflammatory 3E00X3Z
    Antineoplastic 3E00X0
    Destructive Agent 3E00XTZ
    Diagnostic Substance, Other 3E00XKZ
    Hypnotics 3E00XNZ
    Pigment 3E00XMZ
    Sedatives 3E00XNZ
    Serum 3E00X4Z
    Toxoid 3E00X4Z
    Vaccine 3E00X4Z

Introduction of substance in or on (Continued)
  Muscle 3E023GC
    Analgesics 3E023NZ
    Anesthetic, Local 3E023BZ
  ▶Anesthetic Agent 3E023BZ
    Anti-infective 3E0232
    Anti-inflammatory 3E0233Z
    Antineoplastic 3E0230
    Destructive Agent 3E023TZ
    Diagnostic Substance, Other 3E023KZ
    Electrolytic Substance 3E0237Z
    Hypnotics 3E023NZ
    Nutritional Substance 3E0236Z
    Radioactive Substance 3E023HZ
    Sedatives 3E023NZ
    Serum 3E0234Z
    Toxoid 3E0234Z
    Vaccine 3E0234Z
    Water Balance Substance 3E0237Z
  Nerve
    Cranial 3E0X3GC
      Anesthetic
        Local 3E0X3BZ
        Regional 3E0X3CZ
    ▶Anesthetic Agent 3E0X3BZ
      Anti-inflammatory 3E0X33Z
      Destructive Agent 3E0X3TZ
    Peripheral 3E0T3GC
      Anesthetic
        Local 3E0T3BZ
        Regional 3E0T3CZ
    ▶Anesthetic Agent 3E0T3BZ
      Anti-inflammatory 3E0T33Z
      Destructive Agent 3E0T3TZ
    Plexus 3E0T3GC
      Anesthetic
        Local 3E0T3BZ
        Regional 3E0T3CZ
    ▶Anesthetic Agent 3E0T3BZ
      Anti-inflammatory 3E0T33Z
      Destructive Agent 3E0T3TZ
  Nose 3E09
    Analgesics 3E09
    Anesthetic, Local 3E09
  ▶Anesthetic Agent 3E09
    Anti-infective 3E09
    Anti-inflammatory 3E09
    Antineoplastic 3E09
    Destructive Agent 3E09
    Diagnostic Substance, Other 3E09
    Hypnotics 3E09
    Radioactive Substance 3E09
    Sedatives 3E09
    Serum 3E09
    Toxoid 3E09
    Vaccine 3E09
  Pancreatic Tract 3E0J
    Analgesics 3E0J
    Anesthetic, Local 3E0J
  ▶Anesthetic Agent 3E0J
    Anti-infective 3E0J
    Anti-inflammatory 3E0J
    Antineoplastic 3E0J
    Destructive Agent 3E0J
    Diagnostic Substance, Other 3E0J
    Electrolytic Substance 3E0J
    Gas 3E0J
    Hypnotics 3E0J
    Islet Cells, Pancreatic 3E0J
    Nutritional Substance 3E0J
    Radioactive Substance 3E0J
    Sedatives 3E0J
    Water Balance Substance 3E0J
  ▬▶Pericardial Cavity 3E0Y
    Analgesics 3E0Y3NZ
    Anesthetic, Local 3E0Y3BZ
  ▶Anesthetic Agent 3E0Y3BZ
    Anti-infective 3E0Y32
    Anti-inflammatory 3E0Y33Z
    Antineoplastic 3E0Y
    Destructive Agent 3E0Y3TZ

Introduction of substance in or on (Continued)
  Pericardial Cavity (Continued)
    Diagnostic Substance, Other 3E0Y3KZ
    Electrolytic Substance 3E0Y37Z
    Gas 3E0Y
    Hypnotics 3E0Y3NZ
    Nutritional Substance 3E0Y36Z
    Radioactive Substance 3E0Y3HZ
    Sedatives 3E0Y3NZ
    Water Balance Substance 3E0Y37Z
  ▬▶Peritoneal Cavity 3E0M
    ▬▶Adhesion Barrier 3E0M
    Analgesics 3E0M3NZ
    Anesthetic, Local 3E0M3BZ
  ▶Anesthetic Agent 3E0M3BZ
    Anti-infective 3E0M32
    Anti-inflammatory 3E0M33Z
    Antineoplastic 3E0M
    Destructive Agent 3E0M3TZ
    Diagnostic Substance, Other 3E0M3KZ
    Electrolytic Substance 3E0M37Z
    Gas 3E0M
    Hypnotics 3E0M3NZ
    Nutritional Substance 3E0M36Z
    Radioactive Substance 3E0M3HZ
    Sedatives 3E0M3NZ
    Water Balance Substance 3E0M37Z
  Pharynx 3E0D
    Analgesics 3E0D
    Anesthetic, Local 3E0D
  ▶Anesthetic Agent 3E0D
    Anti-infective 3E0D
    Anti-inflammatory 3E0D
    Antiarrhythmic 3E0D
    Antineoplastic 3E0D
    Destructive Agent 3E0D
    Diagnostic Substance, Other 3E0D
    Electrolytic Substance 3E0D
    Hypnotics 3E0D
    Nutritional Substance 3E0D
    Radioactive Substance 3E0D
    Sedatives 3E0D
    Serum 3E0D
    Toxoid 3E0D
    Vaccine 3E0D
    Water Balance Substance 3E0D
  ▬▶Pleural Cavity 3E0L
    ▬▶Adhesion Barrier 3E0L
    Analgesics 3E0L3NZ
    Anesthetic, Local 3E0L3BZ
  ▶Anesthetic Agent 3E0L3BZ
    Anti-infective 3E0L32
    Anti-inflammatory 3E0L33Z
    Antineoplastic 3E0L
    Destructive Agent 3E0L3TZ
    Diagnostic Substance, Other 3E0L3KZ
    Electrolytic Substance 3E0L37Z
    Gas 3E0L
    Hypnotics 3E0L3NZ
    Nutritional Substance 3E0L36Z
    Radioactive Substance 3E0L3HZ
    Sedatives 3E0L3NZ
    Water Balance Substance 3E0L37Z
  Products of Conception 3E0E
    Analgesics 3E0E
    Anesthetic, Local 3E0E
  ▶Anesthetic Agent 3E0E
    Anti-infective 3E0E
    Anti-inflammatory 3E0E
    Antineoplastic 3E0E
    Destructive Agent 3E0E
    Diagnostic Substance, Other 3E0E
    Electrolytic Substance 3E0E
    Gas 3E0E
    Hypnotics 3E0E
    Nutritional Substance 3E0E
    Radioactive Substance 3E0E
    Sedatives 3E0E
    Water Balance Substance 3E0E

▶ New ▬▶ Revised ~~deleted~~ Deleted

Introduction of substance in or on *(Continued)*
Reproductive
Female 3E0P
➠Adhesion Barrier 3E0P
Analgesics 3E0P
~~Anesthetic, Local 3E0P~~
▶Anesthetic Agent 3E0P
Anti-infective 3E0P
Anti-inflammatory 3E0P
Antineoplastic 3E0P
Destructive Agent 3E0P
Diagnostic Substance, Other 3E0P
Electrolytic Substance 3E0P
Gas 3E0P
▶Hormone 3E0P
Hypnotics 3E0P
Nutritional Substance 3E0P
Ovum, Fertilized 3E0P
Radioactive Substance 3E0P
Sedatives 3E0P
Sperm 3E0P
Water Balance Substance 3E0P
Male 3E0N
Analgesics 3E0N
~~Anesthetic, Local 3E0N~~
▶Anesthetic Agent 3E0N
Anti-infective 3E0N
Anti-inflammatory 3E0N
Antineoplastic 3E0N
Destructive Agent 3E0N
Diagnostic Substance, Other 3E0N
Electrolytic Substance 3E0N
Gas 3E0N
Hypnotics 3E0N
Nutritional Substance 3E0N
Radioactive Substance 3E0N
Sedatives 3E0N
Water Balance Substance 3E0N
Respiratory Tract 3E0F
Analgesics 3E0F
~~Anesthetic~~
~~Inhalation 3E0F~~
~~Local 3E0F~~
▶Anesthetic Agent 3E0F
Anti-infective 3E0F
Anti-inflammatory 3E0F
Antineoplastic 3E0F
Destructive Agent 3E0F
Diagnostic Substance, Other 3E0F
Electrolytic Substance 3E0F
Gas 3E0F
Hypnotics 3E0F
Nutritional Substance 3E0F
Radioactive Substance 3E0F
Sedatives 3E0F
Water Balance Substance 3E0F
Skin 3E00XGC
Analgesics 3E00XNZ
~~Anesthetic, Local 3E00XBZ~~
▶Anesthetic Agent 3E00XBZ
Anti-infective 3E00X2
Anti-inflammatory 3E00X3Z
Antineoplastic 3E00X0
Destructive Agent 3E00XTZ
Diagnostic Substance, Other 3E00XKZ
Hypnotics 3E00XNZ
Pigment 3E00XMZ
Sedatives 3E00XNZ
Serum 3E00X4Z
Toxoid 3E00X4Z
Vaccine 3E00X4Z
Spinal Canal 3E0R3GC
Analgesics 3E0R3NZ
~~Anesthetic~~
~~Local 3E0R3BZ~~
~~Regional 3E0R3CZ~~
▶Anesthetic Agent 3E0R3BZ

Introduction of substance in or on *(Continued)*
Spinal Canal *(Continued)*
Anti-infective 3E0R32
Anti-inflammatory 3E0R33Z
Antineoplastic 3E0R30
Destructive Agent 3E0R3TZ
Diagnostic Substance, Other 3E0R3KZ
Electrolytic Substance 3E0R37Z
Gas 3E0R
Hypnotics 3E0R3NZ
Nutritional Substance 3E0R36Z
Radioactive Substance 3E0R3HZ
Sedatives 3E0R3NZ
Stem Cells
Embryonic 3E0R
Somatic 3E0R
Water Balance Substance 3E0R37Z
Subcutaneous Tissue 3E013GC
Analgesics 3E013NZ
~~Anesthetic, Local 3E013BZ~~
▶Anesthetic Agent 3E013BZ
Anti-infective 3E01
Anti-inflammatory 3E0133Z
Antineoplastic 3E0130
Destructive Agent 3E013TZ
Diagnostic Substance, Other 3E013KZ
Electrolytic Substance 3E0137Z
Hormone 3E013V
Hypnotics 3E013NZ
Nutritional Substance 3E0136Z
Radioactive Substance 3E013HZ
Sedatives 3E013NZ
Serum 3E0134Z
Toxoid 3E0134Z
Vaccine 3E0134Z
Water Balance Substance 3E0137Z
Vein
Central 3E04
Analgesics 3E04
Anesthetic, Intracirculatory 3E04
Anti-infective 3E04
Anti-inflammatory 3E04
Antiarrhythmic 3E04
Antineoplastic 3E04
Destructive Agent 3E04
Diagnostic Substance, Other 3E04
Electrolytic Substance 3E04
Hormone 3E04
Hypnotics 3E04
Immunotherapeutic 3E04
Nutritional Substance 3E04
Platelet Inhibitor 3E04
Radioactive Substance 3E04
Sedatives 3E04
Serum 3E04
Thrombolytic 3E04
Toxoid 3E04
Vaccine 3E04
Vasopressor 3E04
Water Balance Substance 3E04
Peripheral 3E03
Analgesics 3E03
Anesthetic, Intracirculatory 3E03
Anti-infective 3E03
Anti-inflammatory 3E03
Antiarrhythmic 3E03
Antineoplastic 3E03
Destructive Agent 3E03
Diagnostic Substance, Other 3E03
Electrolytic Substance 3E03
Hormone 3E03
Hypnotics 3E03
Immunotherapeutic 3E03
Islet Cells, Pancreatic 3E03
Nutritional Substance 3E03
Platelet Inhibitor 3E03
Radioactive Substance 3E03

Introduction of substance in or on *(Continued)*
Vein *(Continued)*
Peripheral *(Continued)*
Sedatives 3E03
Serum 3E03
Thrombolytic 3E03
Toxoid 3E03
Vaccine 3E03
Vasopressor 3E03
Water Balance Substance 3E03
Intubation
Airway
see Insertion of device in, Trachea 0BH1
see Insertion of device in, Mouth and Throat 0CHY
see Insertion of device in, Esophagus 0DH5
Drainage device *see* Drainage
Feeding Device *see* Insertion of device in, Gastrointestinal System 0DH
INTUITY Elite valve system, EDWARDS *use* Zooplastic Tissue, Rapid Deployment Technique in New Technology
IPPB (intermittent positive pressure breathing) *see* Assistance, Respiratory 5A09
Iridectomy
see Excision, Eye 08B
see Resection, Eye 08T
Iridoplasty
see Repair, Eye 08Q
see Replacement, Eye 08R
see Supplement, Eye 08U
Iridotomy *see* Drainage, Eye 089
Irrigation
Biliary Tract, Irrigating Substance 3E1J
Brain, Irrigating Substance 3E1Q38Z
Cranial Cavity, Irrigating Substance 3E1Q38Z
Ear, Irrigating Substance 3E1B
Epidural Space, Irrigating Substance 3E1S38Z
Eye, Irrigating Substance 3E1C
Gastrointestinal Tract
Lower, Irrigating Substance 3E1H
Upper, Irrigating Substance 3E1G
Genitourinary Tract, Irrigating Substance 3E1K
Irrigating Substance 3C1ZX8Z
Joint, Irrigating Substance 3E1U38Z
Mucous Membrane, Irrigating Substance 3E10
Nose, Irrigating Substance 3E19
Pancreatic Tract, Irrigating Substance 3E1J
Pericardial Cavity, Irrigating Substance 3E1Y38Z
Peritoneal Cavity
Dialysate 3E1M39Z
Irrigating Substance 3E1M38Z
Pleural Cavity, Irrigating Substance 3E1L38Z
Reproductive
Female, Irrigating Substance 3E1P
Male, Irrigating Substance 3E1N
Respiratory Tract, Irrigating Substance 3E1F
Skin, Irrigating Substance 3E10
Spinal Canal, Irrigating Substance 3E1R38Z
Isavuconazole Anti-infective XW0
Ischiatic nerve *use* Sciatic Nerve
Ischiocavernosus muscle *use* Perineum Muscle
Ischiofemoral ligament
use Hip Bursa and Ligament, Right
use Hip Bursa and Ligament, Left
Ischium
use Pelvic Bone, Right
use Pelvic Bone, Left
Isolation 8E0ZXY6
Isotope Administration, Whole Body DWY5G
Itrel (3) (4) neurostimulator *use* Stimulator Generator, Single Array in 0JH

J

Jejunal artery *use* Superior Mesenteric Artery
Jejunectomy
  see Excision, Jejunum 0DBA
  see Resection, Jejunum 0DTA
Jejunocolostomy
  see Bypass, Gastrointestinal System 0D1
  see Drainage, Gastrointestinal System 0D9
Jejunopexy
  see Repair, Jejunum 0DQA
  see Reposition, Jejunum 0DSA
Jejunostomy
  see Bypass, Jejunum 0D1A
  see Drainage, Jejunum 0D9A
Jejunotomy *see* Drainage, Jejunum 0D9A
Joint fixation plate
  use Internal Fixation Device in Upper Joints
  use Internal Fixation Device in Lower Joints
Joint liner (insert) *use* Liner in Lower Joints
Joint spacer (antibiotic)
  use Spacer in Upper Joints
  use Spacer in Lower Joints
Jugular body *use* Glomus Jugulare
Jugular lymph node
  use Lymphatic, Right Neck
  use Lymphatic, Left Neck

K

Kappa *use* Pacemaker, Dual Chamber in
  0JH
Kcentra *use* 4-Factor Prothrombin Complex
  Concentrate
Keratectomy, kerectomy
  see Excision, Eye 08B
  see Resection, Eye 08T
Keratocentesis *see* Drainage, Eye 089
Keratoplasty
  see Repair, Eye 08Q
  see Replacement, Eye 08R
  see Supplement, Eye 08U
Keratotomy
  see Drainage, Eye 089
  see Repair, Eye 08Q
Kirschner wire (K-wire)
  use Internal Fixation Device in Head and
    Facial Bones
  use Internal Fixation Device in Upper Bones
  use Internal Fixation Device in Lower Bones
  use Internal Fixation Device in Upper Joints
  use Internal Fixation Device in Lower Joints
Knee (implant) insert *use* Liner in Lower Joints
KUB x-ray *see* Plain Radiography, Kidney,
  Ureter and Bladder BT04
Kuntscher nail
  use Internal Fixation Device, Intramedullary
    in Upper Bones
  use Internal Fixation Device, Intramedullary
    in Lower Bones

L

Labia majora *use* Vulva
Labia minora *use* Vulva
Labial gland
  use Upper Lip
  use Lower Lip
Labiectomy
  see Excision, Female Reproductive System 0UB
  see Resection, Female Reproductive System
    0UT
Lacrimal canaliculus
  use Lacrimal Duct, Right
  use Lacrimal Duct, Left
Lacrimal punctum
  use Lacrimal Duct, Right
  use Lacrimal Duct, Left
Lacrimal sac
  use Lacrimal Duct, Right
  use Lacrimal Duct, Left

▶**LAGB (laparoscopic adjustable gastric**
  banding)
▶Adjustment/revision 0DW64CZ
▶Initial procedure 0DV64CZ
Laminectomy
  ~~*see* Release, Central Nervous System 00N~~
  ▶*see* Release, Central Nervous System and
    Cranial Nerves 00N
  see Release, Peripheral Nervous System 01N
  see Excision, Upper Bones 0PB
  see Excision, Lower Bones 0QB
Laminotomy
  see Release, Central Nervous System 00N
  see Release, Peripheral Nervous System 01N
  see Drainage, Upper Bones 0P9
  see Excision, Upper Bones 0PB
  see Release, Upper Bones 0PN
  see Drainage, Lower Bones 0Q9
  see Excision, Lower Bones 0QB
  see Release, Lower Bones 0QN
LAP-BAND® adjustable gastric banding
  system *use* Extraluminal Device
▶**Laparoscopic-assisted transanal pull-through**
  ▶*see* Excision, Gastrointestinal System 0DB
  ▶*see* Resection, Gastrointestinal System 0DT
Laparoscopy *see* Inspection
Laparotomy
  Drainage *see* Drainage, Peritoneal Cavity
    0W9G
  Exploratory *see* Inspection, Peritoneal *use*
    Nerve, Lumbar Plexus 0WJG
Laryngectomy
  see Excision, Larynx 0CBS
  see Resection, Larynx 0CTS
Laryngocentesis *see* Drainage, Larynx 0C9S
Laryngogram *see* Fluoroscopy, Larynx B91J
Laryngopexy
  see Repair, Larynx 0CQS
Laryngopharynx *use* Pharynx
Laryngoplasty
  see Repair, Larynx 0CQS
  see Replacement, Larynx 0CRS
  see Supplement, Larynx 0CUS
Laryngorrhaphy *see* Repair, Larynx 0CQS
Laryngoscopy 0CJS8ZZ
Laryngotomy *see* Drainage, Larynx 0C9S
Laser Interstitial Thermal Therapy
  Adrenal Gland DGY2KZZ
  Anus DDY8KZZ
  Bile Ducts DFY2KZZ
  Brain D0Y0KZZ
  Brain Stem D0Y1KZZ
  Breast
    Left DMY0KZZ
    Right DMY1KZZ
  Bronchus DBY1KZZ
  Chest Wall DBY7KZZ
  Colon DDY5KZZ
  Diaphragm DBY8KZZ
  Duodenum DDY2KZZ
  Esophagus DDY0KZZ
  Gallbladder DFY1KZZ
  Gland
    Adrenal DGY2KZZ
    Parathyroid DGY4KZZ
    Pituitary DGY0KZZ
    Thyroid DGY5KZZ
  Ileum DDY4KZZ
  Jejunum DDY3KZZ
  Liver DFY0KZZ
  Lung DBY2KZZ
  Mediastinum DBY6KZZ
  Nerve, Peripheral D0Y7KZZ
  Pancreas DFY3KZZ
  Parathyroid Gland DGY4KZZ
  Pineal Body DGY1KZZ
  Pituitary Gland DGY0KZZ
  Pleura DBY5KZZ
  Prostate DVY0KZZ
  Rectum DDY7KZZ
  Spinal Cord D0Y6KZZ

Laser Interstitial Thermal Therapy (*Continued*)
  Stomach DDY1KZZ
  Thyroid Gland DGY5KZZ
  Trachea DBY0KZZ
Lateral (brachial) lymph node
  use Lymphatic, Right Axillary
  use Lymphatic, Left Axillary
Lateral canthus
  use Upper Eyelid, Right
  use Upper Eyelid, Left
Lateral collateral ligament (LCL)
  use Knee Bursa and Ligament, Right
  use Knee Bursa and Ligament, Left
Lateral condyle of femur
  use Lower Femur, Right
  use Lower Femur, Left
Lateral condyle of tibia
  use Tibia, Right
  use Tibia, Left
Lateral cuneiform bone
  use Tarsal, Right
  use Tarsal, Left
Lateral epicondyle of femur
  use Lower Femur, Right
  use Lower Femur, Left
Lateral epicondyle of humerus
  use Humeral Shaft, Right
  use Humeral Shaft, Left
Lateral femoral cutaneous nerve *use* Lumbar
  Plexus
Lateral malleolus
  use Fibula, Right
  use Fibula, Left
Lateral meniscus
  use Knee Joint, Right
  use Knee Joint, Left
➡**Lateral nasal cartilage** *use* Nasal Mucosa and
  Soft Tissue
Lateral plantar artery
  use Foot Artery, Right
  use Foot Artery, Left
Lateral plantar nerve *use* Tibial Nerve
Lateral rectus muscle
  use Extraocular Muscle, Right
  use Extraocular Muscle, Left
Lateral sacral artery
  use Internal Iliac Artery, Right
  use Internal Iliac Artery, Left
Lateral sacral vein
  use Hypogastric Vein, Right
  use Hypogastric Vein, Left
Lateral sural cutaneous nerve *use* Peroneal
  Nerve
Lateral tarsal artery
  use Foot Artery, Right
  use Foot Artery, Left
Lateral temporomandibular ligament *use* Head
  and Neck Bursa and Ligament
Lateral thoracic artery
  use Axillary Artery, Right
  use Axillary Artery, Left
Latissimus dorsi muscle
  use Trunk Muscle, Right
  use Trunk Muscle, Left
Latissimus Dorsi Myocutaneous Flap
  ~~Bilateral 0HRV075~~
  ~~Left 0HRU075~~
  ~~Right 0HRT075~~
  ▶Replacement
    ▶Bilateral 0HRV075
    ▶Left 0HRU075
    ▶Right 0HRT075
  ▶Transfer
    ▶Left 0KXG
    ▶Right 0KXF
Lavage
  see Irrigation
  bronchial alveolar, diagnostic *see* Drainage,
    Respiratory System 0B9
Least splanchnic nerve *use* Thoracic
  Sympathetic Nerve

▶ New   ➡ Revised   ~~deleted~~ Deleted

Left ascending lumbar vein *use* Hemiazygos Vein

Left atrioventricular valve *use* Mitral Valve

Left auricular appendix *use* Atrium, Left

Left colic vein *use* Colic Vein

Left coronary sulcus *use* Heart, Left

Left gastric artery *use* Gastric Artery

Left gastroepiploic artery *use* Splenic Artery

Left gastroepiploic vein *use* Splenic Vein

Left inferior phrenic vein *use* Renal Vein, Left

Left inferior pulmonary vein *use* Pulmonary Vein, Left

Left jugular trunk *use* Thoracic Duct

Left lateral ventricle *use* Cerebral Ventricle

Left ovarian vein *use* Renal Vein, Left

Left second lumbar vein *use* Renal Vein, Left

Left subclavian trunk *use* Thoracic Duct

Left subcostal vein *use* Hemiazygos Vein

Left superior pulmonary vein *use* Pulmonary Vein, Left

Left suprarenal vein *use* Renal Vein, Left

Left testicular vein *use* Renal Vein, Left

Lengthening
  Bone, with device *see* Insertion of Limb Lengthening Device
  Muscle, by incision *see* Division, Muscles ØK8
  Tendon, by incision *see* Division, Tendons ØL8

Leptomeninges, intracranial *use* Cerebral Meninges

Leptomeninges, spinal *use* Spinal Meninges

➡**Lesser alar cartilage** *use* Nasal Mucosa and Soft Tissue

Lesser occipital nerve *use* Cervical Plexus

▶**Lesser Omentum** *use* Omentum

▶**Lesser saphenous vein**
  ▶*use* Saphenous Vein, Right
  ▶*use* Saphenous Vein, Left

Lesser splanchnic nerve *use* Thoracic Sympathetic Nerve

Lesser trochanter
  use Upper Femur, Right
  use Upper Femur, Left

Lesser tuberosity
  use Humeral Head, Right
  use Humeral Head, Left

➡**Lesser wing** *use* Sphenoid Bone
  ~~*use* Sphenoid Bone, Right~~
  ~~*use* Sphenoid Bone, Left~~

Leukopheresis, therapeutic *see* Pheresis, Circulatory 6A55

Levator anguli oris muscle *use* Facial Muscle

Levator ani muscle *use* Perineum Muscle

Levator labii superioris alaeque nasi muscle *use* Facial Muscle

Levator labii superioris muscle *use* Facial Muscle

Levator palpebrae superioris muscle
  use Upper Eyelid, Right
  use Upper Eyelid, Left

Levator scapulae muscle
  use Neck Muscle, Right
  use Neck Muscle, Left

Levator veli palatini muscle *use* Tongue, Palate, Pharynx Muscle

Levatores costarum muscle
  use Thorax Muscle, Right
  use Thorax Muscle, Left

LifeStent® (Flexstar) (XL) Vascular Stent System *use* Intraluminal Device

Ligament of head of fibula
  use Knee Bursa and Ligament, Right
  use Knee Bursa and Ligament, Left

Ligament of the lateral malleolus
  use Ankle Bursa and Ligament, Right
  use Ankle Bursa and Ligament, Left

Ligamentum flavum
  ~~*use* Trunk Bursa and Ligament, Right~~
  ~~*use* Trunk Bursa and Ligament, Left~~
  ▶*use* Upper Spine Bursa and Ligament
  ▶*use* Lower Spine Bursa and Ligament

Ligation *see* Occlusion

Ligation, hemorrhoid *see* Occlusion, Lower Veins, Hemorrhoidal Plexus

Light Therapy GZJZZZZ

Liner
  Removal of device from
    Hip
      Left ØSPBØ9Z
      Right ØSP9Ø9Z
    Knee
      Left ØSPDØ9Z
      Right ØSPCØ9Z
  Revision of device in
    Hip
      Left ØSWBØ9Z
      Right ØSW9Ø9Z
    Knee
      Left ØSWDØ9Z
      Right ØSWCØ9Z
  Supplement
    Hip
      Left ØSUBØ9Z
        Acetabular Surface ØSUEØ9Z
        Femoral Surface ØSUSØ9Z
      Right ØSU9Ø9Z
        Acetabular Surface ØSUAØ9Z
        Femoral Surface ØSURØ9Z
    Knee
      Left ØSUDØ9
        Femoral Surface ØSUUØ9Z
        Tibial Surface ØSUWØ9Z
      Right ØSUCØ9
        Femoral Surface ØSUTØ9Z
        Tibial Surface ØSUVØ9Z

Lingual artery
  use Artery, External Carotid, Right
  use Artery, External Carotid, Left

➡**Lingual tonsil** *use* Pharynx

Lingulectomy, lung
  see Excision, Lung Lingula ØBBH
  see Resection, Lung Lingula ØBTH

Lithotripsy
  see Fragmentation
  with removal of fragments *see* Extirpation

LITT (laser interstitial thermal therapy) *see* Laser Interstitial Thermal Therapy

LIVIAN™ CRT-D *use* Cardiac Resynchronization Defibrillator Pulse Generator in ØJH

Lobectomy
  ~~*see* Excision, Central Nervous System ØØB~~
  ▶*see* Excision, Central Nervous System and Cranial Nerves ØØB
  see Excision, Respiratory System ØBB
  see Resection, Respiratory System ØBT
  see Excision, Hepatobiliary System and Pancreas ØFB
  see Resection, Hepatobiliary System and Pancreas ØFT
  see Excision, Endocrine System ØGB
  see Resection, Endocrine System ØGT

Lobotomy *see* Division, Brain ØØ8Ø

Localization
  see Map
  see Imaging

Locus ceruleus *use* Pons

Long thoracic nerve *use* Brachial Plexus

Loop ileostomy *see* Bypass, Ileum ØD1B

Loop recorder, implantable *use* Monitoring Device

Lower GI series *see* Fluoroscopy, Colon BD14

Lumbar artery *use* Abdominal Aorta

Lumbar facet joint *use* Lumbar Vertebral Joint

Lumbar ganglion *use* Lumbar Sympathetic Nerve

Lumbar lymph node *use* Lymphatic, Aortic

Lumbar lymphatic trunk *use* Cisterna Chyli

Lumbar splanchnic nerve *use* Lumbar Sympathetic Nerve

Lumbosacral facet joint *use* Lumbosacral Joint

Lumbosacral trunk *use* Lumbar Nerve

Lumpectomy
  see Excision

Lunate bone
  use Carpal, Right
  use Carpal, Left

Lunotriquetral ligament
  use Hand Bursa and Ligament, Right
  use Hand Bursa and Ligament, Left

Lymphadenectomy
  see Excision, Lymphatic and Hemic Systems Ø7B
  see Resection, Lymphatic and Hemic Systems Ø7T

Lymphadenotomy *see* Drainage, Lymphatic and Hemic Systems Ø79

Lymphangiectomy
  see Excision, Lymphatic and Hemic Systems Ø7B
  see Resection, Lymphatic and Hemic Systems Ø7T

Lymphangiogram *see* Plain Radiography, Lymphatic System B7Ø

Lymphangioplasty
  see Repair, Lymphatic and Hemic Systems Ø7Q
  see Supplement, Lymphatic and Hemic Systems Ø7U

Lymphangiorrhaphy *see* Repair, Lymphatic and Hemic Systems Ø7Q

Lymphangiotomy *see* Drainage, Lymphatic and Hemic Systems Ø79

Lysis *see* Release

M

Macula
  use Retina, Right
  use Retina, Left
MAGEC® Spinal Bracing and Distraction System *use* Magnetically Controlled Growth Rod(s) in New Technology
Magnet extraction, ocular foreign body *see* Extirpation, Eye Ø8C
Magnetic Resonance Imaging (MRI)
  Abdomen BW3Ø
  Ankle
    Left BQ3H
    Right BQ3G
  Aorta
    Abdominal B43Ø
    Thoracic B33Ø
  Arm
    Left BP3F
    Right BP3E
  Artery
    Celiac B431
    Cervico-Cerebral Arch B33Q
    Common Carotid, Bilateral B335
    Coronary
      Bypass Graft, Multiple B233
      Multiple B231
    Internal Carotid, Bilateral B338
    Intracranial B33R
    Lower Extremity
      Bilateral B43H
      Left B43G
      Right B43F
    Pelvic B43C
    Renal, Bilateral B438
    Spinal B33M
    Superior Mesenteric B434
    Upper Extremity
      Bilateral B33K
      Left B33J
      Right B33H
    Vertebral, Bilateral B33G
  Bladder BT3Ø
  Brachial Plexus BW3P
  Brain BØ3Ø
  Breast
    Bilateral BH32
    Left BH31
    Right BH3Ø
  Calcaneus
    Left BQ3K
    Right BQ3J
  Chest BW33Y
  Coccyx BR3F
  Connective Tissue
    Lower Extremity BL31
    Upper Extremity BL3Ø
  Corpora Cavernosa BV3Ø
  Disc
    Cervical BR31
    Lumbar BR33
    Thoracic BR32
  Ear B93Ø
  Elbow
    Left BP3H
    Right BP3G
  Eye
    Bilateral B837
    Left B836
    Right B835
  Femur
    Left BQ34
    Right BQ33
  Fetal Abdomen BY33
  Fetal Extremity BY35
  Fetal Head BY3Ø
  Fetal Heart BY31
  Fetal Spine BY34
  Fetal Thorax BY32
  Fetus, Whole BY36

Magnetic Resonance Imaging (MRI)
  (Continued)
  Foot
    Left BQ3M
    Right BQ3L
  Forearm
    Left BP3K
    Right BP3J
  Gland
    Adrenal, Bilateral BG32
    Parathyroid BG33
    Parotid, Bilateral B936
    Salivary, Bilateral B93D
    Submandibular, Bilateral B939
    Thyroid BG34
  Head BW38
  Heart, Right and Left B236
  Hip
    Left BQ31
    Right BQ3Ø
  Intracranial Sinus B532
  Joint
    Finger
      Left BP3D
      Right BP3C
    Hand
      Left BP3D
      Right BP3C
    Temporomandibular, Bilateral BN39
  Kidney
    Bilateral BT33
    Left BT32
    Right BT31
    Transplant BT39
  Knee
    Left BQ38
    Right BQ37
  Larynx B93J
  Leg
    Left BQ3F
    Right BQ3D
  Liver BF35
  Liver and Spleen BF36
  Lung Apices BB3G
  Nasopharynx B93F
  Neck BW3F
  Nerve
    Acoustic BØ3C
    Brachial Plexus BW3P
  Oropharynx B93F
  Ovary
    Bilateral BU35
    Left BU34
    Right BU33
  Ovary and Uterus BU3C
  Pancreas BF37
  Patella
    Left BQ3W
    Right BQ3V
  Pelvic Region BW3G
  Pelvis BR3C
  Pituitary Gland BØ39
  Plexus, Brachial BW3P
  Prostate BV33
  Retroperitoneum BW3H
  Sacrum BR3F
  Scrotum BV34
  Sella Turcica BØ39
  Shoulder
    Left BP39
    Right BP38
  Sinus
    Intracranial B532
    Paranasal B932
  Spinal Cord BØ3B
  Spine
    Cervical BR3Ø
    Lumbar BR39
    Thoracic BR37
  Spleen and Liver BF36

Magnetic Resonance Imaging (MRI)
  (Continued)
  Subcutaneous Tissue
    Abdomen BH3H
    Extremity
      Lower BH3J
      Upper BH3F
    Head BH3D
    Neck BH3D
    Pelvis BH3H
    Thorax BH3G
  Tendon
    Lower Extremity BL33
    Upper Extremity BL32
  Testicle
    Bilateral BV37
    Left BV36
    Right BV35
  Toe
    Left BQ3Q
    Right BQ3P
  Uterus BU36
    Pregnant BU3B
  Uterus and Ovary BU3C
  Vagina BU39
  Vein
    Cerebellar B531
    Cerebral B531
    Jugular, Bilateral B535
    Lower Extremity
      Bilateral B53D
      Left B53C
      Right B53B
    Other B53V
    Pelvic (Iliac) Bilateral B53H
    Portal B53T
    Pulmonary, Bilateral B53S
    Renal, Bilateral B53L
    Spanchnic B53T
    Upper Extremity
      Bilateral B53P
      Left B53N
      Right B53M
  Vena Cava
    Inferior B539
    Superior B538
  Wrist
    Left BP3M
    Right BP3L
Magnetically Controlled Growth Rod(s)
  Cervical XNS3
  Lumbar XNSØ
  Thoracic XNS4
Malleotomy *see* Drainage, Ear, Nose, Sinus Ø99
Malleus
  use Auditory Ossicle, Right
  use Auditory Ossicle, Left
Mammaplasty, mammoplasty
  see Alteration, Skin and Breast ØHØ
  see Repair, Skin and Breast ØHQ
  see Replacement, Skin and Breast ØHR
  see Supplement, Skin and Breast ØHU
Mammary duct
  use Breast, Right
  use Breast, Left
  use Breast, Bilateral
Mammary gland
  use Breast, Right
  use Breast, Left
  use Breast, Bilateral
Mammectomy
  see Excision, Skin and Breast ØHB
  see Resection, Skin and Breast ØHT
Mammillary body *use* Hypothalamus
Mammography *see* Plain Radiography, Skin, Subcutaneous Tissue and Breast BHØ
Mammotomy *see* Drainage, Skin and Breast ØH9
Mandibular nerve *use* Trigeminal Nerve
Mandibular notch
  use Mandible, Right
  use Mandible, Left

▶ New   ⇒ Revised   ~~deleted~~ Deleted

Mandibulectomy
  see Excision, Head and Facial Bones 0NB
  see Resection, Head and Facial Bones 0NT
Manipulation
  Adhesions *see* Release
  Chiropractic *see* Chiropractic Manipulation
▶**Manual removal, retained placenta** *see*
    Extraction, Products of Conception,
    Retained 10D1
Manubrium *use* Sternum
Map
  Basal Ganglia 00K8
  Brain 00K0
  Cerebellum 00KC
  Cerebral Hemisphere 00K7
  Conduction Mechanism 02K8
  Hypothalamus 00KA
  Medulla Oblongata 00KD
  Pons 00KB
  Thalamus 00K9
Mapping
  Doppler ultrasound *see* Ultrasonography
  Electrocardiogram only *see* Measurement,
    Cardiac 4A02
Mark IV Breathing Pacemaker System *use*
    Stimulator Generator in Subcutaneous
    Tissue and Fascia
Marsupialization
  see Drainage
  see Excision
Massage, cardiac
  External 5A12012
  Open 02QA0ZZ
Masseter muscle *use* Head Muscle
Masseteric fascia *use* Subcutaneous Tissue and
  Fascia, Face
Mastectomy
  see Excision, Skin and Breast 0HB
  see Resection, Skin and Breast 0HT
Mastoid (postauricular) lymph node
  use Lymphatic, Right Neck
  use Lymphatic, Left Neck
Mastoid air cells
  use Mastoid Sinus, Right
  use Mastoid Sinus, Left
Mastoid process
  use Temporal Bone, Right
  use Temporal Bone, Left
Mastoidectomy
  see Excision, Ear, Nose, Sinus 09B
  see Resection, Ear, Nose, Sinus 09T
Mastoidotomy *see* Drainage, Ear, Nose, Sinus
  099
Mastopexy
  see Reposition, Skin and Breast 0HS
  see Repair, Skin and Breast 0HQ
Mastorrhaphy *see* Repair, Skin and Breast 0HQ
Mastotomy *see* Drainage, Skin and Breast 0H9
Maxillary artery
  use External Carotid Artery, Right
  use External Carotid Artery, Left
Maxillary nerve *use* Trigeminal Nerve
Maximo II DR (VR) *use* Defibrillator Generator
  in 0JH
Maximo II DR CRT-D *use* Cardiac
  Resynchronization Defibrillator Pulse
  Generator in 0JH
Measurement
  Arterial
    Flow
      Coronary 4A03
      Peripheral 4A03
      Pulmonary 4A03
    Pressure
      Coronary 4A03
      Peripheral 4A03
      Pulmonary 4A03
      Thoracic, Other 4A03
    Pulse
      Coronary 4A03
      Peripheral 4A03
      Pulmonary 4A03

Measurement *(Continued)*
  Arterial *(Continued)*
    Saturation, Peripheral 4A03
    Sound, Peripheral 4A03
  Biliary
    Flow 4A0C
    Pressure 4A0C
  Cardiac
    Action Currents 4A02
    Defibrillator 4B02XTZ
    Electrical Activity 4A02
      Guidance 4A02X4A
      No Qualifier 4A02X4Z
    Output 4A02
    Pacemaker 4B02XSZ
    Rate 4A02
    Rhythm 4A02
    Sampling and Pressure
      Bilateral 4A02
      Left Heart 4A02
      Right Heart 4A02
    Sound 4A02
    Total Activity, Stress 4A02XM4
  Central Nervous
    Conductivity 4A00
    Electrical Activity 4A00
    Pressure 4A000BZ
      Intracranial 4A00
    Saturation, Intracranial 4A00
    Stimulator 4B00XVZ
    Temperature, Intracranial 4A00
  Circulatory, Volume 4A05XLZ
  Gastrointestinal
    Motility 4A0B
    Pressure 4A0B
    Secretion 4A0B
  Lymphatic
    Flow 4A06
    Pressure 4A06
  Metabolism 4A0Z
  Musculoskeletal
    Contractility 4A0F
    Stimulator 4B0FXVZ
  Olfactory, Acuity 4A08X0Z
  Peripheral Nervous
    Conductivity
      Motor 4A01
      Sensory 4A01
    Electrical Activity 4A01
    Stimulator 4B01XVZ
  Products of Conception
    Cardiac
      Electrical Activity 4A0H
      Rate 4A0H
      Rhythm 4A0H
      Sound 4A0H
    Nervous
      Conductivity 4A0J
      Electrical Activity 4A0J
      Pressure 4A0J
  Respiratory
    Capacity 4A09
    Flow 4A09
    Pacemaker 4B09XSZ
    Rate 4A09
    Resistance 4A09
    Total Activity 4A09
    Volume 4A09
  Sleep 4A0ZXQZ
  Temperature 4A0Z
  Urinary
  ➡ Contractility 4A0D
  ➡ Flow 4A0D
  ➡ Pressure 4A0D
  ➡ Resistance 4A0D
  ➡ Volume 4A0D
  Venous
    Flow
      Central 4A04
      Peripheral 4A04
      Portal 4A04
      Pulmonary 4A04

Measurement *(Continued)*
  Venous *(Continued)*
    Pressure
      Central 4A04
      Peripheral 4A04
      Portal 4A04
      Pulmonary 4A04
    Pulse
      Central 4A04
      Peripheral 4A04
      Portal 4A04
      Pulmonary 4A04
    Saturation, Peripheral 4A04
    Visual
      Acuity 4A07X0Z
      Mobility 4A07X7Z
      Pressure 4A07XBZ
Meatoplasty, urethra *see* Repair, Urethra 0TQD
Meatotomy *see* Drainage, Urinary System 0T9
Mechanical ventilation *see* Performance,
  Respiratory 5A19
Medial canthus
  use Lower Eyelid, Right
  use Lower Eyelid, Left
Medial collateral ligament (MCL)
  use Knee Bursa and Ligament, Right
  use Knee Bursa and Ligament, Left
Medial condyle of femur
  use Lower Femur, Right
  use Lower Femur, Left
Medial condyle of tibia
  use Tibia, Right
  use Tibia, Left
Medial cuneiform bone
  use Tarsal, Right
  use Tarsal, Left
Medial epicondyle of femur
  use Lower Femur, Right
  use Lower Femur, Left
Medial epicondyle of humerus
  use Humeral Shaft, Right
  use Humeral Shaft, Left
Medial malleolus
  use Tibia, Right
  use Tibia, Left
Medial meniscus
  use Knee Joint, Right
  use Knee Joint, Left
Medial plantar artery
  use Foot Artery, Right
  use Foot Artery, Left
Medial plantar nerve *use* Tibial Nerve
Medial popliteal nerve *use* Tibial Nerve
Medial rectus muscle
  use Extraocular Muscle, Right
  use Extraocular Muscle, Left
Medial sural cutaneous nerve *use* Tibial Nerve
Median antebrachial vein
  use Basilic Vein, Right
  use Basilic Vein, Left
Median cubital vein
  use Basilic Vein, Right
  use Basilic Vein, Left
Median sacral artery *use* Abdominal Aorta
Mediastinal lymph node *use* Lymphatic,
  Thorax
Mediastinoscopy 0WJC4ZZ
Medication Management GZ3ZZZZ
  for substance abuse
    Antabuse HZ83ZZZ
    Bupropion HZ87ZZZ
    Clonidine HZ86ZZZ
    Levo-alpha-acetyl-methadol (LAAM)
      HZ82ZZZ
    Methadone Maintenance HZ81ZZZ
    Naloxone HZ85ZZZ
    Naltrexone HZ84ZZZ
    Nicotine Replacement HZ80ZZZ
    Other Replacement Medication HZ89ZZZ
    Psychiatric Medication HZ88ZZZ
Meditation 8E0ZXY5

▶ New   ➡ Revised   ~~deleted~~ Deleted

Medtronic Endurant® II AAA stent graft system *use* Intraluminal Device

Meissner's (submucous) plexus *use* Abdominal Sympathetic Nerve

Melody® transcatheter pulmonary valve *use* Zooplastic Tissue in Heart and Great Vessels

Membranous urethra *use* Urethra

Meningeorrhaphy
see Repair, Cerebral Meninges 00Q1
see Repair, Spinal Meninges 00QT

Meniscectomy, knee
see Excision, Joint, Knee, Right 0SBC
see Excision, Joint, Knee, Left 0SBD

Mental foramen
use Mandible, Right
use Mandible, Left

Mentalis muscle *use* Facial Muscle

Mentoplasty *see* Alteration, Jaw, Lower 0W05

Mesenterectomy *see* Excision, Mesentery 0DBV

Mesenteriorrhaphy, mesenterorrhaphy *see* Repair, Mesentery 0DQV

Mesenteriplication *see* Repair, Mesentery 0DQV

Mesoappendix *use* Mesentery

Mesocolon *use* Mesentery

Metacarpal ligament
use Hand Bursa and Ligament, Right
use Hand Bursa and Ligament, Left

Metacarpophalangeal ligament
use Hand Bursa and Ligament, Right
use Hand Bursa and Ligament, Left

Metal on metal bearing surface *use* Synthetic Substitute, Metal in 0SR

Metatarsal ligament
use Foot Bursa and Ligament, Right
use Foot Bursa and Ligament, Left

Metatarsectomy
see Excision, Lower Bones 0QB
see Resection, Lower Bones 0QT

Metatarsophalangeal (MTP) joint
use Metatarsal-Phalangeal Joint, Right
use Metatarsal-Phalangeal Joint, Left

Metatarsophalangeal ligament
use Foot Bursa and Ligament, Right
use Foot Bursa and Ligament, Left

Metathalamus *use* Thalamus

Micro-Driver stent (RX) (OTW) *use* Intraluminal Device

MicroMed HeartAssist *use* Implantable Heart Assist System in Heart and Great Vessels

Micrus CERECYTE microcoil *use* Intraluminal Device, Bioactive in Upper Arteries

Midcarpal joint
use Carpal Joint, Right
use Carpal Joint, Left

Middle cardiac nerve *use* Thoracic Sympathetic Nerve

Middle cerebral artery *use* Intracranial Artery

Middle cerebral vein *use* Intracranial Vein

Middle colic vein *use* Colic Vein

Middle genicular artery
use Popliteal Artery, Right
use Popliteal Artery, Left

Middle hemorrhoidal vein
use Hypogastric Vein, Right
use Hypogastric Vein, Left

Middle rectal artery
use Internal Iliac Artery, Right
use Internal Iliac Artery, Left

Middle suprarenal artery *use* Abdominal Aorta

Middle temporal artery
use Temporal Artery, Right
use Temporal Artery, Left

Middle turbinate *use* Nasal Turbinate

MIRODERM™ Biologic Wound Matrix *use* Skin Substitute, Porcine Liver Derived in New Technology

MitraClip valve repair system *use* Synthetic Substitute

Mitral annulus *use* Mitral Valve

Mitroflow® Aortic Pericardial Heart Valve *use* Zooplastic Tissue in Heart and Great Vessels

Mobilization, adhesions *see* Release

Molar gland *use* Buccal Mucosa

Monitoring
Arterial
Flow
Coronary 4A13
Peripheral 4A13
Pulmonary 4A13
Pressure
Coronary 4A13
Peripheral 4A13
Pulmonary 4A13
Pulse
Coronary 4A13
Peripheral 4A13
Pulmonary 4A13
Saturation, Peripheral 4A13
Sound, Peripheral 4A13
Cardiac
Electrical Activity 4A12
Ambulatory 4A12X45
No Qualifier 4A12X4Z
Output 4A12
Rate 4A12
Rhythm 4A12
Sound 4A12
Total Activity, Stress 4A12XM4
Vascular Perfusion, Indocyanine Green Dye 4A12XSH
Central Nervous
Conductivity 4A10
Electrical Activity
Intraoperative 4A10
No Qualifier 4A10
Pressure 4A100BZ
Intracranial 4A10
Saturation, Intracranial 4A10
Temperature, Intracranial 4A10
Gastrointestinal
Motility 4A1B
Pressure 4A1B
Secretion 4A1B
Vascular Perfusion, Indocyanine Green Dye 4A1BXSH
Intraoperative Knee Replacement Sensor XR2
Lymphatic
Flow 4A16
Pressure 4A16
Peripheral Nervous
Conductivity
Motor 4A11
Sensory 4A11
Electrical Activity Intraoperative 4A11
No Qualifier 4A11
Products of Conception
Cardiac
Electrical Activity 4A1H
Rate 4A1H
Rhythm 4A1H
Sound 4A1H
Nervous
Conductivity 4A1J
Electrical Activity 4A1J
Pressure 4A1J
Respiratory
Capacity 4A19
Flow 4A19
Rate 4A19
Resistance 4A19
Volume 4A19
Skin and Breast, Vascular Perfusion, Indocyanine Green Dye 4A1GXSH
Sleep 4A1ZXQZ

Temperature 4A1Z
Urinary
➡Contractility 4A1D
➡Flow 4A1D
➡Pressure 4A1D
➡Resistance 4A1D
➡Volume 4A1D
Venous
Flow
Central 4A14
Peripheral 4A14
Portal 4A14
Pulmonary 4A14
Pressure
Central 4A14
Peripheral 4A14
Portal 4A14
Pulmonary 4A14
Pulse
Central 4A14
Peripheral 4A14
Portal 4A14
Pulmonary 4A14
Saturation
Central 4A14
Portal 4A14
Pulmonary 4A14

Monitoring Device, Hemodynamic
Abdomen 0JH8
Chest 0JH6

Mosaic Bioprosthesis (aortic) (mitral) valve *use* Zooplastic Tissue in Heart and Great Vessels

Motor Function Assessment F01

Motor Treatment F07

MR Angiography
see Magnetic Resonance Imaging (MRI), Heart B23
see Magnetic Resonance Imaging (MRI), Upper Arteries B33
see Magnetic Resonance Imaging (MRI), Lower Arteries B43

MULTI-LINK (VISION)(MINI-VISION) (ULTRA) Coronary Stent System *use* Intraluminal Device

Multiple sleep latency test 4A0ZXQZ

Musculocutaneous nerve *use* Brachial Plexus Nerve

Musculopexy
see Repair, Muscles 0KQ
see Reposition, Muscles 0KS

Musculophrenic artery
use Internal Mammary Artery, Right
use Internal Mammary Artery, Left

Musculoplasty
see Repair, Muscles 0KQ
see Supplement, Muscles 0KU

Musculorrhaphy *see* Repair, Muscles 0KQ

Musculospiral nerve *use* Radial Nerve

Myectomy
see Excision, Muscles 0KB
see Resection, Muscles 0KT

Myelencephalon *use* Medulla Oblongata

Myelogram
CT *see* Computerized Tomography (CT Scan), Central Nervous System B02
MRI *see* Magnetic Resonance Imaging (MRI), Central Nervous System B03

Myenteric (Auerbach's) plexus *use* Abdominal Sympathetic Nerve

▶**Myocardial Bridge Release** *see* Release, Artery, Coronary

Myomectomy *see* Excision, Female Reproductive System 0UB

Myometrium *use* Uterus

Myopexy
see Repair, Muscles 0KQ
see Reposition, Muscles 0KS

▶ New   ➡ Revised   ~~deleted~~ Deleted

Myoplasty
 see Repair, Muscles ØKQ
 see Supplement, Muscles ØKU
Myorrhaphy *see* Repair, Muscles ØKQ
Myoscopy *see* Inspection, Muscles ØKJ
Myotomy
 see Division, Muscles ØK8
 see Drainage, Muscles ØK9

Myringectomy
 see Excision, Ear, Nose, Sinus Ø9B
 see Resection, Ear, Nose, Sinus Ø9T
Myringoplasty
 see Repair, Ear, Nose, Sinus Ø9Q
 see Replacement, Ear, Nose, Sinus Ø9R
 see Supplement, Ear, Nose, Sinus Ø9U

Myringostomy *see* Drainage, Ear, Nose, Sinus Ø99
Myringotomy *see* Drainage, Ear, Nose, Sinus Ø99

N

Nail bed
use Finger Nail
use Toe Nail
Nail plate
use Finger Nail
use Toe Nail
nanoLOCK™ interbody fusion device *use* Interbody Fusion Device, Nanotextured Surface in New Technology
Narcosynthesis GZGZZZZ
➧ **Nasal cavity** *use* Nasal Mucosa and Soft Tissue
Nasal concha *use* Nasal Turbinate
Nasalis muscle *use* Facial Muscle
Nasolacrimal duct
use Lacrimal Duct, Right
use Lacrimal Duct, Left
Nasopharyngeal airway (NPA) *use* Intraluminal Device, Airway in Ear, Nose, Sinus
Navicular bone
use Tarsal, Right
use Tarsal, Left
Near Infrared Spectroscopy, Circulatory System 8E023DZ
Neck of femur
use Upper Femur, Right
use Upper Femur, Left
Neck of humerus (anatomical)(surgical)
use Humeral Head, Right
use Humeral Head, Left
Nephrectomy
see Excision, Urinary System ØTB
see Resection, Urinary System ØTT
Nephrolithotomy *see* Extirpation, Urinary System ØTC
Nephrolysis *see* Release, Urinary System ØTN
Nephropexy
see Repair, Urinary System ØTQ
see Reposition, Urinary System ØTS
Nephroplasty
see Repair, Urinary System ØTQ
see Supplement, Urinary System ØTU
Nephropyeloureterostomy
see Bypass, Urinary System ØT1
see Drainage, Urinary System ØT9
Nephrorrhaphy *see* Repair, Urinary System ØTQ
Nephroscopy, transurethral ØTJ58ZZ
Nephrostomy
see Bypass, Urinary System ØT1
see Drainage, Urinary System ØT9
Nephrotomography
see Plain Radiography, Urinary System BTØ
see Fluoroscopy, Urinary System BT1
Nephrotomy
see Division, Urinary System ØT8
see Drainage, Urinary System ØT9
Nerve conduction study
see Measurement, Central Nervous 4AØØ
see Measurement, Peripheral Nervous 4AØ1
Nerve Function Assessment FØ1
Nerve to the stapedius *use* Facial Nerve
Nesiritide *use* Human B-type Natriuretic Peptide
Neurectomy
~~*see* Excision, Central Nervous System ØØB~~
➧*see* Excision, Central Nervous System and Cranial Nerves ØØB
see Excision, Peripheral Nervous System Ø1B
Neurexeresis
~~*see* Extraction, Central Nervous System ØØD~~
➧*see* Extraction, Central Nervous System and Cranial Nerves ØØD
see Extraction, Peripheral Nervous System Ø1D
Neurohypophysis *use* Gland, Pituitary
Neurolysis
~~*see* Release, Central Nervous System ØØN~~
➧*see* Release, Central Nervous System and Cranial Nerves ØØN
see Release, Peripheral Nervous System Ø1N

Neuromuscular electrical stimulation (NEMS) lead *use* Stimulator Lead in Muscles
Neurophysiologic monitoring *see* Monitoring, Central Nervous 4A1Ø
Neuroplasty
~~*see* Repair, Central Nervous System ØØQ~~
~~*see* Supplement, Central Nervous System ØØU~~
➧*see* Repair, Central Nervous System and Cranial Nerves ØØQ
➧*see* Supplement, Central Nervous System and Cranial Nerves ØØU
see Repair, Peripheral Nervous System Ø1Q
see Supplement, Peripheral Nervous System Ø1U
Neurorrhaphy
~~*see* Repair, Central Nervous System ØØQ~~
➧*see* Repair, Central Nervous System and Cranial Nerves ØØQ
see Repair, Peripheral Nervous System Ø1Q
Neurostimulator Generator
Insertion of device in, Skull ØNHØØNZ
Removal of device from, Skull ØNPØØNZ
Revision of device in, Skull ØNWØØNZ
Neurostimulator generator, multiple channel *use* Stimulator Generator, Multiple Array in ØJH
Neurostimulator generator, multiple channel rechargeable *use* Stimulator Generator, Multiple Array Rechargeable in ØJH
Neurostimulator generator, single channel *use* Stimulator Generator, Single Array in ØJH
Neurostimulator generator, single channel rechargeable *use* Stimulator Generator, Single Array Rechargeable in ØJH
Neurostimulator Lead
Insertion of device in
Brain ØØHØ
Canal, Spinal ØØHU
Cerebral Ventricle ØØH6
Nerve
Cranial ØØHE
Peripheral Ø1HY
Spinal Canal ØØHU
Spinal Cord ØØHV
Vein
Azygos Ø5HØ
Innominate
Left Ø5H4
Right Ø5H3
Removal of device from
Brain ØØPØ
Cerebral Ventricle ØØP6
Nerve
Cranial ØØPE
Peripheral Ø1PY
Spinal Canal ØØPU
Spinal Cord ØØPV
Vein
Azygos Ø5PØ
Innominate
Left Ø5P4
Right Ø5P3
Revision of device in
Brain ØØWØ
Cerebral Ventricle ØØW6
Nerve
Cranial ØØWE
Peripheral Ø1WY
Spinal Canal ØØWU
Spinal Cord ØØWV
Vein
Azygos Ø5WØ
Innominate
Left Ø5W4
Right Ø5W3
Neurotomy
~~*see* Division, Central Nervous System ØØ8~~
➧*see* Division, Central Nervous System and Cranial Nerves ØØ8
see Division, Peripheral Nervous System Ø18

Neurotripsy
~~*see* Destruction, Central Nervous System ØØ5~~
➧*see* Destruction, Central Nervous System and Cranial Nerves ØØ5
see Destruction, Peripheral Nervous System Ø15
Neutralization plate
use Internal Fixation Device in Head and Facial Bones
use Internal Fixation Device in Upper Bones
use Internal Fixation Device in Lower Bones
New Technology
Andexanet Alfa, Factor Xa Inhibitor Reversal Agent XWØ
Blinatumomab Antineoplastic Immunotherapy XWØ
➧Bezlotoxumab Monoclonal Antibody XWØ
Ceftazidime-Avibactam Anti-infective XWØ
Cerebral Embolic Filtration, Dual Filter X2A5312
➧Concentrated Bone Marrow Aspirate XKØ23Ø3
➧Cytarabine and Daunorubicin Liposome Antineoplastic XWØ
Defibrotide Sodium Anticoagulant XWØ
➧Endothelial Damage Inhibitor XYØVX83
➧Engineered Autologous Chimeric Antigen Receptor T-cell Immunotherapy XWØ
Fusion
Cervical Vertebral
~~2 or more, Interbody Fusion Device, Nanotextured Surface XRG2Ø92~~
~~Interbody Fusion Device, Nanotextured Surface XRG1Ø92~~
➧2 or more
➧Nanotextured Surface XRG2Ø92
➧Radiolucent Porous XRG2ØF3
➧Interbody Fusion Device
➧Nanotextured Surface XRG1Ø92
➧Radiolucent Porous XRG1ØF3
~~Cervicothoracic Vertebral, Interbody Fusion Device, Nanotextured Surface XRG4Ø92~~
➧Cervicothoracic Vertebral
➧Nanotextured Surface XRG4Ø92
➧Radiolucent Porous XRG4ØF3
Lumbar Vertebral
~~2 or more, Interbody Fusion Device, Nanotextured Surface XRGCØ92~~
~~Interbody Fusion Device, Nanotextured Surface XRGBØ92~~
➧2 or more
➧Nanotextured Surface XRGCØ92
➧Radiolucent Porous XRGCØF3
➧Interbody Fusion Device
➧Nanotextured Surface XRGBØ92
➧Radiolucent Porous XRGBØF3
~~Lumbosacral, Interbody Fusion Device, Nanotextured Surface XRGDØ92~~
➧Lumbosacral
➧Nanotextured Surface XRGDØ92
➧Radiolucent Porous XRGDØF3
~~Occipital-cervical, Interbody Fusion Device, Nanotextured Surface XRGØØ92~~
➧Occipital-cervical
➧Nanotextured Surface XRGØØ92
➧Radiolucent Porous XRGØØF3
Thoracic Vertebral
~~2 to 7, Interbody Fusion Device, Nanotextured Surface XRG7Ø92~~
~~8 or more, Interbody Fusion Device, Nanotextured Surface XRG8Ø92~~
~~Interbody Fusion Device, Nanotextured Surface XRG6Ø92~~
➧2 to 7
➧Nanotextured Surface XRG7Ø92
➧Radiolucent Porous XRG7ØF3
➧8 or more
➧Nanotextured Surface XRG8Ø92
➧Radiolucent Porous XRG8ØF3

➤ New ➠ Revised ~~deleted~~ Deleted

New Technology *(Continued)*
  Fusion *(Continued)*
    Thoracic Vertebral *(Continued)*
    ▶ Interbody Fusion Device
      ▶ Nanotextured Surface XRG6092
      ▶ Radiolucent Porous XRG60F3
    ~~Thoracolumbar Vertebral, Interbody~~
      ~~Fusion Device, Nanotextured Surface~~
      ~~XRGA09~~
    ▶ Thoracolumbar Vertebral
      ▶ Nanotextured Surface XRGA092
      ▶ Radiolucent Porous XRGA0F3
  Idarucizumab, Dabigatran Reversal Agent
    XW0
  Intraoperative Knee Replacement Sensor XR2
  Isavuconazole Anti-infective XW0
  Orbital Atherectomy Technology X2C
  ▶ Other New Technology Therapeutic
    Substance XW0
  Replacement
    Skin Substitute, Porcine Liver Derived
      XHRPXL2
    Zooplastic Tissue, Rapid Deployment
      Technique X2RF
  Reposition
    Cervical, Magnetically Controlled Growth
      Rod(s) XNS3
    Lumbar, Magnetically Controlled Growth
      Rod(s) XNS0
    Thoracic, Magnetically Controlled Growth
      Rod(s) XNS4
  Uridine Triacetate XW0DX82
Ninth cranial nerve *use* Glossopharyngeal
  Nerve
Nitinol framed polymer mesh *use* Synthetic
  Substitute

Non-tunneled central venous catheter *use*
  Infusion Device
Nonimaging Nuclear Medicine Assay
  Bladder, Kidneys and Ureters CT63
  Blood C763
  Kidneys, Ureters and Bladder CT63
  Lymphatics and Hematologic System
    C76YYZZ
  Ureters, Kidneys and Bladder CT63
  Urinary System CT6YYZZ
Nonimaging Nuclear Medicine Probe
  Abdomen CW50
  Abdomen and Chest CW54
  Abdomen and Pelvis CW51
  Brain C050
  Central Nervous System C05YYZZ
  Chest CW53
  Chest and Abdomen CW54
  Chest and Neck CW56
  Extremity
    Lower CP5PZZZ
    Upper CP5NZZZ
  Head and Neck CW5B
  Heart C25YYZZ
    Right and Left C256
  Lymphatics
    Head C75J
    Head and Neck C755
    Lower Extremity C75P
    Neck C75K
    Pelvic C75D
    Trunk C75M
    Upper Chest C75L
    Upper Extremity C75N
  Lymphatics and Hematologic System
    C75YYZZ

Nonimaging Nuclear Medicine Probe
  (Continued)
  Musculoskeletal System, Other CP5YYZZ
  Neck and Chest CW56
  Neck and Head CW5B
  Pelvic Region CW5J
  Pelvis and Abdomen CW51
  Spine CP55ZZZ
Nonimaging Nuclear Medicine Uptake
  Endocrine System CG4YYZZ
  Gland, Thyroid CG42
▶ **Nostril** *use* Nasal Mucosa and Soft Tissue
Novacor Left Ventricular Assist Device *use*
  Implantable Heart Assist System in Heart
  and Great Vessels
Novation® Ceramic AHS® (Articulation Hip
  System) *use* Synthetic Substitute, Ceramic
  in 0SR
Nuclear medicine
  see Planar Nuclear Medicine Imaging
  see Tomographic (Tomo) Nuclear Medicine
    Imaging
  see Positron Emission Tomographic (PET)
    Imaging
  see Nonimaging Nuclear Medicine Uptake
  see Nonimaging Nuclear Medicine Probe
  see Nonimaging Nuclear Medicine Assay
  see Systemic Nuclear Medicine Therapy
Nuclear scintigraphy *see* Nuclear Medicine
Nutrition, concentrated substances
  Enteral infusion 3E0G36Z
  Parenteral (peripheral) infusion *see*
    Introduction of Nutritional Substance

O

Obliteration *see* Destruction
Obturator artery
  use Internal Iliac Artery, Right
  use Internal Iliac Artery, Left
Obturator lymph node *use* Lymphatic, Pelvis
Obturator muscle
  use Hip Muscle, Right
  use Hip Muscle, Left
Obturator nerve *use* Lumbar Plexus
Obturator vein
  use Hypogastric Vein, Right
  use Hypogastric Vein, Left
Obtuse margin *use* Heart, Left
Occipital artery
  use External Carotid Artery, Right
  use External Carotid Artery, Left
Occipital lobe *use* Cerebral Hemisphere
Occipital lymph node
  use Lymphatic, Right Neck
  use Lymphatic, Left Neck
Occipitofrontalis muscle *use* Facial Muscle
Occlusion
  Ampulla of Vater ØFLC
  Anus ØDLQ
  ~~Aorta, Abdominal 04L0~~
  ▶Aorta
    ▶Abdominal 04L0
    ▶Thoracic, Descending 02LW3DJ
  Artery
    Anterior Tibial
      Left 04LQ
      Right 04LP
    Axillary
      Left 03L6
      Right 03L5
    Brachial
      Left 03L8
      Right 03L7
    Celiac 04L1
    Colic
      Left 04L7
      Middle 04L8
      Right 04L6
    Common Carotid
      Left 03LJ
      Right 03LH
    Common Iliac
      Left 04LD
      Right 04LC
    External Carotid
      Left 03LN
      Right 03LM
    External Iliac
      Left 04LJ
      Right 04LH
    Face 03LR
    Femoral
      Left 04LL
      Right 04LK
    Foot
      Left 04LW
      Right 04LV
    Gastric 04L2
    Hand
      Left 03LF
      Right 03LD
    Hepatic 04L3
    Inferior Mesenteric 04LB
    Innominate 03L2
    Internal Carotid
      Left 03LL
      Right 03LK
    Internal Iliac
      Left 04LF
      Right 04LE
    Internal Mammary
      Left 03L1
      Right 03L0
    Intracranial 03LG

Occlusion *(Continued)*
  Artery *(Continued)*
    Lower 04LY
    Peroneal
      Left 04LU
      Right 04LT
    Popliteal
      Left 04LN
      Right 04LM
    Posterior Tibial
      Left 04LS
      Right 04LR
    ~~Pulmonary, Left 02LR~~
    ▶Pulmonary
      ▶Left 02LR
      ▶Right 02LQ
    ▶Pulmonary Trunk 02LP
    Radial
      Left 03LC
      Right 03LB
    Renal
      Left 04LA
      Right 04L9
    Splenic 04L4
    Subclavian
      Left 03L4
      Right 03L3
    Superior Mesenteric 04L5
    Temporal
      Left 03LT
      Right 03LS
    Thyroid
      Left 03LV
      Right 03LU
    Ulnar
      Left 03LA
      Right 03L9
    Upper 03LY
    Vertebral
      Left 03LQ
      Right 03LP
  Atrium, Left 02L7
  Bladder 0TLB
  Bladder Neck 0TLC
  Bronchus
    Lingula 0BL9
    Lower Lobe
      Left 0BLB
      Right 0BL6
    Main
      Left 0BL7
      Right 0BL3
    Middle Lobe, Right 0BL5
    Upper Lobe
      Left 0BL8
      Right 0BL4
  Carina 0BL2
  Cecum 0DLH
  Cisterna Chyli 07LL
  Colon
    Ascending 0DLK
    Descending 0DLM
    Sigmoid 0DLN
    Transverse 0DLL
  Cord
    Bilateral 0VLH
    Left 0VLG
    Right 0VLF
  Cul-de-sac 0ULF
  Duct
    Common Bile 0FL9
    Cystic 0FL8
    Hepatic
      ▶Common 0FL7
      Left 0FL6
      Right 0FL5
    Lacrimal
      Left 08LY
      Right 08LX
    Pancreatic 0FLD
      Accessory 0FLF

Occlusion *(Continued)*
  Duct *(Continued)*
    Parotid
      Left 0CLC
      Right 0CLB
    Duodenum 0DL9
    Esophagogastric Junction 0DL4
    Esophagus 0DL5
      Lower 0DL3
      Middle 0DL2
      Upper 0DL1
    Fallopian Tube
      Left 0UL6
      Right 0UL5
    Fallopian Tubes, Bilateral 0UL7
    Ileocecal Valve 0DLC
    Ileum 0DLB
    Intestine
      Large 0DLE
        Left 0DLG
        Right 0DLF
      Small 0DL8
    Jejunum 0DLA
    Kidney Pelvis
      Left 0TL4
      Right 0TL3
    Left atrial appendage (LAA) *see* Occlusion,
      Atrium, Left 02L7
    Lymphatic
      Aortic 07LD
      Axillary
        Left 07L6
        Right 07L5
      Head 07L0
      Inguinal
        Left 07LJ
        Right 07LH
      Internal Mammary
        Left 07L9
        Right 07L8
      Lower Extremity
        Left 07LG
        Right 07LF
      Mesenteric 07LB
      Neck
        Left 07L2
        Right 07L1
      Pelvis 07LC
      Thoracic Duct 07LK
      Thorax 07L7
      Upper Extremity
        Left 07L4
        Right 07L3
    Rectum 0DLP
    Stomach 0DL6
      Pylorus 0DL7
    Trachea 0BL1
    Ureter
      Left 0TL7
      Right 0TL6
    Urethra 0TLD
    Vagina 0ULG
    Valve, Pulmonary 02LH
    Vas Deferens
      Bilateral 0VLQ
      Left 0VLP
      Right 0VLN
    Vein
      Axillary
        Left 05L8
        Right 05L7
      Azygos 05L0
      Basilic
        Left 05LC
        Right 05LB
      Brachial
        Left 05LA
        Right 05L9
      Cephalic
        Left 05LF
        Right 05LD

▶ New   ⇒ Revised   ~~deleted~~ Deleted

Occlusion *(Continued)*
  Vein *(Continued)*
    Colic 06L7
    Common Iliac
      Left 06LD
      Right 06LC
    Esophageal 06L3
    External Iliac
      Left 06LG
      Right 06LF
    External Jugular
      Left 05LQ
      Right 05LP
    Face
      Left 05LV
      Right 05LT
    Femoral
      Left 06LN
      Right 06LM
    Foot
      Left 06LV
      Right 06LT
    Gastric 06L2
    ~~Greater Saphenous~~
      ~~Left 06LQ~~
      ~~Right 06LP~~
    Hand
      Left 05LH
      Right 05LG
    Hemiazygos 05L1
    Hepatic 06L4
    Hypogastric
      Left 06LJ
      Right 06LH
    Inferior Mesenteric 06L6
    Innominate
      Left 05L4
      Right 05L3
    Internal Jugular
      Left 05LN
      Right 05LM
    Intracranial 05LL
    ~~Lesser Saphenous~~
      ~~Left 06LS~~
      ~~Right 06LR~~
    Lower 06LY
    Portal 06L8
    Pulmonary
      Left 02LT
      Right 02LS
    Renal
      Left 06LB
      Right 06L9
    ▶ Saphenous
      ▶ Left 06LQ
      ▶ Right 06LP
    Splenic 06L1
    Subclavian
      Left 05L6
      Right 05L5
    Superior Mesenteric 06L5
    Upper 05LY
    Vertebral
      Left 05LS
      Right 05LR
  Vena Cava
    Inferior 06L0
    Superior 02LV
▶ **Occlusion, REBOA (resuscitative endovascular balloon occlusion of the aorta)**
  ▶ 02LW3DJ
  ▶ 04L03DJ
Occupational therapy *see* Activities of Daily Living Treatment, Rehabilitation F08
Odentectomy
  see Excision, Mouth and Throat 0CB
  see Resection, Mouth and Throat 0CT
▶ **Odontoid process** *use* Cervical Vertebra
Olecranon bursa
  use Elbow Bursa and Ligament, Right
  use Elbow Bursa and Ligament, Left

Olecranon process
  use Ulna, Right
  use Ulna, Left
Olfactory bulb *use* Olfactory Nerve
Omentectomy, omentumectomy
  see Excision, Gastrointestinal System 0DB
  see Resection, Gastrointestinal System 0DT
Omentofixation *see* Repair, Gastrointestinal System 0DQ
Omentoplasty
  see Repair, Gastrointestinal System 0DQ
  see Replacement, Gastrointestinal System 0DR
  see Supplement, Gastrointestinal System 0DU
Omentorrhaphy *see* Repair, Gastrointestinal System 0DQ
Omentotomy *see* Drainage, Gastrointestinal System 0D9
Omnilink Elite Vascular Balloon Expandable Stent System *use* Intraluminal Device
Onychectomy
  see Excision, Skin and Breast 0HB
  see Resection, Skin and Breast 0HT
Onychoplasty
  see Repair, Skin and Breast 0HQ
  see Replacement, Skin and Breast 0HR
Onychotomy *see* Drainage, Skin and Breast 0H9
Oophorectomy
  see Excision, Female Reproductive System 0UB
  see Resection, Female Reproductive System 0UT
Oophoropexy
  see Repair, Female Reproductive System 0UQ
  see Reposition, Female Reproductive System 0US
Oophoroplasty
  see Repair, Female Reproductive System 0UQ
  see Supplement, Female Reproductive System 0UU
Oophororrhaphy *see* Repair, Female Reproductive System 0UQ
Oophorostomy *see* Drainage, Female Reproductive System 0U9
Oophorotomy
  see Division, Female Reproductive System 0U8
  see Drainage, Female Reproductive System 0U9
Oophorrhaphy *see* Repair, Female Reproductive System 0UQ
Open Pivot (mechanical) valve *use* Synthetic Substitute
Open Pivot Aortic Valve Graft (AVG) *use* Synthetic Substitute
Ophthalmic artery *use* Intracranial Artery
Ophthalmic nerve *use* Trigeminal Nerve
Ophthalmic vein *use* Intracranial Vein
Opponensplasty
  Tendon replacement *see* Replacement, Tendons 0LR
  Tendon transfer *see* Transfer, Tendons 0LX
Optic chiasma *use* Optic Nerve
Optic disc
  use Retina, Right
  use Retina, Left
➡ **Optic foramen** *use* Sphenoid Bone
  ~~*use* Sphenoid Bone, Right~~
  ~~*use* Sphenoid Bone, Left~~
Optical coherence tomography, intravascular *see* Computerized Tomography (CT Scan)
Optimizer™ III implantable pulse generator *use* Contractility Modulation Device in 0JH
Orbicularis oculi muscle
  use Upper Eyelid, Right
  use Upper Eyelid, Left
Orbicularis oris muscle *use* Facial Muscle
Orbital Atherectomy Technology X2C
Orbital fascia *use* Subcutaneous Tissue and Fascia, Face

Orbital portion of ethmoid bone
  use Orbit, Right
  use Orbit, Left
Orbital portion of frontal bone
  use Orbit, Right
  use Orbit, Left
Orbital portion of lacrimal bone
  use Orbit, Right
  use Orbit, Left
Orbital portion of maxilla
  use Orbit, Right
  use Orbit, Left
Orbital portion of palatine bone
  use Orbit, Right
  use Orbit, Left
Orbital portion of sphenoid bone
  use Orbit, Right
  use Orbit, Left
Orbital portion of zygomatic bone
  use Orbit, Right
  use Orbit, Left
Orchectomy, orchidectomy, orchiectomy
  see Excision, Male Reproductive System 0VB
  see Resection, Male Reproductive System 0VT
Orchidoplasty, orchioplasty
  see Repair, Male Reproductive System 0VQ
  see Replacement, Male Reproductive System 0VR
  see Supplement, Male Reproductive System 0VU
Orchidorrhaphy, orchiorrhaphy *see* Repair, Male Reproductive System 0VQ
Orchidotomy, orchiotomy, orchotomy *see* Drainage, Male Reproductive System 0V9
Orchiopexy
  see Repair, Male Reproductive System 0VQ
  see Reposition, Male Reproductive System 0VS
Oropharyngeal airway (OPA) *use* Intraluminal Device, Airway in Mouth and Throat
Oropharynx *use* Pharynx
Ossiculectomy
  see Excision, Ear, Nose, Sinus 09B
  see Resection, Ear, Nose, Sinus 09T
Ossiculotomy *see* Drainage, Ear, Nose, Sinus 099
Ostectomy
  see Excision, Head and Facial Bones 0NB
  see Resection, Head and Facial Bones 0NT
  see Excision, Upper Bones 0PB
  see Resection, Upper Bones 0PT
  see Excision, Lower Bones 0QB
  see Resection, Lower Bones 0QT
Osteoclasis
  see Division, Head and Facial Bones 0N8
  see Division, Upper Bones 0P8
  see Division, Lower Bones 0Q8
Osteolysis
  see Release, Head and Facial Bones 0NN
  see Release, Upper Bones 0PN
  see Release, Lower Bones 0QN
Osteopathic Treatment
  Abdomen 7W09X
  Cervical 7W01X
  Extremity
    Lower 7W06X
    Upper 7W07X
  Head 7W00X
  Lumbar 7W03X
  Pelvis 7W05X
  Rib Cage 7W08X
  Sacrum 7W04X
  Thoracic 7W02X
Osteopexy
  see Repair, Head and Facial Bones 0NQ
  see Reposition, Head and Facial Bones 0NS
  see Repair, Upper Bones 0PQ
  see Reposition, Upper Bones 0PS
  see Repair, Lower Bones 0QQ
  see Reposition, Lower Bones 0QS

Osteoplasty
see Repair, Head and Facial Bones ØNQ
see Replacement, Head and Facial Bones ØNR
see Supplement, Head and Facial Bones ØNU
see Repair, Upper Bones ØPQ
see Replacement, Upper Bones ØPR
see Supplement, Upper Bones ØPU
see Repair, Lower Bones ØQQ
see Replacement, Lower Bones ØQR
see Supplement, Lower Bones ØQU

Osteorrhaphy
see Repair, Head and Facial Bones ØNQ
see Repair, Upper Bones ØPQ
see Repair, Lower Bones ØQQ

Osteotomy, ostotomy
see Division, Head and Facial Bones ØN8
see Drainage, Head and Facial Bones ØN9
see Division, Upper Bones ØP8
see Drainage, Upper Bones ØP9
see Division, Lower Bones ØQ8
see Drainage, Lower Bones ØQ9

Otic ganglion use Head and Neck Sympathetic Nerve

Otoplasty
see Repair, Ear, Nose, Sinus Ø9Q
see Replacement, Ear, Nose, Sinus Ø9R
see Supplement, Ear, Nose, Sinus Ø9U

Otoscopy see Inspection, Ear, Nose, Sinus Ø9J

Oval window
use Middle Ear, Right
use Middle Ear, Left

Ovarian artery use Abdominal Aorta

Ovarian ligament use Uterine Supporting Structure

Ovariectomy
see Excision, Female Reproductive System ØUB
see Resection, Female Reproductive System ØUT

Ovariocentesis see Drainage, Female Reproductive System ØU9

Ovariopexy
see Repair, Female Reproductive System ØUQ
see Reposition, Female Reproductive System ØUS

Ovariotomy
see Division, Female Reproductive System ØU8
see Drainage, Female Reproductive System ØU9

Ovatio™ CRT-D use Cardiac Resynchronization Defibrillator Pulse Generator in ØJH

Oversewing
Gastrointestinal ulcer see Repair, Gastrointestinal System ØDQ
Pleural bleb see Repair, Respiratory System ØBQ

Oviduct
use Fallopian Tube, Right
use Fallopian Tube, Left

~~Oxidized zirconium ceramic hip bearing surface use Synthetic Substitute, Ceramic on Polyethylene in ØSR~~

Oximetry, Fetal pulse 1ØHØ73Z

▶**OXINIUM** use Synthetic Substitute, Oxidized Zirconium on Polyethylene in ØSR

Oxygenation
Extracorporeal membrane (ECMO) see Performance, Circulatory 5A15
Hyperbaric see Assistance, Circulatory 5AØ5
Supersaturated see Assistance, Circulatory 5AØ5

▶ New   ⟹ Revised   ~~deleted~~ Deleted

P

Pacemaker
Dual Chamber
Abdomen ØJH8
Chest ØJH6
Intracardiac
Insertion of device in
Atrium
Left 02H7
Right 02H6
Vein, Coronary 02H4
Ventricle
Left 02HL
Right 02HK
Removal of device from, Heart 02PA
Revision of device in, Heart 02WA
Single Chamber
Abdomen ØJH8
Chest ØJH6
Single Chamber Rate Responsive
Abdomen ØJH8
Chest ØJH6
Packing
Abdominal Wall 2W43X5Z
Anorectal 2Y43X5Z
Arm
Lower
Left 2W4DX5Z
Right 2W4CX5Z
Upper
Left 2W4BX5Z
Right 2W4AX5Z
Back 2W45X5Z
Chest Wall 2W44X5Z
Ear 2Y42X5Z
Extremity
Lower
Left 2W4MX5Z
Right 2W4LX5Z
Upper
Left 2W49X5Z
Right 2W48X5Z
Face 2W41X5Z
Finger
Left 2W4KX5Z
Right 2W4JX5Z
Foot
Left 2W4TX5Z
Right 2W4SX5Z
Genital Tract, Female 2Y44X5Z
Hand
Left 2W4FX5Z
Right 2W4EX5Z
Head 2W40X5Z
Inguinal Region
Left 2W47X5Z
Right 2W46X5Z
Leg
Lower
Left 2W4RX5Z
Right 2W4QX5Z
Upper
Left 2W4PX5Z
Right 2W4NX5Z
Mouth and Pharynx 2Y40X5Z
Nasal 2Y41X5Z
Neck 2W42X5Z
Thumb
Left 2W4HX5Z
Right 2W4GX5Z
Toe
Left 2W4VX5Z
Right 2W4UX5Z
Urethra 2Y45X5Z
Paclitaxel-eluting coronary stent
use Intraluminal Device, Drug-eluting in Heart and Great Vessels

Paclitaxel-eluting peripheral stent
use Intraluminal Device, Drug-eluting in Upper Arteries
use Intraluminal Device, Drug-eluting in Lower Arteries
Palatine gland *use* Buccal Mucosa
Palatine tonsil *use* Tonsils
Palatine uvula *use* Uvula
Palatoglossal muscle *use* Tongue, Palate, Pharynx Muscle
Palatopharyngeal muscle *use* Tongue, Palate, Pharynx Muscle
Palatoplasty
see Repair, Mouth and Throat ØCQ
see Replacement, Mouth and Throat ØCR
see Supplement, Mouth and Throat ØCU
Palatorrhaphy *see* Repair, Mouth and Throat ØCQ
Palmar (volar) digital vein
use Hand Vein, Right
use Hand Vein, Left
Palmar (volar) metacarpal vein
use Hand Vein, Right
use Hand Vein, Left
Palmar cutaneous nerve
use Radial Nerve
use Median Nerve
Palmar fascia (aponeurosis)
use Subcutaneous Tissue and Fascia, Right Hand
use Subcutaneous Tissue and Fascia, Left Hand
Palmar interosseous muscle
use Hand Muscle, Right
use Hand Muscle, Left
Palmar ulnocarpal ligament
use Wrist Bursa and Ligament, Right
use Wrist Bursa and Ligament, Left
Palmaris longus muscle
use Lower Arm and Wrist Muscle, Right
use Lower Arm and Wrist Muscle, Left
Pancreatectomy
see Excision, Pancreas ØFBG
see Resection, Pancreas ØFTG
Pancreatic artery *use* Splenic Artery
Pancreatic plexus *use* Abdominal Sympathetic Nerve
Pancreatic vein *use* Splenic Vein
Pancreaticoduodenostomy *see* Bypass, Hepatobiliary System and Pancreas ØF1
Pancreaticosplenic lymph node *use* Lymphatic, Aortic
Pancreatogram, endoscopic retrograde *see* Fluoroscopy, Pancreatic Duct BF18
Pancreatolithotomy *see* Extirpation, Pancreas ØFCG
Pancreatotomy
see Division, Pancreas ØF8G
see Drainage, Pancreas ØF9G
Panniculectomy
see Excision, Skin, Abdomen ØHB7
see Excision, Abdominal Wall ØWBF
Paraaortic lymph node *use* Lymphatic, Aortic
Paracentesis
Eye *see* Drainage, Eye Ø89
Peritoneal Cavity *see* Drainage, Peritoneal Cavity ØW9G
Tympanum *see* Drainage, Ear, Nose, Sinus Ø99
Pararectal lymph node *use* Lymphatic, Mesenteric
Parasternal lymph node *use* Lymphatic, Thorax
Parathyroidectomy
see Excision, Endocrine System ØGB
see Resection, Endocrine System ØGT
Paratracheal lymph node *use* Lymphatic, Thorax
Paraurethral (Skene's) gland *use* Vestibular Gland
Parenteral nutrition, total *see* Introduction of Nutritional Substance
Parietal lobe *use* Cerebral Hemisphere
Parotid lymph node *use* Lymphatic, Head
Parotid plexus *use* Facial Nerve

Parotidectomy
see Excision, Mouth and Throat ØCB
see Resection, Mouth and Throat ØCT
Pars flaccida
use Tympanic Membrane, Right
use Tympanic Membrane, Left
Partial joint replacement
Hip *see* Replacement, Lower Joints ØSR
Knee *see* Replacement, Lower Joints ØSR
Shoulder *see* Replacement, Upper Joints ØRR
Partially absorbable mesh *use* Synthetic Substitute
Patch, blood, spinal 3EØS3GC
Patellapexy
see Repair, Lower Bones ØQQ
see Reposition, Lower Bones ØQS
Patellaplasty
see Repair, Lower Bones ØQQ
see Replacement, Lower Bones ØQR
see Supplement, Lower Bones ØQU
Patellar ligament
use Knee Bursa and Ligament, Right
use Knee Bursa and Ligament, Left
Patellar tendon
use Knee Tendon, Right
use Knee Tendon, Left
Patellectomy
see Excision, Lower Bones ØQB
see Resection, Lower Bones ØQT
Patellofemoral joint
use Knee Joint, Right
use Knee Joint, Left
use Knee Joint, Femoral Surface, Right
use Knee Joint, Femoral Surface, Left
Pectineus muscle
use Upper Leg Muscle, Right
use Upper Leg Muscle, Left
Pectoral (anterior) lymph node
use Lymphatic, Right Axillary
use Lymphatic, Left Axillary
Pectoral fascia *use* Subcutaneous Tissue and Fascia, Chest
Pectoralis major muscle
use Thorax Muscle, Right
use Thorax Muscle, Left
Pectoralis minor muscle
use Thorax Muscle, Right
use Thorax Muscle, Left
Pedicle-based dynamic stabilization device
use Spinal Stabilization Device, Pedicle-Based in ØRH
use Spinal Stabilization Device, Pedicle-Based in ØSH
PEEP (positive end expiratory pressure) *see* Assistance, Respiratory 5AØ9
PEG (percutaneous endoscopic gastrostomy) ØDH63UZ
PEJ (percutaneous endoscopic jejunostomy) ØDHA3UZ
Pelvic splanchnic nerve
use Abdominal Sympathetic Nerve
use Sacral Sympathetic Nerve
Penectomy
see Excision, Male Reproductive System ØVB
see Resection, Male Reproductive System ØVT
Penile urethra *use* Urethra
Perceval sutureless valve *use* Zooplastic Tissue, Rapid Deployment Technique in New Technology
Percutaneous endoscopic gastrojejunostomy (PEG/J) tube *use* Feeding Device in Gastrointestinal System
Percutaneous endoscopic gastrostomy (PEG) tube *use* Feeding Device in Gastrointestinal System
Percutaneous nephrostomy catheter *use* Drainage Device
Percutaneous transluminal coronary angioplasty (PTCA) *see* Dilation, Heart and Great Vessels Ø27

▶ New   ⇒ Revised   ~~deleted~~ Deleted

Performance
  Biliary
    Multiple, Filtration 5A1C60Z
    Single, Filtration 5A1C00Z
  Cardiac
    Continuous
        Output 5A1221Z
        Pacing 5A1223Z
      Intermittent, Pacing 5A1213Z
      Single, Output, Manual 5A12012
    Circulatory, Continuous, Oxygenation,
      Membrane 5A15223
  Respiratory
    24-96 Consecutive Hours, Ventilation
      5A1945Z
    Greater than 96 Consecutive Hours,
      Ventilation 5A1955Z
    Less than 24 Consecutive Hours,
      Ventilation 5A1935Z
    Single, Ventilation, Nonmechanical
      5A19054
  Urinary
    ~~Multiple, Filtration 5A1D60Z~~
    ~~Single, Filtration 5A1D00Z~~
    ▶ Continuous, Greater than 18 hours per day,
      Filtration 5A1D90Z
    ▶ Intermittent, Less than 6 Hours Per Day,
      Filtration 5A1D70Z
    ▶ Prolonged Intermittent, 6-18 hours per day,
      Filtration 5A1D80Z
Perfusion *see* Introduction of substance in or on
Perfusion, donor organ
  Heart 6AB50BZ
  Kidney(s) 6ABT0BZ
  Liver 6ABF0BZ
  Lung(s) 6ABB0BZ
Pericardiectomy
  see Excision, Pericardium 02BN
  see Resection, Pericardium 02TN
Pericardiocentesis
  see Drainage, Cavity, Pericardial 0W9D
Pericardiolysis *see* Release, Pericardium
  02NN
Pericardiophrenic artery
  use Internal Mammary Artery, Right
  use Internal Mammary Artery, Left
Pericardioplasty
  see Repair, Pericardium 02QN
  see Replacement, Pericardium 02RN
  see Supplement, Pericardium 02UN
Pericardiorrhaphy *see* Repair, Pericardium
  02QN
Pericardiostomy *see* Drainage, Cavity,
  Pericardial 0W9D
Pericardiotomy *see* Drainage, Cavity, Pericardial
  0W9D
Perimetrium *use* Uterus
Peripheral parenteral nutrition *see* Introduction
  of Nutritional Substance
Peripherally inserted central catheter (PICC)
  use Infusion Device
Peritoneal dialysis 3E1M39Z
Peritoneocentesis
  see Drainage, Peritoneum 0D9W
  see Drainage, Cavity, Peritoneal 0W9G
Peritoneoplasty
  see Repair, Peritoneum 0DQW
  see Replacement, Peritoneum 0DRW
  see Supplement, Peritoneum 0DUW
Peritoneoscopy 0DJW4ZZ
Peritoneotomy *see* Drainage, Peritoneum 0D9W
Peritoneumectomy
  see Excision, Peritoneum 0DBW
Peroneus brevis muscle
  use Lower Leg Muscle, Right
  use Lower Leg Muscle, Left
Peroneus longus muscle
  use Lower Leg Muscle, Right
  use Lower Leg Muscle, Left
Pessary ring *use* Intraluminal Device, Pessary in
  Female Reproductive System

PET scan *see* Positron Emission Tomographic
  (PET) Imaging
Petrous part of temoporal bone
  use Temporal Bone, Right
  use Temporal Bone, Left
Phacoemulsification, lens
  With IOL implant *see* Replacement, Eye 08R
  Without IOL implant *see* Extraction, Eye 08D
Phalangectomy
  see Excision, Upper Bones 0PB
  see Resection, Upper Bones 0PT
  see Excision, Lower Bones 0QB
  see Resection, Lower Bones 0QT
Phallectomy
  see Excision, Penis 0VBS
  see Resection, Penis 0VTS
Phalloplasty
  see Repair, Penis 0VQS
  see Supplement, Penis 0VUS
Phallotomy *see* Drainage, Penis 0V9S
Pharmacotherapy, for substance abuse
  Antabuse HZ93ZZZ
  Bupropion HZ97ZZZ
  Clonidine HZ96ZZZ
  Levo-alpha-acetyl-methadol (LAAM)
    HZ92ZZZ
  Methadone Maintenance HZ91ZZZ
  Naloxone HZ95ZZZ
  Naltrexone HZ94ZZZ
  Nicotine Replacement HZ90ZZZ
  Psychiatric Medication HZ98ZZZ
  Replacement Medication, Other HZ99ZZZ
Pharyngeal constrictor muscle *use* Tongue,
  Palate, Pharynx Muscle
Pharyngeal plexus *use* Vagus Nerve
Pharyngeal recess *use* Nasopharynx
Pharyngeal tonsil *use* Adenoids
Pharyngogram *see* Fluoroscopy, Pharynx B91G
Pharyngoplasty
  see Repair, Mouth and Throat 0CQ
  see Replacement, Mouth and Throat 0CR
  see Supplement, Mouth and Throat 0CU
Pharyngorrhaphy *see* Repair, Mouth and Throat
  0CQ
Pharyngotomy *see* Drainage, Mouth and Throat
  0C9
Pharyngotympanic tube
  use Eustachian Tube, Right
  use Eustachian Tube, Left
Pheresis
  Erythrocytes 6A55
  Leukocytes 6A55
  Plasma 6A55
  Platelets 6A55
  Stem Cells
    Cord Blood 6A55
    Hematopoietic 6A55
Phlebectomy
  see Excision, Upper Veins 05B
  see Extraction, Upper Veins 05D
  see Excision, Lower Veins 06B
  see Extraction, Lower Veins 06D
Phlebography
  see Plain Radiography, Veins B50
  Impedance 4A04X51
Phleborrhaphy
  see Repair, Upper Veins 05Q
  see Repair, Lower Veins 06Q
Phlebotomy
  see Drainage, Upper Veins 059
  see Drainage, Lower Veins 069
Photocoagulation
  for Destruction *see* Destruction
  for Repair *see* Repair
Photopheresis, therapeutic *see* Phototherapy,
  Circulatory 6A65
Phototherapy
  Circulatory 6A65
  Skin 6A60
  ▶ Ultraviolet light *see* Ultraviolet Light
    Therapy, Physiological Systems 6A8

Phrenectomy, phrenoneurectomy *see* Excision,
  Nerve, Phrenic 01B2
Phrenemphraxis *see* Destruction, Nerve,
  Phrenic 0152
Phrenic nerve stimulator generator *use*
  Stimulator Generator in Subcutaneous
  Tissue and Fascia
Phrenic nerve stimulator lead *use*
  Diaphragmatic Pacemaker Lead in
  Respiratory System
Phreniclasis *see* Destruction, Nerve, Phrenic
  0152
Phrenicoexeresis *see* Extraction, Nerve, Phrenic
  01D2
Phrenicotomy *see* Division, Nerve, Phrenic 0182
Phrenicotripsy *see* Destruction, Nerve, Phrenic
  0152
Phrenoplasty
  see Repair, Respiratory System 0BQ
  see Supplement, Respiratory System 0BU
Phrenotomy *see* Drainage, Respiratory System
  0B9
Physiatry *see* Motor Treatment, Rehabilitation F07
Physical medicine *see* Motor Treatment,
  Rehabilitation F07
Physical therapy *see* Motor Treatment,
  Rehabilitation F07
PHYSIOMESH™ Flexible Composite Mesh *use*
  Synthetic Substitute
Pia mater, intracranial *use* Cerebral Meninges
Pia mater, spinal *use* Spinal Meninges
Pinealectomy
  see Excision, Pineal Body 0GB1
  see Resection, Pineal Body 0GT1
Pinealoscopy 0GJ14ZZ
Pinealotomy *see* Drainage, Pineal Body 0G91
Pinna
  use External Ear, Right
  use External Ear, Left
  use External Ear, Bilateral
Pipeline™ Embolization device (PED) *use*
  Intraluminal Device
Piriform recess (sinus) *use* Pharynx
Piriformis muscle
  use Hip Muscle, Right
  use Hip Muscle, Left
▶**PIRRT (Prolonged intermittent renal**
  replacement therapy) 5A1D80Z
Pisiform bone
  use Carpal, Right
  use Carpal, Left
Pisohamate ligament
  use Hand Bursa and Ligament, Right
  use Hand Bursa and Ligament, Left
Pisometacarpal ligament
  use Hand Bursa and Ligament, Right
  use Hand Bursa and Ligament, Left
Pituitectomy
  see Excision, Gland, Pituitary 0GB0
  see Resection, Gland, Pituitary 0GT0
Plain film radiology *see* Plain Radiography
Plain Radiography
  Abdomen BW00ZZZ
  Abdomen and Pelvis BW01ZZZ
  Abdominal Lymphatic
    Bilateral B701
    Unilateral B700
  Airway, Upper BB0DZZZ
  Ankle
    Left BQ0H
    Right BQ0G
  Aorta
    Abdominal B400
    Thoracic B300
    Thoraco-Abdominal B30P
  Aorta and Bilateral Lower Extremity Arteries
    B40D
  Arch
    Bilateral BN0DZZZ
    Left BN0CZZZ
    Right BN0BZZZ

▶ New   ⇒ Revised   ~~deleted~~ Deleted

Plain Radiography *(Continued)*
Arm
  Left BP0FZZZ
  Right BP0EZZZ
Artery
  Brachiocephalic-Subclavian, Right
    B301
  Bronchial B30L
  Bypass Graft, Other B20F
  Cervico-Cerebral Arch B30Q
  Common Carotid
    Bilateral B305
    Left B304
    Right B303
  Coronary
    Bypass Graft
      Multiple B203
      Single B202
    Multiple B201
    Single B200
  External Carotid
    Bilateral B30C
    Left B30B
    Right B309
  Hepatic B402
  Inferior Mesenteric B405
  Intercostal B30L
  Internal Carotid
    Bilateral B308
    Left B307
    Right B306
  Internal Mammary Bypass Graft
    Left B208
    Right B207
  Intra-Abdominal, Other B40B
  Intracranial B30R
  Lower, Other B40J
  Lower Extremity
    Bilateral and Aorta B40D
    Left B40G
    Right B40F
  Lumbar B409
  Pelvic B40C
  Pulmonary
    Left B30T
    Right B30S
  Renal
    Bilateral B408
    Left B407
    Right B406
    Transplant B40M
  Spinal B30M
  Splenic B403
  Subclavian, Left B302
  Superior Mesenteric B404
  Upper, Other B30N
  Upper Extremity
    Bilateral B30K
    Left B30J
    Right B30H
  Vertebral
    Bilateral B30G
    Left B30F
    Right B30D
Bile Duct BF00
Bile Duct and Gallbladder BF03
Bladder BT00
  Kidney and Ureter BT04
Bladder and Urethra BT0B
Bone
  Facial BN05ZZZ
  Nasal BN04ZZZ
Bones, Long, All BW0BZZZ
Breast
  Bilateral BH02ZZZ
  Left BH01ZZZ
  Right BH00ZZZ
Calcaneus
  Left BQ0KZZZ
  Right BQ0JZZZ
Chest BW03ZZZ

Plain Radiography *(Continued)*
Clavicle
  Left BP05ZZZ
  Right BP04ZZZ
Coccyx BR0FZZZ
Corpora Cavernosa BV00
Dialysis Fistula B50W
Dialysis Shunt B50W
Disc
  Cervical BR01
  Lumbar BR03
  Thoracic BR02
Duct
  Lacrimal
    Bilateral B802
    Left B801
    Right B800
  Mammary
    Multiple
      Left BH06
      Right BH05
    Single
      Left BH04
      Right BH03
Elbow
  Left BP0H
  Right BP0G
Epididymis
  Left BV02
  Right BV01
Extremity
  Lower BW0CZZZ
  Upper BW0JZZZ
Eye
  Bilateral B807ZZZ
  Left B806ZZZ
  Right B805ZZZ
Facet Joint
  Cervical BR04
  Lumbar BR06
  Thoracic BR05
Fallopian Tube
  Bilateral BU02
  Left BU01
  Right BU00
Fallopian Tube and Uterus BU08
Femur
  Left, Densitometry BQ04ZZ1
  Right, Densitometry BQ03ZZ1
Finger
  Left BP0SZZZ
  Right BP0RZZZ
Foot
  Left BQ0MZZZ
  Right BQ0LZZZ
Forearm
  Left BP0KZZZ
  Right BP0JZZZ
Gallbladder and Bile Duct BF03
Gland
  Parotid
    Bilateral B906
    Left B905
    Right B904
  Salivary
    Bilateral B90D
    Left B90C
    Right B90B
  Submandibular
    Bilateral B909
    Left B908
    Right B907
Hand
  Left BP0PZZZ
  Right BP0NZZZ
Heart
  Left B205
  Right B204
  Right and Left B206
Hepatobiliary System, All BF0C

Plain Radiography *(Continued)*
Hip
  Left BQ01
    Densitometry BQ01ZZ1
  Right BQ00
    Densitometry BQ00ZZ1
Humerus
  Left BP0BZZZ
  Right BP0AZZZ
Ileal Diversion Loop BT0C
Intracranial Sinus B502
Joint
  Acromioclavicular, Bilateral BP03ZZZ
  Finger
    Left BP0D
    Right BP0C
  Foot
    Left BQ0Y
    Right BQ0X
  Hand
    Left BP0D
    Right BP0C
  Lumbosacral BR0BZZZ
  Sacroiliac BR0D
  Sternoclavicular
    Bilateral BP02ZZZ
    Left BP01ZZZ
    Right BP00ZZZ
  Temporomandibular
    Bilateral BN09
    Left BN08
    Right BN07
  Thoracolumbar BR08ZZZ
  Toe
    Left BQ0Y
    Right BQ0X
Kidney
  Bilateral BT03
  Left BT02
  Right BT01
  Ureter and Bladder BT04
Knee
  Left BQ08
  Right BQ07
Leg
  Left BQ0FZZZ
  Right BQ0DZZZ
Lymphatic
  Head B704
  Lower Extremity
    Bilateral B70B
    Left B709
    Right B708
  Neck B704
  Pelvic B70C
  Upper Extremity
    Bilateral B707
    Left B706
    Right B705
Mandible BN06ZZZ
Mastoid B90HZZZ
Nasopharynx B90FZZZ
Optic Foramina
  Left B804ZZZ
  Right B803ZZZ
Orbit
  Bilateral BN03ZZZ
  Left BN02ZZZ
  Right BN01ZZZ
Oropharynx B90FZZZ
Patella
  Left BQ0WZZZ
  Right BQ0VZZZ
Pelvis BR0CZZZ
Pelvis and Abdomen BW01ZZZ
Prostate BV03
Retroperitoneal Lymphatic
  Bilateral B701
  Unilateral B700
Ribs
  Left BP0YZZZ
  Right BP0XZZZ

Plain Radiography *(Continued)*

Sacrum BR0FZZZ
Scapula
  Left BP07ZZZ
  Right BP06ZZZ
Shoulder
  Left BP09
  Right BP08
Sinus
  Intracranial B502
  Paranasal B902ZZZ
Skull BN00ZZZ
Spinal Cord B00B
Spine
  Cervical, Densitometry BR00ZZ1
  Lumbar, Densitometry BR09ZZ1
  Thoracic, Densitometry BR07ZZ1
  Whole, Densitometry BR0GZZ1
Sternum BR0HZZZ
Teeth
  All BN0JZZZ
  Multiple BN0HZZZ
Testicle
  Left BV06
  Right BV05
Toe
  Left BQ0QZZZ
  Right BQ0PZZZ
Tooth, Single BN0GZZZ
Tracheobronchial Tree
  Bilateral BB09YZZ
  Left BB08YZZ
  Right BB07YZZ
Ureter
  Bilateral BT08
  Kidney and Bladder BT04
  Left BT07
  Right BT06
Urethra BT05
Urethra and Bladder BT0B
Uterus BU06
Uterus and Fallopian Tube BU08
Vagina BU09
Vasa Vasorum BV08
Vein
  Cerebellar B501
  Cerebral B501
  Epidural B500
  Jugular
    Bilateral B505
    Left B504
    Right B503
  Lower Extremity
    Bilateral B50D
    Left B50C
    Right B50B
  Other B50V
  Pelvic (Iliac)
    Left B50G
    Right B50F
  Pelvic (Iliac) Bilateral B50H
  Portal B50T
  Pulmonary
    Bilateral B50S
    Left B50R
    Right B50Q
  Renal
    Bilateral B50L
    Left B50K
    Right B50J
  Spanchnic B50T
  Subclavian
    Left B507
    Right B506
  Upper Extremity
    Bilateral B50P
    Left B50N
    Right B50M
Vena Cava
  Inferior B509
  Superior B508

Plain Radiography *(Continued)*

Whole Body BW0KZZZ
  Infant BW0MZZZ
Whole Skeleton BW0LZZZ
Wrist
  Left BP0M
  Right BP0L

Planar Nuclear Medicine Imaging

Abdomen CW10
Abdomen and Chest CW14
Abdomen and Pelvis CW11
Anatomical Region, Other CW1ZZZZ
Anatomical Regions, Multiple CW1YYZZ
Bladder, Kidneys and Ureters CT13
Bladder and Ureters CT1H
Blood C713
Bone Marrow C710
Brain C010
Breast CH1YYZZ
  Bilateral CH12
  Left CH11
  Right CH10
Bronchi and Lungs CB12
Central Nervous System C01YYZZ
Cerebrospinal Fluid C015
Chest CW13
Chest and Abdomen CW14
Chest and Neck CW16
Digestive System CD1YYZZ
Ducts, Lacrimal, Bilateral C819
Ear, Nose, Mouth and Throat C91YYZZ
Endocrine System CG1YYZZ
Extremity
  Lower CW1D
    Bilateral CP1F
    Left CP1D
    Right CP1C
  Upper CW1M
    Bilateral CP1B
    Left CP19
    Right CP18
Eye C81YYZZ
Gallbladder CF14
Gastrointestinal Tract CD17
  Upper CD15
Gland
  Adrenal, Bilateral CG14
  Parathyroid CG11
  Thyroid CG12
Glands, Salivary, Bilateral C91B
Head and Neck CW1B
Heart C21YYZZ
  Right and Left C216
Hepatobiliary System, All CF1C
Hepatobiliary System and Pancreas CF1YYZZ
Kidneys, Ureters and Bladder CT13
Liver CF15
Liver and Spleen CF16
Lungs and Bronchi CB12
Lymphatics
  Head C71J
  Head and Neck C715
  Lower Extremity C71P
  Neck C71K
  Pelvic C71D
  Trunk C71M
  Upper Chest C71L
  Upper Extremity C71N
Lymphatics and Hematologic System
  C71YYZZ
Musculoskeletal System
  All CP1Z
  Other CP1YYZZ
Myocardium C21G
Neck and Chest CW16
Neck and Head CW1B
Pancreas and Hepatobiliary System
  CF1YYZZ
Pelvic Region CW1J
Pelvis CP16
Pelvis and Abdomen CW11

Planar Nuclear Medicine Imaging *(Continued)*

Pelvis and Spine CP17
Reproductive System, Male CV1YYZZ
Respiratory System CB1YYZZ
Skin CH1YYZZ
Skull CP11
Spine CP15
Spine and Pelvis CP17
Spleen C712
Spleen and Liver CF16
Subcutaneous Tissue CH1YYZZ
Testicles, Bilateral CV19
Thorax CP14
Ureters, Kidneys and Bladder CT13
Ureters and Bladder CT1H
Urinary System CT1YYZZ
Veins C51YYZZ
  Central C51R
  Lower Extremity
    Bilateral C51D
    Left C51C
    Right C51B
  Upper Extremity
    Bilateral C51Q
    Left C51P
    Right C51N
Whole Body CW1N

Plantar digital vein
  use Foot Vein, Right
  use Foot Vein, Left

Plantar fascia (aponeurosis)
  use Foot Subcutaneous Tissue and Fascia, Right
  use Foot Subcutaneous Tissue and Fascia, Left

Plantar metatarsal vein
  use Foot Vein, Right
  use Foot Vein, Left

Plantar venous arch
  use Foot Vein, Right
  use Foot Vein, Left

Plaque Radiation
Abdomen DWY3FZZ
Adrenal Gland DGY2FZZ
Anus DDY8FZZ
Bile Ducts DFY2FZZ
Bladder DTY2FZZ
Bone, Other DPYCFZZ
Bone Marrow D7Y0FZZ
Brain D0Y0FZZ
Brain Stem D0Y1FZZ
Breast
  Left DMY0FZZ
  Right DMY1FZZ
Bronchus DBY1FZZ
Cervix DUY1FZZ
Chest DWY2FZZ
Chest Wall DBY7FZZ
Colon DDY5FZZ
Diaphragm DBY8FZZ
Duodenum DDY2FZZ
Ear D9Y0FZZ
Esophagus DDY0FZZ
Eye D8Y0FZZ
Femur DPY9FZZ
Fibula DPYBFZZ
Gallbladder DFY1FZZ
Gland
  Adrenal DGY2FZZ
  Parathyroid DGY4FZZ
  Pituitary DGY0FZZ
  Thyroid DGY5FZZ
Glands, Salivary D9Y6FZZ
Head and Neck DWY1FZZ
Hemibody DWY4FZZ
Humerus DPY6FZZ
Ileum DDY4FZZ
Jejunum DDY3FZZ
Kidney DTY0FZZ
Larynx D9YBFZZ
Liver DFY0FZZ

► New   ➡ Revised   ~~deleted~~ Deleted

Plaque Radiation *(Continued)*
  Lung DBY2FZZ
  Lymphatics
    Abdomen D7Y6FZZ
    Axillary D7Y4FZZ
    Inguinal D7Y8FZZ
    Neck D7Y3FZZ
    Pelvis D7Y7FZZ
    Thorax D7Y5FZZ
  Mandible DPY3FZZ
  Maxilla DPY2FZZ
  Mediastinum DBY6FZZ
  Mouth D9Y4FZZ
  Nasopharynx D9YDFZZ
  Neck and Head DWY1FZZ
  Nerve, Peripheral D0Y7FZZ
  Nose D9Y1FZZ
  Ovary DUY0FZZ
  Palate
    Hard D9Y8FZZ
    Soft D9Y9FZZ
  Pancreas DFY3FZZ
  Parathyroid Gland DGY4FZZ
  Pelvic Bones DPY8FZZ
  Pelvic Region DWY6FZZ
  Pharynx D9YCFZZ
  Pineal Body DGY1FZZ
  Pituitary Gland DGY0FZZ
  Pleura DBY5FZZ
  Prostate DVY0FZZ
  Radius DPY7FZZ
  Rectum DDY7FZZ
  Rib DPY5FZZ
  Sinuses D9Y7FZZ
  Skin
    Abdomen DHY8FZZ
    Arm DHY4FZZ
    Back DHY7FZZ
    Buttock DHY9FZZ
    Chest DHY6FZZ
    Face DHY2FZZ
    Foot DHYCFZZ
    Hand DHY5FZZ
    Leg DHYBFZZ
    Neck DHY3FZZ
  Skull DPY0FZZ
  Spinal Cord D0Y6FZZ
  Spleen D7Y2FZZ
  Sternum DPY4FZZ
  Stomach DDY1FZZ
  Testis DVY1FZZ
  Thymus D7Y1FZZ
  Thyroid Gland DGY5FZZ
  Tibia DPYBFZZ
  Tongue D9Y5FZZ
  Trachea DBY0FZZ
  Ulna DPY7FZZ
  Ureter DTY1FZZ
  Urethra DTY3FZZ
  Uterus DUY2FZZ
  Whole Body DWY5FZZ
➡**Plasmapheresis, therapeutic** *see* Pheresis,
    Physiological Systems 6A5
➡**Plateletpheresis, therapeutic** *see* Pheresis,
    Physiological Systems 6A5
Platysma muscle
  use Neck Muscle, Right
  use Neck Muscle, Left
Pleurectomy
  see Excision, Respiratory System ØBB
  see Resection, Respiratory System ØBT
Pleurocentesis *see* Drainage, Anatomical
    Regions, General ØW9
Pleurodesis, pleurosclerosis
  Chemical Injection *see* Introduction of
    substance in or on, Pleural Cavity 3EØL
  Surgical *see* Destruction, Respiratory System
    ØB5
Pleurolysis *see* Release, Respiratory System
    ØBN
Pleuroscopy ØBJQ4ZZ

Pleurotomy *see* Drainage, Respiratory System
    ØB9
Plica semilunaris
  use Conjunctiva, Right
  use Conjunctiva, Left
Plication *see* Restriction
Pneumectomy
  see Excision, Respiratory System ØBB
  see Resection, Respiratory System ØBT
Pneumocentesis *see* Drainage, Respiratory
    System ØB9
Pneumogastric nerve *use* Vagus Nerve
Pneumolysis *see* Release, Respiratory System
    ØBN
Pneumonectomy *see* Resection, Respiratory
    System ØBT
Pneumonolysis *see* Release, Respiratory System
    ØBN
Pneumonopexy
  see Repair, Respiratory System ØBQ
  see Reposition, Respiratory System ØBS
Pneumonorrhaphy *see* Repair, Respiratory
    System ØBQ
Pneumonotomy *see* Drainage, Respiratory
    System ØB9
Pneumotaxic center *use* Pons
Pneumotomy *see* Drainage, Respiratory System
    ØB9
Pollicization *see* Transfer, Anatomical Regions,
    Upper Extremities ØXX
Polyethylene socket *use* Synthetic Substitute,
    Polyethylene in ØSR
Polymethylmethacrylate (PMMA) *use*
    Synthetic Substitute
Polypectomy, gastrointestinal *see* Excision,
    Gastrointestinal System ØDB
Polypropylene mesh *use* Synthetic Substitute
Polysomnogram 4A1ZXQZ
Pontine tegmentum *use* Pons
Popliteal ligament
  use Knee Bursa and Ligament, Right
  use Knee Bursa and Ligament, Left
Popliteal lymph node
  use Lymphatic, Right Lower Extremity
  use Lymphatic, Left Lower Extremity
Popliteal vein
  use Femoral Vein, Right
  use Femoral Vein, Left
Popliteus muscle
  use Lower Leg Muscle, Right
  use Lower Leg Muscle, Left
Porcine (bioprosthetic) valve *use* Zooplastic
    Tissue in Heart and Great Vessels
Positive end expiratory pressure *see*
    Performance, Respiratory 5A19
Positron Emission Tomographic (PET)
    Imaging
  Brain CØ3Ø
  Bronchi and Lungs CB32
  Central Nervous System CØ3YYZZ
  Heart C23YYZZ
  Lungs and Bronchi CB32
  Myocardium C23G
  Respiratory System CB3YYZZ
  Whole Body CW3NYZZ
Positron emission tomography *see* Positron
    Emission Tomographic (PET) Imaging
Postauricular (mastoid) lymph node
  use Lymphatic, Right Neck
  use Lymphatic, Left Neck
Postcava *use* Inferior Vena Cava
Posterior (subscapular) lymph node
  use Lymphatic, Right Axillary
  use Lymphatic, Left Axillary
Posterior auricular artery
  use External Carotid Artery, Right
  use External Carotid Artery, Left
Posterior auricular nerve *use* Facial Nerve
Posterior auricular vein
  use External Jugular Vein, Right
  use External Jugular Vein, Left

Posterior cerebral artery *use* Intracranial
    Artery
Posterior chamber
  use Eye, Right
  use Eye, Left
Posterior circumflex humeral artery
  use Axillary Artery, Right
  use Axillary Artery, Left
Posterior communicating artery *use* Intracranial
    Artery
Posterior cruciate ligament (PCL)
  use Knee Bursa and Ligament, Right
  use Knee Bursa and Ligament, Left
Posterior facial (retromandibular) vein
  use Face Vein, Right
  use Face Vein, Left
Posterior femoral cutaneous nerve *use* Sacral
    Plexus Nerve
Posterior inferior cerebellar artery (PICA) *use*
    Intracranial Artery
Posterior interosseous nerve *use* Radial Nerve
Posterior labial nerve *use* Pudendal Nerve
Posterior scrotal nerve *use* Pudendal Nerve
Posterior spinal artery
  use Vertebral Artery, Right
  use Vertebral Artery, Left
Posterior tibial recurrent artery
  use Anterior Tibial Artery, Right
  use Anterior Tibial Artery, Left
Posterior ulnar recurrent artery
  use Ulnar Artery, Right
  use Ulnar Artery, Left
Posterior vagal trunk *use* Vagus Nerve
PPN (peripheral parenteral nutrition) *see*
    Introduction of Nutritional Substance
Preauricular lymph node *use* Lymphatic,
    Head
Precava *use* Superior Vena Cava
Prepatellar bursa
  use Knee Bursa and Ligament, Right
  use Knee Bursa and Ligament, Left
Preputiotomy *see* Drainage, Male Reproductive
    System ØV9
Pressure support ventilation *see* Performance,
    Respiratory 5A19
PRESTIGE® Cervical Disc *use* Synthetic
    Substitute
➡**Pretracheal fascia**
  ▶*use* Subcutaneous Tissue and Fascia, Right
    Neck
  ▶*use* Subcutaneous Tissue and Fascia, Left
    Neck
➡**Prevertebral fascia**
  ▶*use* Subcutaneous Tissue and Fascia, Right
    Neck
  ▶*use* Subcutaneous Tissue and Fascia, Left
    Neck
PrimeAdvanced neurostimulator (SureScan)
    (MRI Safe) *use* Stimulator Generator,
    Multiple Array in ØJH
Princeps pollicis artery
  use Hand Artery, Right
  use Hand Artery, Left
Probing, duct
  Diagnostic *see* Inspection
  Dilation *see* Dilation
PROCEED™ Ventral Patch *use* Synthetic
    Substitute
Procerus muscle *use* Facial Muscle
Proctectomy
  see Excision, Rectum ØDBP
  see Resection, Rectum ØDTP
Proctoclysis *see* Introduction of substance in or
    on, Gastrointestinal Tract, Lower 3EØH
Proctocolectomy
  see Excision, Gastrointestinal System ØDB
  see Resection, Gastrointestinal System ØDT
Proctocolpoplasty
  see Repair, Gastrointestinal System ØDQ
  see Supplement, Gastrointestinal System ØDU

Proctoperineoplasty
see Repair, Gastrointestinal System 0DQ
see Supplement, Gastrointestinal System 0DU
Proctoperineorrhaphy see Repair, Gastrointestinal System 0DQ
Proctopexy
see Repair, Rectum 0DQP
see Reposition, Rectum 0DSP
Proctoplasty
see Repair, Rectum 0DQP
see Supplement, Rectum 0DUP
Proctorrhaphy see Repair, Rectum 0DQP
Proctoscopy 0DJD8ZZ
Proctosigmoidectomy
see Excision, Gastrointestinal System 0DB
see Resection, Gastrointestinal System 0DT
Proctosigmoidoscopy 0DJD8ZZ
Proctostomy see Drainage, Rectum 0D9P
Proctotomy see Drainage, Rectum 0D9P
Prodisc-C use Synthetic Substitute
Prodisc-L use Synthetic Substitute
Production, atrial septal defect see Excision, Septum, Atrial 02B5
Profunda brachii
use Brachial Artery, Right
use Brachial Artery, Left
Profunda femoris (deep femoral) vein
use Femoral Vein, Right
use Femoral Vein, Left
PROLENE Polypropylene Hernia System (PHS) use Synthetic Substitute
Pronator quadratus muscle
use Lower Arm and Wrist Muscle, Right
use Lower Arm and Wrist Muscle, Left
Pronator teres muscle
use Lower Arm and Wrist Muscle, Right
use Lower Arm and Wrist Muscle, Left
Prostatectomy
see Excision, Prostate 0VB0
see Resection, Prostate 0VT0
Prostatic urethra use Urethra
Prostatomy, prostatotomy see Drainage, Prostate 0V90
Protecta XT CRT-D use Cardiac Resynchronization Defibrillator Pulse Generator in 0JH
Protecta XT DR (XT VR) use Defibrillator Generator in 0JH
Protégé® RX Carotid Stent System use Intraluminal Device
Proximal radioulnar joint
use Elbow Joint, Right
use Elbow Joint, Left
Psoas muscle
use Hip Muscle, Right
use Hip Muscle, Left
PSV (pressure support ventilation) see Performance, Respiratory 5A19
Psychoanalysis GZ54ZZZ
Psychological Tests
Cognitive Status GZ14ZZZ
Developmental GZ10ZZZ
Intellectual and Psychoeducational GZ12ZZZ
Neurobehavioral Status GZ14ZZZ
Neuropsychological GZ13ZZZ
Personality and Behavioral GZ11ZZZ

Psychotherapy
Family, Mental Health Services GZ72ZZZ
Group
GZHZZZZ
Mental Health Services GZHZZZZ
Individual
see Psychotherapy, Individual, Mental Health Services
for substance abuse
12-Step HZ53ZZZ
Behavioral HZ51ZZZ
Cognitive HZ50ZZZ
Cognitive-Behavioral HZ52ZZZ
Confrontational HZ58ZZZ
Interactive HZ55ZZZ
Interpersonal HZ54ZZZ
Motivational Enhancement HZ57ZZZ
Psychoanalysis HZ5BZZZ
Psychodynamic HZ5CZZZ
Psychoeducation HZ56ZZZ
Psychophysiological HZ5DZZZ
Supportive HZ59ZZZ
Mental Health Services
Behavioral GZ51ZZZ
Cognitive GZ52ZZZ
Cognitive-Behavioral GZ58ZZZ
Interactive GZ50ZZZ
Interpersonal GZ53ZZZ
Psychoanalysis GZ54ZZZ
Psychodynamic GZ55ZZZ
Psychophysiological GZ59ZZZ
Supportive GZ56ZZZ
PTCA (percutaneous transluminal coronary angioplasty) see Dilation, Heart and Great Vessels 027
Pterygoid muscle use Head Muscle
➡ **Pterygoid process** use Sphenoid Bone
~~use Sphenoid Bone, Right~~
~~use Sphenoid Bone, Left~~
Pterygopalatine (sphenopalatine) ganglion use Head and Neck Sympathetic Nerve
~~Pubic ligament~~
~~use Trunk Bursa and Ligament, Right~~
~~use Trunk Bursa and Ligament, Left~~
Pubis
use Pelvic Bone, Right
use Pelvic Bone, Left
Pubofemoral ligament
use Hip Bursa and Ligament, Right
use Hip Bursa and Ligament, Left
Pudendal nerve use Sacral Plexus
▶ **Pull-through, laparoscopic-assisted transanal**
▶ see Excision, Gastrointestinal System 0DB
▶ see Resection, Gastrointestinal System 0DT
Pull-through, rectal see Resection, Rectum 0DTP
Pulmoaortic canal use Pulmonary Artery, Left
Pulmonary annulus use Pulmonary Valve
Pulmonary artery wedge monitoring see Monitoring, Arterial 4A13
Pulmonary plexus
use Vagus Nerve
use Thoracic Sympathetic Nerve
Pulmonic valve use Pulmonary Valve
Pulpectomy see Excision, Mouth and Throat 0CB

Pulverization see Fragmentation
Pulvinar use Thalamus
Pump reservoir use Infusion Device, Pump in Subcutaneous Tissue and Fascia
Punch biopsy see Excision with qualifier Diagnostic
Puncture see Drainage
Puncture, lumbar see Drainage, Spinal Canal 009U
Pyelography
see Plain Radiography, Urinary System BT0
see Fluoroscopy, Urinary System BT1
Pyeloileostomy, urinary diversion see Bypass, Urinary System 0T1
Pyeloplasty
see Repair, Urinary System 0TQ
see Replacement, Urinary System 0TR
see Supplement, Urinary System 0TU
Pyelorrhaphy see Repair, Urinary System 0TQ
Pyeloscopy 0TJ58ZZ
Pyelostomy
see Bypass, Urinary System 0T1
see Drainage, Urinary System 0T9
Pyelotomy see Drainage, Urinary System 0T9
Pylorectomy
see Excision, Stomach, Pylorus 0DB7
see Resection, Stomach, Pylorus 0DT7
Pyloric antrum use Stomach, Pylorus
Pyloric canal use Stomach, Pylorus
Pyloric sphincter use Stomach, Pylorus
Pylorodiosis see Dilation, Stomach, Pylorus 0D77
Pylorogastrectomy
see Excision, Gastrointestinal System 0DB
see Resection, Gastrointestinal System 0DT
Pyloroplasty
see Repair, Stomach, Pylorus 0DQ7
see Supplement, Stomach, Pylorus 0DU7
Pyloroscopy 0DJ68ZZ
Pylorotomy see Drainage, Stomach, Pylorus 0D97
Pyramidalis muscle
use Abdomen Muscle, Right
use Abdomen Muscle, Left

Q

Quadrangular cartilage use Nasal Septum
Quadrant resection of breast see Excision, Skin and Breast 0HB
Quadrate lobe use Liver
Quadratus femoris muscle
use Hip Muscle, Right
use Hip Muscle, Left
Quadratus lumborum muscle
use Trunk Muscle, Right
use Trunk Muscle, Left
Quadratus plantae muscle
use Foot Muscle, Right
use Foot Muscle, Left
Quadriceps (femoris)
use Upper Leg Muscle, Right
use Upper Leg Muscle, Left
Quarantine 8E0ZXY6

▶ New ➡ Revised ~~deleted~~ Deleted

R

Radial collateral carpal ligament
  use Wrist Bursa and Ligament, Right
  use Wrist Bursa and Ligament, Left
Radial collateral ligament
  use Elbow Bursa and Ligament, Right
  use Elbow Bursa and Ligament, Left
Radial notch
  use Ulna, Right
  use Ulna, Left
Radial recurrent artery
  use Radial Artery, Right
  use Radial Artery, Left
Radial vein
  use Brachial Vein, Right
  use Brachial Vein, Left
Radialis indicis
  use Hand Artery, Right
  use Hand Artery, Left
Radiation Therapy
  see Beam Radiation
  see Brachytherapy
  see Stereotactic Radiosurgery
Radiation treatment *see* Radiation
    Therapy
Radiocarpal joint
  use Wrist Joint, Right
  use Wrist Joint, Left
Radiocarpal ligament
  use Wrist Bursa and Ligament, Right
  use Wrist Bursa and Ligament, Left
Radiography *see* Plain Radiography
Radiology, analog *see* Plain Radiography
Radiology, diagnostic *see* Imaging,
    Diagnostic
Radioulnar ligament
  use Wrist Bursa and Ligament, Right
  use Wrist Bursa and Ligament, Left
Range of motion testing *see* Motor
    Function Assessment, Rehabilitation
    F01
REALIZE® Adjustable Gastric Band *use*
    Extraluminal Device
Reattachment
  Abdominal Wall 0WMF0ZZ
  Ampulla of Vater 0FMC
  Ankle Region
    Left 0YML0ZZ
    Right 0YMK0ZZ
  Arm
    Lower
      Left 0XMF0ZZ
      Right 0XMD0ZZ
    Upper
      Left 0XM90ZZ
      Right 0XM80ZZ
  Axilla
    Left 0XM50ZZ
    Right 0XM40ZZ
  Back
    Lower 0WML0ZZ
    Upper 0WMK0ZZ
  Bladder 0TMB
  Bladder Neck 0TMC
  Breast
    Bilateral 0HMVXZZ
    Left 0HMUXZZ
    Right 0HMTXZZ
  Bronchus
    Lingula 0BM90ZZ
    Lower Lobe
      Left 0BMB0ZZ
      Right 0BM60ZZ
    Main
      Left 0BM70ZZ
      Right 0BM30ZZ
    Middle Lobe, Right 0BM50ZZ
    Upper Lobe
      Left 0BM80ZZ
      Right 0BM40ZZ

Reattachment *(Continued)*
  Bursa and Ligament
    Abdomen
      Left 0MMJ
      Right 0MMH
    Ankle
      Left 0MMR
      Right 0MMQ
    Elbow
      Left 0MM4
      Right 0MM3
    Foot
      Left 0MMT
      Right 0MMS
    Hand
      Left 0MM8
      Right 0MM7
    Head and Neck 0MM0
    Hip
      Left 0MMM
      Right 0MML
    Knee
      Left 0MMP
      Right 0MMN
    Lower Extremity
      Left 0MMW
      Right 0MMV
    Perineum 0MMK
    ▶Rib(s) 0MMG
    Shoulder
      Left 0MM2
      Right 0MM1
    ▶Spine
      ▶Lower 0MMD
      ▶Upper 0MMC
    ▶Sternum 0MMF
    ~~Thorax~~
      ~~Left 0MMG~~
      ~~Right 0MMF~~
    ~~Trunk~~
      ~~Left 0MMD~~
      ~~Right 0MMC~~
    Upper Extremity
      Left 0MMB
      Right 0MM9
    Wrist
      Left 0MM6
      Right 0MM5
  Buttock
    Left 0YM10ZZ
    Right 0YM00ZZ
  Carina 0BM20ZZ
  Cecum 0DMH
  Cervix 0UMC
  Chest Wall 0WM80ZZ
  Clitoris 0UMJXZZ
  Colon
    Ascending 0DMK
    Descending 0DMM
    Sigmoid 0DMN
    Transverse 0DML
  Cord
    Bilateral 0VMH
    Left 0VMG
    Right 0VMF
  Cul-de-sac 0UMF
  ⇒Diaphragm 0BMT0ZZ
    ~~Left 0BMS0ZZ~~
    ~~Right 0BMR0ZZ~~
  Duct
    Common Bile 0FM9
    Cystic 0FM8
    Hepatic
      ▶Common 0FM7
      Left 0FM6
      Right 0FM5
    Pancreatic 0FMD
      Accessory 0FMF
  Duodenum 0DM9
  Ear
    Left 09M1XZZ
    Right 09M0XZZ

Reattachment *(Continued)*
  Elbow Region
    Left 0XMC0ZZ
    Right 0XMB0ZZ
  Esophagus 0DM5
  Extremity
    Lower
      Left 0YMB0ZZ
      Right 0YM90ZZ
    Upper
      Left 0XM70ZZ
      Right 0XM60ZZ
  Eyelid
    Lower
      Left 08MRXZZ
      Right 08MQXZZ
    Upper
      Left 08MPXZZ
      Right 08MNXZZ
  Face 0WM20ZZ
  Fallopian Tube
    Left 0UM6
    Right 0UM5
  Fallopian Tubes, Bilateral 0UM7
  Femoral Region
    Left 0YM80ZZ
    Right 0YM70ZZ
  Finger
    Index
      Left 0XMP0ZZ
      Right 0XMN0ZZ
    Little
      Left 0XMW0ZZ
      Right 0XMV0ZZ
    Middle
      Left 0XMR0ZZ
      Right 0XMQ0ZZ
    Ring
      Left 0XMT0ZZ
      Right 0XMS0ZZ
  Foot
    Left 0YMN0ZZ
    Right 0YMM0ZZ
  Forequarter
    Left 0XM10ZZ
    Right 0XM00ZZ
  Gallbladder 0FM4
  Gland
    Adrenal
      Left 0GM2
      Right 0GM3
  Hand
    Left 0XMK0ZZ
    Right 0XMJ0ZZ
  Hindquarter
    Bilateral 0YM40ZZ
    Left 0YM30ZZ
    Right 0YM20ZZ
  Hymen 0UMK
  Ileum 0DMB
  Inguinal Region
    Left 0YM60ZZ
    Right 0YM50ZZ
  Intestine
    Large 0DME
      Left 0DMG
      Right 0DMF
    Small 0DM8
  Jaw
    Lower 0WM50ZZ
    Upper 0WM40ZZ
  Jejunum 0DMA
  Kidney
    Left 0TM1
    Right 0TM0
  Kidney Pelvis
    Left 0TM4
    Right 0TM3
  Kidneys, Bilateral 0TM2
  Knee Region
    Left 0YMG0ZZ
    Right 0YMF0ZZ

Reattachment *(Continued)*
  Leg
    Lower
      Left 0YMJ0ZZ
      Right 0YMH0ZZ
    Upper
      Left 0YMD0ZZ
      Right 0YMC0ZZ
  Lip
    Lower 0CM10ZZ
    Upper 0CM00ZZ
  Liver 0FM0
    Left Lobe 0FM2
    Right Lobe 0FM1
  Lung
    Left 0BML0ZZ
    Lower Lobe
      Left 0BMJ0ZZ
      Right 0BMF0ZZ
    Middle Lobe, Right 0BMD0ZZ
    Right 0BMK0ZZ
    Upper Lobe
      Left 0BMG0ZZ
      Right 0BMC0ZZ
  Lung Lingula 0BMH0ZZ
  Muscle
    Abdomen
      Left 0KML
      Right 0KMK
    Facial 0KM1
    Foot
      Left 0KMW
      Right 0KMV
    Hand
      Left 0KMD
      Right 0KMC
    Head 0KM0
    Hip
      Left 0KMP
      Right 0KMN
    Lower Arm and Wrist
      Left 0KMB
      Right 0KM9
    Lower Leg
      Left 0KMT
      Right 0KMS
    Neck
      Left 0KM3
      Right 0KM2
    Perineum 0KMM
    Shoulder
      Left 0KM6
      Right 0KM5
    Thorax
      Left 0KMJ
      Right 0KMH
    Tongue, Palate, Pharynx 0KM4
    Trunk
      Left 0KMG
      Right 0KMF
    Upper Arm
      Left 0KM8
      Right 0KM7
    Upper Leg
      Left 0KMR
      Right 0KMQ
  ▶ Nasal Mucosa and Soft Tissue 09MKXZZ
  Neck 0WM60ZZ
  Nipple
    Left 0HMXXZZ
    Right 0HMWXZZ
  ~~Nose 09MKXZZ~~
  Ovary
    Bilateral 0UM2
    Left 0UM1
    Right 0UM0
  Palate, Soft 0CM30ZZ
  Pancreas 0FMG
  Parathyroid Gland 0GMR
    Inferior
      Left 0GMP
      Right 0GMN

Reattachment *(Continued)*
  Parathyroid Gland *(Continued)*
    Multiple 0GMQ
    Superior
      Left 0GMM
      Right 0GML
  Penis 0VMSXZZ
  Perineum
    Female 0WMN0ZZ
    Male 0WMM0ZZ
  Rectum 0DMP
  Scrotum 0VM5XZZ
  Shoulder Region
    Left 0XM30ZZ
    Right 0XM20ZZ
  Skin
    Abdomen 0HM7XZZ
    Back 0HM6XZZ
    Buttock 0HM8XZZ
    Chest 0HM5XZZ
    Ear
      Left 0HM3XZZ
      Right 0HM2XZZ
    Face 0HM1XZZ
    Foot
      Left 0HMNXZZ
      Right 0HMMXZZ
    ~~Genitalia 0HMAXZZ~~
    Hand
      Left 0HMGXZZ
      Right 0HMFXZZ
    ▶ Inguinal 0HMAXZZ
    Lower Arm
      Left 0HMEXZZ
      Right 0HMDXZZ
    Lower Leg
      Left 0HMLXZZ
      Right 0HMKXZZ
    Neck 0HM4XZZ
    Perineum 0HM9XZZ
    Scalp 0HM0XZZ
    Upper Arm
      Left 0HMCXZZ
      Right 0HMBXZZ
    Upper Leg
      Left 0HMJXZZ
      Right 0HMHXZZ
  Stomach 0DM6
  Tendon
    Abdomen
      Left 0LMG
      Right 0LMF
    Ankle
      Left 0LMT
      Right 0LMS
    Foot
      Left 0LMW
      Right 0LMV
    Hand
      Left 0LM8
      Right 0LM7
    Head and Neck 0LM0
    Hip
      Left 0LMK
      Right 0LMJ
    Knee
      Left 0LMR
      Right 0LMQ
    Lower Arm and Wrist
      Left 0LM6
      Right 0LM5
    Lower Leg
      Left 0LMP
      Right 0LMN
    Perineum 0LMH
    Shoulder
      Left 0LM2
      Right 0LM1
    Thorax
      Left 0LMD
      Right 0LMC

Reattachment *(Continued)*
  Tendon *(Continued)*
    Trunk
      Left 0LMB
      Right 0LM9
    Upper Arm
      Left 0LM4
      Right 0LM3
    Upper Leg
      Left 0LMM
      Right 0LML
  Testis
    Bilateral 0VMC
    Left 0VMB
    Right 0VM9
  Thumb
    Left 0XMM0ZZ
    Right 0XML0ZZ
  Thyroid Gland
    Left Lobe 0GMG
    Right Lobe 0GMH
  Toe
    1st
      Left 0YMQ0ZZ
      Right 0YMP0ZZ
    2nd
      Left 0YMS0ZZ
      Right 0YMR0ZZ
    3rd
      Left 0YMU0ZZ
      Right 0YMT0ZZ
    4th
      Left 0YMW0ZZ
      Right 0YMV0ZZ
    5th
      Left 0YMY0ZZ
      Right 0YMX0ZZ
  Tongue 0CM70ZZ
  Tooth
    Lower 0CMX
    Upper 0CMW
  Trachea 0BM10ZZ
  Tunica Vaginalis
    Left 0VM7
    Right 0VM6
  Ureter
    Left 0TM7
    Right 0TM6
  Ureters, Bilateral 0TM8
  Urethra 0TMD
  Uterine Supporting Structure 0UM4
  Uterus 0UM9
  Uvula 0CMN0ZZ
  Vagina 0UMG
  Vulva 0UMMXZZ
  Wrist Region
    Left 0XMH0ZZ
    Right 0XMG0ZZ
▶ **REBOA (resuscitative endovascular balloon occlusion of the aorta)**
▶   02LW3DJ
▶   04L03DJ
Rebound HRD® (Hernia Repair Device) *use*
  Synthetic Substitute
Recession
  see Repair
  see Reposition
Reclosure, disrupted abdominal wall
  0WQFXZZ
Reconstruction
  see Repair
  see Replacement
  see Supplement
Rectectomy
  see Excision, Rectum 0DBP
  see Resection, Rectum 0DTP
Rectocele repair
  see Repair, Subcutaneous Tissue and Fascia, Pelvic Region 0JQC
Rectopexy
  see Repair, Gastrointestinal System 0DQ
  see Reposition, Gastrointestinal System 0DS

▶ New   ➡ Revised   ~~deleted~~ Deleted

Rectoplasty
    see Repair, Gastrointestinal System 0DQ
    see Supplement, Gastrointestinal System 0DU
Rectorrhaphy *see* Repair, Gastrointestinal System 0DQ
Rectoscopy 0DJD8ZZ
Rectosigmoid junction *use* Colon, Sigmoid
Rectosigmoidectomy
    see Excision, Gastrointestinal System 0DB
    see Resection, Gastrointestinal System 0DT
Rectostomy *see* Drainage, Rectum 0D9P
Rectotomy *see* Drainage, Rectum 0D9P
Rectus abdominis muscle
    use Abdomen Muscle, Right
    use Abdomen Muscle, Left
Rectus femoris muscle
    use Upper Leg Muscle, Right
    use Upper Leg Muscle, Left
Recurrent laryngeal nerve *use* Vagus Nerve
Reduction
    Dislocation *see* Reposition
    Fracture *see* Reposition
    Intussusception, intestinal *see* Reposition, Gastrointestinal System 0DS
    Mammoplasty *see* Excision, Skin and Breast 0HB
    Prolapse *see* Reposition
    Torsion *see* Reposition
    Volvulus, gastrointestinal *see* Reposition, Gastrointestinal System 0DS
Refusion *see* Fusion
Rehabilitation
    see Speech Assessment, Rehabilitation F00
    see Motor Function Assessment, Rehabilitation F01
    see Activities of Daily Living Assessment, Rehabilitation F02
    see Speech Treatment, Rehabilitation F06
    see Motor Treatment, Rehabilitation F07
    see Activities of Daily Living Treatment, Rehabilitation F08
    see Hearing Treatment, Rehabilitation F09
    see Cochlear Implant Treatment, Rehabilitation F0B
    see Vestibular Treatment, Rehabilitation F0C
    see Device Fitting, Rehabilitation F0D
    see Caregiver Training, Rehabilitation F0F
Reimplantation
    see Reattachment
    see Reposition
    see Transfer
Reinforcement
    see Repair
    see Supplement
Relaxation, scar tissue *see* Release
Release
    Acetabulum
        Left 0QN5
        Right 0QN4
    Adenoids 0CNQ
    Ampulla of Vater 0FNC
    Anal Sphincter 0DNR
    Anterior Chamber
        Left 08N33ZZ
        Right 08N23ZZ
    Anus 0DNQ
    Aorta
        Abdominal 04N0
        Thoracic
            Ascending/Arch 02NX
            Descending 02NW
    Aortic Body 0GND
    Appendix 0DNJ
    Artery
        Anterior Tibial
            Left 04NQ
            Right 04NP
        Axillary
            Left 03N6
            Right 03N5

Release *(Continued)*
    Artery *(Continued)*
        Brachial
            Left 03N8
            Right 03N7
        Celiac 04N1
        Colic
            Left 04N7
            Middle 04N8
            Right 04N6
        Common Carotid
            Left 03NJ
            Right 03NH
        Common Iliac
            Left 04ND
            Right 04NC
    ▶ Coronary
        ▶ Four or More Arteries 02N3
        ▶ One Artery 02N0
        ▶ Three Arteries 02N2
        ▶ Two Arteries 02N1
        External Carotid
            Left 03NN
            Right 03NM
        External Iliac
            Left 04NJ
            Right 04NH
        Face 03NR
        Femoral
            Left 04NL
            Right 04NK
        Foot
            Left 04NW
            Right 04NV
        Gastric 04N2
        Hand
            Left 03NF
            Right 03ND
        Hepatic 04N3
        Inferior Mesenteric 04NB
        Innominate 03N2
        Internal Carotid
            Left 03NL
            Right 03NK
        Internal Iliac
            Left 04NF
            Right 04NE
        Internal Mammary
            Left 03N1
            Right 03N0
        Intracranial 03NG
        Lower 04NY
        Peroneal
            Left 04NU
            Right 04NT
        Popliteal
            Left 04NN
            Right 04NM
        Posterior Tibial
            Left 04NS
            Right 04NR
        Pulmonary
            Left 02NR
            Right 02NQ
        Pulmonary Trunk 02NP
        Radial
            Left 03NC
            Right 03NB
        Renal
            Left 04NA
            Right 04N9
        Splenic 04N4
        Subclavian
            Left 03N4
            Right 03N3
        Superior Mesenteric 04N5
        Temporal
            Left 03NT
            Right 03NS
        Thyroid
            Left 03NV
            Right 03NU

Release *(Continued)*
    Artery *(Continued)*
        Ulnar
            Left 03NA
            Right 03N9
        Upper 03NY
        Vertebral
            Left 03NQ
            Right 03NP
    Atrium
        Left 02N7
        Right 02N6
    Auditory Ossicle
    ➡ Left 09NA
    ➡ Right 09N9
    Basal Ganglia 00N8
    Bladder 0TNB
    Bladder Neck 0TNC
    Bone
        Ethmoid
            Left 0NNG
            Right 0NNF
    ➡ Frontal 0NN1
        ~~Left 0NN2~~
        ~~Right 0NN1~~
        Hyoid 0NNX
        Lacrimal
            Left 0NNJ
            Right 0NNH
        Nasal 0NNB
    ➡ Occipital 0NN7
        ~~Left 0NN8~~
        ~~Right 0NN7~~
        Palatine
            Left 0NNL
            Right 0NNK
        Parietal
            Left 0NN4
            Right 0NN3
        Pelvic
            Left 0QN3
            Right 0QN2
    ➡ Sphenoid 0NNC
        ~~Left 0NND~~
        ~~Right 0NNC~~
        Temporal
            Left 0NN6
            Right 0NN5
        Zygomatic
            Left 0NNN
            Right 0NNM
    Brain 00N0
    Breast
        Bilateral 0HNV
        Left 0HNU
        Right 0HNT
    Bronchus
        Lingula 0BN9
        Lower Lobe
            Left 0BNB
            Right 0BN6
        Main
            Left 0BN7
            Right 0BN3
        Middle Lobe, Right 0BN5
        Upper Lobe
            Left 0BN8
            Right 0BN4
    Buccal Mucosa 0CN4
    Bursa and Ligament
        Abdomen
            Left 0MNJ
            Right 0MNH
        Ankle
            Left 0MNR
            Right 0MNQ
        Elbow
            Left 0MN4
            Right 0MN3
        Foot
            Left 0MNT
            Right 0MNS

Release *(Continued)*
  Bursa and Ligament *(Continued)*
    Hand
      Left 0MN8
      Right 0MN7
    Head and Neck 0MN0
    Hip
      Left 0MNM
      Right 0MNL
    Knee
      Left 0MNP
      Right 0MNN
    Lower Extremity
      Left 0MNW
      Right 0MNV
    Perineum 0MNK
    ▶Rib(s) 0MNG
    Shoulder
      Left 0MN2
      Right 0MN1
    ▶Spine
      ▶Lower 0MND
      ▶Upper 0MNC
    ▶Sternum 0MNF
    ~~Thorax~~
      ~~Left 0MNG~~
      ~~Right 0MNF~~
    ~~Trunk~~
      ~~Left 0MND~~
      ~~Right 0MNC~~
    Upper Extremity
      Left 0MNB
      Right 0MN9
    Wrist
      Left 0MN6
      Right 0MN5
  Carina 0BN2
  Carotid Bodies, Bilateral 0GN8
  Carotid Body
    Left 0GN6
    Right 0GN7
  Carpal
    Left 0PNN
    Right 0PNM
  Cecum 0DNH
  Cerebellum 00NC
  Cerebral Hemisphere 00N7
  Cerebral Meninges 00N1
  Cerebral Ventricle 00N6
  Cervix 0UNC
  Chordae Tendineae 02N9
  Choroid
    Left 08NB
    Right 08NA
  Cisterna Chyli 07NL
  Clavicle
    Left 0PNB
    Right 0PN9
  Clitoris 0UNJ
  Coccygeal Glomus 0GNB
  Coccyx 0QNS
  Colon
    Ascending 0DNK
    Descending 0DNM
    Sigmoid 0DNN
    Transverse 0DNL
  Conduction Mechanism 02N8
  Conjunctiva
    Left 08NTXZZ
    Right 08NSXZZ
  Cord
    Bilateral 0VNH
    Left 0VNG
    Right 0VNF
  Cornea
    Left 08N9XZZ
    Right 08N8XZZ
  Cul-de-sac 0UNF
  ➠Diaphragm 0BNT
    ~~Left 0BNS~~
    ~~Right 0BNR~~

Release *(Continued)*
  Disc
    Cervical Vertebral 0RN3
    Cervicothoracic Vertebral 0RN5
    Lumbar Vertebral 0SN2
    Lumbosacral 0SN4
    Thoracic Vertebral 0RN9
    Thoracolumbar Vertebral 0RNB
  Duct
    Common Bile 0FN9
    Cystic 0FN8
    Hepatic
      ▶Common 0FN7
      Left 0FN6
      Right 0FN5
    Lacrimal
      Left 08NY
      Right 08NX
    Pancreatic 0FND
      Accessory 0FNF
    Parotid
      Left 0CNC
      Right 0CNB
  Duodenum 0DN9
  Dura Mater 00N2
  Ear
    External
      Left 09N1
      Right 09N0
    External Auditory Canal
      Left 09N4
      Right 09N3
    Inner
      ➠Left 09NE
      ➠Right 09ND
    Middle
      ➠Left 09N6
      ➠Right 09N5
  Epididymis
    Bilateral 0VNL
    Left 0VNK
    Right 0VNJ
  Epiglottis 0CNR
  Esophagogastric Junction 0DN4
  Esophagus 0DN5
    Lower 0DN3
    Middle 0DN2
    Upper 0DN1
  Eustachian Tube
    Left 09NG
    Right 09NF
  Eye
    Left 08N1XZZ
    Right 08N0XZZ
  Eyelid
    Lower
      Left 08NR
      Right 08NQ
    Upper
      Left 08NP
      Right 08NN
  Fallopian Tube
    Left 0UN6
    Right 0UN5
  Fallopian Tubes, Bilateral 0UN7
  Femoral Shaft
    Left 0QN9
    Right 0QN8
  Femur
    Lower
      Left 0QNC
      Right 0QNB
    Upper
      Left 0QN7
      Right 0QN6
  Fibula
    Left 0QNK
    Right 0QNJ
  Finger Nail 0HNQXZZ
  Gallbladder 0FN4

Release *(Continued)*
  Gingiva
    Lower 0CN6
    Upper 0CN5
  Gland
    Adrenal
      Bilateral 0GN4
      Left 0GN2
      Right 0GN3
    Lacrimal
      Left 08NW
      Right 08NV
    Minor Salivary 0CNJ
    Parotid
      Left 0CN9
      Right 0CN8
    Pituitary 0GN0
    Sublingual
      Left 0CNF
      Right 0CND
    Submaxillary
      Left 0CNH
      Right 0CNG
    Vestibular 0UNL
  Glenoid Cavity
    Left 0PN8
    Right 0PN7
  Glomus Jugulare 0GNC
  Humeral Head
    Left 0PND
    Right 0PNC
  Humeral Shaft
    Left 0PNG
    Right 0PNF
  Hymen 0UNK
  Hypothalamus 00NA
  Ileocecal Valve 0DNC
  Ileum 0DNB
  Intestine
    Large 0DNE
      Left 0DNG
      Right 0DNF
    Small 0DN8
  Iris
    Left 08ND3ZZ
    Right 08NC3ZZ
  Jejunum 0DNA
  Joint
    Acromioclavicular
      Left 0RNH
      Right 0RNG
    Ankle
      Left 0SNG
      Right 0SNF
    Carpal
      Left 0RNR
      Right 0RNQ
    ▶Carpometacarpal
      ▶Left 0RNT
      ▶Right 0RNS
    Cervical Vertebral 0RN1
    Cervicothoracic Vertebral 0RN4
    Coccygeal 0SN6
    Elbow
      Left 0RNM
      Right 0RNL
    Finger Phalangeal
      Left 0RNX
      Right 0RNW
    Hip
      Left 0SNB
      Right 0SN9
    Knee
      Left 0SND
      Right 0SNC
    Lumbar Vertebral 0SN0
    Lumbosacral 0SN3
    ~~Metacarpocarpal~~
      ~~Left 0RNT~~
      ~~Right 0RNS~~

▶ New   ➠ Revised   ~~deleted~~ Deleted

Release (Continued)
Joint (Continued)
Metacarpophalangeal
Left 0RNV
Right 0RNU
Metatarsal-Phalangeal
Left 0SNN
Right 0SNM
Metatarsal-Tarsal
Left 0SNL
Right 0SNK
Occipital-cervical 0RN0
Sacrococcygeal 0SN5
Sacroiliac
Left 0SN8
Right 0SN7
Shoulder
Left 0RNK
Right 0RNJ
Sternoclavicular
Left 0RNF
Right 0RNE
Tarsal
Left 0SNJ
Right 0SNH
▶Tarsometatarsal
▶Left 0SNL
▶Right 0SNK
Temporomandibular
Left 0RND
Right 0RNC
Thoracic Vertebral 0RN6
Thoracolumbar Vertebral 0RNA
Toe Phalangeal
Left 0SNQ
Right 0SNP
Wrist
Left 0RNP
Right 0RNN
Kidney
Left 0TN1
Right 0TN0
Kidney Pelvis
Left 0TN4
Right 0TN3
Larynx 0CNS
Lens
Left 08NK3ZZ
Right 08NJ3ZZ
Lip
Lower 0CN1
Upper 0CN0
Liver 0FN0
Left Lobe 0FN2
Right Lobe 0FN1
Lung
Bilateral 0BNM
Left 0BNL
Lower Lobe
Left 0BNJ
Right 0BNF
Middle Lobe, Right 0BND
Right 0BNK
Upper Lobe
Left 0BNG
Right 0BNC
Lung Lingula 0BNH
Lymphatic
Aortic 07ND
Axillary
Left 07N6
Right 07N5
Head 07N0
Inguinal
Left 07NJ
Right 07NH
Internal Mammary
Left 07N9
Right 07N8
Lower Extremity
Left 07NG
Right 07NF

Release (Continued)
Lymphatic (Continued)
Mesenteric 07NB
Neck
Left 07N2
Right 07N1
Pelvis 07NC
Thoracic Duct 07NK
Thorax 07N7
Upper Extremity
Left 07N4
Right 07N3
Mandible
Left 0NNV
Right 0NNT
➡Maxilla 0NNR
Left 0NNS
Right 0NNR
Medulla Oblongata 00ND
Mesentery 0DNV
Metacarpal
Left 0PNQ
Right 0PNP
Metatarsal
Left 0QNP
Right 0QNN
Muscle
Abdomen
Left 0KNL
Right 0KNK
Extraocular
Left 08NM
Right 08NL
Facial 0KN1
Foot
Left 0KNW
Right 0KNV
Hand
Left 0KND
Right 0KNC
Head 0KN0
Hip
Left 0KNP
Right 0KNN
Lower Arm and Wrist
Left 0KNB
Right 0KN9
Lower Leg
Left 0KNT
Right 0KNS
Neck
Left 0KN3
Right 0KN2
Papillary 02ND
Perineum 0KNM
Shoulder
Left 0KN6
Right 0KN5
Thorax
Left 0KNJ
Right 0KNH
Tongue, Palate, Pharynx 0KN4
Trunk
Left 0KNG
Right 0KNF
Upper Arm
Left 0KN8
Right 0KN7
Upper Leg
Left 0KNR
Right 0KNQ
▶Myocardial Bridge see Release, Artery, Coronary
▶Nasal Mucosa and Soft Tissue 09NK
Nasopharynx 09NN
Nerve
Abdominal Sympathetic 01NM
Abducens 00NL
Accessory 00NR
Acoustic 00NN
Brachial Plexus 01N3

Release (Continued)
Nerve (Continued)
Cervical 01N1
Cervical Plexus 01N0
Facial 00NM
Femoral 01ND
Glossopharyngeal 00NP
Head and Neck Sympathetic 01NK
Hypoglossal 00NS
Lumbar 01NB
Lumbar Plexus 01N9
Lumbar Sympathetic 01NN
Lumbosacral Plexus 01NA
Median 01N5
Oculomotor 00NH
Olfactory 00NF
Optic 00NG
Peroneal 01NH
Phrenic 01N2
Pudendal 01NC
Radial 01N6
Sacral 01NR
Sacral Plexus 01NQ
Sacral Sympathetic 01NP
Sciatic 01NF
Thoracic 01N8
Thoracic Sympathetic 01NL
Tibial 01NG
Trigeminal 00NK
Trochlear 00NJ
Ulnar 01N4
Vagus 00NQ
Nipple
Left 0HNX
Right 0HNW
Nose 09NK
➡Omentum 0DNU
Greater 0DNS
Lesser 0DNT
Orbit
Left 0NNQ
Right 0NNP
Ovary
Bilateral 0UN2
Left 0UN1
Right 0UN0
Palate
Hard 0CN2
Soft 0CN3
Pancreas 0FNG
Para-aortic Body 0GN9
Paraganglion Extremity 0GNF
Parathyroid Gland 0GNR
Inferior
Left 0GNP
Right 0GNN
Multiple 0GNQ
Superior
Left 0GNM
Right 0GNL
Patella
Left 0QNF
Right 0QND
Penis 0VNS
Pericardium 02NN
Peritoneum 0DNW
Phalanx
Finger
Left 0PNV
Right 0PNT
Thumb
Left 0PNS
Right 0PNR
Toe
Left 0QNR
Right 0QNQ
Pharynx 0CNM
Pineal Body 0GN1
Pleura
Left 0BNP
Right 0BNN

Release (*Continued*)
Pons 00NB
Prepuce 0VNT
Prostate 0VN0
Radius
   Left 0PNJ
   Right 0PNH
Rectum 0DNP
Retina
   Left 08NF3ZZ
   Right 08NE3ZZ
Retinal Vessel
   Left 08NH3ZZ
   Right 08NG3ZZ
~~Rib~~
   ~~Left 0PN2~~
   ~~Right 0PN1~~
▶Ribs
   ▶1 to 2 0PN1
   ▶3 or More 0PN2
Sacrum 0QN1
Scapula
   Left 0PN6
   Right 0PN5
Sclera
   Left 08N7XZZ
   Right 08N6XZZ
Scrotum 0VN5
Septum
   Atrial 02N5
   Nasal 09NM
   Ventricular 02NM
Sinus
   Accessory 09NP
   Ethmoid
      Left 09NV
      Right 09NU
   Frontal
      Left 09NT
      Right 09NS
   Mastoid
      Left 09NC
      Right 09NB
   Maxillary
      Left 09NR
      Right 09NQ
   Sphenoid
      Left 09NX
      Right 09NW
Skin
   Abdomen 0HN7XZZ
   Back 0HN6XZZ
   Buttock 0HN8XZZ
   Chest 0HN5XZZ
   Ear
      Left 0HN3XZZ
      Right 0HN2XZZ
   Face 0HN1XZZ
   Foot
      Left 0HNNXZZ
      Right 0HNMXZZ
   ~~Genitalia 0HNAXZZ~~
   Hand
      Left 0HNGXZZ
      Right 0HNFXZZ
   ▶Inguinal 0HNAXZZ
   Lower Arm
      Left 0HNEXZZ
      Right 0HNDXZZ
   Lower Leg
      Left 0HNLXZZ
      Right 0HNKXZZ
   Neck 0HN4XZZ
   Perineum 0HN9XZZ
   Scalp 0HN0XZZ
   Upper Arm
      Left 0HNCXZZ
      Right 0HNBXZZ
   Upper Leg
      Left 0HNJXZZ
      Right 0HNHXZZ

Release (*Continued*)
Spinal Cord
   Cervical 00NW
   Lumbar 00NY
   Thoracic 00NX
Spinal Meninges 00NT
Spleen 07NP
Sternum 0PN0
Stomach 0DN6
   Pylorus 0DN7
Subcutaneous Tissue and Fascia
   Abdomen 0JN8
   Back 0JN7
   Buttock 0JN9
   Chest 0JN6
   Face 0JN1
   Foot
      Left 0JNR
      Right 0JNQ
   Hand
      Left 0JNK
      Right 0JNJ
   Lower Arm
      Left 0JNH
      Right 0JNG
   Lower Leg
      Left 0JNP
      Right 0JNN
   Neck
      ~~Anterior 0JN4~~
      ~~Posterior 0JN5~~
      ▶Left 0JN5
      ▶Right 0JN4
   Pelvic Region 0JNC
   Perineum 0JNB
   Scalp 0JN0
   Upper Arm
      Left 0JNF
      Right 0JND
   Upper Leg
      Left 0JNM
      Right 0JNL
Tarsal
   Left 0QNM
   Right 0QNL
Tendon
   Abdomen
      Left 0LNG
      Right 0LNF
   Ankle
      Left 0LNT
      Right 0LNS
   Foot
      Left 0LNW
      Right 0LNV
   Hand
      Left 0LN8
      Right 0LN7
   Head and Neck 0LN0
   Hip
      Left 0LNK
      Right 0LNJ
   Knee
      Left 0LNR
      Right 0LNQ
   Lower Arm and Wrist
      Left 0LN6
      Right 0LN5
   Lower Leg
      Left 0LNP
      Right 0LNN
   Perineum 0LNH
   Shoulder
      Left 0LN2
      Right 0LN1
   Thorax
      Left 0LND
      Right 0LNC
   Trunk
      Left 0LNB
      Right 0LN9

Release (*Continued*)
   Tendon (*Continued*)
   Upper Arm
      Left 0LN4
      Right 0LN3
   Upper Leg
      Left 0LNM
      Right 0LNL
Testis
   Bilateral 0VNC
   Left 0VNB
   Right 0VN9
Thalamus 00N9
Thymus 07NM
Thyroid Gland 0GNK
   Left Lobe 0GNG
   Right Lobe 0GNH
Tibia
   Left 0QNH
   Right 0QNG
Toe Nail 0HNRXZZ
Tongue 0CN7
Tonsils 0CNP
Tooth
   Lower 0CNX
   Upper 0CNW
Trachea 0BN1
Tunica Vaginalis
   Left 0VN7
   Right 0VN6
Turbinate, Nasal 09NL
Tympanic Membrane
   Left 09N8
   Right 09N7
Ulna
   Left 0PNL
   Right 0PNK
Ureter
   Left 0TN7
   Right 0TN6
Urethra 0TND
Uterine Supporting Structure 0UN4
Uterus 0UN9
Uvula 0CNN
Vagina 0UNG
Valve
   Aortic 02NF
   Mitral 02NG
   Pulmonary 02NH
   Tricuspid 02NJ
Vas Deferens
   Bilateral 0VNQ
   Left 0VNP
   Right 0VNN
Vein
   Axillary
      Left 05N8
      Right 05N7
   Azygos 05N0
   Basilic
      Left 05NC
      Right 05NB
   Brachial
      Left 05NA
      Right 05N9
   Cephalic
      Left 05NF
      Right 05ND
   Colic 06N7
   Common Iliac
      Left 06ND
      Right 06NC
   Coronary 02N4
   Esophageal 06N3
   External Iliac
      Left 06NG
      Right 06NF
   External Jugular
      Left 05NQ
      Right 05NP

▶ New   ⇒ Revised   ~~deleted~~ Deleted

Release (Continued)
  Vein (Continued)
    Face
      Left 05NV
      Right 05NT
    Femoral
      Left 06NN
      Right 06NM
    Foot
      Left 06NV
      Right 06NT
    Gastric 06N2
    ~~Greater Saphenous~~
      ~~Left 06NQ~~
      ~~Right 06NP~~
    Hand
      Left 05NH
      Right 05NG
    Hemiazygos 05N1
    Hepatic 06N4
    Hypogastric
      Left 06NJ
      Right 06NH
    Inferior Mesenteric 06N6
    Innominate
      Left 05N4
      Right 05N3
    Internal Jugular
      Left 05NN
      Right 05NM
    Intracranial 05NL
    Lesser Saphenous
      Left 06NS
      Right 06NR
    Lower 06NY
    Portal 06N8
    Pulmonary
      Left 02NT
      Right 02NS
    Renal
      Left 06NB
      Right 06N9
    ▶Saphenous
      ▶Left 06NQ
      ▶Right 06NP
    Splenic 06N1
    Subclavian
      Left 05N6
      Right 05N5
    Superior Mesenteric 06N5
    Upper 05NY
    Vertebral
      Left 05NS
      Right 05NR
  Vena Cava
    Inferior 06N0
    Superior 02NV
  Ventricle
    Left 02NL
    Right 02NK
  Vertebra
    Cervical 0PN3
    Lumbar 0QN0
    Thoracic 0PN4
  Vesicle
    Bilateral 0VN3
    Left 0VN2
    Right 0VN1
  Vitreous
    Left 08N53ZZ
    Right 08N43ZZ
  Vocal Cord
    Left 0CNV
    Right 0CNT
  Vulva 0UNM
Relocation see Reposition
Removal
  Abdominal Wall 2W53X
  Anorectal 2Y53X5Z

Removal (Continued)
  Arm
    Lower
      Left 2W5DX
      Right 2W5CX
    Upper
      Left 2W5BX
      Right 2W5AX
  Back 2W55X
  Chest Wall 2W54X
  Ear 2Y52X5Z
  Extremity
    Lower
      Left 2W5MX
      Right 2W5LX
    Upper
      Left 2W59X
      Right 2W58X
  Face 2W51X
  Finger
    Left 2W5KX
    Right 2W5JX
  Foot
    Left 2W5TX
    Right 2W5SX
  Genital Tract, Female 2Y54X5Z
  Hand
    Left 2W5FX
    Right 2W5EX
  Head 2W50X
  Inguinal Region
    Left 2W57X
    Right 2W56X
  Leg
    Lower
      Left 2W5RX
      Right 2W5QX
    Upper
      Left 2W5PX
      Right 2W5NX
  Mouth and Pharynx 2Y50X5Z
  Nasal 2Y51X5Z
  Neck 2W52X
  Thumb
    Left 2W5HX
    Right 2W5GX
  Toe
    Left 2W5VX
    Right 2W5UX
  Urethra 2Y55X5Z
Removal of device from
  Abdominal Wall 0WPF
  Acetabulum
    Left 0QP5
    Right 0QP4
  Anal Sphincter 0DPR
  Anus 0DPQ
  Artery
    Lower 04PY
    Upper 03PY
  Back
    Lower 0WPL
    Upper 0WPK
  Bladder 0TPB
  Bone
    Facial 0NPW
    Lower 0QPY
    Nasal 0NPB
    Pelvic
      Left 0QP3
      Right 0QP2
    Upper 0PPY
  Bone Marrow 07PT
  Brain 00P0
  Breast
    Left 0HPU
    Right 0HPT
  Bursa and Ligament
    Lower 0MPY
    Upper 0MPX

Removal of device from (Continued)
  Carpal
    Left 0PPN
    Right 0PPM
  Cavity, Cranial 0WP1
  Cerebral Ventricle 00P6
  Chest Wall 0WP8
  Cisterna Chyli 07PL
  Clavicle
    Left 0PPB
    Right 0PP9
  Coccyx 0QPS
  Diaphragm 0BPT
  Disc
    Cervical Vertebral 0RP3
    Cervicothoracic Vertebral 0RP5
    Lumbar Vertebral 0SP2
    Lumbosacral 0SP4
    Thoracic Vertebral 0RP9
    Thoracolumbar Vertebral 0RPB
  Duct
    Hepatobiliary 0FPB
    Pancreatic 0FPD
  Ear
    Inner
      Left 09PE
      Right 09PD
    Left 09PJ
    Right 09PH
  Epididymis and Spermatic Cord 0VPM
  Esophagus 0DP5
  Extremity
    Lower
      Left 0YPB
      Right 0YP9
    Upper
      Left 0XP7
      Right 0XP6
  Eye
    Left 08P1
    Right 08P0
  Face 0WP2
  Fallopian Tube 0UP8
  Femoral Shaft
    Left 0QP9
    Right 0QP8
  Femur
    Lower
      Left 0QPC
      Right 0QPB
    Upper
      Left 0QP7
      Right 0QP6
  Fibula
    Left 0QPK
    Right 0QPJ
  Finger Nail 0HPQX
  Gallbladder 0FP4
  Gastrointestinal Tract 0WPP
  Genitourinary Tract 0WPR
  Gland
    Adrenal 0GP5
    Endocrine 0GPS
    Pituitary 0GP0
    Salivary 0CPA
  Glenoid Cavity
    Left 0PP8
    Right 0PP7
  Great Vessel 02PY
  Hair 0HPSX
  Head 0WP0
  Heart 02PA
  Humeral Head
    Left 0PPD
    Right 0PPC
  Humeral Shaft
    Left 0PPG
    Right 0PPF
  Intestinal Tract
    Lower 0DPD
    Upper 0DP0

Removal of device from (Continued)
Jaw
  Lower 0WP5
  Upper 0WP4
Joint
  Acromioclavicular
    Left 0RPH
    Right 0RPG
  Ankle
    Left 0SPG
    Right 0SPF
  Carpal
    Left 0RPR
    Right 0RPQ
▶ Carpometacarpal
  ▶ Left 0RPT
  ▶ Right 0RPS
  Cervical Vertebral 0RP1
  Cervicothoracic Vertebral 0RP4
  Coccygeal 0SP6
  Elbow
    Left 0RPM
    Right 0RPL
  Finger Phalangeal
    Left 0RPX
    Right 0RPW
  Hip
    Left 0SPB
      Acetabular Surface 0SPE
      Femoral Surface 0SPS
    Right 0SP9
      Acetabular Surface 0SPA
      Femoral Surface 0SPR
  Knee
    Left 0SPD
      Femoral Surface 0SPU
      Tibial Surface 0SPW
    Right 0SPC
      Femoral Surface 0SPT
      Tibial Surface 0SPV
  Lumbar Vertebral 0SP0
  Lumbosacral 0SP3
  ~~Metacarpocarpal~~
    ~~Left 0RPT~~
    ~~Right 0RPS~~
  Metacarpophalangeal
    Left 0RPV
    Right 0RPU
  Metatarsal-Phalangeal
    Left 0SPN
    Right 0SPM
  ~~Metatarsal-Tarsal~~
    ~~Left 0SPL~~
    ~~Right 0SPK~~
  Occipital-cervical 0RP0
  Sacrococcygeal 0SP5
  Sacroiliac
    Left 0SP8
    Right 0SP7
  Shoulder
    Left 0RPK
    Right 0RPJ
  Sternoclavicular
    Left 0RPF
    Right 0RPE
  Tarsal
    Left 0SPJ
    Right 0SPH
▶ Tarsometatarsal
  ▶ Left 0SPL
  ▶ Right 0SPK
  Temporomandibular
    Left 0RPD
    Right 0RPC
  Thoracic Vertebral 0RP6
  Thoracolumbar Vertebral 0RPA
  Toe Phalangeal
    Left 0SPQ
    Right 0SPP
  Wrist
    Left 0RPP
    Right 0RPN

Removal of device from (Continued)
Kidney 0TP5
Larynx 0CPS
Lens
▷ Left 08PK3
▷ Right 08PJ3
Liver 0FP0
Lung
  Left 0BPL
  Right 0BPK
Lymphatic 07PN
  Thoracic Duct 07PK
Mediastinum 0WPC
Mesentery 0DPV
Metacarpal
  Left 0PPQ
  Right 0PPP
Metatarsal
  Left 0QPP
  Right 0QPN
Mouth and Throat 0CPY
Muscle
  Extraocular
    Left 08PM
    Right 08PL
  Lower 0KPY
  Upper 0KPX
▶ Nasal Mucosa and Soft Tissue 09PK
Neck 0WP6
Nerve
  Cranial 00PE
  Peripheral 01PY
~~Nose 09PK~~
Omentum 0DPU
Ovary 0UP3
Pancreas 0FPG
Parathyroid Gland 0GPR
Patella
  Left 0QPF
  Right 0QPD
Pelvic Cavity 0WPJ
Penis 0VPS
Pericardial Cavity 0WPD
Perineum
  Female 0WPN
  Male 0WPM
Peritoneal Cavity 0WPG
Peritoneum 0DPW
Phalanx
  Finger
    Left 0PPV
    Right 0PPT
  Thumb
    Left 0PPS
    Right 0PPR
  Toe
    Left 0QPR
    Right 0QPQ
Pineal Body 0GP1
Pleura 0BPQ
Pleural Cavity
  Left 0WPB
  Right 0WP9
Products of Conception 10P0
Prostate and Seminal Vesicles 0VP4
Radius
  Left 0PPJ
  Right 0PPH
Rectum 0DPP
Respiratory Tract 0WPQ
Retroperitoneum 0WPH
~~Rib~~
  ~~Left 0PP2~~
  ~~Right 0PP1~~
▶ Ribs
  ▶ 1 to 2 0PP1
  ▶ 3 or More 0PP2
Sacrum 0QP1
Scapula
  Left 0PP6
  Right 0PP5

Removal of device from (Continued)
Scrotum and Tunica Vaginalis 0VP8
Sinus 09PY
Skin 0HPPX
Skull 0NP0
Spinal Canal 00PU
Spinal Cord 00PV
Spleen 07PP
Sternum 0PP0
Stomach 0DP6
Subcutaneous Tissue and Fascia
  Head and Neck 0JPS
  Lower Extremity 0JPW
  Trunk 0JPT
  Upper Extremity 0JPV
Tarsal
  Left 0QPM
  Right 0QPL
Tendon
  Lower 0LPY
  Upper 0LPX
Testis 0VPD
Thymus 07PM
Thyroid Gland 0GPK
Tibia
  Left 0QPH
  Right 0QPG
Toe Nail 0HPRX
Trachea 0BP1
Tracheobronchial Tree 0BP0
Tympanic Membrane
  Left 09P8
  Right 09P7
Ulna
  Left 0PPL
  Right 0PPK
Ureter 0TP9
Urethra 0TPD
Uterus and Cervix 0UPD
Vagina and Cul-de-sac 0UPH
Vas Deferens 0VPR
Vein
  Azygos 05P0
  Innominate
    Left 05P4
    Right 05P3
  Lower 06PY
  Upper 05PY
Vertebra
  Cervical 0PP3
  Lumbar 0QP0
  Thoracic 0PP4
Vulva 0UPM
Renal calyx
  use Kidney, Right
  use Kidney, Left
  use Kidneys, Bilateral
  use Kidney
Renal capsule
  use Kidney, Right
  use Kidney, Left
  use Kidneys, Bilateral
  use Kidney
Renal cortex
  use Kidney, Right
  use Kidney, Left
  use Kidneys, Bilateral
  use Kidney
Renal dialysis *see* Performance, Urinary 5A1D
Renal plexus *use* Abdominal Sympathetic Nerve
Renal segment
  use Kidney, Right
  use Kidney, Left
  use Kidneys, Bilateral
  use Kidney
Renal segmental artery
  use Renal Artery, Right
  use Renal Artery, Left
Reopening, operative site
  Control of bleeding *see* Control bleeding in
  Inspection only *see* Inspection

▶ New   ▷ Revised   ~~deleted~~ Deleted

Repair
Abdominal Wall 0WQF
Acetabulum
  Left 0QQ5
  Right 0QQ4
Adenoids 0CQQ
Ampulla of Vater 0FQC
Anal Sphincter 0DQR
Ankle Region
  Left 0YQL
  Right 0YQK
Anterior Chamber
  Left 08Q33ZZ
  Right 08Q23ZZ
Anus 0DQQ
Aorta
  Abdominal 04Q0
  Thoracic
    Ascending/Arch 02QX
    Descending 02QW
Aortic Body 0GQD
Appendix 0DQJ
Arm
  Lower
    Left 0XQF
    Right 0XQD
  Upper
    Left 0XQ9
    Right 0XQ8
Artery
  Anterior Tibial
    Left 04QQ
    Right 04QP
  Axillary
    Left 03Q6
    Right 03Q5
  Brachial
    Left 03Q8
    Right 03Q7
  Celiac 04Q1
  Colic
    Left 04Q7
    Middle 04Q8
    Right 04Q6
  Common Carotid
    Left 03QJ
    Right 03QH
  Common Iliac
    Left 04QD
    Right 04QC
  Coronary
    Four or More Arteries 02Q3
    One Artery 02Q0
    Three Arteries 02Q2
    Two Arteries 02Q1
  External Carotid
    Left 03QN
    Right 03QM
  External Iliac
    Left 04QJ
    Right 04QH
  Face 03QR
  Femoral
    Left 04QL
    Right 04QK
  Foot
    Left 04QW
    Right 04QV
  Gastric 04Q2
  Hand
    Left 03QF
    Right 03QD
  Hepatic 04Q3
  Inferior Mesenteric 04QB
  Innominate 03Q2
  Internal Carotid
    Left 03QL
    Right 03QK
  Internal Iliac
    Left 04QF
    Right 04QE

Repair *(Continued)*
  Artery *(Continued)*
  Internal Mammary
    Left 03Q1
    Right 03Q0
  Intracranial 03QG
  Lower 04QY
  Peroneal
    Left 04QU
    Right 04QT
  Popliteal
    Left 04QN
    Right 04QM
  Posterior Tibial
    Left 04QS
    Right 04QR
  Pulmonary
    Left 02QR
    Right 02QQ
  Pulmonary Trunk 02QP
  Radial
    Left 03QC
    Right 03QB
  Renal
    Left 04QA
    Right 04Q9
  Splenic 04Q4
  Subclavian
    Left 03Q4
    Right 03Q3
  Superior Mesenteric 04Q5
  Temporal
    Left 03QT
    Right 03QS
  Thyroid
    Left 03QV
    Right 03QU
  Ulnar
    Left 03QA
    Right 03Q9
  Upper 03QY
  Vertebral
    Left 03QQ
    Right 03QP
Atrium
  Left 02Q7
  Right 02Q6
Auditory Ossicle
➠ Left 09QA
➠ Right 09Q9
Axilla
  Left 0XQ5
  Right 0XQ4
Back
  Lower 0WQL
  Upper 0WQK
Basal Ganglia 00Q8
Bladder 0TQB
Bladder Neck 0TQC
Bone
  Ethmoid
    Left 0NQG
    Right 0NQF
➠ Frontal 0NQ1
    Left 0NQ2
    Right 0NQ1
  Hyoid 0NQX
  Lacrimal
    Left 0NQJ
    Right 0NQH
  Nasal 0NQB
➠ Occipital 0NQ7
    Left 0NQ8
    Right 0NQ7
  Palatine
    Left 0NQL
    Right 0NQK
  Parietal
    Left 0NQ4
    Right 0NQ3

Repair *(Continued)*
  Bone *(Continued)*
  Pelvic
    Left 0QQ3
    Right 0QQ2
➠ Sphenoid 0NQC
    Left 0NQD
    Right 0NQC
  Temporal
    Left 0NQ6
    Right 0NQ5
  Zygomatic
    Left 0NQN
    Right 0NQM
Brain 00Q0
Breast
  Bilateral 0HQV
  Left 0HQU
  Right 0HQT
  Supernumerary 0HQY
Bronchus
  Lingula 0BQ9
  Lower Lobe
    Left 0BQB
    Right 0BQ6
  Main
    Left 0BQ7
    Right 0BQ3
  Middle Lobe, Right 0BQ5
  Upper Lobe
    Left 0BQ8
    Right 0BQ4
Buccal Mucosa 0CQ4
Bursa and Ligament
  Abdomen
    Left 0MQJ
    Right 0MQH
  Ankle
    Left 0MQR
    Right 0MQQ
  Elbow
    Left 0MQ4
    Right 0MQ3
  Foot
    Left 0MQT
    Right 0MQS
  Hand
    Left 0MQ8
    Right 0MQ7
  Head and Neck 0MQ0
  Hip
    Left 0MQM
    Right 0MQL
  Knee
    Left 0MQP
    Right 0MQN
  Lower Extremity
    Left 0MQW
    Right 0MQV
  Perineum 0MQK
▶ Rib(s) 0MQG
  Shoulder
    Left 0MQ2
    Right 0MQ1
▶ Spine
  ▶ Lower 0MQD
  ▶ Upper 0MQC
▶ Sternum 0MQF
  Thorax
    Left 0MQG
    Right 0MQF
  Trunk
    Left 0MQD
    Right 0MQC
  Upper Extremity
    Left 0MQB
    Right 0MQ9
  Wrist
    Left 0MQ6
    Right 0MQ5

▶ New   ➠ Revised   ~~deleted~~ Deleted

Repair *(Continued)*
  Buttock
    Left 0YQ1
    Right 0YQ0
  Carina 0BQ2
  Carotid Bodies, Bilateral 0GQ8
  Carotid Body
    Left 0GQ6
    Right 0GQ7
  Carpal
    Left 0PQN
    Right 0PQM
  Cecum 0DQH
  Cerebellum 00QC
  Cerebral Hemisphere 00Q7
  Cerebral Meninges 00Q1
  Cerebral Ventricle 00Q6
  Cervix 0UQC
  Chest Wall 0WQ8
  Chordae Tendineae 02Q9
  Choroid
    Left 08QB
    Right 08QA
  Cisterna Chyli 07QL
  Clavicle
    Left 0PQB
    Right 0PQ9
  Clitoris 0UQJ
  Coccygeal Glomus 0GQB
  Coccyx 0QQS
  Colon
    Ascending 0DQK
    Descending 0DQM
    Sigmoid 0DQN
    Transverse 0DQL
  Conduction Mechanism
    02Q8
  Conjunctiva
    Left 08QTXZZ
    Right 08QSXZZ
  Cord
    Bilateral 0VQH
    Left 0VQG
    Right 0VQF
  Cornea
    Left 08Q9XZZ
    Right 08Q8XZZ
  Cul-de-sac 0UQF
  ➡Diaphragm 0BQT
    ~~Left 0BQS~~
    ~~Right 0BQR~~
  Disc
    Cervical Vertebral 0RQ3
    Cervicothoracic Vertebral
      0RQ5
    Lumbar Vertebral 0SQ2
    Lumbosacral 0SQ4
    Thoracic Vertebral 0RQ9
    Thoracolumbar Vertebral 0RQB
  Duct
    Common Bile 0FQ9
    Cystic 0FQ8
    Hepatic
    ▶Common 0FQ7
      Left 0FQ6
      Right 0FQ5
    Lacrimal
      Left 08QY
      Right 08QX
    Pancreatic 0FQD
      Accessory 0FQF
    Parotid
      Left 0CQC
      Right 0CQB
  Duodenum 0DQ9
  Dura Mater 00Q2
  Ear
    External
      Bilateral 09Q2
      Left 09Q1
      Right 09Q0

Repair *(Continued)*
  Ear *(Continued)*
    External Auditory Canal
      Left 09Q4
      Right 09Q3
    Inner
      ➡Left 09QE
      ➡Right 09QD
    Middle
      ➡Left 09Q6
      ➡Right 09Q5
  Elbow Region
    Left 0XQC
    Right 0XQB
  Epididymis
    Bilateral 0VQL
    Left 0VQK
    Right 0VQJ
  Epiglottis 0CQR
  Esophagogastric Junction 0DQ4
  Esophagus 0DQ5
    Lower 0DQ3
    Middle 0DQ2
    Upper 0DQ1
  Eustachian Tube
    Left 09QG
    Right 09QF
  Extremity
    Lower
      Left 0YQB
      Right 0YQ9
    Upper
      Left 0XQ7
      Right 0XQ6
  Eye
    Left 08Q1XZZ
    Right 08Q0XZZ
  Eyelid
    Lower
      Left 08QR
      Right 08QQ
    Upper
      Left 08QP
      Right 08QN
  Face 0WQ2
  Fallopian Tube
    Left 0UQ6
    Right 0UQ5
  Fallopian Tubes, Bilateral 0UQ7
  Femoral Region
    Bilateral 0YQE
    Left 0YQ8
    Right 0YQ7
  Femoral Shaft
    Left 0QQ9
    Right 0QQ8
  Femur
    Lower
      Left 0QQC
      Right 0QQB
    Upper
      Left 0QQ7
      Right 0QQ6
  Fibula
    Left 0QQK
    Right 0QQJ
  Finger
    Index
      Left 0XQP
      Right 0XQN
    Little
      Left 0XQW
      Right 0XQV
    Middle
      Left 0XQR
      Right 0XQQ
    Ring
      Left 0XQT
      Right 0XQS
  Finger Nail 0HQQXZZ

Repair *(Continued)*
  ▶Floor of mouth *see* Repair, Oral Cavity and
    Throat 0WQ3
  Foot
    Left 0YQN
    Right 0YQM
  Gallbladder 0FQ4
  Gingiva
    Lower 0CQ6
    Upper 0CQ5
  Gland
    Adrenal
      Bilateral 0GQ4
      Left 0GQ2
      Right 0GQ3
    Lacrimal
      Left 08QW
      Right 08QV
    Minor Salivary 0CQJ
    Parotid
      Left 0CQ9
      Right 0CQ8
    Pituitary 0GQ0
    Sublingual
      Left 0CQF
      Right 0CQD
    Submaxillary
      Left 0CQH
      Right 0CQG
    Vestibular 0UQL
  Glenoid Cavity
    Left 0PQ8
    Right 0PQ7
  Glomus Jugulare 0GQC
  Hand
    Left 0XQK
    Right 0XQJ
  Head 0WQ0
  Heart 02QA
    Left 02QC
    Right 02QB
  Humeral Head
    Left 0PQD
    Right 0PQC
  Humeral Shaft
    Left 0PQG
    Right 0PQF
  Hymen 0UQK
  Hypothalamus 00QA
  Ileocecal Valve 0DQC
  Ileum 0DQB
  Inguinal Region
    Bilateral 0YQA
    Left 0YQ6
    Right 0YQ5
  Intestine
    Large 0DQE
      Left 0DQG
      Right 0DQF
    Small 0DQ8
  Iris
    Left 08QD3ZZ
    Right 08QC3ZZ
  Jaw
    Lower 0WQ5
    Upper 0WQ4
  Jejunum 0DQA
  Joint
    Acromioclavicular
      Left 0RQH
      Right 0RQG
    Ankle
      Left 0SQG
      Right 0SQF
    Carpal
      Left 0RQR
      Right 0RQQ
    ▶Carpometacarpal
      ▶Left 0RQT
      ▶Right 0RQS
    Cervical Vertebral 0RQ1

▶ New   ➡ Revised   ~~deleted~~ Deleted

Repair *(Continued)*
  Joint *(Continued)*
    Cervicothoracic Vertebral 0RQ4
    Coccygeal 0SQ6
    Elbow
      Left 0RQM
      Right 0RQL
    Finger Phalangeal
      Left 0RQX
      Right 0RQW
    Hip
      Left 0SQB
      Right 0SQ9
    Knee
      Left 0SQD
      Right 0SQC
    Lumbar Vertebral 0SQ0
    Lumbosacral 0SQ3
    ~~Metacarpocarpal~~
      ~~Left 0RQT~~
      ~~Right 0RQS~~
    Metacarpophalangeal
      Left 0RQV
      Right 0RQU
    Metatarsal-Phalangeal
      Left 0SQN
      Right 0SQM
    ~~Metatarsal-Tarsal~~
      ~~Left 0SQL~~
      ~~Right 0SQK~~
    Occipital-cervical 0RQ0
    Sacrococcygeal 0SQ5
    Sacroiliac
      Left 0SQ8
      Right 0SQ7
    Shoulder
      Left 0RQK
      Right 0RQJ
    Sternoclavicular
      Left 0RQF
      Right 0RQE
    Tarsal
      Left 0SQJ
      Right 0SQH
    ▶ Tarsometatarsal
      ▶ Left 0SQL
      ▶ Right 0SQK
    Temporomandibular
      Left 0RQD
      Right 0RQC
    Thoracic Vertebral 0RQ6
    Thoracolumbar Vertebral 0RQA
    Toe Phalangeal
      Left 0SQQ
      Right 0SQP
    Wrist
      Left 0RQP
      Right 0RQN
  Kidney
    Left 0TQ1
    Right 0TQ0
  Kidney Pelvis
    Left 0TQ4
    Right 0TQ3
  Knee Region
    Left 0YQG
    Right 0YQF
  Larynx 0CQS
  Leg
    Lower
      Left 0YQJ
      Right 0YQH
    Upper
      Left 0YQD
      Right 0YQC
  Lens
    Left 08QK3ZZ
    Right 08QJ3ZZ
  Lip
    Lower 0CQ1
    Upper 0CQ0

Repair *(Continued)*
  Liver 0FQ0
    Left Lobe 0FQ2
    Right Lobe 0FQ1
  Lung
    Bilateral 0BQM
    Left 0BQL
    Lower Lobe
      Left 0BQJ
      Right 0BQF
    Middle Lobe, Right 0BQD
    Right 0BQK
    Upper Lobe
      Left 0BQG
      Right 0BQC
  Lung Lingula 0BQH
  Lymphatic
    Aortic 07QD
    Axillary
      Left 07Q6
      Right 07Q5
    Head 07Q0
    Inguinal
      Left 07QJ
      Right 07QH
    Internal Mammary
      Left 07Q9
      Right 07Q8
    Lower Extremity
      Left 07QG
      Right 07QF
    Mesenteric 07QB
    Neck
      Left 07Q2
      Right 07Q1
    Pelvis 07QC
    Thoracic Duct 07QK
    Thorax 07Q7
    Upper Extremity
      Left 07Q4
      Right 07Q3
  Mandible
    Left 0NQV
    Right 0NQT
  ➡ Maxilla 0NQR
    ~~Left 0NQS~~
    ~~Right 0NQR~~
  Mediastinum 0WQC
  Medulla Oblongata 00QD
  Mesentery 0DQV
  Metacarpal
    Left 0PQQ
    Right 0PQP
  Metatarsal
    Left 0QQP
    Right 0QQN
  Muscle
    Abdomen
      Left 0KQL
      Right 0KQK
    Extraocular
      Left 08QM
      Right 08QL
    Facial 0KQ1
    Foot
      Left 0KQW
      Right 0KQV
    Hand
      Left 0KQD
      Right 0KQC
    Head 0KQ0
    Hip
      Left 0KQP
      Right 0KQN
    Lower Arm and Wrist
      Left 0KQB
      Right 0KQ9
    Lower Leg
      Left 0KQT
      Right 0KQS

Repair *(Continued)*
  Muscle *(Continued)*
    Neck
      Left 0KQ3
      Right 0KQ2
    Papillary 02QD
    Perineum 0KQM
    Shoulder
      Left 0KQ6
      Right 0KQ5
    Thorax
      Left 0KQJ
      Right 0KQH
    Tongue, Palate, Pharynx 0KQ4
    Trunk
      Left 0KQG
      Right 0KQF
    Upper Arm
      Left 0KQ8
      Right 0KQ7
    Upper Leg
      Left 0KQR
      Right 0KQQ
  ▶ Nasal Mucosa and Soft Tissue 09QK
  Nasopharynx 09QN
  Neck 0WQ6
  Nerve
    Abdominal Sympathetic 01QM
    Abducens 00QL
    Accessory 00QR
    Acoustic 00QN
    Brachial Plexus 01Q3
    Cervical 01Q1
    Cervical Plexus 01Q0
    Facial 00QM
    Femoral 01QD
    Glossopharyngeal 00QP
    Head and Neck Sympathetic 01QK
    Hypoglossal 00QS
    Lumbar 01QB
    Lumbar Plexus 01Q9
    Lumbar Sympathetic 01QN
    Lumbosacral Plexus 01QA
    Median 01Q5
    Oculomotor 00QH
    Olfactory 00QF
    Optic 00QG
    Peroneal 01QH
    Phrenic 01Q2
    Pudendal 01QC
    Radial 01Q6
    Sacral 01QR
    Sacral Plexus 01QQ
    Sacral Sympathetic 01QP
    Sciatic 01QF
    Thoracic 01Q8
    Thoracic Sympathetic 01QL
    Tibial 01QG
    Trigeminal 00QK
    Trochlear 00QJ
    Ulnar 01Q4
    Vagus 00QQ
  Nipple
    Left 0HQX
    Right 0HQW
  ~~Nose 09QK~~
  ➡ Omentum 0DQU
    ~~Greater 0DQS~~
    ~~Lesser 0DQT~~
  Orbit
    Left 0NQQ
    Right 0NQP
  Ovary
    Bilateral 0UQ2
    Left 0UQ1
    Right 0UQ0
  Palate
    Hard 0CQ2
    Soft 0CQ3
  Pancreas 0FQG
  Para-aortic Body 0GQ9

▶ New   ➡ Revised   ~~deleted~~ Deleted

Repair *(Continued)*
Paraganglion Extremity 0GQF
Parathyroid Gland 0GQR
  Inferior
    Left 0GQP
    Right 0GQN
  Multiple 0GQQ
  Superior
    Left 0GQM
    Right 0GQL
Patella
  Left 0QQF
  Right 0QQD
Penis 0VQS
Pericardium 02QN
Perineum
  Female 0WQN
  Male 0WQM
Peritoneum 0DQW
Phalanx
  Finger
    Left 0PQV
    Right 0PQT
  Thumb
    Left 0PQS
    Right 0PQR
  Toe
    Left 0QQR
    Right 0QQQ
Pharynx 0CQM
Pineal Body 0GQ1
Pleura
  Left 0BQP
  Right 0BQN
Pons 00QB
Prepuce 0VQT
Products of Conception 10Q0
Prostate 0VQ0
Radius
  Left 0PQJ
  Right 0PQH
Rectum 0DQP
Retina
  Left 08QF3ZZ
  Right 08QE3ZZ
Retinal Vessel
  Left 08QH3ZZ
  Right 08QG3ZZ
~~Rib~~
  ~~Left 0PQ2~~
  ~~Right 0PQ1~~
▶Ribs
  ▶1 to 2 0PQ1
  ▶3 or More 0PQ2
Sacrum 0QQ1
Scapula
  Left 0PQ6
  Right 0PQ5
Sclera
  Left 08Q7XZZ
  Right 08Q6XZZ
Scrotum 0VQ5
Septum
  Atrial 02Q5
  Nasal 09QM
  Ventricular 02QM
Shoulder Region
  Left 0XQ3
  Right 0XQ2
Sinus
  Accessory 09QP
  Ethmoid
    Left 09QV
    Right 09QU
  Frontal
    Left 09QT
    Right 09QS
  Mastoid
    Left 09QC
    Right 09QB

Repair *(Continued)*
Sinus *(Continued)*
  Maxillary
    Left 09QR
    Right 09QQ
  Sphenoid
    Left 09QX
    Right 09QW
Skin
  Abdomen 0HQ7XZZ
  Back 0HQ6XZZ
  Buttock 0HQ8XZZ
  Chest 0HQ5XZZ
  Ear
    Left 0HQ3XZZ
    Right 0HQ2XZZ
  Face 0HQ1XZZ
  Foot
    Left 0HQNXZZ
    Right 0HQMXZZ
  ~~Genitalia 0HQAXZZ~~
  Hand
    Left 0HQGXZZ
    Right 0HQFXZZ
  ▶Inguinal 0HQAXZZ
  Lower Arm
    Left 0HQEXZZ
    Right 0HQDXZZ
  Lower Leg
    Left 0HQLXZZ
    Right 0HQKXZZ
  Neck 0HQ4XZZ
  Perineum 0HQ9XZZ
  Scalp 0HQ0XZZ
  Upper Arm
    Left 0HQCXZZ
    Right 0HQBXZZ
  Upper Leg
    Left 0HQJXZZ
    Right 0HQHXZZ
Skull 0NQ0
Spinal Cord
  Cervical 00QW
  Lumbar 00QY
  Thoracic 00QX
Spinal Meninges 00QT
Spleen 07QP
Sternum 0PQ0
Stomach 0DQ6
  Pylorus 0DQ7
Subcutaneous Tissue and Fascia
  Abdomen 0JQ8
  Back 0JQ7
  Buttock 0JQ9
  Chest 0JQ6
  Face 0JQ1
  Foot
    Left 0JQR
    Right 0JQQ
  Hand
    Left 0JQK
    Right 0JQJ
  Lower Arm
    Left 0JQH
    Right 0JQG
  Lower Leg
    Left 0JQP
    Right 0JQN
  Neck
    ~~Anterior 0JQ4~~
    ~~Posterior 0JQ5~~
    ▶Left 0JQ5
    ▶Right 0JQ4
  Pelvic Region 0JQC
  Perineum 0JQB
  Scalp 0JQ0
  Upper Arm
    Left 0JQF
    Right 0JQD
  Upper Leg
    Left 0JQM
    Right 0JQL

Repair *(Continued)*
Tarsal
  Left 0QQM
  Right 0QQL
Tendon
  Abdomen
    Left 0LQG
    Right 0LQF
  Ankle
    Left 0LQT
    Right 0LQS
  Foot
    Left 0LQW
    Right 0LQV
  Hand
    Left 0LQ8
    Right 0LQ7
  Head and Neck 0LQ0
  Hip
    Left 0LQK
    Right 0LQJ
  Knee
    Left 0LQR
    Right 0LQQ
  Lower Arm and Wrist
    Left 0LQ6
    Right 0LQ5
  Lower Leg
    Left 0LQP
    Right 0LQN
  Perineum 0LQH
  Shoulder
    Left 0LQ2
    Right 0LQ1
  Thorax
    Left 0LQD
    Right 0LQC
  Trunk
    Left 0LQB
    Right 0LQ9
  Upper Arm
    Left 0LQ4
    Right 0LQ3
  Upper Leg
    Left 0LQM
    Right 0LQL
Testis
  Bilateral 0VQC
  Left 0VQB
  Right 0VQ9
Thalamus 00Q9
Thumb
  Left 0XQM
  Right 0XQL
Thymus 07QM
Thyroid Gland 0GQK
  Left Lobe 0GQG
  Right Lobe 0GQH
Thyroid Gland Isthmus 0GQJ
Tibia
  Left 0QQH
  Right 0QQG
Toe
  1st
    Left 0YQQ
    Right 0YQP
  2nd
    Left 0YQS
    Right 0YQR
  3rd
    Left 0YQU
    Right 0YQT
  4th
    Left 0YQW
    Right 0YQV
  5th
    Left 0YQY
    Right 0YQX
Toe Nail 0HQRXZZ
Tongue 0CQ7
Tonsils 0CQP

▶ New   ⇒ Revised   ~~deleted~~ Deleted

Repair *(Continued)*
Tooth
  Lower 0CQX
  Upper 0CQW
Trachea 0BQ1
Tunica Vaginalis
  Left 0VQ7
  Right 0VQ6
Turbinate, Nasal 09QL
Tympanic Membrane
  Left 09Q8
  Right 09Q7
Ulna
  Left 0PQL
  Right 0PQK
Ureter
  Left 0TQ7
  Right 0TQ6
Urethra 0TQD
Uterine Supporting Structure 0UQ4
Uterus 0UQ9
Uvula 0CQN
Vagina 0UQG
Valve
  Aortic 02QF
  Mitral 02QG
  Pulmonary 02QH
  Tricuspid 02QJ
Vas Deferens
  Bilateral 0VQQ
  Left 0VQP
  Right 0VQN
Vein
  Axillary
    Left 05Q8
    Right 05Q7
  Azygos 05Q0
  Basilic
    Left 05QC
    Right 05QB
  Brachial
    Left 05QA
    Right 05Q9
  Cephalic
    Left 05QF
    Right 05QD
  Colic 06Q7
  Common Iliac
    Left 06QD
    Right 06QC
  Coronary 02Q4
  Esophageal 06Q3
  External Iliac
    Left 06QG
    Right 06QF
  External Jugular
    Left 05QQ
    Right 05QP
  Face
    Left 05QV
    Right 05QT
  Femoral
    Left 06QN
    Right 06QM
  Foot
    Left 06QV
    Right 06QT
  Gastric 06Q2
  ~~Greater Saphenous~~
    ~~Left 06QQ~~
    ~~Right 06QP~~
  Hand
    Left 05QH
    Right 05QG
  Hemiazygos 05Q1
  Hepatic 06Q4
  Hypogastric
    Left 06QJ
    Right 06QH
  Inferior Mesenteric 06Q6

Repair *(Continued)*
Vein *(Continued)*
  Innominate
    Left 05Q4
    Right 05Q3
  Internal Jugular
    Left 05QN
    Right 05QM
  Intracranial 05QL
  ~~Lesser Saphenous~~
    ~~Left 06QS~~
    ~~Right 06QR~~
  Lower 06QY
  Portal 06Q8
  Pulmonary
    Left 02QT
    Right 02QS
  Renal
    Left 06QB
    Right 06Q9
  ▶Saphenous
    ▶Left 06QQ
    ▶Right 06QP
  Splenic 06Q1
  Subclavian
    Left 05Q6
    Right 05Q5
  Superior Mesenteric 06Q5
  Upper 05QY
  Vertebral
    Left 05QS
    Right 05QR
Vena Cava
  Inferior 06Q0
  Superior 02QV
Ventricle
  Left 02QL
  Right 02QK
Vertebra
  Cervical 0PQ3
  Lumbar 0QQ0
  Thoracic 0PQ4
Vesicle
  Bilateral 0VQ3
  Left 0VQ2
  Right 0VQ1
Vitreous
  Left 08Q53ZZ
  Right 08Q43ZZ
Vocal Cord
  Left 0CQV
  Right 0CQT
Vulva 0UQM
Wrist Region
  Left 0XQH
  Right 0XQG

Repair, obstetric laceration, periurethral
  0UQMXZZ
Replacement
Acetabulum
  Left 0QR5
  Right 0QR4
Ampulla of Vater 0FRC
Anal Sphincter 0DRR
Aorta
  Abdominal 04R0
  Thoracic
    Ascending/Arch 02RX
    Descending 02RW
Artery
  Anterior Tibial
    Left 04RQ
    Right 04RP
  Axillary
    Left 03R6
    Right 03R5
  Brachial
    Left 03R8
    Right 03R7
  Celiac 04R1

Replacement *(Continued)*
Artery *(Continued)*
  Colic
    Left 04R7
    Middle 04R8
    Right 04R6
  Common Carotid
    Left 03RJ
    Right 03RH
  Common Iliac
    Left 04RD
    Right 04RC
  External Carotid
    Left 03RN
    Right 03RM
  External Iliac
    Left 04RJ
    Right 04RH
  Face 03RR
  Femoral
    Left 04RL
    Right 04RK
  Foot
    Left 04RW
    Right 04RV
  Gastric 04R2
  Hand
    Left 03RF
    Right 03RD
  Hepatic 04R3
  Inferior Mesenteric 04RB
  Innominate 03R2
  Internal Carotid
    Left 03RL
    Right 03RK
  Internal Iliac
    Left 04RF
    Right 04RE
  Internal Mammary
    Left 03R1
    Right 03R0
  Intracranial 03RG
  Lower 04RY
  Peroneal
    Left 04RU
    Right 04RT
  Popliteal
    Left 04RN
    Right 04RM
  Posterior Tibial
    Left 04RS
    Right 04RR
  Pulmonary
    Left 02RR
    Right 02RQ
  Pulmonary Trunk 02RP
  Radial
    Left 03RC
    Right 03RB
  Renal
    Left 04RA
    Right 04R9
  Splenic 04R4
  Subclavian
    Left 03R4
    Right 03R3
  Superior Mesenteric 04R5
  Temporal
    Left 03RT
    Right 03RS
  Thyroid
    Left 03RV
    Right 03RU
  Ulnar
    Left 03RA
    Right 03R9
  Upper 03RY
  Vertebral
    Left 03RQ
    Right 03RP

▶ New   ⇒ Revised   ~~deleted~~ Deleted

Replacement *(Continued)*
  Atrium
    Left 02R7
    Right 02R6
  Auditory Ossicle
    Left 09RA0
    Right 09R90
  Bladder 0TRB
  Bladder Neck 0TRC
  Bone
    Ethmoid
      Left 0NRG
      Right 0NRF
    ➡ Frontal 0NR1
      ~~Left 0NR2~~
      ~~Right 0NR1~~
    Hyoid 0NRX
    Lacrimal
      Left 0NRJ
      Right 0NRH
    Nasal 0NRB
    ➡ Occipital 0NR7
      ~~Left 0NR8~~
      ~~Right 0NR7~~
    Palatine
      Left 0NRL
      Right 0NRK
    Parietal
      Left 0NR4
      Right 0NR3
    Pelvic
      Left 0QR3
      Right 0QR2
    ➡ Sphenoid 0NRC
      ~~Left 0NRD~~
      ~~Right 0NRC~~
    Temporal
      Left 0NR6
      Right 0NR5
    Zygomatic
      Left 0NRN
      Right 0NRM
  Breast
    Bilateral 0HRV
    Left 0HRU
    Right 0HRT
  ▶ Bronchus
    ▶ Lingula 0BR9
    ▶ Lower Lobe
      ▶ Left 0BRB
      ▶ Right 0BR6
    ▶ Main
      ▶ Left 0BR7
      ▶ Right 0BR3
    ▶ Middle Lobe, Right 0BR5
    ▶ Upper Lobe
      ▶ Left 0BR8
      ▶ Right 0BR4
  Buccal Mucosa 0CR4
  ▶ Bursa and Ligament
    ▶ Abdomen
      ▶ Left 0MRJ
      ▶ Right 0MRH
    ▶ Ankle
      ▶ Left 0MRR
      ▶ Right 0MRQ
    ▶ Elbow
      ▶ Left 0MR4
      ▶ Right 0MR3
    ▶ Foot
      ▶ Left 0MRT
      ▶ Right 0MRS
    ▶ Hand
      ▶ Left 0MR8
      ▶ Right 0MR7
    ▶ Head and Neck 0MR0
    ▶ Hip
      ▶ Left 0MRM
      ▶ Right 0MRL
    ▶ Knee
      ▶ Left 0MRP
      ▶ Right 0MRN

Replacement *(Continued)*
  Bursa and Ligament *(Continued)*
    ▶ Lower Extremity
      ▶ Left 0MRW
      ▶ Right 0MRV
    ▶ Perineum 0MRK
    ▶ Rib(s) 0MRG
    ▶ Shoulder
      ▶ Left 0MR2
      ▶ Right 0MR1
    ▶ Spine
      ▶ Lower 0MRD
      ▶ Upper 0MRC
    ▶ Sternum 0MRF
    ▶ Upper Extremity
      ▶ Left 0MRB
      ▶ Right 0MR9
    ▶ Wrist
      ▶ Left 0MR6
      ▶ Right 0MR5
  ▶ Carina 0BR2
  Carpal
    Left 0PRN
    Right 0PRM
  ▶ Cerebral Meninges 00R1
  ▶ Cerebral Ventricle 00R6
  Chordae Tendineae 02R9
  Choroid
    Left 08RB
    Right 08RA
  Clavicle
    Left 0PRB
    Right 0PR9
  Coccyx 0QRS
  Conjunctiva
    Left 08RTX
    Right 08RSX
  Cornea
    Left 08R9
    Right 08R8
  ▶ Diaphragm 0BRT
  Disc
    Cervical Vertebral 0RR30
    Cervicothoracic Vertebral 0RR50
    Lumbar Vertebral 0SR20
    Lumbosacral 0SR40
    Thoracic Vertebral 0RR90
    Thoracolumbar Vertebral 0RRB0
  Duct
    Common Bile 0FR9
    Cystic 0FR8
    Hepatic
      ▶ Common 0FR7
      Left 0FR6
      Right 0FR5
    Lacrimal
      Left 08RY
      Right 08RX
    Pancreatic 0FRD
      Accessory 0FRF
    Parotid
      Left 0CRC
      Right 0CRB
  ▶ Dura Mater 00R2
  Ear
    External
      Bilateral 09R2
      Left 09R1
      Right 09R0
    Inner
      Left 09RE0
      Right 09RD0
    Middle
      Left 09R60
      Right 09R50
  Epiglottis 0CRR
  Esophagus 0DR5
  Eye
    Left 08R1
    Right 08R0

Replacement *(Continued)*
  Eyelid
    Lower
      Left 08RR
      Right 08RQ
    Upper
      Left 08RP
      Right 08RN
  Femoral Shaft
    Left 0QR9
    Right 0QR8
  Femur
    Lower
      Left 0QRC
      Right 0QRB
    Upper
      Left 0QR7
      Right 0QR6
  Fibula
    Left 0QRK
    Right 0QRJ
  Finger Nail 0HRQX
  Gingiva
    Lower 0CR6
    Upper 0CR5
  Glenoid Cavity
    Left 0PR8
    Right 0PR7
  Hair 0HRSX
  Humeral Head
    Left 0PRD
    Right 0PRC
  Humeral Shaft
    Left 0PRG
    Right 0PRF
  Iris
    Left 08RD3
    Right 08RC3
  Joint
    Acromioclavicular
      Left 0RRH0
      Right 0RRG0
    Ankle
      Left 0SRG
      Right 0SRF
    Carpal
      Left 0RRR0
      Right 0RRQ0
    ▶ Carpometacarpal
      ▶ Left 0RRT0
      ▶ Right 0RRS0
    Cervical Vertebral 0RR10
    Cervicothoracic Vertebral 0RR40
    Coccygeal 0SR60
    Elbow
      Left 0RRM0
      Right 0RRL0
    Finger Phalangeal
      Left 0RRX0
      Right 0RRW0
    Hip
      Left 0SRB
        Acetabular Surface 0SRE
        Femoral Surface 0SRS
      Right 0SR9
        Acetabular Surface 0SRA
        Femoral Surface 0SRR
    Knee
      Left 0SRD
        Femoral Surface 0SRU
        Tibial Surface 0SRW
      Right 0SRC
        Femoral Surface 0SRT
        Tibial Surface 0SRV
    Lumbar Vertebral 0SR00
    Lumbosacral 0SR30
    ~~Metacarpocarpal~~
      ~~Left 0RRT0~~
      ~~Right 0RRS0~~
    Metacarpophalangeal
      Left 0RRV0
      Right 0RRU0

▶ New   ➡ Revised   ~~deleted~~ Deleted

Replacement *(Continued)*
Joint *(Continued)*
Metatarsal-Phalangeal
Left ØSRNØ
Right ØSRMØ
Metatarsal-Tarsal
Left ØSRLØ
Right ØSRKØ
Occipital-cervical ØRR00
Sacrococcygeal ØSR5Ø
Sacroiliac
Left ØSR8Ø
Right ØSR7Ø
Shoulder
Left ØRRK
Right ØRRJ
Sternoclavicular
Left ØRRFØ
Right ØRREØ
Tarsal
Left ØSRJØ
Right ØSRHØ
▶ Tarsometatarsal
▶ Left ØSRLØ
▶ Right ØSRKØ
Temporomandibular
Left ØRRDØ
Right ØRRCØ
Thoracic Vertebral ØRR6Ø
Thoracolumbar Vertebral ØRRAØ
Toe Phalangeal
Left ØSRQØ
Right ØSRPØ
Wrist
Left ØRRPØ
Right ØRRNØ
Kidney Pelvis
Left ØTR4
Right ØTR3
Larynx ØCRS
Lens
Left 08RK30Z
Right 08RJ30Z
Lip
Lower ØCR1
Upper ØCRØ
Mandible
Left ØNRV
Right ØNRT
⇒ Maxilla ØNRR
Left ØNRS
Right ØNRR
Mesentery ØDRV
Metacarpal
Left ØPRQ
Right ØPRP
Metatarsal
Left ØQRP
Right ØQRN
Muscle, Papillary 02RD
▶ Muscle
▶ Abdomen
▶ Left ØKRL
▶ Right ØKRK
▶ Facial ØKR1
▶ Foot
▶ Left ØKRW
▶ Right ØKRV
▶ Hand
▶ Left ØKRD
▶ Right ØKRC
▶ Head ØKRØ
▶ Hip
▶ Left ØKRP
▶ Right ØKRN
▶ Lower Arm and Wrist
▶ Left ØKRB
▶ Right ØKR9
▶ Lower Leg
▶ Left ØKRT
▶ Right ØKRS

Replacement *(Continued)*
Muscle *(Continued)*
▶ Neck
▶ Left ØKR3
▶ Right ØKR2
▶ Papillary 02RD
▶ Perineum ØKRM
▶ Shoulder
▶ Left ØKR6
▶ Right ØKR5
▶ Thorax
▶ Left ØKRJ
▶ Right ØKRH
▶ Tongue, Palate, Pharynx ØKR4
▶ Trunk
▶ Left ØKRG
▶ Right ØKRF
▶ Upper Arm
▶ Left ØKR8
▶ Right ØKR7
▶ Upper Leg
▶ Left ØKRR
▶ Right ØKRQ
▶ Nasal Mucosa and Soft Tissue
09RK
Nasopharynx 09RN
▶ Nerve
▶ Abducens 00RL
▶ Accessory 00RR
▶ Acoustic 00RN
▶ Cervical 01R1
▶ Facial 00RM
▶ Femoral 01RD
▶ Glossopharyngeal 00RP
▶ Hypoglossal 00RS
▶ Lumbar 01RB
▶ Median 01R5
▶ Oculomotor 00RH
▶ Olfactory 00RF
▶ Optic 00RG
▶ Peroneal 01RH
▶ Phrenic 01R2
▶ Pudendal 01RC
▶ Radial 01R6
▶ Sacral 01RR
▶ Sciatic 01RF
▶ Thoracic 01R8
▶ Tibial 01RG
▶ Trigeminal 00RK
▶ Trochlear 00RJ
▶ Ulnar 01R4
▶ Vagus 00RQ
Nipple
Left ØHRX
Right ØHRW
Nose 09RK
⇒ Omentum ØDRU
Greater ØDRS
Lesser ØDRT
Orbit
Left ØNRQ
Right ØNRP
Palate
Hard ØCR2
Soft ØCR3
Patella
Left ØQRF
Right ØQRD
Pericardium 02RN
Peritoneum ØDRW
Phalanx
Finger
Left ØPRV
Right ØPRT
Thumb
Left ØPRS
Right ØPRR
Toe
Left ØQRR
Right ØQRQ

Replacement *(Continued)*
Pharynx ØCRM
Radius
Left ØPRJ
Right ØPRH
Retinal Vessel
Left 08RH3
Right 08RG3
Rib
Left ØPR2
Right ØPR1
▶ Ribs
▶ 1 to 2 ØPR1
▶ 3 or More ØPR2
Sacrum ØQR1
Scapula
Left ØPR6
Right ØPR5
Sclera
Left 08R7X
Right 08R6X
Septum
Atrial 02R5
Nasal 09RM
Ventricular 02RM
Skin
Abdomen ØHR7
Back ØHR6
Buttock ØHR8
Chest ØHR5
Ear
Left ØHR3
Right ØHR2
Face ØHR1
Foot
Left ØHRN
Right ØHRM
Genitalia ØHRA
Hand
Left ØHRG
Right ØHRF
▶ Inguinal ØHRA
Lower Arm
Left ØHRE
Right ØHRD
Lower Leg
Left ØHRL
Right ØHRK
Neck ØHR4
Perineum ØHR9
Scalp ØHRØ
Upper Arm
Left ØHRC
Right ØHRB
Upper Leg
Left ØHRJ
Right ØHRH
Skin Substitute, Porcine Liver Derived
XHRPXL2
Skull ØNRØ
▶ Spinal Meninges 00RT
Sternum ØPRØ
Subcutaneous Tissue and Fascia
Abdomen ØJR8
Back ØJR7
Buttock ØJR9
Chest ØJR6
Face ØJR1
Foot
Left ØJRR
Right ØJRQ
Hand
Left ØJRK
Right ØJRJ
Lower Arm
Left ØJRH
Right ØJRG
Lower Leg
Left ØJRP
Right ØJRN

Replacement (*Continued*)
Subcutaneous Tissue and Fascia (*Continued*)
Neck
Anterior 0JR4
Posterior 0JR5
▶Left 0JR5
▶Right 0JR4
Pelvic Region 0JRC
Perineum 0JRB
Scalp 0JR0
Upper Arm
Left 0JRF
Right 0JRD
Upper Leg
Left 0JRM
Right 0JRL
Tarsal
Left 0QRM
Right 0QRL
Tendon
Abdomen
Left 0LRG
Right 0LRF
Ankle
Left 0LRT
Right 0LRS
Foot
Left 0LRW
Right 0LRV
Hand
Left 0LR8
Right 0LR7
Head and Neck 0LR0
Hip
Left 0LRK
Right 0LRJ
Knee
Left 0LRR
Right 0LRQ
Lower Arm and Wrist
Left 0LR6
Right 0LR5
Lower Leg
Left 0LRP
Right 0LRN
Perineum 0LRH
Shoulder
Left 0LR2
Right 0LR1
Thorax
Left 0LRD
Right 0LRC
Trunk
Left 0LRB
Right 0LR9
Upper Arm
Left 0LR4
Right 0LR3
Upper Leg
Left 0LRM
Right 0LRL
Testis
Bilateral 0VRC0JZ
Left 0VRB0JZ
Right 0VR90JZ
Thumb
Left 0XRM
Right 0XRL
Tibia
Left 0QRH
Right 0QRG
Toe Nail 0HRRX
Tongue 0CR7
Tooth
Lower 0CRX
Upper 0CRW
▶Trachea 0BR1
Turbinate, Nasal 09RL
Tympanic Membrane
Left 09R8
Right 09R7

Replacement (*Continued*)
Ulna
Left 0PRL
Right 0PRK
Ureter
Left 0TR7
Right 0TR6
Urethra 0TRD
Uvula 0CRN
Valve
Aortic 02RF
Mitral 02RG
Pulmonary 02RH
Tricuspid 02RJ
Vein
Axillary
Left 05R8
Right 05R7
Azygos 05R0
Basilic
Left 05RC
Right 05RB
Brachial
Left 05RA
Right 05R9
Cephalic
Left 05RF
Right 05RD
Colic 06R7
Common Iliac
Left 06RD
Right 06RC
Esophageal 06R3
External Iliac
Left 06RG
Right 06RF
External Jugular
Left 05RQ
Right 05RP
Face
Left 05RV
Right 05RT
Femoral
Left 06RN
Right 06RM
Foot
Left 06RV
Right 06RT
Gastric 06R2
Greater Saphenous
Left 06RQ
Right 06RP
Hand
Left 05RH
Right 05RG
Hemiazygos 05R1
Hepatic 06R4
Hypogastric
Left 06RJ
Right 06RH
Inferior Mesenteric 06R6
Innominate
Left 05R4
Right 05R3
Internal Jugular
Left 05RN
Right 05RM
Intracranial 05RL
Lesser Saphenous
Left 06RS
Right 06RR
Lower 06RY
Portal 06R8
Pulmonary
Left 02RT
Right 02RS
Renal
Left 06RB
Right 06R9
▶Saphenous
▶Left 06RQ
▶Right 06RP

Replacement (*Continued*)
Vein (*Continued*)
Splenic 06R1
Subclavian
Left 05R6
Right 05R5
Superior Mesenteric 06R5
Upper 05RY
Vertebral
Left 05RS
Right 05RR
Vena Cava
Inferior 06R0
Superior 02RV
Ventricle
Left 02RL
Right 02RK
Vertebra
Cervical 0PR3
Lumbar 0QR0
Thoracic 0PR4
Vitreous
Left 08R53
Right 08R43
Vocal Cord
Left 0CRV
Right 0CRT
Zooplastic Tissue, Rapid Deployment
Technique X2RF
Replacement, hip
Partial or total *see* Replacement, Lower Joints
0SR
Resurfacing only *see* Supplement, Lower
Joints 0SU
Replantation *see* Reposition
Replantation, scalp *see* Reattachment, Skin,
Scalp 0HM0
Reposition
Acetabulum
Left 0QS5
Right 0QS4
Ampulla of Vater 0FSC
Anus 0DSQ
Aorta
Abdominal 04S0
Thoracic
Ascending/Arch 02SX0ZZ
Descending 02SW0ZZ
Artery
Anterior Tibial
Left 04SQ
Right 04SP
Axillary
Left 03S6
Right 03S5
Brachial
Left 03S8
Right 03S7
Celiac 04S1
Colic
Left 04S7
Middle 04S8
Right 04S6
Common Carotid
Left 03SJ
Right 03SH
Common Iliac
Left 04SD
Right 04SC
Coronary
One Artery 02S00ZZ
Two Arteries 02S10ZZ
External Carotid
Left 03SN
Right 03SM
External Iliac
Left 04SJ
Right 04SH
Face 03SR
Femoral
Left 04SL
Right 04SK

Reposition *(Continued)*
  Artery *(Continued)*
    Foot
      Left 04SW
      Right 04SV
    Gastric 04S2
    Hand
      Left 03SF
      Right 03SD
    Hepatic 04S3
    Inferior Mesenteric 04SB
    Innominate 03S2
    Internal Carotid
      Left 03SL
      Right 03SK
    Internal Iliac
      Left 04SF
      Right 04SE
    Internal Mammary
      Left 03S1
      Right 03S0
    Intracranial 03SG
    Lower 04SY
    Peroneal
      Left 04SU
      Right 04ST
    Popliteal
      Left 04SN
      Right 04SM
    Posterior Tibial
      Left 04SS
      Right 04SR
    Pulmonary
      Left 02SR0ZZ
      Right 02SQ0ZZ
    Pulmonary Trunk 02SP0ZZ
    Radial
      Left 03SC
      Right 03SB
    Renal
      Left 04SA
      Right 04S9
    Splenic 04S4
    Subclavian
      Left 03S4
      Right 03S3
    Superior Mesenteric 04S5
    Temporal
      Left 03ST
      Right 03SS
    Thyroid
      Left 03SV
      Right 03SU
    Ulnar
      Left 03SA
      Right 03S9
    Upper 03SY
    Vertebral
      Left 03SQ
      Right 03SP
  Auditory Ossicle
    Left 09SA
    Right 09S9
  Bladder 0TSB
  Bladder Neck 0TSC
  Bone
    Ethmoid
      Left 0NSG
      Right 0NSF
  ➡ Frontal 0NS1
      ~~Left 0NS2~~
      ~~Right 0NS1~~
    Hyoid 0NSX
    Lacrimal
      Left 0NSJ
      Right 0NSH
    Nasal 0NSB
  ➡ Occipital 0NS7
      ~~Left 0NS8~~
      ~~Right 0NS7~~

Reposition *(Continued)*
  Bone *(Continued)*
    Palatine
      Left 0NSL
      Right 0NSK
    Parietal
      Left 0NS4
      Right 0NS3
    Pelvic
      Left 0QS3
      Right 0QS2
  ➡ Sphenoid 0NSC
      ~~Left 0NSD~~
      ~~Right 0NSC~~
    Temporal
      Left 0NS6
      Right 0NS5
    Zygomatic
      Left 0NSN
      Right 0NSM
  Breast
    Bilateral 0HSV0ZZ
    Left 0HSU0ZZ
    Right 0HST0ZZ
  Bronchus
    Lingula 0BS90ZZ
    Lower Lobe
      Left 0BSB0ZZ
      Right 0BS60ZZ
    Main
      Left 0BS70ZZ
      Right 0BS30ZZ
    Middle Lobe, Right 0BS50ZZ
    Upper Lobe
      Left 0BS80ZZ
      Right 0BS40ZZ
  Bursa and Ligament
    Abdomen
      Left 0MSJ
      Right 0MSH
    Ankle
      Left 0MSR
      Right 0MSQ
    Elbow
      Left 0MS4
      Right 0MS3
    Foot
      Left 0MST
      Right 0MSS
    Hand
      Left 0MS8
      Right 0MS7
    Head and Neck 0MS0
    Hip
      Left 0MSM
      Right 0MSL
    Knee
      Left 0MSP
      Right 0MSN
    Lower Extremity
      Left 0MSW
      Right 0MSV
    Perineum 0MSK
  ▶ Rib(s) 0MSG
    Shoulder
      Left 0MS2
      Right 0MS1
  ▶ Spine
    ▶ Lower 0MSD
    ▶ Upper 0MSC
  ▶ Sternum 0MSF
    ~~Thorax~~
      ~~Left 0MSG~~
      ~~Right 0MSF~~
    ~~Trunk~~
      ~~Left 0MSD~~
      ~~Right 0MSC~~
    Upper Extremity
      Left 0MSB
      Right 0MS9

Reposition *(Continued)*
  Bursa and Ligament *(Continued)*
    Wrist
      Left 0MS6
      Right 0MS5
  Carina 0BS20ZZ
  Carpal
    Left 0PSN
    Right 0PSM
  Cecum 0DSH
  Cervix 0USC
  Clavicle
    Left 0PSB
    Right 0PS9
  Coccyx 0QSS
  Colon
    Ascending 0DSK
    Descending 0DSM
    Sigmoid 0DSN
    Transverse 0DSL
  Cord
    Bilateral 0VSH
    Left 0VSG
    Right 0VSF
  Cul-de-sac 0USF
  ➡ Diaphragm 0BST0ZZ
    ~~Left 0BSS0ZZ~~
    ~~Right 0BSR0ZZ~~
  Duct
    Common Bile 0FS9
    Cystic 0FS8
    Hepatic
    ▶ Common 0FS7
      Left 0FS6
      Right 0FS5
    Lacrimal
      Left 08SY
      Right 08SX
    Pancreatic 0FSD
      Accessory 0FSF
    Parotid
      Left 0CSC
      Right 0CSB
  Duodenum 0DS9
  Ear
    Bilateral 09S2
    Left 09S1
    Right 09S0
  Epiglottis 0CSR
  Esophagus 0DS5
  Eustachian Tube
    Left 09SG
    Right 09SF
  Eyelid
    Lower
      Left 08SR
      Right 08SQ
    Upper
      Left 08SP
      Right 08SN
  Fallopian Tube
    Left 0US6
    Right 0US5
  Fallopian Tubes, Bilateral 0US7
  Femoral Shaft
    Left 0QS9
    Right 0QS8
  Femur
    Lower
      Left 0QSC
      Right 0QSB
    Upper
      Left 0QS7
      Right 0QS6
  Fibula
    Left 0QSK
    Right 0QSJ
  Gallbladder 0FS4
  Gland
    Adrenal
      Left 0GS2
      Right 0GS3

▶ New   ➡ Revised   ~~deleted~~ Deleted

Reposition *(Continued)*
  Gland *(Continued)*
    Lacrimal
      Left 08SW
      Right 08SV
    Glenoid Cavity
      Left 0PS8
      Right 0PS7
    Hair 0HSSXZZ
    Humeral Head
      Left 0PSD
      Right 0PSC
    Humeral Shaft
      Left 0PSG
      Right 0PSF
    Ileum 0DSB
  ▶Intestine
    ▶Large 0DSE
    ▶Small 0DS8
    Iris
      Left 08SD3ZZ
      Right 08SC3ZZ
    Jejunum 0DSA
    Joint
      Acromioclavicular
        Left 0RSH
        Right 0RSG
      Ankle
        Left 0SSG
        Right 0SSF
      Carpal
        Left 0RSR
        Right 0RSQ
      ▶Carpometacarpal
        ▶Left 0RST
        ▶Right 0RSS
      Cervical Vertebral 0RS1
      Cervicothoracic Vertebral 0RS4
      Coccygeal 0SS6
      Elbow
        Left 0RSM
        Right 0RSL
      Finger Phalangeal
        Left 0RSX
        Right 0RSW
      Hip
        Left 0SSB
        Right 0SS9
      Knee
        Left 0SSD
        Right 0SSC
      Lumbar Vertebral 0SS0
      Lumbosacral 0SS3
      ~~Metacarpocarpal~~
        ~~Left 0RST~~
        ~~Right 0RSS~~
      Metacarpophalangeal
        Left 0RSV
        Right 0RSU
      Metatarsal-Phalangeal
        Left 0SSN
        Right 0SSM
      ~~Metatarsal-Tarsal~~
        ~~Left 0SSL~~
        ~~Right 0SSK~~
      Occipital-cervical 0RS0
      Sacrococcygeal 0SS5
      Sacroiliac
        Left 0SS8
        Right 0SS7
      Shoulder
        Left 0RSK
        Right 0RSJ
      Sternoclavicular
        Left 0RSF
        Right 0RSE
      Tarsal
        Left 0SSJ
        Right 0SSH
      ▶Tarsometatarsal
        ▶Left 0SSL
        ▶Right 0SSK

Reposition *(Continued)*
  Joint *(Continued)*
    Temporomandibular
      Left 0RSD
      Right 0RSC
    Thoracic Vertebral 0RS6
    Thoracolumbar Vertebral 0RSA
    Toe Phalangeal
      Left 0SSQ
      Right 0SSP
    Wrist
      Left 0RSP
      Right 0RSN
  Kidney
    Left 0TS1
    Right 0TS0
  Kidney Pelvis
    Left 0TS4
    Right 0TS3
  Kidneys, Bilateral 0TS2
  Lens
    Left 08SK3ZZ
    Right 08SJ3ZZ
  Lip
    Lower 0CS1
    Upper 0CS0
  Liver 0FS0
  Lung
    Left 0BSL0ZZ
    Lower Lobe
      Left 0BSJ0ZZ
      Right 0BSF0ZZ
    Middle Lobe, Right 0BSD0ZZ
    Right 0BSK0ZZ
    Upper Lobe
      Left 0BSG0ZZ
      Right 0BSC0ZZ
  Lung Lingula 0BSH0ZZ
  Mandible
    Left 0NSV
    Right 0NST
  ➡Maxilla 0NSR
    ~~Left 0NSS~~
    ~~Right 0NSR~~
  Metacarpal
    Left 0PSQ
    Right 0PSP
  Metatarsal
    Left 0QSP
    Right 0QSN
  Muscle
    Abdomen
      Left 0KSL
      Right 0KSK
    Extraocular
      Left 08SM
      Right 08SL
    Facial 0KS1
    Foot
      Left 0KSW
      Right 0KSV
    Hand
      Left 0KSD
      Right 0KSC
    Head 0KS0
    Hip
      Left 0KSP
      Right 0KSN
    Lower Arm and Wrist
      Left 0KSB
      Right 0KS9
    Lower Leg
      Left 0KST
      Right 0KSS
    Neck
      Left 0KS3
      Right 0KS2
    Perineum 0KSM
    Shoulder
      Left 0KS6
      Right 0KS5

Reposition *(Continued)*
  Muscle *(Continued)*
    Thorax
      Left 0KSJ
      Right 0KSH
    Tongue, Palate, Pharynx 0KS4
    Trunk
      Left 0KSG
      Right 0KSF
    Upper Arm
      Left 0KS8
      Right 0KS7
    Upper Leg
      Left 0KSR
      Right 0KSQ
  ▶Nasal Mucosa and Soft Tissue 09SK
  Nerve
    Abducens 00SL
    Accessory 00SR
    Acoustic 00SN
    Brachial Plexus 01S3
    Cervical 01S1
    Cervical Plexus 01S0
    Facial 00SM
    Femoral 01SD
    Glossopharyngeal 00SP
    Hypoglossal 00SS
    Lumbar 01SB
    Lumbar Plexus 01S9
    Lumbosacral Plexus 01SA
    Median 01S5
    Oculomotor 00SH
    Olfactory 00SF
    Optic 00SG
    Peroneal 01SH
    Phrenic 01S2
    Pudendal 01SC
    Radial 01S6
    Sacral 01SR
    Sacral Plexus 01SQ
    Sciatic 01SF
    Thoracic 01S8
    Tibial 01SG
    Trigeminal 00SK
    Trochlear 00SJ
    Ulnar 01S4
    Vagus 00SQ
  Nipple
    Left 0HSXXZZ
    Right 0HSWXZZ
  ~~Nose 09SK~~
  Orbit
    Left 0NSQ
    Right 0NSP
  Ovary
    Bilateral 0US2
    Left 0US1
    Right 0US0
  Palate
    Hard 0CS2
    Soft 0CS3
  Pancreas 0FSG
  Parathyroid Gland 0GSR
    Inferior
      Left 0GSP
      Right 0GSN
    Multiple 0GSQ
    Superior
      Left 0GSM
      Right 0GSL
  Patella
    Left 0QSF
    Right 0QSD
  Phalanx
    Finger
      Left 0PSV
      Right 0PST
    Thumb
      Left 0PSS
      Right 0PSR

▶ New   ➡ Revised   ~~deleted~~ Deleted

Reposition (Continued)
  Phalanx (Continued)
    Toe
      Left 0QSR
      Right 0QSQ
  Products of Conception 10S0
    Ectopic 10S2
  Radius
    Left 0PSJ
    Right 0PSH
  Rectum 0DSP
  Retinal Vessel
    Left 08SH3ZZ
    Right 08SG3ZZ
  ~~Rib~~
    ~~Left 0PS2~~
    ~~Right 0PS1~~
  ▶Ribs
    ▶1 to 2 0PS1
    ▶3 or More 0PS2
  Sacrum 0QS1
  Scapula
    Left 0PS6
    Right 0PS5
  Septum, Nasal 09SM
  ▶Sesamoid Bone(s) 1st Toe
    ▶see Reposition, Metatarsal, Right 0QSN
    ▶see Reposition, Metatarsal, Left 0QSP
  Skull 0NS0
  Spinal Cord
    Cervical 00SW
    Lumbar 00SY
    Thoracic 00SX
  Spleen 07SP0ZZ
  Sternum 0PS0
  Stomach 0DS6
  Tarsal
    Left 0QSM
    Right 0QSL
  Tendon
    Abdomen
      Left 0LSG
      Right 0LSF
    Ankle
      Left 0LST
      Right 0LSS
    Foot
      Left 0LSW
      Right 0LSV
    Hand
      Left 0LS8
      Right 0LS7
    Head and Neck 0LS0
    Hip
      Left 0LSK
      Right 0LSJ
    Knee
      Left 0LSR
      Right 0LSQ
    Lower Arm and Wrist
      Left 0LS6
      Right 0LS5
    Lower Leg
      Left 0LSP
      Right 0LSN
    Perineum 0LSH
    Shoulder
      Left 0LS2
      Right 0LS1
    Thorax
      Left 0LSD
      Right 0LSC
    Trunk
      Left 0LSB
      Right 0LS9
    Upper Arm
      Left 0LS4
      Right 0LS3
    Upper Leg
      Left 0LSM
      Right 0LSL

Reposition (Continued)
  Testis
    Bilateral 0VSC
      Left 0VSB
      Right 0VS9
  Thymus 07SM0ZZ
  Thyroid Gland
    Left Lobe 0GSG
    Right Lobe 0GSH
  Tibia
    Left 0QSH
    Right 0QSG
  Tongue 0CS7
  Tooth
    Lower 0CSX
    Upper 0CSW
  Trachea 0BS10ZZ
  Turbinate, Nasal 09SL
  Tympanic Membrane
    Left 09S8
    Right 09S7
  Ulna
    Left 0PSL
    Right 0PSK
  Ureter
    Left 0TS7
    Right 0TS6
  Ureters, Bilateral 0TS8
  Urethra 0TSD
  Uterine Supporting Structure 0US4
  Uterus 0US9
  Uvula 0CSN
  Vagina 0USG
  Vein
    Axillary
      Left 05S8
      Right 05S7
    Azygos 05S0
    Basilic
      Left 05SC
      Right 05SB
    Brachial
      Left 05SA
      Right 05S9
    Cephalic
      Left 05SF
      Right 05SD
    Colic 06S7
    Common Iliac
      Left 06SD
      Right 06SC
    Esophageal 06S3
    External Iliac
      Left 06SG
      Right 06SF
    External Jugular
      Left 05SQ
      Right 05SP
    Face
      Left 05SV
      Right 05ST
    Femoral
      Left 06SN
      Right 06SM
    Foot
      Left 06SV
      Right 06ST
    Gastric 06S2
    ~~Greater Saphenous~~
      ~~Left 06SQ~~
      ~~Right 06SP~~
    Hand
      Left 05SH
      Right 05SG
    Hemiazygos 05S1
    Hepatic 06S4
    Hypogastric
      Left 06SJ
      Right 06SH
    Inferior Mesenteric 06S6

Reposition (Continued)
  Vein (Continued)
    Innominate
      Left 05S4
      Right 05S3
    Internal Jugular
      Left 05SN
      Right 05SM
    Intracranial 05SL
    ~~Lesser Saphenous~~
      ~~Left 06SS~~
      ~~Right 06SR~~
    Lower 06SY
    Portal 06S8
    Pulmonary
      Left 02ST0ZZ
      Right 02SS0ZZ
    Renal
      Left 06SB
      Right 06S9
    ▶Saphenous
      ▶Left 06SQ
      ▶Right 06SP
    Splenic 06S1
    Subclavian
      Left 05S6
      Right 05S5
    Superior Mesenteric 06S5
    Upper 05SY
    Vertebral
      Left 05SS
      Right 05SR
  Vena Cava
    Inferior 06S0
    Superior 02SV0ZZ
  Vertebra
    Cervical 0PS3
      Magnetically Controlled Growth Rod(s) XNS3
    Lumbar 0QS0
      Magnetically Controlled Growth Rod(s) XNS0
    Thoracic 0PS4
      Magnetically Controlled Growth Rod(s) XNS4
  Vocal Cord
    Left 0CSV
    Right 0CST

Resection
  Acetabulum
    Left 0QT50ZZ
    Right 0QT40ZZ
  Adenoids 0CTQ
  Ampulla of Vater 0FTC
  Anal Sphincter 0DTR
  Anus 0DTQ
  Aortic Body 0GTD
  Appendix 0DTJ
  Auditory Ossicle
    ➡Left 09TA
    ➡Right 09T9
  Bladder 0TTB
  Bladder Neck 0TTC
  Bone
    Ethmoid
      Left 0NTG0ZZ
      Right 0NTF0ZZ
    ➡Frontal 0NT10ZZ
      ~~Left 0NT20ZZ~~
      ~~Right 0NT10ZZ~~
    Hyoid 0NTX0ZZ
    Lacrimal
      Left 0NTJ0ZZ
      Right 0NTH0ZZ
    Nasal 0NTB0ZZ
    ➡Occipital 0NT70ZZ
      ~~Left 0NT80ZZ~~
      ~~Right 0NT70ZZ~~
    Palatine
      Left 0NTL0ZZ
      Right 0NTK0ZZ

Resection *(Continued)*
  Bone *(Continued)*
    Parietal
      Left 0NT40ZZ
      Right 0NT30ZZ
    Pelvic
      Left 0QT30ZZ
      Right 0QT20ZZ
    ➠Sphenoid 0NTC0ZZ
      Left 0NTD0ZZ
      Right 0NTC0ZZ
    Temporal
      Left 0NT60ZZ
      Right 0NT50ZZ
    Zygomatic
      Left 0NTN0ZZ
      Right 0NTM0ZZ
  Breast
    Bilateral 0HTV0ZZ
      Left 0HTU0ZZ
      Right 0HTT0ZZ
    Supernumerary 0HTY0ZZ
  Bronchus
    Lingula 0BT9
    Lower Lobe
      Left 0BTB
      Right 0BT6
    Main
      Left 0BT7
      Right 0BT3
    Middle Lobe, Right 0BT5
    Upper Lobe
      Left 0BT8
      Right 0BT4
  Bursa and Ligament
    Abdomen
      Left 0MTJ
      Right 0MTH
    Ankle
      Left 0MTR
      Right 0MTQ
    Elbow
      Left 0MT4
      Right 0MT3
    Foot
      Left 0MTT
      Right 0MTS
    Hand
      Left 0MT8
      Right 0MT7
    Head and Neck 0MT0
    Hip
      Left 0MTM
      Right 0MTL
    Knee
      Left 0MTP
      Right 0MTN
    Lower Extremity
      Left 0MTW
      Right 0MTV
    Perineum 0MTK
    ▶Rib(s) 0MTG
    Shoulder
      Left 0MT2
      Right 0MT1
    ▶Spine
      ▶Lower 0MTD
      ▶Upper 0MTC
    ▶Sternum 0MTF
    Thorax
      Left 0MTG
      Right 0MTF
    Trunk
      Left 0MTD
      Right 0MTC
    Upper Extremity
      Left 0MTB
      Right 0MT9
    Wrist
      Left 0MT6
      Right 0MT5

Resection *(Continued)*
  Carina 0BT2
  Carotid Bodies, Bilateral 0GT8
  Carotid Body
    Left 0GT6
    Right 0GT7
  Carpal
    Left 0PTN0ZZ
    Right 0PTM0ZZ
  Cecum 0DTH
  Cerebral Hemisphere 00T7
  Cervix 0UTC
  Chordae Tendineae 02T9
  Cisterna Chyli 07TL
  Clavicle
    Left 0PTB0ZZ
    Right 0PT90ZZ
  Clitoris 0UTJ
  Coccygeal Glomus 0GTB
  Coccyx 0QTS0ZZ
  Colon
    Ascending 0DTK
    Descending 0DTM
    Sigmoid 0DTN
    Transverse 0DTL
  Conduction Mechanism
    02T8
  Cord
    Bilateral 0VTH
    Left 0VTG
    Right 0VTF
  Cornea
    Left 08T9XZZ
    Right 08T8XZZ
  Cul-de-sac 0UTF
  ➠Diaphragm 0BTT
    Left 0BTS
    Right 0BTR
  Disc
    Cervical Vertebral 0RT30ZZ
    Cervicothoracic Vertebral 0RT50ZZ
    Lumbar Vertebral 0ST20ZZ
    Lumbosacral 0ST40ZZ
    Thoracic Vertebral 0RT90ZZ
    Thoracolumbar Vertebral 0RTB0ZZ
  Duct
    Common Bile 0FT9
    Cystic 0FT8
    Hepatic
      ▶Common 0FT7
      Left 0FT6
      Right 0FT5
    Lacrimal
      Left 08TY
      Right 08TX
    Pancreatic 0FTD
      Accessory 0FTF
    Parotid
      Left 0CTC0ZZ
      Right 0CTB0ZZ
  Duodenum 0DT9
  Ear
    External
      Left 09T1
      Right 09T0
    Inner
      ➠Left 09TE
      ➠Right 09TD
    Middle
      ➠Left 09T6
      ➠Right 09T5
  Epididymis
    Bilateral 0VTL
    Left 0VTK
    Right 0VTJ
  Epiglottis 0CTR
  Esophagogastric Junction 0DT4
  Esophagus 0DT5
    Lower 0DT3
    Middle 0DT2
    Upper 0DT1

Resection *(Continued)*
  Eustachian Tube
    Left 09TG
    Right 09TF
  Eye
    Left 08T1XZZ
    Right 08T0XZZ
  Eyelid
    Lower
      Left 08TR
      Right 08TQ
    Upper
      Left 08TP
      Right 08TN
  Fallopian Tube
    Left 0UT6
    Right 0UT5
  Fallopian Tubes, Bilateral 0UT7
  Femoral Shaft
    Left 0QT90ZZ
    Right 0QT80ZZ
  Femur
    Lower
      Left 0QTC0ZZ
      Right 0QTB0ZZ
    Upper
      Left 0QT70ZZ
      Right 0QT60ZZ
  Fibula
    Left 0QTK0ZZ
    Right 0QTJ0ZZ
  Finger Nail 0HTQXZZ
  Gallbladder 0FT4
  Gland
    Adrenal
      Bilateral 0GT4
      Left 0GT2
      Right 0GT3
    Lacrimal
      Left 08TW
      Right 08TV
    Minor Salivary 0CTJ0ZZ
    Parotid
      Left 0CT90ZZ
      Right 0CT80ZZ
    Pituitary 0GT0
    Sublingual
      Left 0CTF0ZZ
      Right 0CTD0ZZ
    Submaxillary
      Left 0CTH0ZZ
      Right 0CTG0ZZ
    Vestibular 0UTL
  Glenoid Cavity
    Left 0PT80ZZ
    Right 0PT70ZZ
  Glomus Jugulare 0GTC
  Humeral Head
    Left 0PTD0ZZ
    Right 0PTC0ZZ
  Humeral Shaft
    Left 0PTG0ZZ
    Right 0PTF0ZZ
  Hymen 0UTK
  Ileocecal Valve 0DTC
  Ileum 0DTB
  Intestine
    Large 0DTE
      Left 0DTG
      Right 0DTF
    Small 0DT8
  Iris
    Left 08TD3ZZ
    Right 08TC3ZZ
  Jejunum 0DTA
  Joint
    Acromioclavicular
      Left 0RTH0ZZ
      Right 0RTG0ZZ
    Ankle
      Left 0STG0ZZ
      Right 0STF0ZZ

▶ New   ➠ Revised   ~~deleted~~ Deleted

Resection *(Continued)*
 Joint *(Continued)*
  Carpal
   Left 0RTR0ZZ
   Right 0RTQ0ZZ
  ▶Carpometacarpal
   ▶Left 0RTT0ZZ
   ▶Right 0RTS0ZZ
  Cervicothoracic Vertebral 0RT40ZZ
  Coccygeal 0ST60ZZ
  Elbow
   Left 0RTM0ZZ
   Right 0RTL0ZZ
  Finger Phalangeal
   Left 0RTX0ZZ
   Right 0RTW0ZZ
  Hip
   Left 0STB0ZZ
   Right 0ST90ZZ
  Knee
   Left 0STD0ZZ
   Right 0STC0ZZ
  ~~Metacarpocarpal~~
   ~~Left 0RTT0ZZ~~
   ~~Right 0RTS0ZZ~~
  Metacarpophalangeal
   Left 0RTV0ZZ
   Right 0RTU0ZZ
  Metatarsal-Phalangeal
   Left 0STN0ZZ
   Right 0STM0ZZ
  ~~Metatarsal-Tarsal~~
   ~~Left 0STL0ZZ~~
   ~~Right 0STK0ZZ~~
  Sacrococcygeal 0ST50ZZ
  Sacroiliac
   Left 0ST80ZZ
   Right 0ST70ZZ
  Shoulder
   Left 0RTK0ZZ
   Right 0RTJ0ZZ
  Sternoclavicular
   Left 0RTF0ZZ
   Right 0RTE0ZZ
  Tarsal
   Left 0STJ0ZZ
   Right 0STH0ZZ
  ▶Tarsometatarsal
   ▶Left 0STL0ZZ
   ▶Right 0STK0ZZ
  Temporomandibular
   Left 0RTD0ZZ
   Right 0RTC0ZZ
  Toe Phalangeal
   Left 0STQ0ZZ
   Right 0STP0ZZ
  Wrist
   Left 0RTP0ZZ
   Right 0RTN0ZZ
 Kidney
  Left 0TT1
  Right 0TT0
 Kidney Pelvis
  Left 0TT4
  Right 0TT3
 Kidneys, Bilateral 0TT2
 Larynx 0CTS
 Lens
  Left 08TK3ZZ
  Right 08TJ3ZZ
 Lip
  Lower 0CT1
  Upper 0CT0
 Liver 0FT0
  Left Lobe 0FT2
  Right Lobe 0FT1
 Lung
  Bilateral 0BTM
  Left 0BTL
  Lower Lobe
   Left 0BTJ
   Right 0BTF

Resection *(Continued)*
 Lung *(Continued)*
  Middle Lobe, Right 0BTD
  Right 0BTK
  Upper Lobe
   Left 0BTG
   Right 0BTC
 Lung Lingula 0BTH
 Lymphatic
  Aortic 07TD
  Axillary
   Left 07T6
   Right 07T5
  Head 07T0
  Inguinal
   Left 07TJ
   Right 07TH
  Internal Mammary
   Left 07T9
   Right 07T8
  Lower Extremity
   Left 07TG
   Right 07TF
  Mesenteric 07TB
  Neck
   Left 07T2
   Right 07T1
  Pelvis 07TC
  Thoracic Duct 07TK
  Thorax 07T7
  Upper Extremity
   Left 07T4
   Right 07T3
 Mandible
  Left 0NTV0ZZ
  Right 0NTT0ZZ
 ➡Maxilla 0NTR0ZZ
  ~~Left 0NTS0ZZ~~
  ~~Right 0NTR0ZZ~~
 Metacarpal
  Left 0PTQ0ZZ
  Right 0PTP0ZZ
 Metatarsal
  Left 0QTP0ZZ
  Right 0QTN0ZZ
 Muscle
  Abdomen
   Left 0KTL
   Right 0KTK
  Extraocular
   Left 08TM
   Right 08TL
  Facial 0KT1
  Foot
   Left 0KTW
   Right 0KTV
  Hand
   Left 0KTD
   Right 0KTC
  Head 0KT0
  Hip
   Left 0KTP
   Right 0KTN
  Lower Arm and Wrist
   Left 0KTB
   Right 0KT9
  Lower Leg
   Left 0KTT
   Right 0KTS
  Neck
   Left 0KT3
   Right 0KT2
  Papillary 02TD
  Perineum 0KTM
  Shoulder
   Left 0KT6
   Right 0KT5
  Thorax
   Left 0KTJ
   Right 0KTH
 Tongue, Palate, Pharynx 0KT4

Resection *(Continued)*
 Muscle *(Continued)*
  Trunk
   Left 0KTG
   Right 0KTF
  Upper Arm
   Left 0KT8
   Right 0KT7
  Upper Leg
   Left 0KTR
   Right 0KTQ
 ▶Nasal Mucosa and Soft Tissue
  09TK
 Nasopharynx 09TN
 Nipple
  Left 0HTXXZZ
  Right 0HTWXZZ
 ~~Nose 09TK~~
 ➡Omentum 0DTU
  ~~Greater 0DTS~~
  ~~Lesser 0DTT~~
 Orbit
  Left 0NTQ0ZZ
  Right 0NTP0ZZ
 Ovary
  Bilateral 0UT2
  Left 0UT1
  Right 0UT0
 Palate
  Hard 0CT2
  Soft 0CT3
 Pancreas 0FTG
 Para-aortic Body 0GT9
 Paraganglion Extremity 0GTF
 Parathyroid Gland 0GTR
  Inferior
   Left 0GTP
   Right 0GTN
  Multiple 0GTQ
  Superior
   Left 0GTM
   Right 0GTL
 Patella
  Left 0QTF0ZZ
  Right 0QTD0ZZ
 Penis 0VTS
 Pericardium 02TN
 Phalanx
  Finger
   Left 0PTV0ZZ
   Right 0PTT0ZZ
  Thumb
   Left 0PTS0ZZ
   Right 0PTR0ZZ
  Toe
   Left 0QTR0ZZ
   Right 0QTQ0ZZ
 Pharynx 0CTM
 Pineal Body 0GT1
 Prepuce 0VTT
 Products of Conception, Ectopic
  10T2
 Prostate 0VT0
 Radius
  Left 0PTJ0ZZ
  Right 0PTH0ZZ
 Rectum 0DTP
 ~~Rib~~
  ~~Left 0PT20ZZ~~
  ~~Right 0PT10ZZ~~
 ▶Ribs
  ▶1 to 2 0PT10ZZ
  ▶3 or More 0PT20ZZ
 Scapula
  Left 0PT60ZZ
  Right 0PT50ZZ
 Scrotum 0VT5
 Septum
  Atrial 02T5
  Nasal 09TM
  Ventricular 02TM

Resection (Continued)
Sinus
Accessory 09TP
Ethmoid
Left 09TV
Right 09TU
Frontal
Left 09TT
Right 09TS
Mastoid
Left 09TC
Right 09TB
Maxillary
Left 09TR
Right 09TQ
Sphenoid
Left 09TX
Right 09TW
Spleen 07TP
Sternum 0PT00ZZ
Stomach 0DT6
Pylorus 0DT7
Tarsal
Left 0QTM0ZZ
Right 0QTL0ZZ
Tendon
Abdomen
Left 0LTG
Right 0LTF
Ankle
Left 0LTT
Right 0LTS
Foot
Left 0LTW
Right 0LTV
Hand
Left 0LT8
Right 0LT7
Head and Neck 0LT0
Hip
Left 0LTK
Right 0LTJ
Knee
Left 0LTR
Right 0LTQ
Lower Arm and Wrist
Left 0LT6
Right 0LT5
Lower Leg
Left 0LTP
Right 0LTN
Perineum 0LTH
Shoulder
Left 0LT2
Right 0LT1
Thorax
Left 0LTD
Right 0LTC
Trunk
Left 0LTB
Right 0LT9
Upper Arm
Left 0LT4
Right 0LT3
Upper Leg
Left 0LTM
Right 0LTL
Testis
Bilateral 0VTC
Left 0VTB
Right 0VT9
Thymus 07TM
Thyroid Gland 0GTK
Left Lobe 0GTG
Right Lobe 0GTH
▶Thyroid Gland Isthmus 0GTJ
Tibia
Left 0QTH0ZZ
Right 0QTG0ZZ
Toe Nail 0HTRXZZ
Tongue 0CT7

Resection (Continued)
Tonsils 0CTP
Tooth
Lower 0CTX0Z
Upper 0CTW0Z
Trachea 0BT1
Tunica Vaginalis
Left 0VT7
Right 0VT6
Turbinate, Nasal 09TL
Tympanic Membrane
Left 09T8
Right 09T7
Ulna
Left 0PTL0ZZ
Right 0PTK0ZZ
Ureter
Left 0TT7
Right 0TT6
Urethra 0TTD
Uterine Supporting Structure 0UT4
Uterus 0UT9
Uvula 0CTN
Vagina 0UTG
Valve, Pulmonary 02TH
Vas Deferens
Bilateral 0VTQ
Left 0VTP
Right 0VTN
Vesicle
Bilateral 0VT3
Left 0VT2
Right 0VT1
Vitreous
Left 08T53ZZ
Right 08T43ZZ
Vocal Cord
Left 0CTV
Right 0CTT
Vulva 0UTM
▶**Resection, Left ventricular outflow tract obstruction (LVOT)** *see* Dilation, Ventricle, Left 027L
▶**Resection, Subaortic membrane (Left ventricular outflow tract obstruction)** *see* Dilation, Ventricle, Left 027L
Restoration, Cardiac, Single, Rhythm 5A2204Z
RestoreAdvanced neurostimulator (SureScan) (MRI Safe) *use* Stimulator Generator, Multiple Array Rechargeable in 0JH
RestoreSensor neurostimulator (SureScan) (MRI Safe) *use* Stimulator Generator, Multiple Array Rechargeable in 0JH
RestoreUltra neurostimulator (SureScan) (MRI Safe) *use* Stimulator Generator, Multiple Array Rechargeable in 0JH
Restriction
Ampulla of Vater 0FVC
Anus 0DVQ
Aorta
Abdominal 04V0
Ascending/Arch, Intraluminal Device, Branched or Fenestrated 02VX
Descending, Intraluminal Device, Branched or Fenestrated 02VW
Thoracic
Intraluminal Device, Branched or Fenestrated 04V0
Artery
Anterior Tibial
Left 04VQ
Right 04VP
Axillary
Left 03V6
Right 03V5
Brachial
Left 03V8
Right 03V7
Celiac 04V1

Restriction (Continued)
Artery (Continued)
Colic
Left 04V7
Middle 04V8
Right 04V6
Common Carotid
Left 03VJ
Right 03VH
Common Iliac
~~Left, Intraluminal Device, Branched or Fenestrated 04VD~~
~~Right, Intraluminal Device, Branched or Fenestrated 04VC~~
▶Left 04VD
▶Right 04VC
External Carotid
Left 03VN
Right 03VM
External Iliac
Left 04VJ
Right 04VH
Face 03VR
Femoral
Left 04VL
Right 04VK
Foot
Left 04VW
Right 04VV
Gastric 04V2
Hand
Left 03VF
Right 03VD
Hepatic 04V3
Inferior Mesenteric 04VB
Innominate 03V2
Internal Carotid
Left 03VL
Right 03VK
Internal Iliac
Left 04VF
Right 04VE
Internal Mammary
Left 03V1
Right 03V0
Intracranial 03VG
Lower 04VY
Peroneal
Left 04VU
Right 04VT
Popliteal
Left 04VN
Right 04VM
Posterior Tibial
Left 04VS
Right 04VR
Pulmonary
Left 02VR
Right 02VQ
Pulmonary Trunk 02VP
Radial
Left 03VC
Right 03VB
Renal
Left 04VA
Right 04V9
Splenic 04V4
Subclavian
Left 03V4
Right 03V3
Superior Mesenteric 04V5
Temporal
Left 03VT
Right 03VS
Thyroid
Left 03VV
Right 03VU
Ulnar
Left 03VA
Right 03V9
Upper 03VY

Restriction *(Continued)*
  Artery *(Continued)*
    Vertebral
      Left 03VQ
      Right 03VP
  Bladder 0TVB
  Bladder Neck 0TVC
  Bronchus
    Lingula 0BV9
    Lower Lobe
      Left 0BVB
      Right 0BV6
    Main
      Left 0BV7
      Right 0BV3
    Middle Lobe, Right 0BV5
    Upper Lobe
      Left 0BV8
      Right 0BV4
  Carina 0BV2
  Cecum 0DVH
  Cervix 0UVC
  Cisterna Chyli 07VL
  Colon
    Ascending 0DVK
    Descending 0DVM
    Sigmoid 0DVN
    Transverse 0DVL
  Duct
    Common Bile 0FV9
    Cystic 0FV8
    Hepatic
    ▶ Common 0FV7
      Left 0FV6
      Right 0FV5
    Lacrimal
      Left 08VY
      Right 08VX
    Pancreatic 0FVD
      Accessory 0FVF
    Parotid
      Left 0CVC
      Right 0CVB
  Duodenum 0DV9
  Esophagogastric Junction 0DV4
  Esophagus 0DV5
    Lower 0DV3
    Middle 0DV2
    Upper 0DV1
  Heart 02VA
  Ileocecal Valve 0DVC
  Ileum 0DVB
  Intestine
    Large 0DVE
      Left 0DVG
      Right 0DVF
    Small 0DV8
  Jejunum 0DVA
  Kidney Pelvis
    Left 0TV4
    Right 0TV3
  Lymphatic
    Aortic 07VD
    Axillary
      Left 07V6
      Right 07V5
    Head 07V0
    Inguinal
      Left 07VJ
      Right 07VH
    Internal Mammary
      Left 07V9
      Right 07V8
    Lower Extremity
      Left 07VG
      Right 07VF
    Mesenteric 07VB
    Neck
      Left 07V2
      Right 07V1
    Pelvis 07VC

Restriction *(Continued)*
  Lymphatic *(Continued)*
    Thoracic Duct 07VK
    Thorax 07V7
    Upper Extremity
      Left 07V4
      Right 07V3
  Rectum 0DVP
  Stomach 0DV6
    Pylorus 0DV7
  Trachea 0BV1
  Ureter
    Left 0TV7
    Right 0TV6
  Urethra 0TVD
  ▶ Valve, Mitral 02VG
  Vein
    Axillary
      Left 05V8
      Right 05V7
    Azygos 05V0
    Basilic
      Left 05VC
      Right 05VB
    Brachial
      Left 05VA
      Right 05V9
    Cephalic
      Left 05VF
      Right 05VD
    Colic 06V7
    Common Iliac
      Left 06VD
      Right 06VC
    Esophageal 06V3
    External Iliac
      Left 06VG
      Right 06VF
    External Jugular
      Left 05VQ
      Right 05VP
    Face
      Left 05VV
      Right 05VT
    Femoral
      Left 06VN
      Right 06VM
    Foot
      Left 06VV
      Right 06VT
    Gastric 06V2
    ~~Greater Saphenous~~
      ~~Left 06VQ~~
      ~~Right 06VP~~
    Hand
      Left 05VH
      Right 05VG
    Hemiazygos 05V1
    Hepatic 06V4
    Hypogastric
      Left 06VJ
      Right 06VH
    Inferior Mesenteric 06V6
    Innominate
      Left 05V4
      Right 05V3
    Internal Jugular
      Left 05VN
      Right 05VM
    Intracranial 05VL
    ~~Lesser Saphenous~~
      ~~Left 06VS~~
      ~~Right 06VR~~
    Lower 06VY
    Portal 06V8
    Pulmonary
      Left 02VT
      Right 02VS
    Renal
      Left 06VB
      Right 06V9

Restriction *(Continued)*
  Vein *(Continued)*
    ▶ Saphenous
      ▶ Left 06VQ
      ▶ Right 06VP
    Splenic 06V1
    Subclavian
      Left 05V6
      Right 05V5
    Superior Mesenteric 06V5
    Upper 05VY
    Vertebral
      Left 05VS
      Right 05VR
    Vena Cava
      Inferior 06V0
      Superior 02VV
Resurfacing Device
  Removal of device from
    Left 0SPB0BZ
    Right 0SP90BZ
  Revision of device in
    Left 0SWB0BZ
    Right 0SW90BZ
  Supplement
    Left 0SUB0BZ
      Acetabular Surface 0SUE0BZ
      Femoral Surface 0SUS0BZ
    Right 0SU90BZ
      Acetabular Surface 0SUA0BZ
      Femoral Surface 0SUR0BZ
Resuscitation
  Cardiopulmonary *see* Assistance, Cardiac 5A02
  Cardioversion 5A2204Z
  Defibrillation 5A2204Z
  Endotracheal intubation *see* Insertion of device in, Trachea 0BH1
  External chest compression 5A12012
  Pulmonary 5A19054
▶ **Resuscitative endovascular balloon occlusion of the aorta (REBOA)**
  ▶ 02LW3DJ
  ▶ 04L03DJ
Resuture, Heart valve prosthesis *see* Revision of device in, Heart and Great Vessels 02W
▶ **Retained placenta, manual removal** *see* Extraction, Products of Conception, Retained 10D1
Retraining
  Cardiac *see* Motor Treatment, Rehabilitation F07
  Vocational *see* Activities of Daily Living Treatment, Rehabilitation F08
Retrogasserian rhizotomy *see* Division, Nerve, Trigeminal 008K
Retroperitoneal lymph node *use* Lymphatic, Aortic
Retroperitoneal space *use* Retroperitoneum
Retropharyngeal lymph node
  use Lymphatic, Right Neck
  use Lymphatic, Left Neck
Retropubic space *use* Pelvic Cavity
Reveal (DX) (XT) *use* Monitoring Device
Reverse total shoulder replacement *see* Replacement, Upper Joints 0RR
Reverse® Shoulder Prosthesis *use* Synthetic Substitute, Reverse Ball and Socket in 0RR
Revision
  Correcting a portion of existing device *see* Revision of device in
  Removal of device without replacement *see* Removal of device from
  Replacement of existing device
    see Removal of device from
    see Root operation to place new device, e.g., Insertion, Replacement, Supplement
Revision of device in
  Abdominal Wall 0WWF
  Acetabulum
    Left 0QW5
    Right 0QW4

▶ New   ⇒ Revised   ~~deleted~~ Deleted

Revision of device in (Continued)

Anal Sphincter 0DWR
Anus 0DWQ
Artery
   Lower 04WY
   Upper 03WY
Auditory Ossicle
   Left 09WA
   Right 09W9
Back
   Lower 0WWL
   Upper 0WWK
Bladder 0TWB
Bone
   Facial 0NWW
   Lower 0QWY
   Nasal 0NWB
   Pelvic
      Left 0QW3
      Right 0QW2
   Upper 0PWY
Bone Marrow 07WT
Brain 00W0
Breast
   Left 0HWU
   Right 0HWT
Bursa and Ligament
   Lower 0MWY
   Upper 0MWX
Carpal
   Left 0PWN
   Right 0PWM
Cavity, Cranial 0WW1
Cerebral Ventricle 00W6
Chest Wall 0WW8
Cisterna Chyli 07WL
Clavicle
   Left 0PWB
   Right 0PW9
Coccyx 0QWS
Diaphragm 0BWT
Disc
   Cervical Vertebral 0RW3
   Cervicothoracic Vertebral 0RW5
   Lumbar Vertebral 0SW2
   Lumbosacral 0SW4
   Thoracic Vertebral 0RW9
   Thoracolumbar Vertebral 0RWB
Duct
   Hepatobiliary 0FWB
   Pancreatic 0FWD
   Thoracic 07WK
Ear
   Inner
      Left 09WE
      Right 09WD
   Left 09WJ
   Right 09WH
Epididymis and Spermatic Cord 0VWM
Esophagus 0DW5
Extremity
   Lower
      Left 0YWB
      Right 0YW9
   Upper
      Left 0XW7
      Right 0XW6
Eye
   Left 08W1
   Right 08W0
Face 0WW2
Fallopian Tube 0UW8
Femoral Shaft
   Left 0QW9
   Right 0QW8
Femur
   Lower
      Left 0QWC
      Right 0QWB
   Upper
      Left 0QW7
      Right 0QW6

Revision of device in (Continued)

Fibula
   Left 0QWK
   Right 0QWJ
Finger Nail 0HWQX
Gallbladder 0FW4
Gastrointestinal Tract 0WWP
Genitourinary Tract 0WWR
Gland
   Adrenal 0GW5
   Endocrine 0GWS
   Pituitary 0GW0
   Salivary 0CWA
Glenoid Cavity
   Left 0PW8
   Right 0PW7
Great Vessel 02WY
Hair 0HWSX
Head 0WW0
Heart 02WA
Humeral Head
   Left 0PWD
   Right 0PWC
Humeral Shaft
   Left 0PWG
   Right 0PWF
Intestinal Tract
   Lower 0DWD
   Upper 0DW0
Intestine
   Large 0DWE
   Small 0DW8
Jaw
   Lower 0WW5
   Upper 0WW4
Joint
   Acromioclavicular
      Left 0RWH
      Right 0RWG
   Ankle
      Left 0SWG
      Right 0SWF
   Carpal
      Left 0RWR
      Right 0RWQ
   ▶Carpometacarpal
      ▶Left 0RWT
      ▶Right 0RWS
   Cervical Vertebral 0RW1
   Cervicothoracic Vertebral 0RW4
   Coccygeal 0SW6
   Elbow
      Left 0RWM
      Right 0RWL
   Finger Phalangeal
      Left 0RWX
      Right 0RWW
   Hip
      Left 0SWB
         Acetabular Surface 0SWE
         Femoral Surface 0SWS
      Right 0SW9
         Acetabular Surface 0SWA
         Femoral Surface 0SWR
   Knee
      Left 0SWD
         Femoral Surface 0SWU
         Tibial Surface 0SWW
      Right 0SWC
         Femoral Surface 0SWT
         Tibial Surface 0SWV
   Lumbar Vertebral 0SW0
   Lumbosacral 0SW3
   ~~Metacarpocarpal~~
      ~~Left 0RWT~~
      ~~Right 0RWS~~
   Metacarpophalangeal
      Left 0RWV
      Right 0RWU
   Metatarsal-Phalangeal
      Left 0SWN
      Right 0SWM

Revision of device in (Continued)

Joint (Continued)
   ~~Metatarsal-Tarsal~~
      ~~Left 0SWL~~
      ~~Right 0SWK~~
   Occipital-cervical 0RW0
   Sacrococcygeal 0SW5
   Sacroiliac
      Left 0SW8
      Right 0SW7
   Shoulder
      Left 0RWK
      Right 0RWJ
   Sternoclavicular
      Left 0RWF
      Right 0RWE
   Tarsal
      Left 0SWJ
      Right 0SWH
   ▶Tarsometatarsal
      ▶Left 0SWL
      ▶Right 0SWK
   Temporomandibular
      Left 0RWD
      Right 0RWC
   Thoracic Vertebral 0RW6
   Thoracolumbar Vertebral 0RWA
   Toe Phalangeal
      Left 0SWQ
      Right 0SWP
   Wrist
      Left 0RWP
      Right 0RWN
Kidney 0TW5
Larynx 0CWS
Lens
   Left 08WK
   Right 08WJ
Liver 0FW0
Lung
   Left 0BWL
   Right 0BWK
Lymphatic 07WN
   Thoracic Duct 07WK
Mediastinum 0WWC
Mesentery 0DWV
Metacarpal
   Left 0PWQ
   Right 0PWP
Metatarsal
   Left 0QWP
   Right 0QWN
Mouth and Throat 0CWY
Muscle
   Extraocular
      Left 08WM
      Right 08WL
   Lower 0KWY
   Upper 0KWX
▶Nasal Mucosa and Soft Tissue 09WK
Neck 0WW6
Nerve
   Cranial 00WE
   Peripheral 01WY
~~Nose 09WK~~
Omentum 0DWU
Ovary 0UW3
Pancreas 0FWG
Parathyroid Gland 0GWR
Patella
   Left 0QWF
   Right 0QWD
Pelvic Cavity 0WWJ
Penis 0VWS
Pericardial Cavity 0WWD
Perineum
   Female 0WWN
   Male 0WWM
Peritoneal Cavity 0WWG
Peritoneum 0DWW

▶ New   ➡ Revised   ~~deleted~~ Deleted

Revision of device in (*Continued*)
 Phalanx
  Finger
   Left 0PWV
   Right 0PWT
  Thumb
   Left 0PWS
   Right 0PWR
  Toe
   Left 0QWR
   Right 0QWQ
 Pineal Body 0GW1
 Pleura 0BWQ
 Pleural Cavity
  Left 0WWB
  Right 0WW9
 Prostate and Seminal Vesicles 0VW4
 Radius
  Left 0PWJ
  Right 0PWH
 Respiratory Tract 0WWQ
 Retroperitoneum 0WWH
 ~~Rib~~
  ~~Left 0PW2~~
  ~~Right 0PW1~~
 ▶Ribs
  ▶1 to 2 0PW1
  ▶3 or More 0PW2
 Sacrum 0QW1
 Scapula
  Left 0PW6
  Right 0PW5
 Scrotum and Tunica Vaginalis 0VW8
 Septum
  Atrial 02W5
  Ventricular 02WM
 Sinus 09WY
 Skin 0HWPX
 Skull 0NW0
 Spinal Canal 00WU
 Spinal Cord 00WV
 Spleen 07WP
 Sternum 0PW0
 Stomach 0DW6
 Subcutaneous Tissue and Fascia
  Head and Neck 0JWS
  Lower Extremity 0JWW
  Trunk 0JWT
  Upper Extremity 0JWV
 Tarsal
  Left 0QWM
  Right 0QWL
 Tendon
  Lower 0LWY
  Upper 0LWX
 Testis 0VWD
 Thymus 07WM
 Thyroid Gland 0GWK
 Tibia
  Left 0QWH
  Right 0QWG
 Toe Nail 0HWRX
 Trachea 0BW1

Revision of device in (*Continued*)
 Tracheobronchial Tree 0BW0
 Tympanic Membrane
  Left 09W8
  Right 09W7
 Ulna
  Left 0PWL
  Right 0PWK
 Ureter 0TW9
 Urethra 0TWD
 Uterus and Cervix 0UWD
 Vagina and Cul-de-sac 0UWH
 Valve
  Aortic 02WF
  Mitral 02WG
  Pulmonary 02WH
  Tricuspid 02WJ
 Vas Deferens 0VWR
 Vein
  Azygos 05W0
  Innominate
   Left 05W4
   Right 05W3
  Lower 06WY
  Upper 05WY
 Vertebra
  Cervical 0PW3
  Lumbar 0QW0
  Thoracic 0PW4
 Vulva 0UWM
Revo MRI™ SureScan® pacemaker *use*
  Pacemaker, Dual Chamber in 0JH
rhBMP-2 *use* Recombinant Bone Morphogenetic
  Protein
Rheos® System device *use* Stimulator Generator
  in Subcutaneous Tissue and Fascia
Rheos® System lead *use* Stimulator Lead in
  Upper Arteries
Rhinopharynx *use* Nasopharynx
Rhinoplasty
  ~~see Alteration, Nose 090K~~
  ~~see Repair, Nose 09QK~~
  ~~see Replacement, Nose 09RK~~
  ~~see Supplement, Nose 09UK~~
  ▶*see* Alteration, Nasal Mucosa and Soft Tissue
   090K
  ▶*see* Repair, Nasal Mucosa and Soft Tissue
   09QK
  ▶*see* Replacement, Nasal Mucosa and Soft
   Tissue 09RK
  ▶*see* Supplement, Nasal Mucosa and Soft
   Tissue 09UK
➠**Rhinorrhaphy** *see* Repair, Nasal Mucosa and
  Soft Tissue 09QK
Rhinoscopy 09JKXZZ
Rhizotomy
  ~~see Division, Central Nervous System 008~~
  ▶*see* Division, Central Nervous System and
   Cranial Nerves 008
  see Division, Peripheral Nervous System 018
Rhomboid major muscle
  use Trunk Muscle, Right
  use Trunk Muscle, Left

Rhomboid minor muscle
  use Trunk Muscle, Right
  use Trunk Muscle, Left
Rhythm electrocardiogram *see* Measurement,
  Cardiac 4A02
Rhytidectomy *see* Face lift
Right ascending lumbar vein *use* Azygos Vein
Right atrioventricular valve *use* Tricuspid Valve
Right auricular appendix *use* Atrium, Right
Right colic vein *use* Colic Vein
Right coronary sulcus *use* Heart, Right
Right gastric artery *use* Gastric Artery
Right gastroepiploic vein *use* Superior
  Mesenteric Vein
Right inferior phrenic vein *use* Inferior Vena
  Cava
Right inferior pulmonary vein *use* Pulmonary
  Vein, Right
Right jugular trunk *use* Lymphatic, Right
  Neck
Right lateral ventricle *use* Cerebral Ventricle
Right lymphatic duct *use* Lymphatic, Right
  Neck
Right ovarian vein *use* Inferior Vena Cava
Right second lumbar vein *use* Inferior Vena
  Cava
Right subclavian trunk *use* Lymphatic, Right
  Neck
Right subcostal vein *use* Azygos Vein
Right superior pulmonary vein *use* Pulmonary
  Vein, Right
Right suprarenal vein *use* Inferior Vena Cava
Right testicular vein *use* Inferior Vena Cava
Rima glottidis *use* Larynx
Risorius muscle *use* Facial Muscle
➠**RNS System lead** *use* Neurostimulator Lead in
  Central Nervous System and Cranial
  Nerves
RNS system neurostimulator generator *use*
  Neurostimulator Generator in Head and
  Facial Bones
Robotic Assisted Procedure
  Extremity
   Lower 8E0Y
   Upper 8E0X
  Head and Neck Region 8E09
  Trunk Region 8E0W
Rotation of fetal head
  Forceps 10S07ZZ
  Manual 10S0XZZ
Round ligament of uterus *use* Uterine
  Supporting Structure
Round window
  use Inner Ear, Right
  use Inner Ear, Left
Roux-en-Y operation
  see Bypass, Gastrointestinal System 0D1
  see Bypass, Hepatobiliary System and
   Pancreas 0F1
Rupture
  Adhesions *see* Release
  Fluid collection *see* Drainage

S

Sacral ganglion *use* Sacral Sympathetic Nerve
Sacral lymph node *use* Lymphatic, Pelvis
Sacral nerve modulation (SNM) lead *use* Stimulator Lead in Urinary System
Sacral neuromodulation lead *use* Stimulator Lead in Urinary System
Sacral splanchnic nerve *use* Sacral Sympathetic Nerve
Sacrectomy *see* Excision, Lower Bones ØQB
➡**Sacrococcygeal ligament** *use* Lower Spine Bursa and Ligament
~~*use* Trunk Bursa and Ligament, Right~~
~~*use* Trunk Bursa and Ligament, Left~~
Sacrococcygeal symphysis *use* Sacrococcygeal Joint
➡**Sacroiliac ligament** *use* Lower Spine Bursa and Ligament
~~*use* Trunk Bursa and Ligament, Right~~
~~*use* Trunk Bursa and Ligament, Left~~
➡**Sacrospinous ligament** *use* Lower Spine Bursa and Ligament
~~*use* Trunk Bursa and Ligament, Right~~
~~*use* Trunk Bursa and Ligament, Left~~
➡**Sacrotuberous ligament** *use* Lower Spine Bursa and Ligament
~~*use* Trunk Bursa and Ligament, Right~~
~~*use* Trunk Bursa and Ligament, Left~~
Salpingectomy
see Excision, Female Reproductive System ØUB
see Resection, Female Reproductive System ØUT
Salpingolysis *see* Release, Female Reproductive System ØUN
Salpingopexy
see Repair, Female Reproductive System ØUQ
see Reposition, Female Reproductive System ØUS
Salpingopharyngeus muscle *use* Tongue, Palate, Pharynx Muscle
Salpingoplasty
see Repair, Female Reproductive System ØUQ
see Supplement, Female Reproductive System ØUU
Salpingorrhaphy *see* Repair, Female Reproductive System ØUQ
Salpingoscopy ØUJ88ZZ
Salpingostomy *see* Drainage, Female Reproductive System ØU9
Salpingotomy *see* Drainage, Female Reproductive System ØU9
Salpinx
use Fallopian Tube, Right
use Fallopian Tube, Left
Saphenous nerve *use* Femoral Nerve
SAPIEN transcatheter aortic valve *use* Zooplastic Tissue in Heart and Great Vessels
Sartorius muscle
use Upper Leg Muscle, Right
use Upper Leg Muscle, Left
Scalene muscle
use Neck Muscle, Right
use Neck Muscle, Left
Scan
Computerized Tomography (CT) *see* Computerized Tomography (CT Scan)
Radioisotope *see* Planar Nuclear Medicine Imaging
Scaphoid bone
use Carpal, Right
use Carpal, Left
Scapholunate ligament
use Hand Bursa and Ligament, Right
use Hand Bursa and Ligament, Left
Scaphotrapezium ligament
use Hand Bursa and Ligament, Right
use Hand Bursa and Ligament, Left

Scapulectomy
see Excision, Upper Bones ØPB
see Resection, Upper Bones ØPT
Scapulopexy
see Repair, Upper Bones ØPQ
see Reposition, Upper Bones ØPS
Scarpa's (vestibular) ganglion *use* Acoustic Nerve
Sclerectomy *see* Excision, Eye Ø8B
Sclerotherapy, mechanical *see* Destruction
Sclerotomy *see* Drainage, Eye Ø89
Scrotectomy
see Excision, Male Reproductive System ØVB
see Resection, Male Reproductive System ØVT
Scrotoplasty
see Repair, Male Reproductive System ØVQ
see Supplement, Male Reproductive System ØVU
Scrotorrhaphy *see* Repair, Male Reproductive System ØVQ
Scrototomy *see* Drainage, Male Reproductive System ØV9
Sebaceous gland *use* Skin
Second cranial nerve *use* Optic Nerve
Section, cesarean *see* Extraction, Pregnancy 10D
Secura (DR) (VR) *use* Defibrillator Generator in ØJH
➡**Sella turcica** *use* Sphenoid Bone
~~*use* Sphenoid Bone, Right~~
~~*use* Sphenoid Bone, Left~~
Semicircular canal
use Inner Ear, Right
use Inner Ear, Left
Semimembranosus muscle
use Upper Leg Muscle, Right
use Upper Leg Muscle, Left
Semitendinosus muscle
use Upper Leg Muscle, Right
use Upper Leg Muscle, Left
Seprafilm *use* Adhesion Barrier
Septal cartilage *use* Nasal Septum
Septectomy
see Excision, Heart and Great Vessels Ø2B
see Resection, Heart and Great Vessels Ø2T
see Excision, Ear, Nose, Sinus Ø9B
see Resection, Ear, Nose, Sinus Ø9T
Septoplasty
see Repair, Heart and Great Vessels Ø2Q
see Replacement, Heart and Great Vessels Ø2R
see Supplement, Heart and Great Vessels Ø2U
see Repair, Ear, Nose, Sinus Ø9Q
see Replacement, Ear, Nose, Sinus Ø9R
see Reposition, Ear, Nose, Sinus Ø9S
see Supplement, Ear, Nose, Sinus Ø9U
▶**Septostomy, balloon atrial** Ø2163Z7
Septotomy *see* Drainage, Ear, Nose, Sinus Ø99
Sequestrectomy, bone *see* Extirpation
Serratus anterior muscle
use Thorax Muscle, Right
use Thorax Muscle, Left
Serratus posterior muscle
use Trunk Muscle, Right
use Trunk Muscle, Left
Seventh cranial nerve *use* Facial Nerve
Sheffield hybrid external fixator
use External Fixation Device, Hybrid in ØPH
use External Fixation Device, Hybrid in ØPS
use External Fixation Device, Hybrid in ØQH
use External Fixation Device, Hybrid in ØQS
Sheffield ring external fixator
use External Fixation Device, Ring in ØPH
use External Fixation Device, Ring in ØPS
use External Fixation Device, Ring in ØQH
use External Fixation Device, Ring in ØQS
Shirodkar cervical cerclage ØUVC7ZZ
Shock Wave Therapy, Musculoskeletal 6A93
Short gastric artery *use* Splenic Artery
Shortening
see Excision
see Repair
see Reposition

Shunt creation *see* Bypass
Sialoadenectomy
Complete *see* Resection, Mouth and Throat ØCT
Partial *see* Excision, Mouth and Throat ØCB
Sialodochoplasty
see Repair, Mouth and Throat ØCQ
see Replacement, Mouth and Throat ØCR
see Supplement, Mouth and Throat ØCU
Sialoectomy
see Excision, Mouth and Throat ØCB
see Resection, Mouth and Throat ØCT
Sialography *see* Plain Radiography, Ear, Nose, Mouth and Throat B90
Sialolithotomy *see* Extirpation, Mouth and Throat ØCC
Sigmoid artery *use* Inferior Mesenteric Artery
Sigmoid flexure *use* Sigmoid Colon
Sigmoid vein *use* Inferior Mesenteric Vein
Sigmoidectomy
see Excision, Gastrointestinal System ØDB
see Resection, Gastrointestinal System ØDT
Sigmoidorrhaphy *see* Repair, Gastrointestinal System ØDQ
Sigmoidoscopy ØDJD8ZZ
Sigmoidotomy *see* Drainage, Gastrointestinal System ØD9
Single lead pacemaker (atrium) (ventricle) *use* Pacemaker, Single Chamber in ØJH
Single lead rate responsive pacemaker (atrium) (ventricle) *use* Pacemaker, Single Chamber Rate Responsive in ØJH
Sinoatrial node *use* Conduction Mechanism
Sinogram
Abdominal Wall *see* Fluoroscopy, Abdomen and Pelvis BW11
Chest Wall *see* Plain Radiography, Chest BW03
Retroperitoneum *see* Fluoroscopy, Abdomen and Pelvis BW11
Sinus venosus *use* Atrium, Right
Sinusectomy
see Excision, Ear, Nose, Sinus Ø9B
see Resection, Ear, Nose, Sinus Ø9T
Sinusoscopy Ø9JY4ZZ
Sinusotomy *see* Drainage, Ear, Nose, Sinus Ø99
Sirolimus-eluting coronary stent *use* Intraluminal Device, Drug-eluting in Heart and Great Vessels
Sixth cranial nerve *use* Abducens Nerve
Size reduction, breast *see* Excision, Skin and Breast ØHB
SJM Biocor® Stented Valve System *use* Zooplastic Tissue in Heart and Great Vessels
Skene's (paraurethral) gland *use* Vestibular Gland
Skin Substitute, Porcine Liver Derived, Replacement XHRPXL2
Sling
Fascial, orbicularis muscle (mouth) *see* Supplement, Muscle, Facial ØKU1
Levator muscle, for urethral suspension *see* Reposition, Bladder Neck ØTSC
Pubococcygeal, for urethral suspension *see* Reposition, Bladder Neck ØTSC
Rectum *see* Reposition, Rectum ØDSP
Small bowel series *see* Fluoroscopy, Bowel, Small BD13
Small saphenous vein
~~*use* Lesser Saphenous Vein, Right~~
~~*use* Lesser Saphenous Vein, Left~~
▶*use* Saphenous Vein, Right
▶*use* Saphenous Vein, Left
Snaring, polyp, colon *see* Excision, Gastrointestinal System ØDB
Solar (celiac) plexus *use* Abdominal Sympathetic Nerve
Soleus muscle
use Lower Leg Muscle, Right
use Lower Leg Muscle, Left

▶ New   ➡ Revised   ~~deleted~~ Deleted

Spacer
　Insertion of device in
　　Disc
　　　Lumbar Vertebral 0SH2
　　　Lumbosacral 0SH4
　　Joint
　　　Acromioclavicular
　　　　Left 0RHH
　　　　Right 0RHG
　　　Ankle
　　　　Left 0SHG
　　　　Right 0SHF
　　　Carpal
　　　　Left 0RHR
　　　　Right 0RHQ
　　　▶Carpometacarpal
　　　　▶Left 0RHT
　　　　▶Right 0RHS
　　　Cervical Vertebral 0RH1
　　　Cervicothoracic Vertebral 0RH4
　　　Coccygeal 0SH6
　　　Elbow
　　　　Left 0RHM
　　　　Right 0RHL
　　　Finger Phalangeal
　　　　Left 0RHX
　　　　Right 0RHW
　　　Hip
　　　　Left 0SHB
　　　　Right 0SH9
　　　Knee
　　　　Left 0SHD
　　　　Right 0SHC
　　　Lumbar Vertebral 0SH0
　　　Lumbosacral 0SH3
　　　Metacarpocarpal
　　　　Left 0RHT
　　　　Right 0RHS
　　　Metacarpophalangeal
　　　　Left 0RHV
　　　　Right 0RHU
　　　Metatarsal-Phalangeal
　　　　Left 0SHN
　　　　Right 0SHM
　　　Metatarsal-Tarsal
　　　　Left 0SHL
　　　　Right 0SHK
　　　Occipital-cervical 0RH0
　　　Sacrococcygeal 0SH5
　　　Sacroiliac
　　　　Left 0SH8
　　　　Right 0SH7
　　　Shoulder
　　　　Left 0RHK
　　　　Right 0RHJ
　　　Sternoclavicular
　　　　Left 0RHF
　　　　Right 0RHE
　　　Tarsal
　　　　Left 0SHJ
　　　　Right 0SHH
　　　▶Tarsometatarsal
　　　　▶Left 0SHL
　　　　▶Right 0SHK
　　　Temporomandibular
　　　　Left 0RHD
　　　　Right 0RHC
　　　Thoracic Vertebral 0RH6
　　　Thoracolumbar Vertebral 0RHA
　　　Toe Phalangeal
　　　　Left 0SHQ
　　　　Right 0SHP
　　　Wrist
　　　　Left 0RHP
　　　　Right 0RHN
　Removal of device from
　　Acromioclavicular
　　　Left 0RPH
　　　Right 0RPG
　　Ankle
　　　Left 0SPG
　　　Right 0SPF

Spacer *(Continued)*
　Removal of device from *(Continued)*
　　Carpal
　　　Left 0RPR
　　　Right 0RPQ
　　▶Carpometacarpal
　　　▶Left 0RPT
　　　▶Right 0RPS
　　Cervical Vertebral 0RP1
　　Cervicothoracic Vertebral 0RP4
　　Coccygeal 0SP6
　　Elbow
　　　Left 0RPM
　　　Right 0RPL
　　Finger Phalangeal
　　　Left 0RPX
　　　Right 0RPW
　　Hip
　　　Left 0SPB
　　　Right 0SP9
　　Knee
　　　Left 0SPD
　　　Right 0SPC
　　Lumbar Vertebral 0SP0
　　Lumbosacral 0SP3
　　Metacarpocarpal
　　　Left 0RPT
　　　Right 0RPS
　　Metacarpophalangeal
　　　Left 0RPV
　　　Right 0RPU
　　Metatarsal-Phalangeal
　　　Left 0SPN
　　　Right 0SPM
　　Metatarsal-Tarsal
　　　Left 0SPL
　　　Right 0SPK
　　Occipital-cervical 0RP0
　　Sacrococcygeal 0SP5
　　Sacroiliac
　　　Left 0SP8
　　　Right 0SP7
　　Shoulder
　　　Left 0RPK
　　　Right 0RPJ
　　Sternoclavicular
　　　Left 0RPF
　　　Right 0RPE
　　Tarsal
　　　Left 0SPJ
　　　Right 0SPH
　　▶Tarsometatarsal
　　　▶Left 0SPL
　　　▶Right 0SPK
　　Temporomandibular
　　　Left 0RPD
　　　Right 0RPC
　　Thoracic Vertebral 0RP6
　　Thoracolumbar Vertebral 0RPA
　　Toe Phalangeal
　　　Left 0SPQ
　　　Right 0SPP
　　Wrist
　　　Left 0RPP
　　　Right 0RPN
　Revision of device in
　　Acromioclavicular
　　　Left 0RWH
　　　Right 0RWG
　　Ankle
　　　Left 0SWG
　　　Right 0SWF
　　Carpal
　　　Left 0RWR
　　　Right 0RWQ
　　▶Carpometacarpal
　　　▶Left 0RWT
　　　▶Right 0RWS
　　Cervical Vertebral 0RW1
　　Cervicothoracic Vertebral 0RW4
　　Coccygeal 0SW6

Spacer *(Continued)*
　Revision of device in *(Continued)*
　　Elbow
　　　Left 0RWM
　　　Right 0RWL
　　Finger Phalangeal
　　　Left 0RWX
　　　Right 0RWW
　　Hip
　　　Left 0SWB
　　　Right 0SW9
　　Knee
　　　Left 0SWD
　　　Right 0SWC
　　Lumbar Vertebral 0SW0
　　Lumbosacral 0SW3
　　Metacarpocarpal
　　　Left 0RWT
　　　Right 0RWS
　　Metacarpophalangeal
　　　Left 0RWV
　　　Right 0RWU
　　Metatarsal-Phalangeal
　　　Left 0SWN
　　　Right 0SWM
　　Metatarsal-Tarsal
　　　Left 0SWL
　　　Right 0SWK
　　Occipital-cervical 0RW0
　　Sacrococcygeal 0SW5
　　Sacroiliac
　　　Left 0SW8
　　　Right 0SW7
　　Shoulder
　　　Left 0RWK
　　　Right 0RWJ
　　Sternoclavicular
　　　Left 0RWF
　　　Right 0RWE
　　Tarsal
　　　Left 0SWJ
　　　Right 0SWH
　　▶Tarsometatarsal
　　　▶Left 0SWL
　　　▶Right 0SWK
　　Temporomandibular
　　　Left 0RWD
　　　Right 0RWC
　　Thoracic Vertebral 0RW6
　　Thoracolumbar Vertebral 0RWA
　　Toe Phalangeal
　　　Left 0SWQ
　　　Right 0SWP
　　Wrist
　　　Left 0RWP
　　　Right 0RWN
Spectroscopy
　Intravascular 8E023DZ
　Near infrared 8E023DZ
Speech Assessment F00
Speech therapy *see* Speech Treatment,
　Rehabilitation F06
Speech Treatment F06
Sphenoidectomy
　see Excision, Ear, Nose, Sinus 09B
　see Resection, Ear, Nose, Sinus 09T
　see Excision, Head and Facial Bones 0NB
　see Resection, Head and Facial Bones 0NT
Sphenoidotomy *see* Drainage, Ear, Nose,
　Sinus 099
Sphenomandibular ligament *use* Head and
　Neck Bursa and Ligament
Sphenopalatine (pterygopalatine) ganglion *use*
　Head and Neck Sympathetic Nerve
Sphincterorrhaphy, anal *see* Repair, Sphincter,
　Anal 0DQR
Sphincterotomy, anal
　see Division, Sphincter, Anal 0D8R
　see Drainage, Sphincter, Anal 0D9R
⟹**Spinal cord neurostimulator lead** *use*
　Neurostimulator Lead in Central Nervous
　System and Cranial Nerves

S

Spinal growth rods, magnetically controlled
   use Magnetically Controlled Growth Rod(s) in New Technology
Spinal nerve, cervical *use* Cervical Nerve
Spinal nerve, lumbar *use* Lumbar Nerve
Spinal nerve, sacral *use* Sacral Nerve
Spinal nerve, thoracic *use* Thoracic Nerve
Spinal Stabilization Device
   Facet Replacement
      Cervical Vertebral ØRH1
      Cervicothoracic Vertebral ØRH4
      Lumbar Vertebral ØSHØ
      Lumbosacral ØSH3
      Occipital-cervical ØRHØ
      Thoracic Vertebral ØRH6
      Thoracolumbar Vertebral ØRHA
   Interspinous Process
      Cervical Vertebral ØRH1
      Cervicothoracic Vertebral ØRH4
      Lumbar Vertebral ØSHØ
      Lumbosacral ØSH3
      Occipital-cervical ØRHØ
      Thoracic Vertebral ØRH6
      Thoracolumbar Vertebral ØRHA
   Pedicle-Based
      Cervical Vertebral ØRH1
      Cervicothoracic Vertebral ØRH4
      Lumbar Vertebral ØSHØ
      Lumbosacral ØSH3
      Occipital-cervical ØRHØ
      Thoracic Vertebral ØRH6
      Thoracolumbar Vertebral ØRHA
Spinous process
   use Cervical Vertebra
   use Thoracic Vertebra
   use Lumbar Vertebra
Spiral ganglion *use* Acoustic Nerve
Spiration IBV™ Valve System *use* Intraluminal Device, Endobronchial Valve in Respiratory System
Splenectomy
   see Excision, Lymphatic and Hemic Systems Ø7B
   see Resection, Lymphatic and Hemic Systems Ø7T
Splenic flexure *use* Transverse Colon
Splenic plexus *use* Abdominal Sympathetic Nerve
Splenius capitis muscle *use* Head Muscle
Splenius cervicis muscle
   use Neck Muscle, Right
   use Neck Muscle, Left
Splenolysis *see* Release, Lymphatic and Hemic Systems Ø7N
Splenopexy
   see Repair, Lymphatic and Hemic Systems Ø7Q
   see Reposition, Lymphatic and Hemic Systems Ø7S
Splenoplasty *see* Repair, Lymphatic and Hemic Systems Ø7Q
Splenorrhaphy *see* Repair, Lymphatic and Hemic Systems Ø7Q
Splenotomy *see* Drainage, Lymphatic and Hemic Systems Ø79
Splinting, musculoskeletal *see* Immobilization, Anatomical Regions 2W3
SPY system intravascular fluorescence angiography *see* Monitoring, Physiological Systems 4A1
Stapedectomy
   see Excision, Ear, Nose, Sinus Ø9B
   see Resection, Ear, Nose, Sinus Ø9T
Stapediolysis *see* Release, Ear, Nose, Sinus Ø9N
Stapedioplasty
   see Repair, Ear, Nose, Sinus Ø9Q
   see Replacement, Ear, Nose, Sinus Ø9R
   see Supplement, Ear, Nose, Sinus Ø9U
Stapedotomy *see* Drainage, Ear, Nose, Sinus Ø99
Stapes
   use Auditory Ossicle, Right
   use Auditory Ossicle, Left

▶**STELARA®** *use* Other New Technology Therapeutic Substance
Stellate ganglion *use* Head and Neck Sympathetic Nerve
Stem cell transplant *see* Transfusion, Circulatory 3Ø2
Stensen's duct
   use Parotid Duct, Right
   use Parotid Duct, Left
Stent, intraluminal (cardiovascular) (gastrointestinal)(hepatobiliary)(urinary)
   use Intraluminal Device
Stented tissue valve *use* Zooplastic Tissue in Heart and Great Vessels
Stereotactic Radiosurgery
   Abdomen DW23
   Adrenal Gland DG22
   Bile Ducts DF22
   Bladder DT22
   Bone Marrow D72Ø
   Brain DØ2Ø
   Brain Stem DØ21
   Breast
      Left DM2Ø
      Right DM21
   Bronchus DB21
   Cervix DU21
   Chest DW22
   Chest Wall DB27
   Colon DD25
   Diaphragm DB28
   Duodenum DD22
   Ear D92Ø
   Esophagus DD2Ø
   Eye D82Ø
   Gallbladder DF21
   Gamma Beam
      Abdomen DW23JZZ
      Adrenal Gland DG22JZZ
      Bile Ducts DF22JZZ
      Bladder DT22JZZ
      Bone Marrow D72ØJZZ
      Brain DØ2ØJZZ
      Brain Stem DØ21JZZ
      Breast
         Left DM2ØJZZ
         Right DM21JZZ
      Bronchus DB21JZZ
      Cervix DU21JZZ
      Chest DW22JZZ
      Chest Wall DB27JZZ
      Colon DD25JZZ
      Diaphragm DB28JZZ
      Duodenum DD22JZZ
      Ear D92ØJZZ
      Esophagus DD2ØJZZ
      Eye D82ØJZZ
      Gallbladder DF21JZZ
      Gland
         Adrenal DG22JZZ
         Parathyroid DG24JZZ
         Pituitary DG2ØJZZ
         Thyroid DG25JZZ
      Glands, Salivary D926JZZ
      Head and Neck DW21JZZ
      Ileum DD24JZZ
      Jejunum DD23JZZ
      Kidney DT2ØJZZ
      Larynx D92BJZZ
      Liver DF2ØJZZ
      Lung DB22JZZ
      Lymphatics
         Abdomen D726JZZ
         Axillary D724JZZ
         Inguinal D728JZZ
         Neck D723JZZ
         Pelvis D727JZZ
         Thorax D725JZZ
      Mediastinum DB26JZZ
      Mouth D924JZZ
      Nasopharynx D92DJZZ
      Neck and Head DW21JZZ

Stereotactic Radiosurgery *(Continued)*
   Gamma Beam *(Continued)*
      Nerve, Peripheral DØ27JZZ
      Nose D921JZZ
      Ovary DU2ØJZZ
      Palate
         Hard D928JZZ
         Soft D929JZZ
      Pancreas DF23JZZ
      Parathyroid Gland DG24JZZ
      Pelvic Region DW26JZZ
      Pharynx D92CJZZ
      Pineal Body DG21JZZ
      Pituitary Gland DG2ØJZZ
      Pleura DB25JZZ
      Prostate DV2ØJZZ
      Rectum DD27JZZ
      Sinuses D927JZZ
      Spinal Cord DØ26JZZ
      Spleen D722JZZ
      Stomach DD21JZZ
      Testis DV21JZZ
      Thymus D721JZZ
      Thyroid Gland DG25JZZ
      Tongue D925JZZ
      Trachea DB2ØJZZ
      Ureter DT21JZZ
      Urethra DT23JZZ
      Uterus DU22JZZ
   Gland
      Adrenal DG22
      Parathyroid DG24
      Pituitary DG2Ø
      Thyroid DG25
   Glands, Salivary D926
   Head and Neck DW21
   Ileum DD24
   Jejunum DD23
   Kidney DT2Ø
   Larynx D92B
   Liver DF2Ø
   Lung DB22
   Lymphatics
      Abdomen D726
      Axillary D724
      Inguinal D728
      Neck D723
      Pelvis D727
      Thorax D725
   Mediastinum DB26
   Mouth D924
   Nasopharynx D92D
   Neck and Head DW21
   Nerve, Peripheral DØ27
   Nose D921
   Other Photon
      Abdomen DW23DZZ
      Adrenal Gland DG22DZZ
      Bile Ducts DF22DZZ
      Bladder DT22DZZ
      Bone Marrow D72ØDZZ
      Brain DØ2ØDZZ
      Brain Stem DØ21DZZ
      Breast
         Left DM2ØDZZ
         Right DM21DZZ
      Bronchus DB21DZZ
      Cervix DU21DZZ
      Chest DW22DZZ
      Chest Wall DB27DZZ
      Colon DD25DZZ
      Diaphragm DB28DZZ
      Duodenum DD22DZZ
      Ear D92ØDZZ
      Esophagus DD2ØDZZ
      Eye D82ØDZZ
      Gallbladder DF21DZZ
      Gland
         Adrenal DG22DZZ
         Parathyroid DG24DZZ
         Pituitary DG2ØDZZ
         Thyroid DG25DZZ

▶ New   ⇒ Revised   ~~deleted~~ Deleted

Stereotactic Radiosurgery (Continued)
  Other Photon (Continued)
    Glands, Salivary D926DZZ
    Head and Neck DW21DZZ
    Ileum DD24DZZ
    Jejunum DD23DZZ
    Kidney DT20DZZ
    Larynx D92BDZZ
    Liver DF20DZZ
    Lung DB22DZZ
    Lymphatics
      Abdomen D726DZZ
      Axillary D724DZZ
      Inguinal D728DZZ
      Neck D723DZZ
      Pelvis D727DZZ
      Thorax D725DZZ
    Mediastinum DB26DZZ
    Mouth D924DZZ
    Nasopharynx D92DDZZ
    Neck and Head DW21DZZ
    Nerve, Peripheral D027DZZ
    Nose D921DZZ
    Ovary DU20DZZ
    Palate
      Hard D928DZZ
      Soft D929DZZ
    Pancreas DF23DZZ
    Parathyroid Gland DG24DZZ
    Pelvic Region DW26DZZ
    Pharynx D92CDZZ
    Pineal Body DG21DZZ
    Pituitary Gland DG20DZZ
    Pleura DB25DZZ
    Prostate DV20DZZ
    Rectum DD27DZZ
    Sinuses D927DZZ
    Spinal Cord D026DZZ
    Spleen D722DZZ
    Stomach DD21DZZ
    Testis DV21DZZ
    Thymus D721DZZ
    Thyroid Gland DG25DZZ
    Tongue D925DZZ
    Trachea DB20DZZ
    Ureter DT21DZZ
    Urethra DT23DZZ
    Uterus DU22DZZ
  Ovary DU20
  Palate
    Hard D928
    Soft D929
  Pancreas DF23
  Parathyroid Gland DG24
  Particulate
    Abdomen DW23HZZ
    Adrenal Gland DG22HZZ
    Bile Ducts DF22HZZ
    Bladder DT22HZZ
    Bone Marrow D720HZZ
    Brain D020HZZ
    Brain Stem D021HZZ
    Breast
      Left DM20HZZ
      Right DM21HZZ
    Bronchus DB21HZZ
    Cervix DU21HZZ
    Chest DW22HZZ
    Chest Wall DB27HZZ
    Colon DD25HZZ
    Diaphragm DB28HZZ
    Duodenum DD22HZZ
    Ear D920HZZ
    Esophagus DD20HZZ
    Eye D820HZZ
    Gallbladder DF21HZZ
    Gland
      Adrenal DG22HZZ
      Parathyroid DG24HZZ
      Pituitary DG20HZZ
      Thyroid DG25HZZ

Stereotactic Radiosurgery (Continued)
  Particulate (Continued)
    Glands, Salivary D926HZZ
    Head and Neck DW21HZZ
    Ileum DD24HZZ
    Jejunum DD23HZZ
    Kidney DT20HZZ
    Larynx D92BHZZ
    Liver DF20HZZ
    Lung DB22HZZ
    Lymphatics
      Abdomen D726HZZ
      Axillary D724HZZ
      Inguinal D728HZZ
      Neck D723HZZ
      Pelvis D727HZZ
      Thorax D725HZZ
    Mediastinum DB26HZZ
    Mouth D924HZZ
    Nasopharynx D92DHZZ
    Neck and Head DW21HZZ
    Nerve, Peripheral D027HZZ
    Nose D921HZZ
    Ovary DU20HZZ
    Palate
      Hard D928HZZ
      Soft D929HZZ
    Pancreas DF23HZZ
    Parathyroid Gland DG24HZZ
    Pelvic Region DW26HZZ
    Pharynx D92CHZZ
    Pineal Body DG21HZZ
    Pituitary Gland DG20HZZ
    Pleura DB25HZZ
    Prostate DV20HZZ
    Rectum DD27HZZ
    Sinuses D927HZZ
    Spinal Cord D026HZZ
    Spleen D722HZZ
    Stomach DD21HZZ
    Testis DV21HZZ
    Thymus D721HZZ
    Thyroid Gland DG25HZZ
    Tongue D925HZZ
    Trachea DB20HZZ
    Ureter DT21HZZ
    Urethra DT23HZZ
    Uterus DU22HZZ
  Pelvic Region DW26
  Pharynx D92C
  Pineal Body DG21
  Pituitary Gland DG20
  Pleura DB25
  Prostate DV20
  Rectum DD27
  Sinuses D927
  Spinal Cord D026
  Spleen D722
  Stomach DD21
  Testis DV21
  Thymus D721
  Thyroid Gland DG25
  Tongue D925
  Trachea DB20
  Ureter DT21
  Urethra DT23
  Uterus DU22
Sternoclavicular ligament
  use Shoulder Bursa and Ligament, Right
  use Shoulder Bursa and Ligament, Left
Sternocleidomastoid artery
  use Thyroid Artery, Right
  use Thyroid Artery, Left
Sternocleidomastoid muscle
  use Neck Muscle, Right
  use Neck Muscle, Left
Sternocostal ligament
  ~~use Thorax Bursa and Ligament, Right~~
  ~~use Thorax Bursa and Ligament, Left~~
  ▶ use Sternum Bursa and Ligament
  ▶ use Rib(s) Bursa and Ligament

Sternotomy
  see Division, Sternum 0P80
  see Drainage, Sternum 0P90
Stimulation, cardiac
  Cardioversion 5A2204Z
  Electrophysiologic testing see Measurement,
    Cardiac 4A02
Stimulator Generator
  Insertion of device in
    Abdomen 0JH8
    Back 0JH7
    Chest 0JH6
    Multiple Array
      Abdomen 0JH8
      Back 0JH7
      Chest 0JH6
    Multiple Array Rechargeable
      Abdomen 0JH8
      Back 0JH7
      Chest 0JH6
  Removal of device from, Subcutaneous Tissue
    and Fascia, Trunk 0JPT
  Revision of device in, Subcutaneous Tissue
    and Fascia, Trunk 0JWT
  Single Array
    Abdomen 0JH8
    Back 0JH7
    Chest 0JH6
  Single Array Rechargeable
    Abdomen 0JH8
    Back 0JH7
    Chest 0JH6
Stimulator Lead
  Insertion of device in
    Anal Sphincter 0DHR
    Artery
      Left 03HL
      Right 03HK
    Bladder 0THB
    Muscle
      Lower 0KHY
      Upper 0KHX
    Stomach 0DH6
    Ureter 0TH9
  Removal of device from
    Anal Sphincter 0DPR
    Artery, Upper 03PY
    Bladder 0TPB
    Muscle
      Lower 0KPY
      Upper 0KPX
    Stomach 0DP6
    Ureter 0TP9
  Revision of device in
    Anal Sphincter 0DWR
    Artery, Upper 03WY
    Bladder 0TWB
    Muscle
      Lower 0KWY
      Upper 0KWX
    Stomach 0DW6
    Ureter 0TW9
Stoma
  Excision
    Abdominal Wall 0WBFXZ2
    Neck 0WB6XZ2
  Repair
    Abdominal Wall 0WQFXZ2
    Neck 0WQ6XZ2
Stomatoplasty
  see Repair, Mouth and Throat 0CQ
  see Replacement, Mouth and Throat 0CR
  see Supplement, Mouth and Throat 0CU
Stomatorrhaphy see Repair, Mouth and Throat
    0CQ
Stratos LV use Cardiac Resynchronization
    Pacemaker Pulse Generator in 0JH
Stress test
  4A02XM4
  4A12XM4
Stripping see Extraction

S

▶ New   ⇒ Revised   ~~deleted~~ Deleted

Study

Electrophysiologic stimulation, cardiac *see*
    Measurement, Cardiac 4A02
Ocular motility 4A07X7Z
Pulmonary airway flow measurement *see*
    Measurement, Respiratory 4A09
Visual acuity 4A07X0Z
Styloglossus muscle *use* Tongue, Palate,
    Pharynx Muscle
Stylomandibular ligament *use* Head and Neck
    Bursa and Ligament
Stylopharyngeus muscle *use* Tongue, Palate,
    Pharynx Muscle
Subacromial bursa
    use Shoulder Bursa and Ligament, Right
    use Shoulder Bursa and Ligament, Left
Subaortic (common iliac) lymph node *use*
    Lymphatic, Pelvis
~~Subarachnoid space, intracranial use~~
~~Subarachnoid Space~~
Subarachnoid space, spinal *use* Spinal Canal
Subclavicular (apical) lymph node
    use Lymphatic, Right Axillary
    use Lymphatic, Left Axillary
Subclavius muscle
    use Thorax Muscle, Right
    use Thorax Muscle, Left
Subclavius nerve *use* Brachial Plexus Nerve
Subcostal artery *use* Upper Artery
Subcostal muscle
    use Thorax Muscle, Right
    use Thorax Muscle, Left
Subcostal nerve *use* Thoracic Nerve
➡**Subcutaneous injection reservoir, port** *use*
    Vascular Access Device, Totally
    Implantable in Subcutaneous Tissue and
    Fascia
Subcutaneous injection reservoir, pump *use*
    Infusion Device, Pump in Subcutaneous
    Tissue and Fascia
Subdermal progesterone implant *use*
    Contraceptive Device in Subcutaneous
    Tissue and Fascia
~~Subdural space, intracranial use Subdural~~
~~Space~~
Subdural space, spinal *use* Spinal Canal
Submandibular ganglion
    use Head and Neck Sympathetic Nerve
    use Facial Nerve
Submandibular gland
    use Submaxillary Gland, Right
    use Submaxillary Gland, Left
Submandibular lymph node *use* Lymphatic,
    Head
Submaxillary ganglion *use* Head and Neck
    Sympathetic Nerve
Submaxillary lymph node *use* Lymphatic,
    Head
Submental artery *use* Face Artery
Submental lymph node *use* Lymphatic, Head
Submucous (Meissner's) plexus *use* Abdominal
    Sympathetic Nerve
Suboccipital nerve *use* Cervical Nerve
Suboccipital venous plexus
    use Vertebral Vein, Right
    use Vertebral Vein, Left
Subparotid lymph node *use* Lymphatic, Head
Subscapular (posterior) lymph node
    use Lymphatic, Right Axillary
    use Lymphatic, Left Axillary
Subscapular aponeurosis
    use Subcutaneous Tissue and Fascia, Right
        Upper Arm
    use Subcutaneous Tissue and Fascia, Left
        Upper Arm
Subscapular artery
    use Axillary Artery, Right
    use Axillary Artery, Left
Subscapularis muscle
    use Shoulder Muscle, Right
    use Shoulder Muscle, Left

Substance Abuse Treatment

Counseling
    Family, for substance abuse, Other Family
        Counseling HZ63ZZZ
    Group
        12-Step HZ43ZZZ
        Behavioral HZ41ZZZ
        Cognitive HZ40ZZZ
        Cognitive-Behavioral HZ42ZZZ
        Confrontational HZ48ZZZ
        Continuing Care HZ49ZZZ
        Infectious Disease
            Post-Test HZ4CZZZ
            Pre-Test HZ4CZZZ
        Interpersonal HZ44ZZZ
        Motivational Enhancement HZ47ZZZ
        Psychoeducation HZ46ZZZ
        Spiritual HZ4BZZZ
        Vocational HZ45ZZZ
    Individual
        12-Step HZ33ZZZ
        Behavioral HZ31ZZZ
        Cognitive HZ30ZZZ
        Cognitive-Behavioral HZ32ZZZ
        Confrontational HZ38ZZZ
        Continuing Care HZ39ZZZ
        Infectious Disease
            Post-Test HZ3CZZZ
            Pre-Test HZ3CZZZ
        Interpersonal HZ34ZZZ
        Motivational Enhancement HZ37ZZZ
        Psychoeducation HZ36ZZZ
        Spiritual HZ3BZZZ
        Vocational HZ35ZZZ
    Detoxification Services, for substance abuse
        HZ2ZZZZ
    Medication Management
        Antabuse HZ83ZZZ
        Bupropion HZ87ZZZ
        Clonidine HZ86ZZZ
        Levo-alpha-acetyl-methadol (LAAM)
            HZ82ZZZ
        Methadone Maintenance HZ81ZZZ
        Naloxone HZ85ZZZ
        Naltrexone HZ84ZZZ
        Nicotine Replacement HZ80ZZZ
        Other Replacement Medication HZ89ZZZ
        Psychiatric Medication HZ88ZZZ
    Pharmacotherapy
        Antabuse HZ93ZZZ
        Bupropion HZ97ZZZ
        Clonidine HZ96ZZZ
        Levo-alpha-acetyl-methadol (LAAM)
            HZ92ZZZ
        Methadone Maintenance HZ91ZZZ
        Naloxone HZ95ZZZ
        Naltrexone HZ94ZZZ
        Nicotine Replacement HZ90ZZZ
        Psychiatric Medication HZ98ZZZ
        Replacement Medication, Other HZ99ZZZ
    Psychotherapy
        12-Step HZ53ZZZ
        Behavioral HZ51ZZZ
        Cognitive HZ50ZZZ
        Cognitive-Behavioral HZ52ZZZ
        Confrontational HZ58ZZZ
        Interactive HZ55ZZZ
        Interpersonal HZ54ZZZ
        Motivational Enhancement HZ57ZZZ
        Psychoanalysis HZ5BZZZ
        Psychodynamic HZ5CZZZ
        Psychoeducation HZ56ZZZ
        Psychophysiological HZ5DZZZ
        Supportive HZ59ZZZ
Substantia nigra *use* Basal Ganglia
Subtalar (talocalcaneal) joint
    use Tarsal Joint, Right
    use Tarsal Joint, Left
Subtalar ligament
    use Foot Bursa and Ligament, Right
    use Foot Bursa and Ligament, Left

Subthalamic nucleus *use* Basal Ganglia
Suction curettage (D&C), nonobstetric *see*
    Extraction, Endometrium 0UDB
Suction curettage, obstetric post-delivery
    see Extraction, Products of Conception,
    Retained 10D1
Superficial circumflex iliac vein
    ~~use Greater Saphenous Vein, Right~~
    ~~use Greater Saphenous Vein, Left~~
▶*use* Saphenous Vein, Right
▶*use* Saphenous Vein, Left
Superficial epigastric artery
    use Femoral Artery, Right
    use Femoral Artery, Left
Superficial epigastric vein
    ~~use Greater Saphenous Vein, Right~~
    ~~use Greater Saphenous Vein, Left~~
▶*use* Saphenous Vein, Right
▶*use* Saphenous Vein, Left
Superficial Inferior Epigastric Artery Flap
    ~~Bilateral 0HRV078~~
    ~~Left 0HRU078~~
    ~~Right 0HRT078~~
▶Replacement
    ▶Bilateral 0HRV078
    ▶Left 0HRU078
    ▶Right 0HRT078
▶Transfer
    ▶Left 0KXG
    ▶Right 0KXF
Superficial palmar arch
    use Hand Artery, Right
    use Hand Artery, Left
Superficial palmar venous arch
    use Hand Vein, Right
    use Hand Vein, Left
Superficial temporal artery
    use Temporal Artery, Right
    use Temporal Artery, Left
Superficial transverse perineal muscle *use*
    Perineum Muscle
Superior cardiac nerve *use* Thoracic
    Sympathetic Nerve
Superior cerebellar vein *use* Intracranial Vein
Superior cerebral vein *use* Intracranial Vein
Superior clunic (cluneal) nerve *use* Lumbar
    Nerve
Superior epigastric artery
    use Internal Mammary Artery, Right
    use Internal Mammary Artery, Left
Superior genicular artery
    use Popliteal Artery, Right
    use Popliteal Artery, Left
Superior gluteal artery
    use Internal Iliac Artery, Right
    use Internal Iliac Artery, Left
Superior gluteal nerve *use* Lumbar Plexus Nerve
Superior hypogastric plexus *use* Abdominal
    Sympathetic Nerve
Superior labial artery *use* Face Artery
Superior laryngeal artery
    use Thyroid Artery, Right
    use Thyroid Artery, Left
Superior laryngeal nerve *use* Vagus Nerve
Superior longitudinal muscle *use* Tongue,
    Palate, Pharynx Muscle
Superior mesenteric ganglion *use* Abdominal
    Sympathetic Nerve
Superior mesenteric lymph node *use*
    Lymphatic, Mesenteric
Superior mesenteric plexus *use* Abdominal
    Sympathetic Nerve
Superior oblique muscle
    use Extraocular Muscle, Right
    use Extraocular Muscle, Left
Superior olivary nucleus *use* Pons
Superior rectal artery *use* Inferior Mesenteric
    Artery
Superior rectal vein *use* Inferior Mesenteric Vein
Superior rectus muscle
    use Extraocular Muscle, Right
    use Extraocular Muscle, Left

▶ New   ➡ Revised   ~~deleted~~ Deleted

Superior tarsal plate
  use Upper Eyelid, Right
  use Upper Eyelid, Left
Superior thoracic artery
  use Axillary Artery, Right
  use Axillary Artery, Left
Superior thyroid artery
  use External Carotid Artery, Right
  use External Carotid Artery, Left
  use Thyroid Artery, Right
  use Thyroid Artery, Left
Superior turbinate *use* Nasal Turbinate
Superior ulnar collateral artery
  use Brachial Artery, Right
  use Brachial Artery, Left
Supplement
  Abdominal Wall 0WUF
  Acetabulum
    Left 0QU5
    Right 0QU4
  Ampulla of Vater 0FUC
  Anal Sphincter 0DUR
  Ankle Region
    Left 0YUL
    Right 0YUK
  Anus 0DUQ
  Aorta
    Abdominal 04U0
    Thoracic
      Ascending/Arch 02UX
      Descending 02UW
  Arm
    Lower
      Left 0XUF
      Right 0XUD
    Upper
      Left 0XU9
      Right 0XU8
  Artery
    Anterior Tibial
      Left 04UQ
      Right 04UP
    Axillary
      Left 03U6
      Right 03U5
    Brachial
      Left 03U8
      Right 03U7
    Celiac 04U1
    Colic
      Left 04U7
      Middle 04U8
      Right 04U6
    Common Carotid
      Left 03UJ
      Right 03UH
    Common Iliac
      Left 04UD
      Right 04UC
    External Carotid
      Left 03UN
      Right 03UM
    External Iliac
      Left 04UJ
      Right 04UH
    Face 03UR
    Femoral
      Left 04UL
      Right 04UK
    Foot
      Left 04UW
      Right 04UV
    Gastric 04U2
    Hand
      Left 03UF
      Right 03UD
    Hepatic 04U3
    Inferior Mesenteric 04UB
    Innominate 03U2
    Internal Carotid
      Left 03UL
      Right 03UK

Supplement *(Continued)*
  Artery *(Continued)*
    Internal Iliac
      Left 04UF
      Right 04UE
    Internal Mammary
      Left 03U1
      Right 03U0
    Intracranial 03UG
    Lower 04UY
    Peroneal
      Left 04UU
      Right 04UT
    Popliteal
      Left 04UN
      Right 04UM
    Posterior Tibial
      Left 04US
      Right 04UR
    Pulmonary
      Left 02UR
      Right 02UQ
    Pulmonary Trunk 02UP
    Radial
      Left 03UC
      Right 03UB
    Renal
      Left 04UA
      Right 04U9
    Splenic 04U4
    Subclavian
      Left 03U4
      Right 03U3
    Superior Mesenteric 04U5
    Temporal
      Left 03UT
      Right 03US
    Thyroid
      Left 03UV
      Right 03UU
    Ulnar
      Left 03UA
      Right 03U9
    Upper 03UY
    Vertebral
      Left 03UQ
      Right 03UP
  Atrium
    Left 02U7
    Right 02U6
  Auditory Ossicle
  ➠Left 09UA
  ➠Right 09U9
  Axilla
    Left 0XU5
    Right 0XU4
  Back
    Lower 0WUL
    Upper 0WUK
  Bladder 0TUB
  Bladder Neck 0TUC
  Bone
    Ethmoid
      Left 0NUG
      Right 0NUF
    ➠Frontal 0NU1
      ~~Left 0NU2~~
      ~~Right 0NU1~~
    Hyoid 0NUX
    Lacrimal
      Left 0NUJ
      Right 0NUH
    Nasal 0NUB
    ➠Occipital 0NU7
      ~~Left 0NU8~~
      ~~Right 0NU7~~
    Palatine
      Left 0NUL
      Right 0NUK
    Parietal
      Left 0NU4
      Right 0NU3

Supplement *(Continued)*
  Bone *(Continued)*
    Pelvic
      Left 0QU3
      Right 0QU2
    ➠Sphenoid 0NUC
      ~~Left 0NUD~~
      ~~Right 0NUC~~
    Temporal
      Left 0NU6
      Right 0NU5
    Zygomatic
      Left 0NUN
      Right 0NUM
  Breast
    Bilateral 0HUV
    Left 0HUU
    Right 0HUT
  Bronchus
    Lingula 0BU9
    Lower Lobe
      Left 0BUB
      Right 0BU6
    Main
      Left 0BU7
      Right 0BU3
    Middle Lobe, Right 0BU5
    Upper Lobe
      Left 0BU8
      Right 0BU4
  Buccal Mucosa 0CU4
  Bursa and Ligament
    Abdomen
      Left 0MUJ
      Right 0MUH
    Ankle
      Left 0MUR
      Right 0MUQ
    Elbow
      Left 0MU4
      Right 0MU3
    Foot
      Left 0MUT
      Right 0MUS
    Hand
      Left 0MU8
      Right 0MU7
    Head and Neck 0MU0
    Hip
      Left 0MUM
      Right 0MUL
    Knee
      Left 0MUP
      Right 0MUN
    Lower Extremity
      Left 0MUW
      Right 0MUV
    Perineum 0MUK
    ▶Rib(s) 0MUG
    Shoulder
      Left 0MU2
      Right 0MU1
    ▶Spine
      ▶Lower 0MUD
      ▶Upper 0MUC
    ▶Sternum 0MUF
    ~~Thorax~~
      ~~Left 0MUG~~
      ~~Right 0MUF~~
    ~~Trunk~~
      ~~Left 0MUD~~
      ~~Right 0MUC~~
    Upper Extremity
      Left 0MUB
      Right 0MU9
    Wrist
      Left 0MU6
      Right 0MU5
  Buttock
    Left 0YU1
    Right 0YU0

▶ New   ➠ Revised   ~~deleted~~ Deleted

Supplement *(Continued)*
Carina 0BU2
Carpal
  Left 0PUN
  Right 0PUM
Cecum 0DUH
Cerebral Meninges 00U1
▶Cerebral Ventricle 00U6
Chest Wall 0WU8
Chordae Tendineae 02U9
Cisterna Chyli 07UL
Clavicle
  Left 0PUB
  Right 0PU9
Clitoris 0UUJ
Coccyx 0QUS
Colon
  Ascending 0DUK
  Descending 0DUM
  Sigmoid 0DUN
  Transverse 0DUL
Cord
  Bilateral 0VUH
  Left 0VUG
  Right 0VUF
Cornea
  Left 08U9
  Right 08U8
Cul-de-sac 0UUF
⟹Diaphragm 0BUT
  ~~Left 0BUS~~
  ~~Right 0BUR~~
Disc
  Cervical Vertebral 0RU3
  Cervicothoracic Vertebral 0RU5
  Lumbar Vertebral 0SU2
  Lumbosacral 0SU4
  Thoracic Vertebral 0RU9
  Thoracolumbar Vertebral 0RUB
Duct
  Common Bile 0FU9
  Cystic 0FU8
  Hepatic
   ▶Common 0FU7
   Left 0FU6
   Right 0FU5
  Lacrimal
   Left 08UY
   Right 08UX
  Pancreatic 0FUD
   Accessory 0FUF
Duodenum 0DU9
Dura Mater 00U2
Ear
  External
   Bilateral 09U2
   Left 09U1
   Right 09U0
  Inner
   ⟹Left 09UE
   ⟹Right 09UD
  Middle
   ⟹Left 09U6
   ⟹Right 09U5
Elbow Region
  Left 0XUC
  Right 0XUB
Epididymis
  Bilateral 0VUL
  Left 0VUK
  Right 0VUJ
Epiglottis 0CUR
Esophagogastric Junction 0DU4
Esophagus 0DU5
  Lower 0DU3
  Middle 0DU2
  Upper 0DU1
Extremity
  Lower
   Left 0YUB
   Right 0YU9

Supplement *(Continued)*
Extremity *(Continued)*
  Upper
   Left 0XU7
   Right 0XU6
Eye
  Left 08U1
  Right 08U0
Eyelid
  Lower
   Left 08UR
   Right 08UQ
  Upper
   Left 08UP
   Right 08UN
Face 0WU2
Fallopian Tube
  Left 0UU6
  Right 0UU5
Fallopian Tubes, Bilateral 0UU7
Femoral Region
  Bilateral 0YUE
  Left 0YU8
  Right 0YU7
Femoral Shaft
  Left 0QU9
  Right 0QU8
Femur
  Lower
   Left 0QUC
   Right 0QUB
  Upper
   Left 0QU7
   Right 0QU6
Fibula
  Left 0QUK
  Right 0QUJ
Finger
  Index
   Left 0XUP
   Right 0XUN
  Little
   Left 0XUW
   Right 0XUV
  Middle
   Left 0XUR
   Right 0XUQ
  Ring
   Left 0XUT
   Right 0XUS
Foot
  Left 0YUN
  Right 0YUM
Gingiva
  Lower 0CU6
  Upper 0CU5
Glenoid Cavity
  Left 0PU8
  Right 0PU7
Hand
  Left 0XUK
  Right 0XUJ
Head 0WU0
Heart 02UA
Humeral Head
  Left 0PUD
  Right 0PUC
Humeral Shaft
  Left 0PUG
  Right 0PUF
Hymen 0UUK
Ileocecal Valve 0DUC
Ileum 0DUB
Inguinal Region
  Bilateral 0YUA
  Left 0YU6
  Right 0YU5
Intestine
  Large 0DUE
   Left 0DUG
   Right 0DUF
  Small 0DU8

Supplement *(Continued)*
Iris
  Left 08UD
  Right 08UC
Jaw
  Lower 0WU5
  Upper 0WU4
Jejunum 0DUA
Joint
  Acromioclavicular
   Left 0RUH
   Right 0RUG
  Ankle
   Left 0SUG
   Right 0SUF
  Carpal
   Left 0RUR
   Right 0RUQ
  ▶Carpometacarpal
   ▶Left 0RUT
   ▶Right 0RUS
  Cervical Vertebral 0RU1
  Cervicothoracic Vertebral 0RU4
  Coccygeal 0SU6
  Elbow
   Left 0RUM
   Right 0RUL
  Finger Phalangeal
   Left 0RUX
   Right 0RUW
  Hip
   Left 0SUB
    Acetabular Surface 0SUE
    Femoral Surface 0SUS
   Right 0SU9
    Acetabular Surface 0SUA
    Femoral Surface 0SUR
  Knee
   Left 0SUD
    Femoral Surface 0SUU09Z
    Tibial Surface 0SUW09Z
   Right 0SUC
    Femoral Surface 0SUT09Z
    Tibial Surface 0SUV09Z
  Lumbar Vertebral 0SU0
  Lumbosacral 0SU3
  ~~Metacarpocarpal~~
   ~~Left 0RUT~~
   ~~Right 0RUS~~
  Metacarpophalangeal
   Left 0RUV
   Right 0RUU
  Metatarsal-Phalangeal
   Left 0SUN
   Right 0SUM
  ~~Metatarsal-Tarsal~~
   ~~Left 0SUL~~
   ~~Right 0SUK~~
  Occipital-cervical 0RU0
  Sacrococcygeal 0SU5
  Sacroiliac
   Left 0SU8
   Right 0SU7
  Shoulder
   Left 0RUK
   Right 0RUJ
  Sternoclavicular
   Left 0RUF
   Right 0RUE
  Tarsal
   Left 0SUJ
   Right 0SUH
  ▶Tarsometatarsal
   ▶Left 0SUL
   ▶Right 0SUK
  Temporomandibular
   Left 0RUD
   Right 0RUC
  Thoracic Vertebral 0RU6
  Thoracolumbar Vertebral 0RUA

▶ New   ⟹ Revised   ~~deleted~~ Deleted

Supplement *(Continued)*
Joint *(Continued)*
Toe Phalangeal
Left 0SUQ
Right 0SUP
Wrist
Left 0RUP
Right 0RUN
Kidney Pelvis
Left 0TU4
Right 0TU3
Knee Region
Left 0YUG
Right 0YUF
Larynx 0CUS
Leg
Lower
Left 0YUJ
Right 0YUH
Upper
Left 0YUD
Right 0YUC
Lip
Lower 0CU1
Upper 0CU0
Lymphatic
Aortic 07UD
Axillary
Left 07U6
Right 07U5
Head 07U0
Inguinal
Left 07UJ
Right 07UH
Internal Mammary
Left 07U9
Right 07U8
Lower Extremity
Left 07UG
Right 07UF
Mesenteric 07UB
Neck
Left 07U2
Right 07U1
Pelvis 07UC
Thoracic Duct 07UK
Thorax 07U7
Upper Extremity
Left 07U4
Right 07U3
Mandible
Left 0NUV
Right 0NUT
➥Maxilla 0NUR
~~Left 0NUS~~
~~Right 0NUR~~
Mediastinum 0WUC
Mesentery 0DUV
Metacarpal
Left 0PUQ
Right 0PUP
Metatarsal
Left 0QUP
Right 0QUN
Muscle
Abdomen
Left 0KUL
Right 0KUK
Extraocular
Left 08UM
Right 08UL
Facial 0KU1
Foot
Left 0KUW
Right 0KUV
Hand
Left 0KUD
Right 0KUC
Head 0KU0
Hip
Left 0KUP
Right 0KUN

Supplement *(Continued)*
Muscle *(Continued)*
Lower Arm and Wrist
Left 0KUB
Right 0KU9
Lower Leg
Left 0KUT
Right 0KUS
Neck
Left 0KU3
Right 0KU2
Papillary 02UD
Perineum 0KUM
Shoulder
Left 0KU6
Right 0KU5
Thorax
Left 0KUJ
Right 0KUH
Tongue, Palate, Pharynx 0KU4
Trunk
Left 0KUG
Right 0KUF
Upper Arm
Left 0KU8
Right 0KU7
Upper Leg
Left 0KUR
Right 0KUQ
▶Nasal Mucosa and Soft Tissue 09UK
Nasopharynx 09UN
Neck 0WU6
Nerve
Abducens 00UL
Accessory 00UR
Acoustic 00UN
Cervical 01U1
Facial 00UM
Femoral 01UD
Glossopharyngeal 00UP
Hypoglossal 00US
Lumbar 01UB
Median 01U5
Oculomotor 00UH
Olfactory 00UF
Optic 00UG
Peroneal 01UH
Phrenic 01U2
Pudendal 01UC
Radial 01U6
Sacral 01UR
Sciatic 01UF
Thoracic 01U8
Tibial 01UG
Trigeminal 00UK
Trochlear 00UJ
Ulnar 01U4
Vagus 00UQ
Nipple
Left 0HUX
Right 0HUW
~~Nose 09UK~~
➥Omentum 0DUU
~~Greater 0DUS~~
~~Lesser 0DUT~~
Orbit
Left 0NUQ
Right 0NUP
Palate
Hard 0CU2
Soft 0CU3
Patella
Left 0QUF
Right 0QUD
Penis 0VUS
Pericardium 02UN
Perineum
Female 0WUN
Male 0WUM
Peritoneum 0DUW

Supplement *(Continued)*
Phalanx
Finger
Left 0PUV
Right 0PUT
Thumb
Left 0PUS
Right 0PUR
Toe
Left 0QUR
Right 0QUQ
Pharynx 0CUM
Prepuce 0VUT
Radius
Left 0PUJ
Right 0PUH
Rectum 0DUP
Retina
Left 08UF
Right 08UE
Retinal Vessel
Left 08UH
Right 08UG
~~Rib~~
~~Left 0PU2~~
~~Right 0PU1~~
▶Ribs
▶1 to 2 0PU1
▶3 or More 0PU2
Sacrum 0QU1
Scapula
Left 0PU6
Right 0PU5
Scrotum 0VU5
Septum
Atrial 02U5
Nasal 09UM
Ventricular 02UM
Shoulder Region
Left 0XU3
Right 0XU2
Skull 0NU0
Spinal Meninges 00UT
Sternum 0PU0
Stomach 0DU6
Pylorus 0DU7
Subcutaneous Tissue and Fascia
Abdomen 0JU8
Back 0JU7
Buttock 0JU9
Chest 0JU6
Face 0JU1
Foot
Left 0JUR
Right 0JUQ
Hand
Left 0JUK
Right 0JUJ
Lower Arm
Left 0JUH
Right 0JUG
Lower Leg
Left 0JUP
Right 0JUN
Neck
~~Anterior 0JU4~~
~~Posterior 0JU5~~
▶Left 0JU5
▶Right 0JU4
Pelvic Region 0JUC
Perineum 0JUB
Scalp 0JU0
Upper Arm
Left 0JUF
Right 0JUD
Upper Leg
Left 0JUM
Right 0JUL
Tarsal
Left 0QUM
Right 0QUL

▶ New   ➥ Revised   ~~deleted~~ Deleted

Supplement *(Continued)*
Tendon
  Abdomen
    Left 0LUG
    Right 0LUF
  Ankle
    Left 0LUT
    Right 0LUS
  Foot
    Left 0LUW
    Right 0LUV
  Hand
    Left 0LU8
    Right 0LU7
  Head and Neck 0LU0
  Hip
    Left 0LUK
    Right 0LUJ
  Knee
    Left 0LUR
    Right 0LUQ
  Lower Arm and Wrist
    Left 0LU6
    Right 0LU5
  Lower Leg
    Left 0LUP
    Right 0LUN
  Perineum 0LUH
  Shoulder
    Left 0LU2
    Right 0LU1
  Thorax
    Left 0LUD
    Right 0LUC
  Trunk
    Left 0LUB
    Right 0LU9
  Upper Arm
    Left 0LU4
    Right 0LU3
  Upper Leg
    Left 0LUM
    Right 0LUL
Testis
  Bilateral 0VUC0
  Left 0VUB0
  Right 0VU90
Thumb
  Left 0XUM
  Right 0XUL
Tibia
  Left 0QUH
  Right 0QUG
Toe
  1st
    Left 0YUQ
    Right 0YUP
  2nd
    Left 0YUS
    Right 0YUR
  3rd
    Left 0YUU
    Right 0YUT
  4th
    Left 0YUW
    Right 0YUV
  5th
    Left 0YUY
    Right 0YUX
Tongue 0CU7
Trachea 0BU1
Tunica Vaginalis
  Left 0VU7
  Right 0VU6
Turbinate, Nasal 09UL
Tympanic Membrane
  Left 09U8
  Right 09U7
Ulna
  Left 0PUL
  Right 0PUK

Supplement *(Continued)*
Ureter
  Left 0TU7
  Right 0TU6
Urethra 0TUD
Uterine Supporting Structure 0UU4
Uvula 0CUN
Vagina 0UUG
Valve
  Aortic 02UF
  Mitral 02UG
  Pulmonary 02UH
  Tricuspid 02UJ
Vas Deferens
  Bilateral 0VUQ
  Left 0VUP
  Right 0VUN
Vein
  Axillary
    Left 05U8
    Right 05U7
  Azygos 05U0
  Basilic
    Left 05UC
    Right 05UB
  Brachial
    Left 05UA
    Right 05U9
  Cephalic
    Left 05UF
    Right 05UD
  Colic 06U7
  Common Iliac
    Left 06UD
    Right 06UC
  Esophageal 06U3
  External Iliac
    Left 06UG
    Right 06UF
  External Jugular
    Left 05UQ
    Right 05UP
  Face
    Left 05UV
    Right 05UT
  Femoral
    Left 06UN
    Right 06UM
  Foot
    Left 06UV
    Right 06UT
  Gastric 06U2
  ~~Greater Saphenous~~
    ~~Left 06UQ~~
    ~~Right 06UP~~
  Hand
    Left 05UH
    Right 05UG
  Hemiazygos 05U1
  Hepatic 06U4
  Hypogastric
    Left 06UJ
    Right 06UH
  Inferior Mesenteric 06U6
  Innominate
    Left 05U4
    Right 05U3
  Internal Jugular
    Left 05UN
    Right 05UM
  Intracranial 05UL
  ~~Lesser Saphenous~~
    ~~Left 06US~~
    ~~Right 06UR~~
  Lower 06UY
  Portal 06U8
  Pulmonary
    Left 02UT
    Right 02US
  Renal
    Left 06UB
    Right 06U9

Supplement *(Continued)*
Vein *(Continued)*
  ▶Saphenous
    ▶Left 06UQ
    ▶Right 06UP
  Splenic 06U1
  Subclavian
    Left 05U6
    Right 05U5
  Superior Mesenteric 06U5
  Upper 05UY
  Vertebral
    Left 05US
    Right 05UR
Vena Cava
  Inferior 06U0
  Superior 02UV
Ventricle
  Left 02UL
  Right 02UK
Vertebra
  Cervical 0PU3
  Lumbar 0QU0
  Thoracic 0PU4
Vesicle
  Bilateral 0VU3
  Left 0VU2
  Right 0VU1
Vocal Cord
  Left 0CUV
  Right 0CUT
Vulva 0UUM
Wrist Region
  Left 0XUH
  Right 0XUG
Supraclavicular (Virchow's) lymph node
  use Lymphatic, Right Neck
  use Lymphatic, Left Neck
Supraclavicular nerve *use* Cervical Plexus
Suprahyoid lymph node *use* Lymphatic, Head
Suprahyoid muscle
  use Neck Muscle, Right
  use Neck Muscle, Left
Suprainguinal lymph node *use* Lymphatic, Pelvis
Supraorbital vein
  use Face Vein, Right
  use Face Vein, Left
Suprarenal gland
  use Adrenal Gland, Left
  use Adrenal Gland, Right
  use Adrenal Gland, Bilateral
  use Adrenal Gland
Suprarenal plexus *use* Abdominal Sympathetic Nerve
Suprascapular nerve *use* Brachial Plexus Nerve
Supraspinatus fascia
  use Subcutaneous Tissue and Fascia, Right Upper Arm
  use Subcutaneous Tissue and Fascia, Left Upper Arm
Supraspinatus muscle
  use Shoulder Muscle, Right
  use Shoulder Muscle, Left
Supraspinous ligament
  ~~use Trunk Bursa and Ligament, Right~~
  ~~use Trunk Bursa and Ligament, Left~~
  ▶*use* Upper Spine Bursa and Ligament
  ▶*use* Lower Spine Bursa and Ligament
Suprasternal notch *use* Sternum
Supratrochlear lymph node
  use Lymphatic, Right Upper Extremity
  use Lymphatic, Left Upper Extremity
Sural artery
  use Popliteal Artery, Right
  use Popliteal Artery, Left
Suspension
  Bladder Neck *see* Reposition, Bladder Neck 0TSC
  Kidney *see* Reposition, Urinary System 0TS
  Urethra *see* Reposition, Urinary System 0TS

▶ New   ⟹ Revised   ~~deleted~~ Deleted

Suspension *(Continued)*
    Urethrovesical *see* Reposition, Bladder Neck
        ØTSC
    Uterus *see* Reposition, Uterus ØUS9
    Vagina *see* Reposition, Vagina ØUSG
Suture
    Laceration repair *see* Repair
    Ligation *see* Occlusion
Suture Removal
    Extremity
        Lower 8EØYXY8
        Upper 8EØXXY8
    Head and Neck Region 8EØ9XY8
    Trunk Region 8EØWXY8

Sutureless valve, Perceval *use* Zooplastic
    Tissue, Rapid Deployment Technique in
    New Technology
Sweat gland *use* Skin
Sympathectomy
    see Excision, Peripheral Nervous System Ø1B
SynCardia Total Artificial Heart *use* Synthetic
    Substitute
Synchra CRT-P *use* Cardiac Resynchronization
    Pacemaker Pulse Generator in ØJH
SynchroMed pump *use* Infusion Device, Pump
    in Subcutaneous Tissue and Fascia

Synechiotomy, iris *see* Release, Eye Ø8N
Synovectomy
    Lower joint *see* Excision, Lower Joints ØSB
    Upper joint *see* Excision, Upper Joints ØRB
Systemic Nuclear Medicine Therapy
    Abdomen CW7Ø
    Anatomical Regions, Multiple CW7YYZZ
    Chest CW73
    Thyroid CW7G
    Whole Body CW7N

T

Takedown
  Arteriovenous shunt *see* Removal of device from, Upper Arteries Ø3P
  Arteriovenous shunt, with creation of new shunt *see* Bypass, Upper Arteries Ø31
➡**Stoma**
  ▶*see* Excision
  ▶*see* Reposition
Talent® Converter *use* Intraluminal Device
Talent® Occluder *use* Intraluminal Device
Talent® Stent Graft (abdominal) (thoracic) *use* Intraluminal Device
Talocalcaneal (subtalar) joint
  use Tarsal Joint, Right
  use Tarsal Joint, Left
Talocalcaneal ligament
  use Foot Bursa and Ligament, Right
  use Foot Bursa and Ligament, Left
Talocalcaneonavicular joint
  use Tarsal Joint, Right
  use Tarsal Joint, Left
Talocalcaneonavicular ligament
  use Foot Bursa and Ligament, Right
  use Foot Bursa and Ligament, Left
Talocrural joint
  use Ankle Joint, Right
  use Ankle Joint, Left
Talofibular ligament
  use Ankle Bursa and Ligament, Right
  use Ankle Bursa and Ligament, Left
Talus bone
  use Tarsal, Right
  use Tarsal, Left
➡**TandemHeart® System** *use* Short-term External Heart Assist System in Heart and Great Vessels
Tarsectomy
  see Excision, Lower Bones ØQB
  see Resection, Lower Bones ØQT
~~Tarsometatarsal joint~~
  ~~use Metatarsal-Tarsal Joint, Right~~
  ~~use Metatarsal-Tarsal Joint, Left~~
Tarsometatarsal ligament
  use Foot Bursa and Ligament, Right
  use Foot Bursa and Ligament, Left
Tarsorrhaphy *see* Repair, Eye Ø8Q
Tattooing
  Cornea 3EØCXMZ
  Skin *see* Introduction of substance in or on Skin 3EØØ
TAXUS® Liberté® Paclitaxel-eluting Coronary Stent System *use* Intraluminal Device, Drug-eluting in Heart and Great Vessels
TBNA (transbronchial needle aspiration) *see* Drainage, Respiratory System ØB9
Telemetry
  4A12X4Z
  Ambulatory 4A12X45
Temperature gradient study 4AØZXKZ
Temporal lobe *use* Cerebral Hemisphere
Temporalis muscle *use* Head Muscle
Temporoparietalis muscle *use* Head Muscle
Tendolysis *see* Release, Tendons ØLN
Tendonectomy
  see Excision, Tendons ØLB
  see Resection, Tendons ØLT
Tendonoplasty, tenoplasty
  see Repair, Tendons ØLQ
  see Replacement, Tendons ØLR
  see Supplement, Tendons ØLU
Tendorrhaphy *see* Repair, Tendons ØLQ
Tendototomy
  see Division, Tendons ØL8
  see Drainage, Tendons ØL9
Tenectomy, tenonectomy
  see Excision, Tendons ØLB
  see Resection, Tendons ØLT
Tenolysis *see* Release, Tendons ØLN
Tenontorrhaphy *see* Repair, Tendons ØLQ

Tenontotomy
  see Division, Tendons ØL8
  see Drainage, Tendons ØL9
Tenorrhaphy *see* Repair, Tendons ØLQ
Tenosynovectomy
  see Excision, Tendons ØLB
  see Resection, Tendons ØLT
Tenotomy
  see Division, Tendons ØL8
  see Drainage, Tendons ØL9
Tensor fasciae latae muscle
  use Hip Muscle, Right
  use Hip Muscle, Left
Tensor veli palatini muscle *use* Tongue, Palate, Pharynx Muscle
Tenth cranial nerve *use* Vagus Nerve
Tentorium cerebelli *use* Dura Mater
Teres major muscle
  use Shoulder Muscle, Right
  use Shoulder Muscle, Left
Teres minor muscle
  use Shoulder Muscle, Right
  use Shoulder Muscle, Left
Termination of pregnancy
  Aspiration curettage 10A07ZZ
  Dilation and curettage 10A07ZZ
  Hysterotomy 10A00ZZ
  Intra-amniotic injection 10A03ZZ
  Laminaria 10A07ZW
  Vacuum 10A07Z6
Testectomy
  see Excision, Male Reproductive System ØVB
  see Resection, Male Reproductive System ØVT
Testicular artery *use* Abdominal Aorta
Testing
  Glaucoma 4A07XBZ
  Hearing *see* Hearing Assessment, Diagnostic Audiology F13
  Mental health *see* Psychological Tests
  Muscle function, electromyography (EMG) *see* Measurement, Musculoskeletal 4A0F
  Muscle function, manual *see* Motor Function Assessment, Rehabilitation F01
  Neurophysiologic monitoring, intra-operative *see* Monitoring, Physiological Systems 4A1
  Range of motion *see* Motor Function Assessment, Rehabilitation F01
  Vestibular function *see* Vestibular Assessment, Diagnostic Audiology F15
Thalamectomy *see* Excision, Thalamus 00B9
Thalamotomy
  see Drainage, Thalamus 0099
Thenar muscle
  use Hand Muscle, Right
  use Hand Muscle, Left
Therapeutic Massage
  Musculoskeletal System 8E0KX1Z
  Reproductive System
    Prostate 8E0VX1C
    Rectum 8E0VX1D
Therapeutic occlusion coil(s) *use* Intraluminal Device
Thermography 4A0ZXKZ
Thermotherapy, prostate *see* Destruction, Prostate 0V50
Third cranial nerve *use* Oculomotor Nerve
Third occipital nerve *use* Cervical Nerve
Third ventricle *use* Cerebral Ventricle
Thoracectomy *see* Excision, Anatomical Regions, General ØWB
Thoracentesis *see* Drainage, Anatomical Regions, General ØW9
Thoracic aortic plexus *use* Thoracic Sympathetic Nerve
Thoracic esophagus *use* Esophagus, Middle
Thoracic facet joint *use* Thoracic Vertebral Joint
Thoracic ganglion *use* Thoracic Sympathetic Nerve
Thoracoacromial artery
  use Axillary Artery, Right
  use Axillary Artery, Left

Thoracocentesis *see* Drainage, Anatomical Regions, General ØW9
Thoracolumbar facet joint *use* Thoracolumbar Vertebral Joint
Thoracoplasty
  see Repair, Anatomical Regions, General ØWQ
  see Supplement, Anatomical Regions, General ØWU
Thoracostomy tube *use* Drainage Device
Thoracostomy, for lung collapse *see* Drainage, Respiratory System ØB9
Thoracotomy *see* Drainage, Anatomical Regions, General ØW9
Thoratec IVAD (Implantable Ventricular Assist Device) *use* Implantable Heart Assist System in Heart and Great Vessels
➡**Thoratec Paracorporeal Ventricular Assist Device** *use* Short-term External Heart Assist System in Heart and Great Vessels
Thrombectomy *see* Extirpation
Thymectomy
  see Excision, Lymphatic and Hemic Systems 07B
  see Resection, Lymphatic and Hemic Systems 07T
Thymopexy
  see Repair, Lymphatic and Hemic Systems 07Q
  see Reposition, Lymphatic and Hemic Systems 07S
Thymus gland *use* Thymus
Thyroarytenoid muscle
  use Neck Muscle, Right
  use Neck Muscle, Left
Thyrocervical trunk
  use Thyroid Artery, Right
  use Thyroid Artery, Left
Thyroid cartilage *use* Larynx
Thyroidectomy
  see Excision, Endocrine System ØGB
  see Resection, Endocrine System ØGT
Thyroidorrhaphy *see* Repair, Endocrine System ØGQ
Thyroidoscopy ØGJK4ZZ
Thyroidotomy *see* Drainage, Endocrine System ØG9
Tibial insert *use* Liner in Lower Joints
Tibialis anterior muscle
  use Lower Leg Muscle, Right
  use Lower Leg Muscle, Left
Tibialis posterior muscle
  use Lower Leg Muscle, Right
  use Lower Leg Muscle, Left
Tibiofemoral joint
  use Knee Joint, Right
  use Knee Joint, Left
  use Knee Joint, Tibial Surface, Right
  use Knee Joint, Tibial Surface, Left
~~TigerPaw® system for closure of left atrial appendage use Extraluminal Device~~
Tissue bank graft *use* Nonautologous Tissue Substitute
Tissue Expander
  Insertion of device in
    Breast
      Bilateral ØHHV
      Left ØHHU
      Right ØHHT
    Nipple
      Left ØHHX
      Right ØHHW
    Subcutaneous Tissue and Fascia
      Abdomen ØJH8
      Back ØJH7
      Buttock ØJH9
      Chest ØJH6
      Face ØJH1
      Foot
        Left ØJHR
        Right ØJHQ
      Hand
        Left ØJHK
        Right ØJHJ

▶ New   ➡ Revised   ~~deleted~~ Deleted

Tissue Expander *(Continued)*
Insertion of device in *(Continued)*
Subcutaneous Tissue and Fascia
(Continued)
Lower Arm
Left ØJHH
Right ØJHG
Lower Leg
Left ØJHP
Right ØJHN
Neck
~~Anterior ØJH4~~
~~Posterior ØJH5~~
▶Left ØJH5
▶Right ØJH4
Pelvic Region ØJHC
Perineum ØJHB
Scalp ØJHØ
Upper Arm
Left ØJHF
Right ØJHD
Upper Leg
Left ØJHM
Right ØJHL
Removal of device from
Breast
Left ØHPU
Right ØHPT
Subcutaneous Tissue and Fascia
Head and Neck ØJPS
Lower Extremity ØJPW
Trunk ØJPT
Upper Extremity ØJPV
Revision of device in
Breast
Left ØHWU
Right ØHWT
Subcutaneous Tissue and Fascia
Head and Neck ØJWS
Lower Extremity ØJWW
Trunk ØJWT
Upper Extremity ØJWV
Tissue expander (inflatable) (injectable)
use Tissue Expander in Skin and Breast
use Tissue Expander in Subcutaneous Tissue and Fascia
Tissue Plasminogen Activator (tPA)(r-tPA) *use*
Thrombolytic, Other
Titanium Sternal Fixation System (TSFS)
use Internal Fixation Device, Rigid Plate in ØPS
use Internal Fixation Device, Rigid Plate in ØPH
Tomographic (Tomo) Nuclear Medicine Imaging
Abdomen CW2Ø
Abdomen and Chest CW24
Abdomen and Pelvis CW21
Anatomical Regions, Multiple CW2YYZZ
Bladder, Kidneys and Ureters CT23
Brain CØ2Ø
Breast CH2YYZZ
Bilateral CH22
Left CH21
Right CH2Ø
Bronchi and Lungs CB22
Central Nervous System CØ2YYZZ
Cerebrospinal Fluid CØ25
Chest CW23
Chest and Abdomen CW24
Chest and Neck CW26
Digestive System CD2YYZZ
Endocrine System CG2YYZZ
Extremity
Lower CW2D
Bilateral CP2F
Left CP2D
Right CP2C
Upper CW2M
Bilateral CP2B
Left CP29
Right CP28
Gallbladder CF24

Tomographic (Tomo) Nuclear Medicine Imaging *(Continued)*
Gastrointestinal Tract CD27
Gland, Parathyroid CG21
Head and Neck CW2B
Heart C22YYZZ
Right and Left C226
Hepatobiliary System and Pancreas CF2YYZZ
Kidneys, Ureters and Bladder CT23
Liver CF25
Liver and Spleen CF26
Lungs and Bronchi CB22
Lymphatics and Hematologic System C72YYZZ
Musculoskeletal System, Other CP2YYZZ
Myocardium C22G
Neck and Chest CW26
Neck and Head CW2B
Pancreas and Hepatobiliary System CF2YYZZ
Pelvic Region CW2J
Pelvis CP26
Pelvis and Abdomen CW21
Pelvis and Spine CP27
Respiratory System CB2YYZZ
Skin CH2YYZZ
Skull CP21
Skull and Cervical Spine CP23
Spine
Cervical CP22
Cervical and Skull CP23
Lumbar CP2H
Thoracic CP2G
Thoracolumbar CP2J
Spine and Pelvis CP27
Spleen C722
Spleen and Liver CF26
Subcutaneous Tissue CH2YYZZ
Thorax CP24
Ureters, Kidneys and Bladder CT23
Urinary System CT2YYZZ
Tomography, computerized *see* Computerized Tomography (CT Scan)
Tongue, base of *use* Pharynx
Tonometry 4AØ7XBZ
Tonsillectomy
see Excision, Mouth and Throat ØCB
see Resection, Mouth and Throat ØCT
Tonsillotomy *see* Drainage, Mouth and Throat ØC9
Total Anomalous Pulmonary Venous Return (TAPVR) repair
see Bypass, Atrium, Left Ø217
see Bypass, Vena Cava, Superior Ø21V
Total artificial (replacement) heart *use* Synthetic Substitute
Total parenteral nutrition (TPN) *see* Introduction of Nutritional Substance
Trachectomy
see Excision, Trachea ØBB1
see Resection, Trachea ØBT1
Trachelectomy
see Excision, Cervix ØUBC
see Resection, Cervix ØUTC
Trachelopexy
see Repair, Cervix ØUQC
see Reposition, Cervix ØUSC
Tracheloplasty
see Repair, Cervix ØUQC
Trachelorrhaphy *see* Repair, Cervix ØUQC
Trachelotomy *see* Drainage, Cervix ØU9C
Tracheobronchial lymph node *see* Lymphatic, Thorax
Tracheoesophageal fistulization ØB11ØD6
Tracheolysis *see* Release, Respiratory System ØBN
Tracheoplasty
see Repair, Respiratory System ØBQ
see Supplement, Respiratory System ØBU
Tracheorrhaphy *see* Repair, Respiratory System ØBQ
Tracheoscopy ØBJ18ZZ
Tracheostomy *see* Bypass, Respiratory System ØB1

Tracheostomy Device
Bypass, Trachea ØB11
Change device in, Trachea ØB21XFZ
Removal of device from, Trachea ØBP1
Revision of device in, Trachea ØBW1
Tracheostomy tube *use* Tracheostomy Device in Respiratory System
Tracheotomy *see* Drainage, Respiratory System ØB9
Traction
Abdominal Wall 2W63X
Arm
Lower
Left 2W6DX
Right 2W6CX
Upper
Left 2W6BX
Right 2W6AX
Back 2W65X
Chest Wall 2W64X
Extremity
Lower
Left 2W6MX
Right 2W6LX
Upper
Left 2W69X
Right 2W68X
Face 2W61X
Finger
Left 2W6KX
Right 2W6JX
Foot
Left 2W6TX
Right 2W6SX
Hand
Left 2W6FX
Right 2W6EX
Head 2W6ØX
Inguinal Region
Left 2W67X
Right 2W66X
Leg
Lower
Left 2W6RX
Right 2W6QX
Upper
Left 2W6PX
Right 2W6NX
Neck 2W62X
Thumb
Left 2W6HX
Right 2W6GX
Toe
Left 2W6VX
Right 2W6UX
➡**Tractotomy** *see* Division, Central Nervous System and Cranial Nerves ØØ8
Tragus
use External Ear, Right
use External Ear, Left
use External Ear, Bilateral
Training, caregiver *see* Caregiver Training
TRAM (transverse rectus abdominis myocutaneous) flap reconstruction
Free *see* Replacement, Skin and Breast ØHR
Pedicled *see* Transfer, Muscles ØKX
Transection *see* Division
Transfer
Buccal Mucosa ØCX4
Bursa and Ligament
Abdomen
Left ØMXJ
Right ØMXH
Ankle
Left ØMXR
Right ØMXQ
Elbow
Left ØMX4
Right ØMX3
Foot
Left ØMXT
Right ØMXS

Transfer (Continued)
  Bursa and Ligament (Continued)
    Hand
      Left ØMX8
      Right ØMX7
    Head and Neck ØMXØ
    Hip
      Left ØMXM
      Right ØMXL
    Knee
      Left ØMXP
      Right ØMXN
    Lower Extremity
      Left ØMXW
      Right ØMXV
    Perineum ØMXK
    ▶Rib(s) ØMXG
    Shoulder
      Left ØMX2
      Right ØMX1
    ▶Spine
      ▶Lower ØMXD
      ▶Upper ØMXC
    ▶Sternum ØMXF
    Thorax
      Left ØMXG
      Right ØMXF
    Trunk
      Left ØMXD
      Right ØMXC
    Upper Extremity
      Left ØMXB
      Right ØMX9
    Wrist
      Left ØMX6
      Right ØMX5
  Finger
    Left ØXXPØZM
    Right ØXXNØZL
  Gingiva
    Lower ØCX6
    Upper ØCX5
  Intestine
    Large ØDXE
    Small ØDX8
  Lip
    Lower ØCX1
    Upper ØCXØ
  Muscle
    Abdomen
      Left ØKXL
      Right ØKXK
    Extraocular
      Left Ø8XM
      Right Ø8XL
    Facial ØKX1
    Foot
      Left ØKXW
      Right ØKXV
    Hand
      Left ØKXD
      Right ØKXC
    Head ØKXØ
    Hip
      Left ØKXP
      Right ØKXN
    Lower Arm and Wrist
      Left ØKXB
      Right ØKX9
    Lower Leg
      Left ØKXT
      Right ØKXS
    Neck
      Left ØKX3
      Right ØKX2
    Perineum ØKXM
    Shoulder
      Left ØKX6
      Right ØKX5
    Thorax
      Left ØKXJ
      Right ØKXH

Transfer (Continued)
  Muscle (Continued)
    Tongue, Palate, Pharynx ØKX4
    Trunk
      Left ØKXG
      Right ØKXF
    Upper Arm
      Left ØKX8
      Right ØKX7
    Upper Leg
      Left ØKXR
      Right ØKXQ
  Nerve
    Abducens ØØXL
    Accessory ØØXR
    Acoustic ØØXN
    Cervical Ø1X1
    Facial ØØXM
    Femoral Ø1XD
    Glossopharyngeal ØØXP
    Hypoglossal ØØXS
    Lumbar Ø1XB
    Median Ø1X5
    Oculomotor ØØXH
    Olfactory ØØXF
    Optic ØØXG
    Peroneal Ø1XH
    Phrenic Ø1X2
    Pudendal Ø1XC
    Radial Ø1X6
    Sciatic Ø1XF
    Thoracic Ø1X8
    Tibial Ø1XG
    Trigeminal ØØXK
    Trochlear ØØXJ
    Ulnar Ø1X4
    Vagus ØØXQ
  Palate, Soft ØCX3
  Skin
    Abdomen ØHX7XZZ
    Back ØHX6XZZ
    Buttock ØHX8XZZ
    Chest ØHX5XZZ
    Ear
      Left ØHX3XZZ
      Right ØHX2XZZ
    Face ØHX1XZZ
    Foot
      Left ØHXNXZZ
      Right ØHXMXZZ
    Genitalia ØHXAXZZ
    Hand
      Left ØHXGXZZ
      Right ØHXFXZZ
    ▶Inguinal ØHXAXZZ
    Lower Arm
      Left ØHXEXZZ
      Right ØHXDXZZ
    Lower Leg
      Left ØHXLXZZ
      Right ØHXKXZZ
    Neck ØHX4XZZ
    Perineum ØHX9XZZ
    Scalp ØHXØXZZ
    Upper Arm
      Left ØHXCXZZ
      Right ØHXBXZZ
    Upper Leg
      Left ØHXJXZZ
      Right ØHXHXZZ
  Stomach ØDX6
  Subcutaneous Tissue and Fascia
    Abdomen ØJX8
    Back ØJX7
    Buttock ØJX9
    Chest ØJX6
    Face ØJX1
    Foot
      Left ØJXR
      Right ØJXQ

Transfer (Continued)
  Subcutaneous Tissue and Fascia (Continued)
    Hand
      Left ØJXK
      Right ØJXJ
    Lower Arm
      Left ØJXH
      Right ØJXG
    Lower Leg
      Left ØJXP
      Right ØJXN
    Neck
      Anterior ØJX4
      Posterior ØJX5
      ▶Left ØJX5
      ▶Right ØJX4
    Pelvic Region ØJXC
    Perineum ØJXB
    Scalp ØJXØ
    Upper Arm
      Left ØJXF
      Right ØJXD
    Upper Leg
      Left ØJXM
      Right ØJXL
  Tendon
    Abdomen
      Left ØLXG
      Right ØLXF
    Ankle
      Left ØLXT
      Right ØLXS
    Foot
      Left ØLXW
      Right ØLXV
    Hand
      Left ØLX8
      Right ØLX7
    Head and Neck ØLXØ
    Hip
      Left ØLXK
      Right ØLXJ
    Knee
      Left ØLXR
      Right ØLXQ
    Lower Arm and Wrist
      Left ØLX6
      Right ØLX5
    Lower Leg
      Left ØLXP
      Right ØLXN
    Perineum ØLXH
    Shoulder
      Left ØLX2
      Right ØLX1
    Thorax
      Left ØLXD
      Right ØLXC
    Trunk
      Left ØLXB
      Right ØLX9
    Upper Arm
      Left ØLX4
      Right ØLX3
    Upper Leg
      Left ØLXM
      Right ØLXL
  Tongue ØCX7
Transfusion
  Artery
    Central
      Antihemophilic Factors 3Ø26
      Blood
        Platelets 3Ø26
        Red Cells 3Ø26
          Frozen 3Ø26
        White Cells 3Ø26
        Whole 3Ø26
      Bone Marrow 3Ø26
      Factor IX 3Ø26
      Fibrinogen 3Ø26
      Globulin 3Ø26

▶ New ⇒ Revised ~~deleted~~ Deleted

Transfusion *(Continued)*
  Artery *(Continued)*
    Central *(Continued)*
      Plasma
        Fresh 3026
        Frozen 3026
      Plasma Cryoprecipitate 3026
      Serum Albumin 3026
    Stem Cells
      Cord Blood 3026
      Hematopoietic 3026
    Peripheral
      Antihemophilic Factors 3025
      Blood
        Platelets 3025
        Red Cells 3025
          Frozen 3025
        White Cells 3025
        Whole 3025
      Bone Marrow 3025
      Factor IX 3025
      Fibrinogen 3025
      Globulin 3025
      Plasma
        Fresh 3025
        Frozen 3025
      Plasma Cryoprecipitate 3025
      Serum Albumin 3025
      Stem Cells
        Cord Blood 3025
        Hematopoietic 3025
  Products of Conception
    Antihemophilic Factors 3027
    Blood
      Platelets 3027
      Red Cells 3027
        Frozen 3027
      White Cells 3027
      Whole 3027
    Factor IX 3027
    Fibrinogen 3027
    Globulin 3027
    Plasma
      Fresh 3027
      Frozen 3027
    Plasma Cryoprecipitate 3027
    Serum Albumin 3027
  Vein
    4-Factor Prothrombin Complex
      Concentrate 3028[03]B1
    Central
      Antihemophilic Factors 3024
      Blood
        Platelets 3024
        Red Cells 3024
          Frozen 3024
        White Cells 3024
        Whole 3024
      Bone Marrow 3024
      Factor IX 3024
      Fibrinogen 3024
      Globulin 3024
      Plasma
        Fresh 3024
        Frozen 3024
      Plasma Cryoprecipitate 3024
      Serum Albumin 3024
      Stem Cells
        Cord Blood 3024
        Embryonic 3024
        Hematopoietic 3024
    Peripheral
      Antihemophilic Factors 3023
      Blood
        Platelets 3023
        Red Cells 3023
          Frozen 3023
        White Cells 3023
        Whole 3023
      Bone Marrow 3023
      Factor IX 3023
      Fibrinogen 3023

Transfusion *(Continued)*
  Vein *(Continued)*
    Peripheral *(Continued)*
      Globulin 3023
      Plasma
        Fresh 3023
        Frozen 3023
      Plasma Cryoprecipitate 3023
      Serum Albumin 3023
      Stem Cells
        Cord Blood 3023
        Embryonic 3023
        Hematopoietic 3023
Transplant *see* Transplantation
Transplantation
  Bone marrow *see* Transfusion, Circulatory 302
  Esophagus 0DY50Z
  Face 0WY20Z
  Hand
    Left 0XYK0Z
    Right 0XYJ0Z
  Heart 02YA0Z
  Hematopoietic cell *see* Transfusion,
    Circulatory 302
  Intestine
    Large 0DYE0Z
    Small 0DY80Z
  Kidney
    Left 0TY10Z
    Right 0TY00Z
  Liver 0FY00Z
  Lung
    Bilateral 0BYM0Z
    Left 0BYL0Z
    Lower Lobe
      Left 0BYJ0Z
      Right 0BYF0Z
    Middle Lobe, Right 0BYD0Z
    Right 0BYK0Z
    Upper Lobe
      Left 0BYG0Z
      Right 0BYC0Z
  Lung Lingula 0BYH0Z
  Ovary
    Left 0UY10Z
    Right 0UY00Z
  Pancreas 0FYG0Z
  Products of Conception 10Y0
  Spleen 07YP0Z
  Stem cell *see* Transfusion, Circulatory
    302
  Stomach 0DY60Z
  Thymus 07YM0Z
Transposition
  ▶*see* Bypass
  see Reposition
  see Transfer
Transversalis fascia *use* Subcutaneous Tissue
  and Fascia, Trunk
Transverse (cutaneous) cervical nerve *use*
  Cervical Plexus
Transverse acetabular ligament
  use Hip Bursa and Ligament, Right
  use Hip Bursa and Ligament, Left
Transverse facial artery
  use Temporal Artery, Right
  use Temporal Artery, Left
▶**Transverse foramen** *use* Cervical Vertebra
Transverse humeral ligament
  use Shoulder Bursa and Ligament, Right
  use Shoulder Bursa and Ligament, Left
Transverse ligament of atlas *use* Head and
  Neck Bursa and Ligament
▶**Transverse process**
  ▶*use* Cervical Vertebra
  ▶*use* Thoracic Vertebra
  ▶*use* Lumbar Vertebra
Transverse Rectus Abdominis Myocutaneous
  Flap
  Replacement
    Bilateral 0HRV076
    Left 0HRU076
    Right 0HRT076

Transverse Rectus Abdominis Myocutaneous
  Flap *(Continued)*
  Transfer
    Left 0KXL
    Right 0KXK
Transverse scapular ligament
  use Shoulder Bursa and Ligament, Right
  use Shoulder Bursa and Ligament, Left
Transverse thoracis muscle
  use Thorax Muscle, Right
  use Thorax Muscle, Left
Transversospinalis muscle
  use Trunk Muscle, Right
  use Trunk Muscle, Left
Transversus abdominis muscle
  use Abdomen Muscle, Right
  use Abdomen Muscle, Left
Trapezium bone
  use Carpal, Right
  use Carpal, Left
Trapezius muscle
  use Trunk Muscle, Right
  use Trunk Muscle, Left
Trapezoid bone
  use Carpal, Right
  use Carpal, Left
Triceps brachii muscle
  use Upper Arm Muscle, Right
  use Upper Arm Muscle, Left
Tricuspid annulus *use* Tricuspid Valve
Trifacial nerve *use* Trigeminal Nerve
Trifecta™ Valve (aortic) *use* Zooplastic Tissue in
  Heart and Great Vessels
Trigone of bladder *use* Bladder
Trimming, excisional *see* Excision
Triquetral bone
  use Carpal, Right
  use Carpal, Left
Trochanteric bursa
  use Hip Bursa and Ligament, Right
  use Hip Bursa and Ligament, Left
TUMT (Transurethral microwave
  thermotherapy of prostate) 0V507ZZ
TUNA (transurethral needle ablation of
  prostate) 0V507ZZ
➡**Tunneled central venous catheter** *use* Vascular
  Access Device, Tunneled in Subcutaneous
  Tissue and Fascia
Tunneled spinal (intrathecal) catheter *use*
  Infusion Device
Turbinectomy
  see Excision, Ear, Nose, Sinus 09B
  see Resection, Ear, Nose, Sinus 09T
Turbinoplasty
  see Repair, Ear, Nose, Sinus 09Q
  see Replacement, Ear, Nose, Sinus 09R
  see Supplement, Ear, Nose, Sinus 09U
Turbinotomy
  see Division, Ear, Nose, Sinus 098
  see Drainage, Ear, Nose, Sinus 099
TURP (transurethral resection of prostate)
  see Excision, Prostate 0VB0
  see Resection, Prostate 0VT0
Twelfth cranial nerve *use* Hypoglossal Nerve
Two lead pacemaker *use* Pacemaker, Dual
  Chamber in 0JH
Tympanic cavity
  use Middle Ear, Right
  use Middle Ear, Left
Tympanic nerve *use* Glossopharyngeal Nerve
Tympanic part of temoporal bone
  use Temporal Bone, Right
  use Temporal Bone, Left
Tympanogram *see* Hearing Assessment,
  Diagnostic Audiology F13
Tympanoplasty
  see Repair, Ear, Nose, Sinus 09Q
  see Replacement, Ear, Nose, Sinus 09R
  see Supplement, Ear, Nose, Sinus 09U
Tympanosympathectomy *see* Excision, Nerve,
  Head and Neck Sympathetic 01BK
Tympanotomy *see* Drainage, Ear, Nose, Sinus 099

U

Ulnar collateral carpal ligament
  use Wrist Bursa and Ligament, Right
  use Wrist Bursa and Ligament, Left
Ulnar collateral ligament
  use Elbow Bursa and Ligament, Right
  use Elbow Bursa and Ligament, Left
Ulnar notch
  use Radius, Right
  use Radius, Left
Ulnar vein
  use Brachial Vein, Right
  use Brachial Vein, Left
Ultrafiltration
  Hemodialysis *see* Performance, Urinary 5A1D
  Therapeutic plasmapheresis *see* Pheresis, Circulatory 6A55
Ultraflex™ Precision Colonic Stent System *use* Intraluminal Device
ULTRAPRO Hernia System (UHS) *use* Synthetic Substitute
ULTRAPRO Partially Absorbable Lightweight Mesh *use* Synthetic Substitute
ULTRAPRO Plug *use* Synthetic Substitute
Ultrasonic osteogenic stimulator
  use Bone Growth Stimulator in Head and Facial Bones
  use Bone Growth Stimulator in Upper Bones
  use Bone Growth Stimulator in Lower Bones
Ultrasonography
  Abdomen BW40ZZZ
  Abdomen and Pelvis BW41ZZZ
  Abdominal Wall BH49ZZZ
  Aorta
    Abdominal, Intravascular B440ZZ3
    Thoracic, Intravascular B340ZZ3
  Appendix BD48ZZZ
  Artery
    Brachiocephalic-Subclavian, Right, Intravascular B341ZZ3
    Celiac and Mesenteric, Intravascular B44KZZ3
    Common Carotid
      Bilateral, Intravascular B345ZZ3
      Left, Intravascular B344ZZ3
      Right, Intravascular B343ZZ3
    Coronary
      Multiple B241YZZ
        Intravascular B241ZZ3
        Transesophageal B241ZZ4
      Single B240YZZ
        Intravascular B240ZZ3
        Transesophageal B240ZZ4
    Femoral, Intravascular B44LZZ3
    Inferior Mesenteric, Intravascular B445ZZ3
    Internal Carotid
      Bilateral, Intravascular B348ZZ3
      Left, Intravascular B347ZZ3
      Right, Intravascular B346ZZ3
    Intra-Abdominal, Other, Intravascular B44BZZ3
    Intracranial, Intravascular B34RZZ3
    Lower Extremity
      Bilateral, Intravascular B44HZZ3
      Left, Intravascular B44GZZ3
      Right, Intravascular B44FZZ3
    Mesenteric and Celiac, Intravascular B44KZZ3
    Ophthalmic, Intravascular B34VZZ3
    Penile, Intravascular B44NZZ3
    Pulmonary
      Left, Intravascular B34TZZ3
      Right, Intravascular B34SZZ3
    Renal
      Bilateral, Intravascular B448ZZ3
      Left, Intravascular B447ZZ3
      Right, Intravascular B446ZZ3
    Subclavian, Left, Intravascular B342ZZ3
    Superior Mesenteric, Intravascular B444ZZ3

Ultrasonography *(Continued)*
  Artery *(Continued)*
    Upper Extremity
      Bilateral, Intravascular B34KZZ3
      Left, Intravascular B34JZZ3
      Right, Intravascular B34HZZ3
  Bile Duct BF40ZZZ
  Bile Duct and Gallbladder BF43ZZZ
  Bladder BT40ZZZ
    and Kidney BT4JZZZ
  Brain B040ZZZ
  Breast
    Bilateral BH42ZZZ
    Left BH41ZZZ
    Right BH40ZZZ
  Chest Wall BH4BZZZ
  Coccyx BR4FZZZ
  Connective Tissue
    Lower Extremity BL41ZZZ
    Upper Extremity BL40ZZZ
  Duodenum BD49ZZZ
  Elbow
    Left, Densitometry BP4HZZ1
    Right, Densitometry BP4GZZ1
  Esophagus BD41ZZZ
  Extremity
    Lower BH48ZZZ
    Upper BH47ZZZ
  Eye
    Bilateral B847ZZZ
    Left B846ZZZ
    Right B845ZZZ
  Fallopian Tube
    Bilateral BU42
    Left BU41
    Right BU40
  Fetal Umbilical Cord BY47ZZZ
  Fetus
    First Trimester, Multiple Gestation BY4BZZZ
    Second Trimester, Multiple Gestation BY4DZZZ
    Single
      First Trimester BY49ZZZ
      Second Trimester BY4CZZZ
      Third Trimester BY4FZZZ
    Third Trimester, Multiple Gestation BY4GZZZ
  Gallbladder BF42ZZZ
  Gallbladder and Bile Duct BF43ZZZ
  Gastrointestinal Tract BD47ZZZ
  Gland
    Adrenal
      Bilateral BG42ZZZ
      Left BG41ZZZ
      Right BG40ZZZ
    Parathyroid BG43ZZZ
    Thyroid BG44ZZZ
  Hand
    Left, Densitometry BP4PZZ1
    Right, Densitometry BP4NZZ1
  Head and Neck BH4CZZZ
  Heart
    Left B245YZZ
      Intravascular B245ZZ3
      Transesophageal B245ZZ4
    Pediatric B24DYZZ
      Intravascular B24DZZ3
      Transesophageal B24DZZ4
    Right B244YZZ
      Intravascular B244ZZ3
      Transesophageal B244ZZ4
    Right and Left B246YZZ
      Intravascular B246ZZ3
      Transesophageal B246ZZ4
  Heart with Aorta B24BYZZ
    Intravascular B24BZZ3
    Transesophageal B24BZZ4
  Hepatobiliary System, All BF4CZZZ
  Hip
    Bilateral BQ42ZZZ
    Left BQ41ZZZ
    Right BQ40ZZZ

Ultrasonography *(Continued)*
  Kidney
    and Bladder BT4JZZZ
    Bilateral BT43ZZZ
    Left BT42ZZZ
    Right BT41ZZZ
    Transplant BT49ZZZ
  Knee
    Bilateral BQ49ZZZ
    Left BQ48ZZZ
    Right BQ47ZZZ
  Liver BF45ZZZ
  Liver and Spleen BF46ZZZ
  Mediastinum BB4CZZZ
  Neck BW4FZZZ
  Ovary
    Bilateral BU45
    Left BU44
    Right BU43
  Ovary and Uterus BU4C
  Pancreas BF47ZZZ
  Pelvic Region BW4GZZZ
  Pelvis and Abdomen BW41ZZZ
  Penis BV4BZZZ
  Pericardium B24CYZZ
    Intravascular B24CZZ3
    Transesophageal B24CZZ4
  Placenta BY48ZZZ
  Pleura BB4BZZZ
  Prostate and Seminal Vesicle BV49ZZZ
  Rectum BD4CZZZ
  Sacrum BR4FZZZ
  Scrotum BV44ZZZ
  Seminal Vesicle and Prostate BV49ZZZ
  Shoulder
    Left, Densitometry BP49ZZ1
    Right, Densitometry BP48ZZ1
  Spinal Cord B04BZZZ
  Spine
    Cervical BR40ZZZ
    Lumbar BR49ZZZ
    Thoracic BR47ZZZ
  Spleen and Liver BF46ZZZ
  Stomach BD42ZZZ
  Tendon
    Lower Extremity BL43ZZZ
    Upper Extremity BL42ZZZ
  Ureter
    Bilateral BT48ZZZ
    Left BT47ZZZ
    Right BT46ZZZ
  Urethra BT45ZZZ
  Uterus BU46
  Uterus and Ovary BU4C
  Vein
    Jugular
      Left, Intravascular B544ZZ3
      Right, Intravascular B543ZZ3
    Lower Extremity
      Bilateral, Intravascular B54DZZ3
      Left, Intravascular B54CZZ3
      Right, Intravascular B54BZZ3
    Portal, Intravascular B54TZZ3
    Renal
      Bilateral, Intravascular B54LZZ3
      Left, Intravascular B54KZZ3
      Right, Intravascular B54JZZ3
    Spanchnic, Intravascular B54TZZ3
    Subclavian
      Left, Intravascular B547ZZ3
      Right, Intravascular B546ZZ3
    Upper Extremity
      Bilateral, Intravascular B54PZZ3
      Left, Intravascular B54NZZ3
      Right, Intravascular B54MZZ3
  Vena Cava
    Inferior, Intravascular B549ZZ3
    Superior, Intravascular B548ZZ3
  Wrist
    Left, Densitometry BP4MZZ1
    Right, Densitometry BP4LZZ1

▶ New   ⇒ Revised   ~~deleted~~ Deleted

Ultrasound bone healing system
 use Bone Growth Stimulator in Head and
  Facial Bones
 use Bone Growth Stimulator in Upper Bones
 use Bone Growth Stimulator in Lower Bones
Ultrasound Therapy
 Heart 6A75
 No Qualifier 6A75
 Vessels
  Head and Neck 6A75
  Other 6A75
  Peripheral 6A75
Ultraviolet Light Therapy, Skin 6A80
Umbilical artery
 use Internal Iliac Artery, Right
 use Internal Iliac Artery, Left
 ▶ *use* Lower Artery
Uniplanar external fixator
 use External Fixation Device, Monoplanar in
  0PH
 use External Fixation Device, Monoplanar
  in 0PS
 use External Fixation Device, Monoplanar in
  0QH
 use External Fixation Device, Monoplanar
  in 0QS
Upper GI series *see* Fluoroscopy,
 Gastrointestinal, Upper BD15
Ureteral orifice
 use Ureter, Left
 use Ureter
 use Ureter, Right
 use Ureters, Bilateral
Ureterectomy
 see Excision, Urinary System 0TB
 see Resection, Urinary System 0TT
Ureterocolostomy *see* Bypass, Urinary System
 0T1
Ureterocystostomy *see* Bypass, Urinary System
 0T1
Ureteroenterostomy *see* Bypass, Urinary System
 0T1
Ureteroileostomy *see* Bypass, Urinary System 0T1
Ureterolithotomy *see* Extirpation, Urinary
 System 0TC
Ureterolysis *see* Release, Urinary System 0TN
Ureteroneocystostomy
 see Bypass, Urinary System 0T1
 see Reposition, Urinary System 0TS
Ureteropelvic junction (UPJ)
 use Kidney Pelvis, Right
 use Kidney Pelvis, Left
Ureteropexy
 see Repair, Urinary System 0TQ
 see Reposition, Urinary System 0TS
Ureteroplasty
 see Repair, Urinary System 0TQ
 see Replacement, Urinary System 0TR
 see Supplement, Urinary System 0TU
Ureteroplication *see* Restriction, Urinary
 System 0TV
Ureteropyelography *see* Fluoroscopy, Urinary
 System BT1
Ureterorrhaphy *see* Repair, Urinary System 0TQ
Ureteroscopy 0TJ98ZZ
Ureterostomy
 see Bypass, Urinary System 0T1
 see Drainage, Urinary System 0T9
Ureterotomy *see* Drainage, Urinary System 0T9
Ureteroureterostomy *see* Bypass, Urinary
 System 0T1
Ureterovesical orifice
 use Ureter, Right
 use Ureter, Left
 use Ureters, Bilateral
 use Ureter
Urethral catheterization, indwelling 0T9B70Z
Urethrectomy
 see Excision, Urethra 0TBD
 see Resection, Urethra 0TTD
Urethrolithotomy *see* Extirpation, Urethra 0TCD
Urethrolysis *see* Release, Urethra 0TND

Urethropexy
 see Repair, Urethra 0TQD
 see Reposition, Urethra 0TSD
Urethroplasty
 see Repair, Urethra 0TQD
 see Replacement, Urethra 0TRD
 see Supplement, Urethra 0TUD
Urethrorrhaphy *see* Repair, Urethra 0TQD
Urethroscopy 0TJD8ZZ
Urethrotomy *see* Drainage, Urethra 0T9D
Uridine Triacetate XW0DX82
Urinary incontinence stimulator lead *use*
 Stimulator Lead in Urinary System
Urography *see* Fluoroscopy, Urinary System BT1
▶**Ustekinumab** *use* Other New Technology
 Therapeutic Substance
Uterine Artery
 use Internal Iliac Artery, Right
 use Internal Iliac Artery, Left
Uterine artery embolization (UAE) *see*
 Occlusion, Lower Arteries 04L
Uterine cornu *use* Uterus
Uterine tube
 use Fallopian Tube, Right
 use Fallopian Tube, Left
Uterine vein
 use Hypogastric Vein, Right
 use Hypogastric Vein, Left
Uvulectomy
 see Excision, Uvula 0CBN
 see Resection, Uvula 0CTN
Uvulorrhaphy *see* Repair, Uvula 0CQN
Uvulotomy *see* Drainage, Uvula 0C9N

V

Vaccination *see* Introduction of Serum, Toxoid,
 and Vaccine
Vacuum extraction, obstetric 10D07Z6
Vaginal artery
 use Internal Iliac Artery, Right
 use Internal Iliac Artery, Left
Vaginal pessary *use* Intraluminal Device,
 Pessary in Female Reproductive System
Vaginal vein
 use Hypogastric Vein, Right
 use Hypogastric Vein, Left
Vaginectomy
 see Excision, Vagina 0UBG
 see Resection, Vagina 0UTG
Vaginofixation
 see Repair, Vagina 0UQG
 see Reposition, Vagina 0USG
Vaginoplasty
 see Repair, Vagina 0UQG
 see Supplement, Vagina 0UUG
Vaginorrhaphy *see* Repair, Vagina 0UQG
Vaginoscopy 0UJH8ZZ
Vaginotomy *see* Drainage, Female Reproductive
 System 0U9
Vagotomy *see* Division, Nerve, Vagus 008Q
Valiant Thoracic Stent Graft *use* Intraluminal
 Device
Valvotomy, valvulotomy
 see Division, Heart and Great Vessels 028
 see Release, Heart and Great Vessels 02N
Valvuloplasty
 see Repair, Heart and Great Vessels 02Q
 see Replacement, Heart and Great Vessels 02R
 see Supplement, Heart and Great Vessels 02U
▶**Valvuloplasty, Alfieri Stitch** *see* Restriction,
 Valve, Mitral 02VG
Vascular Access Device
 Insertion of device in
  Abdomen 0JH8
  Chest 0JH6
  Lower Arm
   Left 0JHH
   Right 0JHG
  Lower Leg
   Left 0JHP
   Right 0JHN

Vascular Access Device *(Continued)*
 Insertion of device in *(Continued)*
  Upper Arm
   Left 0JHF
   Right 0JHD
  Upper Leg
   Left 0JHM
   Right 0JHL
 Removal of device from
  Lower Extremity 0JPW
  Trunk 0JPT
  Upper Extremity 0JPV
 Reservoir
  Insertion of device in
   Abdomen 0JH8
   Chest 0JH6
   Lower Arm
    Left 0JHH
    Right 0JHG
   Lower Leg
    Left 0JHP
    Right 0JHN
   Upper Arm
    Left 0JHF
    Right 0JHD
   Upper Leg
    Left 0JHM
    Right 0JHL
  Removal of device from
   Lower Extremity 0JPW
   Trunk 0JPT
   Upper Extremity 0JPV
  Revision of device in
   Lower Extremity 0JWW
   Trunk 0JWT
   Upper Extremity 0JWV
  Revision of device in
   Lower Extremity 0JWW
   Trunk 0JWT
   Upper Extremity 0JWV
 ▶ Totally Implantable
  ▶ Insertion of device in
   ▶ Abdomen 0JH8
   ▶ Chest 0JH6
   ▶ Lower Arm
    ▶ Left 0JHH
    ▶ Right 0JHG
   ▶ Lower Leg
    ▶ Left 0JHP
    ▶ Right 0JHN
   ▶ Upper Arm
    ▶ Left 0JHF
    ▶ Right 0JHD
   ▶ Upper Leg
    ▶ Left 0JHM
    ▶ Right 0JHL
  ▶ Removal of device from
   ▶ Lower Extremity 0JPW
   ▶ Trunk 0JPT
   ▶ Upper Extremity 0JPV
  ▶ Revision of device in
   ▶ Lower Extremity 0JWW
   ▶ Trunk 0JWT
   ▶ Upper Extremity 0JWV
 ▶ Tunneled
  ▶ Insertion of device in
   ▶ Abdomen 0JH8
   ▶ Chest 0JH6
   ▶ Lower Arm
    ▶ Left 0JHH
    ▶ Right 0JHG
   ▶ Lower Leg
    ▶ Left 0JHP
    ▶ Right 0JHN
   ▶ Upper Arm
    ▶ Left 0JHF
    ▶ Right 0JHD
   ▶ Upper Leg
    ▶ Left 0JHM
    ▶ Right 0JHL

Vascular Access Device (*Continued*)
Tunneled (*Continued*)
▶Removal of device from
▶Lower Extremity 0JPW
▶Trunk 0JPT
▶Upper Extremity 0JPV
▶Revision of device in
▶Lower Extremity 0JWW
▶Trunk 0JWT
▶Upper Extremity 0JWV
Vasectomy *see* Excision, Male Reproductive System 0VB
Vasography
see Plain Radiography, Male Reproductive System BV0
see Fluoroscopy, Male Reproductive System BV1
Vasoligation *see* Occlusion, Male Reproductive System 0VL
Vasorrhaphy *see* Repair, Male Reproductive System 0VQ
Vasostomy *see* Bypass, Male Reproductive System 0V1
Vasotomy
Drainage *see* Drainage, Male Reproductive System 0V9
With ligation *see* Occlusion, Male Reproductive System 0VL
Vasovasostomy *see* Repair, Male Reproductive System 0VQ
Vastus intermedius muscle
use Upper Leg Muscle, Right
use Upper Leg Muscle, Left
Vastus lateralis muscle
use Upper Leg Muscle, Right
use Upper Leg Muscle, Left
Vastus medialis muscle
use Upper Leg Muscle, Right
use Upper Leg Muscle, Left
VCG (vectorcardiogram) *see* Measurement, Cardiac 4A02
➡**Vectra® Vascular Access Graft** *use* Vascular Access Device, Tunneled in Subcutaneous Tissue and Fascia
Venectomy
see Excision, Upper Veins 05B
see Excision, Lower Veins 06B
Venography
see Plain Radiography, Veins B50
see Fluoroscopy, Veins B51
Venorrhaphy
see Repair, Upper Veins 05Q
see Repair, Lower Veins 06Q
Venotripsy
see Occlusion, Upper Veins 05L
see Occlusion, Lower Veins 06L
Ventricular fold *use* Larynx
➡**Ventriculoatriostomy** *see* Bypass, Central Nervous System and Cranial Nerves 001
➡**Ventriculocisternostomy** *see* Bypass, Central Nervous System and Cranial Nerves 001
Ventriculogram, cardiac
Combined left and right heart *see* Fluoroscopy, Heart, Right and Left B216
Left ventricle *see* Fluoroscopy, Heart, Left B215
Right ventricle *see* Fluoroscopy, Heart, Right B214
Ventriculopuncture, through previously implanted catheter 8C01X6J
Ventriculoscopy 00J04ZZ
Ventriculostomy
External drainage *see* Drainage, Cerebral Ventricle 0096
Internal shunt *see* Bypass, Cerebral Ventricle 0016
Ventriculovenostomy *see* Bypass, Cerebral Ventricle 0016
Ventrio™ Hernia Patch *use* Synthetic Substitute
VEP (visual evoked potential) 4A07X0Z
Vermiform appendix *use* Appendix
Vermilion border
use Upper Lip
use Lower Lip

Versa *use* Pacemaker, Dual Chamber in 0JH
Version, obstetric
External 10S0XZZ
Internal 10S07ZZ
Vertebral arch
use Cervical Vertebra
use Thoracic Vertebra
use Lumbar Vertebra
▶**Vertebral body**
▶*use* Cervical Vertebra
▶*use* Thoracic Vertebra
▶*use* Lumbar Vertebra
Vertebral canal *use* Spinal Canal
Vertebral foramen
use Cervical Vertebra
use Thoracic Vertebra
use Lumbar Vertebra
Vertebral lamina
use Cervical Vertebra
use Thoracic Vertebra
use Lumbar Vertebra
Vertebral pedicle
use Cervical Vertebra
use Thoracic Vertebra
use Lumbar Vertebra
Vesical vein
use Hypogastric Vein, Right
use Hypogastric Vein, Left
Vesicotomy *see* Drainage, Urinary System 0T9
Vesiculectomy
see Excision, Male Reproductive System 0VB
see Resection, Male Reproductive System 0VT
Vesiculogram, seminal *see* Plain Radiography, Male Reproductive System BV0
Vesiculotomy *see* Drainage, Male Reproductive System 0V9
Vestibular (Scarpa's) ganglion *use* Acoustic Nerve
Vestibular Assessment F15Z
Vestibular nerve *use* Acoustic Nerve
Vestibular Treatment F0C
Vestibulocochlear nerve *use* Acoustic Nerve
VH-IVUS (virtual histology intravascular ultrasound) *see* Ultrasonography, Heart B24
Virchow's (supraclavicular) lymph node
use Lymphatic, Right Neck
use Lymphatic, Left Neck
Virtuoso (II) (DR) (VR) *use* Defibrillator Generator in 0JH
Vistogard® *use* Uridine Triacetate
Vitrectomy
see Excision, Eye 08B
see Resection, Eye 08T
Vitreous body
use Vitreous, Right
use Vitreous, Left
Viva (XT)(S) *use* Cardiac Resynchronization Defibrillator Pulse Generator in 0JH
Vocal fold
use Vocal Cord, Right
use Vocal Cord, Left
Vocational
Assessment *see* Activities of Daily Living Assessment, Rehabilitation F02
Retraining *see* Activities of Daily Living Treatment, Rehabilitation F08
Volar (palmar) digital vein
use Hand Vein, Right
use Hand Vein, Left
Volar (palmar) metacarpal vein
use Hand Vein, Right
use Hand Vein, Left
Vomer bone *use* Nasal Septum
Vomer of nasal septum *use* Nasal Bone
Voraxaze *use* Glucarpidase
Vulvectomy
see Excision, Female Reproductive System 0UB
see Resection, Female Reproductive System 0UT
▶**VYXEOS™** *use* Cytarabine and Daunorubicin Liposome Antineoplastic

W

WALLSTENT® Endoprosthesis *use* Intraluminal Device
Washing *see* Irrigation
Wedge resection, pulmonary *see* Excision, Respiratory System 0BB
Window *see* Drainage
Wiring, dental 2W31X9Z

X

Xact Carotid Stent System *use* Intraluminal Device
X-ray *see* Plain Radiography
X-STOP® Spacer
use Spinal Stabilization Device, Interspinous Process in 0RH
use Spinal Stabilization Device, Interspinous Process in 0SH
Xenograft *use* Zooplastic Tissue in Heart and Great Vessels
XIENCE Everolimus Eluting Coronary Stent System *use* Intraluminal Device, Drug-eluting in Heart and Great Vessels
Xiphoid process *use* Sternum
XLIF® System *use* Interbody Fusion Device in Lower Joints

Y

Yoga Therapy 8E0ZXY4

Z

Z-plasty, skin for scar contracture *see* Release, Skin and Breast 0HN
Zenith AAA Endovascular Graft
use Intraluminal Device, Branched or Fenestrated, One or Two Arteries in 04V
use Intraluminal Device, Branched or Fenestrated, Three or More Arteries in 04V
use Intraluminal Device
Zenith Flex® AAA Endovascular Graft *use* Intraluminal Device
Zenith TX2® TAA Endovascular Graft *use* Intraluminal Device
Zenith® Renu™ AAA Ancillary Graft *use* Intraluminal Device
Zilver® PTX® (paclitaxel) Drug-Eluting Peripheral Stent
use Intraluminal Device, Drug-eluting in Upper Arteries
use Intraluminal Device, Drug-eluting in Lower Arteries
Zimmer® NexGen® LPS Mobile Bearing Knee *use* Synthetic Substitute
Zimmer® NexGen® LPS-Flex Mobile Knee *use* Synthetic Substitute
▶**ZINPLAVA™** *use* Bezlotoxumab Monoclonal Antibody
Zonule of Zinn
use Lens, Right
use Lens, Left
Zooplastic Tissue, Rapid Deployment Technique, Replacement X2RF
Zotarolimus-eluting coronary stent *use* Intraluminal Device, Drug-eluting in Heart and Great Vessels
➡**Zygomatic process of frontal bone** *use* Frontal Bone
~~*use* Frontal Bone, Right~~
~~*use* Frontal Bone, Left~~
Zygomatic process of temporal bone
use Temporal Bone, Right
use Temporal Bone, Left
Zygomaticus muscle *use* Facial Muscle
Zyvox *use* Oxazolidinones

▶ New   ➡ Revised   ~~deleted~~ Deleted

KEYS

Appendices

DEFINITIONS
SECTION-CHARACTER

Ø 3   Medical and Surgical - Operation 803
Ø 4   Medical and Surgical - Body Part 805
Ø 5   Medical and Surgical - Approach 821
Ø 6   Medical and Surgical - Device 822
1 3   Obstetrics - Operation 828
1 5   Obstetrics - Approach 829
2 3   Placement - Operation 829
2 5   Placement - Approach 830
3 3   Administration - Operation 830
3 5   Administration - Approach 830
3 6   Administration - Substance 830
4 3   Measurement and Monitoring - Operation 831
4 5   Measurement and Monitoring - Approach 831
5 3   Extracorporeal Assistance and Performance - Operation 831
6 3   Extracorporeal Therapies - Operation 831
7 3   Osteopathic - Operation 832
7 5   Osteopathic - Approach 832
8 3   Other Procedures - Operation 832
8 5   Other Procedures - Approach 832
9 3   Chiropractic - Operation 832
9 5   Chiropractic - Approach 833
B 3   Imaging - Type 833
C 3   Nuclear Medicine - Type 833
F 3   Physical Rehabilitation and Diagnostic Audiology - Type 834
F 5   Physical Rehabilitation and Diagnostic Audiology - Type Qualifier 834
G 3   Mental Health - Type 842
G 4   Mental Health - Qualifier 843
H 3   Substance Abuse Treatment - Type 844
X 3   New Technology - Operation 844
X 5   New Technology - Approach 845
X 6   New Technology - Device/Substance/Technology 845

SECTION Ø - MEDICAL AND SURGICAL
CHARACTER 3 - OPERATION

Alteration	**Definition:** Modifying the anatomic structure of a body part without affecting the function of the body part **Explanation:** Principal purpose is to improve appearance **Includes/Examples:** Face lift, breast augmentation
Bypass	**Definition:** Altering the route of passage of the contents of a tubular body part **Explanation:** Rerouting contents of a body part to a downstream area of the normal route, to a similar route and body part, or to an abnormal route and dissimilar body part. Includes one or more anastomoses, with or without the use of a device **Includes/Examples:** Coronary artery bypass, colostomy formation
Change	**Definition:** Taking out or off a device from a body part and putting back an identical or similar device in or on the same body part without cutting or puncturing the skin or a mucous membrane **Explanation:** All CHANGE procedures are coded using the approach EXTERNAL **Includes/Examples:** Urinary catheter change, gastrostomy tube change
Control	**Definition:** Stopping, or attempting to stop, postprocedural or other acute bleeding **Explanation:** The site of the bleeding is coded as an anatomical region and not to a specific body part **Includes/Examples:** Control of post-prostatectomy hemorrhage, control of intracranial subdural hemorrhage, control of bleeding duodenal ulcer, control of retroperitoneal hemorrhage
Creation	**Definition:** Putting in or on biological or synthetic material to form a new body part that to the extent possible replicates the anatomic structure or function of an absent body part **Explanation:** Used for gender reassignment surgery and corrective procedures in individuals with congenital anomalies **Includes/Examples:** Creation of vagina in a male, creation of right and left atrioventricular valve from common atrioventricular valve
Destruction	**Definition:** Physical eradication of all or a portion of a body part by the direct use of energy, force, or a destructive agent **Explanation:** None of the body part is physically taken out **Includes/Examples:** Fulguration of rectal polyp, cautery of skin lesion

Detachment	**Definition:** Cutting off all or a portion of the upper or lower extremities **Explanation:** The body part value is the site of the detachment, with a qualifier if applicable to further specify the level where the extremity was detached **Includes/Examples:** Below knee amputation, disarticulation of shoulder
Dilation	**Definition:** Expanding an orifice or the lumen of a tubular body part **Explanation:** The orifice can be a natural orifice or an artificially created orifice. Accomplished by stretching a tubular body part using intraluminal pressure or by cutting part of the orifice or wall of the tubular body part **Includes/Examples:** Percutaneous transluminal angioplasty, internal urethrotomy
Division	**Definition:** Cutting into a body part, without draining fluids and/or gases from the body part, in order to separate or transect a body part **Explanation:** All or a portion of the body part is separated into two or more portions **Includes/Examples:** Spinal cordotomy, osteotomy
Drainage	**Definition:** Taking or letting out fluids and/or gases from a body part **Explanation:** The qualifier DIAGNOSTIC is used to identify drainage procedures that are biopsies **Includes/Examples:** Thoracentesis, incision and drainage
Excision	**Definition:** Cutting out or off, without replacement, a portion of a body part **Explanation:** The qualifier DIAGNOSTIC is used to identify excision procedures that are biopsies **Includes/Examples:** Partial nephrectomy, liver biopsy
Extirpation	**Definition:** Taking or cutting out solid matter from a body part **Explanation:** The solid matter may be an abnormal byproduct of a biological function or a foreign body; it may be imbedded in a body part or in the lumen of a tubular body part. The solid matter may or may not have been previously broken into pieces **Includes/Examples:** Thrombectomy, choledocholithotomy
Extraction	**Definition:** Pulling or stripping out or off all or a portion of a body part by the use of force **Explanation:** The qualifier DIAGNOSTIC is used to identify extraction procedures that are biopsies **Includes/Examples:** Dilation and curettage, vein stripping

SECTION Ø - MEDICAL AND SURGICAL
CHARACTER 3 - OPERATION

Fragmentation	**Definition:** Breaking solid matter in a body part into pieces **Explanation:** Physical force (e.g., manual, ultrasonic) applied directly or indirectly is used to break the solid matter into pieces. The solid matter may be an abnormal byproduct of a biological function or a foreign body. The pieces of solid matter are not taken out **Includes/Examples:** Extracorporeal shockwave lithotripsy, transurethral lithotripsy
Fusion	**Definition:** Joining together portions of an articular body part rendering the articular body part immobile **Explanation:** The body part is joined together by fixation device, bone graft, or other means **Includes/Examples:** Spinal fusion, ankle arthrodesis
Insertion	**Definition:** Putting in a nonbiological appliance that monitors, assists, performs, or prevents a physiological function but does not physically take the place of a body part **Includes/Examples:** Insertion of radioactive implant, insertion of central venous catheter
Inspection	**Definition:** Visually and/or manually exploring a body part **Explanation:** Visual exploration may be performed with or without optical instrumentation. Manual exploration may be performed directly or through intervening body layers **Includes/Examples:** Diagnostic arthroscopy, exploratory laparotomy
Map	**Definition:** Locating the route of passage of electrical impulses and/or locating functional areas in a body part **Explanation:** Applicable only to the cardiac conduction mechanism and the central nervous system **Includes/Examples:** Cardiac mapping, cortical mapping
Occlusion	**Definition:** Completely closing an orifice or the lumen of a tubular body part **Explanation:** The orifice can be a natural orifice or an artificially created orifice **Includes/Examples:** Fallopian tube ligation, ligation of inferior vena cava
Reattachment	**Definition:** Putting back in or on all or a portion of a separated body part to its normal location or other suitable location **Explanation:** Vascular circulation and nervous pathways may or may not be reestablished **Includes/Examples:** Reattachment of hand, reattachment of avulsed kidney

Release	**Definition:** Freeing a body part from an abnormal physical constraint by cutting or by the use of force **Explanation:** Some of the restraining tissue may be taken out but none of the body part is taken out **Includes/Examples:** Adhesiolysis, carpal tunnel release
Removal	**Definition:** Taking out or off a device from a body part **Explanation:** If a device is taken out and a similar device put in without cutting or puncturing the skin or mucous membrane, the procedure is coded to the root operation CHANGE. Otherwise, the procedure for taking out a device is coded to the root operation REMOVAL **Includes/Examples:** Drainage tube removal, cardiac pacemaker removal
Repair	**Definition:** Restoring, to the extent possible, a body part to its normal anatomic structure and function **Explanation:** Used only when the method to accomplish the repair is not one of the other root operations **Includes/Examples:** Colostomy takedown, suture of laceration
Replacement	**Definition:** Putting in or on biological or synthetic material that physically takes the place and/or function of all or a portion of a body part **Explanation:** The body part may have been taken out or replaced, or may be taken out, physically eradicated, or rendered nonfunctional during the Replacement procedure. A Removal procedure is coded for taking out the device used in a previous replacement procedure **Includes/Examples:** Total hip replacement, bone graft, free skin graft
Reposition	**Definition:** Moving to its normal location, or other suitable location, all or a portion of a body part **Explanation:** The body part is moved to a new location from an abnormal location, or from a normal location where it is not functioning correctly. The body part may or may not be cut out or off to be moved to the new location **Includes/Examples:** Reposition of undescended testicle, fracture reduction
Resection	**Definition:** Cutting out or off, without replacement, all of a body part **Includes/Examples:** Total nephrectomy, total lobectomy of lung

SECTION 0 - MEDICAL AND SURGICAL
CHARACTER 3 - OPERATION

Restriction	**Definition:** Partially closing an orifice or the lumen of a tubular body part **Explanation:** The orifice can be a natural orifice or an artificially created orifice **Includes/Examples:** Esophagogastric fundoplication, cervical cerclage
Revision	**Definition:** Correcting, to the extent possible, a portion of a malfunctioning device or the position of a displaced device **Explanation:** Revision can include correcting a malfunctioning or displaced device by taking out or putting in components of the device such as a screw or pin **Includes/Examples:** Adjustment of position of pacemaker lead, recementing of hip prosthesis
Supplement	**Definition:** Putting in or on biological or synthetic material that physically reinforces and/or augments the function of a portion of a body part **Explanation:** The biological material is non-living, or is living and from the same individual. The body part may have been previously replaced, and the Supplement procedure is performed to physically reinforce and/or augment the function of the replaced body part **Includes/Examples:** Herniorrhaphy using mesh, free nerve graft, mitral valve ring annuloplasty, put a new acetabular liner in a previous hip replacement

Transfer	**Definition:** Moving, without taking out, all or a portion of a body part to another location to take over the function of all or a portion of a body part **Explanation:** The body part transferred remains connected to its vascular and nervous supply **Includes/Examples:** Tendon transfer, skin pedicle flap transfer
Transplantation	**Definition:** Putting in or on all or a portion of a living body part taken from another individual or animal to physically take the place and/or function of all or a portion of a similar body part **Explanation:** The native body part may or may not be taken out, and the transplanted body part may take over all or a portion of its function **Includes/Examples:** Kidney transplant, heart transplant

SECTION 0 - MEDICAL AND SURGICAL
CHARACTER 4 - BODY PART

1st Toe, Left 1st Toe, Right	**Includes:** Hallux
Abdomen Muscle, Left Abdomen Muscle, Right	**Includes:** External oblique muscle Internal oblique muscle Pyramidalis muscle Rectus abdominis muscle Transversus abdominis muscle
Abdominal Aorta	**Includes:** Inferior phrenic artery Lumbar artery Median sacral artery Middle suprarenal artery Ovarian artery Testicular artery

Abdominal Sympathetic Nerve	**Includes:** Abdominal aortic plexus Auerbach's (myenteric) plexus Celiac (solar) plexus Celiac ganglion Gastric plexus Hepatic plexus Inferior hypogastric plexus Inferior mesenteric ganglion Inferior mesenteric plexus Meissner's (submucous) plexus Myenteric (Auerbach's) plexus Pancreatic plexus Pelvic splanchnic nerve Renal plexus Solar (celiac) plexus Splenic plexus Submucous (Meissner's) plexus Superior hypogastric plexus Superior mesenteric ganglion Superior mesenteric plexus Suprarenal plexus

SECTION Ø - MEDICAL AND SURGICAL
CHARACTER 4 - BODY PART

Abducens Nerve	**Includes:** Sixth cranial nerve
Accessory Nerve	**Includes:** Eleventh cranial nerve
Acoustic Nerve	**Includes:** Cochlear nerve Eighth cranial nerve Scarpa's (vestibular) ganglion Spiral ganglion Vestibular (Scarpa's) ganglion Vestibular nerve Vestibulocochlear nerve
Adenoids	**Includes:** Pharyngeal tonsil
Adrenal Gland Adrenal Gland, Left Adrenal Gland, Right Adrenal Glands, Bilateral	**Includes:** Suprarenal gland
Ampulla of Vater	**Includes:** Duodenal ampulla Hepatopancreatic ampulla
Anal Sphincter	**Includes:** External anal sphincter Internal anal sphincter
Ankle Bursa and Ligament, Left Ankle Bursa and Ligament, Right	**Includes:** Calcaneofibular ligament Deltoid ligament Ligament of the lateral malleolus Talofibular ligament
Ankle Joint, Left Ankle Joint, Right	**Includes:** Inferior tibiofibular joint Talocrural joint
Anterior Chamber, Left Anterior Chamber, Right	**Includes:** Aqueous humour
Anterior Tibial Artery, Left Anterior Tibial Artery, Right	**Includes:** Anterior lateral malleolar artery Anterior medial malleolar artery Anterior tibial recurrent artery Dorsalis pedis artery Posterior tibial recurrent artery
Anus	**Includes:** Anal orifice

Aortic Valve	**Includes:** Aortic annulus
Appendix	**Includes:** Vermiform appendix
Atrial Septum	**Includes:** Interatrial septum
Atrium, Left	**Includes:** Atrium pulmonale Left auricular appendix
Atrium, Right	**Includes:** Atrium dextrum cordis Right auricular appendix Sinus venosus
Auditory Ossicle, Left Auditory Ossicle, Right	**Includes:** Incus Malleus Stapes
Axillary Artery, Left Axillary Artery, Right	**Includes:** Anterior circumflex humeral artery Lateral thoracic artery Posterior circumflex humeral artery Subscapular artery Superior thoracic artery Thoracoacromial artery
Azygos Vein	**Includes:** Right ascending lumbar vein Right subcostal vein
Basal Ganglia	**Includes:** Basal nuclei Claustrum Corpus striatum Globus pallidus Substantia nigra Subthalamic nucleus
Basilic Vein, Left Basilic Vein, Right	**Includes:** Median antebrachial vein Median cubital vein
Bladder	**Includes:** Trigone of bladder
Brachial Artery, Left Brachial Artery, Right	**Includes:** Inferior ulnar collateral artery Profunda brachii Superior ulnar collateral artery

SECTION Ø - MEDICAL AND SURGICAL
CHARACTER 4 - BODY PART

Brachial Plexus	**Includes:** Axillary nerve Dorsal scapular nerve First intercostal nerve Long thoracic nerve Musculocutaneous nerve Subclavius nerve Suprascapular nerve
Brachial Vein, Left Brachial Vein, Right	**Includes:** Radial vein Ulnar vein
Brain	**Includes:** Cerebrum Corpus callosum Encephalon
Breast, Bilateral Breast, Left Breast, Right	**Includes:** Mammary duct Mammary gland
Buccal Mucosa	**Includes:** Buccal gland Molar gland Palatine gland
Carotid Bodies, Bilateral Carotid Body, Left Carotid Body, Right	**Includes:** Carotid glomus
Carpal Joint, Left Carpal Joint, Right	**Includes:** Intercarpal joint Midcarpal joint
Carpal, Left Carpal, Right	**Includes:** Capitate bone Hamate bone Lunate bone Pisiform bone Scaphoid bone Trapezium bone Trapezoid bone Triquetral bone
Celiac Artery	**Includes:** Celiac trunk
Cephalic Vein, Left Cephalic Vein, Right	**Includes:** Accessory cephalic vein
Cerebellum	**Includes:** Culmen
Cerebral Hemisphere	**Includes:** Frontal lobe Occipital lobe Parietal lobe Temporal lobe

Cerebral Meninges	**Includes:** Arachnoid mater, intracranial Leptomeninges, intracranial Pia mater, intracranial
Cerebral Ventricle	**Includes:** Aqueduct of Sylvius Cerebral aqueduct (Sylvius) Choroid plexus Ependyma Foramen of Monro (intraventricular) Fourth ventricle Interventricular foramen (Monro) Left lateral ventricle Right lateral ventricle Third ventricle
Cervical Nerve	**Includes:** Greater occipital nerve Spinal nerve, cervical Suboccipital nerve Third occipital nerve
Cervical Plexus	**Includes:** Ansa cervicalis Cutaneous (transverse) cervical nerve Great auricular nerve Lesser occipital nerve Supraclavicular nerve Transverse (cutaneous) cervical nerve
Cervical Vertebra	**Includes:** Dens Odontoid process Spinous process Transverse foramen Transverse process Vertebral body Vertebral arch Vertebral foramen Vertebral lamina Vertebral pedicle
Cervical Vertebral Joint	**Includes:** Atlantoaxial joint Cervical facet joint
Cervical Vertebral Joints, 2 or more	**Includes:** Cervical facet joint
Cervicothoracic Vertebral Joint	**Includes:** Cervicothoracic facet joint
Cisterna Chyli	**Includes:** Intestinal lymphatic trunk Lumbar lymphatic trunk
Coccygeal Glomus	**Includes:** Coccygeal body

SECTION Ø - MEDICAL AND SURGICAL
CHARACTER 4 - BODY PART

Body Part	Includes
Colic Vein	**Includes:** Ileocolic vein Left colic vein Middle colic vein Right colic vein
Conduction Mechanism	**Includes:** Atrioventricular node Bundle of His Bundle of Kent Sinoatrial node
Conjunctiva, Left Conjunctiva, Right	**Includes:** Plica semilunaris
Dura Mater	**Includes:** Diaphragma sellae Dura mater, intracranial Falx cerebri Tentorium cerebelli
Elbow Bursa and Ligament, Left Elbow Bursa and Ligament, Right	**Includes:** Annular ligament Olecranon bursa Radial collateral ligament Ulnar collateral ligament
Elbow Joint, Left Elbow Joint, Right	**Includes:** Distal humerus, involving joint Humeroradial joint Humeroulnar joint Proximal radioulnar joint
Epidural Space, Intracranial	**Includes:** Extradural space, intracranial
Epiglottis	**Includes:** Glossoepiglottic fold
Esophagogastric Junction	**Includes:** Cardia Cardioesophageal junction Gastroesophageal (GE) junction
Esophagus, Lower	**Includes:** Abdominal esophagus
Esophagus, Middle	**Includes:** Thoracic esophagus
Esophagus, Upper	**Includes:** Cervical esophagus
Ethmoid Bone, Left Ethmoid Bone, Right	**Includes:** Cribriform plate
Ethmoid Sinus, Left Ethmoid Sinus, Right	**Includes:** Ethmoidal air cell

Body Part	Includes
Eustachian Tube, Left Eustachian Tube, Right	**Includes:** Auditory tube Pharyngotympanic tube
External Auditory Canal, Left External Auditory Canal, Right	**Includes:** External auditory meatus
External Carotid Artery, Left External Carotid Artery, Right	**Includes:** Ascending pharyngeal artery Internal maxillary artery Lingual artery Maxillary artery Occipital artery Posterior auricular artery Superior thyroid artery
External Ear, Bilateral External Ear, Left External Ear, Right	**Includes:** Antihelix Antitragus Auricle Earlobe Helix Pinna Tragus
External Iliac Artery, Left External Iliac Artery, Right	**Includes:** Deep circumflex iliac artery Inferior epigastric artery
External Jugular Vein, Left External Jugular Vein, Right	**Includes:** Posterior auricular vein
Extraocular Muscle, Left Extraocular Muscle, Right	**Includes:** Inferior oblique muscle Inferior rectus muscle Lateral rectus muscle Medial rectus muscle Superior oblique muscle Superior rectus muscle
Eye, Left Eye, Right	**Includes:** Ciliary body Posterior chamber
Face Artery	**Includes:** Angular artery Ascending palatine artery External maxillary artery Facial artery Inferior labial artery Submental artery Superior labial artery

SECTION Ø - MEDICAL AND SURGICAL
CHARACTER 4 - BODY PART

Face Vein, Left **Face Vein, Right**	**Includes:** Angular vein Anterior facial vein Common facial vein Deep facial vein Frontal vein Posterior facial (retromandibular) vein Supraorbital vein
Facial Muscle	**Includes:** Buccinator muscle Corrugator supercilii muscle Depressor anguli oris muscle Depressor labii inferioris muscle Depressor septi nasi muscle Depressor supercilii muscle Levator anguli oris muscle Levator labii superioris alaeque nasi muscle Levator labii superioris muscle Mentalis muscle Nasalis muscle Occipitofrontalis muscle Orbicularis oris muscle Procerus muscle Risorius muscle Zygomaticus muscle
Facial Nerve	**Includes:** Chorda tympani Geniculate ganglion Greater superficial petrosal nerve Nerve to the stapedius Parotid plexus Posterior auricular nerve Seventh cranial nerve Submandibular ganglion
Fallopian Tube, Left **Fallopian Tube, Right**	**Includes:** Oviduct Salpinx Uterine tube
Femoral Artery, Left **Femoral Artery, Right**	**Includes:** Circumflex iliac artery Deep femoral artery Descending genicular artery External pudendal artery Superficial epigastric artery
Femoral Nerve	**Includes:** Anterior crural nerve Saphenous nerve
Femoral Shaft, Left **Femoral Shaft, Right**	**Includes:** Body of femur

Femoral Vein, Left **Femoral Vein, Right**	**Includes:** Deep femoral (profunda femoris) vein Popliteal vein Profunda femoris (deep femoral) vein
Fibula, Left **Fibula, Right**	**Includes:** Body of fibula Head of fibula Lateral malleolus
Finger Nail	**Includes:** Nail bed Nail plate
Finger Phalangeal Joint, Left **Finger Phalangeal Joint, Right**	**Includes:** Interphalangeal (IP) joint
Foot Artery, Left **Foot Artery, Right**	**Includes:** Arcuate artery Dorsal metatarsal artery Lateral plantar artery Lateral tarsal artery Medial plantar artery
Foot Bursa and Ligament, Left **Foot Bursa and Ligament, Right**	**Includes:** Calcaneocuboid ligament Cuneonavicular ligament Intercuneiform ligament Interphalangeal ligament Metatarsal ligament Metatarsophalangeal ligament Subtalar ligament Talocalcaneal ligament Talocalcaneonavicular ligament Tarsometatarsal ligament
Foot Muscle, Left **Foot Muscle, Right**	**Includes:** Abductor hallucis muscle Adductor hallucis muscle Extensor digitorum brevis muscle Extensor hallucis brevis muscle Flexor digitorum brevis muscle Flexor hallucis brevis muscle Quadratus plantae muscle
Foot Vein, Left **Foot Vein, Right**	**Includes:** Common digital vein Dorsal metatarsal vein Dorsal venous arch Plantar digital vein Plantar metatarsal vein Plantar venous arch
Frontal Bone	**Includes:** Zygomatic process of frontal bone

SECTION Ø - MEDICAL AND SURGICAL
CHARACTER 4 - BODY PART

Gastric Artery	**Includes:** Left gastric artery Right gastric artery
Glenoid Cavity, Left Glenoid Cavity, Right	**Includes:** Glenoid fossa (of scapula)
Glomus Jugulare	**Includes:** Jugular body
Glossopharyngeal Nerve	**Includes:** Carotid sinus nerve Ninth cranial nerve Tympanic nerve
Hand Artery, Left Hand Artery, Right	**Includes:** Deep palmar arch Princeps pollicis artery Radialis indicis Superficial palmar arch
Hand Bursa and Ligament, Left Hand Bursa and Ligament, Right	**Includes:** Carpometacarpal ligament Intercarpal ligament Interphalangeal ligament Lunotriquetral ligament Metacarpal ligament Metacarpophalangeal ligament Pisohamate ligament Pisometacarpal ligament Scapholunate ligament Scaphotrapezium ligament
Hand Muscle, Left Hand Muscle, Right	**Includes:** Hypothenar muscle Palmar interosseous muscle Thenar muscle
Hand Vein, Left Hand Vein, Right	**Includes:** Dorsal metacarpal vein Palmar (volar) digital vein Palmar (volar) metacarpal vein Superficial palmar venous arch Volar (palmar) digital vein Volar (palmar) metacarpal vein
Head and Neck Bursa and Ligament	**Includes:** Alar ligament of axis Cervical interspinous ligament Cervical intertransverse ligament Cervical ligamentum flavum Interspinous ligament Lateral temporomandibular ligament Sphenomandibular ligament Stylomandibular ligament Transverse ligament of atlas
Head and Neck Sympathetic Nerve	**Includes:** Cavernous plexus Cervical ganglion Ciliary ganglion Internal carotid plexus Otic ganglion Pterygopalatine (sphenopalatine) ganglion Sphenopalatine (pterygopalatine) ganglion Stellate ganglion Submandibular ganglion Submaxillary ganglion
Head Muscle	**Includes:** Auricularis muscle Masseter muscle Pterygoid muscle Splenius capitis muscle Temporalis muscle Temporoparietalis muscle
Heart, Left	**Includes:** Left coronary sulcus Obtuse margin
Heart, Right	**Includes:** Right coronary sulcus
Hemiazygos Vein	**Includes** Left ascending lumbar vein Left subcostal vein
Hepatic Artery	**Includes:** Common hepatic artery Gastroduodenal artery Hepatic artery proper
Hip Bursa and Ligament, Left Hip Bursa and Ligament, Right	**Includes:** Iliofemoral ligament Ischiofemoral ligament Pubofemoral ligament Transverse acetabular ligament Trochanteric bursa
Hip Joint, Left Hip Joint, Right	**Includes:** Acetabulofemoral joint
Hip Muscle, Left Hip Muscle, Right	**Includes:** Gemellus muscle Gluteus maximus muscle Gluteus medius muscle Gluteus minimus muscle Iliacus muscle Obturator muscle Piriformis muscle Psoas muscle Quadratus femoris muscle Tensor fasciae latae muscle

SECTION 0 - MEDICAL AND SURGICAL
CHARACTER 4 - BODY PART

Humeral Head, Left Humeral Head, Right	**Includes:** Greater tuberosity Lesser tuberosity Neck of humerus (anatomical) (surgical)
Humeral Shaft, Left Humeral Shaft, Right	**Includes:** Distal humerus Humerus, distal Lateral epicondyle of humerus Medial epicondyle of humerus
Hypogastric Vein, Left Hypogastric Vein, Right	**Includes:** Gluteal vein Internal iliac vein Internal pudendal vein Lateral sacral vein Middle hemorrhoidal vein Obturator vein Uterine vein Vaginal vein Vesical vein
Hypoglossal Nerve	**Includes:** Twelfth cranial nerve
Hypothalamus	**Includes:** Mammillary body
Inferior Mesenteric Artery	**Includes:** Sigmoid artery Superior rectal artery
Inferior Mesenteric Vein	**Includes:** Sigmoid vein Superior rectal vein
Inferior Vena Cava	**Includes:** Postcava Right inferior phrenic vein Right ovarian vein Right second lumbar vein Right suprarenal vein Right testicular vein
Inguinal Region, Bilateral Inguinal Region, Left Inguinal Region, Right	**Includes:** Inguinal canal Inguinal triangle
Inner Ear, Left Inner Ear, Right	**Includes:** Bony labyrinth Bony vestibule Cochlea Round window Semicircular canal

Innominate Artery	**Includes:** Brachiocephalic artery Brachiocephalic trunk
Innominate Vein, Left Innominate Vein, Right	**Includes:** Brachiocephalic vein Inferior thyroid vein
Internal Carotid Artery, Left Internal Carotid Artery, Right	**Includes:** Caroticotympanic artery Carotid sinus
Internal Iliac Artery, Left Internal Iliac Artery, Right	**Includes:** Deferential artery Hypogastric artery Iliolumbar artery Inferior gluteal artery Inferior vesical artery Internal pudendal artery Lateral sacral artery Middle rectal artery Obturator artery Superior gluteal artery Umbilical artery Uterine Artery Vaginal artery
Internal Mammary Artery, Left Internal Mammary Artery, Right	**Includes:** Anterior intercostal artery Internal thoracic artery Musculophrenic artery Pericardiophrenic artery Superior epigastric artery
Intracranial Artery	**Includes:** Anterior cerebral artery Anterior choroidal artery Anterior communicating artery Basilar artery Circle of Willis Internal carotid artery, intracranial portion Middle cerebral artery Ophthalmic artery Posterior cerebral artery Posterior communicating artery Posterior inferior cerebellar artery (PICA)

APPENDIX A

SECTION Ø - MEDICAL AND SURGICAL
CHARACTER 4 - BODY PART

Intracranial Vein	**Includes:** Anterior cerebral vein Basal (internal) cerebral vein Dural venous sinus Great cerebral vein Inferior cerebellar vein Inferior cerebral vein Internal (basal) cerebral vein Middle cerebral vein Ophthalmic vein Superior cerebellar vein Superior cerebral vein
Jejunum	**Includes:** Duodenojejunal flexure
Kidney	**Includes:** Renal calyx Renal capsule Renal cortex Renal segment
Kidney Pelvis, Left Kidney Pelvis, Right	**Includes:** Ureteropelvic junction (UPJ)
Kidney, Left Kidney, Right Kidneys, Bilateral	**Includes:** Renal calyx Renal capsule Renal cortex Renal segment
Knee Bursa and Ligament, Left Knee Bursa and Ligament, Right	**Includes:** Anterior cruciate ligament (ACL) Lateral collateral ligament (LCL) Ligament of head of fibula Medial collateral ligament (MCL) Patellar ligament Popliteal ligament Posterior cruciate ligament (PCL) Prepatellar bursa
Knee Joint, Femoral Surface, Left Knee Joint, Femoral Surface, Right	**Includes:** Femoropatellar joint Patellofemoral joint
Knee Joint, Left Knee Joint, Right	**Includes:** Femoropatellar joint Femorotibial joint Lateral meniscus Medial meniscus Patellofemoral joint Tibiofemoral joint

Knee Joint, Tibial Surface, Left Knee Joint, Tibial Surface, Right	**Includes:** Femorotibial joint Tibiofemoral joint
Knee Tendon, Left Knee Tendon, Right	**Includes:** Patellar tendon
Lacrimal Duct, Left Lacrimal Duct, Right	**Includes:** Lacrimal canaliculus Lacrimal punctum Lacrimal sac Nasolacrimal duct
Larynx	**Includes:** Aryepiglottic fold Arytenoid cartilage Corniculate cartilage ~~Cricoid cartilage~~ Cuneiform cartilage False vocal cord Glottis Rima glottidis Thyroid cartilage Ventricular fold
Lens, Left Lens, Right	**Includes:** Zonule of Zinn
Liver	**Includes:** Quadrate lobe
Lower Arm and Wrist Muscle, Left Lower Arm and Wrist Muscle, Right	**Includes:** Anatomical snuffbox Brachioradialis muscle Extensor carpi radialis muscle Extensor carpi ulnaris muscle Flexor carpi radialis muscle Flexor carpi ulnaris muscle Flexor pollicis longus muscle Palmaris longus muscle Pronator quadratus muscle Pronator teres muscle
Lower Artery	**Includes:** Umbilical artery
Lower Eyelid, Left Lower Eyelid, Right	**Includes:** Inferior tarsal plate Medial canthus
Lower Femur, Left Lower Femur, Right	**Includes:** Lateral condyle of femur Lateral epicondyle of femur Medial condyle of femur Medial epicondyle of femur

SECTION Ø - MEDICAL AND SURGICAL
CHARACTER 4 - BODY PART

Lower Leg Muscle, Left Lower Leg Muscle, Right	**Includes:** Extensor digitorum longus muscle Extensor hallucis longus muscle Fibularis brevis muscle Fibularis longus muscle Flexor digitorum longus muscle Flexor hallucis longus muscle Gastrocnemius muscle Peroneus brevis muscle Peroneus longus muscle Popliteus muscle Soleus muscle Tibialis anterior muscle Tibialis posterior muscle
Lower Leg Tendon, Left Lower Leg Tendon, Right	**Includes:** Achilles tendon
Lower Lip	**Includes:** Frenulum labii inferioris Labial gland Vermilion border
Lower Spine Bursa and Ligament	**Includes:** Iliolumbar ligament Interspinous ligament Intertransverse ligament Ligamentum flavum Sacrococcygeal ligament Sacroiliac ligament Sacrospinous ligament Sacrotuberous ligament Supraspinous ligament
Lumbar Nerve	**Includes:** Lumbosacral trunk Spinal nerve, lumbar Superior clunic (cluneal) nerve
Lumbar Plexus	**Includes:** Accessory obturator nerve Genitofemoral nerve Iliohypogastric nerve Ilioinguinal nerve Lateral femoral cutaneous nerve Obturator nerve Superior gluteal nerve
Lumbar Spinal Cord	**Includes:** Cauda equina Conus medullaris
Lumbar Sympathetic Nerve	**Includes:** Lumbar ganglion Lumbar splanchnic nerve

Lumbar Vertebra	**Includes:** Spinous process Transverse process Vertebral arch Vertebral body Vertebral foramen Vertebral lamina Vertebral pedicle
Lumbar Vertebral Joint	**Includes:** Lumbar facet joint
Lumbosacral Joint	**Includes:** Lumbosacral facet joint
Lymphatic, Aortic	**Includes:** Celiac lymph node Gastric lymph node Hepatic lymph node Lumbar lymph node Pancreaticosplenic lymph node Paraaortic lymph node Retroperitoneal lymph node
Lymphatic, Head	**Includes:** Buccinator lymph node Infraauricular lymph node Infraparotid lymph node Parotid lymph node Preauricular lymph node Submandibular lymph node Submaxillary lymph node Submental lymph node Subparotid lymph node Suprahyoid lymph node
Lymphatic, Left Axillary	**Includes:** Anterior (pectoral) lymph node Apical (subclavicular) lymph node Brachial (lateral) lymph node Central axillary lymph node Lateral (brachial) lymph node Pectoral (anterior) lymph node Posterior (subscapular) lymph node Subclavicular (apical) lymph node Subscapular (posterior) lymph node
Lymphatic, Left Lower Extremity	**Includes:** Femoral lymph node Popliteal lymph node
Lymphatic, Left Neck	**Includes:** Cervical lymph node Jugular lymph node Mastoid (postauricular) lymph node Occipital lymph node Postauricular (mastoid) lymph node Retropharyngeal lymph node Supraclavicular (Virchow's) lymph node Virchow's (supraclavicular) lymph node

813

SECTION Ø - MEDICAL AND SURGICAL
CHARACTER 4 - BODY PART

Lymphatic, Left Upper Extremity	**Includes:** Cubital lymph node Deltopectoral (infraclavicular) lymph node Epitrochlear lymph node Infraclavicular (deltopectoral) lymph node Supratrochlear lymph node
Lymphatic, Mesenteric	**Includes:** Inferior mesenteric lymph node Pararectal lymph node Superior mesenteric lymph node
Lymphatic, Pelvis	**Includes:** Common iliac (subaortic) lymph node Gluteal lymph node Iliac lymph node Inferior epigastric lymph node Obturator lymph node Sacral lymph node Subaortic (common iliac) lymph node Suprainguinal lymph node
Lymphatic, Right Axillary	**Includes:** Anterior (pectoral) lymph node Apical (subclavicular) lymph node Brachial (lateral) lymph node Central axillary lymph node Lateral (brachial) lymph node Pectoral (anterior) lymph node Posterior (subscapular) lymph node Subclavicular (apical) lymph node Subscapular (posterior) lymph node
Lymphatic, Right Lower Extremity	**Includes:** Femoral lymph node Popliteal lymph node
Lymphatic, Right Neck	**Includes:** Cervical lymph node Jugular lymph node Mastoid (postauricular) lymph node Occipital lymph node Postauricular (mastoid) lymph node Retropharyngeal lymph node Right jugular trunk Right lymphatic duct Right subclavian trunk Supraclavicular (Virchow's) lymph node Virchow's (supraclavicular) lymph node
Lymphatic, Right Upper Extremity	**Includes:** Cubital lymph node Deltopectoral (infraclavicular) lymph node Epitrochlear lymph node Infraclavicular (deltopectoral) lymph node Supratrochlear lymph node

Lymphatic, Thorax	**Includes:** Intercostal lymph node Mediastinal lymph node Parasternal lymph node Paratracheal lymph node Tracheobronchial lymph node
Main Bronchus, Right	**Includes:** Bronchus Intermedius Intermediate bronchus
Mandible, Left Mandible, Right	**Includes:** Alveolar process of mandible Condyloid process Mandibular notch Mental foramen
Mastoid Sinus, Left Mastoid Sinus, Right	**Includes:** Mastoid air cells
Maxilla	**Includes:** Alveolar process of maxilla
Maxillary Sinus, Left Maxillary Sinus, Right	**Includes:** Antrum of Highmore
Median Nerve	**Includes:** Anterior interosseous nerve Palmar cutaneous nerve
Medulla Oblongata	**Includes:** Myelencephalon
Mesentery	**Includes:** Mesoappendix Mesocolon
Metatarsal-Phalangeal Joint, Left Metatarsal-Phalangeal Joint, Right	**Includes:** Metatarsophalangeal (MTP) joint
Middle Ear, Left Middle Ear, Right	**Includes:** Oval window Tympanic cavity
Minor Salivary Gland	**Includes:** Anterior lingual gland
Mitral Valve	**Includes:** Bicuspid valve Left atrioventricular valve Mitral annulus
Nasal Bone	**Includes:** Vomer of nasal septum

SECTION 0 - MEDICAL AND SURGICAL
CHARACTER 4 - BODY PART

Nasal Mucosa and Soft Tissue	**Includes:** Columella External naris Greater alar cartilage Internal naris Lateral nasal cartilage Lesser alar cartilage Nasal cavity Nostril
Nasal Septum	**Includes:** Quadrangular cartilage Septal cartilage Vomer bone
Nasal Turbinate	**Includes:** Inferior turbinate Middle turbinate Nasal concha Superior turbinate
Nasopharynx	**Includes:** Choana Fossa of Rosenmuller Pharyngeal recess Rhinopharynx
Neck Muscle, Left Neck Muscle, Right	**Includes:** Anterior vertebral muscle Arytenoid muscle Cricothyroid muscle Infrahyoid muscle Levator scapulae muscle Platysma muscle Scalene muscle Splenius cervicis muscle Sternocleidomastoid muscle Suprahyoid muscle Thyroarytenoid muscle
Nipple, Left Nipple, Right	**Includes:** Areola
Occipital Bone	**Includes:** Foramen magnum
Oculomotor Nerve	**Includes:** Third cranial nerve
Olfactory Nerve	**Includes:** First cranial nerve Olfactory bulb
Omentum	**Includes:** Gastrocolic ligament Gastrocolic omentum Gastrohepatic omentum Gastrophrenic ligament Gastrosplenic ligament Greater Omentum Hepatogastric ligament Lesser Omentum

Optic Nerve	**Includes:** Optic chiasma Second cranial nerve
Orbit, Left Orbit, Right	**Includes:** Bony orbit Orbital portion of ethmoid bone Orbital portion of frontal bone Orbital portion of lacrimal bone Orbital portion of maxilla Orbital portion of palatine bone Orbital portion of sphenoid bone Orbital portion of zygomatic bone
Pancreatic Duct	**Includes:** Duct of Wirsung
Pancreatic Duct, Accessory	**Includes:** Duct of Santorini
Parotid Duct, Left Parotid Duct, Right	**Includes:** Stensen's duct
Pelvic Bone, Left Pelvic Bone, Right	**Includes:** Iliac crest Ilium Ischium Pubis
Pelvic Cavity	**Includes:** Retropubic space
Penis	**Includes:** Corpus cavernosum Corpus spongiosum
Perineum Muscle	**Includes:** Bulbospongiosus muscle Cremaster muscle Deep transverse perineal muscle Ischiocavernosus muscle Levator ani muscle Superficial transverse perineal muscle
Peritoneum	**Includes:** Epiploic foramen
Peroneal Artery, Left Peroneal Artery, Right	**Includes:** Fibular artery
Peroneal Nerve	**Includes:** Common fibular nerve Common peroneal nerve External popliteal nerve Lateral sural cutaneous nerve

SECTION Ø - MEDICAL AND SURGICAL
CHARACTER 4 - BODY PART

Pharynx	**Includes:** Base of Tongue Hypopharynx Laryngopharynx Lingual tonsil Oropharynx Piriform recess (sinus) Tongue, base of
Phrenic Nerve	**Includes:** Accessory phrenic nerve
Pituitary Gland	**Includes:** Adenohypophysis Hypophysis Neurohypophysis
Pons	**Includes:** Apneustic center Basis pontis Locus ceruleus Pneumotaxic center Pontine tegmentum Superior olivary nucleus
Popliteal Artery, Left Popliteal Artery, Right	**Includes:** Inferior genicular artery Middle genicular artery Superior genicular artery Sural artery
Portal Vein	**Includes:** Hepatic portal vein
Prepuce	**Includes:** Foreskin Glans penis
Pudendal Nerve	**Includes:** Posterior labial nerve Posterior scrotal nerve
Pulmonary Artery, Left	**Includes:** Arterial canal (duct) Botallo's duct Pulmoaortic canal
Pulmonary Valve	**Includes:** Pulmonary annulus Pulmonic valve
Pulmonary Vein, Left	**Includes:** Left inferior pulmonary vein Left superior pulmonary vein
Pulmonary Vein, Right	**Includes:** Right inferior pulmonary vein Right superior pulmonary vein
Radial Artery, Left Radial Artery, Right	**Includes:** Radial recurrent artery

Radial Nerve	**Includes:** Dorsal digital nerve Musculospiral nerve Palmar cutaneous nerve Posterior interosseous nerve
Radius, Left Radius, Right	**Includes:** Ulnar notch
Rectum	**Includes:** Anorectal junction
Renal Artery, Left Renal Artery, Right	**Includes:** Inferior suprarenal artery Renal segmental artery
Renal Vein, Left	**Includes:** Left inferior phrenic vein Left ovarian vein Left second lumbar vein Left suprarenal vein Left testicular vein
Retina, Left Retina, Right	**Includes:** Fovea Macula Optic disc
Retroperitoneum	**Includes:** Retroperitoneal space
Rib(s) Bursa and Ligament	**Includes:** Costotransverse ligament Costoxiphoid ligament Sternocostal ligament
Sacral Nerve	**Includes:** Spinal nerve, sacral
Sacral Plexus	**Includes:** Inferior gluteal nerve Posterior femoral cutaneous nerve Pudendal nerve
Sacral Sympathetic Nerve	**Includes:** Ganglion impar (ganglion of Walther) Pelvic splanchnic nerve Sacral ganglion Sacral splanchnic nerve
Sacrococcygeal Joint	**Includes:** Sacrococcygeal symphysis
Saphenous Vein, Left Saphenous Vein, Right	**Includes:** External pudendal vein Great(er) saphenous vein Lesser saphenous vein Small saphenous vein Superficial circumflex iliac vein Superficial epigastric vein

SECTION Ø - MEDICAL AND SURGICAL
CHARACTER 4 - BODY PART

Scapula, Left Scapula, Right	**Includes:** Acromion (process) Coracoid process
Sciatic Nerve	**Includes:** Ischiatic nerve
Shoulder Bursa and Ligament, Left Shoulder Bursa and Ligament, Right	**Includes:** Acromioclavicular ligament Coracoacromial ligament Coracoclavicular ligament Coracohumeral ligament Costoclavicular ligament Glenohumeral ligament Interclavicular ligament Sternoclavicular ligament Subacromial bursa Transverse humeral ligament Transverse scapular ligament
Shoulder Joint, Left Shoulder Joint, Right	**Includes:** Glenohumeral joint Glenoid ligament (labrum)
Shoulder Muscle, Left Shoulder Muscle, Right	**Includes:** Deltoid muscle Infraspinatus muscle Subscapularis muscle Supraspinatus muscle Teres major muscle Teres minor muscle
Sigmoid Colon	**Includes:** Rectosigmoid junction Sigmoid flexure
Skin	**Includes:** Dermis Epidermis Sebaceous gland Sweat gland
Sphenoid Bone	**Includes:** Greater wing Lesser wing Optic foramen Pterygoid process Sella turcica
Spinal Canal	**Includes:** Epidural space, spinal Extradural space, spinal Subarachnoid space, spinal Subdural space, spinal Vertebral canal
Spinal Meninges	**Includes:** Arachnoid mater, spinal Denticulate (dentate) ligament Dura mater, spinal Filum terminale Leptomeninges, spinal Pia mater, spinal
Spleen	**Includes:** Accessory spleen
Splenic Artery	**Includes:** Left gastroepiploic artery Pancreatic artery Short gastric artery
Splenic Vein	**Includes:** Left gastroepiploic vein Pancreatic vein
Sternum	**Includes:** Manubrium Suprasternal notch Xiphoid process
Sternum Bursa and Ligament	**Includes:** Costotransverse ligament Costoxiphoid ligament Sternocostal ligament
Stomach, Pylorus	**Includes:** Pyloric antrum Pyloric canal Pyloric sphincter
Subclavian Artery, Left Subclavian Artery, Right	**Includes:** Costocervical trunk Dorsal scapular artery Internal thoracic artery
Subcutaneous Tissue and Fascia, Chest	**Includes:** Pectoral fascia
Subcutaneous Tissue and Fascia, Face	**Includes:** Masseteric fascia Orbital fascia
Subcutaneous Tissue and Fascia, Left Foot	**Includes:** Plantar fascia (aponeurosis)
Subcutaneous Tissue and Fascia, Left Hand	**Includes:** Palmar fascia (aponeurosis)
Subcutaneous Tissue and Fascia, Left Lower Arm	**Includes:** Antebrachial fascia Bicipital aponeurosis

SECTION Ø - MEDICAL AND SURGICAL
CHARACTER 4 - BODY PART

SECTION Ø, CHARACTER 4

Subcutaneous Tissue and Fascia, Left Neck	**Includes:** Deep cervical fascia Pretracheal fascia Prevertebral fascia
Subcutaneous Tissue and Fascia, Left Upper Arm	**Includes:** Axillary fascia Deltoid fascia Infraspinatus fascia Subscapular aponeurosis Supraspinatus fascia
Subcutaneous Tissue and Fascia, Left Upper Leg	**Includes:** Crural fascia Fascia lata Iliac fascia Iliotibial tract (band)
Subcutaneous Tissue and Fascia, Right Foot	**Includes:** Plantar fascia (aponeurosis)
Subcutaneous Tissue and Fascia, Right Hand	**Includes:** Palmar fascia (aponeurosis)
Subcutaneous Tissue and Fascia, Right Lower Arm	**Includes:** Antebrachial fascia Bicipital aponeurosis
Subcutaneous Tissue and Fascia, Right Neck	**Includes:** Deep cervical fascia Pretracheal fascia Prevertebral fascia
Subcutaneous Tissue and Fascia, Right Upper Arm	**Includes:** Axillary fascia Deltoid fascia Infraspinatus fascia Subscapular aponeurosis Supraspinatus fascia
Subcutaneous Tissue and Fascia, Right Upper Leg	**Includes:** Crural fascia Fascia lata Iliac fascia Iliotibial tract (band)
Subcutaneous Tissue and Fascia, Scalp	**Includes:** Galea aponeurotica
Subcutaneous Tissue and Fascia, Trunk	**Includes:** External oblique aponeurosis Transversalis fascia
Submaxillary Gland, Left Submaxillary Gland, Right	**Includes:** Submandibular gland

Superior Mesenteric Artery	**Includes:** Ileal artery Ileocolic artery Inferior pancreaticoduodenal artery Jejunal artery
Superior Mesenteric Vein	**Includes:** Right gastroepiploic vein
Superior Vena Cava	**Includes:** Precava
Tarsal Joint, Left Tarsal Joint, Right	**Includes:** Calcaneocuboid joint Cuboideonavicular joint Cuneonavicular joint Intercuneiform joint Subtalar (talocalcaneal) joint Talocalcaneal (subtalar) joint Talocalcaneonavicular joint
Tarsal, Left Tarsal, Right	**Includes:** Calcaneus Cuboid bone Intermediate cuneiform bone Lateral cuneiform bone Medial cuneiform bone Navicular bone Talus bone
Temporal Artery, Left Temporal Artery, Right	**Includes:** Middle temporal artery Superficial temporal artery Transverse facial artery
Temporal Bone, Left Temporal Bone, Right	**Includes:** Mastoid process Petrous part of temporal bone Tympanic part of temporal bone Zygomatic process of temporal bone
Thalamus	**Includes:** Epithalamus Geniculate nucleus Metathalamus Pulvinar
Thoracic Aorta, Ascending/Arch	**Includes:** Aortic arch Ascending aorta
Thoracic Duct	**Includes:** Left jugular trunk Left subclavian trunk
Thoracic Nerve	**Includes:** Intercostal nerve Intercostobrachial nerve Spinal nerve, thoracic Subcostal nerve

SECTION Ø - MEDICAL AND SURGICAL
CHARACTER 4 - BODY PART

Thoracic Sympathetic Nerve	**Includes:** Cardiac plexus Esophageal plexus Greater splanchnic nerve Inferior cardiac nerve Least splanchnic nerve Lesser splanchnic nerve Middle cardiac nerve Pulmonary plexus Superior cardiac nerve Thoracic aortic plexus Thoracic ganglion
Thoracic Vertebra	**Includes:** Spinous process Transverse process Vertebral arch Vertebral body Vertebral foramen Vertebral lamina Vertebral pedicle
Thoracic Vertebral Joint	**Includes:** Costotransverse joint Costovertebral joint Thoracic facet joint
Thoracolumbar Vertebral Joint	**Includes:** Thoracolumbar facet joint
Thorax Muscle, Left Thorax Muscle, Right	**Includes:** Intercostal muscle Levatores costarum muscle Pectoralis major muscle Pectoralis minor muscle Serratus anterior muscle Subclavius muscle Subcostal muscle Transverse thoracis muscle
Thymus	**Includes:** Thymus gland
Thyroid Artery, Left Thyroid Artery, Right	**Includes:** Cricothyroid artery Hyoid artery Sternocleidomastoid artery Superior laryngeal artery Superior thyroid artery Thyrocervical trunk
Tibia, Left Tibia, Right	**Includes:** Lateral condyle of tibia Medial condyle of tibia Medial malleolus

Tibial Nerve	**Includes:** Lateral plantar nerve Medial plantar nerve Medial popliteal nerve Medial sural cutaneous nerve
Toe Nail	**Includes:** Nail bed Nail plate
Toe Phalangeal Joint, Left Toe Phalangeal Joint, Right	**Includes:** Interphalangeal (IP) joint
Tongue	**Includes:** Frenulum linguae
Tongue, Palate, Pharynx Muscle	**Includes:** Chrondroglossus muscle Genioglossus muscle Hyoglossus muscle Inferior longitudinal muscle Levator veli palatini muscle Palatoglossal muscle Palatopharyngeal muscle Pharyngeal constrictor muscle Salpingopharyngeus muscle Styloglossus muscle Stylopharyngeus muscle Superior longitudinal muscle Tensor veli palatini muscle
Tonsils	**Includes:** Palatine tonsil
Trachea	**Includes:** Cricoid cartilage
Transverse Colon	**Includes:** Hepatic flexure Splenic flexure
Tricuspid Valve	**Includes:** Right atrioventricular valve Tricuspid annulus
Trigeminal Nerve	**Includes:** Fifth cranial nerve Gasserian ganglion Mandibular nerve Maxillary nerve Ophthalmic nerve Trifacial nerve
Trochlear Nerve	**Includes:** Fourth cranial nerve

APPENDIX A

SECTION Ø - MEDICAL AND SURGICAL
CHARACTER 4 - BODY PART

Trunk Muscle, Left Trunk Muscle, Right	**Includes:** Coccygeus muscle Erector spinae muscle Interspinalis muscle Intertransversarius muscle Latissimus dorsi muscle Quadratus lumborum muscle Rhomboid major muscle Rhomboid minor muscle Serratus posterior muscle Transversospinalis muscle Trapezius muscle
Tympanic Membrane, Left Tympanic Membrane, Right	**Includes:** Pars flaccida
Ulna, Left Ulna, Right	**Includes:** Olecranon process Radial notch
Ulnar Artery, Left Ulnar Artery, Right	**Includes:** Anterior ulnar recurrent artery Common interosseous artery Posterior ulnar recurrent artery
Ulnar Nerve	**Includes:** Cubital nerve
Upper Arm Muscle, Left Upper Arm Muscle, Right	**Includes:** Biceps brachii muscle Brachialis muscle Coracobrachialis muscle Triceps brachii muscle
Upper Artery	**Includes:** Aortic intercostal artery Bronchial artery Esophageal artery Subcostal artery
Upper Eyelid, Left Upper Eyelid, Right	**Includes:** Lateral canthus Levator palpebrae superioris muscle Orbicularis oculi muscle Superior tarsal plate
Upper Femur, Left Upper Femur, Right	**Includes:** Femoral head Greater trochanter Lesser trochanter Neck of femur

Upper Leg Muscle, Left Upper Leg Muscle, Right	**Includes:** Adductor brevis muscle Adductor longus muscle Adductor magnus muscle Biceps femoris muscle Gracilis muscle Pectineus muscle Quadriceps (femoris) Rectus femoris muscle Sartorius muscle Semimembranosus muscle Semitendinosus muscle Vastus intermedius muscle Vastus lateralis muscle Vastus medialis muscle
Upper Lip	**Includes:** Frenulum labii superioris Labial gland Vermilion border
Upper Spine Bursa and Ligament	**Includes:** Interspinous ligament Intertransverse ligament Ligamentum flavum Supraspinous ligament
Ureter Ureter, Left Ureter, Right Ureters, Bilateral	**Includes:** Ureteral orifice Ureterovesical orifice
Urethra	**Includes:** Bulbourethral (Cowper's) gland Cowper's (bulbourethral) gland External urethral sphincter Internal urethral sphincter Membranous urethra Penile urethra Prostatic urethra
Uterine Supporting Structure	**Includes:** Broad ligament Infundibulopelvic ligament Ovarian ligament Round ligament of uterus
Uterus	**Includes:** Fundus uteri Myometrium Perimetrium Uterine cornu
Uvula	**Includes:** Palatine uvula

SECTION Ø - MEDICAL AND SURGICAL
CHARACTER 4 - BODY PART

Vagus Nerve	**Includes:** Anterior vagal trunk Pharyngeal plexus Pneumogastric nerve Posterior vagal trunk Pulmonary plexus Recurrent laryngeal nerve Superior laryngeal nerve Tenth cranial nerve
Vas Deferens Vas Deferens, Bilateral Vas Deferens, Left Vas Deferens, Right	**Includes:** Ductus deferens Ejaculatory duct
Ventricle, Right	**Includes:** Conus arteriosus
Ventricular Septum	**Includes:** Interventricular septum
Vertebral Artery, Left Vertebral Artery, Right	**Includes:** Anterior spinal artery Posterior spinal artery
Vertebral Vein, Left Vertebral Vein, Right	**Includes:** Deep cervical vein Suboccipital venous plexus

Vestibular Gland	**Includes:** Bartholin's (greater vestibular) gland Greater vestibular (Bartholin's) gland Paraurethral (Skene's) gland Skene's (paraurethral) gland
Vitreous, Left Vitreous, Right	**Includes:** Vitreous body
Vocal Cord, Left Vocal Cord, Right	**Includes:** Vocal fold
Vulva	**Includes:** Labia majora Labia minora
Wrist Bursa and Ligament, Left Wrist Bursa and Ligament, Right	**Includes:** Palmar ulnocarpal ligament Radial collateral carpal ligament Radiocarpal ligament Radioulnar ligament Ulnar collateral carpal ligament
Wrist Joint, Left Wrist Joint, Right	**Includes:** Distal radioulnar joint Radiocarpal joint

SECTION Ø - MEDICAL AND SURGICAL
CHARACTER 5 - APPROACH

External	**Definition:** Procedures performed directly on the skin or mucous membrane and procedures performed indirectly by the application of external force through the skin or mucous membrane
Open	**Definition:** Cutting through the skin or mucous membrane and any other body layers necessary to expose the site of the procedure
Percutaneous	**Definition:** Entry, by puncture or minor incision, of instrumentation through the skin or mucous membrane and any other body layers necessary to reach the site of the procedure
Percutaneous Endoscopic	**Definition:** Entry, by puncture or minor incision, of instrumentation through the skin or mucous membrane and any other body layers necessary to reach and visualize the site of the procedure

Via Natural or Artificial Opening	**Definition:** Entry of instrumentation through a natural or artificial external opening to reach the site of the procedure
Via Natural or Artificial Opening Endoscopic	**Definition:** Entry of instrumentation through a natural or artificial external opening to reach and visualize the site of the procedure
Via Natural or Artificial Opening With Percutaneous Endoscopic Assistance	**Definition:** Entry of instrumentation through a natural or artificial external opening and entry, by puncture or minor incision, of instrumentation through the skin or mucous membrane and any other body layers necessary to aid in the performance of the procedure

SECTION Ø - MEDICAL AND SURGICAL
CHARACTER 6 - DEVICE

Artificial Sphincter in Gastrointestinal System	**Includes:** Artificial anal sphincter (AAS) Artificial bowel sphincter (neosphincter)
Artificial Sphincter in Urinary System	**Includes:** AMS 8ØØ® Urinary Control System Artificial urinary sphincter (AUS)
Autologous Arterial Tissue in Heart and Great Vessels	**Includes:** Autologous artery graft
Autologous Arterial Tissue in Lower Arteries	**Includes:** Autologous artery graft
Autologous Arterial Tissue in Lower Veins	**Includes:** Autologous artery graft
Autologous Arterial Tissue in Upper Arteries	**Includes:** Autologous artery graft
Autologous Arterial Tissue in Upper Veins	**Includes:** Autologous artery graft
Autologous Tissue Substitute	**Includes:** Autograft Cultured epidermal cell autograft Epicel® cultured epidermal autograft
Autologous Venous Tissue in Heart and Great Vessels	**Includes:** Autologous vein graft
Autologous Venous Tissue in Lower Arteries	**Includes:** Autologous vein graft
Autologous Venous Tissue in Lower Veins	**Includes:** Autologous vein graft
Autologous Venous Tissue in Upper Arteries	**Includes:** Autologous vein graft
Autologous Venous Tissue in Upper Veins	**Includes:** Autologous vein graft
Bone Growth Stimulator in Head and Facial Bones	**Includes:** Electrical bone growth stimulator (EBGS) Ultrasonic osteogenic stimulator Ultrasound bone healing system
Bone Growth Stimulator in Lower Bones	**Includes:** Electrical bone growth stimulator (EBGS) Ultrasonic osteogenic stimulator Ultrasound bone healing system
Bone Growth Stimulator in Upper Bones	**Includes:** Electrical bone growth stimulator (EBGS) Ultrasonic osteogenic stimulator Ultrasound bone healing system
Cardiac Lead in Heart and Great Vessels	**Includes:** Cardiac contractility modulation lead
Cardiac Lead, Defibrillator for Insertion in Heart and Great Vessels	**Includes:** ACUITY™ Steerable Lead Attain Ability® lead Attain StarFix® (OTW) lead Cardiac resynchronization therapy (CRT) lead Corox (OTW) Bipolar Lead Durata® Defibrillation Lead ENDOTAK RELIANCE® (G) Defibrillation Lead
Cardiac Lead, Pacemaker for Insertion in Heart and Great Vessels	**Includes:** ACUITY™ Steerable Lead Attain Ability® Lead Attain StarFix® (OTW) lead Cardiac resynchronization therapy (CRT) lead Corox (OTW) Bipolar Lead
Cardiac Resynchronization Defibrillator Pulse Generator for Insertion in Subcutaneous Tissue and Fascia	**Includes:** COGNIS® CRT-D Concerto II CRT-D Consulta CRT-D CONTAK RENEWAL® 3 RF (HE) CRT-D LIVIAN™ CRT-D Maximo II DR CRT-D Ovatio™ CRT-D Protecta XT CRT-D Viva (XT)(S)
Cardiac Resynchronization Pacemaker Pulse Generator for Insertion in Subcutaneous Tissue and Fascia	**Includes:** Consulta CRT-P Stratos LV Synchra CRT-P
Contraceptive Device in Female Reproductive System	**Includes:** Intrauterine device (IUD)
Contraceptive Device in Subcutaneous Tissue and Fascia	**Includes:** Subdermal progesterone implant
Contractility Modulation Device for Insertion in Subcutaneous Tissue and Fascia	**Includes:** Optimizer™ III implantable pulse generator

SECTION Ø - MEDICAL AND SURGICAL
CHARACTER 6 - DEVICE

Defibrillator Generator for Insertion in Subcutaneous Tissue and Fascia	**Includes:** Implantable cardioverter-defibrillator (ICD) Maximo II DR (VR) Protecta XT DR (XT VR) Secura (DR) (VR) Evera (XT)(S)(DR/VR) Virtuoso (II) (DR) (VR)
Diaphragmatic Pacemaker Lead in Respiratory System	**Includes:** Phrenic nerve stimulator lead
Drainage Device	**Includes:** Cystostomy tube Foley catheter Percutaneous nephrostomy catheter Thoracostomy tube
External Fixation Device in Head and Facial Bones	**Includes:** External fixator
External Fixation Device in Lower Bones	**Includes:** External fixator
External Fixation Device in Lower Joints	**Includes:** External fixator
External Fixation Device in Upper Bones	**Includes:** External fixator
External Fixation Device in Upper Joints	**Includes:** External fixator
External Fixation Device, Hybrid for Insertion in Upper Bones	**Includes:** Delta frame external fixator Sheffield hybrid external fixator
External Fixation Device, Hybrid for Insertion in Lower Bones	**Includes:** Delta frame external fixator Sheffield hybrid external fixator
External Fixation Device, Hybrid for Reposition in Upper Bones	**Includes:** Delta frame external fixator Sheffield hybrid external fixator
External Fixation Device, Hybrid for Reposition in Lower Bones	**Includes:** Delta frame external fixator Sheffield hybrid external fixator

External Fixation Device, Limb Lengthening for Insertion in Upper Bones	**Includes:** Ilizarov-Vecklich device
External Fixation Device, Limb Lengthening for Insertion in Lower Bones	**Includes:** Ilizarov-Vecklich device
External Fixation Device, Monoplanar for Insertion in Upper Bones	**Includes:** Uniplanar external fixator
External Fixation Device, Monoplanar for Insertion in Lower Bones	**Includes:** Uniplanar external fixator
External Fixation Device, Monoplanar for Reposition in Upper Bones	**Includes:** Uniplanar external fixator
External Fixation Device, Monoplanar for Reposition in Lower Bones	**Includes:** Uniplanar external fixator
External Fixation Device, Ring for Insertion in Upper Bones	**Includes:** Ilizarov external fixator Sheffield ring external fixator
External Fixation Device, Ring for Insertion in Lower Bones	**Includes:** Ilizarov external fixator Sheffield ring external fixator
External Fixation Device, Ring for Reposition in Upper Bones	**Includes:** Ilizarov external fixator Sheffield ring external fixator
External Fixation Device, Ring for Reposition in Lower Bones	**Includes:** Ilizarov external fixator Sheffield ring external fixator
Extraluminal Device	**Includes:** AtriClip LAA Exclusion System LAP-BAND® adjustable gastric banding system REALIZE® Adjustable Gastric Band
Feeding Device in Gastrointestinal System	**Includes:** Percutaneous endoscopic gastrojejunostomy (PEG/J) tube Percutaneous endoscopic gastrostomy (PEG) tube

SECTION Ø - MEDICAL AND SURGICAL
CHARACTER 6 - DEVICE

Hearing Device in Ear, Nose, Sinus	**Includes:** Esteem® implantable hearing system
Hearing Device in Head and Facial Bones	**Includes:** Bone anchored hearing device
Hearing Device, Bone Conduction for Insertion in Ear, Nose, Sinus	**Includes:** Bone anchored hearing device
Hearing Device, Multiple Channel Cochlear Prosthesis for Insertion in Ear, Nose, Sinus	**Includes:** Cochlear implant (CI), multiple channel (electrode)
Hearing Device, Single Channel Cochlear Prosthesis for Insertion in Ear, Nose, Sinus	**Includes:** Cochlear implant (CI), single channel (electrode)
Implantable Heart Assist System in Heart and Great Vessels	**Includes:** Berlin Heart Ventricular Assist Device DeBakey Left Ventricular Assist Device DuraHeart Left Ventricular Assist System HeartMate 3™ LVAS HeartMate II® Left Ventricular Assist Device (LVAD) HeartMate XVE® Left Ventricular Assist Device (LVAD) MicroMed HeartAssist Novacor Left Ventricular Assist Device Thoratec IVAD (Implantable Ventricular Assist Device)
Infusion Device	**Includes:** Ascenda Intrathecal Catheter InDura, intrathecal catheter (1P) (spinal) Non-tunneled central venous catheter Peripherally inserted central catheter (PICC) Tunneled spinal (intrathecal) catheter
Infusion Device, Pump in Subcutaneous Tissue and Fascia	**Includes:** Implantable drug infusion pump (anti-spasmodic) (chemotherapy) (pain) Injection reservoir, pump Pump reservoir Subcutaneous injection reservoir, pump SynchroMed pump
Interbody Fusion Device in Lower Joints	**Includes:** Axial Lumbar Interbody Fusion System AxiaLIF® System CoRoent® XL Direct Lateral Interbody Fusion (DLIF) device EXtreme Lateral Interbody Fusion (XLIF) device Interbody fusion (spine) cage XLIF® System
Interbody Fusion Device in Upper Joints	**Includes:** BAK/C® Interbody Cervical Fusion System Interbody fusion (spine) cage
Internal Fixation Device in Head and Facial Bones	**Includes:** Bone screw (interlocking) (lag) (pedicle) (recessed) Kirschner wire (K-wire) Neutralization plate
Internal Fixation Device in Lower Bones	**Includes:** Bone screw (interlocking) (lag) (pedicle) (recessed) Clamp and rod internal fixation system (CRIF) Kirschner wire (K-wire) Neutralization plate
Internal Fixation Device in Lower Joints	**Includes:** Fusion screw (compression) (lag) (locking) Joint fixation plate Kirschner wire (K-wire)
Internal Fixation Device in Upper Bones	**Includes:** Bone screw (interlocking) (lag) (pedicle) (recessed) Clamp and rod internal fixation system (CRIF) Kirschner wire (K-wire) Neutralization plate
Internal Fixation Device in Upper Joints	**Includes:** Fusion screw (compression) (lag) (locking) Joint fixation plate Kirschner wire (K-wire)
Internal Fixation Device, Intramedullary in Lower Bones	**Includes:** Intramedullary (IM) rod (nail) Intramedullary skeletal kinetic distractor (ISKD) Kuntscher nail
Internal Fixation Device, Intramedullary in Upper Bones	**Includes:** Intramedullary (IM) rod (nail) Intramedullary skeletal kinetic distractor (ISKD) Kuntscher nail
Internal Fixation Device, Rigid Plate for Insertion in Upper Bones	**Includes:** Titanium Sternal Fixation System (TSFS)
Internal Fixation Device, Rigid Plate for Reposition in Upper Bones	**Includes:** Titanium Sternal Fixation System (TSFS)

SECTION Ø - MEDICAL AND SURGICAL
CHARACTER 6 - DEVICE

Intraluminal Device	**Includes:** Absolute Pro Vascular (OTW) Self-Expanding Stent System Acculink (RX) Carotid Stent System AFX® Endovascular AAA System AneuRx® AAA Advantage® Assurant (Cobalt) stent Carotid WALLSTENT® Monorail® Endoprosthesis CoAxia NeuroFlo catheter Colonic Z-Stent® Complete (SE) stent Cook Zenith AAA Endovascular Graft Driver stent (RX) (OTW) E-Luminexx™ (Biliary) (Vascular) Stent Embolization coil(s) Endologix AFX® Endovascular AAA System Endurant® Endovascular Stent Graft Endurant® II AAA stent graft system EXCLUDER® AAA Endoprosthesis Express® (LD) Premounted Stent System Express® Biliary SD Monorail® Premounted Stent System Express® SD Renal Monorail® Premounted Stent System FLAIR® Endovascular Stent Graft Formula™ Balloon-Expandable Renal Stent System GORE EXCLUDER® AAA Endoprosthesis GORE TAG® Thoracic Endoprosthesis Herculink (RX) Elite Renal Stent System LifeStent® (Flexstar) (XL) Vascular Stent System Medtronic Endurant® II AAA stent graft system Micro-Driver stent (RX) (OTW) MULTI-LINK (VISION)(MINI-VISION)(ULTRA) Coronary Stent System Omnilink Elite Vascular Balloon Expandable Stent System Pipeline™ Embolization device (PED) Protégé® RX Carotid Stent System Stent, intraluminal (cardiovascular) (gastrointestinal)(hepatobiliary)(urinary) Talent® Converter Talent® Occluder Talent® Stent Graft (abdominal) (thoracic) Therapeutic occlusion coil(s) Ultraflex™ Precision Colonic Stent System Valiant Thoracic Stent Graft WALLSTENT® Endoprosthesis Xact Carotid Stent System Zenith AAA Endovascular Graft Zenith Flex® AAA Endovascular Graft Zenith® Renu™ AAA Ancillary Graft Zenith TX2® TAA Endovascular Graft
Intraluminal Device, Airway in Ear, Nose, Sinus	**Includes:** Nasopharyngeal airway (NPA)
Intraluminal Device, Airway in Gastrointestinal System	**Includes:** Esophageal obturator airway (EOA)
Intraluminal Device, Airway in Mouth and Throat	**Includes:** Guedel airway Oropharyngeal airway (OPA)
Intraluminal Device, Bioactive in Upper Arteries	**Includes:** Bioactive embolization coil(s) Micrus CERECYTE microcoil
Intraluminal Device, Branched or Fenestrated, One or Two Arteries for Restriction in Lower Arteries	**Includes:** Cook Zenith AAA Endovascular Graft EXCLUDER® AAA Endoprosthesis EXCLUDER® IBE Endoprosthesis GORE EXCLUDER® AAA Endoprosthesis GORE EXCLUDER® IBE Endoprosthesis Zenith AAA Endovascular Graft
Intraluminal Device, Branched or Fenestrated, Three or More Arteries for Restriction in Lower Arteries	**Includes:** Cook Zenith AAA Endovascular Graft EXCLUDER® AAA Endoprosthesis GORE EXCLUDER® AAA Endoprosthesis Zenith AAA Endovascular Graft
Intraluminal Device, Drug-eluting in Heart and Great Vessels	**Includes:** CYPHER® Stent Endeavor® (III) (IV) (Sprint) Zotarolimus-eluting Coronary Stent System Everolimus-eluting coronary stent Paclitaxel-eluting coronary stent Sirolimus-eluting coronary stent TAXUS® Liberté® Paclitaxel-eluting Coronary Stent System XIENCE Everolimus Eluting Coronary Stent System Zotarolimus-eluting coronary stent
Intraluminal Device, Drug-eluting in Lower Arteries	**Includes:** Paclitaxel-eluting peripheral stent Zilver® PTX® (paclitaxel) Drug-Eluting Peripheral Stent
Intraluminal Device, Drug-eluting in Upper Arteries	**Includes:** Paclitaxel-eluting peripheral stent Zilver® PTX® (paclitaxel) Drug-Eluting Peripheral Stent
Intraluminal Device, Endobronchial Valve in Respiratory System	**Includes:** Spiration IBV™ Valve System
Intraluminal Device, Endotracheal Airway in Respiratory System	**Includes:** Endotracheal tube (cuffed) (double-lumen)

SECTION Ø - MEDICAL AND SURGICAL
CHARACTER 6 - DEVICE

Intraluminal Device, Pessary in Female Reproductive System	**Includes:** Pessary ring Vaginal pessary
Liner in Lower Joints	**Includes:** Acetabular cup Hip (joint) liner Joint liner (insert) Knee (implant) insert Tibial insert
Monitoring Device	**Includes:** Blood glucose monitoring system Cardiac event recorder Continuous Glucose Monitoring (CGM) device Implantable glucose monitoring device Loop recorder, implantable Reveal (DX) (XT)
Monitoring Device, Hemodynamic for Insertion in Subcutaneous Tissue and Fascia	**Includes:** Implantable hemodynamic monitor (IHM) Implantable hemodynamic monitoring system (IHMS)
Monitoring Device, Pressure Sensor for Insertion in Heart and Great Vessels	**Includes:** CardioMEMS® pressure sensor EndoSure® sensor
Neurostimulator Lead in Central Nervous System and Cranial Nerves	**Includes:** Cortical strip neurostimulator lead DBS lead Deep brain neurostimulator lead RNS System lead Spinal cord neurostimulator lead
Neurostimulator Lead in Peripheral Nervous System	**Includes:** InterStim® Therapy lead
Neurostimulator Generator in Head and Facial Bones	**Includes:** RNS system neurostimulator generator
Nonautologous Tissue Substitute	**Includes:** Acellular Hydrated Dermis Bone bank bone graft Cook Biodesign® Fistula Plug(s) Cook Biodesign® Hernia Graft(s) Cook Biodesign® Layered Graft(s) Cook Zenapro™ Layered Graft(s) Tissue bank graft
Pacemaker, Dual Chamber for Insertion in Subcutaneous Tissue and Fascia	**Includes:** Advisa (MRI) EnRhythm Kappa Revo MRI™ SureScan® pacemaker Two lead pacemaker Versa
Pacemaker, Single Chamber for Insertion in Subcutaneous Tissue and Fascia	**Includes:** Single lead pacemaker (atrium) (ventricle)
Pacemaker, Single Chamber Rate Responsive for Insertion in Subcutaneous Tissue and Fascia	**Includes:** Single lead rate responsive pacemaker (atrium) (ventricle)
Radioactive Element	**Includes:** Brachytherapy seeds
Radioactive Element, Cesium-131 Collagen Implant for Insertion in Central Nervous System and Cranial Nerves	Cesium-131 Collagen Implant GammaTile™
Resurfacing Device in Lower Joints	**Includes:** CONSERVE® PLUS Total Resurfacing Hip System Cormet Hip Resurfacing System
Short-term External Heart Assist System in Heart and Great Vessels	Biventricular external heart assist system BVS 5ØØØ Ventricular Assist Device Centrimag® Blood Pump Impella® heart pump TandemHeart® System Thoratec Paracorporeal Ventricular Assist Device
Spacer in Lower Joints	**Includes:** Joint spacer (antibiotic)
Spacer in Upper Joints	**Includes:** Joint spacer (antibiotic)
Spinal Stabilization Device, Facet Replacement for Insertion in Upper Joints	**Includes:** Facet replacement spinal stabilization device
Spinal Stabilization Device, Facet Replacement for Insertion in Lower Joints	**Includes:** Facet replacement spinal stabilization device

SECTION Ø - MEDICAL AND SURGICAL
CHARACTER 6 - DEVICE

Spinal Stabilization Device, Interspinous Process for Insertion in Upper Joints	**Includes:** Interspinous process spinal stabilization device X-STOP® Spacer
Spinal Stabilization Device, Interspinous Process for Insertion in Lower Joints	**Includes:** Interspinous process spinal stabilization device X-STOP® Spacer
Spinal Stabilization Device, Pedicle-Based for Insertion in Upper Joints	**Includes:** Dynesys® Dynamic Stabilization System Pedicle-based dynamic stabilization device
Spinal Stabilization Device, Pedicle-Based for Insertion in Lower Joints	**Includes:** Dynesys® Dynamic Stabilization System Pedicle-based dynamic stabilization device
Stimulator Generator in Subcutaneous Tissue and Fascia	**Includes:** Baroreflex Activation Therapy® (BAT®) Diaphragmatic pacemaker generator Mark IV Breathing Pacemaker System Phrenic nerve stimulator generator Rheos® System device
Stimulator Generator, Multiple Array for Insertion in Subcutaneous Tissue and Fascia	**Includes:** Activa PC neurostimulator Enterra gastric neurostimulator Neurostimulator generator, multiple channel PrimeAdvanced neurostimulator (SureScan) (MRI Safe)
Stimulator Generator, Multiple Array Rechargeable for Insertion in Subcutaneous Tissue and Fascia	**Includes:** Activa RC neurostimulator Neurostimulator generator, multiple channel rechargeable RestoreAdvanced neurostimulator (SureScan) (MRI Safe) RestoreSensor neurostimulator (SureScan) (MRI Safe) RestoreUltra neurostimulator (SureScan) (MRI Safe)
Stimulator Generator, Single Array for Insertion in Subcutaneous Tissue and Fascia	**Includes:** Activa SC neurostimulator InterStim® Therapy neurostimulator Itrel (3) (4) neurostimulator Neurostimulator generator, single channel
Stimulator Generator, Single Array Rechargeable for Insertion in Subcutaneous Tissue and Fascia	**Includes:** Neurostimulator generator, single channel rechargeable

Stimulator Lead in Gastrointestinal System	**Includes:** Gastric electrical stimulation (GES) lead Gastric pacemaker lead
Stimulator Lead in Muscles	**Includes:** Electrical muscle stimulation (EMS) lead Electronic muscle stimulator lead Neuromuscular electrical stimulation (NEMS) lead
Stimulator Lead in Upper Arteries	**Includes:** Baroreflex Activation Therapy® (BAT®) Carotid (artery) sinus (baroreceptor) lead Rheos® System lead
Stimulator Lead in Urinary System	**Includes:** Sacral nerve modulation (SNM) lead Sacral neuromodulation lead Urinary incontinence stimulator lead
Synthetic Substitute	**Includes:** AbioCor® Total Replacement Heart AMPLATZER® Muscular VSD Occluder Annuloplasty ring Bard® Composix® (E/X) (LP) mesh Bard® Composix® Kugel® patch Bard® Dulex™ mesh Bard® Ventralex™ hernia patch BRYAN® Cervical Disc System Ex-PRESS™ mini glaucoma shunt Flexible Composite Mesh GORE® DUALMESH® Holter valve ventricular shunt MitraClip valve repair system Nitinol framed polymer mesh Open Pivot (mechanical) valve Open Pivot Aortic Valve Graft (AVG) Partially absorbable mesh PHYSIOMESH™ Flexible Composite Mesh Polymethylmethacrylate (PMMA) Polypropylene mesh PRESTIGE® Cervical Disc PROCEED™ Ventral Patch Prodisc-C Prodisc-L PROLENE Polypropylene Hernia System (PHS) Rebound HRD® (Hernia Repair Device) SynCardia Total Artificial Heart Total artificial (replacement) heart ULTRAPRO Hernia System (UHS) ULTRAPRO Partially Absorbable Lightweight Mesh ULTRAPRO Plug Ventrio™ Hernia Patch Zimmer® NexGen® LPS Mobile Bearing Knee Zimmer® NexGen® LPS-Flex Mobile Knee

APPENDIX A

SECTION Ø - MEDICAL AND SURGICAL
CHARACTER 6 - DEVICE

Synthetic Substitute, Ceramic for Replacement in Lower Joints	**Includes:** Ceramic on ceramic bearing surface Novation® Ceramic AHS® (Articulation Hip System)
Synthetic Substitute, Intraocular Telescope for Replacement in Eye	**Includes:** Implantable Miniature Telescope™ (IMT)
Synthetic Substitute, Metal for Replacement in Lower Joints	**Includes:** Cobalt/chromium head and socket Metal on metal bearing surface
Synthetic Substitute, Metal on Polyethylene for Replacement in Lower Joints	**Includes:** Cobalt/chromium head and polyethylene socket
Synthetic Substitute, Oxidized Zirconium on Polyethylene for Replacement in Lower Joints	OXINIUM
Synthetic Substitute, Polyethylene for Replacement in Lower Joints	**Includes:** Polyethylene socket
Synthetic Substitute, Reverse Ball and Socket for Replacement in Upper Joints	**Includes:** Delta III Reverse shoulder prosthesis Reverse® Shoulder Prosthesis
Tissue Expander in Skin and Breast	**Includes:** Tissue expander (inflatable) (injectable)

Tissue Expander in Subcutaneous Tissue and Fascia	**Includes:** Tissue expander (inflatable) (injectable)
Tracheostomy Device in Respiratory System	**Includes:** Tracheostomy tube
Vascular Access Device, Totally Implantable in Subcutaneous Tissue and Fascia	**Includes:** Implanted (venous) (access) port Injection reservoir, port Subcutaneous injection reservoir, port
Vascular Access Device, Tunneled in Subcutaneous Tissue and Fascia	**Includes:** Tunneled central venous catheter Vectra® Vascular Access Graft
Zooplastic Tissue in Heart and Great Vessels	**Includes:** 3f (Aortic) Bioprosthesis valve Bovine pericardial valve Bovine pericardium graft Contegra Pulmonary Valved Conduit CoreValve transcatheter aortic valve Epic™ Stented Tissue Valve (aortic) Freestyle (Stentless) Aortic Root Bioprosthesis Hancock Bioprosthesis (aortic) (mitral) valve Hancock Bioprosthetic Valved Conduit Melody® transcatheter pulmonary valve Mitroflow® Aortic Pericardial Heart Valve Mosaic Bioprosthesis (aortic) (mitral) valve Porcine (bioprosthetic) valve SAPIEN transcatheter aortic valve SJM Biocor® Stented Valve System Stented tissue valve Trifecta™ Valve (aortic) Xenograft

SECTION 1 - OBSTETRICS
CHARACTER 3 - OPERATION

Abortion	**Definition:** Artificially terminating a pregnancy
Change	**Definition:** Taking out or off a device from a body part and putting back an identical or similar device in or on the same body part without cutting or puncturing the skin or a mucous membrane
Delivery	**Definition:** Assisting the passage of the products of conception from the genital canal
Drainage	**Definition:** Taking or letting out fluids and/or gases from a body part by the use of force

Extraction	**Definition:** Pulling or stripping out or off all or a portion of a body part
Insertion	**Definition:** Putting in a nonbiological appliance that monitors, assists, performs, or prevents a physiological function but does not physically take the place of a body part
Inspection	**Definition:** Visually and/or manually exploring a body part **Explanation:** Visual exploration may be performed with or without optical instrumentation. Manual exploration may be performed directly or through intervening body layers

SECTION 1 - OBSTETRICS
CHARACTER 3 - OPERATION

Removal	**Definition:** Taking out or off a device from a body part, region or orifice **Explanation:** If a device is taken out and a similar device put in without cutting or puncturing the skin or mucous membrane, the procedure is coded to the root operation CHANGE. Otherwise, the procedure for taking out a device is coded to the root operation REMOVAL
Repair	**Definition:** Restoring, to the extent possible, a body part to its normal anatomic structure and function **Explanation:** Used only when the method to accomplish the repair is not one of the other root operations

Reposition	**Definition:** Moving to its normal location or other suitable location all or a portion of a body part **Explanation:** The body part is moved to a new location from an abnormal location, or from a normal location where it is not functioning correctly. The body part may or may not be cut out or off to be moved to the new location
Resection	**Definition:** Cutting out or off, without replacement, all of a body part
Transplantation	**Definition:** Putting in or on all or a portion of a living body part taken from another individual or animal to physically take the place and/or function of all or a portion of a similar body part **Explanation:** The native body part may or may not be taken out, and the transplanted body part may take over all or a portion of its function

SECTION 1 - OBSTETRICS
CHARACTER 5 - APPROACH

External	**Definition:** Procedures performed directly on the skin or mucous membrane and procedures performed indirectly by the application of external force through the skin or mucous membrane
Open	**Definition:** Cutting through the skin or mucous membrane and any other body layers necessary to expose the site of the procedure
Percutaneous	**Definition:** Entry, by puncture or minor incision, of instrumentation through the skin or mucous membrane and any other body layers necessary to reach the site of the procedure

Percutaneous Endoscopic	**Definition:** Entry, by puncture or minor incision, of instrumentation through the skin or mucous membrane and any other body layers necessary to reach and visualize the site of the procedure
Via Natural or Artificial Opening	**Definition:** Entry of instrumentation through a natural or artificial external opening to reach the site of the procedure
Via Natural or Artificial Opening Endoscopic	**Definition:** Entry of instrumentation through a natural or artificial external opening to reach and visualize the site of the procedure

SECTION 2 - PLACEMENT
CHARACTER 3 - OPERATION

Change	**Definition:** Taking out or off a device from a body part and putting back an identical or similar device in or on the same body part without cutting or puncturing the skin or a mucous membrane
Compression	**Definition:** Putting pressure on a body region
Dressing	**Definition:** Putting material on a body region for protection

Immobilization	**Definition:** Limiting or preventing motion of a body region
Packing	**Definition:** Putting material in a body region or orifice
Removal	**Definition:** Taking out or off a device from a body part
Traction	**Definition:** Exerting a pulling force on a body region in a distal direction

SECTION 2 - PLACEMENT
CHARACTER 5 - APPROACH

External	**Definition:** Procedures performed directly on the skin or mucous membrane and procedures performed indirectly by the application of external force through the skin or mucous membrane

SECTION 3 - ADMINISTRATION
CHARACTER 3 - OPERATION

Introduction	**Definition:** Putting in or on a therapeutic, diagnostic, nutritional, physiological, or prophylactic substance except blood or blood products

Irrigation	**Definition:** Putting in or on a cleansing substance
Transfusion	**Definition:** Putting in blood or blood products

SECTION 3 - ADMINISTRATION
CHARACTER 5 - APPROACH

External	**Definition:** Procedures performed directly on the skin or mucous membrane and procedures performed indirectly by the application of external force through the skin or mucous membrane
Open	**Definition:** Cutting through the skin or mucous membrane and any other body layers necessary to expose the site of the procedure
Percutaneous	**Definition:** Entry, by puncture or minor incision, of instrumentation through the skin or mucous membrane and any other body layers necessary to reach the site of the procedure

Percutaneous Endoscopic	**Definition:** Entry, by puncture or minor incision, of instrumentation through the skin or mucous membrane and any other body layers necessary to reach and visualize the site of the procedure
Via Natural or Artificial Opening	**Definition:** Entry of instrumentation through a natural or artificial external opening to reach the site of the procedure
Via Natural or Artificial Opening Endoscopic	**Definition:** Entry of instrumentation through a natural or artificial external opening to reach and visualize the site of the procedure

SECTION 3 - ADMINISTRATION
CHARACTER 6 - SUBSTANCE

4-Factor Prothrombin Complex Concentrate	**Includes:** Kcentra
Adhesion Barrier	**Includes:** Seprafilm
Anti-Infective Envelope	**Includes:** AIGISRx Antibacterial Envelope Antimicrobial envelope
Clofarabine	**Includes:** Clolar
Glucarpidase	**Includes:** Voraxaze

Human B-type Natriuretic Peptide	**Includes:** Nesiritide
Other Thrombolytic	**Includes:** Tissue Plasminogen Activator (tPA)(r-tPA)
Oxazolidinones	**Includes:** Zyvox
Recombinant Bone Morphogenetic Protein	**Includes:** Bone morphogenetic protein 2 (BMP 2) rhBMP-2

SECTION 4 - MEASUREMENT AND MONITORING
CHARACTER 3 - OPERATION

Measurement	**Definition:** Determining the level of a physiological or physical function at a point in time	Monitoring	**Definition:** Determining the level of a physiological or physical function repetitively over a period of time

SECTION 4 - MEASUREMENT AND MONITORING
CHARACTER 5 - APPROACH

External	**Definition:** Procedures performed directly on the skin or mucous membrane and procedures performed indirectly by the application of external force through the skin or mucous membrane	Percutaneous Endoscopic	**Definition:** Entry, by puncture or minor incision, of instrumentation through the skin or mucous membrane and any other body layers necessary to reach and visualize the site of the procedure
Open	**Definition:** Cutting through the skin or mucous membrane and any other body layers necessary to expose the site of the procedure	Via Natural or Artificial Opening	**Definition:** Entry of instrumentation through a natural or artificial external opening to reach the site of the procedure
Percutaneous	**Definition:** Entry, by puncture or minor incision, of instrumentation through the skin or mucous membrane and any other body layers necessary to reach the site of the procedure	Via Natural or Artificial Opening Endoscopic	**Definition:** Entry of instrumentation through a natural or artificial external opening to reach and visualize the site of the procedure

SECTION 5 - EXTRACORPOREAL OR SYSTEMIC ASSISTANCE AND PERFORMANCE
CHARACTER 3 - OPERATION

Assistance	**Definition:** Taking over a portion of a physiological function by extracorporeal means	Restoration	**Definition:** Returning, or attempting to return, a physiological function to its original state by extracorporeal means.
Performance	**Definition:** Completely taking over a physiological function by extracorporeal means		

SECTION 6 - EXTRACORPOREAL OR SYSTEMIC THERAPIES
CHARACTER 3 - OPERATION

Atmospheric Control	**Definition:** Extracorporeal control of atmospheric pressure and composition	Pheresis	**Definition:** Extracorporeal separation of blood products
Decompression	**Definition:** Extracorporeal elimination of undissolved gas from body fluids	Phototherapy	**Definition:** Extracorporeal treatment by light rays
Electromagnetic Therapy	**Definition:** Extracorporeal treatment by electromagnetic rays	Shock Wave Therapy	**Definition:** Extracorporeal treatment by shock waves
Hyperthermia	**Definition:** Extracorporeal raising of body temperature	Ultrasound Therapy	**Definition:** Extracorporeal treatment by ultrasound
Hypothermia	**Definition:** Extracorporeal lowering of body temperature	Ultraviolet Light Therapy	**Definition:** Extracorporeal treatment by ultraviolet light
Perfusion	**Definition:** Extracorporeal treatment by diffusion of therapeutic fluid		

APPENDIX A

SECTION 7 - OSTEOPATHIC
CHARACTER 3 - OPERATION

Treatment	**Definition:** Manual treatment to eliminate or alleviate somatic dysfunction and related disorders

SECTION 7 - OSTEOPATHIC
CHARACTER 5 - APPROACH

External	**Definition:** Procedures performed directly on the skin or mucous membrane and procedures performed indirectly by the application of external force through the skin or mucous membrane

SECTION 8 - OTHER PROCEDURES
CHARACTER 3 - OPERATION

Other Procedures	**Definition:** Methodologies which attempt to remediate or cure a disorder or disease

SECTION 8 - OTHER PROCEDURES
CHARACTER 5 - APPROACH

External	**Definition:** Procedures performed directly on the skin or mucous membrane and procedures performed indirectly by the application of external force through the skin or mucous membrane
Percutaneous	**Definition:** Entry, by puncture or minor incision, of instrumentation through the skin or mucous membrane and any other body layers necessary to reach the site of the procedure
Percutaneous Endoscopic	**Definition:** Entry, by puncture or minor incision, of instrumentation through the skin or mucous membrane and any other body layers necessary to reach and visualize the site of the procedure

Via Natural or Artificial Opening	**Definition:** Entry of instrumentation through a natural or artificial external opening to reach the site of the procedure
Via Natural or Artificial Opening Endoscopic	**Definition:** Entry of instrumentation through a natural or artificial external opening to reach and visualize the site of the procedure

SECTION 9 - CHIROPRACTIC
CHARACTER 3 - OPERATION

Manipulation	**Definition:** Manual procedure that involves a directed thrust to move a joint past the physiological range of motion, without exceeding the anatomical limit

SECTION 9 - CHIROPRACTIC
CHARACTER 5 - APPROACH

External	**Definition:** Procedures performed directly on the skin or mucous membrane and procedures performed indirectly by the application of external force through the skin or mucous membrane

SECTION B - IMAGING
CHARACTER 3 - TYPE

Computerized Tomography (CT Scan)	**Definition:** Computer reformatted digital display of multiplanar images developed from the capture of multiple exposures of external ionizing radiation	Plain Radiography	**Definition:** Planar display of an image developed from the capture of external ionizing radiation on photographic or photoconductive plate
Fluoroscopy	**Definition:** Single plane or bi-plane real time display of an image developed from the capture of external ionizing radiation on a fluorescent screen. The image may also be stored by either digital or analog means	Ultrasonography	**Definition:** Real time display of images of anatomy or flow information developed from the capture of reflected and attenuated high frequency sound waves
Magnetic Resonance Imaging (MRI)	**Definition:** Computer reformatted digital display of multiplanar images developed from the capture of radiofrequency signals emitted by nuclei in a body site excited within a magnetic field		

SECTION C - NUCLEAR MEDICINE
CHARACTER 3 - TYPE

Nonimaging Nuclear Medicine Assay	**Definition:** Introduction of radioactive materials into the body for the study of body fluids and blood elements, by the detection of radioactive emissions	Planar Nuclear Medicine Imaging	**Definition:** Introduction of radioactive materials into the body for single plane display of images developed from the capture of radioactive emissions
Nonimaging Nuclear Medicine Probe	**Definition:** Introduction of radioactive materials into the body for the study of distribution and fate of certain substances by the detection of radioactive emissions; or, alternatively, measurement of absorption of radioactive emissions from an external source	Positron Emission Tomographic (PET) Imaging	**Definition:** Introduction of radioactive materials into the body for three dimensional display of images developed from the simultaneous capture, 18Ø degrees apart, of radioactive emissions
Nonimaging Nuclear Medicine Uptake	**Definition:** Introduction of radioactive materials into the body for measurements of organ function, from the detection of radioactive emissions	Systemic Nuclear Medicine Therapy	**Definition:** Introduction of unsealed radioactive materials into the body for treatment
		Tomographic (Tomo) Nuclear Medicine Imaging	**Definition:** Introduction of radioactive materials into the body for three dimensional display of images developed from the capture of radioactive emissions

SECTION F - PHYSICAL REHABILITATION AND DIAGNOSTIC AUDIOLOGY

CHARACTER 3 - TYPE

Activities of Daily Living Assessment	**Definition:** Measurement of functional level for activities of daily living	Hearing Treatment	**Definition:** Application of techniques to improve, augment, or compensate for hearing and related functional impairment
Activities of Daily Living Treatment	**Definition:** Exercise or activities to facilitate functional competence for activities of daily living	Motor and/or Nerve Function Assessment	**Definition:** Measurement of motor, nerve, and related functions
Caregiver Training	**Definition:** Training in activities to support patient's optimal level of function	Motor Treatment	**Definition:** Exercise or activities to increase or facilitate motor function
Cochlear Implant Treatment	**Definition:** Application of techniques to improve the communication abilities of individuals with cochlear implant	Speech Assessment	**Definition:** Measurement of speech and related functions
Device Fitting	**Definition:** Fitting of a device designed to facilitate or support achievement of a higher level of function	Speech Treatment	**Definition:** Application of techniques to improve, augment, or compensate for speech and related functional impairment
Hearing Aid Assessment	**Definition:** Measurement of the appropriateness and/or effectiveness of a hearing device	Vestibular Assessment	**Definition:** Measurement of the vestibular system and related functions
Hearing Assessment	**Definition:** Measurement of hearing and related functions	Vestibular Treatment	**Definition:** Application of techniques to improve, augment, or compensate for vestibular and related functional impairment

SECTION F - PHYSICAL REHABILITATION AND DIAGNOSTIC AUDIOLOGY

CHARACTER 5 - TYPE QUALIFIER

Acoustic Reflex Decay	**Definition:** Measures reduction in size/strength of acoustic reflex over time **Includes/Examples:** Includes site of lesion test	Alternate Binaural or Monaural Loudness Balance	**Definition:** Determines auditory stimulus parameter that yields the same objective sensation **Includes/Examples:** Sound intensities that yield same loudness perception
Acoustic Reflex Patterns	**Definition:** Defines site of lesion based upon presence/absence of acoustic reflexes with ipsilateral vs. contralateral stimulation	Anthropometric Characteristics	**Definition:** Measures edema, body fat composition, height, weight, length and girth
Acoustic Reflex Threshold	**Definition:** Determines minimal intensity that acoustic reflex occurs with ipsilateral and/or contralateral stimulation	Aphasia (Assessment)	**Definition:** Measures expressive and receptive speech and language function including reading and writing
Aerobic Capacity and Endurance	**Definition:** Measures autonomic responses to positional changes; perceived exertion, dyspnea or angina during activity; performance during exercise protocols; standard vital signs; and blood gas analysis or oxygen consumption	Aphasia (Treatment)	**Definition:** Applying techniques to improve, augment, or compensate for receptive/expressive language impairments
		Articulation/Phonology (Assessment)	**Definition:** Measures speech production

SECTION F - PHYSICAL REHABILITATION AND DIAGNOSTIC AUDIOLOGY
CHARACTER 5 - TYPE QUALIFIER

Articulation/Phonology (Treatment)	**Definition:** Applying techniques to correct, improve, or compensate for speech productive impairment	Bathing/Showering	**Includes/Examples:** Includes obtaining and using supplies; soaping, rinsing, and drying body parts; maintaining bathing position; and transferring to and from bathing positions
Assistive Listening Device	**Definition:** Assists in use of effective and appropriate assistive listening device/system	Bathing/Showering Techniques	**Definition:** Activities to facilitate obtaining and using supplies, soaping, rinsing and drying body parts, maintaining bathing position, and transferring to and from bathing positions
Assistive Listening System/Device Selection	**Definition:** Measures the effectiveness and appropriateness of assistive listening systems/devices	Bed Mobility (Assessment)	**Definition:** Transitional movement within bed
Assistive, Adaptive, Supportive or Protective Devices	**Explanation:** Devices to facilitate or support achievement of a higher level of function in wheelchair mobility; bed mobility; transfer or ambulation ability; bath and showering ability; dressing; grooming; personal hygiene; play or leisure	Bed Mobility (Treatment)	**Definition:** Exercise or activities to facilitate transitional movements within bed
Auditory Evoked Potentials	**Definition:** Measures electric responses produced by the VIIIth cranial nerve and brainstem following auditory stimulation	Bedside Swallowing and Oral Function	**Includes/Examples:** Bedside swallowing includes assessment of sucking, masticating, coughing, and swallowing. Oral function includes assessment of musculature for controlled movements, structures and functions to determine coordination and phonation
Auditory Processing (Assessment)	**Definition:** Evaluates ability to receive and process auditory information and comprehension of spoken language		
Auditory Processing (Treatment)	**Definition:** Applying techniques to improve the receiving and processing of auditory information and comprehension of spoken language	Bekesy Audiometry	**Definition:** Uses an instrument that provides a choice of discrete or continuously varying pure tones; choice of pulsed or continuous signal
Augmentative/ Alternative Communication System (Assessment)	**Definition:** Determines the appropriateness of aids, techniques, symbols, and/or strategies to augment or replace speech and enhance communication **Includes/Examples:** Includes the use of telephones, writing equipment, emergency equipment, and TDD	Binaural Electroacoustic Hearing Aid Check	**Definition:** Determines mechanical and electroacoustic function of bilateral hearing aids using hearing aid test box
		Binaural Hearing Aid (Assessment)	**Definition:** Measures the candidacy, effectiveness, and appropriateness of hearing aids **Explanation:** Measures bilateral fit
Augmentative/ Alternative Communication System (Treatment)	**Includes/Examples:** Includes augmentative communication devices and aids	Binaural Hearing Aid (Treatment)	**Explanation:** Assists in achieving maximum understanding and performance
Aural Rehabilitation	**Definition:** Applying techniques to improve the communication abilities associated with hearing loss	Bithermal, Binaural Caloric Irrigation	**Definition:** Measures the rhythmic eye movements stimulated by changing the temperature of the vestibular system
Aural Rehabilitation Status	**Definition:** Measures impact of a hearing loss including evaluation of receptive and expressive communication skills	Bithermal, Monaural Caloric Irrigation	**Definition:** Measures the rhythmic eye movements stimulated by changing the temperature of the vestibular system in one ear

SECTION F - PHYSICAL REHABILITATION AND DIAGNOSTIC AUDIOLOGY

CHARACTER 5 - TYPE QUALIFIER

Brief Tone Stimuli	**Definition:** Measures specific central auditory process
Cerumen Management	**Definition:** Includes examination of external auditory canal and tympanic membrane and removal of cerumen from external ear canal
Cochlear Implant	**Definition:** Measures candidacy for cochlear implant
Cochlear Implant Rehabilitation	**Definition:** Applying techniques to improve the communication abilities of individuals with cochlear implant; includes programming the device, providing patients/families with information
Communicative/ Cognitive Integration Skills (Assessment)	**Definition:** Measures ability to use higher cortical functions **Includes/Examples:** Includes orientation, recognition, attention span, initiation and termination of activity, memory, sequencing, categorizing, concept formation, spatial operations, judgment, problem solving, generalization and pragmatic communication
Communicative/ Cognitive Integration Skills (Treatment)	**Definition:** Activities to facilitate the use of higher cortical functions **Includes/Examples:** Includes level of arousal, orientation, recognition, attention span, initiation and termination of activity, memory sequencing, judgment and problem solving, learning and generalization, and pragmatic communication
Computerized Dynamic Posturography	**Definition:** Measures the status of the peripheral and central vestibular system and the sensory/motor component of balance; evaluates the efficacy of vestibular rehabilitation
Conditioned Play Audiometry	**Definition:** Behavioral measures using nonspeech and speech stimuli to obtain frequency-specific and ear-specific information on auditory status from the patient **Explanation:** Obtains speech reception threshold by having patient point to pictures of spondaic words
Coordination/Dexterity (Assessment)	**Definition:** Measures large and small muscle groups for controlled goal-directed movements **Explanation:** Dexterity includes object manipulation
Coordination/Dexterity (Treatment)	**Definition:** Exercise or activities to facilitate gross coordination and fine coordination
Cranial Nerve Integrity	**Definition:** Measures cranial nerve sensory and motor functions, including tastes, smell and facial expression
Dichotic Stimuli	**Definition:** Measures specific central auditory process
Distorted Speech	**Definition:** Measures specific central auditory process
Dix-Hallpike Dynamic	**Definition:** Measures nystagmus following Dix-Hallpike maneuver
Dressing	**Includes/Examples:** Includes selecting clothing and accessories, obtaining clothing from storage, dressing and, fastening and adjusting clothing and shoes, and applying and removing personal devices, prosthesis or orthosis
Dressing Techniques	**Definition:** Activities to facilitate selecting clothing and accessories, dressing and undressing, adjusting clothing and shoes, applying and removing devices, prostheses or orthoses
Dynamic Orthosis	**Includes/Examples:** Includes customized and prefabricated splints, inhibitory casts, spinal and other braces, and protective devices; allows motion through transfer of movement from other body parts or by use of outside forces
Ear Canal Probe Microphone	**Definition:** Real ear measures
Ear Protector Attentuation	**Definition:** Measures ear protector fit and effectiveness
Electrocochleography	**Definition:** Measures the VIIIth cranial nerve action potential
Environmental, Home and Work Barriers	**Definition:** Measures current and potential barriers to optimal function, including safety hazards, access problems and home or office design

SECTION F - PHYSICAL REHABILITATION AND DIAGNOSTIC AUDIOLOGY
CHARACTER 5 - TYPE QUALIFIER

Ergonomics and Body Mechanics	**Definition:** Ergonomic measurement of job tasks, work hardening or work conditioning needs; functional capacity; and body mechanics
Eustachian Tube Function	**Definition:** Measures eustachian tube function and patency of eustachian tube
Evoked Otoacoustic Emissions, Diagnostic	**Definition:** Measures auditory evoked potentials in a diagnostic format
Evoked Otoacoustic Emissions, Screening	**Definition:** Measures auditory evoked potentials in a screening format
Facial Nerve Function	**Definition:** Measures electrical activity of the VIIth cranial nerve (facial nerve)
Feeding/Eating (Assessment)	**Includes/Examples:** Includes setting up food, selecting and using utensils and tableware, bringing food or drink to mouth, cleaning face, hands, and clothing, and management of alternative methods of nourishment
Feeding/Eating (Treatment)	**Definition:** Exercise or activities to facilitate setting up food, selecting and using utensils and tableware, bringing food or drink to mouth, cleaning face, hands, and clothing, and management of alternative methods of nourishment
Filtered Speech	**Definition:** Uses high or low pass filtered speech stimuli to assess central auditory processing disorders, site of lesion testing
Fluency (Assessment)	**Definition:** Measures speech fluency or stuttering
Fluency (Treatment)	**Definition:** Applying techniques to improve and augment fluent speech
Gait and/or Balance	**Definition:** Measures biomechanical, arthrokinematic and other spatial and temporal characteristics of gait and balance
Gait Training/ Functional Ambulation	**Definition:** Exercise or activities to facilitate ambulation on a variety of surfaces and in a variety of environments
Grooming/Personal Hygiene (Assessment)	**Includes/Examples:** Includes ability to obtain and use supplies in a sequential fashion, general grooming, oral hygiene, toilet hygiene, personal care devices, including care for artificial airways

Grooming/Personal Hygiene (Treatment)	**Definition:** Activities to facilitate obtaining and using supplies in a sequential fashion: general grooming, oral hygiene, toilet hygiene, cleaning body, and personal care devices, including artificial airways
Hearing and Related Disorders Counseling	**Definition:** Provides patients/families/ caregivers with information, support, referrals to facilitate recovery from a communication disorder **Includes/Examples:** Includes strategies for psychosocial adjustment to hearing loss for clients and families/caregivers
Hearing and Related Disorders Prevention	**Definition:** Provides patients/families/ caregivers with information and support to prevent communication disorders
Hearing Screening	**Definition:** Pass/refer measures designed to identify need for further audiologic assessment
Home Management (Assessment)	**Definition:** Obtaining and maintaining personal and household possessions and environment **Includes/Examples:** Includes clothing care, cleaning, meal preparation and cleanup, shopping, money management, household maintenance, safety procedures, and childcare/parenting
Home Management (Treatment)	**Definition:** Activities to facilitate obtaining and maintaining personal household possessions and environment **Includes/Examples:** Includes clothing care, cleaning, meal preparation and clean-up, shopping, money management, household maintenance, safety procedures, childcare/ parenting
Instrumental Swallowing and Oral Function	**Definition:** Measures swallowing function using instrumental diagnostic procedures **Explanation:** Methods include videofluoroscopy, ultrasound, manometry, endoscopy
Integumentary Integrity	**Includes/Examples:** Includes burns, skin conditions, ecchymosis, bleeding, blisters, scar tissue, wounds and other traumas, tissue mobility, turgor and texture

SECTION F - PHYSICAL REHABILITATION AND DIAGNOSTIC AUDIOLOGY
CHARACTER 5 - TYPE QUALIFIER

Manual Therapy Techniques	**Definition:** Techniques in which the therapist uses his/her hands to administer skilled movements **Includes/Examples:** Includes connective tissue massage, joint mobilization and manipulation, manual lymph drainage, manual traction, soft tissue mobilization and manipulation
Masking Patterns	**Definition:** Measures central auditory processing status
Monaural Electroacoustic Hearing Aid Check	**Definition:** Determines mechanical and electroacoustic function of one hearing aid using hearing aid test box
Monaural Hearing Aid (Assessment)	**Definition:** Measures the candidacy, effectiveness, and appropriateness of a hearing aid **Explanation:** Measures unilateral fit
Monaural Hearing Aid (Treatment)	**Explanation:** Assists in achieving maximum understanding and performance
Motor Function (Assessment)	**Definition:** Measures the body's functional and versatile movement patterns **Includes/Examples:** Includes motor assessment scales, analysis of head, trunk and limb movement, and assessment of motor learning
Motor Function (Treatment)	**Definition:** Exercise or activities to facilitate crossing midline, laterality, bilateral integration, praxis, neuromuscular relaxation, inhibition, facilitation, motor function and motor learning
Motor Speech (Assessment)	**Definition:** Measures neurological motor aspects of speech production
Motor Speech (Treatment)	**Definition:** Applying techniques to improve and augment the impaired neurological motor aspects of speech production
Muscle Performance (Assessment)	**Definition:** Measures muscle strength, power and endurance using manual testing, dynamometry or computer-assisted electromechanical muscle test; functional muscle strength, power and endurance; muscle pain, tone, or soreness; or pelvic-floor musculature **Explanation:** Muscle endurance refers to the ability to contract a muscle repeatedly over time
Muscle Performance (Treatment)	**Definition:** Exercise or activities to increase the capacity of a muscle to do work in terms of strength, power, and/or endurance **Explanation:** Muscle strength is the force exerted to overcome resistance in one maximal effort. Muscle power is work produced per unit of time, or the product of strength and speed. Muscle endurance is the ability to contract a muscle repeatedly over time
Neuromotor Development	**Definition:** Measures motor development, righting and equilibrium reactions, and reflex and equilibrium reactions
Non-invasive Instrumental Status	**Definition:** Instrumental measures of oral, nasal, vocal, and velopharyngeal functions as they pertain to speech production
Nonspoken Language (Assessment)	**Definition:** Measures nonspoken language (print, sign, symbols) for communication
Nonspoken Language (Treatment)	**Definition:** Applying techniques that improve, augment, or compensate spoken communication
Oral Peripheral Mechanism	**Definition:** Structural measures of face, jaw, lips, tongue, teeth, hard and soft palate, pharynx as related to speech production
Orofacial Myofunctional (Assessment)	**Definition:** Measures orofacial myofunctional patterns for speech and related functions
Orofacial Myofunctional (Treatment)	**Definition:** Applying techniques to improve, alter, or augment impaired orofacial myofunctional patterns and related speech production errors
Oscillating Tracking	**Definition:** Measures ability to visually track
Pain	**Definition:** Measures muscle soreness, pain and soreness with joint movement, and pain perception **Includes/Examples:** Includes questionnaires, graphs, symptom magnification scales or visual analog scales
Perceptual Processing (Assessment)	**Definition:** Measures stereognosis, kinesthesia, body schema, right-left discrimination, form constancy, position in space, visual closure, figure-ground, depth perception, spatial relations and topographical orientation

SECTION F - PHYSICAL REHABILITATION AND DIAGNOSTIC AUDIOLOGY
CHARACTER 5 - TYPE QUALIFIER

Perceptual Processing (Treatment)	**Definition:** Exercise and activities to facilitate perceptual processing **Explanation:** Includes stereognosis, kinesthesia, body schema, right-left discrimination, form constancy, position in space, visual closure, figure-ground, depth perception, spatial relations, and topographical orientation **Includes/Examples:** Includes stereognosis, kinesthesia, body schema, right-left discrimination, form constancy, position in space, visual closure, figure-ground, depth perception, spatial relations, and topographical orientation
Performance Intensity Phonetically Balanced Speech Discrimination	**Definition:** Measures word recognition over varying intensity levels
Postural Control	**Definition:** Exercise or activities to increase postural alignment and control
Prosthesis	**Definition:** Artificial substitutes for missing body parts that augment performance or function **Includes/Examples:** Limb prosthesis, ocular prosthesis
Psychosocial Skills (Assessment)	**Definition:** The ability to interact in society and to process emotions **Includes/Examples:** Includes psychological (values, interests, self-concept); social (role performance, social conduct, interpersonal skills, self expression); self-management (coping skills, time management, self-control)
Psychosocial Skills (Treatment)	**Definition:** The ability to interact in society and to process emotions **Includes/Examples:** Includes psychological (values, interests, self-concept); social (role performance, social conduct, interpersonal skills, self expression); self-management (coping skills, time management, self-control)
Pure Tone Audiometry, Air	**Definition:** Air-conduction pure tone threshold measures with appropriate masking
Pure Tone Audiometry, Air and Bone	**Definition:** Air-conduction and bone-conduction pure tone threshold measures with appropriate masking

Pure Tone Stenger	**Definition:** Measures unilateral nonorganic hearing loss based on simultaneous presentation of pure tones of differing volume
Range of Motion and Joint Integrity	**Definition:** Measures quantity, quality, grade, and classification of joint movement and/or mobility **Explanation:** Range of Motion is the space, distance or angle through which movement occurs at a joint or series of joints. Joint integrity is the conformance of joints to expected anatomic, biomechanical and kinematic norms
Range of Motion and Joint Mobility	**Definition:** Exercise or activities to increase muscle length and joint mobility
Receptive/Expressive Language (Assessment)	**Definition:** Measures receptive and expressive language
Receptive/Expressive Language (Treatment)	**Definition:** Applying techniques tot improve and augment receptive/expressive language
Reflex Integrity	**Definition:** Measures the presence, absence, or exaggeration of developmentally appropriate, pathologic or normal reflexes
Select Picture Audiometry	**Definition:** Establishes hearing threshold levels for speech using pictures
Sensorineural Acuity Level	**Definition:** Measures sensorineural acuity masking presented via bone conduction
Sensory Aids	**Definition:** Determines the appropriateness of a sensory prosthetic device, other than a hearing aid or assistive listening system/device
Sensory Awareness/Processing/Integrity	**Includes/Examples:** Includes light touch, pressure, temperature, pain, sharp/dull, proprioception, vestibular, visual, auditory, gustatory, and olfactory
Short Increment Sensitivity Index	**Definition:** Measures the ear's ability to detect small intensity changes; site of lesion test requiring a behavioral response
Sinusoidal Vertical Axis Rotational	**Definition:** Measures nystagmus following rotation
Somatosensory Evoked Potentials	**Definition:** Measures neural activity from sites throughout the body

APPENDIX A

SECTION F - PHYSICAL REHABILITATION AND DIAGNOSTIC AUDIOLOGY
CHARACTER 5 - TYPE QUALIFIER

Speech and/or Language Screening	**Definition:** Identifies need for further speech and/or language evaluation
Speech Threshold	**Definition:** Measures minimal intensity needed to repeat spondaic words
Speech-Language Pathology and Related Disorders Counseling	**Definition:** Provides patients/families with information, support, referrals to facilitate recovery from a communication disorder
Speech-Language Pathology and Related Disorders Prevention	**Definition:** Applying techniques to avoid or minimize onset and/or development of a communication disorder
Speech/Word Recognition	**Definition:** Measures ability to repeat/ identify single syllable words; scores given as a percentage; includes word recognition/ speech discrimination
Staggered Spondaic Word	**Definition:** Measures central auditory processing site of lesion based upon dichotic presentation of spondaic words
Static Orthosis	**Includes/Examples:** Includes customized and prefabricated splints, inhibitory casts, spinal and other braces, and protective devices; has no moving parts, maintains joint(s) in desired position
Stenger	**Definition:** Measures unilateral nonorganic hearing loss based on simultaneous presentation of signals of differing volume
Swallowing Dysfunction	**Definition:** Activities to improve swallowing function in coordination with respiratory function **Includes/Examples:** Includes function and coordination of sucking, mastication, coughing, swallowing
Synthetic Sentence Identification	**Definition:** Measures central auditory dysfunction using identification of third order approximations of sentences and competing messages
Temporal Ordering of Stimuli	**Definition:** Measures specific central auditory process

Therapeutic Exercise	**Definition:** Exercise or activities to facilitate sensory awareness, sensory processing, sensory integration, balance training, conditioning, reconditioning **Includes/Examples:** Includes developmental activities, breathing exercises, aerobic endurance activities, aquatic exercises, stretching and ventilatory muscle training
Tinnitus Masker (Assessment)	**Definition:** Determines candidacy for tinnitus masker
Tinnitus Masker (Treatment)	**Explanation:** Used to verify physical fit, acoustic appropriateness, and benefit; assists in achieving maximum benefit
Tone Decay	**Definition:** Measures decrease in hearing sensitivity to a tone; site of lesion test requiring a behavioral response
Transfer	**Definition:** Transitional movement from one surface to another
Transfer Training	**Definition:** Exercise or activities to facilitate movement from one surface to another
Tympanometry	**Definition:** Measures the integrity of the middle ear; measures ease at which sound flows through the tympanic membrane while air pressure against the membrane is varied
Unithermal Binaural Screen	**Definition:** Measures the rhythmic eye movements stimulated by changing the temperature of the vestibular system in both ears using warm water, screening format
Ventilation, Respiration and Circulation	**Definition:** Measures ventilatory muscle strength, power and endurance, pulmonary function and ventilatory mechanics **Includes/Examples:** Includes ability to clear airway, activities that aggravate or relieve edema, pain, dyspnea or other symptoms, chest wall mobility, cardiopulmonary response to performance of ADL and IAD, cough and sputum, standard vital signs

SECTION F - PHYSICAL REHABILITATION AND DIAGNOSTIC AUDIOLOGY

CHARACTER 5 - TYPE QUALIFIER

Vestibular	**Definition:** Applying techniques to compensate for balance disorders; includes habituation, exercise therapy, and balance retraining
Visual Motor Integration (Assessment)	**Definition:** Coordinating the interaction of information from the eyes with body movement during activity
Visual Motor Integration (Treatment)	**Definition:** Exercise or activities to facilitate coordinating the interaction of information from eyes with body movement during activity
Visual Reinforcement Audiometry	**Definition:** Behavioral measures using nonspeech and speech stimuli to obtain frequency/ear-specific information on auditory status **Includes/Examples:** Includes a conditioned response of looking toward a visual reinforcer (e.g., lights, animated toy) every time auditory stimuli are heard
Vocational Activities and Functional Community or Work Reintegration Skills (Assessment)	**Definition:** Measures environmental, home, work (job/school/play) barriers that keep patients from functioning optimally in their environment **Includes/Examples:** Includes assessment of vocational skill and interests, environment of work (job/school/play), injury potential and injury prevention or reduction, ergonomic stressors, transportation skills, and ability to access and use community resources
Vocational Activities and Functional Community or Work Reintegration Skills (Treatment)	**Definition:** Activities to facilitate vocational exploration, body mechanics training, job acquisition, and environmental or work (job/school/play) task adaptation **Includes/Examples:** Includes injury prevention and reduction, ergonomic stressor reduction, job coaching and simulation, work hardening and conditioning, driving training, transportation skills, and use of community resources

Voice (Assessment)	**Definition:** Measures vocal structure, function and production
Voice (Treatment)	**Definition:** Applying techniques to improve voice and vocal function
Voice Prosthetic (Assessment)	**Definition:** Determines the appropriateness of voice prosthetic/adaptive device to enhance or facilitate communication
Voice Prosthetic (Treatment)	**Includes/Examples:** Includes electrolarynx, and other assistive, adaptive, supportive devices
Wheelchair Mobility (Assessment)	**Definition:** Measures fit and functional abilities within wheelchair in a variety of environments
Wheelchair Mobility (Treatment)	**Definition:** Management, maintenance and controlled operation of a wheelchair, scooter or other device, in and on a variety of surfaces and environments
Wound Management	**Includes/Examples:** Includes non-selective and selective debridement (enzymes, autolysis, sharp debridement), dressings (wound coverings, hydrogel, vacuum-assisted closure), topical agents, etc.

SECTION G - MENTAL HEALTH
CHARACTER 3 - TYPE

Biofeedback	**Definition:** Provision of information from the monitoring and regulating of physiological processes in conjunction with cognitive-behavioral techniques to improve patient functioning or well-being **Includes/Examples:** Includes EEG, blood pressure, skin temperature or peripheral blood flow, ECG, electrooculogram, EMG, respirometry or capnometry, GSR/EDR, perineometry to monitor/regulate bowel/bladder activity, electrogastrogram to monitor/regulate gastric motility
Counseling	**Definition:** The application of psychological methods to treat an individual with normal developmental issues and psychological problems in order to increase function, improve well-being, alleviate distress, maladjustment or resolve crises
Crisis Intervention	**Definition:** Treatment of a traumatized, acutely disturbed or distressed individual for the purpose of short-term stabilization **Includes/Examples:** Includes defusing, debriefing, counseling, psychotherapy and/or coordination of care with other providers or agencies
Electroconvulsive Therapy	**Definition:** The application of controlled electrical voltages to treat a mental health disorder **Includes/Examples:** Includes appropriate sedation and other preparation of the individual
Family Psychotherapy	**Definition:** Treatment that includes one or more family members of an individual with a mental health disorder by behavioral, cognitive, psychoanalytic, psychodynamic or psychophysiological means to improve functioning or well-being **Explanation:** Remediation of emotional or behavioral problems presented by one or more family members in cases where psychotherapy with more than one family member is indicated

Group Psychotherapy	**Definition:** Treatment of two or more individuals with a mental health disorder by behavioral, cognitive, psychoanalytic, psychodynamic or psychophysiological means to improve functioning or well-being
Hypnosis	**Definition:** Induction of a state of heightened suggestibility by auditory, visual and tactile techniques to elicit an emotional or behavioral response
Individual Psychotherapy	**Definition:** Treatment of an individual with a mental health disorder by behavioral, cognitive, psychoanalytic, psychodynamic or psychophysiological means to improve functioning or well-being
Light Therapy	**Definition:** Application of specialized light treatments to improve functioning or well-being
Medication Management	**Definition:** Monitoring and adjusting the use of medications for the treatment of a mental health disorder
Narcosynthesis	**Definition:** Administration of intravenous barbiturates in order to release suppressed or repressed thoughts
Psychological Tests	**Definition:** The administration and interpretation of standardized psychological tests and measurement instruments for the assessment of psychological function

SECTION G - MENTAL HEALTH
CHARACTER 4 - QUALIFIER

Behavioral	**Definition:** Primarily to modify behavior **Includes/Examples:** Includes modeling and role playing, positive reinforcement of target behaviors, response cost, and training of self-management skills
Cognitive	**Definition:** Primarily to correct cognitive distortions and errors
Cognitive-Behavioral	**Definition:** Combining cognitive and behavioral treatment strategies to improve functioning **Explanation:** Maladaptive responses are examined to determine how cognitions relate to behavior patterns in response to an event. Uses learning principles and information-processing models
Developmental	**Definition:** Age-normed developmental status of cognitive, social and adaptive behavior skills
Intellectual and Psychoeducational	**Definition:** Intellectual abilities, academic achievement and learning capabilities (including behaviors and emotional factors affecting learning)
Interactive	**Definition:** Uses primarily physical aids and other forms of non-oral interaction with a patient who is physically, psychologically or developmentally unable to use ordinary language for communication **Includes/Examples:** Includes the use of toys in symbolic play
Interpersonal	**Definition:** Helps an individual make changes in interpersonal behaviors to reduce psychological dysfunction **Includes/Examples:** Includes exploratory techniques, encouragement of affective expression, clarification of patient statements, analysis of communication patterns, use of therapy relationship and behavior change techniques
Neurobehavioral and Cognitive Status	**Definition:** Includes neurobehavioral status exam, interview(s), and observation for the clinical assessment of thinking, reasoning and judgment, acquired knowledge, attention, memory, visual spatial abilities, language functions, and planning

Neuropsychological	**Definition:** Thinking, reasoning and judgment, acquired knowledge, attention, memory, visual spatial abilities, language functions, planning
Personality and Behavioral	**Definition:** Mood, emotion, behavior, social functioning, psychopathological conditions, personality traits and characteristics
Psychoanalysis	**Definition:** Methods of obtaining a detailed account of past and present mental and emotional experiences to determine the source and eliminate or diminish the undesirable effects of unconscious conflicts **Explanation:** Accomplished by making the individual aware of their existence, origin, and inappropriate expression in emotions and behavior
Psychodynamic	**Definition:** Exploration of past and present emotional experiences to understand motives and drives using insight-oriented techniques to reduce the undesirable effects of internal conflicts on emotions and behavior **Explanation:** Techniques include empathetic listening, clarifying self-defeating behavior patterns, and exploring adaptive alternatives
Psychophysiological	**Definition:** Monitoring and alteration of physiological processes to help the individual associate physiological reactions combined with cognitive and behavioral strategies to gain improved control of these processes to help the individual cope more effectively
Supportive	**Definition:** Formation of therapeutic relationship primarily for providing emotional support to prevent further deterioration in functioning during periods of particular stress **Explanation:** Often used in conjunction with other therapeutic approaches
Vocational	**Definition:** Exploration of vocational interests, aptitudes and required adaptive behavior skills to develop and carry out a plan for achieving a successful vocational placement **Includes/Examples:** Includes enhancing work related adjustment and/or pursuing viable options in training education or preparation

SECTION H - SUBSTANCE ABUSE TREATMENT
CHARACTER 3 - TYPE

Detoxification Services	**Definition:** Detoxification from alcohol and/or drugs **Explanation:** Not a treatment modality, but helps the patient stabilize physically and psychologically until the body becomes free of drugs and the effects of alcohol	Individual Counseling	**Definition:** The application of psychological methods to treat an individual with addictive behavior **Explanation:** Comprised of several different techniques, which apply various strategies to address drug addiction
Family Counseling	**Definition:** The application of psychological methods that includes one or more family members to treat an individual with addictive behavior **Explanation:** Provides support and education for family members of addicted individuals. Family member participation is seen as a critical area of substance abuse treatment	Individual Psychotherapy	**Definition:** Treatment of an individual with addictive behavior by behavioral, cognitive, psychoanalytic, psychodynamic or psychophysiological means
Group Counseling	**Definition:** The application of psychological methods to treat two or more individuals with addictive behavior **Explanation:** Provides structured group counseling sessions and healing power through the connection with others	Medication Management	**Definition:** Monitoring and adjusting the use of replacement medications for the treatment of addiction
		Pharmacotherapy	**Definition:** The use of replacement medications for the treatment of addiction

SECTION X - NEW TECHNOLOGY
CHARACTER 3 - OPERATION

Assistance	**Definition:** Taking over a portion of a physiological function by extracorporeal means	Replacement	**Definition:** Putting in or on biological or synthetic material that physically takes the place and/or function of all or a portion of a body part **Explanation:** The body part may have been taken out or replaced, or may be taken out, physically eradicated, or rendered nonfunctional during the Replacement procedure. A Removal procedure is coded for taking out the device used in a previous replacement procedure **Includes/Examples:** Total hip replacement, bone graft, free skin graft
Extirpation	**Definition:** Taking or cutting out solid matter from a body part **Explanation:** The solid matter may be an abnormal byproduct of a biological function or foreign body; it may be imbedded in a body part or in the lumen of a tubular body part. The solid matter may or may not have been previously broken into pieces. **Includes/Examples:** Thrombectomy, choledocholithotomy		
Fusion	**Definition:** Joining together portions of an articular body part rendering the articular body part immobile **Explanation:** The body part is joined together by fixation device, bone graft, or other means **Includes/Examples:** Spinal fusion, ankle arthrodesis	Reposition	**Definition:** Moving to its normal location, or other suitable location, all or a portion of a body part **Explanation:** The body part is moved to a new location from an abnormal location, or from a normal location where it is not functioning correctly. The body part may or may not be cut out or off to be moved to the new location **Includes/Examples:** Reposition of undescended testicle, fracture reduction
Introduction	**Definition:** Putting in or on a therapeutic, diagnostic, nutritional, physiological, or prophylactic substance except blood or blood products		
Monitoring	**Definition:** Determining the level of a physiological or physical function repetitively over a period of time		

SECTION X - NEW TECHNOLOGY
CHARACTER 5 - APPROACH

External	**Definition:** Procedures performed directly on the skin or mucous membrane and procedures performed indirectly by the application of external force through the skin or mucous membrane
Open	**Definition:** Cutting through the skin or mucous membrane and any other body layers necessary to expose the site of the procedure

Percutaneous	**Definition:** Entry, by puncture or minor incision, of instrumentation through the skin or mucous membrane and any other body layers necessary to reach the site of the procedure
Percutaneous Endoscopic	**Definition:** Entry, by puncture or minor incision, of instrumentation through the skin or mucous membrane and any other body layers necessary to reach and visualize the site of the procedure

SECTION X - NEW TECHNOLOGY
CHARACTER 6 - DEVICE / SUBSTANCE / TECHNOLOGY

Device/Substance/Technology	Description
Andexanet Alfa, Factor Xa Inhibitor Reversal Agent	Factor Xa Inhibitor Reversal Agent, Andexanet Alfa
Bezlotoxumab Monoclonal Antibody	ZINPLAVA™
Concentrated Bone Marrow Aspirate	CBMA (Concentrated Bone Marrow Aspirate)
Cytarabine and Daunorubicin Liposome Antineoplastic	VYXEOS™
Defibrotide Sodium Anticoagulant	Defitelio
Endothelial Damage Inhibitor	DuraGraft® Endothelial Damage Inhibitor
Engineered Autologous Chimeric Antigen Receptor T-cell Immunotherapy	Axicabtagene Ciloeucel
Interbody Fusion Device, Nanotextured Surface in New Technology	nanoLOCK™ interbody fusion device
Interbody Fusion Device, Radiolucent Porous in New Technology	COALESCE® radiolucent interbody fusion device COHERE® radiolucent interbody fusion device
Magnetically Controlled Growth Rod(s) in New Technology	MAGEC® Spinal Bracing and Distraction System Spinal growth rods, magnetically controlled
Other New Technology Therapeutic Substance	STELARA® Ustekinumab
Skin Substitute, Porcine Liver Derived in New Technology	MIRODERM™ Biologic Wound Matrix
Uridine Triacetate	Vistogard®
Zooplastic Tissue, Rapid Deployment Technique in New Technology	EDWARDS INTUITY Elite valve system INTUITY Elite valve system, EDWARDS Perceval sutureless valve Sutureless valve, Perceval

BODY PART KEY

Abdominal aortic plexus	**Use:** Abdominal Sympathetic Nerve
Abdominal esophagus	**Use:** Esophagus, Lower
Abductor hallucis muscle	**Use:** Foot Muscle, Right Foot Muscle, Left
Accessory cephalic vein	**Use:** Cephalic Vein, Right Cephalic Vein, Left
Accessory obturator nerve	**Use:** Lumbar Plexus
Accessory phrenic nerve	**Use:** Phrenic Nerve
Accessory spleen	**Use:** Spleen
Acetabulofemoral joint	**Use:** Hip Joint, Right Hip Joint, Left
Achilles tendon	**Use:** Lower Leg Tendon, Right Lower Leg Tendon, Left
Acromioclavicular ligament	**Use:** Shoulder Bursa and Ligament, Right Shoulder Bursa and Ligament, Left
Acromion (process)	**Use:** Scapula, Right Scapula, Left
Adductor brevis muscle	**Use:** Upper Leg Muscle, Right Upper Leg Muscle, Left
Adductor hallucis muscle	**Use:** Foot Muscle, Right Foot Muscle, Left
Adductor longus muscle Adductor magnus muscle	**Use:** Upper Leg Muscle, Right Upper Leg Muscle, Left
Adenohypophysis	**Use:** Pituitary Gland
Alar ligament of axis	**Use:** Head and Neck Bursa and Ligament
Alveolar process of mandible	**Use:** Mandible, Right Mandible, Left

Alveolar process of maxilla	**Use:** Maxilla
Anal orifice	**Use:** Anus
Anatomical snuffbox	**Use:** Lower Arm and Wrist Muscle, Right Lower Arm and Wrist Muscle, Left
Angular artery	**Use:** Face Artery
Angular vein	**Use:** Face Vein, Right Face Vein, Left
Annular ligament	**Use:** Elbow Bursa and Ligament, Right Elbow Bursa and Ligament, Left
Anorectal junction	**Use:** Rectum
Ansa cervicalis	**Use:** Cervical Plexus
Antebrachial fascia	**Use:** Subcutaneous Tissue and Fascia, Right Lower Arm Subcutaneous Tissue and Fascia, Left Lower Arm
Anterior (pectoral) lymph node	**Use:** Lymphatic, Right Axillary Lymphatic, Left Axillary
Anterior cerebral artery	**Use:** Intracranial Artery
Anterior cerebral vein	**Use:** Intracranial Vein
Anterior choroidal artery	**Use:** Intracranial Artery
Anterior circumflex humeral artery	**Use:** Axillary Artery, Right Axillary Artery, Left
Anterior communicating artery	**Use:** Intracranial Artery
Anterior cruciate ligament (ACL)	**Use:** Knee Bursa and Ligament, Right Knee Bursa and Ligament, Left
Anterior crural nerve	**Use:** Femoral Nerve

BODY PART KEY

Anterior facial vein	**Use:** Face Vein, Right Face Vein, Left
Anterior intercostal artery	**Use:** Internal Mammary Artery, Right Internal Mammary Artery, Left
Anterior interosseous nerve	**Use:** Median Nerve
Anterior lateral malleolar artery	**Use:** Anterior Tibial Artery, Right Anterior Tibial Artery, Left
Anterior lingual gland	**Use:** Minor Salivary Gland
Anterior medial malleolar artery	**Use:** Anterior Tibial Artery, Right Anterior Tibial Artery, Left
Anterior spinal artery	**Use:** Vertebral Artery, Right Vertebral Artery, Left
Anterior tibial recurrent artery	**Use:** Anterior Tibial Artery, Right Anterior Tibial Artery, Left
Anterior ulnar recurrent artery	**Use:** Ulnar Artery, Right Ulnar Artery, Left
Anterior vagal trunk	**Use:** Vagus Nerve
Anterior vertebral muscle	**Use:** Neck Muscle, Right Neck Muscle, Left
Antihelix Antitragus	**Use:** External Ear, Right External Ear, Left External Ear, Bilateral
Antrum of Highmore	**Use:** Maxillary Sinus, Right Maxillary Sinus, Left
Aortic annulus	**Use:** Aortic Valve
Aortic arch	**Use:** Thoracic Aorta, Ascending/Arch
Aortic intercostal artery	**Use:** Upper Artery
Apical (subclavicular) lymph node	**Use:** Lymphatic, Right Axillary Lymphatic, Left Axillary

Apneustic center	**Use:** Pons
Aqueduct of Sylvius	**Use:** Cerebral Ventricle
Aqueous humour	**Use:** Anterior Chamber, Right Anterior Chamber, Left
Arachnoid mater	**Use:** Cerebral Meninges Spinal Meninges
Arcuate artery	**Use:** Foot Artery, Right Foot Artery, Left
Areola	**Use:** Nipple, Right Nipple, Left
Arterial canal (duct)	**Use:** Pulmonary Artery, Left
Aryepiglottic fold Arytenoid cartilage	**Use:** Larynx
Arytenoid muscle	**Use:** Neck Muscle, Right Neck Muscle, Left
Ascending aorta	**Use:** Thoracic Aorta, Ascending/Arch
Ascending palatine artery	**Use:** Face Artery
Ascending pharyngeal artery	**Use:** External Carotid Artery, Right External Carotid Artery, Left
Atlantoaxial joint	**Use:** Cervical Vertebral Joint
Atrioventricular node	**Use:** Conduction Mechanism
Atrium dextrum cordis	**Use:** Atrium, Right
Atrium pulmonale	**Use:** Atrium, Left
Auditory tube	**Use:** Eustachian Tube, Right Eustachian Tube, Left
Auerbach's (myenteric) plexus	**Use:** Abdominal Sympathetic Nerve

BODY PART KEY

Auricle	**Use:** External Ear, Right External Ear, Left External Ear, Bilateral
Auricularis muscle	**Use:** Head Muscle
Axillary fascia	**Use:** Subcutaneous Tissue and Fascia, Right Upper Arm Subcutaneous Tissue and Fascia, Left Upper Arm
Axillary nerve	**Use:** Brachial Plexus
Bartholin's (greater vestibular) gland	**Use:** Vestibular Gland
Basal (internal) cerebral vein	**Use:** Intracranial Vein
Basal nuclei	**Use:** Basal Ganglia
Base of Tongue	**Use:** Pharynx
Basilar artery	**Use:** Intracranial Artery
Basis pontis	**Use:** Pons
Biceps brachii muscle	**Use:** Upper Arm Muscle, Right Upper Arm Muscle, Left
Biceps femoris muscle	**Use:** Upper Leg Muscle, Right Upper Leg Muscle, Left
Bicipital aponeurosis	**Use:** Subcutaneous Tissue and Fascia, Right Lower Arm Subcutaneous Tissue and Fascia, Left Lower Arm
Bicuspid valve	**Use:** Mitral Valve
Body of femur	**Use:** Femoral Shaft, Right Femoral Shaft, Left
Body of fibula	**Use:** Fibula, Right Fibula, Left
Bony labyrinth	**Use:** Inner Ear, Right Inner Ear, Left

Bony orbit	**Use:** Orbit, Right Orbit, Left
Bony vestibule	**Use:** Inner Ear, Right Inner Ear, Left
Botallo's duct	**Use:** Pulmonary Artery, Left
Brachial (lateral) lymph node	**Use:** Lymphatic, Right Axillary Lymphatic, Left Axillary
Brachialis muscle	**Use:** Upper Arm Muscle, Right Upper Arm Muscle, Left
Brachiocephalic artery Brachiocephalic trunk	**Use:** Innominate Artery
Brachiocephalic vein	**Use:** Innominate Vein, Right Innominate Vein, Left
Brachioradialis muscle	**Use:** Lower Arm and Wrist Muscle, Right Lower Arm and Wrist Muscle, Left
Broad ligament	**Use:** Uterine Supporting Structure
Bronchial artery	**Use:** Upper Artery
Bronchus Intermedius	**Use:** Main Bronchus, Right
Buccal gland	**Use:** Buccal Mucosa
Buccinator lymph node	**Use:** Lymphatic, Head
Buccinator muscle	**Use:** Facial Muscle
Bulbospongiosus muscle	**Use:** Perineum Muscle
Bulbourethral (Cowper's) gland	**Use:** Urethra
Bundle of His Bundle of Kent	**Use:** Conduction Mechanism
Calcaneocuboid joint	**Use:** Tarsal Joint, Right Tarsal Joint, Left
Calcaneocuboid ligament	**Use:** Foot Bursa and Ligament, Right Foot Bursa and Ligament, Left

BODY PART KEY

Calcaneofibular ligament	**Use:** Ankle Bursa and Ligament, Right Ankle Bursa and Ligament, Left
Calcaneus	**Use:** Tarsal, Right Tarsal, Left
Capitate bone	**Use:** Carpal, Right Carpal, Left
Cardia	**Use:** Esophagogastric Junction
Cardiac plexus	**Use:** Thoracic Sympathetic Nerve
Cardioesophageal junction	**Use:** Esophagogastric Junction
Caroticotympanic artery	**Use:** Internal Carotid Artery, Right Internal Carotid Artery, Left
Carotid glomus	**Use:** Carotid Body, Left Carotid Body, Right Carotid Bodies, Bilateral
Carotid sinus	**Use:** Internal Carotid Artery, Right Internal Carotid Artery, Left
Carotid sinus nerve	**Use:** Glossopharyngeal Nerve
Carpometacarpal ligament	**Use:** Hand Bursa and Ligament, Right Hand Bursa and Ligament, Left
Cauda equina	**Use:** Lumbar Spinal Cord
Cavernous plexus	**Use:** Head and Neck Sympathetic Nerve
Celiac (solar) plexus Celiac ganglion	**Use:** Abdominal Sympathetic Nerve
Celiac lymph node	**Use:** Lymphatic, Aortic
Celiac trunk	**Use:** Celiac Artery
Central axillary lymph node	**Use:** Lymphatic, Right Axillary Lymphatic, Left Axillary
Cerebral aqueduct (Sylvius)	**Use:** Cerebral Ventricle

Cerebrum	**Use:** Brain
Cervical esophagus	**Use:** Esophagus, Upper
Cervical facet joint	**Use:** Cervical Vertebral Joint Cervical Vertebral Joints, 2 or more
Cervical ganglion	**Use:** Head and Neck Sympathetic Nerve
Cervical interspinous ligament Cervical intertransverse ligament Cervical ligamentum flavum	**Use:** Head and Neck Bursa and Ligament
Cervical lymph node	**Use:** Lymphatic, Right Neck Lymphatic, Left Neck
Cervicothoracic facet joint	**Use:** Cervicothoracic Vertebral Joint
Choana	**Use:** Nasopharynx
Chondroglossus muscle	**Use:** Tongue, Palate, Pharynx Muscle
Chorda tympani	**Use:** Facial Nerve
Choroid plexus	**Use:** Cerebral Ventricle
Ciliary body	**Use:** Eye, Right Eye, Left
Ciliary ganglion	**Use:** Head and Neck Sympathetic Nerve
Circle of Willis	**Use:** Intracranial Artery
Circumflex iliac artery	**Use:** Femoral Artery, Right Femoral Artery, Left
Claustrum	**Use:** Basal Ganglia
Coccygeal body	**Use:** Coccygeal Glomus
Coccygeus muscle	**Use:** Trunk Muscle, Right Trunk Muscle, Left
Cochlea	**Use:** Inner Ear, Right Inner Ear, Left

BODY PART KEY

Cochlear nerve	**Use:** Acoustic Nerve
Columella	**Use:** Nasal Mucosa and Soft Tissue
Common digital vein	**Use:** Foot Vein, Right Foot Vein, Left
Common facial vein	**Use:** Face Vein, Right Face Vein, Left
Common fibular nerve	**Use:** Peroneal Nerve
Common hepatic artery	**Use:** Hepatic Artery
Common iliac (subaortic) lymph node	**Use:** Lymphatic, Pelvis
Common interosseous artery	**Use:** Ulnar Artery, Right Ulnar Artery, Left
Common peroneal nerve	**Use:** Peroneal Nerve
Condyloid process	**Use:** Mandible, Right Mandible, Left
Conus arteriosus	**Use:** Ventricle, Right
Conus medullaris	**Use:** Lumbar Spinal Cord
Coracoacromial ligament	**Use:** Shoulder Bursa and Ligament, Right Shoulder Bursa and Ligament, Left
Coracobrachialis muscle	**Use:** Upper Arm Muscle, Right Upper Arm Muscle, Left
Coracoclavicular ligament Coracohumeral ligament	**Use:** Shoulder Bursa and Ligament, Right Shoulder Bursa and Ligament, Left
Coracoid process	**Use:** Scapula, Right Scapula, Left
Corniculate cartilage	**Use:** Larynx
Corpus callosum	**Use:** Brain
Corpus cavernosum Corpus spongiosum	**Use:** Penis
Corpus striatum	**Use:** Basal Ganglia
Corrugator supercilii muscle	**Use:** Facial Muscle
Costocervical trunk	**Use:** Subclavian Artery, Right Subclavian Artery, Left
Costoclavicular ligament	**Use:** Shoulder Bursa and Ligament, Right Shoulder Bursa and Ligament, Left
Costotransverse joint	**Use:** Thoracic Vertebral Joint Thoracic Vertebral Joints, 2 to 7 Thoracic Vertebral Joints, 8 or more
Costotransverse ligament	**Use:** Sternum Bursa and Ligament Rib(s) Bursa and Ligament
Costovertebral joint	**Use:** Thoracic Vertebral Joint Thoracic Vertebral Joints, 2 to 7 Thoracic Vertebral Joints, 8 or more
Costoxiphoid ligament	**Use:** Sternum Bursa and Ligament Rib(s) Bursa and Ligament
Cowper's (bulbourethral) gland	**Use:** Urethra
Cremaster muscle	**Use:** Perineum Muscle
Cribriform plate	**Use:** Ethmoid Bone, Right Ethmoid Bone, Left
Cricoid cartilage	**Use:** Trachea
Cricothyroid artery	**Use:** Thyroid Artery, Right Thyroid Artery, Left
Cricothyroid muscle	**Use:** Neck Muscle, Right Neck Muscle, Left

BODY PART KEY

Crural fascia	**Use:** Subcutaneous Tissue and Fascia, Right Upper Leg Subcutaneous Tissue and Fascia, Left Upper Leg
Cubital lymph node	**Use:** Lymphatic, Right Upper Extremity Lymphatic, Left Upper Extremity
Cubital nerve	**Use:** Ulnar Nerve
Cuboid bone	**Use:** Tarsal, Right Tarsal, Left
Cuboideonavicular joint	**Use:** Tarsal Joint, Right Tarsal Joint, Left
Culmen	**Use:** Cerebellum
Cuneiform cartilage	**Use:** Larynx
Cuneonavicular joint	**Use:** Tarsal Joint, Right Tarsal Joint, Left
Cuneonavicular ligament	**Use:** Foot Bursa and Ligament, Right Foot Bursa and Ligament, Left
Cutaneous (transverse) cervical nerve	**Use:** Cervical Plexus
Deep cervical fascia	**Use:** Subcutaneous Tissue and Fascia, Right Neck Subcutaneous Tissue and Fascia, Left Neck
Deep cervical vein	**Use:** Vertebral Vein, Right Vertebral Vein, Left
Deep circumflex iliac artery	**Use:** External Iliac Artery, Right External Iliac Artery, Left
Deep facial vein	**Use:** Face Vein, Right Face Vein, Left
Deep femoral (profunda femoris) vein	**Use:** Femoral Vein, Right Femoral Vein, Left
Deep femoral artery	**Use:** Femoral Artery, Right Femoral Artery, Left

Deep palmar arch	**Use:** Hand Artery, Right Hand Artery, Left
Deep transverse perineal muscle	**Use:** Perineum Muscle
Deferential artery	**Use:** Internal Iliac Artery, Right Internal Iliac Artery, Left
Deltoid fascia	**Use:** Subcutaneous Tissue and Fascia, Right Upper Arm Subcutaneous Tissue and Fascia, Left Upper Arm
Deltoid ligament	**Use:** Ankle Bursa and Ligament, Right Ankle Bursa and Ligament, Left
Deltoid muscle	**Use:** Shoulder Muscle, Right Shoulder Muscle, Left
Deltopectoral (infraclavicular) lymph node	**Use:** Lymphatic, Right Upper Extremity Lymphatic, Left Upper Extremity
Dens	**Use:** Cervical Vertebra
Denticulate (dentate) ligament	**Use:** Spinal Cord
Depressor anguli oris muscle Depressor labii inferioris muscle Depressor septi nasi muscle Depressor supercilii muscle	**Use:** Facial Muscle
Dermis	**Use:** Skin
Descending genicular artery	**Use:** Femoral Artery, Right Femoral Artery, Left
Diaphragma sellae	**Use:** Dura Mater
Distal humerus	**Use:** Humeral Shaft, Right Humeral Shaft, Left
Distal humerus, involving joint	**Use:** Elbow Joint, Right Elbow Joint, Left
Distal radioulnar joint	**Use:** Wrist Joint, Right Wrist Joint, Left
Dorsal digital nerve	**Use:** Radial Nerve

BODY PART KEY

Dorsal metacarpal vein	**Use:** Hand Vein, Right Hand Vein, Left
Dorsal metatarsal artery	**Use:** Foot Artery, Right Foot Artery, Left
Dorsal metatarsal vein	**Use:** Foot Vein, Right Foot Vein, Left
Dorsal scapular artery	**Use:** Subclavian Artery, Right Subclavian Artery, Left
Dorsal scapular nerve	**Use:** Brachial Plexus
Dorsal venous arch	**Use:** Foot Vein, Right Foot Vein, Left
Dorsalis pedis artery	**Use:** Anterior Tibial Artery, Right Anterior Tibial Artery, Left
Duct of Santorini	**Use:** Pancreatic Duct, Accessory
Duct of Wirsung	**Use:** Pancreatic Duct
Ductus deferens	**Use:** Vas Deferens, Right Vas Deferens, Left Vas Deferens, Bilateral Vas Deferens
Duodenal ampulla	**Use:** Ampulla of Vater
Duodenojejunal flexure	**Use:** Jejunum
Dura mater, intracranial	**Use:** Dura Mater
Dura mater, spinal	**Use:** Spinal Meninges
Dural venous sinus	**Use:** Intracranial Vein
Earlobe	**Use:** External Ear, Right External Ear, Left External Ear, Bilateral
Eighth cranial nerve	**Use:** Acoustic Nerve

Ejaculatory duct	**Use:** Vas Deferens, Right Vas Deferens, Left Vas Deferens, Bilateral Vas Deferens
Eleventh cranial nerve	**Use:** Accessory Nerve
Encephalon	**Use:** Brain
Ependyma	**Use:** Cerebral Ventricle
Epidermis	**Use:** Skin
Epidural space, spinal	**Use:** Spinal Canal
Epiploic foramen	**Use:** Peritoneum
Epithalamus	**Use:** Thalamus
Epitrochlear lymph node	**Use:** Lymphatic, Right Upper Extremity Lymphatic, Left Upper Extremity
Erector spinae muscle	**Use:** Trunk Muscle, Right Trunk Muscle, Left
Esophageal artery	**Use:** Upper Artery
Esophageal plexus	**Use:** Thoracic Sympathetic Nerve
Ethmoidal air cell	**Use:** Ethmoid Sinus, Right Ethmoid Sinus, Left
Extensor carpi radialis muscle Extensor carpi ulnaris muscle	**Use:** Lower Arm and Wrist Muscle, Right Lower Arm and Wrist Muscle, Left
Extensor digitorum brevis muscle	**Use:** Foot Muscle, Right Foot Muscle, Left
Extensor digitorum longus muscle	**Use:** Lower Leg Muscle, Right Lower Leg Muscle, Left
Extensor hallucis brevis muscle	**Use:** Foot Muscle, Right Foot Muscle, Left

BODY PART KEY

Extensor hallucis longus muscle	**Use:** Lower Leg Muscle, Right Lower Leg Muscle, Left
External anal sphincter	**Use:** Anal Sphincter
External auditory meatus	**Use:** External Auditory Canal, Right External Auditory Canal, Left
External maxillary artery	**Use:** Face Artery
External naris	**Use:** Nasal Mucosa and Soft Tissue
External oblique aponeurosis	**Use:** Subcutaneous Tissue and Fascia, Trunk
External oblique muscle	**Use:** Abdomen Muscle, Right Abdomen Muscle, Left
External popliteal nerve	**Use:** Peroneal Nerve
External pudendal artery	**Use:** Femoral Artery, Right Femoral Artery, Left
External pudendal vein	**Use:** Saphenous Vein, Right Saphenous Vein, Left
External urethral sphincter	**Use:** Urethra
Extradural space, intracranial	**Use:** Epidural Space, Intracranial
Extradural space, spinal	**Use:** Spinal Canal
Facial artery	**Use:** Face Artery
False vocal cord	**Use:** Larynx
Falx cerebri	**Use:** Dura Mater
Fascia lata	**Use:** Subcutaneous Tissue and Fascia, Right Upper Leg Subcutaneous Tissue and Fascia, Left Upper Leg
Femoral head	**Use:** Upper Femur, Right Upper Femur, Left

Femoral lymph node	**Use:** Lymphatic, Right Lower Extremity Lymphatic, Left Lower Extremity
Femoropatellar joint Femorotibial joint	**Use:** Knee Joint, Right Knee Joint, Left
Fibular artery	**Use:** Peroneal Artery, Right Peroneal Artery, Left
Fibularis brevis muscle Fibularis longus muscle	**Use:** Lower Leg Muscle, Right Lower Leg Muscle, Left
Fifth cranial nerve	**Use:** Trigeminal Nerve
Filum terminale	**Use:** Spinal Meninges
First cranial nerve	**Use:** Olfactory Nerve
First intercostal nerve	**Use:** Brachial Plexus
Flexor carpi radialis muscle Flexor carpi ulnaris muscle	**Use:** Lower Arm and Wrist Muscle, Right Lower Arm and Wrist Muscle, Left
Flexor digitorum brevis muscle	**Use:** Foot Muscle, Right Foot Muscle, Left
Flexor digitorum longus muscle	**Use:** Lower Leg Muscle, Right Lower Leg Muscle, Left
Flexor hallucis brevis muscle	**Use:** Foot Muscle, Right Foot Muscle, Left
Flexor hallucis longus muscle	**Use:** Lower Leg Muscle, Right Lower Leg Muscle, Left
Flexor pollicis longus muscle	**Use:** Lower Arm and Wrist Muscle, Right Lower Arm and Wrist Muscle, Left
Foramen magnum	**Use:** Occipital Bone
Foramen of Monro (intraventricular)	**Use:** Cerebral Ventricle
Foreskin	**Use:** Prepuce
Fossa of Rosenmuller	**Use:** Nasopharynx

BODY PART KEY

Fourth cranial nerve	**Use:** Trochlear Nerve
Fourth ventricle	**Use:** Cerebral Ventricle
Fovea	**Use:** Retina, Right Retina, Left
Frenulum labii inferioris	**Use:** Lower Lip
Frenulum labii superioris	**Use:** Upper Lip
Frenulum linguae	**Use:** Tongue
Frontal lobe	**Use:** Cerebral Hemisphere
Frontal vein	**Use:** Face Vein, Right Face Vein, Left
Fundus uteri	**Use:** Uterus
Galea aponeurotica	**Use:** Subcutaneous Tissue and Fascia, Scalp
Ganglion impar (ganglion of Walther)	**Use:** Sacral Sympathetic Nerve
Gasserian ganglion	**Use:** Trigeminal Nerve
Gastric lymph node	**Use:** Lymphatic, Aortic
Gastric plexus	**Use:** Abdominal Sympathetic Nerve
Gastrocnemius muscle	**Use:** Lower Leg Muscle, Right Lower Leg Muscle, Left
Gastrocolic ligament Gastrocolic omentum	**Use:** Omentum
Gastroduodenal artery	**Use:** Hepatic Artery
Gastroesophageal (GE) junction	**Use:** Esophagogastric Junction
Gastrohepatic omentum Gastrophrenic ligament Gastrosplenic ligament	**Use:** Omentum

Gemellus muscle	**Use:** Hip Muscle, Right Hip Muscle, Left
Geniculate ganglion	**Use:** Facial Nerve
Geniculate nucleus	**Use:** Thalamus
Genioglossus muscle	**Use:** Tongue, Palate, Pharynx Muscle
Genitofemoral nerve	**Use:** Lumbar Plexus
Glans penis	**Use:** Prepuce
Glenohumeral joint	**Use:** Shoulder Joint, Right Shoulder Joint, Left
Glenohumeral ligament	**Use:** Shoulder Bursa and Ligament, Right Shoulder Bursa and Ligament, Left
Glenoid fossa (of scapula)	**Use:** Glenoid Cavity, Right Glenoid Cavity, Left
Glenoid ligament (labrum)	**Use:** Shoulder Bursa and Ligament, Right Shoulder Bursa and Ligament, Left
Globus pallidus	**Use:** Basal Ganglia
Glossoepiglottic fold	**Use:** Epiglottis
Glottis	**Use:** Larynx
Gluteal lymph node	**Use:** Lymphatic, Pelvis
Gluteal vein	**Use:** Hypogastric Vein, Right Hypogastric Vein, Left
Gluteus maximus muscle Gluteus medius muscle Gluteus minimus muscle	**Use:** Hip Muscle, Right Hip Muscle, Left
Gracilis muscle	**Use:** Upper Leg Muscle, Right Upper Leg Muscle, Left

BODY PART KEY

Great auricular nerve	**Use:** Cervical Plexus
Great cerebral vein	**Use:** Intracranial Vein
Greater saphenous vein	**Use:** Saphenous Vein, Right Saphenous Vein, Left
Greater alar cartilage	**Use:** Nasal Mucosa and Soft Tissue
Greater occipital nerve	**Use:** Cervical Nerve
Greater Omentum	**Use:** Omentum
Greater splanchnic nerve	**Use:** Thoracic Sympathetic Nerve
Greater superficial petrosal nerve	**Use:** Facial Nerve
Greater trochanter	**Use:** Upper Femur, Right Upper Femur, Left
Greater tuberosity	**Use:** Humeral Head, Right Humeral Head, Left
Greater vestibular (Bartholin's) gland	**Use:** Vestibular Gland
Greater wing	**Use:** Sphenoid Bone
Hallux	**Use:** 1st Toe, Right 1st Toe, Left
Hamate bone	**Use:** Carpal, Right Carpal, Left
Head of fibula	**Use:** Fibula, Right Fibula, Left
Helix	**Use:** External Ear, Right External Ear, Left External Ear, Bilateral
Hepatic artery proper	**Use:** Hepatic Artery
Hepatic flexure	**Use:** Transverse Colon

Hepatic lymph node	**Use:** Lymphatic, Aortic
Hepatic plexus	**Use:** Abdominal Sympathetic Nerve
Hepatic portal vein	**Use:** Portal Vein
Hepatogastric ligament	**Use:** Omentum
Hepatopancreatic ampulla	**Use:** Ampulla of Vater
Humeroradial joint Humeroulnar joint	**Use:** Elbow Joint, Right Elbow Joint, Left
Humerus, distal	**Use:** Humeral Shaft, Right Humeral Shaft, Left
Hyoglossus muscle	**Use:** Tongue, Palate, Pharynx Muscle
Hyoid artery	**Use:** Thyroid Artery, Right Thyroid Artery, Left
Hypogastric artery	**Use:** Internal Iliac Artery, Right Internal Iliac Artery, Left
Hypopharynx	**Use:** Pharynx
Hypophysis	**Use:** Pituitary Gland
Hypothenar muscle	**Use:** Hand Muscle, Right Hand Muscle, Left
Ileal artery Ileocolic artery	**Use:** Superior Mesenteric Artery
Ileocolic vein	**Use:** Colic Vein
Iliac crest	**Use:** Pelvic Bone, Right Pelvic Bone, Left
Iliac fascia	**Use:** Subcutaneous Tissue and Fascia, Right Upper Leg Subcutaneous Tissue and Fascia, Left Upper Leg

APPENDIX B

BODY PART KEY

Iliac lymph node	**Use:** Lymphatic, Pelvis
Iliacus muscle	**Use:** Hip Muscle, Right Hip Muscle, Left
Iliofemoral ligament	**Use:** Hip Bursa and Ligament, Right Hip Bursa and Ligament, Left
Iliohypogastric nerve Ilioinguinal nerve	**Use:** Lumbar Plexus
Iliolumbar artery	**Use:** Internal Iliac Artery, Right Internal Iliac Artery, Left
Iliolumbar ligament	**Use:** Lower Spine Bursa and Ligament

Iliotibial tract (band)	**Use:**
	Subcutaneous Tissue and Fascia,
	    Right Upper Leg
	Subcutaneous Tissue and Fascia,
	    Left Upper Leg

Ilium	**Use:** Pelvic Bone, Right Pelvic Bone, Left
Incus	**Use:** Auditory Ossicle, Right Auditory Ossicle, Left
Inferior cardiac nerve	**Use:** Thoracic Sympathetic Nerve
Inferior cerebellar vein Inferior cerebral vein	**Use:** Intracranial Vein
Inferior epigastric artery	**Use:** External Iliac Artery, Right External Iliac Artery, Left
Inferior epigastric lymph node	**Use:** Lymphatic, Pelvis
Inferior genicular artery	**Use:** Popliteal Artery, Right Popliteal Artery, Left
Inferior gluteal artery	**Use:** Internal Iliac Artery, Right Internal Iliac Artery, Left
Inferior gluteal nerve	**Use:** Sacral Plexus

Inferior hypogastric plexus	**Use:** Abdominal Sympathetic Nerve
Inferior labial artery	**Use:** Face Artery
Inferior longitudinal muscle	**Use:** Tongue, Palate, Pharynx Muscle
Inferior mesenteric ganglion	**Use:** Abdominal Sympathetic Nerve
Inferior mesenteric lymph node	**Use:** Lymphatic, Mesenteric
Inferior mesenteric plexus	**Use:** Abdominal Sympathetic Nerve
Inferior oblique muscle	**Use:** Extraocular Muscle, Right Extraocular Muscle, Left
Inferior pancreaticoduodenal artery	**Use:** Superior Mesenteric Artery
Inferior phrenic artery	**Use:** Abdominal Aorta
Inferior rectus muscle	**Use:** Extraocular Muscle, Right Extraocular Muscle, Left
Inferior suprarenal artery	**Use:** Renal Artery, Right Renal Artery, Left
Inferior tarsal plate	**Use:** Lower Eyelid, Right Lower Eyelid, Left
Inferior thyroid vein	**Use:** Innominate Vein, Right Innominate Vein, Left
Inferior tibiofibular joint	**Use:** Ankle Joint, Right Ankle Joint, Left
Inferior turbinate	**Use:** Nasal Turbinate
Inferior ulnar collateral artery	**Use:** Brachial Artery, Right Brachial Artery, Left
Inferior vesical artery	**Use:** Internal Iliac Artery, Right Internal Iliac Artery, Left

BODY PART KEY

BODY PART KEY

Infraauricular lymph node	**Use:** Lymphatic, Head
Infraclavicular (deltopectoral) lymph node	**Use:** Lymphatic, Right Upper Extremity Lymphatic, Left Upper Extremity
Infrahyoid muscle	**Use:** Neck Muscle, Right Neck Muscle, Left
Infraparotid lymph node	**Use:** Lymphatic, Head
Infraspinatus fascia	**Use:** Subcutaneous Tissue and Fascia, Right Upper Arm Subcutaneous Tissue and Fascia, Left Upper Arm
Infraspinatus muscle	**Use:** Shoulder Muscle, Right Shoulder Muscle, Left
Infundibulopelvic ligament	**Use:** Uterine Supporting Structure
Inguinal canal Inguinal triangle	**Use:** Inguinal Region, Right Inguinal Region, Left Inguinal Region, Bilateral
Interatrial septum	**Use:** Atrial Septum
Intercarpal joint	**Use:** Carpal Joint, Right Carpal Joint, Left
Intercarpal ligament	**Use:** Hand Bursa and Ligament, Right Hand Bursa and Ligament, Left
Interclavicular ligament	**Use:** Shoulder Bursa and Ligament, Right Shoulder Bursa and Ligament, Left
Intercostal lymph node	**Use:** Lymphatic, Thorax
Intercostal muscle	**Use:** Thorax Muscle, Right Thorax Muscle, Left
Intercostal nerve Intercostobrachial nerve	**Use:** Thoracic Nerve
Intercuneiform joint	**Use:** Tarsal Joint, Right Tarsal Joint, Left

Intercuneiform ligament	**Use:** Foot Bursa and Ligament, Right Foot Bursa and Ligament, Left
Intermediate bronchus	**Use:** Main Bronchus, Right
Intermediate cuneiform bone	**Use:** Tarsal, Right Tarsal, Left
Internal (basal) cerebral vein	**Use:** Intracranial Vein
Internal anal sphincter	**Use:** Anal Sphincter
Internal carotid artery, intracranial portion	**Use:** Intracranial Artery
Internal carotid plexus	**Use:** Head and Neck Sympathetic Nerve
Internal iliac vein	**Use:** Hypogastric Vein, Right Hypogastric Vein, Left
Internal maxillary artery	**Use:** External Carotid Artery, Right External Carotid Artery, Left
Internal naris	**Use:** Nasal Mucosa and Soft Tissue
Internal oblique muscle	**Use:** Abdomen Muscle, Right Abdomen Muscle, Left
Internal pudendal artery	**Use:** Internal Iliac Artery, Right Internal Iliac Artery, Left
Internal pudendal vein	**Use:** Hypogastric Vein, Right Hypogastric Vein, Left
Internal thoracic artery	**Use:** Internal Mammary Artery, Right Internal Mammary Artery, Left Subclavian Artery, Right Subclavian Artery, Left
Internal urethral sphincter	**Use:** Urethra
Interphalangeal (IP) joint	**Use:** Finger Phalangeal Joint, Right Finger Phalangeal Joint, Left Toe Phalangeal Joint, Right Toe Phalangeal Joint, Left

BODY PART KEY

Interphalangeal ligament	**Use:** Hand Bursa and Ligament, Right Hand Bursa and Ligament, Left Foot Bursa and Ligament, Right Foot Bursa and Ligament, Left
Interspinalis muscle	**Use:** Trunk Muscle, Right Trunk Muscle, Left
Interspinous ligament	**Use:** Head and Neck Bursa and Ligament Upper Spine Bursa and Ligament Lower Spine Bursa and Ligament
Intertransversarius muscle	**Use:** Trunk Muscle, Right Trunk Muscle, Left
Intertransverse ligament	**Use:** Upper Spine Bursa and Ligament Lower Spine Bursa and Ligament
Interventricular foramen (Monro)	**Use:** Cerebral Ventricle
Interventricular septum	**Use:** Ventricular Septum
Intestinal lymphatic trunk	**Use:** Cisterna Chyli
Ischiatic nerve	**Use:** Sciatic Nerve
Ischiocavernosus muscle	**Use:** Perineum Muscle
Ischiofemoral ligament	**Use:** Hip Bursa and Ligament, Right Hip Bursa and Ligament, Left
Ischium	**Use:** Pelvic Bone, Right Pelvic Bone, Left
Jejunal artery	**Use:** Superior Mesenteric Artery
Jugular body	**Use:** Glomus Jugulare
Jugular lymph node	**Use:** Lymphatic, Right Neck Lymphatic, Left Neck
Labia majora Labia minora	**Use:** Vulva
Labial gland	**Use:** Upper Lip Lower Lip

Lacrimal canaliculus Lacrimal punctum Lacrimal sac	**Use:** Lacrimal Duct, Right Lacrimal Duct, Left
Laryngopharynx	**Use:** Pharynx
Lateral (brachial) lymph node	**Use:** Lymphatic, Right Axillary Lymphatic, Left Axillary
Lateral canthus	**Use:** Upper Eyelid, Right Upper Eyelid, Left
Lateral collateral ligament (LCL)	**Use:** Knee Bursa and Ligament, Right Knee Bursa and Ligament, Left
Lateral condyle of femur	**Use:** Lower Femur, Right Lower Femur, Left
Lateral condyle of tibia	**Use:** Tibia, Right Tibia, Left
Lateral cuneiform bone	**Use:** Tarsal, Right Tarsal, Left
Lateral epicondyle of femur	**Use:** Lower Femur, Right Lower Femur, Left
Lateral epicondyle of humerus	**Use:** Humeral Shaft, Right Humeral Shaft, Left
Lateral femoral cutaneous nerve	**Use:** Lumbar Plexus
Lateral malleolus	**Use:** Fibula, Right Fibula, Left
Lateral meniscus	**Use:** Knee Joint, Right Knee Joint, Left
Lateral nasal cartilage	**Use:** Nasal Mucosa and Soft Tissue
Lateral plantar artery	**Use:** Foot Artery, Right Foot Artery, Left
Lateral plantar nerve	**Use:** Tibial Nerve
Lateral rectus muscle	**Use:** Extraocular Muscle, Right Extraocular Muscle, Left

BODY PART KEY

Lateral sacral artery	**Use:** Internal Iliac Artery, Right Internal Iliac Artery, Left
Lateral sacral vein	**Use:** Hypogastric Vein, Right Hypogastric Vein, Left
Lateral sural cutaneous nerve	**Use:** Peroneal Nerve
Lateral tarsal artery	**Use:** Foot Artery, Right Foot Artery, Left
Lateral temporomandibular ligament	**Use:** Head and Neck Bursa and Ligament
Lateral thoracic artery	**Use:** Axillary Artery, Right Axillary Artery, Left
Latissimus dorsi muscle	**Use:** Trunk Muscle, Right Trunk Muscle, Left
Least splanchnic nerve	**Use:** Thoracic Sympathetic Nerve
Left ascending lumbar vein	**Use:** Hemiazygos Vein
Left atrioventricular valve	**Use:** Mitral Valve
Left auricular appendix	**Use:** Atrium, Left
Left colic vein	**Use:** Colic Vein
Left coronary sulcus	**Use:** Heart, Left
Left gastric artery	**Use:** Gastric Artery
Left gastroepiploic artery	**Use:** Splenic Artery
Left gastroepiploic vein	**Use:** Splenic Vein
Left inferior phrenic vein	**Use:** Renal Vein, Left
Left inferior pulmonary vein	**Use:** Pulmonary Vein, Left
Left jugular trunk	**Use:** Thoracic Duct

Left lateral ventricle	**Use:** Cerebral Ventricle
Left ovarian vein Left second lumbar vein	**Use:** Renal Vein, Left
Left subclavian trunk	**Use:** Thoracic Duct
Left subcostal vein	**Use:** Hemiazygos Vein
Left superior pulmonary vein	**Use:** Pulmonary Vein, Left
Left suprarenal vein Left testicular vein	**Use:** Renal Vein, Left
Leptomeninges, intracranial	**Use:** Cerebral Meninges
Leptomeninges, spinal	**Use:** Spinal Meninges
Lesser alar cartilage	**Use:** Nasal Mucosa and Soft Tissue
Lesser occipital nerve	**Use:** Cervical Plexus
Lesser Omentum	**Use:** Omentum
Lesser saphenous vein	**Use:** Saphenous Vein, Right Saphenous Vein, Left
Lesser splanchnic nerve	**Use:** Thoracic Sympathetic Nerve
Lesser trochanter	**Use:** Upper Femur, Right Upper Femur, Left
Lesser tuberosity	**Use:** Humeral Head, Right Humeral Head, Left
Lesser wing	**Use:** Sphenoid Bone
Levator anguli oris muscle	**Use:** Facial Muscle
Levator ani muscle	**Use:** Perineum Muscle
Levator labii superioris alaeque nasi muscle Levator labii superioris muscle	**Use:** Facial Muscle

BODY PART KEY

Levator palpebrae superioris muscle	**Use:** Upper Eyelid, Right Upper Eyelid, Left
Levator scapulae muscle	**Use:** Neck Muscle, Right Neck Muscle, Left
Levator veli palatini muscle	**Use:** Tongue, Palate, Pharynx Muscle
Levatores costarum muscle	**Use:** Thorax Muscle, Right Thorax Muscle, Left
Ligament of head of fibula	**Use:** Knee Bursa and Ligament, Right Knee Bursa and Ligament, Left
Ligament of the lateral malleolus	**Use:** Ankle Bursa and Ligament, Right Ankle Bursa and Ligament, Left
Ligamentum flavum	**Use:** Upper Spine Bursa and Ligament Lower Spine Bursa and Ligament
Lingual artery	**Use:** External Carotid Artery, Right External Carotid Artery, Left
Lingual tonsil	**Use:** Pharynx
Locus ceruleus	**Use:** Pons
Long thoracic nerve	**Use:** Brachial Plexus
Lumbar artery	**Use:** Abdominal Aorta
Lumbar facet joint	**Use:** Lumbar Vertebral Joint Lumbar Vertebral Joints, 2 or more
Lumbar ganglion	**Use:** Lumbar Sympathetic Nerve
Lumbar lymph node	**Use:** Lymphatic, Aortic
Lumbar lymphatic trunk	**Use:** Cisterna Chyli
Lumbar splanchnic nerve	**Use:** Lumbar Sympathetic Nerve
Lumbosacral facet joint	**Use:** Lumbosacral Joint

Lumbosacral trunk	**Use:** Lumbar Nerve
Lunate bone	**Use:** Carpal, Right Carpal, Left
Lunotriquetral ligament	**Use:** Hand Bursa and Ligament, Right Hand Bursa and Ligament, Left
Macula	**Use:** Retina, Right Retina, Left
Malleus	**Use:** Auditory Ossicle, Right Auditory Ossicle, Left
Mammary duct Mammary gland	**Use:** Breast, Right Breast, Left Breast, Bilateral
Mammillary body	**Use:** Hypothalamus
Mandibular nerve	**Use:** Trigeminal Nerve
Mandibular notch	**Use:** Mandible, Right Mandible, Left
Manubrium	**Use:** Sternum
Masseter muscle	**Use:** Head Muscle
Masseteric fascia	**Use:** Subcutaneous Tissue and Fascia, Face
Mastoid (postauricular) lymph node	**Use:** Lymphatic, Right Neck Lymphatic, Left Neck
Mastoid air cells	**Use:** Mastoid Sinus, Right Mastoid Sinus, Left
Mastoid process	**Use:** Temporal Bone, Right Temporal Bone, Left
Maxillary artery	**Use:** External Carotid Artery, Right External Carotid Artery, Left
Maxillary nerve	**Use:** Trigeminal Nerve

BODY PART KEY

Medial canthus	**Use:** Lower Eyelid, Right Lower Eyelid, Left
Medial collateral ligament (MCL)	**Use:** Knee Bursa and Ligament, Right Knee Bursa and Ligament, Left
Medial condyle of femur	**Use:** Lower Femur, Right Lower Femur, Left
Medial condyle of tibia	**Use:** Tibia, Right Tibia, Left
Medial cuneiform bone	**Use:** Tarsal, Right Tarsal, Left
Medial epicondyle of femur	**Use:** Lower Femur, Right Lower Femur, Left
Medial epicondyle of humerus	**Use:** Humeral Shaft, Right Humeral Shaft, Left
Medial malleolus	**Use:** Tibia, Right Tibia, Left
Medial meniscus	**Use:** Knee Joint, Right Knee Joint, Left
Medial plantar artery	**Use:** Foot Artery, Right Foot Artery, Left
Medial plantar nerve Medial popliteal nerve	**Use:** Tibial Nerve
Medial rectus muscle	**Use:** Extraocular Muscle, Right Extraocular Muscle, Left
Medial sural cutaneous nerve	**Use:** Tibial Nerve
Median antebrachial vein Median cubital vein	**Use:** Basilic Vein, Right Basilic Vein, Left
Median sacral artery	**Use:** Abdominal Aorta
Mediastinal lymph node	**Use:** Lymphatic, Thorax
Meissner's (submucous) plexus	**Use:** Abdominal Sympathetic Nerve
Membranous urethra	**Use:** Urethra
Mental foramen	**Use:** Mandible, Right Mandible, Left
Mentalis muscle	**Use:** Facial Muscle
Mesoappendix Mesocolon	**Use:** Mesentery
Metacarpal ligament Metacarpophalangeal ligament	**Use:** Hand Bursa and Ligament, Right Hand Bursa and Ligament, Left
Metatarsal ligament	**Use:** Foot Bursa and Ligament, Right Foot Bursa and Ligament, Left
Metatarsophalangeal (MTP) joint	**Use:** Metatarsal-Phalangeal Joint, Right Metatarsal-Phalangeal Joint, Left
Metatarsophalangeal ligament	**Use:** Foot Bursa and Ligament, Right Foot Bursa and Ligament, Left
Metathalamus	**Use:** Thalamus
Midcarpal joint	**Use:** Carpal Joint, Right Carpal Joint, Left
Middle cardiac nerve	**Use:** Thoracic Sympathetic Nerve
Middle cerebral artery	**Use:** Intracranial Artery
Middle cerebral vein	**Use:** Intracranial Vein
Middle colic vein	**Use:** Colic Vein
Middle genicular artery	**Use:** Popliteal Artery, Right Popliteal Artery, Left
Middle hemorrhoidal vein	**Use:** Hypogastric Vein, Right Hypogastric Vein, Left
Middle rectal artery	**Use:** Internal Iliac Artery, Right Internal Iliac Artery, Left
Middle suprarenal artery	**Use:** Abdominal Aorta

BODY PART KEY

Middle temporal artery	**Use:** Temporal Artery, Right Temporal Artery, Left
Middle turbinate	**Use:** Nasal Turbinate
Mitral annulus	**Use:** Mitral Valve
Molar gland	**Use:** Buccal Mucosa
Musculocutaneous nerve	**Use:** Brachial Plexus
Musculophrenic artery	**Use:** Internal Mammary Artery, Right Internal Mammary Artery, Left
Musculospiral nerve	**Use:** Radial Nerve
Myelencephalon	**Use:** Medulla Oblongata
Myenteric (Auerbach's) plexus	**Use:** Abdominal Sympathetic Nerve
Myometrium	**Use:** Uterus
Nail bed Nail plate	**Use:** Finger Nail Toe Nail
Nasal cavity	**Use:** Nasal Mucosa and Soft Tissue
Nasal concha	**Use:** Nasal Turbinate
Nasalis muscle	**Use:** Facial Muscle
Nasolacrimal duct	**Use:** Lacrimal Duct, Right Lacrimal Duct, Left
Navicular bone	**Use:** Tarsal, Right Tarsal, Left
Neck of femur	**Use:** Upper Femur, Right Upper Femur, Left
Neck of humerus (anatomical) (surgical)	**Use:** Humeral Head, Right Humeral Head, Left
Nerve to the stapedius	**Use:** Facial Nerve

Neurohypophysis	**Use:** Pituitary Gland
Ninth cranial nerve	**Use:** Glossopharyngeal Nerve
Nostril	**Use:** Nasal Mucosa and Soft Tissue
Obturator artery	**Use:** Internal Iliac Artery, Right Internal Iliac Artery, Left
Obturator lymph node	**Use:** Lymphatic, Pelvis
Obturator muscle	**Use:** Hip Muscle, Right Hip Muscle, Left
Obturator nerve	**Use:** Lumbar Plexus
Obturator vein	**Use:** Hypogastric Vein, Right Hypogastric Vein, Left
Obtuse margin	**Use:** Heart, Left
Occipital artery	**Use:** External Carotid Artery, Right External Carotid Artery, Left
Occipital lobe	**Use:** Cerebral Hemisphere
Occipital lymph node	**Use:** Lymphatic, Right Neck Lymphatic, Left Neck
Occipitofrontalis muscle	**Use:** Facial Muscle
Odontoid process	**Use:** Cervical Vertebra
Olecranon bursa	**Use:** Elbow Bursa and Ligament, Right Elbow Bursa and Ligament, Left
Olecranon process	**Use:** Ulna, Right Ulna, Left
Olfactory bulb	**Use:** Olfactory Nerve
Ophthalmic artery	**Use:** Intracranial Artery
Ophthalmic nerve	**Use:** Trigeminal Nerve

BODY PART KEY

Ophthalmic vein	**Use:** Intracranial Vein
Optic chiasma	**Use:** Optic Nerve
Optic disc	**Use:** Retina, Right Retina, Left
Optic foramen	**Use:** Sphenoid Bone
Orbicularis oculi muscle	**Use:** Upper Eyelid, Right Upper Eyelid, Left
Orbicularis oris muscle	**Use:** Facial Muscle
Orbital fascia	**Use:** Subcutaneous Tissue and Fascia, Face
Orbital portion of ethmoid bone Orbital portion of frontal bone Orbital portion of lacrimal bone Orbital portion of maxilla Orbital portion of palatine bone Orbital portion of sphenoid bone Orbital portion of zygomatic bone	**Use:** Orbit, Right Orbit, Left
Oropharynx	**Use:** Pharynx
Otic ganglion	**Use:** Head and Neck Sympathetic Nerve
Oval window	**Use:** Middle Ear, Right Middle Ear, Left
Ovarian artery	**Use:** Abdominal Aorta
Ovarian ligament	**Use:** Uterine Supporting Structure
Oviduct	**Use:** Fallopian Tube, Right Fallopian Tube, Left
Palatine gland	**Use:** Buccal Mucosa
Palatine tonsil	**Use:** Tonsils
Palatine uvula	**Use:** Uvula
Palatoglossal muscle Palatopharyngeal muscle	**Use:** Tongue, Palate, Pharynx Muscle

Palmar (volar) digital vein Palmar (volar) metacarpal vein	**Use:** Hand Vein, Right Hand Vein, Left
Palmar cutaneous nerve	**Use:** Median Nerve Radial Nerve
Palmar fascia (aponeurosis)	**Use:** Subcutaneous Tissue and Fascia, Right Hand Subcutaneous Tissue and Fascia, Left Hand
Palmar interosseous muscle	**Use:** Hand Muscle, Right Hand Muscle, Left
Palmar ulnocarpal ligament	**Use:** Wrist Bursa and Ligament, Right Wrist Bursa and Ligament, Left
Palmaris longus muscle	**Use:** Lower Arm and Wrist Muscle, Right Lower Arm and Wrist Muscle, Left
Pancreatic artery	**Use:** Splenic Artery
Pancreatic plexus	**Use:** Abdominal Sympathetic Nerve
Pancreatic vein	**Use:** Splenic Vein
Pancreaticosplenic lymph node Paraaortic lymph node	**Use:** Lymphatic, Aortic
Pararectal lymph node	**Use:** Lymphatic, Mesenteric
Parasternal lymph node Paratracheal lymph node	**Use:** Lymphatic, Thorax
Paraurethral (Skene's) gland	**Use:** Vestibular Gland
Parietal lobe	**Use:** Cerebral Hemisphere
Parotid lymph node	**Use:** Lymphatic, Head
Parotid plexus	**Use:** Facial Nerve
Pars flaccida	**Use:** Tympanic Membrane, Right Tympanic Membrane, Left
Patellar ligament	**Use:** Knee Bursa and Ligament, Right Knee Bursa and Ligament, Left

BODY PART KEY

Patellar tendon	**Use:** Knee Tendon, Right Knee Tendon, Left
Pectineus muscle	**Use:** Upper Leg Muscle, Right Upper Leg Muscle, Left
Pectoral (anterior) lymph node	**Use:** Lymphatic, Right Axillary Lymphatic, Left Axillary
Pectoral fascia	**Use:** Subcutaneous Tissue and Fascia, Chest
Pectoralis major muscle Pectoralis minor muscle	**Use:** Thorax Muscle, Right Thorax Muscle, Left
Pelvic splanchnic nerve	**Use:** Abdominal Sympathetic Nerve Sacral Sympathetic Nerve
Penile urethra	**Use:** Urethra
Pericardiophrenic artery	**Use:** Internal Mammary Artery, Right Internal Mammary Artery, Left
Perimetrium	**Use:** Uterus
Peroneus brevis muscle Peroneus longus muscle	**Use:** Lower Leg Muscle, Right Lower Leg Muscle, Left
Petrous part of temporal bone	**Use:** Temporal Bone, Right Temporal Bone, Left
Pharyngeal constrictor muscle	**Use:** Tongue, Palate, Pharynx Muscle
Pharyngeal plexus	**Use:** Vagus Nerve
Pharyngeal recess	**Use:** Nasopharynx
Pharyngeal tonsil	**Use:** Adenoids
Pharyngotympanic tube	**Use:** Eustachian Tube, Right Eustachian Tube, Left
Pia mater, intracranial	**Use:** Cerebral Meninges
Pia mater, spinal	**Use:** Spinal Meninges

Pinna	**Use:** External Ear, Right External Ear, Left External Ear, Bilateral
Piriform recess (sinus)	**Use:** Pharynx
Piriformis muscle	**Use:** Hip Muscle, Right Hip Muscle, Left
Pisiform bone	**Use:** Carpal, Right Carpal, Left
Pisohamate ligament Pisometacarpal ligament	**Use:** Hand Bursa and Ligament, Right Hand Bursa and Ligament, Left
Plantar digital vein	**Use:** Foot Vein, Right Foot Vein, Left
Plantar fascia (aponeurosis)	**Use:** Subcutaneous Tissue and Fascia, Right Foot Subcutaneous Tissue and Fascia, Left Foot
Plantar metatarsal vein Plantar venous arch	**Use:** Foot Vein, Right Foot Vein, Left
Platysma muscle	**Use:** Neck Muscle, Right Neck Muscle, Left
Plica semilunaris	**Use:** Conjunctiva, Right Conjunctiva, Left
Pneumogastric nerve	**Use:** Vagus Nerve
Pneumotaxic center Pontine tegmentum	**Use:** Pons
Popliteal ligament	**Use:** Knee Bursa and Ligament, Right Knee Bursa and Ligament, Left
Popliteal lymph node	**Use:** Lymphatic, Right Lower Extremity Lymphatic, Left Lower Extremity
Popliteal vein	**Use:** Femoral Vein, Right Femoral Vein, Left
Popliteus muscle	**Use:** Lower Leg Muscle, Right Lower Leg Muscle, Left

BODY PART KEY

Postauricular (mastoid) lymph node	**Use:** Lymphatic, Right Neck Lymphatic, Left Neck
Postcava	**Use:** Inferior Vena Cava
Posterior (subscapular) lymph node	**Use:** Lymphatic, Right Axillary Lymphatic, Left Axillary
Posterior auricular artery	**Use:** External Carotid Artery, Right External Carotid Artery, Left
Posterior auricular nerve	**Use:** Facial Nerve
Posterior auricular vein	**Use:** External Jugular Vein, Right External Jugular Vein, Left
Posterior cerebral artery	**Use:** Intracranial Artery
Posterior chamber	**Use:** Eye, Right Eye, Left
Posterior circumflex humeral artery	**Use:** Axillary Artery, Right Axillary Artery, Left
Posterior communicating artery	**Use:** Intracranial Artery
Posterior cruciate ligament (PCL)	**Use:** Knee Bursa and Ligament, Right Knee Bursa and Ligament, Left
Posterior facial (retromandibular) vein	**Use:** Face Vein, Right Face Vein, Left
Posterior femoral cutaneous nerve	**Use:** Sacral Plexus
Posterior inferior cerebellar artery (PICA)	**Use:** Intracranial Artery
Posterior interosseous nerve	**Use:** Radial Nerve
Posterior labial nerve Posterior scrotal nerve	**Use:** Pudendal Nerve
Posterior spinal artery	**Use:** Vertebral Artery, Right Vertebral Artery, Left
Posterior tibial recurrent artery	**Use:** Anterior Tibial Artery, Right Anterior Tibial Artery, Left

Posterior ulnar recurrent artery	**Use:** Ulnar Artery, Right Ulnar Artery, Left
Posterior vagal trunk	**Use:** Vagus Nerve
Preauricular lymph node	**Use:** Lymphatic, Head
Precava	**Use:** Superior Vena Cava
Prepatellar bursa	**Use:** Knee Bursa and Ligament, Right Knee Bursa and Ligament, Left
Pretracheal fascia Prevertebral fascia	**Use:** Subcutaneous Tissue and Fascia, Right Neck Subcutaneous Tissue and Fascia, Left Neck
Princeps pollicis artery	**Use:** Hand Artery, Right Hand Artery, Left
Procerus muscle	**Use:** Facial Muscle
Profunda brachii	**Use:** Brachial Artery, Right Brachial Artery, Left
Profunda femoris (deep femoral) vein	**Use:** Femoral Vein, Right Femoral Vein, Left
Pronator quadratus muscle Pronator teres muscle	**Use:** Lower Arm and Wrist Muscle, Right Lower Arm and Wrist Muscle, Left
Prostatic urethra	**Use:** Urethra
Proximal radioulnar joint	**Use:** Elbow Joint, Right Elbow Joint, Left
Psoas muscle	**Use:** Hip Muscle, Right Hip Muscle, Left
Pterygoid muscle	**Use:** Head Muscle
Pterygoid process	**Use:** Sphenoid Bone
Pterygopalatine (sphenopalatine) ganglion	**Use:** Head and Neck Sympathetic Nerve

APPENDIX B

BODY PART KEY

Pubis	**Use:** Pelvic Bone, Right Pelvic Bone, Left
Pubofemoral ligament	**Use:** Hip Bursa and Ligament, Right Hip Bursa and Ligament, Left
Pudendal nerve	**Use:** Sacral Plexus
Pulmoaortic canal	**Use:** Pulmonary Artery, Left
Pulmonary annulus	**Use:** Pulmonary Valve
Pulmonary plexus	**Use:** Vagus Nerve Thoracic Sympathetic Nerve
Pulmonic valve	**Use:** Pulmonary Valve
Pulvinar	**Use:** Thalamus
Pyloric antrum Pyloric canal Pyloric sphincter	**Use:** Stomach, Pylorus
Pyramidalis muscle	**Use:** Abdomen Muscle, Right Abdomen Muscle, Left
Quadrangular cartilage	**Use:** Nasal Septum
Quadrate lobe	**Use:** Liver
Quadratus femoris muscle	**Use:** Hip Muscle, Right Hip Muscle, Left
Quadratus lumborum muscle	**Use:** Trunk Muscle, Right Trunk Muscle, Left
Quadratus plantae muscle	**Use:** Foot Muscle, Right Foot Muscle, Left
Quadriceps (femoris)	**Use:** Upper Leg Muscle, Right Upper Leg Muscle, Left
Radial collateral carpal ligament	**Use:** Wrist Bursa and Ligament, Right Wrist Bursa and Ligament, Left
Radial collateral ligament	**Use:** Elbow Bursa and Ligament, Right Elbow Bursa and Ligament, Left

Radial notch	**Use:** Ulna, Right Ulna, Left
Radial recurrent artery	**Use:** Radial Artery, Right Radial Artery, Left
Radial vein	**Use:** Brachial Vein, Right Brachial Vein, Left
Radialis indicis	**Use:** Hand Artery, Right Hand Artery, Left
Radiocarpal joint	**Use:** Wrist Joint, Right Wrist Joint, Left
Radiocarpal ligament Radioulnar ligament	**Use:** Wrist Bursa and Ligament, Right Wrist Bursa and Ligament, Left
Rectosigmoid junction	**Use:** Sigmoid Colon
Rectus abdominis muscle	**Use:** Abdomen Muscle, Right Abdomen Muscle, Left
Rectus femoris muscle	**Use:** Upper Leg Muscle, Right Upper Leg Muscle, Left
Recurrent laryngeal nerve	**Use:** Vagus Nerve
Renal calyx Renal capsule Renal cortex	**Use:** Kidney, Right Kidney, Left Kidneys, Bilateral Kidney
Renal plexus	**Use:** Abdominal Sympathetic Nerve
Renal segment	**Use:** Kidney, Right Kidney, Left Kidneys, Bilateral Kidney
Renal segmental artery	**Use:** Renal Artery, Right Renal Artery, Left
Retroperitoneal lymph node	**Use:** Lymphatic, Aortic
Retroperitoneal space	**Use:** Retroperitoneum

BODY PART KEY

Retropharyngeal lymph node	**Use:** Lymphatic, Right Neck Lymphatic, Left Neck
Retropubic space	**Use:** Pelvic Cavity
Rhinopharynx	**Use:** Nasopharynx
Rhomboid major muscle Rhomboid minor muscle	**Use:** Trunk Muscle, Right Trunk Muscle, Left
Right ascending lumbar vein	**Use:** Azygos Vein
Right atrioventricular valve	**Use:** Tricuspid Valve
Right auricular appendix	**Use:** Atrium, Right
Right colic vein	**Use:** Colic Vein
Right coronary sulcus	**Use:** Heart, Right
Right gastric artery	**Use:** Gastric Artery
Right gastroepiploic vein	**Use:** Superior Mesenteric Vein
Right inferior phrenic vein	**Use:** Inferior Vena Cava
Right inferior pulmonary vein	**Use:** Pulmonary Vein, Right
Right jugular trunk	**Use:** Lymphatic, Right Neck
Right lateral ventricle	**Use:** Cerebral Ventricle
Right lymphatic duct	**Use:** Lymphatic, Right Neck
Right ovarian vein Right second lumbar vein	**Use:** Inferior Vena Cava
Right subclavian trunk	**Use:** Lymphatic, Right Neck
Right subcostal vein	**Use:** Azygos Vein
Right superior pulmonary vein	**Use:** Pulmonary Vein, Right
Right suprarenal vein Right testicular vein	**Use:** Inferior Vena Cava

Rima glottidis	**Use:** Larynx
Risorius muscle	**Use:** Facial Muscle
Round ligament of uterus	**Use:** Uterine Supporting Structure
Round window	**Use:** Inner Ear, Right Inner Ear, Left
Sacral ganglion	**Use:** Sacral Sympathetic Nerve
Sacral lymph node	**Use:** Lymphatic, Pelvis
Sacral splanchnic nerve	**Use:** Sacral Sympathetic Nerve
Sacrococcygeal ligament	**Use:** Lower Spine Bursa and Ligament
Sacrococcygeal symphysis	**Use:** Sacrococcygeal Joint
Sacroiliac ligament Sacrospinous ligament Sacrotuberous ligament	**Use:** Lower Spine Bursa and Ligament
Salpingopharyngeus muscle	**Use:** Tongue, Palate, Pharynx Muscle
Salpinx	**Use:** Fallopian Tube, Right Fallopian Tube, Left
Saphenous nerve	**Use:** Femoral Nerve
Sartorius muscle	**Use:** Upper Leg Muscle, Right Upper Leg Muscle, Left
Scalene muscle	**Use:** Neck Muscle, Right Neck Muscle, Left
Scaphoid bone	**Use:** Carpal, Right Carpal, Left
Scapholunate ligament Scaphotrapezium ligament	**Use:** Hand Bursa and Ligament, Right Hand Bursa and Ligament, Left
Scarpa's (vestibular) ganglion	**Use:** Acoustic Nerve
Sebaceous gland	**Use:** Skin

BODY PART KEY

Second cranial nerve	**Use:** Optic Nerve
Sella turcica	**Use:** Sphenoid Bone
Semicircular canal	**Use:** Inner Ear, Right Inner Ear, Left
Semimembranosus muscle Semitendinosus muscle	**Use:** Upper Leg Muscle, Right Upper Leg Muscle, Left
Septal cartilage	**Use:** Nasal Septum
Serratus anterior muscle	**Use:** Thorax Muscle, Right Thorax Muscle, Left
Serratus posterior muscle	**Use:** Trunk Muscle, Right Trunk Muscle, Left
Seventh cranial nerve	**Use:** Facial Nerve
Short gastric artery	**Use:** Splenic Artery
Sigmoid artery	**Use:** Inferior Mesenteric Artery
Sigmoid flexure	**Use:** Sigmoid Colon
Sigmoid vein	**Use:** Inferior Mesenteric Vein
Sinoatrial node	**Use:** Conduction Mechanism
Sinus venosus	**Use:** Atrium, Right
Sixth cranial nerve	**Use:** Abducens Nerve
Skene's (paraurethral) gland	**Use:** Vestibular Gland
Small saphenous vein	**Use:** Saphenous Vein, Right Saphenous Vein, Left
Solar (celiac) plexus	**Use:** Abdominal Sympathetic Nerve
Soleus muscle	**Use:** Lower Leg Muscle, Right Lower Leg Muscle, Left

Sphenomandibular ligament	**Use:** Head and Neck Bursa and Ligament
Sphenopalatine (pterygopalatine) ganglion	**Use:** Head and Neck Sympathetic Nerve
Spinal nerve, cervical	**Use:** Cervical Nerve
Spinal nerve, lumbar	**Use:** Lumbar Nerve
Spinal nerve, sacral	**Use:** Sacral Nerve
Spinal nerve, thoracic	**Use:** Thoracic Nerve
Spinous process	**Use:** Cervical Vertebra Thoracic Vertebra Lumbar Vertebra
Spiral ganglion	**Use:** Acoustic Nerve
Splenic flexure	**Use:** Transverse Colon
Splenic plexus	**Use:** Abdominal Sympathetic Nerve
Splenius capitis muscle	**Use:** Head Muscle
Splenius cervicis muscle	**Use:** Neck Muscle, Right Neck Muscle, Left
Stapes	**Use:** Auditory Ossicle, Right Auditory Ossicle, Left
Stellate ganglion	**Use:** Head and Neck Sympathetic Nerve
Stensen's duct	**Use:** Parotid Duct, Right Parotid Duct, Left
Sternoclavicular ligament	**Use:** Shoulder Bursa and Ligament, Right Shoulder Bursa and Ligament, Left
Sternocleidomastoid artery	**Use:** Thyroid Artery, Right Thyroid Artery, Left

BODY PART KEY

Sternocleidomastoid muscle	**Use:** Neck Muscle, Right Neck Muscle, Left
Sternocostal ligament	**Use:** Sternum Bursa and Ligament Rib(s) Bursa and Ligament
Styloglossus muscle	**Use:** Tongue, Palate, Pharynx Muscle
Stylomandibular ligament	**Use:** Head and Neck Bursa and Ligament
Stylopharyngeus muscle	**Use:** Tongue, Palate, Pharynx Muscle
Subacromial bursa	**Use:** Shoulder Bursa and Ligament, Right Shoulder Bursa and Ligament, Left
Subaortic (common iliac) lymph node	**Use:** Lymphatic, Pelvis
Subarachnoid space, spinal	**Use:** Spinal Canal
Subclavicular (apical) lymph node	**Use:** Lymphatic, Right Axillary Lymphatic, Left Axillary
Subclavius muscle	**Use:** Thorax Muscle, Right Thorax Muscle, Left
Subclavius nerve	**Use:** Brachial Plexus
Subcostal artery	**Use:** Upper Artery
Subcostal muscle	**Use:** Thorax Muscle, Right Thorax Muscle, Left
Subcostal nerve	**Use:** Thoracic Nerve
Subdural space, spinal	**Use:** Spinal Canal
Submandibular ganglion	**Use:** Facial Nerve Head and Neck Sympathetic Nerve
Submandibular gland	**Use:** Submaxillary Gland, Right Submaxillary Gland, Left
Submandibular lymph node	**Use:** Lymphatic, Head
Submaxillary ganglion	**Use:** Head and Neck Sympathetic Nerve
Submaxillary lymph node	**Use:** Lymphatic, Head
Submental artery	**Use:** Face Artery
Submental lymph node	**Use:** Lymphatic, Head
Submucous (Meissner's) plexus	**Use:** Abdominal Sympathetic Nerve
Suboccipital nerve	**Use:** Cervical Nerve
Suboccipital venous plexus	**Use:** Vertebral Vein, Right Vertebral Vein, Left
Subparotid lymph node	**Use:** Lymphatic, Head
Subscapular (posterior) lymph node	**Use:** Lymphatic, Right Axillary Lymphatic, Left Axillary
Subscapular aponeurosis	**Use:** Subcutaneous Tissue and Fascia, Right Upper Arm Subcutaneous Tissue and Fascia, Left Upper Arm
Subscapular artery	**Use:** Axillary Artery, Right Axillary Artery, Left
Subscapularis muscle	**Use:** Shoulder Muscle, Right Shoulder Muscle, Left
Substantia nigra	**Use:** Basal Ganglia
Subtalar (talocalcaneal) joint	**Use:** Tarsal Joint, Right Tarsal Joint, Left
Subtalar ligament	**Use:** Foot Bursa and Ligament, Right Foot Bursa and Ligament, Left
Subthalamic nucleus	**Use:** Basal Ganglia
Superficial circumflex iliac vein	**Use:** Saphenous Vein, Right Saphenous Vein, Left

BODY PART KEY

Superficial epigastric artery	**Use:** Femoral Artery, Right Femoral Artery, Left
Superficial epigastric vein	**Use:** Saphenous Vein, Right Saphenous Vein, Left
Superficial palmar arch	**Use:** Hand Artery, Right Hand Artery, Left
Superficial palmar venous arch	**Use:** Hand Vein, Right Hand Vein, Left
Superficial temporal artery	**Use:** Temporal Artery, Right Temporal Artery, Left
Superficial transverse perineal muscle	**Use:** Perineum Muscle
Superior cardiac nerve	**Use:** Thoracic Sympathetic Nerve
Superior cerebellar vein Superior cerebral vein	**Use:** Intracranial Vein
Superior clunic (cluneal) nerve	**Use:** Lumbar Nerve
Superior epigastric artery	**Use:** Internal Mammary Artery, Right Internal Mammary Artery, Left
Superior genicular artery	**Use:** Popliteal Artery, Right Popliteal Artery, Left
Superior gluteal artery	**Use:** Internal Iliac Artery, Right Internal Iliac Artery, Left
Superior gluteal nerve	**Use:** Lumbar Plexus
Superior hypogastric plexus	**Use:** Abdominal Sympathetic Nerve
Superior labial artery	**Use:** Face Artery
Superior laryngeal artery	**Use:** Thyroid Artery, Right Thyroid Artery, Left
Superior laryngeal nerve	**Use:** Vagus Nerve
Superior longitudinal muscle	**Use:** Tongue, Palate, Pharynx Muscle

Superior mesenteric ganglion	**Use:** Abdominal Sympathetic Nerve
Superior mesenteric lymph node	**Use:** Lymphatic, Mesenteric
Superior mesenteric plexus	**Use:** Abdominal Sympathetic Nerve
Superior oblique muscle	**Use:** Extraocular Muscle, Right Extraocular Muscle, Left
Superior olivary nucleus	**Use:** Pons
Superior rectal artery	**Use:** Inferior Mesenteric Artery
Superior rectal vein	**Use:** Inferior Mesenteric Vein
Superior rectus muscle	**Use:** Extraocular Muscle, Right Extraocular Muscle, Left
Superior tarsal plate	**Use:** Upper Eyelid, Right Upper Eyelid, Left
Superior thoracic artery	**Use:** Axillary Artery, Right Axillary Artery, Left
Superior thyroid artery	**Use:** External Carotid Artery, Right External Carotid Artery, Left Thyroid Artery, Right Thyroid Artery, Left
Superior turbinate	**Use:** Nasal Turbinate
Superior ulnar collateral artery	**Use:** Brachial Artery, Right Brachial Artery, Left
Supraclavicular (Virchow's) lymph node	**Use:** Lymphatic, Right Neck Lymphatic, Left Neck
Supraclavicular nerve	**Use:** Cervical Plexus
Suprahyoid lymph node	**Use:** Lymphatic, Head
Suprahyoid muscle	**Use:** Neck Muscle, Right Neck Muscle, Left

BODY PART KEY

Suprainguinal lymph node	**Use:** Lymphatic, Pelvis
Supraorbital vein	**Use:** Face Vein, Right Face Vein, Left
Suprarenal gland	**Use:** Adrenal Gland, Left Adrenal Gland, Right Adrenal Glands, Bilateral Adrenal Gland
Suprarenal plexus	**Use:** Abdominal Sympathetic Nerve
Suprascapular nerve	**Use:** Brachial Plexus
Supraspinatus fascia	**Use:** Subcutaneous Tissue and Fascia, Right Upper Arm Subcutaneous Tissue and Fascia, Left Upper Arm
Supraspinatus muscle	**Use:** Shoulder Muscle, Right Shoulder Muscle, Left
Supraspinous ligament	**Use:** Upper Spine Bursa and Ligament Lower Spine Bursa and Ligament
Suprasternal notch	**Use:** Sternum
Supratrochlear lymph node	**Use:** Lymphatic, Right Upper Extremity Lymphatic, Left Upper Extremity
Sural artery	**Use:** Popliteal Artery, Right Popliteal Artery, Left
Sweat gland	**Use:** Skin
Talocalcaneal (subtalar) joint	**Use:** Tarsal Joint, Right Tarsal Joint, Left
Talocalcaneal ligament	**Use:** Foot Bursa and Ligament, Right Foot Bursa and Ligament, Left
Talocalcaneonavicular joint	**Use:** Tarsal Joint, Right Tarsal Joint, Left
Talocalcaneonavicular ligament	**Use:** Foot Bursa and Ligament, Right Foot Bursa and Ligament, Left

Talocrural joint	**Use:** Ankle Joint, Right Ankle Joint, Left
Talofibular ligament	**Use:** Ankle Bursa and Ligament, Right Ankle Bursa and Ligament, Left
Talus bone	**Use:** Tarsal, Right Tarsal, Left
Tarsometatarsal ligament	**Use:** Foot Bursa and Ligament, Right Foot Bursa and Ligament, Left
Temporal lobe	**Use:** Cerebral Hemisphere
Temporalis muscle Temporoparietalis muscle	**Use:** Head Muscle
Tensor fasciae latae muscle	**Use:** Hip Muscle, Right Hip Muscle, Left
Tensor veli palatini muscle	**Use:** Tongue, Palate, Pharynx Muscle
Tenth cranial nerve	**Use:** Vagus Nerve
Tentorium cerebelli	**Use:** Dura Mater
Teres major muscle Teres minor muscle	**Use:** Shoulder Muscle, Right Shoulder Muscle, Left
Testicular artery	**Use:** Abdominal Aorta
Thenar muscle	**Use:** Hand Muscle, Right Hand Muscle, Left
Third cranial nerve	**Use:** Oculomotor Nerve
Third occipital nerve	**Use:** Cervical Nerve
Third ventricle	**Use:** Cerebral Ventricle
Thoracic aortic plexus	**Use:** Thoracic Sympathetic Nerve
Thoracic esophagus	**Use:** Esophagus, Middle

BODY PART KEY

Thoracic facet joint	**Use:** Thoracic Vertebral Joint Thoracic Vertebral Joints, 2 to 7 Thoracic Vertebral Joints, 8 or more
Thoracic ganglion	**Use:** Thoracic Sympathetic Nerve
Thoracoacromial artery	**Use:** Axillary Artery, Right Axillary Artery, Left
Thoracolumbar facet joint	**Use:** Thoracolumbar Vertebral Joint
Thymus gland	**Use:** Thymus
Thyroarytenoid muscle	**Use:** Neck Muscle, Right Neck Muscle, Left
Thyrocervical trunk	**Use:** Thyroid Artery, Right Thyroid Artery, Left
Thyroid cartilage	**Use:** Larynx
Tibialis anterior muscle Tibialis posterior muscle	**Use:** Lower Leg Muscle, Right Lower Leg Muscle, Left
Tibiofemoral joint	**Use:** Knee Joint, Right Knee Joint, Left Knee Joint, Tibial Surface, Right Knee Joint, Tibial Surface, Left
Tongue, base of	**Use:** Pharynx
Tracheobronchial lymph node	**Use:** Lymphatic, Thorax
Tragus	**Use:** External Ear, Right External Ear, Left External Ear, Bilateral
Transversalis fascia	**Use:** Subcutaneous Tissue and Fascia, Trunk
Transverse (cutaneous) cervical nerve	**Use:** Cervical Plexus
Transverse acetabular ligament	**Use:** Hip Bursa and Ligament, Right Hip Bursa and Ligament, Left
Transverse facial artery	**Use:** Temporal Artery, Right Temporal Artery, Left
Transverse foramen	**Use:** Cervical Vertebra
Transverse humeral ligament	**Use:** Shoulder Bursa and Ligament, Right Shoulder Bursa and Ligament, Left
Transverse ligament of atlas	**Use:** Head and Neck Bursa and Ligament
Transverse process	**Use:** Cervical Vertebra Thoracic Vertebra Lumbar Vertebra
Transverse scapular ligament	**Use:** Shoulder Bursa and Ligament, Right Shoulder Bursa and Ligament, Left
Transverse thoracis muscle	**Use:** Thorax Muscle, Right Thorax Muscle, Left
Transversospinalis muscle	**Use:** Trunk Muscle, Right Trunk Muscle, Left
Transversus abdominis muscle	**Use:** Abdomen Muscle, Right Abdomen Muscle, Left
Trapezium bone	**Use:** Carpal, Right Carpal, Left
Trapezius muscle	**Use:** Trunk Muscle, Right Trunk Muscle, Left
Trapezoid bone	**Use:** Carpal, Right Carpal, Left
Triceps brachii muscle	**Use:** Upper Arm Muscle, Right Upper Arm Muscle, Left
Tricuspid annulus	**Use:** Tricuspid Valve
Trifacial nerve	**Use:** Trigeminal Nerve
Trigone of bladder	**Use:** Bladder

BODY PART KEY

BODY PART KEY

Triquetral bone	**Use:** Carpal, Right Carpal, Left
Trochanteric bursa	**Use:** Hip Bursa and Ligament, Right Hip Bursa and Ligament, Left
Twelfth cranial nerve	**Use:** Hypoglossal Nerve
Tympanic cavity	**Use:** Middle Ear, Right Middle Ear, Left
Tympanic nerve	**Use:** Glossopharyngeal Nerve
Tympanic part of temporal bone	**Use:** Temporal Bone, Right Temporal Bone, Left
Ulnar collateral carpal ligament	**Use:** Wrist Bursa and Ligament, Right Wrist Bursa and Ligament, Left
Ulnar collateral ligament	**Use:** Elbow Bursa and Ligament, Right Elbow Bursa and Ligament, Left
Ulnar notch	**Use:** Radius, Right Radius, Left
Ulnar vein	**Use:** Brachial Vein, Right Brachial Vein, Left
Umbilical artery	**Use:** Internal Iliac Artery, Right Internal Iliac Artery, Left Lower Artery
Ureteral orifice	**Use:** Ureter, Right Ureter, Left Ureters, Bilateral Ureter
Ureteropelvic junction (UPJ)	**Use:** Kidney Pelvis, Right Kidney Pelvis, Left
Ureterovesical orifice	**Use:** Ureter, Right Ureter, Left Ureters, Bilateral Ureter

Uterine artery	**Use:** Internal Iliac Artery, Right Internal Iliac Artery, Left
Uterine cornu	**Use:** Uterus
Uterine tube	**Use:** Fallopian Tube, Right Fallopian Tube, Left
Uterine vein	**Use:** Hypogastric Vein, Right Hypogastric Vein, Left
Vaginal artery	**Use:** Internal Iliac Artery, Right Internal Iliac Artery, Left
Vaginal vein	**Use:** Hypogastric Vein, Right Hypogastric Vein, Left
Vastus intermedius muscle Vastus lateralis muscle Vastus medialis muscle	**Use:** Upper Leg Muscle, Right Upper Leg Muscle, Left
Ventricular fold	**Use:** Larynx
Vermiform appendix	**Use:** Appendix
Vermilion border	**Use:** Upper Lip Lower Lip
Vertebral arch Vertebral body	**Use:** Cervical Vertebra Thoracic Vertebra Lumbar Vertebra
Vertebral canal	**Use:** Spinal Canal
Vertebral foramen Vertebral lamina Vertebral pedicle	**Use:** Cervical Vertebra Thoracic Vertebra Lumbar Vertebra
Vesical vein	**Use:** Hypogastric Vein, Right Hypogastric Vein, Left
Vestibular (Scarpa's) ganglion Vestibular nerve Vestibulocochlear nerve	**Use:** Acoustic Nerve
Virchow's (supraclavicular) lymph node	**Use:** Lymphatic, Right Neck Lymphatic, Left Neck

BODY PART KEY

Vitreous body	**Use:** Vitreous, Right Vitreous, Left
Vocal fold	**Use:** Vocal Cord, Right Vocal Cord, Left
Volar (palmar) digital vein Volar (palmar) metacarpal vein	**Use:** Hand Vein, Right Hand Vein, Left
Vomer bone	**Use:** Nasal Septum
Vomer of nasal septum	**Use:** Nasal Bone

Xiphoid process	**Use:** Sternum
Zonule of Zinn	**Use:** Lens, Right Lens, Left
Zygomatic process of frontal bone	**Use:** Frontal Bone
Zygomatic process of temporal bone	**Use:** Temporal Bone, Right Temporal Bone, Left
Zygomaticus muscle	**Use:** Facial Muscle

DEVICE KEY

3f (Aortic) Bioprosthesis valve	**Use:** Zooplastic Tissue in Heart and Great Vessels	Artificial bowel sphincter (neosphincter)	**Use:** Artificial Sphincter in Gastrointestinal System
AbioCor® Total Replacement Heart	**Use:** Synthetic Substitute	Artificial urinary sphincter (AUS)	**Use:** Artificial Sphincter in Urinary System
Acellular Hydrated Dermis	**Use:** Nonautologous Tissue Substitute	Assurant (Cobalt) stent	**Use:** Intraluminal Device
Acetabular cup	**Use:** Liner in Lower Joints	AtriClip LAA Exclusion System	**Use:** Extraluminal Device
Activa PC neurostimulator	**Use:** Stimulator Generator, Multiple Array for Insertion in Subcutaneous Tissue and Fascia	Attain Ability® lead	**Use:** Cardiac Lead, Pacemaker for Insertion in Heart and Great Vessels Cardiac Lead, Defibrillator for Insertion in Heart and Great Vessels
Activa RC neurostimulator	**Use:** Stimulator Generator, Multiple Array Rechargeable for Insertion in Subcutaneous Tissue and Fascia	Attain StarFix® (OTW) lead	**Use:** Cardiac Lead, Pacemaker for Insertion in Heart and Great Vessels Cardiac Lead, Defibrillator for Insertion in Heart and Great Vessels
Activa SC neurostimulator	**Use:** Stimulator Generator, Single Array for Insertion in Subcutaneous Tissue and Fascia		
ACUITY™ Steerable Lead	**Use:** Cardiac Lead, Pacemaker for Insertion in Heart and Great Vessels Cardiac Lead, Defibrillator for Insertion in Heart and Great Vessels	Autograft	**Use:** Autologous Tissue Substitute
		Autologous artery graft	**Use:** Autologous Arterial Tissue in Heart and Great Vessels Autologous Arterial Tissue in Upper Arteries Autologous Arterial Tissue in Lower Arteries Autologous Arterial Tissue in Upper Veins Autologous Arterial Tissue in Lower Veins
Advisa (MRI)	**Use:** Pacemaker, Dual Chamber for Insertion in Subcutaneous Tissue and Fascia		
AFX® Endovascular AAA System	**Use:** Intraluminal Device		
AMPLATZER® Muscular VSD Occluder	**Use:** Synthetic Substitute	Autologous vein graft	**Use:** Autologous Venous Tissue in Heart and Great Vessels Autologous Venous Tissue in Upper Arteries Autologous Venous Tissue in Lower Arteries Autologous Venous Tissue in Upper Veins Autologous Venous Tissue in Lower Veins
AMS 800® Urinary Control System	**Use:** Artificial Sphincter in Urinary System		
AneuRx® AAA Advantage®	**Use:** Intraluminal Device		
Annuloplasty ring	**Use:** Synthetic Substitute		
Artificial anal sphincter (AAS)	**Use:** Artificial Sphincter in Gastrointestinal System	Axial Lumbar Interbody Fusion System	**Use:** Interbody Fusion Device in Lower Joints

DEVICE KEY

AxiaLIF® System	**Use:** Interbody Fusion Device in Lower Joints
BAK/C® Interbody Cervical Fusion System	**Use:** Interbody Fusion Device in Upper Joints
Bard® Composix® (E/X) (LP) mesh	**Use:** Synthetic Substitute
Bard® Composix® Kugel® patch	**Use:** Synthetic Substitute
Bard® Dulex™ mesh	**Use:** Synthetic Substitute
Bard® Ventralex™ hernia patch	**Use:** Synthetic Substitute
Baroreflex Activation Therapy® (BAT®)	**Use:** Stimulator Lead in Upper Arteries Cardiac Rhythm Related Device in Subcutaneous Tissue and Fascia
Berlin Heart Ventricular Assist Device	**Use:** Implantable Heart Assist System in Heart and Great Vessels
Bioactive embolization coil(s)	**Use:** Intraluminal Device, Bioactive in Upper Arteries
Biventricular external heart assist system	**Use:** Short-term External Heart Assist System in Heart and Great Vessels
Blood glucose monitoring system	**Use:** Monitoring Device
Bone anchored hearing device	**Use:** Hearing Device, Bone Conduction for Insertion in Ear, Nose, Sinus Hearing Device in Head and Facial Bones
Bone bank bone graft	**Use:** Nonautologous Tissue Substitute
Bone screw (interlocking) (lag) (pedicle) (recessed)	**Use:** Internal Fixation Device in Head and Facial Bones Internal Fixation Device in Upper Bones Internal Fixation Device in Lower Bones
Bovine pericardial valve	**Use:** Zooplastic Tissue in Heart and Great Vessels
Bovine pericardium graft	**Use:** Zooplastic Tissue in Heart and Great Vessels
Brachytherapy seeds	**Use:** Radioactive Element
BRYAN® Cervical Disc System	**Use:** Synthetic Substitute
BVS 5000 Ventricular Assist Device	**Use:** Short-term External Heart Assist System in Heart and Great Vessels
Cardiac contractility modulation lead	**Use:** Cardiac Lead in Heart and Great Vessels
Cardiac event recorder	**Use:** Monitoring Device
Cardiac resynchronization therapy (CRT) lead	**Use:** Cardiac Lead, Pacemaker for Insertion in Heart and Great Vessels Cardiac Lead, Defibrillator for Insertion in Heart and Great Vessels
CardioMEMS® pressure sensor	**Use:** Monitoring Device, Pressure Sensor for Insertion in Heart and Great Vessels
Carotid (artery) sinus (baroreceptor) lead	**Use:** Stimulator Lead in Upper Arteries
Carotid WALLSTENT® Monorail® Endoprosthesis	**Use:** Intraluminal Device
Centrimag® Blood Pump	**Use:** Short-term External Heart Assist System in Heart and Great Vessels
Ceramic on ceramic bearing surface	**Use:** Synthetic Substitute, Ceramic for Replacement in Lower Joints
Cesium-131 Collagen Implant	**Use:** Radioactive Element, Cesium-131 Collagen Implant for Insertion in Central Nervous System and Cranial Nerves
Clamp and rod internal fixation system (CRIF)	**Use:** Internal Fixation Device in Upper Bones Internal Fixation Device in Lower Bones

DEVICE KEY

COALESCE® radiolucent interbody fusion device	**Use:** Interbody Fusion Device, Radiolucent Porous in New Technology
CoAxia NeuroFlo catheter	**Use:** Intraluminal Device
Cobalt/chromium head and polyethylene socket	**Use:** Synthetic Substitute, Metal on Polyethylene for Replacement in Lower Joints
Cobalt/chromium head and socket	**Use:** Synthetic Substitute, Metal for Replacement in Lower Joints
Cochlear implant (CI), multiple channel (electrode)	**Use:** Hearing Device, Multiple Channel Cochlear Prosthesis for Insertion in Ear, Nose, Sinus
Cochlear implant (CI), single channel (electrode)	**Use:** Hearing Device, Single Channel Cochlear Prosthesis for Insertion in Ear, Nose, Sinus
COGNIS® CRT-D	**Use:** Cardiac Resynchronization Defibrillator Pulse Generator for Insertion in Subcutaneous Tissue and Fascia
COHERE® radiolucent interbody fusion device	**Use:** Interbody Fusion Device, Radiolucent Porous in New Technology
Colonic Z-Stent®	**Use:** Intraluminal Device
Complete (SE) stent	**Use:** Intraluminal Device
Concerto II CRT-D	**Use:** Cardiac Resynchronization Defibrillator Pulse Generator for Insertion in Subcutaneous Tissue and Fascia
CONSERVE® PLUS Total Resurfacing Hip System	**Use:** Resurfacing Device in Lower Joints
Consulta CRT-D	**Use:** Cardiac Resynchronization Defibrillator Pulse Generator for Insertion in Subcutaneous Tissue and Fascia
Consulta CRT-P	**Use:** Cardiac Resynchronization Pacemaker Pulse Generator for Insertion in Subcutaneous Tissue and Fascia
CONTAK RENEWAL® 3 RF (HE) CRT-D	**Use:** Cardiac Resynchronization Defibrillator Pulse Generator for Insertion in Subcutaneous Tissue and Fascia
Contegra Pulmonary Valved Conduit	**Use:** Zooplastic Tissue in Heart and Great Vessels
Continuous Glucose Monitoring (CGM) device	**Use:** Monitoring Device
Cook Biodesign® Fistula Plug(s)	**Use:** Nonautologous Tissue Substitute
Cook Biodesign® Hernia Graft(s)	**Use:** Nonautologous Tissue Substitute
Cook Biodesign® Layered Graft(s)	**Use:** Nonautologous Tissue Substitute
Cook Zenapro™ Layered Graft(s)	**Use:** Nonautologous Tissue Substitute
Cook Zenith AAA Endovascular Graft	**Use:** Intraluminal Device, Branched or Fenestrated, One or Two Arteries for Restriction in Lower Arteries; Intraluminal Device, Branched or Fenestrated, Three or More Arteries for Restriction in Lower Arteries; Intraluminal Device
CoreValve transcatheter aortic valve	**Use:** Zooplastic Tissue in Heart and Great Vessels
Cormet Hip Resurfacing System	**Use:** Resurfacing Device in Lower Joints
CoRoent® XL	**Use:** Interbody Fusion Device in Lower Joints
Corox (OTW) Bipolar Lead	**Use:** Cardiac Lead, Pacemaker for Insertion in Heart and Great Vessels; Cardiac Lead, Defibrillator for Insertion in Heart and Great Vessels

DEVICE KEY

Cortical strip neurostimulator lead	**Use:** Neurostimulator Lead in Central Nervous System and Cranial Nerves
Cultured epidermal cell autograft	**Use:** Autologous Tissue Substitute
CYPHER® Stent	**Use:** Intraluminal Device, Drug-eluting in Heart and Great Vessels
Cystostomy tube	**Use:** Drainage Device
DBS lead	**Use:** Neurostimulator Lead in Central Nervous System and Cranial Nerves
DeBakey Left Ventricular Assist Device	**Use:** Implantable Heart Assist System in Heart and Great Vessels
Deep brain neurostimulator lead	**Use:** Neurostimulator Lead in Central Nervous System and Cranial Nerves
Delta frame external fixator	**Use:** External Fixation Device, Hybrid for Insertion in Upper Bones External Fixation Device, Hybrid for Reposition in Upper Bones External Fixation Device, Hybrid for Insertion in Lower Bones External Fixation Device, Hybrid for Reposition in Lower Bones
Delta III Reverse shoulder prosthesis	**Use:** Synthetic Substitute, Reverse Ball and Socket for Replacement in Upper Joints
Diaphragmatic pacemaker generator	**Use:** Stimulator Generator in Subcutaneous Tissue and Fascia
Direct Lateral Interbody Fusion (DLIF) device	**Use:** Interbody Fusion Device in Lower Joints
Driver stent (RX) (OTW)	**Use:** Intraluminal Device
DuraHeart Left Ventricular Assist System	**Use:** Implantable Heart Assist System in Heart and Great Vessels

Durata® Defibrillation Lead	**Use:** Cardiac Lead, Defibrillator for Insertion in Heart and Great Vessels
Dynesys® Dynamic Stabilization System	**Use:** Spinal Stabilization Device, Pedicle-Based for Insertion in Upper Joints Spinal Stabilization Device, Pedicle-Based for Insertion in Lower Joints
E-Luminexx™ (Biliary) (Vascular) Stent	**Use:** Intraluminal Device
EDWARDS INTUITY Elite valve system	**Use:** Zooplastic Tissue, Rapid Deployment Technique in New Technology
Electrical bone growth stimulator (EBGS)	**Use:** Bone Growth Stimulator in Head and Facial Bones Bone Growth Stimulator in Upper Bones Bone Growth Stimulator in Lower Bones
Electrical muscle stimulation (EMS) lead	**Use:** Stimulator Lead in Muscles
Electronic muscle stimulator lead	**Use:** Stimulator Lead in Muscles
Embolization coil(s)	**Use:** Intraluminal Device
Endeavor® (III) (IV) (Sprint) Zotarolimus-eluting Coronary Stent System	**Use:** Intraluminal Device, Drug-eluting in Heart and Great Vessels
Endologix AFX® Endovascular AAA System	**Use:** Intraluminal Device
EndoSure® sensor	**Use:** Monitoring Device, Pressure Sensor for Insertion in Heart and Great Vessels
ENDOTAK RELIANCE® (G) Defibrillation Lead	**Use:** Cardiac Lead, Defibrillator for Insertion in Heart and Great Vessels
Endotracheal tube (cuffed) (double-lumen)	**Use:** Intraluminal Device, Endotracheal Airway in Respiratory System
Endurant® Endovascular Stent Graft	**Use:** Intraluminal Device

DEVICE KEY

Endurant® II AAA stent graft system	**Use:** Intraluminal Device
EnRhythm	**Use:** Pacemaker, Dual Chamber for Insertion in Subcutaneous Tissue and Fascia
Enterra gastric neurostimulator	**Use:** Stimulator Generator, Multiple Array for Insertion in Subcutaneous Tissue and Fascia
Epic™ Stented Tissue Valve (aortic)	**Use:** Zooplastic Tissue in Heart and Great Vessels
Epicel® cultured epidermal autograft	**Use:** Autologous Tissue Substitute
Esophageal obturator airway (EOA)	**Use:** Intraluminal Device, Airway in Gastrointestinal System
Esteem® implantable hearing system	**Use:** Hearing Device in Ear, Nose, Sinus
Everolimus-eluting coronary stent	**Use:** Intraluminal Device, Drug-eluting in Heart and Great Vessels
Ex-PRESS™ mini glaucoma shunt	**Use:** Synthetic Substitute
EXCLUDER® AAA Endoprosthesis	**Use:** Intraluminal Device, Branched or Fenestrated, One or Two Arteries for Restriction in Lower Arteries; Intraluminal Device, Branched or Fenestrated, Three or More Arteries for Restriction in Lower Arteries
EXCLUDER® IBE Endoprosthesis	**Use:** Intraluminal Device, Branched or Fenestrated, One or Two Arteries for Restriction in Lower Arteries
Express® (LD) Premounted Stent System	**Use:** Intraluminal Device
Express® Biliary SD Monorail® Premounted Stent System	**Use:** Intraluminal Device
Express® SD Renal Monorail® Premounted Stent System	**Use:** Intraluminal Device

External fixator	**Use:** External Fixation Device in Head and Facial Bones; External Fixation Device in Upper Bones; External Fixation Device in Lower Bones; External Fixation Device in Upper Joints; External Fixation Device in Lower Joints
EXtreme Lateral Interbody Fusion (XLIF) device	**Use:** Interbody Fusion Device in Lower Joints
Facet replacement spinal stabilization device	**Use:** Spinal Stabilization Device, Facet Replacement for Insertion in Upper Joints; Spinal Stabilization Device, Facet Replacement for Insertion in Lower Joints
FLAIR® Endovascular Stent Graft	**Use:** Intraluminal Device
Flexible Composite Mesh	**Use:** Synthetic Substitute
Foley catheter	**Use:** Drainage Device
Formula™ Balloon-Expandable Renal Stent System	**Use:** Intraluminal Device
Freestyle (Stentless) Aortic Root Bioprosthesis	**Use:** Zooplastic Tissue in Heart and Great Vessels
Fusion screw (compression) (lag) (locking)	**Use:** Internal Fixation Device in Upper Joints; Internal Fixation Device in Lower Joints
GammaTile™	**Use:** Radioactive Element, Cesium-131 Collagen Implant for Insertion in Central Nervous System and Cranial Nerves
Gastric electrical stimulation (GES) lead	**Use:** Stimulator Lead in Gastrointestinal System
Gastric pacemaker lead	**Use:** Stimulator Lead in Gastrointestinal System

DEVICE KEY

Device	Use
GORE EXCLUDER® AAA Endoprosthesis	**Use:** Intraluminal Device, Branched or Fenestrated, One or Two Arteries for Restriction in Lower Arteries
GORE EXCLUDER® IBE Endoprosthesis	**Use:** Intraluminal Device, Branched or Fenestrated, One or Two Arteries for Restriction in Lower Arteries
GORE TAG® Thoracic Endoprosthesis	**Use:** Intraluminal Device
GORE® DUALMESH®	**Use:** Synthetic Substitute
Guedel airway	**Use:** Intraluminal Device, Airway in Mouth and Throat
Hancock Bioprosthesis (aortic) (mitral) valve	**Use:** Zooplastic Tissue in Heart and Great Vessels
Hancock Bioprosthetic Valved Conduit	**Use:** Zooplastic Tissue in Heart and Great Vessels
HeartMate 3™ LVAS	**Use:** Implantable Heart Assist System in Heart and Great Vessels
HeartMate II® Left Ventricular Assist Device (LVAD)	**Use:** Implantable Heart Assist System in Heart and Great Vessels
HeartMate XVE® Left Ventricular Assist Device (LVAD)	**Use:** Implantable Heart Assist System in Heart and Great Vessels
Hip (joint) liner	**Use:** Liner in Lower Joints
Holter valve ventricular shunt	**Use:** Synthetic Substitute
Ilizarov external fixator	**Use:** External Fixation Device, Ring for Insertion in Upper Bones. External Fixation Device, Ring for Reposition in Upper Bones. External Fixation Device, Ring for Insertion in Lower Bones. External Fixation Device, Ring for Reposition in Lower Bones
Ilizarov-Vecklich device	**Use:** External Fixation Device, Limb Lengthening for Insertion in Upper Bones. External Fixation Device, Limb Lengthening for Insertion in Lower Bones
Impella® heart pump	**Use:** Short-term External Heart Assist System in Heart and Great Vessels
Implantable cardioverter-defibrillator (ICD)	**Use:** Defibrillator Generator for Insertion in Subcutaneous Tissue and Fascia
Implantable drug infusion pump (anti-spasmodic) (chemotherapy) (pain)	**Use:** Infusion Device, Pump in Subcutaneous Tissue and Fascia
Implantable glucose monitoring device	**Use:** Monitoring Device
Implantable hemodynamic monitor (IHM)	**Use:** Monitoring Device, Hemodynamic for Insertion in Subcutaneous Tissue and Fascia
Implantable hemodynamic monitoring system (IHMS)	**Use:** Monitoring Device, Hemodynamic for Insertion in Subcutaneous Tissue and Fascia
Implantable Miniature Telescope™ (IMT)	**Use:** Synthetic Substitute, Intraocular Telescope for Replacement in Eye
Implanted (venous) (access) port	**Use:** Vascular Access Device, Totally Implantable in Subcutaneous Tissue and Fascia
InDura, intrathecal catheter (1P) (spinal)	**Use:** Infusion Device
Injection reservoir, port	**Use:** Vascular Access Device, Totally Implantable in Subcutaneous Tissue and Fascia
Injection reservoir, pump	**Use:** Infusion Device, Pump in Subcutaneous Tissue and Fascia

DEVICE KEY

Interbody fusion (spine) cage	**Use:** Interbody Fusion Device in Upper Joints Interbody Fusion Device in Lower Joints
Interspinous process spinal stabilization device	**Use:** Spinal Stabilization Device, Interspinous Process for Insertion in Upper Joints Spinal Stabilization Device, Interspinous Process for Insertion in Lower Joints
InterStim® Therapy lead	**Use:** Neurostimulator Lead in Peripheral Nervous System
InterStim® Therapy neurostimulator	**Use:** Stimulator Generator, Single Array for Insertion in Subcutaneous Tissue and Fascia
Intramedullary (IM) rod (nail)	**Use:** Internal Fixation Device, Intramedullary in Upper Bones Internal Fixation Device, Intramedullary in Lower Bones
Intramedullary skeletal kinetic distractor (ISKD)	**Use:** Internal Fixation Device, Intramedullary in Upper Bones Internal Fixation Device, Intramedullary in Lower Bones
Intrauterine device (IUD)	**Use:** Contraceptive Device in Female Reproductive System
INTUITY Elite valve system, EDWARDS	**Use:** Zooplastic Tissue, Rapid Deployment Technique in New Technology
Itrel (3) (4) neurostimulator	**Use:** Stimulator Generator, Single Array for Insertion in Subcutaneous Tissue and Fascia
Joint fixation plate	**Use:** Internal Fixation Device in Upper Joints Internal Fixation Device in Lower Joints
Joint liner (insert)	**Use:** Liner in Lower Joints
Joint spacer (antibiotic)	**Use:** Spacer in Upper Joints Spacer in Lower Joints

Kappa	**Use:** Pacemaker, Dual Chamber for Insertion in Subcutaneous Tissue and Fascia
Kinetra® neurostimulator	**Use:** Stimulator Generator, Multiple Array for Insertion in Subcutaneous Tissue and Fascia
Kirschner wire (K-wire)	**Use:** Internal Fixation Device in Head and Facial Bones Internal Fixation Device in Upper Bones Internal Fixation Device in Lower Bones Internal Fixation Device in Upper Joints Internal Fixation Device in Lower Joints
Knee (implant) insert	**Use:** Liner in Lower Joints
Kuntscher nail	**Use:** Internal Fixation Device, Intramedullary in Upper Bones Internal Fixation Device, Intramedullary in Lower Bones
LAP-BAND® adjustable gastric banding system	**Use:** Extraluminal Device
LifeStent® (Flexstar) (XL) Vascular Stent System	**Use:** Intraluminal Device
LIVIAN™ CRT-D	**Use:** Cardiac Resynchronization Defibrillator Pulse Generator for Insertion in Subcutaneous Tissue and Fascia
Loop recorder, implantable	**Use:** Monitoring Device
MAGEC® Spinal Bracing and Distraction System	**Use:** Magnetically Controlled Growth Rod(s) in New Technology
Mark IV Breathing Pacemaker System	Stimulator Generator in Subcutaneous Tissue and Fascia
Maximo II DR (VR)	**Use:** Defibrillator Generator for Insertion in Subcutaneous Tissue and Fascia
Maximo II DR CRT-D	**Use:** Cardiac Resynchronization Defibrillator Pulse Generator for Insertion in Subcutaneous Tissue and Fascia

DEVICE KEY

Device	Use
Medtronic Endurant® II AAA stent graft system	**Use:** Intraluminal Device
Melody® transcatheter pulmonary valve	**Use:** Zooplastic Tissue in Heart and Great Vessels
Metal on metal bearing surface	**Use:** Synthetic Substitute, Metal for Replacement in Lower Joints
Micro-Driver stent (RX) (OTW)	**Use:** Intraluminal Device
Micrus CERECYTE microcoil	**Use:** Intraluminal Device, Bioactive in Upper Arteries
MIRODERM™ Biologic Wound Matrix	**Use:** Skin Substitute, Porcine Liver Derived in New Technology
MitraClip valve repair system	**Use:** Synthetic Substitute
Mitroflow® Aortic Pericardial Heart Valve	**Use:** Zooplastic Tissue in Heart and Great Vessels
Mosaic Bioprosthesis (aortic) (mitral) valve	**Use:** Zooplastic Tissue in Heart and Great Vessels
MULTI-LINK (VISION)(MINIVISION) (ULTRA) Coronary Stent System	**Use:** Intraluminal Device
nanoLOCK™ interbody fusion device	**Use:** Interbody Fusion Device, Nanotextured Surface in New Technology
Nasopharyngeal airway (NPA)	**Use:** Intraluminal Device, Airway in Ear, Nose, Sinus
Neuromuscular electrical stimulation (NEMS) lead	**Use:** Stimulator Lead in Muscles
Neurostimulator generator, multiple channel	**Use:** Stimulator Generator, Multiple Array for Insertion in Subcutaneous Tissue and Fascia
Neurostimulator generator, multiple channel rechargeable	**Use:** Stimulator Generator, Multiple Array Rechargeable for Insertion in Subcutaneous Tissue and Fascia
Neurostimulator generator, single channel	**Use:** Stimulator Generator, Single Array for Insertion in Subcutaneous Tissue and Fascia
Neurostimulator generator, single channel rechargeable	**Use:** Stimulator Generator, Single Array Rechargeable for Insertion in Subcutaneous Tissue and Fascia
Neutralization plate	**Use:** Internal Fixation Device in Head and Facial Bones; Internal Fixation Device in Upper Bones; Internal Fixation Device in Lower Bones
Nitinol framed polymer mesh	**Use:** Synthetic Substitute
Non-tunneled central venous catheter	**Use:** Infusion Device
Novacor Left Ventricular Assist Device	**Use:** Implantable Heart Assist System in Heart and Great Vessels
Novation® Ceramic AHS® (Articulation Hip System)	**Use:** Synthetic Substitute, Ceramic for Replacement in Lower Joints
Optimizer™ III implantable pulse generator	**Use:** Contractility Modulation Device for Insertion in Subcutaneous Tissue and Fascia
Oropharyngeal airway (OPA)	**Use:** Intraluminal Device, Airway in Mouth and Throat
Ovatio™ CRT-D	**Use:** Cardiac Resynchronization Defibrillator Pulse Generator for Insertion in Subcutaneous Tissue and Fascia
OXINIUM	**Use:** Synthetic Substitute, Oxidized Zirconium on Polyethylene for Replacement in Lower Joints
Paclitaxel-eluting coronary stent	**Use:** Intraluminal Device, Drug-eluting in Heart and Great Vessels
Paclitaxel-eluting peripheral stent	**Use:** Intraluminal Device, Drug-eluting in Upper Arteries; Intraluminal Device, Drug-eluting in Lower Arteries

DEVICE KEY

Partially absorbable mesh	**Use:** Synthetic Substitute
Pedicle-based dynamic stabilization device	**Use:** Spinal Stabilization Device, Pedicle-Based for Insertion in Upper Joints Spinal Stabilization Device, Pedicle-Based for Insertion in Lower Joints
Perceval sutureless valve	**Use:** Zooplastic Tissue, Rapid Deployment Technique in New Technology
Percutaneous endoscopic gastrojejunostomy (PEG/J) tube	**Use:** Feeding Device in Gastrointestinal System
Percutaneous endoscopic gastrostomy (PEG) tube	**Use:** Feeding Device in Gastrointestinal System
Percutaneous nephrostomy catheter	**Use:** Drainage Device
Peripherally inserted central catheter (PICC)	**Use:** Infusion Device
Pessary ring	**Use:** Intraluminal Device, Pessary in Female Reproductive System
Phrenic nerve stimulator generator	**Use:** Stimulator Generator in Subcutaneous Tissue and Fascia
Phrenic nerve stimulator lead	**Use:** Diaphragmatic Pacemaker Lead in Respiratory System
PHYSIOMESH™ Flexible Composite Mesh	**Use:** Synthetic Substitute
Pipeline™ Embolization device (PED)	**Use:** Intraluminal Device
Polyethylene socket	**Use:** Synthetic Substitute, Polyethylene for Replacement in Lower Joints
Polymethylmethacrylate (PMMA)	**Use:** Synthetic Substitute
Polypropylene mesh	**Use:** Synthetic Substitute
Porcine (bioprosthetic) valve	**Use:** Zooplastic Tissue in Heart and Great Vessels

PRESTIGE® Cervical Disc	**Use:** Synthetic Substitute
PrimeAdvanced neurostimulator	**Use:** Stimulator Generator, Multiple Array for Insertion in Subcutaneous Tissue and Fascia
PROCEED™ Ventral Patch	**Use:** Synthetic Substitute
Prodisc-C	**Use:** Synthetic Substitute
Prodisc-L	**Use:** Synthetic Substitute
PROLENE Polypropylene Hernia System (PHS)	**Use:** Synthetic Substitute
Protecta XT CRT-D	**Use:** Cardiac Resynchronization Defibrillator Pulse Generator for Insertion in Subcutaneous Tissue and Fascia
Protecta XT DR (XT VR)	**Use:** Defibrillator Generator for Insertion in Subcutaneous Tissue and Fascia
Protégé® RX Carotid Stent System	**Use:** Intraluminal Device
Pump reservoir	**Use:** Infusion Device, Pump in Subcutaneous Tissue and Fascia
PVAD™ Ventricular Assist Device	**Use:** External Heart Assist System in Heart and Great Vessels
REALIZE® Adjustable Gastric Band	**Use:** Extraluminal Device
Rebound HRD® (Hernia Repair Device)	**Use:** Synthetic Substitute
RestoreAdvanced neurostimulator	**Use:** Stimulator Generator, Multiple Array Rechargeable for Insertion in Subcutaneous Tissue and Fascia
RestoreSensor neurostimulator	**Use:** Stimulator Generator, Multiple Array Rechargeable for Insertion in Subcutaneous Tissue and Fascia

DEVICE KEY

RestoreUltra neurostimulator	**Use:** Stimulator Generator, Multiple Array Rechargeable for Insertion in Subcutaneous Tissue and Fascia
Reveal (DX) (XT)	**Use:** Monitoring Device
Reverse® Shoulder Prosthesis	**Use:** Synthetic Substitute, Reverse Ball and Socket for Replacement in Upper Joints
Revo MRI™ SureScan® pacemaker	**Use:** Pacemaker, Dual Chamber for Insertion in Subcutaneous Tissue and Fascia
Rheos® System device	**Use:** Cardiac Rhythm Related Device in Subcutaneous Tissue and Fascia
Rheos® System lead	**Use:** Stimulator Lead in Upper Arteries
RNS System lead	**Use:** Neurostimulator Lead in Central Nervous System and Cranial Nerves
RNS system neurostimulator generator	**Use:** Neurostimulator Generator in Head and Facial Bones
Sacral nerve modulation (SNM) lead	**Use:** Stimulator Lead in Urinary System
Sacral neuromodulation lead	**Use:** Stimulator Lead in Urinary System
SAPIEN transcatheter aortic valve	**Use:** Zooplastic Tissue in Heart and Great Vessels
Secura (DR) (VR)	**Use:** Defibrillator Generator for Insertion in Subcutaneous Tissue and Fascia
Sheffield hybrid external fixator	**Use:** External Fixation Device, Hybrid for Insertion in Upper Bones External Fixation Device, Hybrid for Reposition in Upper Bones External Fixation Device, Hybrid for Insertion in Lower Bones External Fixation Device, Hybrid for Reposition in Lower Bones

Sheffield ring external fixator	**Use:** External Fixation Device, Ring for Insertion in Upper Bones External Fixation Device, Ring for Reposition in Upper Bones External Fixation Device, Ring for Insertion in Lower Bones External Fixation Device, Ring for Reposition in Lower Bones
Single lead pacemaker (atrium) (ventricle)	**Use:** Pacemaker, Single Chamber for Insertion in Subcutaneous Tissue and Fascia
Single lead rate responsive pacemaker (atrium) (ventricle)	**Use:** Pacemaker, Single Chamber Rate Responsive for Insertion in Subcutaneous Tissue and Fascia
Sirolimus-eluting coronary stent	**Use:** Intraluminal Device, Drug-eluting in Heart and Great Vessels
SJM Biocor® Stented Valve System	**Use:** Zooplastic Tissue in Heart and Great Vessels
Soletra® neurostimulator	**Use:** Stimulator Generator, Single Array for Insertion in Subcutaneous Tissue and Fascia
Spinal cord neurostimulator lead	**Use:** Neurostimulator Lead in Central Nervous System and Cranial Nerves
Spinal growth rods, magnetically controlled	**Use:** Magnetically Controlled Growth Rod(s) in New Technology
Spiration IBV™ Valve System	**Use:** Intraluminal Device, Endobronchial Valve in Respiratory System
Stent (angioplasty) (embolization)	**Use:** Intraluminal Device
Stented tissue valve	**Use:** Zooplastic Tissue in Heart and Great Vessels
Stratos LV	**Use:** Cardiac Resynchronization Pacemaker Pulse Generator for Insertion in Subcutaneous Tissue and Fascia

DEVICE KEY

Subcutaneous injection reservoir, port	**Use:** Vascular Access Device, Totally Implantable in Subcutaneous Tissue and Fascia
Subcutaneous injection reservoir, pump	**Use:** Infusion Device, Pump in Subcutaneous Tissue and Fascia
Subdermal progesterone implant	**Use:** Contraceptive Device in Subcutaneous Tissue and Fascia
Sutureless valve, Perceval	**Use:** Zooplastic Tissue, Rapid Deployment Technique in New Technology
SynCardia Total Artificial Heart	**Use:** Synthetic Substitute
Synchra CRT-P	**Use:** Cardiac Resynchronization Pacemaker Pulse Generator for Insertion in Subcutaneous Tissue and Fascia
Talent® Converter	**Use:** Intraluminal Device
Talent® Occluder	**Use:** Intraluminal Device
Talent® Stent Graft (abdominal) (thoracic)	**Use:** Intraluminal Device
TandemHeart® System	**Use:** Short-term External Heart Assist System in Heart and Great Vessels
TAXUS® Liberté® Paclitaxel-eluting Coronary Stent System	**Use:** Intraluminal Device, Drug-eluting in Heart and Great Vessels
Therapeutic occlusion coil(s)	**Use:** Intraluminal Device
Thoracostomy tube	**Use:** Drainage Device
Thoratec IVAD (Implantable Ventricular Assist Device)	**Use:** Implantable Heart Assist System in Heart and Great Vessels
Thoratec Paracorporeal Ventricular Assist Device	**Use:** Short-term External Heart Assist System in Heart and Great Vessels
Tibial insert	**Use:** Liner in Lower Joints

Tissue bank graft	**Use:** Nonautologous Tissue Substitute
Tissue expander (inflatable) (injectable)	**Use:** Tissue Expander in Skin and Breast Tissue Expander in Subcutaneous Tissue and Fascia
Titanium Sternal Fixation System (TSFS)	**Use:** Internal Fixation Device, Rigid Plate for Insertion in Upper Bones Internal Fixation Device, Rigid Plate for Reposition in Upper Bones
Total artificial (replacement) heart	**Use:** Synthetic Substitute
Tracheostomy tube	**Use:** Tracheostomy Device in Respiratory System
Trifecta™ Valve (aortic)	**Use:** Zooplastic Tissue in Heart and Great Vessels
Tunneled central venous catheter	**Use:** Vascular Access Device, Tunneled in Subcutaneous Tissue and Fascia
Tunneled spinal (intrathecal) catheter	**Use:** Infusion Device
Two lead pacemaker	**Use:** Pacemaker, Dual Chamber for Insertion in Subcutaneous Tissue and Fascia
Ultraflex™ Precision Colonic Stent System	**Use:** Intraluminal Device
ULTRAPRO Hernia System (UHS)	**Use:** Synthetic Substitute
ULTRAPRO Partially Absorbable Lightweight Mesh	**Use:** Synthetic Substitute
ULTRAPRO Plug	**Use:** Synthetic Substitute
Ultrasonic osteogenic stimulator	**Use:** Bone Growth Stimulator in Head and Facial Bones Bone Growth Stimulator in Upper Bones Bone Growth Stimulator in Lower Bones

DEVICE KEY

Ultrasound bone healing system	**Use:** Bone Growth Stimulator in Head and Facial Bones Bone Growth Stimulator in Upper Bones Bone Growth Stimulator in Lower Bones
Uniplanar external fixator	**Use:** External Fixation Device, Monoplanar for Insertion in Upper Bones External Fixation Device, Monoplanar for Reposition in Upper Bones External Fixation Device, Monoplanar for Insertion in Lower Bones External Fixation Device, Monoplanar for Reposition in Lower Bones
Urinary incontinence stimulator lead	**Use:** Stimulator Lead in Urinary System
Vaginal pessary	**Use:** Intraluminal Device, Pessary in Female Reproductive System
Valiant Thoracic Stent Graft	**Use:** Intraluminal Device
Vectra® Vascular Access Graft	**Use:** Vascular Access Device, Tunneled in Subcutaneous Tissue and Fascia
Ventrio™ Hernia Patch	**Use:** Synthetic Substitute
Versa	**Use:** Pacemaker, Dual Chamber for Insertion in Subcutaneous Tissue and Fascia
Virtuoso (II) (DR) (VR)	**Use:** Defibrillator Generator for Insertion in Subcutaneous Tissue and Fascia

WALLSTENT® Endoprosthesis	**Use:** Intraluminal Device
X-STOP® Spacer	**Use:** Spinal Stabilization Device, Interspinous Process for Insertion in Upper Joints Spinal Stabilization Device, Interspinous Process for Insertion in Lower Joints
Xenograft	**Use:** Zooplastic Tissue in Heart and Great Vessels
XIENCE V Everolimus Eluting Coronary Stent System	**Use:** Intraluminal Device, Drug-eluting in Heart and Great Vessels
XLIF® System	**Use:** Interbody Fusion Device in Lower Joints
Zenith Flex® AAA Endovascular Graft	**Use:** Intraluminal Device
Zenith TX2® TAA Endovascular Graft	**Use:** Intraluminal Device
Zenith® Renu™ AAA Ancillary Graft	**Use:** Intraluminal Device
Zilver® PTX® (paclitaxel) Drug-Eluting Peripheral Stent	**Use:** Intraluminal Device, Drug-eluting in Upper Arteries Intraluminal Device, Drug-eluting in Lower Arteries
Zimmer® NexGen® LPS Mobile Bearing Knee	**Use:** Synthetic Substitute
Zimmer® NexGen® LPS-Flex Mobile Knee	**Use:** Synthetic Substitute
Zotarolimus-eluting coronary stent	**Use:** Intraluminal Device, Drug-eluting in Heart and Great Vessels

SUBSTANCE KEY

Term	ICD-10-PCS Value
AIGISRx Antibacterial Envelope Antimicrobial envelope	**Use:** Anti-Infective Envelope
Axicabtagene Ciloeucel	**Use:** Engineered Autologous Chimeric Antigen Receptor T-cell Immunotherapy
Bone morphogenetic protein 2 (BMP 2)	**Use:** Recombinant Bone Morphogenetic Protein
CBMA (Concentrated Bone Marrow Aspirate)	**Use:** Concentrated Bone Marrow Aspirate
Clolar	**Use:** Clofarabine
Defitelio	**Use:** Defibrotide Sodium Anticoagulant
DuraGraft® Endothelial Damage Inhibitor	**Use:** Endothelial Damage Inhibitor
Factor Xa Inhibitor Reversal Agent, Andexanet Alfa	**Use:** Andexanet Alfa, Factor Xa Inhibitor Reversal Agent
Kcentra	**Use:** 4-Factor Prothrombin Complex Concentrate
Nesiritide	**Use:** Human B-type Natriuretic Peptide

Term	ICD-10-PCS Value
rhBMP-2	**Use:** Recombinant Bone Morphogenetic Protein
Seprafilm	**Use:** Adhesion Barrier
STELARA®	**Use:** Other New Technology Therapeutic Substance
Tissue Plasminogen Activator (tPA) (rtPA)	**Use:** Other Thrombolytic
Ustekinumab	**Use:** Other New Technology Therapeutic Substance
Vistogard®	**Use:** Uridine Triacetate
Voraxaze	**Use:** Glucarpidase
VYXEOS™	**Use:** Cytarabine and Daunorubicin Liposome Antineoplastic
ZINPLAVA™	**Use:** Bezlotoxumab Monoclonal Antibody
Zyvox	**Use:** Oxazolidinones

Appendix D: Substance Key

DEVICE AGGREGATION TABLE

Specific Device	for Operation	in Body System	General Device
Autologous Arterial Tissue	All applicable	Heart and Great Vessels Lower Arteries Lower Veins Upper Arteries Upper Veins	**7** Autologous Tissue Substitute
Autologous Venous Tissue	All applicable	Heart and Great Vessels Lower Arteries Lower Veins Upper Arteries Upper Veins	**7** Autologous Tissue Substitute
Cardiac Lead, Defibrillator	Insertion	Heart and Great Vessels	**M** Cardiac Lead
Cardiac Lead, Pacemaker	Insertion	Heart and Great Vessels	**M** Cardiac Lead
Cardiac Resynchronization Defibrillator Pulse Generator	Insertion	Subcutaneous Tissue and Fascia	**P** Cardiac Rhythm Related Device
Cardiac Resynchronization Pacemaker Pulse Generator	Insertion	Subcutaneous Tissue and Fascia	**P** Cardiac Rhythm Related Device
Contractility Modulation Device	Insertion	Subcutaneous Tissue and Fascia	**P** Cardiac Rhythm Related Device
Defibrillator Generator	Insertion	Subcutaneous Tissue and Fascia	**P** Cardiac Rhythm Related Device
Epiretinal Visual Prosthesis	All applicable	Eye	**J** Synthetic Substitute
External Fixation Device, Hybrid	Insertion	Lower Bones Upper Bones	**5** External Fixation Device
External Fixation Device, Hybrid	Reposition	Lower Bones Upper Bones	**5** External Fixation Device
External Fixation Device, Limb Lengthening	Insertion	Lower Bones Upper Bones	**5** External Fixation Device
External Fixation Device, Monoplanar	Insertion	Lower Bones Upper Bones	**5** External Fixation Device
External Fixation Device, Monoplanar	Reposition	Lower Bones Upper Bones	**5** External Fixation Device
External Fixation Device, Ring	Insertion	Lower Bones Upper Bones	**5** External Fixation Device
External Fixation Device, Ring	Reposition	Lower Bones Upper Bones	**5** External Fixation Device
Hearing Device, Bone Conduction	Insertion	Ear, Nose, Sinus	**S** Hearing Device
Hearing Device, Multiple Channel Cochlear Prosthesis	Insertion	Ear, Nose, Sinus	**S** Hearing Device
Hearing Device, Single Channel Cochlear Prosthesis	Insertion	Ear, Nose, Sinus	**S** Hearing Device
Internal Fixation Device, Intramedullary	All applicable	Lower Bones Upper Bones	**4** Internal Fixation Device
Internal Fixation Device, Rigid Plate	Insertion	Upper Bones	**4** Internal Fixation Device
Internal Fixation Device, Rigid Plate	Reposition	Upper Bones	**4** Internal Fixation Device
Intraluminal Device, Pessary	All applicable	Female Reproductive System	**D** Intraluminal Device

DEVICE AGGREGATION TABLE

Specific Device	for Operation	in Body System	General Device
Intraluminal Device, Airway	All applicable	Ear, Nose, Sinus Gastrointestinal System Mouth and Throat	**D** Intraluminal Device
Intraluminal Device, Bioactive	All applicable	Upper Arteries	**D** Intraluminal Device
Intraluminal Device, Branched or Fenestrated, One or Two Arteries	Restriction	Heart and Great Vessels Lower Arteries	**D** Intraluminal Device
Intraluminal Device, Branched or Fenestrated, Three or More Arteries	Restriction	Heart and Great Vessels Lower Arteries	**D** Intraluminal Device
Intraluminal Device, Drug-eluting	All applicable	Heart and Great Vessels Lower Arteries Upper Arteries	**D** Intraluminal Device
Intraluminal Device, Drug-eluting, Four or More	All applicable	Heart and Great Vessels Lower Arteries Upper Arteries	**D** Intraluminal Device
Intraluminal Device, Drug-eluting, Three	All applicable	Heart and Great Vessels Lower Arteries Upper Arteries	**D** Intraluminal Device
Intraluminal Device, Drug-eluting, Two	All applicable	Heart and Great Vessels Lower Arteries Upper Arteries	**D** Intraluminal Device
Intraluminal Device, Endobronchial Valve	All applicable	Respiratory System	**D** Intraluminal Device
Intraluminal Device, Endotracheal Airway	All applicable	Respiratory System	**D** Intraluminal Device
Intraluminal Device, Four or More	All applicable	Heart and Great Vessels Lower Arteries Upper Arteries	**D** Intraluminal Device
Intraluminal Device, Radioactive	All applicable	Heart and Great Vessels	**D** Intraluminal Device
Intraluminal Device, Three	All applicable	Heart and Great Vessels Lower Arteries Upper Arteries	**D** Intraluminal Device
Intraluminal Device, Two	All applicable	Heart and Great Vessels Lower Arteries Upper Arteries	**D** Intraluminal Device
Monitoring Device, Hemodynamic	Insertion	Subcutaneous Tissue and Fascia	**2** Monitoring Device
Monitoring Device, Pressure Sensor	Insertion	Heart and Great Vessels	**2** Monitoring Device
Pacemaker, Dual Chamber	Insertion	Subcutaneous Tissue and Fascia	**P** Cardiac Rhythm Related Device
Pacemaker, Single Chamber	Insertion	Subcutaneous Tissue and Fascia	**P** Cardiac Rhythm Related Device
Pacemaker, Single Chamber Rate Responsive	Insertion	Subcutaneous Tissue and Fascia	**P** Cardiac Rhythm Related Device
Spinal Stabilization Device, Facet Replacement	Insertion	Lower Joints Upper Joints	**4** Internal Fixation Device
Spinal Stabilization Device, Interspinous Process	Insertion	Lower Joints Upper Joints	**4** Internal Fixation Device
Spinal Stabilization Device, Pedicle-Based	Insertion	Lower Joints Upper Joints	**4** Internal Fixation Device

DEVICE AGGREGATION TABLE

Specific Device	for Operation	in Body System	General Device
Stimulator Generator, Multiple Array	Insertion	Subcutaneous Tissue and Fascia	**M** Stimulator Generator
Stimulator Generator, Multiple Array Rechargeable	Insertion	Subcutaneous Tissue and Fascia	**M** Stimulator Generator
Stimulator Generator, Single Array	Insertion	Subcutaneous Tissue and Fascia	**M** Stimulator Generator
Stimulator Generator, Single Array Rechargeable	Insertion	Subcutaneous Tissue and Fascia	**M** Stimulator Generator
Synthetic Substitute, Ceramic	Replacement	Lower Joints	**J** Synthetic Substitute
Synthetic Substitute, Ceramic on Polyethylene	Replacement	Lower Joints	**J** Synthetic Substitute
Synthetic Substitute, Intraocular Telescope	Replacement	Eye	**J** Synthetic Substitute
Synthetic Substitute, Metal	Replacement	Lower Joints	**J** Synthetic Substitute
Synthetic Substitute, Metal on Polyethylene	Replacement	Lower Joints	**J** Synthetic Substitute
Synthetic Substitute, Oxidized Zirconium on Polyethylene	Replacement	Lower Joints	J Synthetic Substitute
Synthetic Substitute, Polyethylene	Replacement	Lower Joints	**J** Synthetic Substitute
Synthetic Substitute, Reverse Ball and Socket	Replacement	Upper Joints	**J** Synthetic Substitute
Synthetic Substitute, Unicondylar	Replacement	Lower Joints	**J** Synthetic Substitute

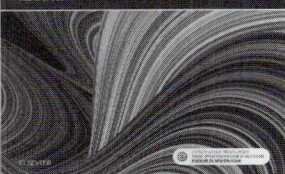

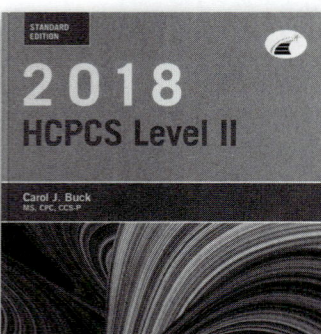
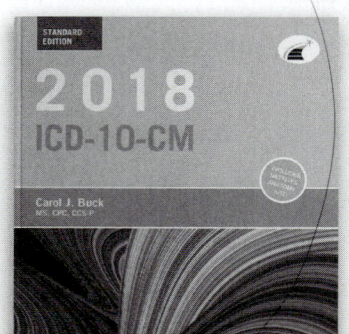
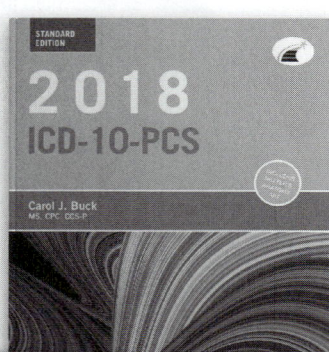
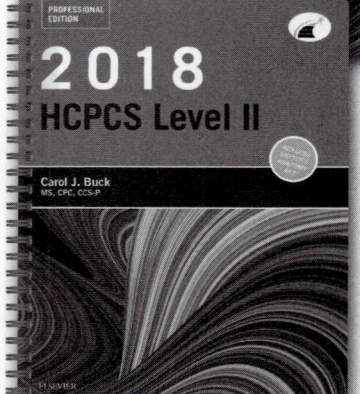
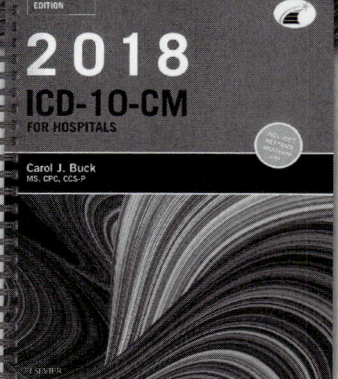
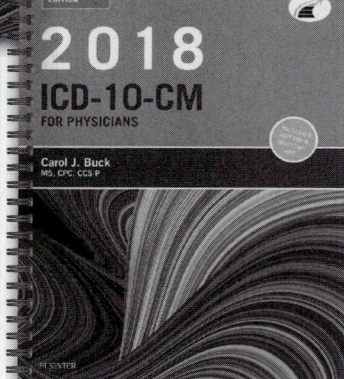
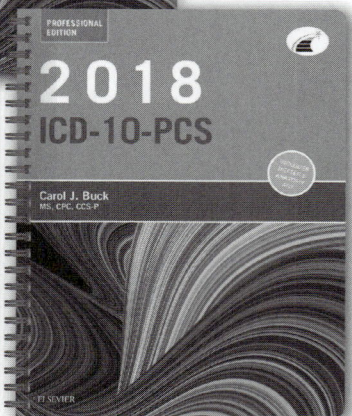

STEP **4**: PROFESSIONAL

> *"Nothing is particularly hard if you divide it into small jobs."*
> — HENRY FORD

WE WANT TO APPLAUD YOU FOR TAKING THIS STEP IN YOUR CAREER.
Medical coding is a fine profession that has the ability to intrigue and captivate you for a lifetime. Practice your craft carefully, with due diligence, patience for the process, and always the highest ethical standards.

TRACK YOUR PROGRESS!

See the checklist in the front of this book to learn more about your next step toward coding success!

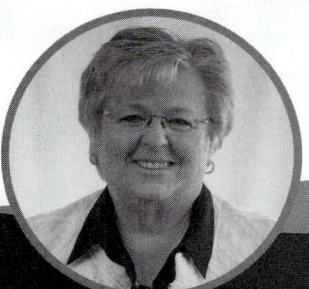

Author and Educator
Carol J. Buck, MS, CPC, CCS-P

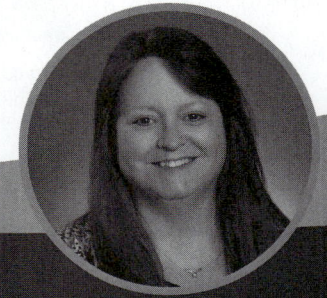

Lead Technical Collaborator
Jackie Grass Koesterman, CPC

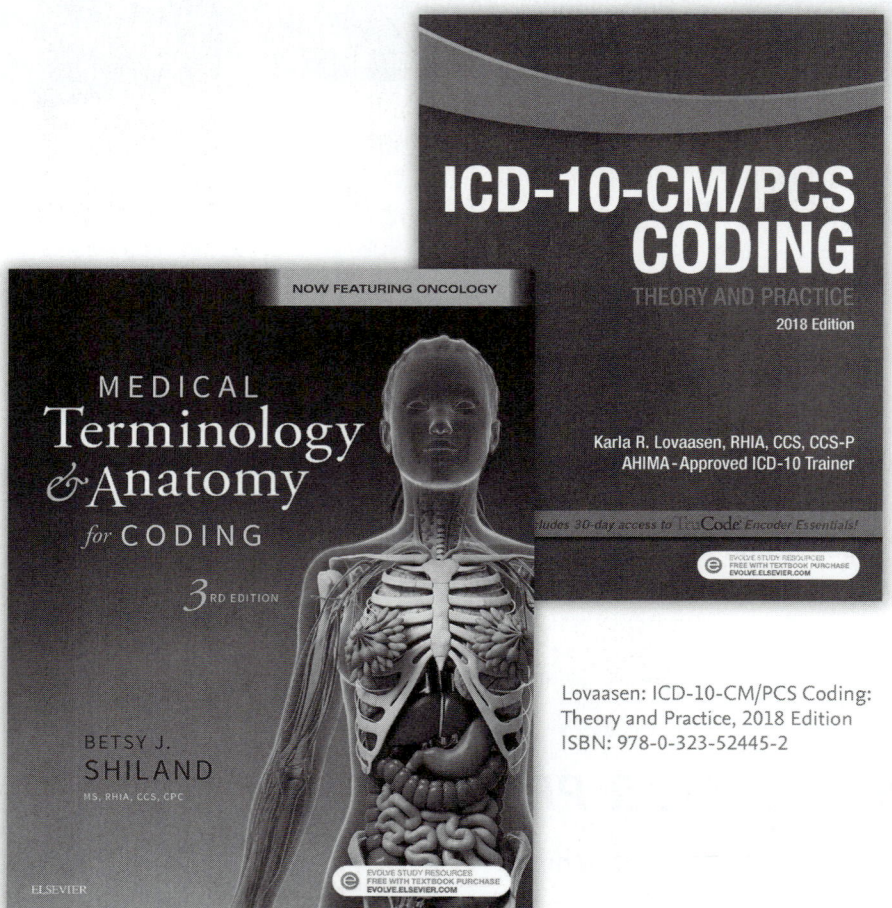

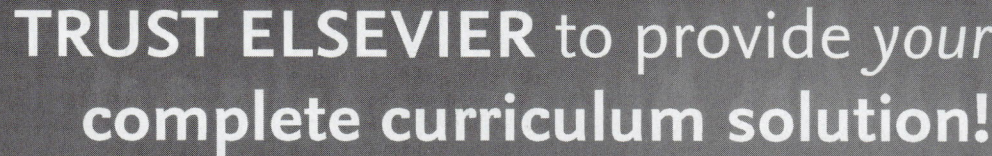

TRUST ELSEVIER to provide *your* complete curriculum solution!

ELSEVIER

CONTENT

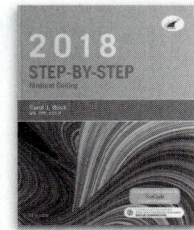

978-0-323-43081-4

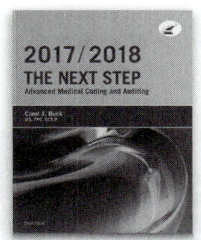

978-0-323-43077-7

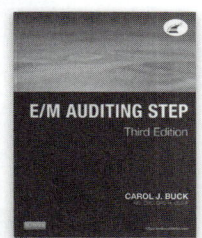

978-1-4557-5199-0

STUDY TOOLS

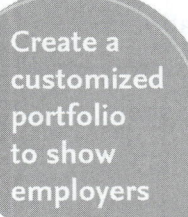

Create a customized portfolio to show employers

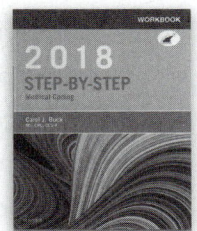

978-0-323-43079-1

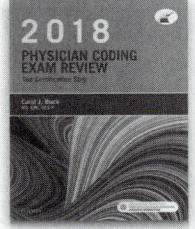

978-0-323-43078-4

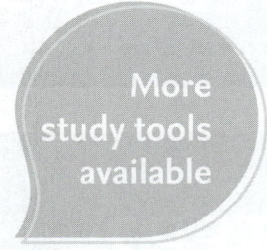

More study tools available

SIMULATIONS

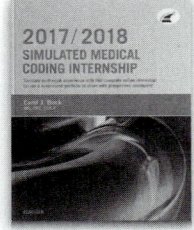

978-0-323-49772-5

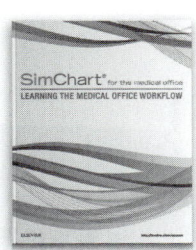

978-0-323-49791-6

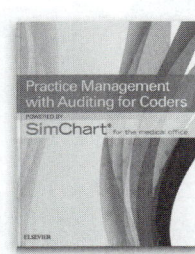

978-0-323-43011-1

COURSES

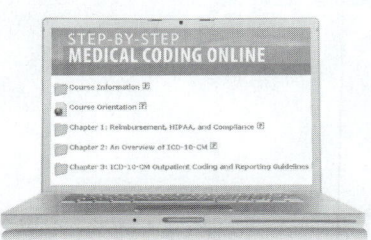

978-0-323-56672-8

Trust Carol J. Buck and Elsevier to take you through the **levels** *of* **CODING SUCCESS**

STEP4:
PROFESSIONAL

STEP3: CERTIFY

STEP2: PRACTICE

STEP1: LEARN

With the resources you need for every level of coding success, Carol J. Buck and Elsevier are with you every step of your coding career. From beginning to advanced, from the classroom to the workplace, from application to certification, the Step Series products are your guides to greater opportunities and successful career advancement.

Keep climbing with the most trusted names in medical coding.

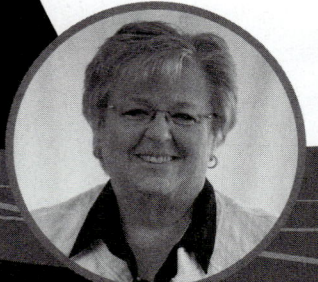

Author and Educator
Carol J. Buck, MS, CPC, CCS-P

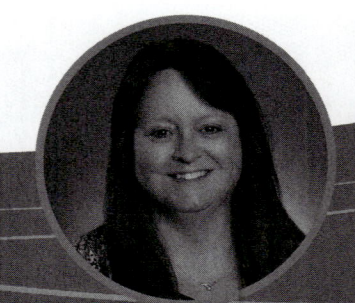

Lead Technical Collaborator
Jackie Grass Koesterman, CPC